GUIDELINES FOR
Critical Care Nursing

GUIDELINES FOR Critical Care Nursing

NANCIE URBAN, MSN, RN, CCRN

Director, Clinical Practice and Research
St. Joseph's Hospital
Milwaukee, Wisconsin

KAY KNOX GREENLEE, MSN, RN, CCRN

Clinical Nurse Specialist—Critical Care
St. Cloud Hospital
St. Cloud, Minnesota

JOANNE KRUMBERGER, MSN, RN, CCRN

Critical Care CNS
Veterans Administration Medical Center
Milwaukee, Wisconsin

CHRIS WINKELMAN, MSN, RN, CCRN

Clinical Nurse 3
MetroHealth Medical Center
Cleveland, Ohio

with 110 *illustrations*

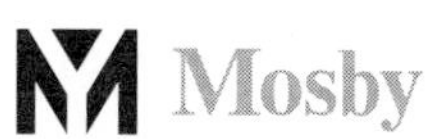

St. Louis Baltimore Boston Carlsbad Chicago Naples New York Philadelphia Portland
London Madrid Mexico City Singapore Sydney Tokyo Toronto Wiesbaden

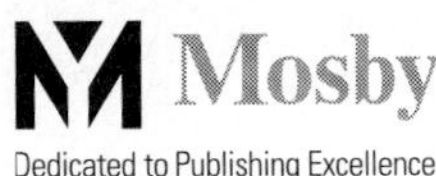

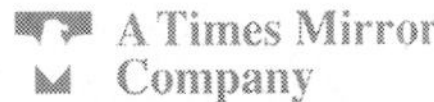

Publisher: Nancy Coon
Editor: Barry Bowlus
Associate Developmental Editor: Brian Morovitz
Project Manager: Linda McKinley
Production Editor: Rich Barber
Designer: Elizabeth Fett

A NOTE TO THE READER

The author and publisher have made every attempt to check dosages and nursing content for accuracy. Because the science of pharmacology is continually advancing, our knowledge base continues to expand. Therefore we recommend that the reader always check product information for changes in dosage or administration before administering any medication. This is particularly important with new or rarely used drugs.

Printed in the United States of America
Composition by: Graphic World, Inc.
Printing/binding by: Maple Vail Book Manufacturing Group

Mosby–Year Book, Inc.
11830 Westline Industrial Drive
St. Louis, Missouri 63146

Guidelines for critical care nursing / [edited by] Nancie Urban . . .
[et al.].—1st ed.
p. cm.
Includes bibliographical references and index.
ISBN 0-8016-7840-4
1. Intensive care nursing. I. Urban, Nancie.
[DNLM: 1. Critical Care—standards. 2. Nursing Care—standards.
WY 154 G946 1995]
RT120.I5G85 1995
610.73′61—dc20
DNLM/DLC
for Library of Congress 94-48566
CIP

95 96 97 98 99 / 9 8 7 6 5 4 3 2 1

In grateful memory of my grandmother who raised me to believe in the Lord, embracing responsibility and the value of a sense of humor.

Nancie Urban

Many people have made it possible for me to achieve this personal and professional goal; however, certain individuals helped make this a reality. To Doug, my husband—thank you for loving me through rough times. To Laura and Jesse, my children—thank you for being patient and for your love. To my parents—thanks for believing in me. Finally, to my colleagues at St. Cloud Hospital—thanks for your commitment to nursing and for making the vision of critical care real.

Kay Knox Greenlee

For mom and dad.

Joanne Krumberger

To my husband Craig and my loving family.

Chris Winkelman

Contributors

Nancy Abou-Awdi, MS, RN, CCRN, CCRC
Research Coordinator
Transplant Service
St. Luke's Episcopal Hospital/Texas Heart Institute
Houston, Texas
Guideline 25

Arlene Gordovez Agra, RN, CCRN
Medical ICU
MetroHealth Medical Center
Cleveland, Ohio
Appendix D

Anne Aloi, MSN, RN, CCRN
Clinician 4
Medical Intensive Care Unit
University of Virginia
Charlottesville, Virginia
Guideline 37

Mandy Bass, MS, RN, CCRN, CNN
Clinical Specialist, Transplantation
Intensive Care Nursing Service
Massachusetts General Hospital
Boston, Massachusetts
Guideline 52

Richard A. Beastrom, MN, RN, CPAN
Clinical Nurse 3
Post Anesthesia Care Unit
Saint Cloud Hospital
Saint Cloud, Minnesota
Appendix F

Hilary S. Blackwood, MSN, RN, CCRN
Clinician III
Patient Care Services/Surgical Intensive Care Unit
University of Virginia Health Sciences Center
Charlottesville, Virginia
Guideline 66

Patricia A. Blissitt, MSN, RN, CCRN, CNRN
Neuroscience Clinical Nurse Specialist/Case Manager
Neuroscience Service Line
Baptist Memorial Hospital
Memphis, Tennessee
Guideline 7

Siobhan Bremner, BSN, MPH, RN
Clinical Nurse Specialist
Cardiac Electrophysiology
St. Luke's Medical Center
Milwaukee, Wisconsin
Guideline 18

Anita Bush, PhD, RN, CCRN, CNRN
Affiliate Assistant Professor
Behavioral Science
University of Alaska/Fairbanks
Fairbanks, Alaska
Guideline 28

Karen K. Carlson, MN, RN, CCRN
Critical Care Clinical Specialist
Group Health Central Hospital
Seattle, WA
Guidelines 51, 53, 54, 55, 64

Lisa Cerino-Toth, BSN, RN
Arrhythmia Specialist
Cardiology
Johns Hopkins University
Baltimore, Maryland
Guideline 31

Karen Ann Clark, MS, RN
Clinical Nurse Specialist
Intensive Care
Sarasota Memorial Hospital
Sarasota, Florida
Guidelines 56 and 57

Kathy A. Coburn, RN
Manager
Ernst & Young LLP
Dallas, Texas
Guidelines 5 and 6

Helen A. Cook, MSN, RN
Assistant Nurse Manager
Neuroscience Intensive Care Unit
Duke University Medical Center
Durham, North Carolina
Guideline 3

Elise Dempsey, MS, RN, CCRN
Department Manager
Critical Care Department
Dominican Santa Cruz Hospital
Santa Cruz, California
Guideline 27

Mary A. Doucet, MS, RN, CCRN
Critical Care Clinical Nurse Specialist
Surgical ICU
New England Deaconess Hospital
Boston, Massachusetts
Guideline 47

Myra F. Ellis, MSN, RN, CCRN
Cardiovascular Nurse Coordinator
Aultman Heart Center
Aultman Hospital
Canton, Ohio
Guideline 63

Jocelyn A. Farrar, MS, RN, CCRN
Instructor
University of Maryland School of Nursing
Baltimore, Maryland

Clinical Nurse
Critical Care Float Pool
R Adams Cowley Shock Trauma Center
University of Maryland Medical System
Baltimore, Maryland
Guideline 65

Eleanor R. Fitzpatrick, MSN, RN, CCRN
Clinical Nurse Specialist
Intermediate Surgical Intensive Care Unit
Thomas Jefferson University Hospital
Philadelphia, Pennsylvania
Guideline 49

Patricia J. Forg, BS, RN, CNN
Transplantation Services
University of Washington Medical Center
Seattle, Washington
Guidelines 44 and 45

Jan Whetstone Foster, MSN, RN, CCRN
Nurse Manager
Medical Intensive Care Unit
The University of Texas/M.D. Anderson Cancer Center
Houston, Texas
Guideline 61

Polly E. Gardner, MN, RN, ARNP
Cardiovascular Adult Nurse Practitioner
Cardiology
Northwest Hospital
Seattle, Washington
Guideline 30

Peter A. Gonzalez, BSN, RN
Neurosurgical ICU
University of North Carolina Hospitals
Chapel Hill, North Carolina
Guideline 11

Cynthia A. Goodrich, MS, RN, CCRN
Clinical Instructor
Physiological Nursing
University of Washington
Seattle, Washington

Critical Care Clinical Nurse Specialist
Department of Nursing Education
Harborview Medical Center
Seattle, Washington
Guideline 38

Susan Flewelling Goran, MSN, RN, CCRN
Staff Development Specialist
Department of Nursing Resources
Maine Medical Center
Portland, Maine
Guidelines 26 and 32

Kay Knox Greenlee, MSN, RN, CCRN
Clinical Nurse Specialist
Surgical/Special Care Department
St. Cloud Hospital
St. Cloud, Minnesota
Guidelines 35 and 41

Ann Smith Gregoire, MSN, RN, CRNP, CCRN
Clinical Nurse Specialist
Surgical Intensive Care Unit
Thomas Jefferson University Hospital
Philadelphia, Pennsylvania
Guideline 49

Teresa Heise Halloran, MSN, RN, CCRN
Clinical Care Service Director
Memorial Hospital
Belleville, Illinois
Guideline 10

June Howland-Gradman, MS, RN, CCRN
Care Center Leader
Cardiac Services
University of Chicago Hospital
Chicago, Illinois
Guideline 29

Mary Ann Jarachovic, BSN, RN
Clinical Nurse III
Medical Intensive Care Unit
MetroHealth Medical Center
Cleveland, Ohio
Appendix D

Eileen M. Kelly, MSN, RN, CCRN
Clinical Nurse Specialist
Medical and Surgical Coronary Care Units
Thomas Jefferson University Hospital
Philadelphia, Pennsylvania
Guideline 13

Kathleen Kerber, MSN, RN, CCRN, CS
Clinical Nurse Specialist
Trauma/Critical Care Nursing
MetroHealth Medical Center
Cleveland, Ohio
Guideline 62

Christine Ashley Kessler, MN, RN, CCRN, CS
Critical Care Consultant and Educator
Previous affiliation:
Manager, Clinical Research Division
Inova Institute of Research and Education
Fairfax Hospital
Falls Church, Virginia
Guideline 58

Joanne M. Krumberger, MSN, RN, CCRN
Critical Care Clinical Nurse Specialist
Clement J. Zablocki Veterans Affairs Medical Center
Milwaukee, Wisconsin
Guideline 43 and Appendix B

Sandra A. Kucharski, MS, RN, CCRN
Nurse-in-Charge, Medical Intermediate Unit
Department of Nursing
Brigham and Women's Hospital
Boston, Massachusetts
Guideline 46

Nora E. Ladewig, MSN, RN, CCRN
Clinical Practice Nurse 5
Nursing Division
St. Luke's Medical Center
Milwaukee, Wisconsin
Guideline 2

S. Jill Ley, MS, RN, CCRN
Outcomes Coordinator
Department of Cardiovascular Surgery
California Pacific Medical Center
San Francisco, California
Guideline 33

Joan Littel-Conrad, RN, CCRN, CPTC
Organ Donation Coordinator
Wisconsin Donor Network
Froedtert Memorial Lutheran Hospital
Milwaukee, Wisconsin
Appendix E

Debra Lynn-McHale, MSN, RN, CS, CCRN
Staff Development Coordinator
Thomas Jefferson University Hospital
Philadelphia, Pennsylvania
Guideline 13

Tamera L. Mahaffey, MSN, RN
Cardiovascular Clinical Nurse Specialist
Nebraska Heart Institute
Lincoln, Nebraska
Guideline 14

Karen A. McQuillan, MS, RN, CCRN
Neurotrauma Clinical Nurse Specialist
R. Adams Cowley Shock Trauma Center
University of Maryland Medical Center
Baltimore, Maryland
Guideline 4

Noreen Mocsny, MEd, RN
Neurology Unit
VAMC
Cincinnati, Ohio
Guideline 9

Jacqueline A. Morgan, MSN, RN
Clinical Nurse III
MICU Department
MetroHealth Medical Center
Cleveland, Ohio
Clinical Faculty
School of Nursing
Cleveland State University
Cleveland, Ohio
Guideline 36

Christine C. Morrison, MSN, RN, CCRN
Thoracic Cardiovascular Clinical Coordinator
Heart Center
University of Virginia Health Sciences Center
Charlottesville, Virginia
Guideline 39

Susan O'Brien Norris, MS, RN, CCRN
Cardiovascular Clinical Nurse Specialist
Mercy Medical Center
Oshkosh, Wisconsin
Guideline 24

Susan G. Osguthorpe, MS, RN, CNA
Acting Chief
Nursing Service
Salt Lake City VA Medical Center
Salt Lake City, Utah
Guideline 16

Penny L. Powers, BSN, RN, CCTC
Manager
Transplant Service
St. Luke's Episcopal Hospital
Houston, Texas
Guideline 25

Andrea D'Amato Quinn, MS, RN, CCRN, CS
Clinical Nurse Specialist
Surgical Nursing
Yale New Haven Hospital
New Haven, Connecticut
Guideline 48

Kathleen M. Quinn, BSN, MBA, RN, CCRN
Director of Outpatient Services
Medicine Department
University of Virginia Health Sciences Center
Charlottesville, Virginia
Guideline 39

Kara Lee Rusy, MSN, RN, CCRN
Adult Nurse Practitioner
Neurosurgery
St. Mark's Hospital
Salt Lake City, Utah
Guideline 8

Bev Ryan, MSN, RN, CCRN
Clinician 4
Medical Intensive Care Unit
University of Virginia
Charlottesville, Virginia
Guideline 37

Catherine Ryan, MS, RN, CCRN
Clinical Nurse Specialist
Critical Care
Alexian Brothers Medical Center
Elk Grove Village, Illinois
Guideline 20

Marguerite Scaduto-Philips, MA, RN
Adjunct Faculty
Nursing Department
Bergen Community College
Paramus, New Jersey
Guideline 19

Mary G. Schigoda, MSN, RN, CCRN
Clinical Nurse Specialist/Manager
Thoracic Transplant Intensive Care Unit
St. Luke's Medical Center
Milwaukee, Wisconsin
Guideline 17

Kerri L. Schneider, MSN, RN, CCRN
Staff RN/Intensive Care
Nursing Department
St. Mary's Medical Center
Racine, Wisconsin

Adjunct Clinical Instructor
Nursing Department
Alverno College
Milwaukee, Wisconsin
Guideline 2

Kelly A. Scholz, BSN, RN
Staff Nurse
Cardiac Electrophysiology
St. Luke's Medical Center
Milwaukee, Wisconsin
Guideline 18

Peg Snyder, MN, RN, CCRN
Clinical Nurse Specialist
Critical Care
Northwest Hospital
Seattle, Washington
Guidelines 42 and 59

David Strider, MSN, MSB, RN, CCRN
Vascular Care Coordinator
Heart Center
University of Virginia Health Sciences Center
Charlottesville, Virginia
Guideline 39

Jeanette Torrence Thompson, BSN, RN, CCTC
Lung Transplant Coordinator
Department of Transplantation
University of North Carolina Hospitals
Chapel Hill, North Carolina
Guideline 40

Debbie Tribett, MS, RN, CCRN
Critical Care Nurse Consultant
Edgewater, Maryland
Guideline 60

Nancie Urban, MSN, RN, CCRN
Director
Clinical Practice and Research
St. Joseph's Hospital
Milwaukee, Wisconsin
Guidelines 22 and 31, Appendix A

Patricia Swanson VerMaas, MSN, RN
Cardiovascular Nurse Specialist
Nebraska Heart Institute
Lincoln, Nebraska
Guideline 15

Pamela Becker Weilitz, MSN, RN
Manager
Nursing Care Delivery
Barnes/Jewish Hospital at Washington University Medical Center
St. Louis, Missouri
Guideline 34

Gayle R. Whitman, MSN, RN, FAAN
Director
Cardiac Nursing
Cleveland Clinic Hospital
Cleveland, Ohio
Guideline 23

Chris Winkelman, MSN, RN, CCRN
Staff Nurse
MetroHealth Medical Center
Cleveland, Ohio
Guidelines 1 and 12

Kimberly Woods-McCormick, BSN, RN, CCRN
Emergency Care Services Education Coordinator
Education Department
Poudre Valley Hospital
Ft. Collins, Colorado
Guideline 21

Arlene Yuan, MSN, RN, CCRN
Thoracic Cardiovascular Practitioner Teacher
School of Nursing
University of Virginia Health Sciences Center
Charlottesville, Virginia
Guideline 39

Marge Zerbe, BS, RNC
Nursing Educator
Obstetrical Seminars and Consulting
Dayton, Ohio
Guideline 67

Suzanne Wasch Zimmerman, BSN, RN, CCRN
Nurse Education Clinician
Surgery/Trauma ICU
University of North Carolina Hospitals
Chapel Hill, North Carolina
Guideline 50

Reviewers

Alinthia Allwood-Gallagher, BSN, MA
Clinical Unit Coordinator
MMC Weiler Division
Bronx, New York

Sarah E. Angermuller, ADN, BS, MEd, MSN
Associate Professor
Columbus College, Georgia

Esther Bay, BSN, MSN, CS, CCRN
Nursing Faculty
Henry Ford Community College
Dearborn, Michigan

Tally Bell, AS, BSN, MN
Manager, Clinical Education
HCA Wesley Medical Center
Wichita, Kansas

Joe E. Bierchen, BSN, MSN, EdD
Professor
St. Petersburg Junior College
St. Petersburg, Florida

Kathyrn Bizek, BSN, MSN, CCRN, CS
Clinical Nurse Specialist, Critical Care
Associate Graduate Faculty
Detroit Receiving Hospital & Wayne State University
Detroit, Michigan

Cindy Bogard, MS, RN, CCRN
Clinical Nurse Specialist/Critical Care
Baptist Medical Center
Kansas City, Missouri

Rebecca Butler, RN
Liver Transplant Coordinator
Emory University Hospital
Atlanta, Georgia

Marcia Chorba, BSN, MSN
Professor or Nursing
Mercy Hospital
Pittsburgh, Pennsylvania

Denise A. Coleman, MSN, RN
Hospice Coordinator
Medical College of Virginia
Richmond, Virginia

Rose E. Constantino, BSN, MN, PhD, JD, RN
Associate Professor and Principal Investigator
University of Pittsburgh
Pittsburgh, Pennsylvania

Mary Beth Drangstveit, RN, CCTC
Transplant Coordinator
University of Minnesota
Minneapolis, Minnesota

Leann Eaton, MSN, RN
Assistant Professor
Jewish Hospital College of Nursing & Allied Health
St. Louis, Missouri

Lynn Feeman, BSN, MSN
Clinical Nurse Specialist
Northside Hospital
Atlanta, Georgia

Jeannine Forrest, BSN, MS
Teaching Associate
UIC College of Nursing
Chicago, Illinois

Pamela G. Harrison, MS, RN
Assistant Professor
Indiana Wesleyan University
Marion, Indiana

Linda Heitman, MSN, RNC
Cardiac Clinical Nurse Specialist/Regional Heart Center Coordinator
Southeast Missouri Hospital
Cape Girardeau, Missouri

Cynthia Hermey, MN, CCRN
Clinical Nurse Specialist/Critical Care Services
DePaul Medical Center
Norfolk, Virginia

Rose Hoffman, MSN, RN
Course Coordinator
West Penn Hospital
Pittsburgh, Pennsylvania

Josephine B. Mello Jacavone, BSN, MSN
Assistant Professor of Nursing
Atlantic Union College
South Lancaster, Massachusetts

Susan Kaiser, BSN, RN, CCRN
National Institutes of Health
Bethesda, Maryland

Martha J. Kleindienst, MS, RN
Northwest Memorial Hospital
Division of Organ Transplant
Chicago, Illinois

Larry E. Lancaster, ADN, BSU, MSN, EdD
Associate Professor
Vanderbilt University
Nashville, Tennessee

Paul Langlois, RN, DNSc
Clinical Nurse Researcher
Wilford Hall Medical Center
Lackland Air Force Base, Texas

Marijo Letizia, C, MS, RN
Instructor of Medical Surgical Nursing
Loyola University of Chicago
Chicago, Illinois

Marianne T. Marcus, BSN, MA, MEd, EdD
Chairperson
University of Texas
Houston, Texas

Carol F. Metcalf, MPH, PhD
Nursing Instructor
TMCC
Reno, Nevada

Peggy Norton, MSN, RN
Clinical Nurse Specialist
Loyola University Medical Center
Chicago, Illinois

Elizabeth M. Outlaw, BSN, MA
Per Diem Staff Nurse
Stamford Hospital
Stamford, Connecticut

Tonya Parker, MSN, RN
Assistant Professor of Nursing
Northwestern State University
Shreveport, Louisiana

Christy A. Price, MSN, RN
Nephrology Clinical Specialist
Independent Nursing Consultant
Lake Bluff, Illinois

Claire Raymond, PharmD
Clinical Pharmacist/Critical Care Medicine
The Jewish Hospital of St. Louis
St. Louis, Missouri

Jane Reddell, MSN, RN, CCRN
Instructor
Methodist Hospital School of Nursing
Lubbock, Texas

Cassandra Salvatore, BSN, MeD, MS
Coordinator/Nurse Internship Program
Wilford Hall Medical Center
Lackland Air Force Base, Texas

Sandra Schmid, CSJ, BSN, RN
Coordinator/Abdominal Organ Transplant
St. Louis University Hospital
St. Louis, Missouri

April Sieh, BSN, MSN
Instructor
Delta College
University Center, Michigan

Janyce Streeter, MS, RN
Registered Nurse
Utah Valley Regional Medical Center
Provo, Utah

Gail Taylor, BSN, MSN
Associate Chief/Nursing Education
VA Medical Center
Fort Wayne, Indiana

Robyn Thompson, BA, BSN, MS
Associate Professor of Nursing
Umpqua Community College
Roseburg, Oregon

Elizabeth Thompson, BSN
Critical Care Instructor
Lancaster General Hospital
Lancaster, Pennsylvania

Cesarina Thompson, MSN, PhD
Assistant Professor of Nursing
Southern Connecticut State University
New Haven, Connecticut

Joy Thompson, MSN, RN, CCRN
St. Louis University Hospital
St. Louis, Missouri

Margaret B. Todd, BSN, MSN
Health Careers
Angelina College
Lufkin, Texas

Geraldine Varassi, EdD, RN
Nursing Educator
North Shore University Hospital
Manhasset, New York

Marla Weston, MS, RN, CCRN
Director/Patient Care Systems
Desert Samaritan Medical Center
Mesa, Arizona

Sheila Zielinski, BSN, MN
Clinical Nurse Specialist
Methodist Hospital
Indianapolis, Indiana

Foreword

Nancie Urban, MSN, RN, CCRN
Kay Knox Greenlee, MSN, RN, CCRN
Joanne Krumberger, MSN, RN, CCRN
Chris Winkelman, MSN, RN, CCRN

Guidelines for Critical Care Nursing represents a departure from standards, or from standard care plan books that have been published to date. The format was adapted from the recommendations of the American Nurses Association (ANA) in response to the clinical guideline initiatives of the Agency for Health Care Policy and Research (AHCPR).

GUIDELINES VERSUS STANDARDS

Standards have been defined as authoritative statements that describe competent practice.[1] Standards represent minimum expectations and must be written in broad terms to allow for individual variations in patient presentation. On the other hand, guidelines describe recommendations for care related to specific conditions yet remain sensitive to individual variations. Implicit in any guideline statement or document is the understanding that the recommended interventions are contingent on predefined assessment findings. In the event that assessment reveals a unique presentation of the condition being described, guidelines must be altered to respond to the variance.

GUIDELINES AND STANDARD CARE PLANS

Guidelines are similar to standard care plans. They describe a customary approach to patient care for select conditions. However, *Guidelines for Critical Care Nursing* has departed significantly from other standard care plan resources in three key aspects: (1) description of the condition, (2) specificity of assessment parameters, and (3) presentation of a focused, prioritized plan of care.

Guidelines for Critical Care Nursing presents a concise description of the condition including a definition and description of its prevalence and impact on patients and/or society. In addition, a brief review of pathophysiology, especially as it relates to intervention, is included. The text also discusses management trends and controversies with emphasis on research regarding the condition and related intervention. *Guidelines for Critical Care Nursing* departs from standard guideline format by including discussion regarding the length of stay that may be anticipated for each condition. The emphasis on decreasing length of stay and performing more procedures in the ambulatory setting presents increasing challenges to critical care nurses. Considering each clinical condition in context with an anticipated time frame is both a pragmatic and imperative enhancement to the guideline formats suggested by ANA and AHCPR.

Guideline format places emphasis on assessment specific to each condition. Specific assessment is essential to optimize patient-focused interventions. As a result, the assessment section for each clinical guideline in *Guidelines for Critical Care Nursing* does not include "routine" assessment. Instead, each clinical guideline focuses on appropriate, specific assessment requirements and findings.

Finally, the care plan section of *Guidelines for Critical Care Nursing* departs significantly from previous standard care plan formats. The care plan is divided into three "phases" denoting the relative acuity of the patient rather than the type of unit in which the patient may be located. Patient location in an intensive care unit versus an intermediate/step-down unit or a general unit is as much a function of the size and organization of the facility and physician preference as it may be related to actual patient status. As a result, this book divides the care plan section into an "intensive phase" with emphasis on clinical stabilization and management of complex technologies, condition, or complications; an "intermediate phase" with emphasis on patient education and progression toward greater independence; and a summary comment regarding transition to discharge irrespective of the unit in which the patient might be located. This approach also formally acknowledges the provision of critical care outside the ICU and includes the intermediate care unit and ambulatory settings within the scope of critical care. Patient acuity and intervention needs, not geography, provide the focus for planning care based on the defined phases in *Guidelines for Critical Care Nursing*.

The care plan section for each clinical condition focuses on the priorities of care specific to that condition. Care that applies to all critically ill adults, regardless of specific condition, is described in the introductory chapter and not repeated in the subsequent clinical guidelines. In addition, the care plan is based on **patient** rather than nursing care priorities, with appropriate expected patient outcomes for each. While NANDA-approved nursing diagnoses are used when an appropriate label exists, priorities are not limited to those that can be described by NANDA taxonomy. The most bedside-relevant language, rather than taxonomic language, is used to describe all patient care priorities. Expected patient outcomes are described to serve as the focal point for the interventions that follow.

Interventions are also uniquely presented in *Guidelines for Critical Care Nursing*. Interventions are listed in order of relative priority from a "bedside" perspective. That is, the interventions are listed as a nurse might implement them at the bedside, keeping all of the patient-care priorities and expected patient outcomes holistically in mind. The result is a concise and clinically relevant care plan for each phase of the clinical condition. The support device chapters use a similarly practical approach by concisely listing nursing care requirements including basic troubleshooting actions.

APPLICATION OF GUIDELINES TO CLINICAL PRACTICE

The prioritized approach of *Guidelines for Critical Care Nursing*, with its concise and holistic presentation of interventions, makes this book a logical reference for practicing critical care nurses regardless of their specific practice setting. As a result, ICU, intermediate or step-down unit, ambulatory department, and even home care nurses providing care for patients who require "intensive" nursing care will find this approach to planning care useful. Graduate students in critical care will also find the guideline approach a practical and useful reference. While not specifically intended as a reference for undergraduate students, the bedside orientation of guidelines and their practical, concise format may make this text a valuable adjunct for senior students who experience critical care nursing in their curriculum.

Guidelines may be used as a clinically relevant resource for specific clinical conditions found in various critical care environments. In addition to the background information provided in the description section of the guideline, the length-of-stay information, prioritized patient care requirements, and condition-specific interventions will serve as a useful guide for bedside nursing care. *Guidelines for Critical Care Nursing*, with emphasis on research and expected patient outcomes, will also provide a foundation for quality-improvement monitoring and action. The guidelines may also stimulate ideas for nursing research into interventions that may improve patient outcomes beyond current practice potential.

We hope that all who use this resource will find it a clinically relevant, practical, patient-focused reference.

Enjoy!

REFERENCE

1. Dean-Baar S, Grindel C, Jack J, McGuffin B, Nonemaker SE, Urban N: *Standards for clinical nursing practice*, 1992, American Nurses Association.

Contents

Introduction

Kay Knox Greenlee, MSN, RN, CCRN
Nancie Urban, MSN, RN, CCRN

The scope of nursing care of the critically ill adult is twofold. The first priority is to identify patient needs and priorities associated with the clinical condition or support device(s) that may be needed to ensure optimal patient outcomes. This includes the vital role of nurses in monitoring for complications and evaluating responses to interventions. As nurses, we are additionally responsible for determining human responses to the health problem.[29] While many of these human responses are specific to the clinical condition or support device, others are generic to most if not all critically ill patients. This introductory chapter will describe guidelines for the common responses and issues while subsequent chapters will focus on nursing care guidelines associated with specific clinical conditions or support devices.

HOLISTIC ASSESSMENT

A holistic assessment is required to determine the need for care or treatment and the type of care or treatment to be provided.[1] The first component of this assessment relates to physiologic systems. The second component relates to the functional capacity of the human being in response to the illness or intervention. A head-to-toe physical assessment determines and prioritizes patient care needs and appropriate interventions, monitors for and detects complications, and determines patient response to the treatment plan. A functional health assessment identifies human responses precipitated by the critical illness. Additionally, a holistic assessment determines educational and discharge needs.

Physical Assessment Component

A preliminary physical assessment is necessary to obtain baseline information about the patient's condition upon admission to the critical care environment. While the specific components of this assessment may vary slightly based on the presenting priorities of the patient, a minimum physical assessment would include the following parameters:

System	Normal findings
Neurological	
Level of consciousness	Alert and oriented
General behavior	Appropriate to situation
Motor function	Able to move all extremities with equal, normal strength
Sensory function	Sensation intact
Cardiovascular	
Heart rate	60 to 100/min at rest
Heart rhythm	Regular
Blood pressure	120/60 ± 15, <10 mm Hg difference between arms
Heart sounds	S_1 and S_2
ECG	Normal sinus rhythm
Respiratory	
Respiratory rate	16 to 20 at rest
Respiratory pattern	Regular
Respiratory effort	Nonlabored Chest movement symmetrical
Breath sounds	Vesicular breath sounds posterior and axillary, bronchial over trachea, bronchovesicular near major bronchi, below clavicle and between scapulae
Cough effectiveness	Able to cough effectively
Sputum production	Sputum production minimal, color clear to white
Gastrointestinal	
Abdominal exam	Soft, symmetrical, nontender, without palpable masses or pulsations
Bowel sounds	Present in all quadrants
Genitourinary	
Bladder	Nondistended
Urine	Clear, amber-yellow
Integumentary	Skin intact

Physical systems require reassessment in the critically ill person based on patient status, the type of treatment, and the need to determine patient response to treatment. A complete physical reassessment of the critically ill adult is recommended every 24 hours at minimum, with significant changes in medical diagnosis or patient condition, and/or with any changes in clinical diagnosis. Most patients will require more frequent reassessment of systems directly involved with the clinical condition or support device in use. System assessments specific to a clinical condition or support device are described in the remainder of this book.

Functional Health Pattern Component

Assessment of functional health patterns is a common framework for evaluating the human responses of patients and associated nursing care requirements. It provides necessary historical information about the optimal functioning of the individual patient prior to the critical illness and how that functioning has been or might be affected by the illness. This perspective enables formulation of realistic, individualized expectations regarding patient outcomes. The functional patterns defined by Gordon[14] are one example of this type of assessment framework and are summarized in the preceding Box. This framework is useful in a variety of practice settings including critical care. Use of this type of framework may enhance continuity of care as critically ill patients make transitions between various phases of care.

Like physical systems, functional health patterns require periodic reassessment. A complete functional assessment is recommended on admission to and discharge from the critical care setting. More frequent reassessments of specific patterns are determined by the care priorities of the individual patient.

The following human response/functioning guidelines address selected parameters that are common to all critically ill adults. Similar to the framework by Gordon, these guidelines serve as a foundation for most if not all clinical-condition and support-device guidelines contained in this book. A specific clinical or support-device guideline will address these issues only when they demonstrate particular meaning or risk beyond the challenge that is common to all critically ill adults. When confronting issues not addressed in a specific guideline, the reader may wish to return to this chapter as needed for review of the foundational principles.

In context with the guideline format, a description of the condition, assessment parameters, and the common patient-care priorities associated with each of the general response/functioning guidelines will be identified. However, the etiologies for these priorities are most often specific to the clinical condition or support device. As a result, etiologies will be designated within a specific clinical-condition or support-device guideline where they apply.

Functional Health Pattern Definitions

Health perception/health management
Describes client's perceived pattern of health and well-being and how health is managed

Nutrition metabolic
Describes pattern of food and fluid consumption related to metabolic need and pattern indicators of local nutrient supply

Elimination
Describes patterns of excretory function (bowel, bladder, skin)

Activity exercise
Describes pattern of exercise, activity, leisure, and recreation

Sleep rest
Describes patterns of sleep, rest, and relaxation

Cognitive perceptual
Describes sensory-perceptual and cognitive pattern

Self-perception/self-concept
Describes self-concept pattern and perceptions of self (e.g., body comfort, body image, feeling state)

Role relationship
Describes pattern of role-engagements and relationships

Sexuality reproductive
Describes client's pattern of satisfaction and dissatisfaction with sexuality pattern; describes reproductive patterns

Coping stress tolerance
Describes general coping pattern and effectiveness of the pattern in terms of stress tolerance

Value beliefs
Describes patterns of values, beliefs (including spiritual), or goals that guide choices or decisions

FACILITATING COPING

Description

A critical illness stresses the physical system and the psychoemotional integrity of the individual. The critical care environment can overwhelm and stress the visual, auditory, and tactile senses. The environment further impacts the patient because lack of privacy and dependency may be created. Coping is the human response to all of these stressors. The ability to cope with the stress of a critical illness is dependent upon a person's perception of the situation, resources available, and previous experiences with stressful situations. A patient may respond by modifying the situation, altering or controlling the meaning of the situation, or managing the stress after it has occurred.[40]

Coping with physical and psychological stressors can reduce the physiologic changes that result from stress. Stress can depress the immune system.[22] This may increase the risk of infection. High levels of stress can also compromise wound healing because of increased levels of catecholamines resulting in vasoconstriction.[45] The cardiovascular effects from increased levels of epinephrine and norepinephrine, present during times of stress, include increased myocardial oxygen consumption and cardiac workload.[6] This is of particular concern for a patient with compromised cardiac functioning. Nursing intervention is essential to facilitate coping of the critically ill adult and prevent these physiologic events.

While the patient is the primary concern, the family (as defined by the patient) must also be considered when discussing the stress related to a critical illness. Research has focused on the needs of family members and the responsibility of nurses to meet these needs.[18,20,26] Meeting these needs will greatly enhance the ability of the family to cope. The focus during the intensive phase of care is to facilitate coping with the sudden change in physical and social functioning. Facilitation of coping through the intermediate and transition-to-discharge phases often relates to the realization of surviving a critical illness. In addition, assisting the patient and family to return to a pre-illness state of health and functioning is equally important.

ASSESSMENT

PARAMETER	ANTICIPATED ALTERATION
Physiologic responses to stress	Increased oxygen consumption Increased heart rate, blood pressure, respiratory rate Fatigue Irritability
Past coping behaviors	Effective coping behaviors in evidence Potential that coping behaviors may interfere with care requirements
Support systems	Separated from primary support
Power resources[25] • Physical strength and reserve • Psychological stamina and support network • Positive self-concept • Energy • Knowledge • Motivation • Belief system	Supportive behaviors or deficits in adaptive coping behaviors
Sense of worth, usual religious and cultural practices	May be compromised
General behavior	May withdraw or act out unlike usual behavior pattern
General appearance	Associated with clinical condition and emotional response
Attention/concentration	May be severely impaired
Insight into illness	May be limited
Feelings/mood	Often labile
Usual roles and relationship between roles	May be significantly altered
Feelings related to performance of roles	May be adaptive or maladaptive

PLAN OF CARE

PATIENT CARE PRIORITIES	EXPECTED PATIENT OUTCOMES
Compromised coping	Uses coping strategies
Ineffective coping	Identifies coping strategies
Spiritual distress	Verbalizes spiritual peace
Altered family dynamics	Is able to cope with situation
Grieving	Acknowledges losses
Fear, anxiety, and hopelessness	Verbalizes or demonstrates decreased anxiety, fear, or hopelessness
Powerlessness	Verbalizes feeling of control

Plan of Care (cont'd)

INTERVENTIONS

Provide a calm, safe environment *to minimize external stressors.*

Promote a caring environment. *Families of the critically ill identified the following as characteristics of a caring nurse: uses active listening, evaluates family expectations, and recognizes anxiety.*[23]

Assist to develop coping mechanisms. *This may be the patient's and family's first experience with illness. Guidance by the nurse is needed to determine if coping mechanisms from past experiences are ineffective.*

Provide an opportunity to verbalize concerns.

Support and facilitate relaxation. *Relaxation counters the effects of stress. Relaxation should include positioning, a quiet environment, focus on breathing, and a passive attitude.*[6]

Anxiolytics as necessary. *Pharmacologic intervention may be necessary when the patient is in a state of physiological and psychological stress and unable to concentrate or comprehend in order to realistically use coping strategies.*

Establish a trusting therapeutic relationship. *Patients perceive a caring environment when the nurse speaks in a low, modulated voice, is accepting of messes, is able to smile and joke with the patient, and demonstrates caring about what is happening.*[9]

Include patient and family in planning care.

Encourage self-care *to promote control and hope.*

Incorporate values and beliefs into the plan of care.

Encourage practice of appropriate rituals.

Consult with spiritual care personnel, e.g., hospital chaplain or patient's clergy.

Assist patient and family to use alternative coping strategies.

Assist family to meet nutrition, activity, and sleep needs. *When the family is concerned about the critically ill patient, they sometimes forget to care for themselves.*

Provide accurate, realistic information.

Address plan to meet family needs as listed in the following box.

Assist to balance reality and hope. *Assessment of the family situation is necessary to determine perception. The nurse offers hope or a realistic view based on which one is needed.*

Meet the need for information.

Allow opportunity to grieve by encouraging expression of grief, acknowledging anticipated or actual loss, and providing necessary time to grieve.

Assist to identify support system, including support groups within the local community.

Assess family's need for support related to ability to manage maintenance of home. *While not the initial priority, consideration needs to be given to what is happening outside the hospital. It is important to check with the family and provide support as needed. Concern about the home situation may contribute to the patient's anxiety.*

The Most Important Family Needs[18]

- To have questions answered honestly
- To be assured the best possible care is being given to the patient
- To know the prognosis
- To feel there is hope
- To know specific facts about the patient's progress
- To receive understandable explanations
- To know exactly what is being done for the patient
- To know why things were done for the patient
- To see the patient frequently
- To talk to the doctor every day
- To be told about transfer plans
- To be called at home about changes in the patient's condition
- To know how the patient is being treated medically
- To feel hospital personnel care about the patient
- To receive information about the patient daily

PAIN MANAGEMENT

Description

Pain is a common response to illness and treatment of the critically ill. The pain experienced is usually acute. However, critically ill patients may have a history of chronic pain that also must be managed. The physiological and psychological risks associated with untreated pain are significant. The physiological consequences include increased myocardial oxygen consumption with potential for ischemia, splinting and altered respiratory pattern resulting in decreased volume and flow with potential for ineffective airway clearance, and restricted mobility with potential for contraction and rigidity.[34] The psychological consequences of pain are cognitive emotional and behavioral responses including powerlessness, helplessness, depression, and anxiety.[12]

Assessment of pain is essential to planning appropriate individualized care. Interventions are directed toward preventing, managing, and helping the patient express and obtain relief from pain.

ASSESSMENT

PARAMETER	ANTICIPATED ALTERATION
Observe Behavior	
Facial expression	Guarding
Protective behaviors	Withdrawal Avoidance of movement
Palliative behaviors	Rubbing area Positioning for comfort Requesting pain medication
Affective behaviors	Crying Moaning Screaming
Subjective Elements	
Qualitative	Burning, sharp, throbbing, aching, cramping
Intensity	0 to 10: none to severe
Emotional component	0 to 10: none to bothersome
Physiologic Responses	
Heart rate	Increased
Blood pressure	Increased
Pupils	Dilated
Skin	Diaphoretic
Source of Pain	
Cutaneous	May be localized to site of origin
Somatic	May be referred to an associated site
Visceral	

PLAN OF CARE

PATIENT CARE PRIORITIES	EXPECTED PATIENT OUTCOMES
Pain, acute	Satisfied with pain management
Pain, chronic	

INTERVENTIONS

Implement pain treatment flowchart described in Figure I-1.[2]
Assess for pain q2h, while awake, and 5 to 30 minutes after interventions.
Consider pharmacologic and nonpharmacologic pain interventions as described in Table I-1.

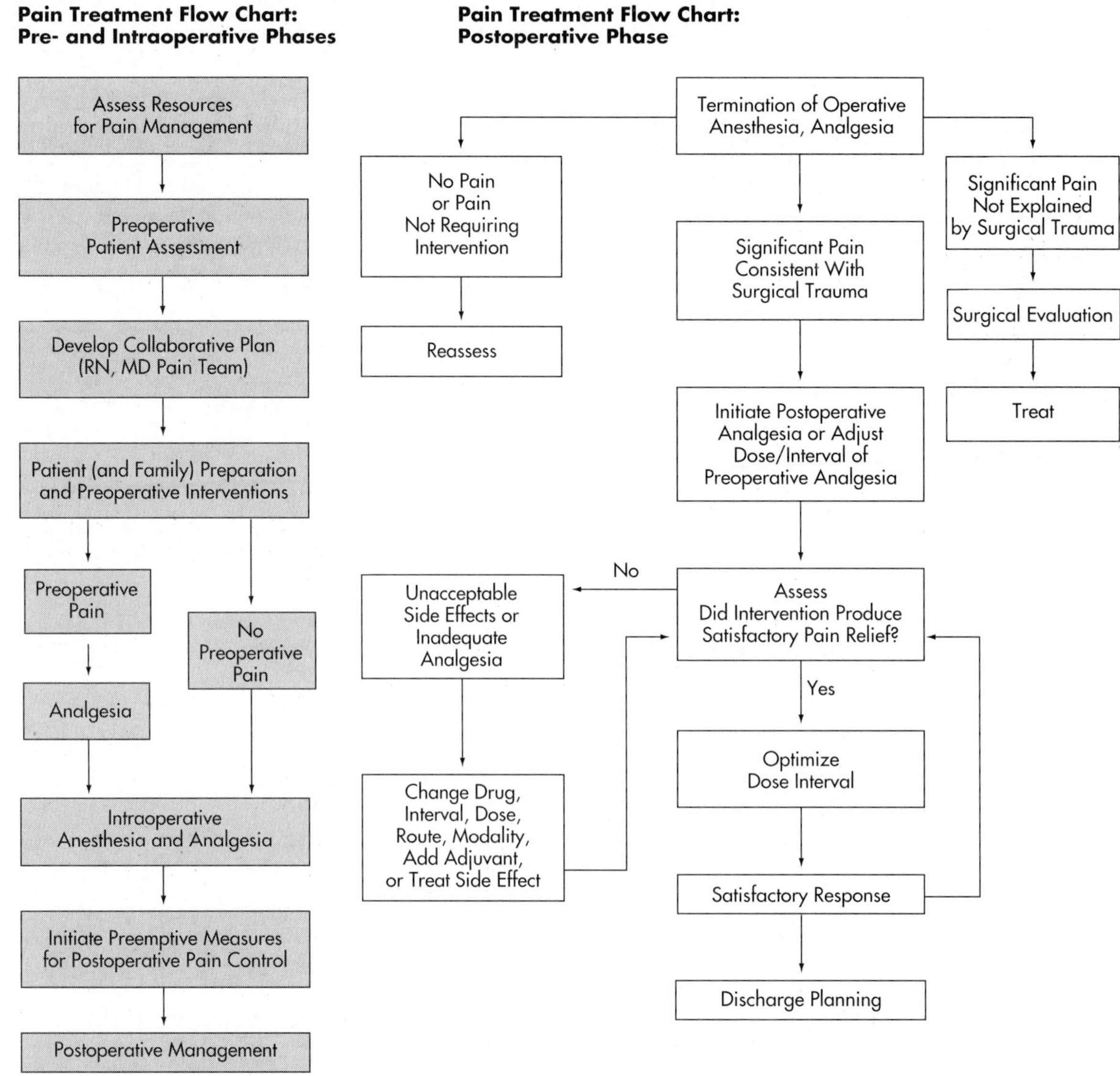

Figure I-1 Pain Treatment Flowchart (AHCPR). From *Acute pain management: operative or medical procedures and trauma,* Clinical Practice Guideline No. 1, AHCPR Publication No. 92-0032, Rockville, Md, February 1992, Agency for Health Care Policy and Research, Public Health Service, U.S. Department of Health and Human Services.

TABLE I-1 Pharmacologic and Nonpharmacologic Interventions

	Pharmacologic interventions*		
	Intervention†	**Type of evidence***	**Comments**
NSAIDs	Oral (alone)	Ib, IV	Effective for mild to moderate pain. Begin preoperatively. Relatively contraindicated in patients with renal disease and risk of or actual coagulopathy. May mask fever.
	Oral (adjunct to opioid)	Ia, IV	Potentiating effect resulting in opioid sparing. Begin preop. Cautions as above.
	Parenteral (ketorolac)	Ib, IV	Effective for moderate to severe pain. Expensive. Useful where opioids contraindicated, especially to avoid respiratory depression and sedation. Advance to opioid.

TABLE I-1 Pharmacologic and Nonpharmacologic Interventions—cont'd

Pharmacologic interventions*

Intervention†		Type of evidence*	Comments
Opioids	Oral	IV	As effective as parenteral in appropriate doses. Use as soon as medication tolerated. Route of choice.
	Intramuscular	Ib, IV	Has been the standard parenteral route, but injections painful and absorption unreliable. Hence, avoid this route when possible.
	Subcutaneous	Ib, IV	Preferable to intramuscular when a low-volume continuous infusion is needed and intravenous access is difficult to maintain. Injections painful and absorption unreliable. Avoid this route for long-term repetitive dosing.
	Intravenous	Ib, IV	Parenteral route of choice after major surgery. Suitable for titrated bolus or continuous administration (including PCA), but requires monitoring. Significant risk of respiratory depression with inappropriate dosing.
	PCA (systemic)	Ia, IV	Intravenous or subcutaneous routes recommended. Good steady level of analgesia. Popular with patients but requires special infusion pumps and staff education. See cautions about opioids above.
	Epidural & intrathecal	Ia, IV	When suitable, provides good analgesia. Significant risk of respiratory depression, sometimes delayed in onset. Requires careful monitoring. Use of infusion pumps requires additional equipment and staff education. Expensive if infusion pumps are employed.
Local anesthetics	Epidural & intrathecal	Ia, IV	Limited indications. Effective regional analgesia. Opioid sparing. Addition of opioid to local anesthetic may improve analgesia. Risks of hypotension, weakness, numbness. Requires careful monitoring. Use of infusion pump requires additional equipment and staff education.
	Peripheral nerve block	Ia, IV	Limited indications and duration of action. Effective regional analgesia. Opioid sparing.
Simple relaxation (begin preoperatively)	Jay relaxation Progressive muscle relaxation Simple imagery	Ia, IIa, IIb, IV	Effective in reducing mild to moderate pain and as an adjunct to analgesic drugs for severe pain. Use when patients express an interest in relaxation. Requires 3-5 minutes of staff time for instructions.
	Music	Ib, IIa, IV	Both patient-preferred and "easy listening" music are effective in reducing mild to moderate pain.
Complex relaxation (begin preoperatively)	Biofeedback	Ib, IIa, IIb, IV	Effective in reducing mild to moderate pain and operative site muscle tension. Requires skilled personnel and special equipment.
	Imagery	Ib, IIa, IV	Effective for reduction of mild to moderate pain. Requires skilled personnel.
Education/instruction (begin preoperatively)		Ia, IIa, IIb, IV	Effective for reduction of pain. Should include sensory and procedural information and instruction aimed at reducing activity related pain. Requires 5-15 minutes of staff time.
TENS		Ia, IIa, III, IV	Effective in reducing pain and improving physical function. Requires skilled personnel and special equipment. May be useful as an adjunct to drug therapy.

Type of Evidence—Key
Ia Evidence obtained from meta-analysis of randomized controlled trials.
b Evidence obtained from at least one randomized controlled trial.
IIa Evidence obtained from at least one well-designed controlled study without randomization.
b Evidence obtained from at least one other type of well-designed quasi-experimental study.
III Evidence obtained from well-designed nonexperimental studies, such as comparative studies, correlational studies, and case studies.
IV Evidence obtained from expert committee reports or opinions and/or clinical experiences of respected authorities.

*From *Acute pain management: operative or medical procedures and trauma,* Clinical Practice Guideline, no 1, AHCPR Publication, no 92-0032, Rockville, Md, February, 1992, Agency for Health Care Policy and Research, Public Health Service, US Department of Health and Human Services.

†From *Accreditation manual for hospitals, 1994,* Section I: Assessment of patients, Chicago, 1993, Joint Commission on the Accreditation of Health Care Organizations.

REST AND SLEEP DEPRIVATION

Description

The average adult sleeps 6 to 8 hours or 25 to 33% of the day.[13] Sleep is often taken for granted, but the inability to sleep is a major concern in the critically ill patient. Sleep deprivation results from the clinical condition including pain and the environment. The suggested functions of sleep include cellular restoration, energy conservation, and reparative, instinctive, protective, and adaptive outcomes.

Sleep deprivation may result from decreased amounts, quality, or consistency of sleep.[37] Lack of sleep should be viewed as a stressor contributing to a situation already overwhelmed with physiological and psychological stress. The symptoms noted include confusion, disorientation, hallucinations, apathy, combativeness, anxiety, decreased concentration, muscle pain, impaired respiratory function, and decreased immune response.[10]

ASSESSMENT

PARAMETER	ANTICIPATED ALTERATION
Usual schedule of sleep Any problems sleeping Routines used to facilitate sleep Sleep latency (time it takes to fall asleep) Periods of wakefulness Frequency of awakenings	All aspects of normal sleep patterns may be disrupted

PLAN OF CARE

PATIENT CARE PRIORITIES	EXPECTED PATIENT OUTCOMES
Sleep pattern disturbance	Uninterrupted 90-minute period of sleep at least twice during usual sleep hours. Two uninterrupted rest periods throughout the day.

INTERVENTIONS

Create environment conducive to sleep and rest.
- Give consideration to lights, noise, temperature, position of comfort, hygiene, elimination.
- Close doors, decrease phone volume, dim lights, keep voices low, and remote alarms, if possible.

Teach relaxation strategies and facilitate use of relaxation *to promote sleep and rest.*

Pain management. *The presence of pain affects a person's ability to sleep. Sleep may be possible with pain, but the quality and duration will be affected.*

Provide reassurance. *Patients are sometimes afraid to go to sleep. Knowing the methods used to monitor sleep and safety measures in place during sleep is often reassuring.*

Provide diversional physical activity during waking hours and avoid naps close to planned period of prolonged sleep *to increase the possibility of achieving REM sleep.*

MOBILITY

Description

Immobility affects multiple body systems and increases the risk of complications. Cardiovascular effects include fluid shifts, decreased work capacity, orthostatic intolerance, and decreased venous flow.[38] Lung volumes are decreased and the ventilation-perfusion relationship may change with immobility, increasing the risk for pulmonary emboli and atelectasis. Immobility contributes to changes in elimination patterns as well. Constipation and urinary stasis result, with urinary stasis increasing the risk for UTI (urinary tract infection). Muscles begin to atrophy resulting in weakness and fatigue. The risk for contracture and nerve injury also increases with immobility. Pressure and friction associated with immobility increase the risk for skin breakdown. Prolonged immobility will also have a psychological effect. Patients associate bed confinement with illness, resulting in feelings of hopelessness and dependence, as well as potential alteration in sensory perception.

Limitations to mobility and usual activity are experienced by every critically ill patient during the intensive phase of care. The limitations may be imposed to protect physiologic functioning or decrease the risk of complications. As the patient progresses to the intermediate phase of care, activity may be limited as result of weakness, discomfort, or prolonged bed rest.

When activity is limited or when the patient is unable to move independently, positioning to optimize ventilation and other physiologic functioning becomes essential. Mobility has a therapeutic impact in that it can enhance healing, prevent complications, and enhance pain management. Since patients associate bed confinement with the illness, the first step of movement may significantly impact the patient's psychological recovery and well-being. Moving the patient from the bed to a chair is a sign of progression and beginning recovery.

Assessment of mobility includes what the patient was able to do prior to the critical illness as well as current functioning. Goals are established to determine if the patient will be able to achieve or in some cases exceed the activities achieved prior to the illness. Mobility is also one of several factors considered when determining the risk for skin breakdown.

ASSESSMENT

PARAMETER	ANTICIPATED ALTERATION
Usual activities of daily living (self care, energy, mobility, exercise program, leisure activities)	May be significantly compromised
Physiologic response to activity	VS and oxygenation may be altered
Ability to bear weight	May be unable to bear weight
Assistive devices	May be required
Assess risk for skin breakdown within 24 to 48 hours of admission and reassess risk q8h to q48h depending on condition and risk.[5] Risk factors include: • Sensory perception • Activity • Immobility • Nutrition • Moisture • Incontinence • Level of consciousness	Areas of skin compromise or overt breakdown may be noted, especially heels and other bony areas

PLAN OF CARE

PATIENT CARE PRIORITIES	EXPECTED PATIENT OUTCOMES
Self-care deficit	Participates in increased self-care activities
Activity intolerance	Demonstrates improved tolerance
Impaired physical mobility	Demonstrates increased strength and mobility
Impaired home maintenance management	Indicates measures taken to maintain home maintenance
High risk for impaired skin integrity	Skin integrity maintained

INTERVENTIONS

Balance rest with activity.

Limit visitors as necessary.

Teach energy-saving techniques. *Keep in mind that patient comfort and cooperation may be enhanced by the presence of family or visitors.*

Teach pursed lipped breathing *to optimize balanced respiration during exertion and minimize risk of Valsalva maneuvers.*

Assess vital signs pre- and post-activity.

Passive or active range of motion q8h.

Maintain proper body alignment.

Pain management prior to activity.

Progress activity as tolerated.

Toileting by commode instead of bedpan. *This improves mobility but also decreases stress and anxiety related to meeting elimination needs while lying in bed.*

Plan of Care (cont'd)

Collaborate with physical therapist and other rehab services *to optimize patient recovery and return to optimal level of functional status.*

Prevention measures as described by the Panel for the Prediction and Prevention of Pressure Ulcers in Adults.[33]

- Keep heels elevated off bed surface at all times using pillows or other devices prn.
- Reposition at least q2h to reduce pressure.
- Use pillows or wedge between bony prominences to prevent direct contact with one another while patient is in bed.
- Protect contact points, use lift sheets or trapeze to decrease friction.
- Use lubricants, protective films, protective dressings, and protective padding to decrease risk of skin injury from friction.
- Avoid massage over bony prominences as this may lead to deep tissue trauma.
- Daily hygiene and peri care, increase frequency with incontinence. Avoid hot water and use mild cleansing agent to decrease irritation and dryness. Minimize force and friction applied to skin.
- Minimize skin exposure to moisture due to incontinence, perspiration, or wound drainage.
- Avoid direct pressure to trochanter when positioned on side.
- Risk of shearing can be decreased by maintaining HOB at lowest degree of elevation consistent with medical condition and other restrictions.
- Use pressure-reducing device (foam, static air, alternating air, gel, water mattress) on bed or chair for individuals at risk.
- Shift pressure point qh while in chair, teach patient to shift weight q15min if able.

SAFETY

Description

Safety is a basic concern to the critically ill patient. The goal is to protect the patient and prevent injury. Within the critical care environment, specific safety issues include risk of falls, electrical sensitivity, risk of infection, and risks related to vulnerabilities. Infection control will be discussed as a separate topic.

The critically ill patient is at risk for falls because of multiple factors including impaired judgement, assistance needed to meet elimination and hygiene needs, sleep deprivation, sensory deficits, immobility, weakness, and the use of certain medications such as narcotics, sedatives, and antihypertensives. Assessing the patient for risk of falls and creating a safe environment are important nursing interventions for preventing falls.[36] Most published risk assessment tools have been developed and tested on elderly patients. However, an awareness of these risk factors can help decrease risk for all critically ill adults. While the incidence of falls in a critical care environment may be less than or comparable to the medical and surgical areas, the risk for falls may increase when patients transfer out of the intensive care setting. Roberts found that adult patients treated in an ICU and transferred to a general medical or surgical unit were nearly three times as likely to fall than those never treated in an ICU.[35] The incidence was greatest for patients treated in a medical and neurological ICU.

When the protective skin barrier is interrupted, such as with a transvenous pacemaker or pulmonary artery catheter, the patient is at risk for microshock and is considered electrically sensitive.[3] Electrical safety in the critical care environment is a shared responsibility of the nurse, biomedical engineer, and hospital administration. An electrically safe environment is created through regulations, routine monitoring and maintenance, and knowledgeable users of electrical equipment.

Screening for vulnerabilities during initial care of the patient will help direct discharge planning and decrease the risk of injury. In addition, an awareness of potential physical, emotional, or sexual abuse or neglect are key categories of assessment. The nurse is not required to treat the problem but must refer suspected patients to a social worker or designated facility or agency for more detailed assessment and follow-up.

Critical illnesses related to drug and chemical abuse may pose special challenges in caring for a patient. The risk of injury during withdrawal requires close observation, early identification, and prompt treatment. It is also important to make referrals so that appropriate follow-up is done, which could possibly prevent a subsequent critical illness.

ASSESSMENT

PARAMETER	ANTICIPATED ALTERATION
Assess Factors Associated with High Risk of Fall[36]	
Mental status *to determine cognitive awareness*	Any/all fall risk factors may be present
Functional health status *to determine level of independence in ADLs*	
History of falls	
Sensory assessment *to determine degree of impairment*	
Emotions *to evaluate mood fluctuations*	
Sleep pattern	
Mobility *to determine gait and balance*	
Recent loss	
Hypotension	
Medications	
Assess for Risk of Electrical Sensitivity	
Transvenous pacemaker	Presence of invasive monitoring or therapeutic devices or lines highly probable
Epicardial pacer wires	
Pulmonary artery catheter	
Indwelling arterial lines	
Vulnerability Assessments	
Signs of physical, emotional, or sexual abuse or neglect	Evidence or suspicion of abuse or neglect must be reported to the appropriate agency as well as clinically managed

PLAN OF CARE

PATIENT CARE PRIORITIES	EXPECTED PATIENT OUTCOMES
High risk for injury	Free of injury

INTERVENTIONS

Call light or means to call for assistance readily available to patient.
Bed in low position with at least two side rails up.
Assist patient to meet elimination and hygiene needs on a planned schedule.
Eliminate clutter in room to create free path for ambulation.
Use electrical safety measures including three-prong plugs, ensure all cords and plugs are grounded, avoid extension cords, do not place liquid or wet items on electrical equipment.
Apply restraints after alternative measures to control patient behavior have failed.
Assess for orthostatic BP changes with initial out-of-bed activity.
Report evidence or suspicion of evidence of abuse or neglect to the appropriate agency.

NUTRITION

Description

Adequate nutritional intake is important for critically ill patients, who are frequently in a state of hypermetabolism requiring increased caloric intake, specifically proteins. Malnutrition contributes to increased length of stay, delayed wound healing, and immunosuppression. Additionally, critically ill patients who are NPO for greater than three days, have nausea and vomiting, or have diarrhea greater than three days are at risk for developing malnutrition.[32] Selecting interventions to achieve the goal of adequate caloric and

TABLE I-2 Enteral versus Parenteral Nutrition

Enteral nutrition	Parenteral nutrition
Indications	**Indications**
• Totally or partially functioning GI tract • Unable or unwilling to take in adequate calories	• GI tract cannot or should not work • Patient able to tolerate only small volumes of enteral nutrition and needs supplement to meet requirements
Nursing care	**Nursing care**
• Check placement q4h, use air insufflation or aspirated GI contents as indication of good placement • Check residual q4h to prevent distention • Administer at room temperature • Flush between feedings • Elevate HOB 30-40° to decrease risk of aspiration and to facilitate gastric emptying	• Filter and tubing changed q24h • Sterile occlusive dressing changed q24h if gauze, q72h if transparent • Monitor site for signs of infection

From Viall CD: Nutrition. In Kinney M, et al, editors: *AACN's clinical reference for critical-care nursing,* ed 3, St Louis, 1993, Mosby, pp 297-328.

protein intake are done in collaboration with the physician and dietician. Monitoring for the presence of complications specific to the type of nutrition provided is also an important nursing intervention.

Providing nutritional support is not without potential complications. Patients receiving enteral feedings are at risk for aspiration and diarrhea. The risk of aspiration can be decreased by using the nursing care guidelines shown in Table I-2. Diarrhea in a patient receiving enteral feeding is multifactorial, including sorbitol-based or hyperosmolar elixirs, antibiotics, albumin <2.6 g/dl, *C. difficele,* and change in rate of administration.[32] Patients receiving parenteral nutrition also are at risk for catheter sepsis.

ASSESSMENT

PARAMETER	ANTICIPATED ALTERATION
Daily food and fluid intake	Significantly changed May be NPO
Weight gain or loss pattern	Losses associated with catabolic states Gains associated with alteration in fluid balance
Ingestion factors: appetite, discomfort, teeth, oral mucosa, allergies	Anorexia common
Religious, ethnic, or cultural preferences	May be difficult to accomodate
Albumin	WNL: 3.2 to 4.5 g/dl
Transferrin level	WNL: >200 mg/dl
Prealbumin level	WNL: >15 mg/dl
Nitrogen balance	WNL: −5 to 0 during catabolic state

PLAN OF CARE

PATIENT CARE PRIORITIES	EXPECTED PATIENT OUTCOMES
Alteration in nutritional intake	Adequate caloric intake to maintain anabolic state
High risk for impaired wound healing	Intact skin or no further breakdown
	Maintenance of goal body weight
	Positive nitrogen balance
	Progressive wound healing

INTERVENTIONS

Consult with dietician *to ensure comprehensive assessment and identification of optimal diet.*

Create environment conducive to eating.

Plan of Care (cont'd)

Provide oral care and rest prior to mealtime *to ensure adequate energy reserves to eat, prevent aspiration, and optimize digestion.*

Determine appropriate route of nutrition for patients unable to tolerate regular diet and provide nursing care according to guidelines.[41] (See Table I-2.)

For patients with diarrhea, select one of the following interventions and evaluate patient response before trying another intervention.[32]

- Add bulk or fiber
- Change elixirs
- Lactobacillus for patient on antibiotics >2 weeks
- Anti-diarrheal medications
- Peptide-based formula
- Albumin replacement
- Decrease rate of feeding

INFECTION CONTROL

Description

Infection control practices are directed toward preventing nosocomial infections in the patient and protecting the health care team from disease transmission. Within the critical care environment, high risk for infection is due to organisms present, multiple invasive procedures and devices used, numerous health care team members, and the type of underlying disease present in the patient.[30] The risk of infection increases with the patient's age and with the use of drugs, such as steroids, antineoplastics, and some antibiotics. Common sites of nosocomial infections in the critically ill include the respiratory system, urinary tract, bloodstream, and surgical wounds.[44] Interventions are directed toward monitoring for and preventing nosocomial infections.

As the prevalence of HIV, HBV, TB and other infectious diseases increases, so does the risk to health care workers. Universal precautions should be instituted to decrease risk of exposure to blood-borne pathogens potentially present in all critically ill patients and in other infectious agents.

ASSESSMENT

TYPE OF INFECTION	HIGH RISK PROFILE
Respiratory	Age >65, nutritional status, COPD, impaired immunity, endotracheal tube.
Urinary	Female gender, Foley catheter, bed rest.
Blood	Invasive lines, age >65, severity of illness, nutritional status, chronic disease such as diabetes or renal failure, immobility, multiple invasions into closed system lines.
Wound	Environmental risk of colonization, remote infection, type and duration of surgery, use of implants, use of drains.

PLAN OF CARE

PATIENT CARE PRIORITIES	EXPECTED PATIENT OUTCOMES
High risk for infection	Free of signs of infection

INTERVENTIONS

General interventions

Protect patient from exposure to infectious pathogens.

Use sterile technique for invasive procedures.

Strict hand washing and glove changes between patients and procedures.

Evaluate the need to continue invasive lines or tubes daily *to ensure their removal as soon as possible.*

Plan of Care (cont'd)

Respiratory-specific interventions	Promote mobility or turn, deep breathe, and cough. Oral care at least q8h, q2h when intubated. Evacuate moisture collected in ventilator circuit. Suction based on assessment.
Urinary-specific interventions	Foley care with soap and water. Maintain a closed system.
Blood-specific interventions	Dressing and tubing changes according to hospital policy. Change IVs started in the field or during codes within 24 hours.
Wound interventions	Change wound dressing when soiled or no longer occlusive.
Universal precautions[39]	Wear gloves when touching blood, body fluids, mucous membranes, or nonintact skin of all patients, and for handling items or surfaces soiled with blood or body fluids. Wear masks and protective eye wear or shields when generation of droplets of blood or other body fluids are likely. Wear gown or apron during procedures that are likely to generate splashing.

DISCHARGE PLANNING

Discharge planning must begin when a patient arrives in the critical care setting. National changes in health care continue to press for ever-faster discharge of patients from the acute care—essentially the critical care—environment. As a result, critical care nurses must become involved in anticipating the discharge needs of their patients. They must also consider the ramifications of their daily clinical care decisions on the need and potential for discharge at the earliest possible time. This consideration must be extended to include discharge from the hospital, not just the ICU. The complexity and, often, the unpredictability of critically ill patients makes discharge planning a very challenging and dynamic process for the critical care nurse; a challenge that tests and stretches the assessment and clinical decision-making skills of even the most expert critical care nurse.

A classification of discharge alternatives is summarized in Table I-3. This classification makes assessment of the home environment and support system of patients a vital component of the admission assessment. Collaboration with internal resources such as social workers, discharge planners, or home care coordinators optimally occurs early in the hospitalization of a critically ill patient. Early planning can be the "magic" that ensures timely transfer or discharge of patients in context with the reality of scarce community resources. Early discharge planning also helps keep the patient and family focused on progressive recovery, facilitates their sense of control and participation, prevents surprises, and may reduce anxiety while facilitating coping.

A high percentage of critically ill patients will be discharged from medical or surgical units where patients have progressed from the intermediate phase of care to transition to discharge. Planning on the part of the critical care nurse will contribute to an easier discharge when the time comes. Concerns identified by patients within four months post-discharge are listed in the following Box. Critical care nurses can begin to address these concerns at the time of transfer, with reinforcement by the discharging unit to increase comprehension on the part of the patient and family members.

Studies have been conducted looking at the effects of discharge planning on length of stay and rehospitalization. These studies are small and age-specific, but they introduce the concept that discharge planning can decrease length of stay and prevent or reduce readmissions.

THE ISSUE OF ETHICS

The Patient Self-Determination Act went into effect December 1, 1991, and requires that Medicate- and Medicaid-funded hospitals provide written information to adult patients about their rights to make treatment decisions and execute advance directives. Decisions may relate to advance directives, resuscitation, and withdrawal of life-support therapy. The algorithmic guide in Figure I-2 was developed to assist the health care team in treatment decisions.[21]

Prior to discharge it is important to address decisions related to advance directives. Advance directives are initiated by the patient and/or family as a way to have their

TABLE I-3 Discharge Levels

Discharge Level 1	Patient to return to prehospital living environment. Routine or standard discharge teaching will prepare patient for discharge.
Discharge Level 2	Patient to return to prehospital living environment. Patient requires discharge teaching above standard or routine, specific to new diagnosis.
Discharge Level 3	Patient to return to prehospital living environment, with assistance. Referral to outside agency is necessary to meet patient's care needs.
Discharge Level 4	Patient is unable to return to prehospital living environment. Alternative living arrangements are necessary.

Data collected from Pelletier E: A quality discharge plan breeds cooperation and success, *The next step: glasrock home health care newsletter,* 7(4):4-6, 1991.

Post-Hospitalization Concerns[4]

Understanding progress
Deciding how much activity is good
Knowing what insurance pays for
Knowing what to expect from medicines
Knowing how to control pain
Knowing when to consult the doctor
Knowing how to take prescribed medications
Understanding the diet to follow
Arranging a way home from the hospital
Getting help with housekeeping or cooking
Getting needed medical equipment
Having a nurse to provide care

Information compiled from Boyle K, Nance J, Passau-Buck S: Post-hospitalization concerns of medical-surgical patients *Applied Nursing Research,* 5(3):122-126, 1992.

values and choices respected. Advance directives include living wills and Durable Power of Attorney for Health Care (DPA). The living will is used when the declarant is terminally ill and unable to make decisions. The DPA authorizes a proxy decision maker for health-related matters. The DPA goes into effect when individuals are unable to make or communicate health care decisions whether or not their condition is imminently terminal.

Nurses play a key role in resuscitation decisions—frequent contact with the patient and family provides the opportunity to understand their concerns and wishes. Nurses are more likely to be there when the time is right to discuss preferences for resuscitation. Appropriate times to ask patients about their wishes include upon admission, prior to major surgery, upon admission to a critical care unit, or when a patient expresses doubt about the current treatment plan.[28] At these times, the nurse is obligated to discuss the information with the physician and other members of the health care team as appropriate. Delay in addressing DNR (do not resuscitate) status and orders without clarification or documentation of rationale create frustration.[24] We should not ask the family to make medical judgements. Rather, we should provide realistic factual information and make recommendations to assist the patient, or the family if the patient is unable to communicate, in reaching a decision.[8] Definition of resuscitation includes CPR, and respiratory and pharmacologic support with cardiac and respiratory arrest. Patients and/or families may choose aggressive intervention up to the point of arrest and then stop.

DNR decisions may be made in conjunction with withdrawal of life-sustaining therapy as well. Withdrawal of or limiting life-support therapies is carried out at the request of the patient and/or family or when the therapy has been deemed futile. As long as the patient is competent, an informed decision can be made by the patient and carried out in collaboration with members of the health care team. In some cases the therapy may be viewed as futile by the health care team but continued at the family's request. Futility is a complex concept that includes an analysis of benefits versus burdens to determine if the benefits produced outweigh the burdens in suffering or financial cost. The patient needs to determine whether the benefits are worth the burdens. Along with benefit-burden analysis, consideration must be given to the patient's goals.[7] Questions such as (1) What purpose is this intervention serving? (2) Is it providing physiologic good or helping the patient in some other way? and (3) Is it harming the patient in some way? should be used to analyze the situation prior to approaching the family regarding such difficult and delicate decisions.[42]

COLLABORATION

Collaboration is essential to optimal patient outcomes in the current health care environment. One discipline, even as holistic a discipline as nursing, simply cannot do it alone. Most research related to collaboration has focused on the nurse and physician. However, it is important to remember

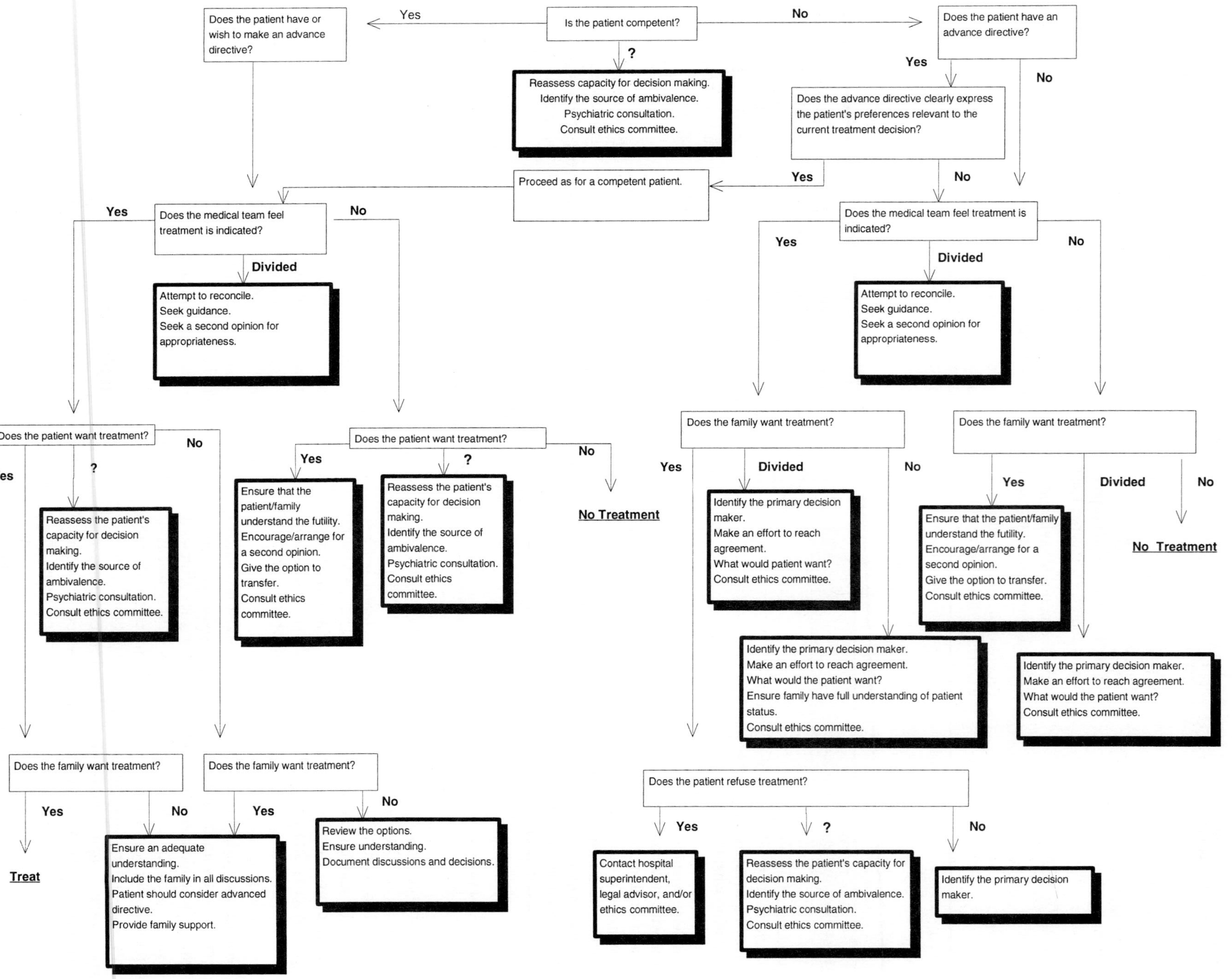

Figure I-2 Algorithm for decision making

Collaboration

Keys to successful collaboration[11,16]

Assign high priority to building collaborative practice
Recognize the benefit
Possess an environment that facilitates the process
Allow time for the process to evolve
Make a commitment to optimal patient outcomes
Value efficiency and clinical competence.

Strategies to enhance collaboration[43]

Regularly scheduled rounds
Joint education
Integrated record
Joint patient-care meeting
Joint practice committee
Collaborative research
Performance improvement
Share with planning and decision making

Factors that foster collaboration[15]

Refrain from rigid divisions of labor and territoriality among health care team
Develop lines of authority that recognize overlapping skills and responsibilities
Avoid sexism and sex role stereotypes
Foster communication
Introduce and orient new members
Recognize individual limits of knowledge and skill
Avoid stereotypes
Avoid erroneous and unsubstantiated assumptions
Initiate change in policy or therapy only after adequate explanation
Incorporate true multidisciplinary approach

that other health care professionals are members of a collaborative team. Early discharge and alternate forms of convalescent care are not realistic without a carefully orchestrated effort by all caregivers, community resources, patients, and their support systems. The nurse is undoubtedly the central coordinator of the effort to bring into operation a complex plan of care for the patient. However, the skill with which critical care nurses use their talents to apply a holistic assessment framework to the involvement of other caregivers, consults, and resources will significantly impact both patient outcome and overall resource utilization. This is a decidedly powerful contribution that reaches far beyond any single bedside or patient.

Effective collaboration has been demonstrated to enhance patient satisfaction and affect mortality and morbidity.[17] Collaborative interactions and communication among physicians and nurses can result in lower than predicted mortality rates.[19] Staff satisfaction also has been shown to be significantly better in critical care environments that foster a high level of collaboration.[27] Strategies to enhance and foster collaboration are summarized in the preceding Box.

SUMMARY

This chapter has provided an overview of the general guidelines for nursing care of all critically ill adults. Subsequent chapters provide nursing care guidelines for specific clinical conditions and support devices commonly associated with critical care. In total, the guidelines provide a resource for critical care nurses with the intent to help them be part of creating "a health care system driven by the needs of patients in which critical care nurses make their optimal contribution."[43]

REFERENCES

1. *Accreditation manual for hospitals, 1994,* Section 1: Assessment of patients, Chicago, 1993, Joint Commission on the Accreditation of Health Care Organizations.
2. *Acute pain management: operative or medical procedures and trauma,* Clinical Practice Guideline, no 1, AHCPR Publication, no 92-0032, Rockville, Md, February, 1992, Agency for Health Care Policy and Research, Public Health Service, US Department of Health and Human Services.
3. Boggs RL, Wooldridge-King M: *AACN procedure manual for critical care,* ed 3, Philadelphia, 1993, WB Saunders.
4. Boyle K, Nance J, Passau-Buck S: Post-hospitalization concerns of medical-surgical patients, *Appl Nurs Res* 5(3):122-126, 1992.
5. Braden B, Bergstrom N: A conceptual schema for the study of the etiology of pressure sores, *Rehabil Nurs* 12(1):8-12, 1987.
6. Clark S: Psychosocial needs of critically ill patients. In Clochesy J, et al, editors: *Critical care nursing,* Philadelphia, 1993, WB Saunders.
7. Daly B: Futility. *AACN Clin Iss Crit Care Nurs* 5(1):77-85, 1994.
8. Daly BJ, Newton B, Montenegro HD, Langdon T: Withdrawal of mechanical ventilation: ethical principles and guidelines for terminal weaning, *Am J Crit Care* 2(3):217-223, 1993.
9. Drew N: Exclusion and confirmation: a phenomenology of patients' experiences with caregivers, *Image J Nurs Sch* 18(2):39-43, 1986.
10. Edward GB, Schuring LM: Sleep protocol: a research-based practice change, *Critical Care Nurse* 13(2):84-88, 1993.
11. Evans SA, Carlson R: Nurse/physician collaboration: solving the nursing shortage crisis, *Am J Crit Care* 1(1):25-32, 1992.
12. Faucett J: Psychological aspects of pain and coping in critical care. In Puntillo KA, editor: *Pain in the critically ill: assessment and management,* Gaithersburg, Md, 1991, Aspen.
13. Fountain D: Effects of sensory alterations. In Clochesy J, et al, editors: *Critical care nursing,* Philadelphia, 1993, WB Saunders.
14. Gordon M: *Nursing diagnosis: process and application,* ed 2, New York, 1987, McGraw-Hill.
15. Harvey MA, et al: Results of the consensus conference on fostering more humane critical care: creating a healing environment, *AACN Clin Iss Crit Care Nurs* 4(3):484-507, 1993.
16. Johnson ND: Collaboration: an environment for optimal outcome, *Crit Care Nurs Q* 15(3):34-43, 1992.
17. King L, Lee JL, Henneman E: A collaborative practice model for critical care, *Am J Crit Care* 2(6):444-449, 1993.
18. Kleinpell RN: Needs of families of critically ill patients: a literature review, *Critical Care Nurse* 11(9):34-40, 1991.
19. Knaus WA, et al: An evaluation of outcomes from intensive care in major medical centers, *Ann Intern Med* 104:410-418, 1986.

20. Leske JS: Internal psycholmetric properties of the critical care family needs inventory, *Heart Lung* 20:236-244, 1991.
21. Levenson JL, Pettrey L: Controversial decisions regarding treatment and DNR: an algorithmic guide for the uncertain in decision-making ethics, *Am J Crit Care* 3(2):87-91, 1994.
22. Lock SE: Stress, adaptation and immunity: studies in humans, *Gen Hosp Psychiatry* 4:49-58, 1982.
23. Long CO, Greeneich DS: Family satisfaction techniques: meeting family expectations, *Dimensions of Critical Care Nursing* 13(2):104-111, 1994.
24. Marsden C: Do-not-resuscitate orders and end-of-life care plan, *Am J Crit Care* 2(2):177-179, 1993.
25. Miller JF: *Coping with chronic illness: overcoming powerlessness.* Philadelphia, 1983, FA Davis.
26. Miracle VA: Needs of families of patients undergoing invasive cardiac procedures, *Am J Crit Care Nurs* 3(2):155-157, 1994.
27. Mitchell P, et al: AACN demonstration project: profile of excellence in critical care nursing, *Heart Lung* 18:219-335, 1989.
28. Moseley MJ, Clark E, Morales C: Identifying opportunities to ask patients about their treatment wishes, *Dimensions of Critical Care Nursing* 12(6):320-322, 1993.
29. *Nursing: a social policy statement,* Kansas City, Mo, American Nurses Association, 1980.
30. Parent PC: Infection control: management strategies for adult patients in the critical care environment, *Crit Care Nurs Q* 15(3):1-9, 1992.
31. Pelletier E: A quality discharge plan breeds cooperation and success, *The next step: Glasrock Home Health Care Newsletter* 7(4):4-6, 1991.
32. Posa PJ: Nutritional support of the critically ill patient: bedside strategies for successful patient outcomes, *Crit Care Nurs Q* 16(4):61-79, 1994.
33. *Pressure ulcers in adults: prediction and prevention,* Clinical Practice Guideline No. 3, AHCPR Publication No. 92-0047, Rockville, Md, May 1992, Agency for Health Care Policy and Research, Public Health Service, U.S. Department of Health and Human Services.
34. Puntillo KA: *Pain in the critically ill: assessment and management,* Gaithersburg, Md, 1991, Aspen.
35. Roberts BL: Is a stay in an ICU unit a risk for falls? *Appl Nurs Res* 6(3):135-136, 1993.
36. Spellbring AM: Assessing elderly patients at high risk for falls: a reliability study, *J Nurs Care Qual* 6(3):30-35, 1992.
37. Spenceley SM: Sleep inquiry: a look with fresh eyes, *Image J Nurs Sch* 25(3):249-256, 1993.
38. Szaflarski NL: Immobility phenomena in critically ill adults. In Clochesy, et al, editors: *Critical Care Nursing,* pp 31-54, Philadelphia, 1993, WB Saunders.
39. Update: universal precautions for prevention of virus, hepatitis B virus, and other bloodborne pathogens in health care settings, *MMWR Morb Mortal Wkly Rep* 37(24):377-383, 387-388, 1988.
40. Urban N: Patient responses to the environment. In Kinney M, et al, editors: *AACN's clinical reference for critical-care nursing,* ed 3, St Louis, 1993, Mosby.
41. Viall CD: Nutrition. In Kinney M, et al, editors: *AACN's clinical reference for critical-care nursing,* ed 3, pp 297-328, St Louis, 1993, Mosby.
42. Villaire M: Margaret L. Campbell: making an end-of-life difference, *Critical Care Nurse* 14(1):111-117, 1994.
43. Vision Statement, AACN, 1992.
44. Weinstien RA: Epidemiology and control of nosocomial infections in adult intensive care units, *Am J Med* 91(3B):179S-183S, 1991.
45. West JM: Wound healing in the surgical patient: influence of perioperative stress response on perfusion, *AACN Clin Iss Crit Care* 1(3):595-601, 1990.

UNIT

I

Neurologic System

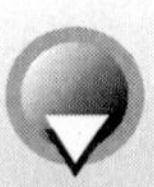

C L I N I C A L G U I D E L I N E

1

Increased Intracranial Pressure

Chris Winkelman, MSN, RN, CCRN

DESCRIPTION

There are many etiologies and pathophysiologic conditions associated with increased intracranial pressure (see Table 1-1). Within the rigid skull, there are three alterable volumes: tissue, blood volume, and cerebrospinal fluid (CSF). An increase in one of these volumes will cause a decrease in one or both of the remaining components. This compensatory decrement is limited. Once the limit is reached, intracranial pressure increases. Mortality associated with intracranial hypertension is as high as 50%,[41] depending on associated pathology,[20] rate of volume expansion,[15] location of mass,[1,19] and effectiveness of compensatory mechanisms.[30]

Normal pressure inside the skull ranges from 0 to 10 mm Hg. Intracranial hypertension is defined as a sustained elevation of ICP greater than 15 mm Hg.[17] The effects of increased intracranial pressure on cerebral tissues depend on the severity and duration of elevation.[41] Intracranial hypertension is clearly associated with adverse patient outcomes such as coma, decreased function, impaired mentation, altered mobility and sensation, and death.[23]

PATHOPHYSIOLOGY

There is a physiologic, compensatory response to intracranial volume increases. Initially, the volume of CSF may be reduced through displacement to the spinal subarachnoid space. There is also evidence of increased CSF reabsorption through subarachnoid villi in the presence of raised ICP.[30] Production of CSF does not appear to decrease unless cerebral blood flow is compromised.[43] The second method of compensation involves displacement of venous blood out of the cranial compartment.[30] At some point, the CSF and venous compensatory mechanisms will be exhausted and ICP will rise (Figure 1-1). The point at which a small increase in volume results in a sharp increase in pressure varies with the patient and underlying condition.

Increased ICP is pathologic because of its effect on cerebral blood flow. Compression of blood vessels results in ischemia and infarction of brain tissue.[42] In addition, autoregulation may be impaired in the presence of intracranial hypertension. Autoregulation refers to the ability to maintain a constant cerebral blood flow by changing the caliber of cerebral blood vessels. Autoregulation is influenced by systemic mean arterial pressures (MAP) and metabolic factors, particularly $Paco_2$ and Pao_2. With a MAP of less than 60 mm Hg or greater than 160 mm Hg, autoregulation may cease to function and cerebral blood flow may become passively dependent on changes in systemic arterial pressure.[30] A Pao_2 of less than 50 mm Hg will result in vasodilation. Cerebral vasodilation also occurs with increasing $Paco_2$ values between 20 and 80 mm Hg. This vasodilation is associated with increased, potentially pathologic blood volume.

Metabolic demands can also affect cerebral blood flow and volume. Blood flow increases with brain activity, fever, and seizure activity. Decreasing metabolic demands by minimizing brain activity, maintaining normothermia, and preventing seizures may decrease cerebral blood flow and mitigate the effects of increased intracranial pressure on blood flow.

Cerebral perfusion pressure (CPP) is a calculated value that may be used as a guide in reflecting the adequacy of cerebral blood flow.[15] A normal range for CPP is 70 to 100 mm Hg.[20,30] Ischemia and neuronal death may be seen when CPP falls below 40 mm Hg.[8] CPP is calculated by subtracting ICP from MAP: $CPP = MAP - ICP$. It is important to note that this value may not reflect local perfusion to injured brain or focal areas of increased intracranial pressure; adequate cerebral blood flow cannot be ensured for all areas of the brain based solely on the calculation of cerebral perfusion pressure. Transcranial Doppler[26] and bedside cerebral blood flow devices[42] are presently being investigated for their utility in evaluating the effects and treatment of ICP on cerebral blood flow.

TABLE 1-1 Conditions Associated with Increased Intracranial Pressure

Intracranial volume	Associated conditions
Brain tissue	Mass lesions Brain tumors Intracranial hematoma Abscess Cerebral edema Metabolic derangements
Intravascular blood volume	Cerebral vasodilation Hypoxia Hypercarbia Brain activity/Metabolic demands Drug effect Venous outflow obstruction Head position: hyperextension, flexion, lateral rotation Circumferential ties at neck pressure Positive end-expiratory pressure (PEEP) Valsalva maneuver Endotracheal suctioning
Cerebrospinal fluid volume	CSF outflow obstruction/ Obstructive hydrocephalus Decreased CSF reabsorption/ Communicating hydrocephalus Increased CSF production (rare)

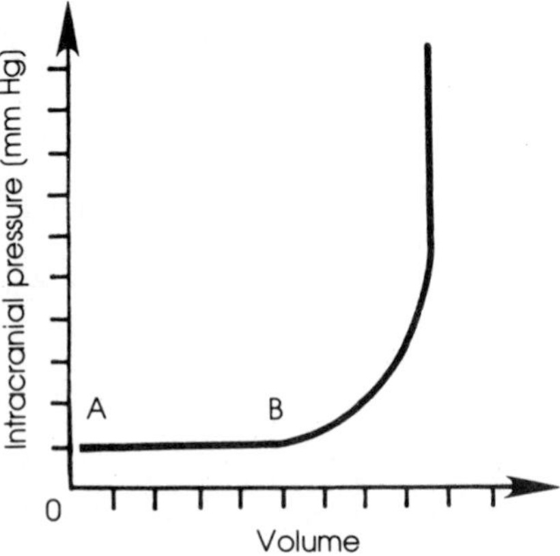

Figure 1-1 Intracranial volume-pressure curve. *A,* At this point fairly large increases in intracranial volume can be tolerated without much rise in intracranial pressure; *B,* At this point comparatively small increases in intracranial volume may cause very large increase in intracranial pressure. (From Rudy EB: *Advanced neurological and neuroscience nursing,* St Louis, 1984, Mosby–Year Book.)

LENGTH OF STAY/ANTICIPATED COURSE

The length of hospitalization for patients with increased intracranial pressure depends on the primary brain injury,[42] the presence of secondary insults,[9,23] and the aggressiveness of treatment.[14] Increased ICP is not a diagnostic related group (DRG).

MANAGEMENT TRENDS AND CONTROVERSIES

There are three major goals in the diagnosis and treatment of intracranial hypertension: (1) discover and remove, if possible, the source of increased intracranial volume; (2) control increased intracranial pressure; and (3) prevent occurrence of secondary injuries.

The diagnosis of increased intracranial volume related to intracranial hypertension was revolutionized by computerized tomography (CT). CT scanning is the major tool in identifying surgical lesions.[20] More recently, magnetic resonance imaging (MRI) is proving useful in demonstrating primary injuries not visualized with CT techniques and may have a role in the diagnosis and treatment of mass/lesions amenable to surgical management.

Control of intracranial hypertension requires a collaborative effort for the most effective prescription and implementation of treatment. The management of increased ICP depends on the underlying patient condition. Usual interventions include: CSF drainage, fluid management, controlled systemic blood pressure, use of hyperventilation, and administration of diuretics and other pharmacologic interventions.

Cerebrospinal fluid drainage is accomplished through placement of an intraventricular catheter that provides a conduit for monitoring intracranial pressures as well as draining CSF. CSF drainage allows for rapid reduction of ICP and is the treatment of choice when intracranial hypertension is caused by hydrocephalus. CSF drainage is regulated by adjusting the height of the drainage system relative to the inferred anatomic level of the foramen of Monro. Too rapid CSF drainage can cause ventricular collapse. A positive back pressure prevents rapid drainage and is accomplished by maintaining the drainage system a specified height above the reference point[8]; e.g., 10 cm above the tip of the ear. A pressure-regulated valve may also be placed in line with the tubing; this technique has the additional advantage of preventing retrograde travel of CSF and bacteria to the ventricles.

Fluid management can assist in controlling ICP and maintaining cerebral perfusion pressure. Fluid administration is guided by systemic blood pressure, central venous and pulmonary artery pressures, and serum osmolarity. The goal is to maintain normal cardiac output and normal ranges of systemic, pulmonary, and central venous pressures, with a serum osmolarity of 305 to 310 mOsm/kg H_2O (normal 285 to 295 mOsm/kg H_2O). There is some evidence that hypertonic solutions may be useful for fluid resuscitation. In several studies, ICP did not increase with administration of 3% hypertonic saline or hydroxyethyl starch; ICP did rise in response to large quantities of lactated Ringer's or other isotonic solutions.[29,40,46] However, these studies did not always incorporate a model of brain injury and increased ICP. Intracranial dynamics may differ in the injured brain, thus results of these studies must be applied cautiously. Because hyperglycemia exacerbates ischemic brain damage in laboratory models,[10,44] the use of glucose-containing solutions is often avoided. Likewise, hypotonic solutions will move passively into the brain and are contraindicated for this population.

Autoregulation is dependent on mean arterial blood pressure. Therefore, avoidance of hypotension and hypertension is valuable in controlling intracranial pressure; a mean systemic arterial pressure of 100 mm Hg is recommended. Systemic hypertension, with systolic blood pressures in excess of 160 mm Hg, increases cerebral blood volume and exacerbates the extravasation of proteins and water into the brain in the presence of a disrupted blood-brain barrier. However, an elevated mean arterial pressure of 150 mm Hg may be useful in anoxic injuries.[35] Systemic hypotension is implicated in secondary brain injuries.

Hyperventilation has been a mainstay in the treatment of intracranial hypertension for two decades. The goal of hyperventilation is to decrease $Pa{CO_2}$ to 27 to 35 mm Hg. This range of $Pa{CO_2}$ constricts cerebral blood vessels and thereby reduces cerebral blood volume which in turn decreases ICP. Also, hyperventilation causes respiratory alkalosis, which may combat tissue acidosis. However, this therapy is not without risks. Respiratory alkalosis may contribute to an internal environment that lowers the seizure threshold. Each millimeter decrease in $Pa{CO_2}$ results in a cerebral blood flow decrease of 2 to 3 ml/100 g of tissue per minute.[42] This reduced flow can cause ischemia in injured brain tissues. Additionally, in patients with severe head injury, the vasoreactivity of cerebral vessels may be reduced, limiting the effectiveness of hyperventilation. The adverse effects of hyperventilation may be mitigated by maintaining a narrow range of decreased $Pa{CO_2}$; values below 25 mm Hg are to be avoided.[39,42]

Diuretic therapy is a useful treatment modality in the presence of increased ICP. Mannitol is the osmotic agent of choice, although some neurosurgeons use glycerol or urea. Osmotic agents remove tissue fluid via the vascular osmotic pressure gradient. To be effective, the blood-brain barrier must be intact so that the drug is contained within the vascular space. Furosemide, a loop diuretic, also may be used to reduce intracranial pressure. Not only does furosemide reduce systemic volume, it may inhibit CSF production and decrease sodium transport within the brain, limiting neuronal damage.[37,41] Presently, the use of dimethyl sulfoxide (DMSO) is under investigation for the control of ICP.[16] A potent diuretic, DMSO is thought to cause cerebral vasodilation, changes in prostaglandin actions, and stabilization of mitochondria during cellular injury.[21] It is essential to maintain adequate circulating intravascular volume in the presence of diuretic therapy; administer fluid replacement therapy to maintain a serum osmolarity below 315 mOsm/kg.

The efficacy of glucocorticosteroids to treat cerebral edema and intracranial hypertension is questionable. A recent secondary analysis of published data reports no beneficial effects.[5] Steroids may stabilize cell membranes, improving cerebral blood flow and restoring autoregulation. However, large doses and prolonged therapy are associated with immunosuppression, hyperglycemia and carbohydrate intolerance, gastric ulceration, and water and sodium retention.

Continuous, high-dose barbiturate therapy can reduce elevated ICP and protect against cerebral hypoxia and ischemia by stabilizing cell membranes, scavenging free radicals, and reducing cerebral metabolism and blood flow through induced coma state.[5,20] This intervention usually is reserved for patients who have not responded to hyperventilation, diuretic therapy, and ventricular drainage.

In head-injured adults, sudden increases in ICP can occur in response to endotracheal suctioning (ETS). There are data to support the use of lidocaine to blunt the ICP response to ETS, especially when administered intratracheally and when coupled with the peak effects of muscle relaxants or other anesthetic agents.[4]

New therapies under investigation include agents to decrease CSF production,[3] drugs to decrease cerebral metabolism, agents to block cell mediators implicated in neuronal damage and destruction, and medications such as tromethamine (THAM) and superoxide dysmutane (SOD) to mitigate the effects of damage to central nervous system cells and blood vessels in the presence of elevated ICP.[2,28] Additional areas of investigation are designed to better understand the mechanisms and pathophysiology of intracranial hypertension and the effect of increased intracranial pressure on patient outcomes.

The final major goal of therapeutic intervention for patients with increased ICP is prevention of secondary injuries to the central nervous system (CNS). Hypoxia, hypercarbia, and hypotension have been identified as significant cause of mortality and morbidity in patients suffering head injury.[9,23] For this reason, patients with severe head injury or suspected pathologic intracranial pressure are intubated and mechanically ventilated to maintain $Pa{O_2}$ 80 to 100 mm Hg and $Pa{CO_2}$ 27 to 35 mm Hg. Hypotension is avoided through adequate fluid replacement therapy as described above, as well as blood replacement for hematocrit less than 26%. Evaluating the effectiveness of oxygen therapy, mechanical hyperventilation, and fluid therapy is key to preventing secondary CNS injury and ischemia in the presence of increased ICP.[20]

ASSESSMENT

PARAMETER	ANTICIPATED ALTERATION
Neurological Status	
Intracranial pressure	Increased: >15 to 20 mm Hg *due to accumulation of blood, CSF, or tissue.*
LOC	Abrupt decrease in arousal and awareness. *LOC is the most sensitive indicator of neurological function. The arousal component of consciousness depends on the function of the reticular system in the brainstem. Awareness is a measure of cortical activity.*[42]
Pupillary response to light	Enlargement. Asymmetry. Irregular shape (oval). Decrease in reactivity. Change from baseline/preresuscitation. *A new unilateral dilated, fixed pupil is a medical emergency, indicating lateral transtentorial herniation and a need for possible surgical intervention.*[20]
Glasgow coma score (GCS)	Decrease of 1 or more points on GCS. A score of 9 to 12 signifies moderate head injury; a score of 8 or less indicates severe head injury. (See Figure 1-2.) *This scale aids clinicians in making meaningful comparisons between patients and practitioners and in predicting head-injury outcomes and mortality.*[37]
Cranial nerve function	Potential loss of protective corneal (cranial nerves V and VII) and gag reflexes (cranial nerves IX and X). *Loss of these reflexes indicates the need for eye protection and airway maintenance.* Potential loss of oculovestibular/cold calorics and oculocephalic/doll's eye reflexes (cranial nerves III, VI, and VIII). *Tests of these reflexes serve to assess brainstem function; absence indicates a poor prognosis.*
Focal motor response	Response can vary in each of the four limbs. *Upper-extremity motor response is the most powerful predictor in patients with severe neurological impairment.*[20] *Each extremity is evaluated and recorded independently; use the same scale as that of the motor component of the GCS.*

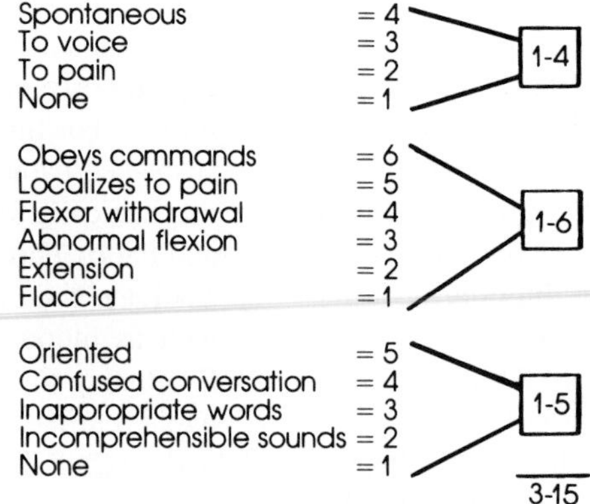

Figure 1-2 Glasgow Coma Scale as modified with addition of "flexor withdrawal" bringing score range to possible high of 15 and retaining a low score of 3. (Used with permission from Jones CJ, *Neurosurg Nurs* 11:94, 1979.)

Physical Examination

Respirations	Abnormal or irregular pattern *due to compression of respiratory control centers.* Rate Increased: >20 *due to neurogenic hyperventilation, a ventilator response associated with brain trauma and intracranial hypertension.*
Pulse	Change of >10 bpm and/or heart rate of <60 bpm *due to the classic Kocher-Cushing response, characterized by a slowing of the pulse and a rise in systemic pressure which usually happens late in the patient's course, providing minimal warning of a catastrophic event.*
Blood pressure	Change in systolic >15 mm Hg and/or widening pulse pressure *due to brain trauma.*
ECG	Progressive bracycardia, junctional escape rhythms, and idioventricular rhythms[42] *due to brain trauma, especially with brainstem injury. ST- and T-wave changes.* Neurogenic T-waves (inverted T-waves with increased amplitude and duration)[6,38] *due to brain trauma, possibly the result of circulating central nervous system hormones or stimulation of myocardial depressant factor.*
Headache	Increasing

Laboratory Data

Serum osmolarity	Increased: >310 mOsm/kg, or Decreased: <285 mOsm/kg *due to complications of diabetes insipidus or syndrome of inappropriate secretion of antidiuretic hormone, both of which are associated with increased ICP and its related pathologies and can lead to hyper- and hypo-osmolar states.*

Diagnostic Procedures for the Cranial Vault

Computerized Tomography (CT)	Space-occupying lesions Contusions Hemorrhage Edema
Magnetic Resonance Imaging (MRI)	Small hemorrhages Diffuse axonal injury patterns Early identification of infarct
Evoked Potential Studies (EPS)	Abnormal or absent response to visual, auditory, or somatosensory stimulation, *EPS studies have become valuable in locating lesions and in clarifying prognosis in head-injured patients.*[42]
Electroencephalogram (EEG)	Changes in the compressed spectral array (CSA). *CSA is a computerized technique that condenses standard EEG data by more than 1000-fold. Changes in CSA patterns have preceded rises in ICP and clinical deterioration. Identification of patterns that may predict ICP increases is underway.*
Doppler ultrasound	Decreased flow velocity in major cerebral vessels.
Continuous cerebral blood flow studies	Absent local or global blood flow. *CBF studies can assist in determining the effect of elevated ICP on blood flow and monitoring the effects of treatment to improve flow in ischemic areas.*

PLAN OF CARE

INTENSIVE PHASE

Treatment of ICP generally occurs in the critical care setting. The focus is on maintaining an ICP less than 15 mm Hg. In some settings, an alternate or additional goal is to regulate cerebral perfusion pressure so that it remains within a therapeutic range of 70 to 120 mm Hg.

Plan of Care (cont'd)

PATIENT CARE PRIORITIES	EXPECTED PATIENT OUTCOMES
Potential for injury *r/t decreased intracranial adaptive capacity*	Normothermic or rapid identification of fever and fever-reducing interventions. Fluid and electrolytes in balance. Absence of seizures and/or injury related to seizure activity.
Decreased cerebral tissue perfusion *r/t injury*	Improved or stable neurologic status. ICP <15 mm Hg. *Some practitioners recommend a minimum CPP >70 to 80 mm Hg.*[22]
Ineffective airway clearance *r/t decreased level of consciousness and possible cranial nerve dysfunction*	Airway patent Free of pulmonary complications such as iatrogenic pneumonia or aspiration. Clear lungs on auscultation. ABG within prescribed limits. *Generally* Pa_{CO_2} *is prescribed at 27 to 35 mm Hg and* Pa_{O_2} *at 80 to 100 mm Hg.* Pa_{CO_2} *<25 mm Hg is not recommended.*

INTERVENTIONS

Monitor neurologic signs continuously and in response to interventions: consciousness; pupillary reaction to light; Glasgow coma score; focal motor response; and blink, cough, and gag reflexes. *Data provided by ICP monitoring must always be interpreted in concert with neurologic examination and multisystem assessment. There are times when neurologic deterioration may not be reflected in ICP values.*[45]

Monitor vital signs with neurologic examination. *Adequate circulating volume is essential to cerebral perfusion.*

Carefully document neurologic assessment *to detect subtle changes or deterioration over time.*

Perform nursing care activities only if CPP >50 mm Hg.[42]

If ICP >15 mm Hg during interventions and ICP ventricular drainage device is placed, leave the drainage system open during intervention.[20,42] If response is consistently pathologic, consider pre-medicating with a short-acting, reversible narcotic *to prevent damaging intracranial hypertension.*

Maintain integrity and accuracy of ICP monitoring system *to prevent complications and ensure appropriate decision making.*

Elevate head of bed 30 degrees *to facilitate intracranial venous drainage and reduce ICP. Some practitioners recommend no head-of-bed elevation to maximize CPP.*[31,32] *Individualize backrest position after analysis of the patient's response to ICP, CPP, and blood-flow velocities to that position.*[18]

Space care activities. *Because activities have a cumulative effect on ICP, intervals of inactivity permit ICP to return to baseline.*[25]

Evaluate all interventions for effect on CPP. *Therapeutic treatment for elevated ICP may reduce MAP and compromise CPP. ICP and CPP must be considered in tandem when caring for the patient with neurologic insult.*[22]

Evaluate intracranial pressure waveform for evidence of reduced compliance. *Early or prophylactic interventions can be initiated in the presence of reduced compliance to prevent ICP elevation. Refer to guidelines for intracranial pressure monitoring in this text for more information and related care.*

Maintain open, unobstructed airway.

Monitor respiratory parameters: rate and pattern of respirations, airway pressures and volumes, breath sounds, arterial blood gas values.

Suction during peak sedation levels, 5 to 15 minutes following intermittent dosing of appropriate medication *to prevent increase in ICP associated with this intervention.*

Plan of Care (cont'd)

Consider use of lidocaine prior to suctioning *to minimize neurogenic response to suctioning and prevent increases in ICP.*[4]

Oxygenate with 100% FiO_2 for 20 to 30 seconds or 3 to 4 lung volumes prior to and after each suctioning effort *to ensure adequate oxygenation and minimize further cerebral insult.*[13]

Hyperventilate for up to 60 seconds after second passage of suction catheter *to reverse stepwise ICP elevation if present.*[7]

Use no more than two passes of 10 seconds each during suctioning episode to minimize ICP elevation and prevent further cerebral hypoxemia.[34]

Secure endotracheal tube with noncirumferential method *as circumferential tape/ties may result in obstruction of cerebral venous return.*

Turn patient q2h *to mobilize pulmonary secretions and maintain patent airway.*

Perform chest physiotherapy as needed *to mobilize pulmonary secretions and maintain patent airway.*

Turn conscious patients passively *to avoid Valsalva maneuver or isometric contractions which may increase ICP.*

Maintain head and body alignment *as hyperextension, flexion, and lateral rotation may increase ICP.*[11,25,27,36]

Avoid positioning with a marked degree of hip flexion *to ensure optimal circulation and prevent potential increase in ICP, thus impairing venous return from the cranial vault.*

Avoid elevations in body temperature *which increase cerebral metabolic rate.*

Assess and document bowel status, maintain regular bowel regimen, and prevent constipation or straining at stool *which may result in Valsalva maneuver and increased ICP.*

Monitor intake and output *to maintain adequate circulating volume and to detect onset of diabetes insipidus or SIADH.*

Provide a quiet environment and avoid unnecessary conversation at the bedside regarding the patient's condition *to control cerebral metabolic rate.*[24]

Monitor electrolytes, serum osmolality, and urine-specific gravity *to detect imbalances caused by ADH excess/deficit or stress response.*

Administer medication to prevent gastric ulceration.

Prevent hazards of immobility through frequent repositioning, the use of pneumatic compression devices on lower extremities, and implementation of range of motion exercises TID.

Provide patient and family with clear, concise information about status and plan, *to minimize anxiety and facilitate coping.*

Teach the family to interact with the patient, especially if consciousness is altered or communication is impaired.

INTERMEDIATE PHASE

A patient experiencing ongoing increased intracranial pressure is not a candidate for transfer to the intermediate or acute care setting. However, with resolution of elevated intracranial pressures, the overall goal of nursing care changes to monitoring and preventing complications specific to the underlying cause of the patient's intracranial hypertension and to promoting neurologic recovery and adaptation.

PATIENT CARE PRIORITIES	EXPECTED PATIENT OUTCOMES
Altered level of responsiveness *r/t brain injury.*	Progress to a higher level of responsiveness.
Uncompensated cognitive deficit *r/t brain injury, especially frontal lobe injury.*	Experience decreased episodes and/or duration of inappropriate behavior and mood. Sustain no injury caused by cognitive deficit. Participate with the family in decisions related to treatment.
Self-care deficit *r/t brain injury; physical disability.*	Meet hygiene, nutrition, and elimination needs (with assistance). Plan with the family realistically for the future.

Plan of Care (cont'd)

Impaired physical mobility *r/t brain injury or deconditioned status.*	Use compensation techniques.
High risk of ventilatory insufficiency or airway occlusion *r/t depressed cough or gag reflexes; impaired swallowing; presence of endotracheal or tracheostomy tube.*	Demonstrate adequate ventilation and airway clearance.
Uncompensated sensory deficit *r/t brain injury.*	Maintain pulse and blood pressure within safe parameters during activity.
Impaired communication *r/t brain injury; presence of endotracheal or tracheostomy tube.*	Establish a defined method of communication.

INTERVENTIONS

Monitor behavioral response *to determine assets and deficits.*
Coordinate a program that includes tactile, gustatory, olfactory, visual, and auditory stimuli *to facilitate optimal return of neurologic function.*
Provide a safe environment *to avoid injury and promote trust.*
Acknowledge behavior in a calm, factual manner *to avoid judgmental attitudes and escalating inappropriate mannerisms.*
Correct misperceptions, delusions, and hallucinations in a calm, factual manner *to facilitate recovery and coping.*
Teach family measures to control inappropriate behavior *to facilitate coping and begin preparation for discharge.*
Provide for feeding, bathing, toileting, and dressing to maintain hygiene.
Provide opportunities for the individual and family to engage in care in order *to increase knowledge about care and promote self-competence.*
Provide information about recovery and community resources in collaboration with social workers or other discharge planning staff.
Collaborate with speech therapist *to optimize assessment and intervention for potential communication or swallowing deficits.*
Provide alternative means of communication.
Provide active and passive ranges of motion, increasing level of activity as endurance improves, *to prevent disuse syndrome and complications from immobility.*
Monitor heart rate and blood pressure before, during, and after activity *to prevent undue stress yet optimize rehabilitation goals.*
Monitor respiratory status *to prevent complications of limited mobility and prevent aspiration.*
Position the individual *to prevent airway obstruction and promote ventilation.*

TRANSITION TO DISCHARGE

After the intermediate phase, the nurse prepares the patient and family for ongoing recovery care. Some patients will need additional care in a rehabilitation setting, perhaps a setting that specializes in neurologic rehabilitation (e.g., coma stimulation). Given the prevalence of subtle and long-lasting effects of even mild head injury,[33] the focus of nursing care at this stage is to prepare the patient and family for ongoing care and vigilance.

REFERENCES

1. Andrews BT, et al: The effect of intracerebral hematoma location on the risk of brainstem compression and clinical outcome, *J Neurosurg* 69:518-522, 1988.
2. Becker DP: Brain acidosis in head injury: a clinical trial. In Becker DP, Povlishick JJ, editors: *Central nervous system trauma report 1985,* pp 229-242, Bethesda, Md, 1985, National Institutes of Health/National Institutes of Neurological Disorders and Stroke.
3. Boyson SJ, Alexander A: Net production of cerebrospinal fluid is decreased by SCH-23390, *Ann Neurol* 27(6):631-635, 1990.
4. Brucia JJ, Owen DC, Rudy EB: The effects of lidocaine on intracranial hypertension, *J Neurosci Nurs* 24(4):205-214, 1992.
5. Chesnut RM, Marshall LF: Treatment of abnormal intracranial pressure, *Neurosurg Clin N Am* 2:267-284, 1991.
6. Conner R: Myocardial damage secondary to brain lesions, *Am Heart J* 78(2):145-148, 1969.

7. Crosby L, Parsons L: Cardiovascular response of closed head-injured patients to standardized endotracheal tube suctioning and manual hyperventilation procedure, *J Neurosci Nurs* 24:40-49, 1992.
8. Deardon NM: Management of raised intracranial pressure after severe head injury, *Br J Hosp Med* 36(2):94-100, 1986.
9. Eisenberg HM, et al: The effects of three potentially preventable complications on outcome after severe head injury. In Ishii S, Nugui H, Brock M, editors: *Intracranial Pressure V*, Berlin, 1983, Springer-Verlag.
10. Ginsberg MD, Welsh FA, Budd WW: Deleterious effect of glucose pretreatment in recovery from diffuse cerebral ischemia in the cat. I: Local cerebral blood flow and glucose utilization, *Stroke*11:347-354, 1980.
11. Hulme A, Cooper R: The effects of head position and jugular vein compression on intracranial pressure. In Beks J, Bosch DA, Brock M, editors: *Intracranial pressure III*, pp 359-363, Berlin, 1976, Springer-Verlag.
12. Jennet WB, Harper AM, Miller JD: Relation between cerebral blood flow and cerebral perfusion pressure, *Br J Surg* 390:57(5), 1970.
13. Kerr ME, et al: Head-injured adults: recommendations for endotracheal suctioning, *J Neurosci Nurs* 25:86-91, 1993.
14. Klauber MR, Marshall LF, Toole BM: Cause of decline in head-injury mortality rate in San Diego County, *J Neurosurg* 62:528-531, 1985.
15. Kraay CR: Intracranial pressure monitoring. In Clochesy JM, et al, editors: *Crit Care Nurs* pp 208-278, Philadelphia, 1992, WB Saunders.
16. Kulah A, Akar M, Baykut L: Dimethyl sulfoxide in the management of patient with brain swelling and increased intracranial pressure after severe closed head injury, *Neurochirurgia (Stuttg)* 33(6):177-180, 1990.
17. Langfitt TW: Increased intracranial pressure and cerebral circulation. In Yoummans JR, editors: *Neurological surgery*, ed 3, Philadelphia, 1990, WB Saunders.
18. March K, et al: Effect of backrest position on intracranial and cerebral perfusion pressures, *J Neurosci Nurs* 226:375-381, 1990.
19. Marshall LF, et al: Pupillary abnormalities, elevated intracranial pressure, and mass lesion location. In Miller JD, et al, editors: *Intracranial pressure VI*, pp 656-660, Berlin, 1986, Springer-Verlag.
20. Marshall SB, et al: *Neuroscience critical care: pathophysiology and patient management*, Philadelphia, 1990, WB Saunders.
21. Martin ML: Pharmacologic therapeutic modalities: phenytoin, dimethyl oxide, and calcium channel blockers, *Crit Care Quarterly* 5(4):72-81, 1983.
22. McQuillan KA: Intracranial monitoring: technical imperatives, *AACN Clin Iss Crit Care Nurs* 2(4):623-636, 1991.
23. Miller JD, Becker DP, Ward JD: Significance of intracranial hypertension in severe head injury, *J Neurosurg* 47:503-516, 1977.
24. Mitchell PH, Mause NK: Relationship of patient-nurse activity to intracranial pressure variations: a pilot study, *Nurs Res* 27(1):4-10, 1978.
25. Mitchell PH, Ozuna J, Lipe HP: Moving the patient in bed: effects on intracranial pressure, *Nurs Res* 30:933-940, 1981.
26. Newell DW, Aaslid R: Transcranial Doppler: clinical and experimental uses, *Cerebrovasc Brain Metab Rev* 4(2):122-43, 1992.
27. Parsons LC, Wilson MM: Cerebrovascular status of severe closed head-injured patients following passive position changes, *Nurs Res* 33:68-75, 1984.
28. Pfenninger E, Linder KH, Ahnefeld FQ: An infusion of THAM as therapy to lower increased intracranial pressure, *Anaesthesist* 38(4):189-92, 1989.
29. Poole GV, et al: Cerebral hemodynamics after hemorrhagic shock: effects of the type of resuscitation fluid, *Crit Care Med* 14:629-633, 1986.
30. Rockoff M, Kennedy S: Physiology and clinical aspects of raised intracranial pressure. In Ropper AH, Kennedy SF, editors: *Neurological and neurosurgical intensive care*, pp 9-21, Rockville, Md, 1988, Aspen Publishers.
31. Rosner MJ, Coley IB: Cerebral perfusion pressure, intracranial pressure, and head elevation, *J Neurosurg* 65:636-641, 1986.
32. Rosner MJ, Daughton S: Cerebral perfusion pressure management in head injury, *J Trauma* 30:933-940, 1990.
33. Rudy EB: *Advanced neurological and neurosurgical nursing*, St Louis, 1984, Mosby.
34. Rudy EB, et al: Endotracheal suctioning in adults with head injury, *Heart Lung* 20(6):667-675, 1991.
35. Safer P: Brain resuscitation. In Tinker IG, and Rapin M, editors: *Care of the critically ill patient*, pp 751-763, Philadelphia, 1983, FA Davis.
36. Snyder M: Relation of nursing activities to increases in intracranial pressure, *J Adv Nurs* 8:273-279, 1983.
37. Spielman GM: Central nervous system I: head injuries. In Cardona VD, Hurn PD, Mason PJB, editors: *Trauma nursing: from resuscitation through rehabilitation*, pp 365-418, Philadelphia, 1988, WB Saunders.
38. Staller AG: Systemic effects of severe head trauma, *Crit Care Quarterly* 10(1):58-68, 1987.
39. Stone JL: Nonsurgical management of increased intracranial pressure, *Semin Neurol* 9(3):218-224, 1989.
40. Todd MM, Tommasino C, Moore S: Cerebral effects of isovolemic hemodilution with a hypertonic solution, *J Neurosurg* 63:944-948, 1985.
41. Walleck CA: Acute head injury. In VonRueden K, Walleck CA, editors: *Crit Care Nurs Quarterly* 10(1):45-57, 1990.
42. Walleck CA: Patients with head injury and brain dysfunction. In Clochesy JM, et al, editors: *Critical care nursing*, Philadelphia, 1992, WB Saunders.
43. Ward JD, et al: Cerebral homeostasis and protection. In Wirth FP, Ratcheson RA, editors: *Neurosurgical critical care* pp 187-213, Baltimore, 1987, Williams & Wilkins.
44. Welsh FA, et al: Deleterious effect of glucose pretreatment on recovery from diffuse cerebral ischemia in the cat. II: Regional metabolite levels, *Stroke* 11:355-363, 1980.
45. Wilkinson HA: Intracranial pressure monitoring: techniques and pitfalls. In Cooper PR, editor: *Head injury*, pp 192-220, Philadelphia, 1987, WB Saunders.
46. Zornow MH, et al: Effect of a hypertonic lactated Ringer's solution on cerebral edema and intracranial pressure following cryogenic brain injury, *Anesthesiology* 67:A654, 1987.

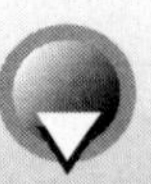

CLINICAL GUIDELINE

2

Subarachnoid Hemorrhage

Nora E. Ladewig, MSN, RN, CCRN
Kerri L. Schneider, MSN, RN, CCRN

DESCRIPTION

A subarachnoid hemorrhage (SAH) occurs when a cerebral vessel leaks or ruptures allowing blood to escape into the subarachnoid space. Annually, 25,000 to 28,000 persons between the ages of 35 to 65 years in North America sustain SAH.[2] Mortality is approximately 50%, with more than one third of the patients dying before hospitalization. Of those surviving SAH, 20% to 50% suffer permanent neurologic disability.[5,13,16]

PATHOPHYSIOLOGY

The most common cause of SAH is a ruptured cerebral aneurysm. Less common causes are arteriovenous malformations, head injury/trauma, hypertensive cerebral hemorrhage, blood dyscrasias, brain tumor hemorrhage, and cocaine use.[4,17] Aneurysms are formed from a weakness in the arterial wall and result in an outpouching or ballooning appearance. This ballooning vessel may cause focal neurological defects without bleeding, allowing early intervention to secure the aneurysm and prevent SAH complications. Aneurysms are most likely to be found along bifurcations within the circle of Willis, especially in the anterior cerebral circulation. Aneurysms rupture when the pressure on the arterial wall exceeds the wall's strength.

Prior to rupture, nearly half of the patients with cerebral aneurysms have a warning leak[10] that presents with similar, milder symptoms than SAH. The high mortality and morbidity associated with SAH may be decreased through community awareness, increasing recognition of warning signs, and early intervention before severe SAH occurs. Signs and symptoms of SAH are listed in Table 2-1, based on the Hunt-Hess classification scheme (1968).

Hemorrhage into the subarachnoid space results in several responses that alter regional blood flow to the cerebrum. These responses include impaired autoregulation, decreased cerebral perfusion pressure, increased intracranial pressure, and arterial vasospasm. Consequently, cerebral ischemia and infarction are common sequelae to SAH and contribute significantly to mortality and morbidity. Cerebral vasospasm is a permanent, abnormal narrowing of the artery, which occurs 3 to 14 days after the original insult. This phenomenon is detailed in a separate guideline.

Two additional complications contribute to delayed mortality and morbidity: rebleeding and hydrocephalus. Onset of these complications is characterized by a decrease in neurologic function. Thus frequency and consistency of neurological assessment and documentation of the patient's status beyond the acute phase of SAH cannot be overemphasized.

Rebleeding can occur within the first two weeks following aneurysm rupture, especially within the first 24 hours.[8] The likelihood of rebleeding significantly affects the neurosurgeon's decisions about surgical intervention.

Hydrocephalus is the result of interruption or impairment of cerebrospinal fluid (CSF) flow in the subarachnoid space, where reabsorption of CSF normally occurs, or in the intraventricular spaces, where CSF is manufactured and distributed. Communicating hydrocephalus usually occurs 4 to 20 days after SAH. Patients may exhibit no symptoms or develop acute neurological deterioration, requiring emergency drainage of CSF.

TABLE 2-1 Hunt and Hess Classification of Aneurysm Patients

Category	Criterion
Grade I	Asymptomatic, or minimal headache and slight nuchal rigidity
Grade II	Moderate to severe headache, nuchal rigidity, no neurological deficit other than cranial nerve palsy
Grade III	Drowsiness, confusion, or mild focal deficit
Grade IV	Stupor, moderate to severe hemiparesis, possible early decerebrate rigidity, and vegetative disturbances
Grade V	Deep coma, decerebrate rigidity, moribund appearance

Used with permission from Hunt WE, Hess RM: Surgical risk as related to time of intervention in the repair of intracranial aneurysms, *Neurosurg* 28:14-20, 1968.

LENGTH OF STAY/ANTICIPATED COURSE

The length of stay for patients with subarachnoid hemorrhage averages 8.7 days for medical management (DRG 14) and 13.9 days for surgical management (DRG 2).[14] Depending on the severity of the SAH, patients may require extensive monitoring in the ICU setting or may require only vigilant observation in a general unit.[14]

MANAGEMENT TRENDS AND CONTROVERSIES

The goal of clinical management is to prevent occurrences that cause abrupt changes in blood pressure and increases in intracranial pressure. The purpose of definitive medical intervention is to surgically secure the leaking vessel. Nursing interventions include bed rest, maintaining a nonstressful environment, normalization of blood pressure, avoidance of Valsalva maneuvers, control of fluid and electrolytes, and evaluating patient response to pain relief measures, sedatives, and prophylactic antiseizure medications.

Short-acting antihypertensives may be used for blood pressure control. Sudden lowering of blood pressure or use of long-acting agents is contraindicated, as hypotension contributes to the sequelae associated with vasospasm. Typically, the goal is to maintain a systemic systolic blood pressure at 150 mm Hg to decrease the risk of rebleeding, yet promote therapeutic cerebral perfusion pressure. Osmotic diuretics and beta-blockers may be used to treat acute episodes of hypertension, defined as systolic blood pressure above 150 mm Hg, or a cerebral perfusion pressure greater than 85 mm Hg.[6]

Steroids also may be given. Preliminary clinical studies have shown that large doses of methylprednisolone can reduce the inflammatory reaction after SAH and possibly limit ischemia.[1]

Current medical management includes early operative intervention. Surgeons advocating intervention before day 4 cite a lower incidence of rebleeding, reduced vasospasm, and more effective management of delayed ischemia.[4] Previously, surgery was postponed until 8 to 10 days after the initial SAH; this delay in surgery does not significantly affect mortality or morbidity. The impact of early surgical intervention on the overall patient outcome remains controversial and is generally recommended for patients with a Hunt-Hess SAH Grade III or less.

A new, alternative approach to securing aneurysms has been developed within the subspecialty, interventional radiology. The procedure entails threading a catheter into the affected cerebral blood vessel and injecting a bonding agent at the stem of the aneurysm, diverting blood flow from the weakened wall. It is useful for berrylike or saccular aneurysmal SAH.

Consistent and frequent neurological exam is the hallmark of care for this vulnerable population.

ASSESSMENT

PARAMETER	ANTICIPATED ALTERATION
Headache	Sudden onset, often described as "the worst ever." Severity peaks and may be related to a feeling of being hit, or that something "popped" inside one's head. The pain may be focal or diffuse.
LOC	May experience a period of unconsciousness or decreased level of awareness and arousal: confusion, restlessness, agitation, or lethargy possible.
Eye signs	Photophobia, diplopia, ovoid pupil(s), sluggish pupillary reaction to light, visual field defects.
Cranial nerves	Focal or generalized deficits.
Reflexes	Abnormal, with decreased movement, abnormal posturing, hemiparesis, hemianesthesia/paresia.

Neurologic signs	Nucchal rigidity *due to blood leaking into the meningeal/subarachnoid space of the spinal column.* Kernig's sign: flex one leg at the hip and knees, then straighten the knee. *Resistance or pain indicates blood in the subarachnoid space.* Brudzinski's sign: with the patient supine, flex neck. *Flexion of hips or knees, resistance, or report of pain indicates blood in the subarachnoid space.*
Focal motor/sensory deficits	Hemiparesis, hemiparalysis, aphasia, sensory disturbances, visual field defects, pain in and around eyes, seizure *due to bleeding extending intracerebrally or compressing brain tissue by hematoma.*
Systemic symptoms	Fever *due to blood in the subarachnoid space which interferes with hypothalamic temperature regulation.* Nausea and vomiting *may be related to intense headache pain, or due to blood in the subarachnoid space.*
CT scan	Blood in the subarachnoid space. Intracerebral extension of SAH. Communicating hydrocephalus. *May help point to area of bleeding.*
MRI	Blood and infarct in the cranial vault. *Usually obtained during the subacute phase to plan discharge as CT and angiography provide definitive location and treatment information.*
Cerebral angiography	Vascular pathology; location of aneurysms, AVM, and degree of vasospasm.
Serum Na^+	Decreased: <136 mEq/L *may be related to onset of inappropriate ADH secretion (SIADH) or sodium wasting as a result of release of a cerebral natriurtic factor. Decreased sodium can lead to intracranial hypertension, seizures, and coma.*[12]
WBC	Increased: >10,000/mm^3 and/or presence in CSF *indicates meningeal irritation.*
Lumbar puncture	Frank blood or presence of fibrinolysis products in CSF. *Performed if CT scan results are nondiagnostic and patient has no signs of increased intracranial pressure.*

PLAN OF CARE

INTENSIVE PHASE

Initial acute care of the patient with SAH focuses on maintaining airway, breathing, and circulation. Close and frequent monitoring is necessary for early detection and treatment of complications such as rebleeding, vasospasm, and hydrocephalus. Additionally, the patient and family may need assistance to prepare for surgical intervention and recurring diagnostic evaluation during this phase.

PATIENT CARE PRIORITIES	EXPECTED PATIENT OUTCOMES
Ineffective airway clearance *r/t altered neurological status*	Patent airway
Altered cerebral perfusion *r/t displacement of blood to the subarachnoid space and potential increased intracranial pressure.*	Neurological stability or improvement ICP <15 to 20 mm Hg
High risk for fluid volume excess *r/t management/therapy*	MAP 70 to 120 mm Hg CVP normal or slightly elevated PA pressures normal or slightly elevated
High risk for injury *r/t decreased intracranial adaptive capacity, seizures, fever, restlessness, agitation*	Body temperature normal Free of seizures and injury
Impaired physical mobility *r/t therapy, neurological deficits*	Nutrition, elimination, and activity needs met

Plan of Care (cont'd)

INTERVENTIONS

Monitor ABG.

Maintain PaO_2 >80 mm Hg *to insure adequate cerebral oxygenation.*

Maintain SaO_2 95% *to insure adequate cerebral oxygenation.*

Maintain $PaCO_2$ at 27 to 37 mm Hg *to prevent cerebral vasodilation and increased ICP.*

Maintain mixed venous oxygen saturation (SvO_2) 60 to 80%, *which indicates safe oxygen consumption systemically.*

Maintain jugular oxygen saturation (SjO_2) 60 to 80%, *which indicates optimal oxygen consumption in the brain.*

Continuously monitor BP and HR.

Maintain SBP and MAP within prescribed range *to provide necessary pressure to prevent sequelae of vasospasm, ischemic events from hypotension, and rebleeding from hypertension.*

Establish neurological baseline and vital signs *to permit early identification of clinically significant changes.*

Monitor neurological status hourly. Increase frequency to q15min for at least one hour and notify MD if deterioration of status is observed.

Provide sedation as needed.

Maintain stable, quiet environment: minimize stimulation, limit unnecessary visitors, reduce activity, control headache pain, prevent straining with defecation and isometric contractions, prevent hip and neck flexion, and prevent lateral rotation of the neck *to prevent transient or sustained increases in intracranial pressure.*

Space interventions 15 to 60 minutes apart *to prevent cumulative increases in ICP.*[3]

Monitor intake and output hourly *to prevent fluid imbalance which can contribute to cerebral hypo- or hyperperfusion.*

Use gentle touch to the patient's forehead, hand, or cheek *to reduce ICP.*[11,15]

Monitor body temperature continuously *to prevent hypermetabolic demands on brain in presence of hyperthermia.* If hyperthermic, provide aggressive cooling therapy but avoid shivering, *which increases oxygen consumption systemically and possibly reduces available oxygen to the cerebrum.*

Institute seizure precautions for high-risk patients. Observe for seizure activity and monitor antiseizure drug levels as indicated.

INTERMEDIATE PHASE

Rarely does the patient who has experienced SAH have a recovery that is unblemished by some alteration in neurological function. Recovery goals help the patient achieve the highest level of functioning; these goals are initiated during the intermediate phase of care.

PATIENT CARE PRIORITIES

Impaired verbal communication *r/t altered neurological status*

Self-care deficit *r/t neurological damage*

High risk for ineffective coping *r/t knowledge deficit of illness and rehabilitation, or uncertainty in prognosis and treatment*

EXPECTED PATIENT OUTCOMES

Begin to understand the disease process and effects on life patterns

Prepare for rehabilitation

Develop a satisfactory means of making needs and desires known

Voice or demonstrate emotional response and coping strategies

INTERVENTIONS

Identify communication deficits and use alternate forms of communication.

Instruct family members in causes and manifestations of communication deficits. Instruct family in alternative forms of communication.

Consult speech therapy to optimize speech abilities and *to evaluate for effective cough, gag, and swallowing abilities.*

Plan of Care (cont'd)

Request bedside physical and occupational therapy *to maximize abilities.*

Provide passive range of motion q4h during waking hours. Maintain functional alignment for all limbs *to preserve musculoskeletal status and optimize rehabilitative potential.*

Provide supportive and assistive devices *to maximize abilities and recreational diversion.* Devices include spence boots, walker, prism glasses, communication board, and easy-touch call light.

Provide information to patient and family about disease process, recovery progress, and follow-up care requirements as indicated by their readiness *to facilitate coping and begin preparation for discharge.*

Provide patient and family time to grieve regarding changes in body image, role performance, and functional ability *to facilitate coping and ability to begin preparing for the future.*

Assist the family and patient to set goals *to enable them to gauge progress.*

Investigate the need for emotional and social support through group activities and lay organizations.

TRANSITION TO DISCHARGE

As the patient's physiological and physical status stabilizes, nursing care focuses on preparing the patient for discharge. If neurological deficits severely impair the ability to carry out daily activities, then inpatient rehabilitation may be required. Other patients may benefit from a discharge to home with home care and outpatient services. Still others may be referred to a long-term-care facility with the expectation that a devastating brain injury precludes rehabilitation. Less than 10% of SAH patients who survive can expect to return to a level of functioning similar to that experienced before SAH.[9] During this transition, the nurse must focus on the patient's abilities and progress and support patient and family efforts to maximize independence.

REFERENCES

1. Adams HP: Prevention of brain ischemia after aneurysmal subarachnoid hemorrhage, *Neurol Clin* 10:251-262, 1992.
2. Awad IA, et al: Clinical vasospasm after subarachnoid hemorrhage: response to hypervolemic hemodilution and arterial hypertension, *Stroke* 18:365-372, 1987.
3. Bruya MA: Planned periods of rest in the intensive care unit: nursing care activities and intracranial pressure, *J Neurosurg Nurs* 13:184-194, 1981.
4. Cook H: Aneurysmal subarachnoid hemorrhage: neurosurgical frontiers and nursing challenges, *AACN Clinical Issues* 2:665-674, 1991.
5. Crowell RM: Management of subarachnoid hemorrhage, *Semin Neurol* 9:210-217, 1989.
6. Hickey JV: *Neurological and neurosurgical nursing,* Philadelphia, 1992, JB Lippincott.
7. Reference deleted in proofs.
8. Kassell NF, Torner JC: Aneurysmal rebleeding: a preliminary report from the cooperative aneurysm study, *J Neurosurg* 13(5):479-481, 1983.
9. Marshall LF, et al: *Neuroscience critical care: pathophysiology and patient management,* Philadelphia, 1990, WB Saunders.
10. Aquillera DC: *Crisis intervention theory and methodology,* St Louis, 1994, Mosby–Year Book.
11. Schneider KL: *The effect of purposeful touch on patient's intracranial pressure,* Unpublished masters thesis, 1991, Marquette University.
12. Segatore M: Hyponatremia after aneurysmal subarachnoid hemorrhage, *J Neurosci Nurs* 25:92-99, 1993.
13. Solomon RA, Fink ME: Current strategies for the management of aneurysmal subarachnoid hemorrhage, *Arch Neurol* 44:769-774, 1987.
14. *St Anthony's DRG guidebook 1995,* Reston, Va, 1994, St Anthony.
15. Walleck C: *The effects of purposeful touch on intracranial pressure,* Master's thesis, 1982, University of Maryland.
16. Weltz TE, Horner TG: Pathophysiology and treatment of subarachnoid hemorrhage, *Clin Pharmacol Ther* 9:35-39, 1990.
17. Willis D, Harbit MD: A fatal attraction: cocaine-related subarachnoid hemorrhage, *J Neurosci Nurs* 21:171, 1989.

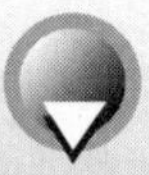

CLINICAL GUIDELINE

3

Cerebral Vasospasm

Helen A. Cook, MSN, RN

DESCRIPTION

Cerebral vasospasm is the luminal narrowing of a cerebral artery or arteries. Demonstrated angiographically, cerebral vasospasm also has been termed cerebral arterial spasm (Figure 3-1). Areas of spasm may be local, segmental, or diffuse.[16,35] Largely manifested as a complication of aneurysmal subarachnoid hemorrhage, cerebral vasospasm also may be associated with toxemia of pregnancy, meningitis, traumatic head injury, postoperative craniotomy, and other causes of spontaneous subarachnoid hemorrhage.[15,31,32,36] Symptomatic vasospasm presents itself as a syndrome of progressive deterioration in neurologic status described as delayed cerebral ischemia.[1,2] Unresolved symptomatic vasospasm results in cerebral infarction, permanent neurologic deficit, and, in severe cases, death.[33]

Any patient with aneurysmal subarachnoid hemorrhage is at risk for developing cerebral vasospasm. Peak incidence for onset of vasospasm occurs between the fourth through eighth days following aneurysmal subarachnoid hemorrhage.[2] Clinically significant vasospasm is rarely seen prior to the fourth day or after the twelfth day. Patients at greatest risk for cerebral vasospasm are those with more severe grades (i.e., higher grades) of subarachnoid hemorrhage and large blood clots in the subarachnoid cisterns. Probability of severe vasospasm is most accurately predicted on the basis of clot size on CT scan obtained within one to two days after hemorrhage.[1,10,17]

Additional prognostic indicators for development of cerebral vasospasm after aneurysmal rupture include the presence of acute hydrocephalus, hyponatremia, focal electroencephalographic changes, electrocardiographic changes, elevated blood leukocyte counts, and administration of antifibrinolytic agents.[2,14,21,28] Approximately 60% of patients surviving initial aneurysmal subarachnoid hemorrhage exhibit angiographic vasospasm.[12,35] However, only 20% to 30% of aneurysmal subarachnoid hemorrhage patients develop symptomatic vasospasm. Residual neurologic deficit and death occur in almost half of those patients with symptomatic cerebral vasospasm.[35] The morbidity and mortality associated with cerebral vasospasm is secondary to progressive ischemia and infarction of brain tissue.

PATHOPHYSIOLOGY

The pathogenesis of cerebral vasospasm is not clearly understood, although several theories regarding its etiology abound. Cerebral vasospasm has been attributed to (1) biochemically mediated contractions of cerebral vasculature; (2) the release of spasmogenic substances from extravasated subarachnoid blood; (3) the release of mitogenic substances from platelets, causing arterial hyperplasia; and (4) an inflammatory response subsequent to subarachnoid hemorrhage.[12] Recent studies are highly suggestive of the role of oxyhemoglobin as the primary spasmogenic substance behind the cascading development of cerebral vasospasm.[19,20] Oxyhemoglobin has many mechanisms of action contributing to spasmogenesis of cerebral arteries. These mechanisms include the release of oxygen-free radicals, the generation of lipid peroxidation, metabolism to bilirubin, and the release of products from the metabolism of arachidonic acid.[6,19,34] Oxyhemoglobin also is known to inhibit endothelium-dependent relaxation of arterial vasculature. Evidence also suggests that oxyhemoglobin potentiates the degeneration of vessel structure.[19,34]

Regardless of etiology, there is a distinct vessel morphology associated with spasm of cerebral arteries. Arter-

A

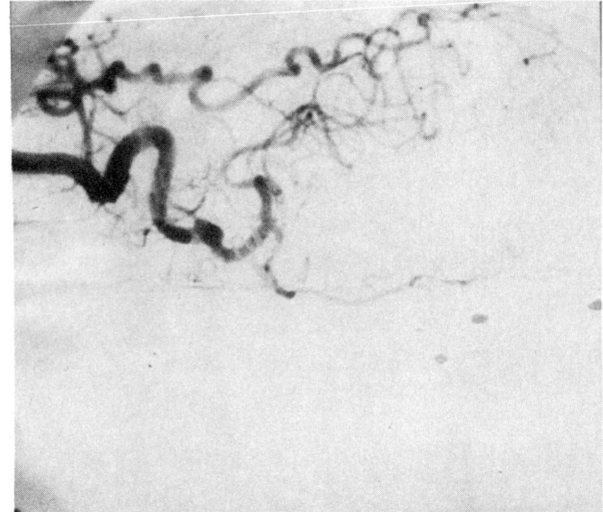

B

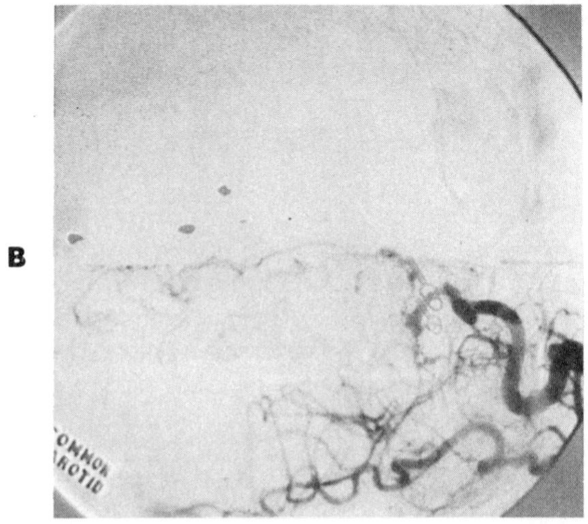

Figure 3-1 A, Anterior-posterior carotid arteriogram with internal carotid artery (ICA). Notice aneurysm is clipped and there is no evidence of vasospasm. **B,** AP carotid arteriogram with middle cerebral artery (MCA). Notice aneurysm is clipped and there is no evidence of vasospasm.

iopathic changes include edema of intimal and medial layers, medial necrosis and fibrosis, and adventitial inflammation.[22]

Consequently, arterial luminal narrowing contributes to an increase in cerebral vascular resistance. Increased cerebral vascular resistance brings about a reduction in cerebral blood flow and subsequent increase in flow velocities. Significant reductions in cerebral blood flow with severe luminal narrowing lead to decreased flow velocities contributing to cerebral ischemia and eventual infarction.[3,24]

Symptomatic vasospasm reflects the severity of angiographic vasospasm. Severity of vasospasm can be classified according to a grading system developed by Fisher and others.[11] The grading system in Table 3-1 defines dimensions of cerebral vasospasm for the proximal segments of the middle and anterior cerebral arteries.

TABLE 3-1 Fisher Scale for Severity of Vasospasm

Grade	Degree of Vasospasm
0	No vessel narrowing
1	Minimal vessel narrowing
2	Vessel narrowing, but columns distinct and at least 1.0 mm wide
3	Vessel narrowing to 0.5 mm, columns indistinct, forward flow delayed
4	Vessel less than 0.5 mm in diameter, forward flow almost nil

Adapted from Fisher CM, Roberson GH, Ojemann RG: Cerebral vasospasm with ruptured saccular aneurysm—the clinical manifestations, *Neurosurg* 1:245-248, 1977.

The course of cerebral vasospasm is self-limiting, although its duration is variable. Angiographic vasospasm usually resolves within a three-week time period.[35]

LENGTH OF STAY/ANTICIPATED COURSE

The length of stay for patients at risk for symptomatic cerebral vasospasm is contingent upon the time frame for onset of vasospasm after subarachnoid hemorrhage, and associated prognostic indicators for development of significant cerebral vasospasm. For patients experiencing the clinical effects of vasospasm, the length of stay is contingent upon the duration and severity of angiographic spasm and stabilization of neurologic status. Ages between 30 and 65 years and gender do not seem to influence incidence or severity of vasospasm.[2,15]

There is not a specific DRG assigned to cerebral vasospasm. Nonspecific cerebrovascular disorders with complications (DRG 16) may be used as a discharge diagnosis. The average length of stay for DRG 16 is 7.8 days.[30]

MANAGEMENT TRENDS AND CONTROVERSIES

The current and conventional treatment for cerebral vasospasm is primarily supportive. Interventions include hemodilutional hyperperfusion and the use of calcium channel blockers. Early surgical obliteration of the offending cerebral aneurysm is preferred prior to institution of aggressive hemodynamic therapy.

The intent of hemodilutional hyperperfusion is to counter the effects of decreased cerebral blood flow associated with vasospasm. Cerebral blood flow is affected by circulating intravascular volume, cardiac function, systemic arterial blood pressure, and blood viscosity.[9,18,29] Hence, the goal of hemodilutional hyperperfusion is to optimize cerebral blood flow through augmentation of pulmonary capillary wedge pressure, cardiac output, and hematocrit. Finn and others.[9] found that neurologic function with symptomatic cerebral vasospasm correlates positively with pulmonary capillary wedge pressure and cardiac index. Deterioration in neurologic status is reflected with decreases in pulmonary capillary wedge pressure and cardiac index. Increases in pulmonary capillary wedge pressure and cardiac index produced improvement in neurologic function. Of note are one-to-two-hour lag periods between changes in neurologic status and wedge pressure.

Thus manipulation of hemodynamic status requires ongoing monitoring of pulmonary artery pressure and cardiac output/cardiac index. The aim of therapy is to achieve and sustain pulmonary capillary wedge pressure with intravascular volume expansion so that cardiac index is at least 4/L/min/m^2.[9] Usually, pulmonary capillary wedge pressures between 14 mm Hg and 18 mm Hg support cardiac indexes in the prescribed range. Intravascular volume expansion is accomplished by infusion of crystalloid, hetastarch, and plasma protein fraction in reference to pulmonary capillary wedge pressure. Additional pharmacologic support to maintain pulmonary capillary wedge pressure within range may be needed using fludrocortisone (Florinef) and vasopressin (Aqueous Pitressin).

Hemodilution is achieved through volume expansion without infusion of whole blood or red blood cell products.[29] Hematocrit is the parameter monitored to assess blood viscosity. Hemodilution is considered adequate when hematocrits are between 30% and 35%.[9,29]

Pharmacologic measures to induce hypertension for enhancement of cerebral blood flow during vasospasm are secondary to intravascular volume expansion.[9] For patients with neurologic deficits unresponsive to hemodilutional volume expansion, inotropic and vasoconstrictive therapy is considered. Pharmacologic agents employed for such purpose include titrated infusions of dopamine, dobutamine, and phenylephrine.

Calcium channel blockers are used to inhibit vascular smooth muscle contraction. The calcium channel blocker nimodipine (Nimotop) has been shown to reduce the severity of ischemia associated with cerebral vasospasm, although the frequency of vasospasm remains unchanged.[23,26] Nimodipine's mechanism of action in reducing the morbidity and mortality of cerebral vasospasm is not clearly understood. It is suggested that nimodipine affects microcirculation either by enhancing collateral cerebral blood flow or by decreasing platelet aggregation. A neuronal protective effect also may play a role.[23] Other calcium antagonists for use in the treatment of cerebral vasospasm, such as nicardipine, are under investigation.

Other therapies in the treatment of cerebral vasospasm also are under investigation. Current investigational interventions include cerebral balloon angioplasty and intrathecal fibrinolytic therapy. High-dose methylprednisolone and magnesium sulfate may also be forthcoming with investigational trials.[27,37]

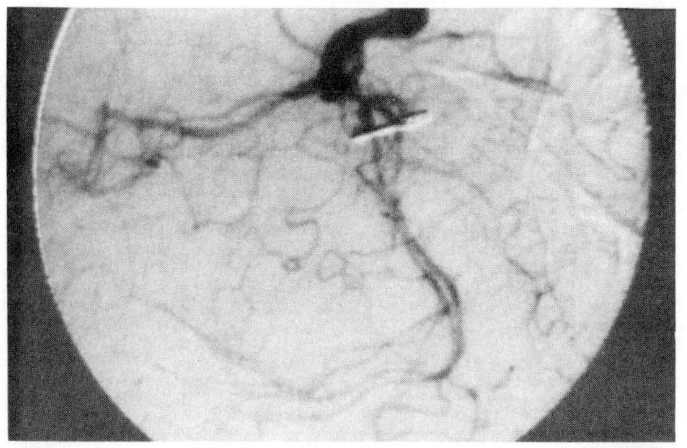

A

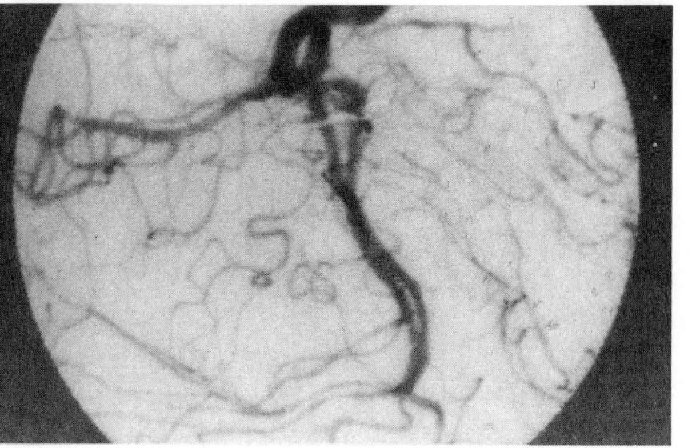

B

Figure 3-2 Same vessels with clips showing vasospasm of **A,** ICA, MCA (M1 segment), and **B,** anterior cerebral artery (ACA, A1 segment).

Cerebral angioplasty has been indicated in the treatment of severe vasospasm refractory to hemodilutional hyperperfusion and calcium antagonists.[4,7,16] Cerebral angioplasty involves angiographic isolation of vasospastic arteries with temporary balloon inflation to dilate cerebral artery segments back to prespasm diameter (Figure 3-2). The balloon angioplasty results in a sustained, permanent resolution of angiographic spasm. Concurrent and subsequent improvements in symptomatic vasospasm have also been reported.[4,7,13,16] Unfortunately, complications associated with cerebral angioplasty are catastrophic. Such complications include hemorrhagic infarction, arterial dissection, and arterial rupture.[4,5,7,16]

Fibrinolytic therapy also has been indicated in the treatment of cerebral vasospasm after subarachnoid hemorrhage. Recombinant tissue plasminogen activator (rt-PA) has been administered via intracisternal and intraventricular routes after surgical clip ligation of offending aneurysms.[8,25,38] Significant improvements in patient outcomes specific to angiographic and symptomatic vasospasm have been documented. Further study is needed to determine appropriate dosing of rt-PA and patient risk. However, rt-PA seems to be an effective way to clear large subarachnoid clots before cerebral arteries develop vasospasm.[8,25,38]

ASSESSMENT

PARAMETER	ANTICIPATED ALTERATION
Neurologic Status	
Clinical signs	Worsening of headache Slight increase in nuchal rigidity
LOC	Lethargy/confusion progressing to more focal neurologic changes *that are dependent upon the area of spasm*
EEG	Focal delta or theta waves *precede changes in arteriogram by 4 days*
Cardiovascular Status	
HR	Slight increase
BP	Slight increase *due to compensatory response to increased cerebral blood flow*
ECG	Elevated ST segment Peaked P and T waves Large U waves Prolonged QT interval *due to catecholamine release associated with subarachnoid bleed and hypothalamic dysfunction*
Temperature	Steady low-grade fever
Laboratory Studies	
Na^+	Hyponatremia *due to hypothalamic dysfunction*
WBC	Elevated $>10{,}000/mm^3$ without infectious source of febrile state
CT scan	No evidence of hydrocephalus, aneurysm rebleed, hematoma, or other cause to account for change in neurologic status *Newly infarcted area on CT scan may be indicative of earlier, sustained ischemia secondary to vasospasm*
Cerebral arteriogram	Focal, segmental, or diffuse narrowing of arterial lumen(s) Increased: 50% narrowing in severe vasospasm
Transcranial Doppler	Increased flow velocities for middle cerebral artery: Increased: 120 cm/sec = moderate spasm Increased: 200 cm/sec = severe spasm
Cerebral blood flow	Increased: 50 cc/100 g/min (20 cc/100 g/min with neurologic dysfunction)

PLAN OF CARE

INTENSIVE PHASE

Cerebral vasospasm is an acute neurologic complication, requiring intensive care management. After a course of treatment, which may last 14 days, the patient will be ready for less-intense assessment and care.

PATIENT CARE PRIORITIES	EXPECTED PATIENT OUTCOMES
Alteration in cerebral tissue perfusion (real or potential) *r/t cerebral vasospasm.*	Maintain/improve neurologic function PCWP $\geq$14 mm Hg (or as prescribed) Cardiac index $\geq$4 $L/min/m^2$ Blood pressure adequate to support cardiac output and neurologic status Hematocrit 30% to 35%

Plan of Care (cont'd)

High-risk for fluid volume excess *r/t hemodilutional hyperperfusion.*	Optimal cardiac output/index with PCWP at beginning of Starling curve plateau Absence of canon *a* and *v* waves on PCWP tracing (if patient has competent mitral valve) Absence of pulmonary edema
Self-care deficit *r/t knowledge about cerebral vasospasm.*	Patient/family demonstrate reduced anxiety/improved coping skills

INTERVENTIONS

Monitor neurologic status hourly and prn.
Concurrently monitor hemodynamic parameters (i.e., BP, PCWP, CO/CI) with neurologic function *to establish relationship between cardiac function and cerebral blood flow.*
Establish relationship between PCWP and CO/CI (i.e., modified Starling curve) *to determine optimal cardiac function.*
Administer crystalloids and colloids as needed *to achieve and maintain PCWP as prescribed and to reduce blood viscosity.*
Administer calcium channel blockers as ordered *to augment cerebral circulation.*
Administer fludrocortisone (Florinef) and vasopressin (Aqueous Pitressin) as needed *to maintain PCWP in prescribed range.*
Administer inotropic agents as needed *to achieve hypertension and/or cardiac output for adequate cerebral blood flow.*
Administer vasoconstrictive agents as needed *to achieve hypertension for adequate cerebral blood flow.*
Avoid administration of whole blood/red blood cell products for hematocrit ≥30% *to achieve/maintain hemodilution.*
Monitor hematocrit and serum chemistries *for evidence of hemodilution.*
Monitor I/O hourly.
Monitor daily weights.
Assess breath sounds q2h to q4h and prn *for evidence of heart failure or fluid overload.*
Analyze PCWP tracings for presence of canon *a* and *v* waves *as a means of early detection of fluid overload.*
Administer diuretics as needed *to reduce excess fluid/pulmonary edema.*
Determine optimal cardiac function in relation to PCWP and CI/CO *to reduce potential for fluid overload.*
Establish satisfactory communication system with patient, family, and/or significant others.
Provide comfort measures including pain relief for headache related to cerebral vasospasm.
Provide information tailored to level of understanding. *Include explanation of potentially prolonged ICU stay without evidence of symptomatic vasospasm.*
Evaluate effectiveness of teaching plan as evidenced by patient/family/significant other understanding of cerebral vasospasm.
Assess need for additional interventions by multidisciplinary team members.

INTERMEDIATE PHASE

The patient enters the intermediate care phase with stabilization of neurologic function and normalization of hemodynamic parameters. Nursing care continues to focus on adequate cerebral tissue perfusion with ongoing, astute assessment of neurologic status.

PATIENT CARE PRIORITIES	EXPECTED PATIENT OUTCOMES
Maintain adequate cerebral tissue perfusion.	Neurologic function maintained
High risk for self-care deficit *r/t understanding of disease process.*	Patient/family able to verbalize understanding of cerebral vasospasm

Plan of Care (cont'd)

INTERVENTIONS

Monitor neurologic status and blood pressure every two to four hours and prn.
Administer nimodipine as ordered *to augment cerebral circulation.*
Supplement intake with volume expanders as ordered *to optimize cerebral blood flow.*
Encourage po intake as tolerated.
Provide for adequate sleep/rest periods *to promote healing and mental integrity.*
Provide and reinforce teaching introduced during intensive care phase *to reduce anxiety and promote understanding.*

TRANSITION TO DISCHARGE

As the patient moves beyond the intermediate phase toward discharge, evaluation and planning for post-hospital care needs is essential. The focus of nursing care during this transition period is the assessment of neurologic function, self-care capability, and home environment. Patients with residual neurologic deficits after cerebral vasospasm may require rehabilitation or skilled care services. Collaboration with social work, physical therapy, occupational therapy, speech therapy, and other disciplines may be necessary to assure that a patient's discharge needs are met.

REFERENCES

1. Adams HP, et al: Predicting cerebral ischemia after aneurysmal subarachnoid hemorrhage: influences of clinical condition, CT results, and antifibrinolytic therapy, *Neurology* 37:1586-1591, 1987.
2. Barker FG, Heros RC: Clinical aspects of vasospasm, *Neurosurg Clin N Am* 1:277-288, 1990.
3. Bell TE, et al: Transcranial Doppler: correlation of blood velocity measurement with clinical status in subarachnoid hemorrhage, *J Neurosci Nurs* 24:215-219, 1992.
4. Brothers MF, Holgate RC: Intracranial angioplasty for treatment of vasospasm after subarachnoid hemorrhage: technique and modifications to improve branch access, *Am J Neuroradiol* 11:239-247, 1990.
5. Cook HA: Cerebral angioplasty: a new treatment for vasospasm secondary to subarachnoid hemorrhage, *J Neurosci Nurs* 22:319-321, 1990.
6. Duff TA, et al: Bilirubin and the induction of intracranial arterial spasm, *J Neurosurg* 69:593-598, 1988.
7. Eskridge JM, Newell DW, Pendleton GA: Transluminal angioplasty for treatment of vasospasm, *Neurosurg Clin N Am* 1:387-400, 1990.
8. Findlay JM, et al: Intracisternal recombinant tissue plasminogen activator after aneurysmal subarachnoid hemorrhage, *J Neurosurg* 75:181-188, 1991.
9. Finn SS, et al: Observations on the perioperative management of aneurysmal subarachnoid hemorrhage, *J Neurosurg* 65:48-62, 1986.
10. Fisher CM, Kistler JP, Davis KM: Relation of cerebral vasospasm to subarachnoid hemorrhage visualized by computerized tomographic scanning, *Neurosurgery* 6:1-8, 1980.
11. Fisher CM, Roberson GH, Ojemann RG: Cerebral vasospasm with ruptured saccular aneurysm—the clinical manifestations, *Neurosurgery* 1:245-248, 1977.
12. Flynn EP: Cerebral vasospasm following intracranial aneurysm rupture: a protocol for detection, *J Neurosci Nurs* 21:348-352, 1989.
13. Grimes CM: Cerebral balloon angioplasty for treatment of vasospasm after subarachnoid hemorrhage, *Heart Lung* 20:431-435, 1991.
14. Haley EC, Torner JC, Kassell NF: Antifibrinolytic therapy and cerebral vasospasm, *Neurosurg Clin N Am* 1:349-356, 1990.
15. Heros RC, Zervas NT, Varsos V: Cerebral vasospasm after subarachnoid hemorrhage: an update, *Ann Neurol* 14:599-608, 1983.
16. Higashida RT, et al: Transluminal angioplasty for treatment of intracranial arterial vasospasm, *J Neurosurg* 71:648-653, 1989.
17. Hijdra A, et al: Prediction of delayed cerebral ischemia, rebleeding, and outcome after aneurysmal subarachnoid hemorrhage, *Stroke* 19:1250-1256, 1988.
18. Kassell NF, et al: Treatment of ischemic deficits from vasospasm with intravascular volume expansion and induced arterial hypertension, *Neurosurgery* 11:337-343, 1982.
19. Macdonald RL, Weir BKA: A review of hemoglobin and the pathogenesis of cerebral vasospasm, *Stroke* 22:971-982, 1991.
20. Macdonald RL, et al: Etiology of cerebral vasospasm in primates, *J Neurosurg* 75:415-424, 1991.
21. Maiuri F, et al: The blood leukocyte count and its prognostic significance in subarachnoid hemorrhage, *J Neurosurg Sci* 31:45-48, 1987.
22. Mayberg MR, Okada T, Bark DH: Morphologic changes in cerebral arteries after subarachnoid hemorrhage, *Neurosurg Clin N Am* 1:417-432, 1990.
23. Meyer FB: Calcium antagonists and vasospasm, *Neurosurg Clin N Am* 1:367-376, 1990.
24. Newell DW, Winn HR: Transcranial Doppler in cerebral vasospasm, *Neurosurg Clin N Am* 1:319-328, 1990.
25. Ohman J, Servo A, Heiskanen O: Effect of intrathecal fibrinolytic therapy on clot lysis and vasospasm in patients with aneurysmal subarachnoid hemorrhage, *J Neurosurg* 75:197-201, 1991.
26. Petruk KC, et al: Nimodipine treatment in poor-grade aneurysm patients, *J Neurosurg* 68:505-517, 1988.
27. Rim Z, et al: Magnesium sulfate reverses experimental delayed cerebral vasospasm after subarachnoid hemorrhage in rats, *Stroke* 22:922-927, 1991.
28. Rivierez M, et al: Value of electroencephalogram in prediction and diagnosis of vasospasm after intracranial aneurysm rupture, *Acta Neurochir (Wien)* 110:17-23, 1991.
29. Stewart-Amidei C: Hypervolemic hemodilution: a new approach to subarachnoid hemorrhage, *Heart Lung* 18:590-598, 1989.
30. *St Anthony's DRG guidebook 1995*, Reston, Va, 1994, St Anthony.
31. Susi EA, Walls SK: Traumatic cerebral vasospasms and secondary head injury, *Critical Care Nursing Clinics of North America* 2(1):15-20, 1990.

32. Trommer BL, Homer D, Mikhael MA: Cerebral vasospasm and eclampsia, *Stroke* 19:326-329, 1988.
33. Welty TE, Horner TG: Pathophysiology and treatment of subarachnoid hemorrhage, *Clinical Pharmacology* 9:35-39, 1990.
34. White RP: Responses of isolated cerebral arteries to vasoactive agents, *Neurosurg Clin N Am* 1:401-416, 1990.
35. Wilkins RH: Attempts at prevention and treatment of delayed ischaemic dysfunction in patients with subarachnoid hemorrhage, *Acta Neurochir (Wien) Suppl* 45:36-40, 1988.
36. Wilkins RH: Cerebral vasospasm in conditions other than subarachnoid hemorrhage, *Neurosurg Cl N Am* 1:329-334, 1990.
37. Yamakawa K, et al: Effect of high-dose methylprednisolone on vasospasm after subarachnoid hemorrhage, *Neurol med Chir (Tokyo):* 31:24-31, 1991.
38. Zabramski JM, et al: Phase I trial of tissue plasminogen activator for the prevention of vasospasm in patients with aneurysmal subarachnoid hemorrhage, *J Neurosurg* 75:189-196, 1991.

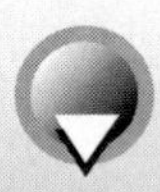

C L I N I C A L G U I D E L I N E

4

Traumatic Brain Injury

Karen A. McQuillan, MS, RN, CCRN

DESCRIPTION

Traumatic brain injury occurs when mechanical forces transmitted to the head result in brain tissue damage. Head injury and craniocerebral trauma are other terms with broader meanings that are used frequently when referring to traumatic brain injury. The term head injury encompasses injury to the scalp, skull, and/or brain, while craniocerebral trauma denotes injury to the cranium and/or brain.[53]

Inconsistencies between definitions for head injury, lack of a central head-injury data base, and varied methods for case findings make accurate determination of traumatic brain injury incidence impossible.[63,73] An analysis of multiple studies conducted in the United States estimates the average incidence of brain injury to be approximately 200 for every 100,000 persons.[63] Each year an estimated 500,000 Americans sustain head injuries severe enough to result in prehospital death or require hospitalization.[29,63] Traumatic brain injury is the cause of death for an estimated 75,000 Americans annually, with approximately two thirds of these deaths occurring in the prehospital setting.[63,73,82] Head injuries constitute the leading cause of death due to trauma. Reported brain injury fatality rates in the United States range from 17 to 30 per 100,000 persons each year.[63,116]

Many of those who survive traumatic brain injury suffer from long-lasting disabilities. Permanent disabilities caused by traumatic brain injury afflict an estimated 70,000 to 90,000 Americans each year, and approximately 2000 individuals remain in a persistent vegetative state.[29] The direct costs of caring for patients with brain injuries, as well as the indirect costs caused by loss of the victim's economic productivity, total billions of dollars each year.[29,82] The high mortality, morbidity, costs, and health-care resource utilization associated with traumatic brain injury make this disease a major public health problem in the United States.

The highest incidence of brain injury occurs in young adults between the ages of 15 and 24. Two additional yet less-significant peaks in incidence occur in children under 4 years of age and the elderly over 75 years of age.[63,69,116] Males are two to three times more likely to sustain traumatic brain injury than females.[63,69,116] Occurrence of traumatic brain injury increases the risk of a second injury twofold, and after two brain injuries caused by trauma the risk for a subsequent head injury is increased eightfold.[42,82]

Motor vehicle crashes cause the overall majority of traumatic brain injuries, followed by falls, assaults, and recreational/sporting activities.[29,63,69] Falls constitute the leading cause of head injury among the elderly, while motor vehicle crashes cause the most brain injuries among adolescents and young adults.[69,116] Alcohol intoxication, a significant contributing factor in traumatic injury, has been reported to be present in approximately 50% of the individuals who suffered traumatic brain injury.[58,117] The incidence of brain injury associated with motor vehicle crashes is increased when vehicle occupants neglect to utilize safety restraints, and with cyclists who do not wear protective helmets.[63,85,91,115,124]

PATHOPHYSIOLOGY

Mechanisms of Injury

Mechanisms that cause trauma-induced brain injury include skull deformation, acceleration-deceleration, rotation, and penetration. Skull deformation usually occurs when there is a direct blow to the head resulting in distortion of the skull contour. Indentation, outward bowing, or fracture of the cranium occurs, which can precipitate contusion or laceration of the underlying brain tissue or result in intracranial hemorrhage.

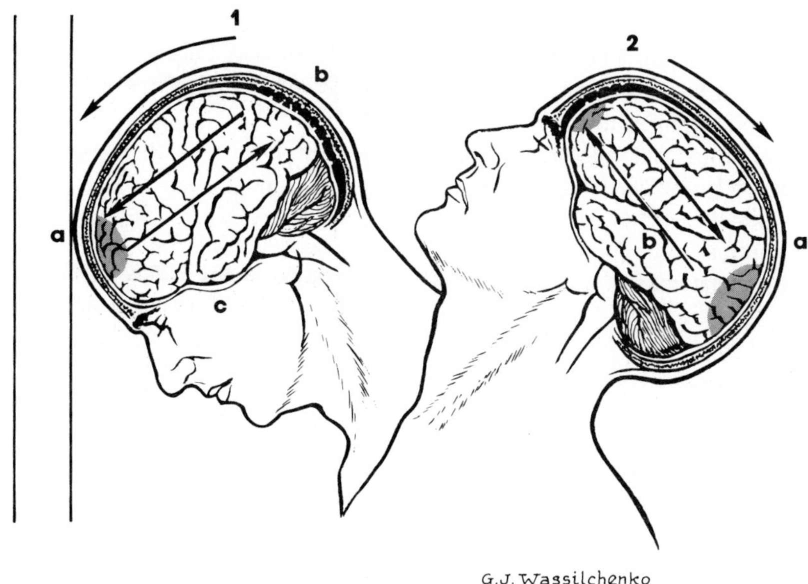

Figure 4-1 Brain injury resulting from acceleration-deceleration and shearing forces. *1a*. Site of impact and direct trauma to the brain (coup injury); *1b*. Shearing of subdural veins; *1c*. Trauma to base of the brain. *2a*. Trauma to the brain hitting the opposite side of the skull (contrecoup injury); *2b*. Shearing forces throughout brain causing diffuse brain injury. (Modified from Rudy EB: *Advanced neurological and neuroscience nursing,* St Louis, 1984, Mosby–Year Book.)

Acceleration-deceleration is a major cause of traumatic brain injury that results when there are rapid alterations in the velocity of skull and brain movement along a straight linear path.[7,53] Acceleration occurs when the head is struck by a moving object (e.g., bat, fist) setting the skull and brain into motion, and deceleration results when the head suddenly hits a stationary object (e.g., windshield). The solid skull moves much faster than the semisolid brain tissue, causing injury to the brain as it makes contact with the rough bony prominences within the skull and collides against the walls of the cranium. Brain injury can occur at the site of head impact (coup injury), as well as adjacent to the site of impact (contrecoup injury) as the brain tissue collides with the contralateral skull surface (Figure 4-1).

The third mechanism, rotation, results when acceleration-deceleration of the brain does not follow a straight linear path. Instead, the brain moves in angular, twisted, or side-to-side directions.[53] Rotation distorts the brain and causes stretching and shearing of brain tissue and potential vascular injury.[53,56] The maximal stress from rotational acceleration forces occurs where tissues of different densities interface (e.g., white and gray matter, fibrous tissue and cerebral tissue). The amount of brain injury sustained will depend on the amount and direction of the angular accelerative force.[53,82]

Penetrating brain injuries include missile injuries, typically caused by gunshots, and impalement injuries that extend through the scalp and skull into the brain tissue. Brain tissue and/or blood vessels are injured by the penetrating object. Bullet velocity, size, shape, and direction, as well as the effect it has once inside the cranium, will determine the extent of damage caused by a penetrating gunshot wound.[53]

Types of Brain Injury

The various types of traumatic brain injuries are generally categorized as diffuse or focal injuries. Diffuse brain injuries are characterized by widespread and nonlocalized brain damage that is sometimes difficult to visualize using macroscopic brain-assessment techniques. The primary mechanism for development of diffuse brain injuries is believed to be rotational acceleration forces that move the brain over a 45 to 60 degree angle within the skull, causing axonal stretching or shearing. The amount and duration of the acceleration forces and the direction of head movement will determine the extent of axonal injury. Different diffuse axonal injuries have essentially the same pathophysiology but varied severity, ranging from concussion, which causes little to no neurologic dysfunction, to severe diffuse axonal injury, which is a major cause of death and disability.[1,36,82]

Focal injuries, which may coexist with diffuse lesions, are characterized by localized areas of brain damage.[73,82] Acceleration-deceleration forces and skull deformation and penetration are mechanisms that can produce focal brain injuries. Brain damage results from localized tissue injury and from the mass effect created by the focal lesion, which increases intracranial pressure (ICP) causing brain compression, shift, and herniation.[36,82] These lesions are associated with focal or lateralizing symptoms, such as hemiparesis, unilateral pupil dilation, cranial nerve dysfunction, speech deficits, or decerebrate posturing.[82] Focal lesions include contusions, epidural hematomas, subdural hematomas, and intracerebral hematomas.

The various types of traumatic brain injuries are reviewed in Table 4-1. Two brain injuries that may result from a traumatic event and frequently require critical care intervention will not be discussed in detail in this chapter; they are intracerebral hematoma and subarachnoid hemorrhage. An intracerebral hematoma is a well-defined collection of blood deep within the brain tissue.[23,82] Intracerebral hematomas may also be caused by cerebrovascular accidents (CVA) and the interested reader is referred to the guideline on CVAs for more information on this type of brain injury. Hemorrhage into the subarachnoid space is a common finding with severe head injury, but may also be caused by aneurysm rupture.[53] The reader interested in subarachnoid hemorrhage is referred to that guideline.

Primary and Secondary Brain Injury

Brain damage that results from trauma can be classified as primary or secondary. The initial brain-tissue and/or vascular injury that occurs at the time of traumatic impact is known as primary brain injury. Currently, no treatment exists to reverse primary brain injury.[73,82] It is well recognized that not all brain injury occurs at the time of impact, but that multiple factors can serve to exacerbate the initial insult causing what is known as secondary brain injury.[19,80,120,130] The events or complications that follow the primary brain injury and result in secondary insult include hypoxia, intracranial hypertension, systemic hypotension, hypercarbia, ischemia, seizures, infections, electrolyte imbalance, and others.[19,53,80,120] Secondary brain injury can continue to occur long after the primary insult, contributing to a poor neurologic outcome and possible death for the patient.[53]

Potential Multisystem Complications

Brain tissue injury and resulting neurologic deficits can serve as a trigger for the onset of a multitude of harmful and potentially lethal complications. Complications may plague not only the injured neurologic system, but may also occur within other body systems as well.* Potential complications that have been associated with traumatic brain injury are listed in the following box. Many of these complications can contribute to secondary brain injury, prolonged hospitalization, and poor patient outcome.

LENGTH OF STAY/ANTICIPATED COURSE

The length of stay and hospital course for patients with traumatic brain injury will vary depending on the severity of the injury, the presence of associated injuries, the onset of complications, and patient factors that existed prior to the traumatic event. The DRGs that may be applied to trau-

*References 5, 9, 20, 28, 73, 81, 82, 98, 137.

Potential Complications Associated with Traumatic Brain Injury

Neurologic

Cerebral edema
Hydrocephalus
Traumatic aneurysm
Arteriovenous fistulae formation
Delayed intracranial hemorrhage
Intracranial hypertension
Cerebral infarction
Brain tissue ischemia
Seizures
Intracranial infections
Hygroma formation
Motor, sensory, cognitive, behavioral, and/or psychosocial deficits

Respiratory

Airway obstruction
Abnormal ventilatory pattern
Hypoxia
Aspiration
Pneumonia
Atelectasis
Acute respiratory distress syndrome (ARDS)
Neurogenic pulmonary edema
Pulmonary embolism

Cardiovascular

Cardiac arrhythmias
Cardiac repolarization abnormalities
Deep-vein thrombosis
Disseminated intravascular coagulation

Fluid and electrolyte disturbances

Syndrome of inappropriate antidiuretic hormone
Cerebral salt wasting
Diabetes insipidus
Sodium retention
Water retention

Gastrointestinal

Ileus
Gastrointestinal mucosal damage
Gastrointestinal bleeding
Constipation

Immunologic

Infections

Metabolic

Protein-calorie malnutrition
Hypoalbuminemia
Hyperglycemia

Musculoskeletal/integumentary

Skin breakdown
Contractures
Heterotopic ossification

TABLE 4-1 Types of Traumatic Brain Injury

Type of injury	Pathophysiology	Specific symptoms	Treatment
Diffuse injuries			
Concussion	Temporary physiologic dysfunction of axons without substantial anatomic or structural disruption[36]	*Mild concussion* No loss of consciousness Disorientation, confusion Possible retrograde or post-traumatic amnesia *Classic* Unconsciousness less than 6 hours Retrograde and post-traumatic amnesia Mild neurologic impairment *General symptoms* CT scan normal Headache Dizziness Visual disturbance Nausea Drowsiness Gait disturbance Difficulty concentrating Memory impairment Personality change Irritability Emotional liability[36,53,82]	Observe Discharge teaching regarding postconcussive syndrome
Diffuse axonal injury (DAI)	Widespread damage to axonal fibers caused by stretching or shearing Diffuse brain swelling may occur in response to severe DAI	Severity of injury is classified as mild, moderate or severe based on clinical presentation *Mild* Immediate loss of consciousness lasting 6-24 hours Stupor or restlessness may persist after awakening Transient decorticate or decerebrate posturing seen in about 30%[36,82] Mild to moderate memory impairment Post-traumatic amnesia lasting hours *Moderate* Immediate loss of consciousness lasting over 24 hours Confusion and amnesia persists after awakening Purposeful movements or withdrawal to pain usually seen Transient decorticate or decerebrate posturing seen in 35%[36] Mild to severe memory, behavioral, cognitive, intellectual, and personality deficits	Prevent and treat intracranial hypertension and other sources of secondary brain injury Prevent and treat systemic complications

Continued.

TABLE 4-1 Types of Traumatic Brain Injury—cont'd

Type of injury	Pathophysiology	Specific symptoms	Treatment
Diffuse injuries—cont'd			
		Severe Immediate prolonged loss of consciousness lasting days to weeks Persistant decorticate or decerebrate posturing Severe motor deficits Specific symptoms of increased ICP Systemic hypertension, hyperthermia, and profuse diaphoresis over face and occasionally neck and upper torso (hyperhidrosis) seen with diencephalic involvement Severe memory, cognitive, intellectual, and personality deficits[36,82] CT scan may appear normal or may show small hemorrhagic lesions of the white matter, usually within the central aspect of the cerebrum and the upper and usually dorsal area of the brainstem, with diffuse cerebral edema MRI better visualizes these lesions, particularly nonhemorrhagic shear injury[37,38,113]	
Focal injuries			
Contusion	Bruising of brain tissue with blood extravasation causing secondary edema formation, and tissue necrosis and infarction[82] Frontal and temporal lobes are most common sites where brain comes in contact with rough bony projections at base of inner skull[41,53,103]	Depend on location and extent of lesion and presence of associated brain insults[23] Focal neurologic deficits (i.e., lesions around speech or motor areas that will cause speech or motor dysfunction) Altered level of consciousness may be seen; unconsciousness is usually secondary to associated concussion or DAI[23,82,100] Signs of elevated ICP with brain compression and possible herniation may occur with large contusions or progressive edema. (Temporal lobe contusions present a particularly high risk for brain herniation that may occur without warning due to the close proximity of the temporal lobe to the tentorial notch and midbrain.)[23,82] Visualized on CT scan and MRI	Large surface contusions may be surgically evacuated[44,73] Prevent and treat intracranial hypertension and other sources of secondary TBI Prevent and treat systemic complications

TABLE 4-1 Types of Traumatic Brain Injury—cont'd

Type of injury	Pathophysiology	Specific symptoms	Treatment
Focal injuries—cont'd			
Epidural hematoma (EDH)	Intracranial collection of blood above the dura mater (Figure 4-2) Brain compression and eventually herniation result as the hematoma enlarges Often little underlying brain injury exists[23] Most commonly associated with a linear fracture of the temoral bone and laceration of the underlying middle meningeal artery or veins	Depends on time since injury, rate of hematoma expansion, and presence of associated lesions[23] 60% present clinical symptoms within six hours[82] "Classic" presentation consists of loss of consciousness followed by a lucid period and subsequent unconsciousness. The lucid interval is not seen in the majority (two thirds) of patients.[22,23] Initial loss of consciousness may occur due to a concussion[23,82] Early presentation may include nausea and vomiting,[22] headache, dizziness, restlessness[73] Continued hematoma expansion causes deteriorating level of consciousness, hemiparesis, pupil dilation, decerebration Possible seizures[53,82] Visualized on CT scan	Majority require prompt surgical evacuation of the hematoma and vessel ligation Prevent and treat any secondary brain injury and systemic complications
Subdural hematoma (SDH)	Collection of blood beneath the dura mater and above the arachnoid lining of the brain (Figure 4-3) Usually associated with contusion of the brain beneath the clot[82] Brain is compressed and may herniate as hematoma expands Most commonly caused by laceration of bridging veins in the subdural space[23,82]	Depend on degree of underlying brain injury and rate of hematoma expansion[23] *Acute SDH* Symptoms present within 24-48 hours of trauma[4,73] Immediate loss of consciousness, an intermittent lucid period, or gradual deterioration in level of consciousness[23,82] Pupil abnormalities (i.e., pupil dilation and inequality) and motor deficits (i.e., hemiparesis, hemiplegia, decerebration) are most common[23] Headache Cranial nerve dysfunction Aphasias Vital sign alterations (i.e. hypertension, bradycardia)[23] Visualized on CT scan	Usually requires prompt surgical evacuation of clot and contused, nonviable brain tissue Control hemorrhage source Prevent and treat intracranial hypertension and other sources of secondary TBI Prevent and treat systemic complications

Continued.

TABLE 4-1 Types of Traumatic Brain Injury—cont'd

Type of injury	Pathophysiology	Specific symptoms	Treatment
Focal injuries—cont'd			
	Subacute SDH generally associated with a less severe underlying contusion[4]	*Subacute SDH* Symptoms similar to an acute SDH that appear two days to two weeks after trauma[4,82]	
	Initial hematoma reorganizes to form an outer membrane that eventually encapsulates the clot As the hematoma slowly expands the brain is compressed causing progressive neurological dysfunction	*Chronic SDH* History of prior low-impact injury is common Symptoms present two weeks to months after trauma[4,53] Presentation varies but may include: headache of increasing severity, impaired consciousness (i.e., confusion), inappropriate behavior, slowed cerebration, amnesia, lethargy, nausea and vomiting, ataxia, incontinence, impaired language skills with dominant hemisphere compression, hemiparesis, pupil dilation, seizures[23,53,73]	Symptomatic patients usually require surgical evacuation of the clot[3] Observe for evidence of rebleed, development of cerebral edema, infection, or seizures postoperatively and treat appropriately

Abbreviations:
TBI—Traumatic Brain Injury
CT Scan—Computerized Tomography Scan
MRI—Magnetic Resonance Imaging

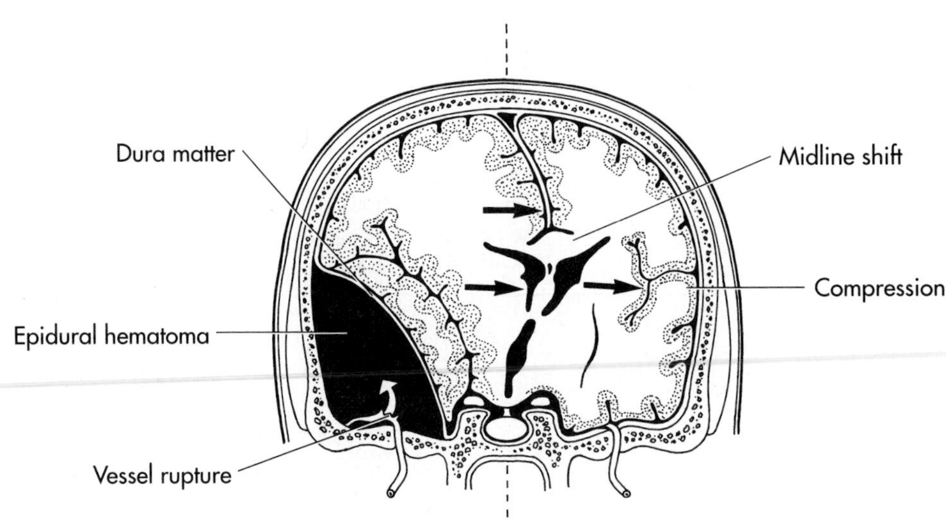

Figure 4-2 Epidural bleeding with hematoma formation.

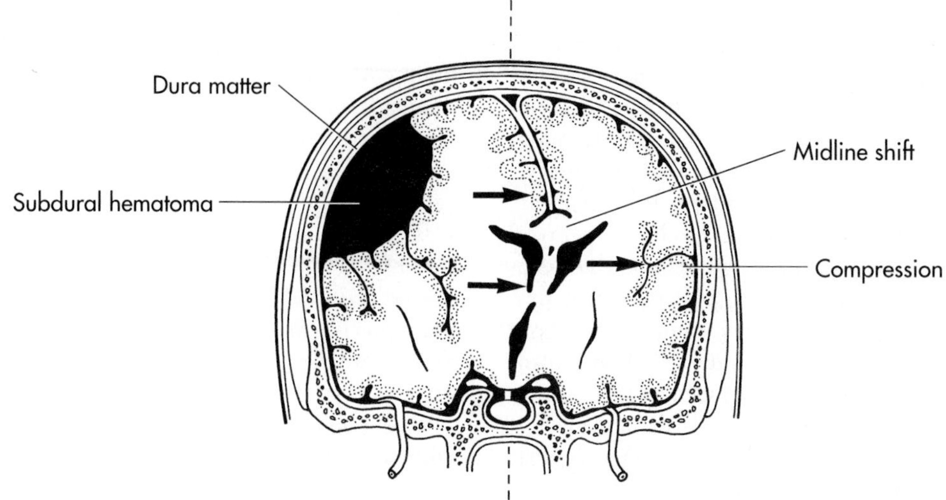

Figure 4-3 Subdural hematoma.

matic brain injury reflect this variability. Possible DRGs are listed in Table 4-2.[117a]

The severity of brain injury (determined by the location, extent, and type of primary brain insult and any subsequent secondary brain injury) is a primary determinant of patient outcome.[73,110,127] The coexistence of extracranial injuries and development of any multisystem complications are likely to complicate the patient's hospital course, prolong length of stay, and adversely affect patient outcome.[19,110,127] Patient factors, such as preexisting disease or advanced age, are additional considerations that may alter the patient's hospital course, lengthen hospitalization, and influence outcome.[127,128]

TABLE 4-2 DRGs Associated With Traumatic Brain Injury

DRG#	Label	LOS
2	Crainiotomy for trauma, age greater than 17	13.9 days
27	Traumatic stupor and coma, coma greater than 1 hour	7.5 days
28	Traumatic stupor and coma, coma greater than 1 hour with complications	8.3 days
31	Concussion, age greater than 17 with complications	5.6 days
32	Concussion, age greater than 17 without complications	3.4 days
484	Crainiotomy for multiple significant trauma	20.6 days
487	Other multiple significant trauma (medical management)	10.2 days

MANAGEMENT TRENDS AND CONTROVERSIES

The primary goal in caring for patients with traumatic brain injury is to prevent or minimize secondary brain insults.[73,79,82,130] Interventions aimed at prevention, early recognition, and aggressive treatment of hypoxia, hypercapnea, intracranial hypertension, hypotension, and other potential sources of secondary brain injury are the priorities for critical care management of the patient with traumatic brain injury.[73,130] It is well established that if these sources of secondary brain insult go unrecognized or untreated the mortality and morbidity of traumatic brain injury increases substantially.*

The first-priority interventions for brain-injured patients, not unlike any other trauma victims, are to secure a patent airway and ensure adequate ventilation to promote adequate gas exchange. Supplemental oxygen is usually necessary, and mechanical ventilation may be required to ensure that the Pa_{O_2} is maintained above 80 mm Hg and mild hyperventilation is attained. Pulmonary toilet, including suctioning and chest physiotherapy, is essential to maintain airway patency and avoid pulmonary complications. Despite the ICP elevations typically initiated by implementation of respiratory care procedures, nursing research has demonstrated that these interventions can be safely administered to brain-injured patients if research-based procedures are followed.[25,77,93,107] Lidocaine administered prior to respiratory care procedures has been suggested as an effective method

*References 19, 72, 73, 80, 101, 120.

of attenuating the ICP-elevation response to these interventions, although further clinical investigation is needed on use of this therapeutic intervention.[8,16,31]

Therapeutic hyperventilation is used to induce cerebral vasoconstriction, reduce cerebral blood flow, and decrease intracranial pressure in patients with traumatic brain injury. This intervention has come under scrutiny. Research has shown that the cerebral vessels adapt to prolonged periods of hyperventilation and allow the cerebral blood flow to return to prehyperventilation levels despite persistent hypocarbia.[2,87] Rebound ICP elevation may result when carbon dioxide levels are normalized too rapidly.[11,48] It has also been suggested that vasoconstriction induced by therapeutic hyperventilation may result in ischemia of the already injured brain.[21,90,133] One recent clinical trial suggests that prophylactic use of prolonged hyperventilation may actually have adverse effects on outcome in certain subsets of brain-injured patients.[86] Therapeutic hyperventilation remains widely used for ICP control in patients with traumatic brain injury, but should be instituted cautiously. Moderate ranges of hypocarbia (28 to 32 mm Hg) and gradual return to a normocapnic state are recommended to help alleviate potential complications associated with this intervention.[11,20,90]

Diuretic therapy is another strategy employed to reduce ICP. Mannitol, a commonly used osmotic diuretic, establishes an osmotic gradient which pulls extracellular fluid from the brain tissue into the intravascular space thereby reducing brain water volume.[82] Furosemide is a loop diuretic that can be used alone to reduce ICP or with mannitol to lower ICP in a synergistic fashion.[73,96,131] Furosemide is thought to be less reliable than mannitol in reducing ICP, and caution must be used if it is administered in conjunction with mannitol since fluid and electrolyte disturbances can be exacerbated.[20,73,129]

Fluids are administered in addition to diuretics to achieve a euvolemic hyperosmolar patient state. The desired serum osmolarity is 300 to 315 mOsm/L. Generally, isotonic fluids, such as normal saline or Plasmalyte-A (Travenol Laboratories, Deerfield, IL), are the crystalloid solutions of choice. Half-normal saline solution may also be used as a maintenance fluid.[73,82] More hypotonic solutions, such as dextrose in water, are usually avoided since these fluids can easily extravasate out of the intravascular space and exacerbate edema.[73,119] Research has suggested that hypertonic saline solutions may be preferable for resuscitation of patients with brain injury since only small amounts are necessary to effectively stabilize hemodynamic parameters, and these solutions may minimize ICP elevations by reducing brain water content.[6,32,45,119] Although hypertonic solutions show promise for use in patients with brain injury, they have many potential adverse effects and further human clinical investigation is required before they are accepted for routine clinical use. Blood and blood products may also be used as replacement fluids when anemia or coagulopathies require correction.

An area of controversy exists concerning the therapeutic merit of using glucocorticoid steroids in an effort to reduce brain edema and stabilize cell membranes in patients with traumatic brain injury.[73,88] Although a few clinical studies have demonstrated that large-dose steroids may improve mortality,[39,40] multiple studies have shown that high and conventional doses of steroids fail to effectively treat intracranial pressure or improve the outcomes of brain-injured patients.[15,24,27,43] Citing weaknesses in the studies supporting steroid use, and based on the findings of the other studies unsupportive of steroid use, it is suggested that glucocorticoid steroids should not be used for treatment of traumatic brain injury.[20,88]

Reduction of cerebral stimulation and metabolic demand with subsequent decrease in cerebral oxygen consumption is another effective method of lowering ICP to prevent secondary brain injury. Minimizing noxious stimuli and maintaining normothermia are two nursing strategies that can reduce cerebral stimulation and metabolic demand. Sedatives or analgesics, which are preferably short-acting or easily reversible (e.g., morphine sulfate, thiopental), can also be used to control pain and agitation, thereby lowering cerebral metabolic requirements and reducing ICP. Extreme caution must be used when administering these pharmacologic agents since the neurologic exam may become unreliable, and, in a patient not being mechanically ventilated, respiratory suppression can result. Paralytic agents used in conjunction with sedation are instituted to achieve muscle relaxation and reduce ICP in intubated patients with severe agitation, posturing, or asynchronous breathing with the ventilator. High doses of barbiturates can be administered to patients on mechanical ventilation with intracranial hypertension that is refractory to all other conventional therapy. Paralytic and high-dose barbiturate therapy nearly obliterates the neurologic examination, making monitored ICP and pupil size the only clinical parameters available to continually assess for potential neurologic deterioration.[20,82] Caution must also be used when administering high doses of barbiturates, since their depressant effect is not exclusive to the neurologic system and myocardial depression and hypotension may result.

Surgical intervention to insert an intraventricular catheter for cerebral spinal fluid removal, evacuate an intracranial hematoma or foreign object, elevate a depressed skull fracture, or remove brain tissue may be necessary to decompress the brain. Research in comatose patients clearly has shown that when removal of an acute subdural hematoma is delayed for over four hours from the time of injury, the mortality rate triples when compared to surgical intervention that takes place within four hours of injury.[109] Controversy still exists concerning the neurosurgical management of certain traumatic brain lesions. Indications for removal of a hemorrhagic contusion and management of chronic subdural hematomas are examples of controversies surrounding neurosurgical care of the brain-injured patient.[23,73,100]

Research regarding nursing interventions has been instrumental in defining the care most appropriate for a patient with traumatic brain injury. Clinical trials have assisted in clarifying anticipated patient responses to various activities and stimuli so that the nurse can plan care appropriately.* Studies have identified activities and interventions that typically elevate ICP so that the nurse can minimize stimuli known to increase ICP (e.g., neck flexion, shivering, posturing) and plan how to space activities.[10,57,83,114,126,134] When the patient is intolerant of procedures known to raise ICP, the nurse may administer prescribed drugs, such as a morphine or lidocaine, prior to initiating such interventions to minimize ICP elevations.[82] Research-based protocols also have been developed for specific nursing interventions such as suctioning[61,93,107] and positioning of patients with brain injury.[60,66,70,77]

Controversy surrounds optimal head-of-the-bed positioning for the patient with traumatic brain injury. Research has generally supported positioning the patient with the head of the bed elevated 30 degrees to minimize ICP.[33,60,95] Although studies have demonstrated that cerebral perfusion pressure (CPP) is not adversely affected at these moderate head-of-the-bed elevations,[33,35,95] one researcher has suggested that positioning the head-injured patient flat is most desirable since the cerebral perfusion is optimized and the severity and frequency of ICP waves are minimized using this position.[105] Other researchers have clearly shown that patients demonstrate highly individualized responses to various positions and suggest each patient be positioned to optimize individual cerebrovascular parameters.[70,102]

Systemic hypotension must also be treated to avoid secondary brain injury and optimize patient outcome.[72,80,120] Adequate intravascular fluid volume must be restored as soon as possible to alleviate systemic hypotension and avoid impaired systemic or cerebral tissue perfusion. Patient clinical assessment findings and hemodynamic parameters should guide the volume of fluid necessary to achieve sufficient intravascular volume while avoiding fluid overload. Once adequate intravascular volume is ensured, inotropic and/or vasopressor agents may be necessary to achieve an adequate systemic blood pressure and cardiac output. Generally, a systolic blood pressure between 100 and 160 mm Hg is desired; this creates a mean arterial blood pressure high enough to keep the cerebral perfusion pressure well over 50 mm Hg.[73,82,130] Ideally, the CPP should be maintained above 70 mm Hg.[18,73,106] Care must be taken when administering drugs to treat intracranial hypertension (e.g., sedatives or diuretics) since these may have a detrimental effect on systemic blood pressure.

Although prevention of secondary brain insult is of paramount importance, other therapeutic goals also require attention in order to optimize the functional outcomes of patients with traumatic brain injury. A second therapeutic goal is prevention, early recognition, and appropriate treatment of multisystem complications associated with traumatic brain injury. This includes such interventions as antacid therapy to prevent gastrointestinal mucosal erosion, pulmonary toilet to prevent respiratory complications, meticulous skin care to avoid skin breakdwon, use of aseptic technique to guard against infection, and provision of sufficient protein and calorie supplementation while avoiding hyperglycemia to prevent malnutrition. Meticulous comprehensive assessment and monitoring of the patient with traumatic brain injury is essential to enable early recognition of complications so that appropriate intervention can be initiated.

Prevention and treatment of potential complications associated with traumatic brain injury is also plagued with areas of controversy. Debate surrounds the effectiveness of prophylactic antibiotics to prevent post-traumatic intracranial infection. Proponents of antibiotic prophylaxis advocate antibiotic treatment when patients have open or penetrating head injuries or basilar skull fractures, to reduce risk of intracranial infection.[14,104] Others argue that use of antibiotic prophylaxis offers no greater protection against infection, while subjecting the patient to potential drug side effects and risk of developing drug-resistant organism superinfections.[51,55] Consensus exists that once an intracranial infection is suspected, a cerebral spinal fluid (CSF) culture should be obtained, if possible, and antibiotics that are able to penetrate the blood-brain barrier and cover the probable or cultured infectious organism(s) should be initiated.[65]

Prophylactic use of anticonvulsants following traumatic brain injury is also a controversial subject. Proponents recommend that anticonvulsants be given routinely, particularly to those patients who have high risk factors present for seizure development (e.g., penetrating head injury, focal intracranial hemorrhagic lesions).[23,50] The efficacy of phenytoin (Dilantin) prophylaxis has been questioned by others, and it has been shown that phenytoin is effective in preventing seizures only for the first week after onset of head injury.[122,136]

Once the patient is stabilized, physical, cognitive, psychosocial, and emotional rehabilitation become a third therapeutic focus. This process of rehabilitation should be initiated upon admission and instituted even while the patient is in the critical care setting.[82,110] The tremendous emotional and psychosocial needs of the patient's family or significant others must not be overlooked, and appropriate interventions to meet these needs should be incorporated into the plan of care.[123] The therapeutic goals for the patient and family are best achieved by a collaborative team approach that employs an organized system of care that is attentive to detail.[73,82]

Current research regarding traumatic brain injury has focused on both improving assessment strategies and developing more effective treatment. Assessment techniques that can provide continuous or frequent information about brain

*References 3, 25, 33, 35, 52, 66, 70, 77, 93-95, 105, 107, 125, 132.

blood flow, function, oxygen delivery, and/or metabolism and warn of impending brain ischemia offer tremendously helpful information for treatment of brain injury and are the focus of much of the current research. Devices that enable continuous monitoring of jugular venous oxygen saturation, allowing calculation of the cerebral extraction of oxygen if the oxygen saturation of arterial blood is known[26,111]; regional cerebral blood flow[30,78]; and cerebral oxygen saturation[75] are examples of assessment strategies recently introduced that indicate progress in this area of brain injury research.

A large amount of research focusing on treatment of traumatic brain injury is also in progress. Controversial aspects of care for the patient with traumatic brain injury will undoubtedly continue to undergo further investigation. Research has also focused on better defining the pathologic alterations occurring at the cellular level so that agents aimed at preventing or reversing these events can be developed.* Pharmacologic agents currently under investigation to target these various biochemical events thought to cause secondary brain injury include antioxidants and free radical scavengers,[46,47] calcium channel antagonists,[74] buffering agents,[71] neurotransmitter antagonists,[17,49,68] and others.[34,76] Finally, agents that may enhance or stimulate neuronal regrowth and reorganization are currently under investigation.[67,108,112,118]

*References 13, 49, 54, 62, 68, 71, 97, 137.

ASSESSMENT

PARAMETER	ANTICIPATED ALTERATION
Patient History	
Prior trauma	Report a history of trauma, usually just prior to symptom onset
Physical Assessment	
Physical assessment findings are dependent on the location, type, and severity of brain injury.	Focal injury typically causes symptoms specific to the anatomic area that is affected. (See Table 4-3.) Areas of ecchymosis, edema, hematoma formation, abrasions, and lacerations, which may be accompanied with perfuse bleeding, may be present on the head indicating where the force directly impacted. *Since brain injury can result from indirect transmission of forces to the brain, without direct impact of the head, these symptoms may not be present.* Entrance/exit wound(s) may be visible *if patient has a penetrating head wound.* Depression of a portion of the skull and palpable bone edge *may be evident if a depressed skull fracture is present.* Ecchymosis of the periorbital area (Raccoon's eyes) or mastoid process (Battle's sign) *due to accompanying basilar skull fracture.* Cerebral spinal fluid or blood leakage from the nose (rhinorrhea) or ear (otorrhea) *due to an accompanying basilar skull fracture with a dural tear.*
LOC	Decreased, ranging from a restless and confused state to coma. *Impaired arousal results from disruption of the reticular activating system responsible for maintaining wakefulness, and decreased awareness results from dysfunction of the cerebral cortex.*[82]
Glasgow coma scale (See Box on page 36, "Glasgow Coma Scale.")	Total score is determined by adding together the scores for three categories: best eye opening, best verbal response, and best motor response. The lower the score the more severe the brain injury and more depressed the level of consciousness.
Motor function	Impaired generalized motor responsiveness *related to a specific level of brain dysfunction.* (See Table 4-4.)
Muscle strength	Unilateral or bilateral deficits (e.g., hemiparesis or hemiplegia) *usually due to damage to or compression of the descending corticospinal or pyramidal tracts.*
Muscle tone	Varies, or may be normal, increased, or decreased. Flaccidity *due to lower brainstem dysfunction and lower motor neuron lesions.* Spasticity *due to upper motor neuron lesions.*[53,82]

TABLE 4-3 Symptoms Related to Focal Lesion Location

Lesion location	Associated focal symptoms
Frontal lobe	Frontal headache Mental function disturbance such as shortened attention span, emotional liability, apathy, inappropriate behavior, memory impairment, flat affect, and impulsiveness Contralateral hemiparesis Expressive aphasia (related to dominant hemisphere dysfunction) Seizures (focal or Jacksonian)
Parietal lobe	Sensory impairment Hyperesthesias and paresthesias Loss of proprioception Inability to recognize body parts or neurologic deficits Inability to localize sensory stimuli Dyslexia Loss of right-left discrimination Inability to calculate Inability to write Visual field deficits Seizures
Temporal lobe	Localized headaches Hearing deficits Contralateral facial weakness Auditory agnosia Receptive aphasia (related to dominant hemisphere dysfunction) Visual field deficits Psychomotor seizures
Occipital lobe	Headache Visual agnosia Visual hallucinations Visual field deficits Focal or generalized seizures (frequently associated with visual aura)
Cerebellum	Headache in the postoccipital region or below the ear Impaired coordination Unsteadiness Ataxia Loss of balance Intention tremors Nystagmus
Pituitary and hypothalamus region	Headaches Hormonal dysfunction Loss of temperature control Visual deficits such as decreased visual acuity and clarity
Brainstem	Cranial nerve (III through XII) dysfunction Loss of corneal, oculocephalic, oculovestibular, gag, and/or swallow reflexes Impairment of motor and/or sensory tracts Cerebellar dysfunction Vomiting Altered respiratory patterns Widened pulse pressure seen with medullary vasomotor compression (hypotension with patient decompensation)

Note: Level of consciousness may be affected with lesions in any of these locations.

TABLE 4-4 Alterations in Motor Response Related to Specific Areas of Brain Dysfunction

Best motor response	Related area of brain dysfunction
Monoparesis or hemiparesis	Hemispheric damage that compresses or damages the contralateral corticospinal tract
Localizes to painful stimuli, but unable to follow commands	Cortical areas
Flexion/withdrawal (pulls extremity away from noxious stimuli)	Damage to the internal capsule or cerebral hemispheres resulting in corticospinal tract disruption
Abnormal flexion or decorticate posturing (characterized by rigid arm, wrist, and finger flexion with leg extension, internal rotation, and plantar flexion)	Extensive cortical dysfunction
Abnormal extension or decerebrate posturing (characterized by rigid arm extension, adduction, and internal rotation, finger and wrist flexion, leg extension, and plantar flexion)	Midbrain or upper pons regions of the brainstem
Flaccidity	Lower brainstem

Used with permission from Hickey JV: *The Clinical Practice of Neurological and Neurosurgical Nursing,* ed 3, Philadelphia, 1992, JB Lippincott, and Mitchell PH: Central nervous system 1: closed head injuries. In Cardona VD et al, editors: *Trauma Nursing from Resuscitation through Rehabilitation,* Philadelphia, 1994, WB Saunders.

Glasgow Coma Scale

Eye opening	
Spontaneous	4
To verbal command	3
To pain	2
None	1
Best motor response	
Obeys verbal commands	6
Localizes pain	5
Flexion/withdrawal	4
Abnormal flexion	3
Abnormal extension	2
None	1
Best verbal response	
Oriented and converses	5
Disoriented and converses	4
Inappropriate words	3
Incomprehensible sounds	2
None	1
Total	3-15

NOTE: Record if one or more parts of the scale are not testable (e.g., endotracheal intubation makes verbal response untestable)

Used with permission from Teasdale G, Jennett B: Assessment of coma and impaired consciousness: a practical scale, *Lancet* 2:81-84, 1974.

Physical Assessment—cont'd

Deep tendon reflexes	Initially may be absent, but then hyperactive *with upper motor neuron lesions.*
Muscle coordination	Impaired coordination and ataxia *usually due to dysfunction of the cerebellum or associated nerve tracts. Sensory and motor deficit can also contribute to ataxia and poor coordination of movements.*
Babinski's reflex	Often, initially absent or hypoactive but later positive, characterized by dorsiflexion of the great toe. *Presence indicates an upper motor neuron lesion.*
Ability to communicate	Expressive and/or receptive aphasias may be present *due to compression or damage to the cortical areas that control the ability to speak, write, or interpret auditory or written communication.*
Sensation	Various sensory deficits may result *due to compression, or damage to sensory pathways or parietal lobe.*
Cranial nerves (CN)	The sensory, motor, and/or reflex dysfunction that occurs will depend on which CN(s) are damaged or compressed (See Table 4-5.) *CN III through CN XII deficits usually indicate compression or injury of the brainstem from which these nerves originate.*

TABLE 4-5 The Cranial Nerves

Number	Name	Origin	Function	Assessment
I	Olfactory	Olfactory bulb	Sensory: Smell	Have patient identify odors Test each nostril separately
II	Optic	Retina	Sensory: Vision	Test visual acuity Test visual fields
III	Oculomotor	Midbrain	Motor: Pupil constriction Elevation of eyelid Extraocular movement	Test direct and consensual pupil reaction to light to assess II and III Assess for ptosis Test fields of gaze to assess III, IV, and VI Test accommodation
IV	Trochlear	Midbrain	Motor: Downward & inward eye movements	Test fields of gaze
V	Trigeminal	Pons to cervical cord	Motor: Temporal & masseter muscles Lateral jaw movement Sensory: Facial (3 divisions) 1. Ophthalmic-forehead 2. Maxillary-cheeks 3. Mandibular-lower jaw and tongue	Test jaw movement—strength and symmetry; assess ability to chew Test corneal reflex to assess V and VII Test touch sensation of forehead, cheeks, and jaw with cotton and water of different temperatures
VI	Abducens	Pons	Motor: Abduction of eye	Test fields of gaze
VII	Facial	Pons	Motor: Muscles of face, including those of forehead, mouth, and around the eyes Sensory: Taste of anterior ⅔ of tongue	Test facial movement—ability to wrinkle forehead, frown, smile, and raise eyebrows symmetrically Test sweet or salty taste on anterior aspect of tongue
VIII	Acoustic	Pons and medulla	Sensory: Hearing (cochlear division); balance (vestibular division)	Test hearing MD can do caloric test to assess III, VI, and VIII Test balance
IX	Glossopharyngeal	Medulla	Motor: Pharynx Sensory: Posterior tongue, soft palate and pharyngeal sensation, taste in posterior tongue, carotid body and sinus receptors with reflex control of respiration, BP and HR	Test taste on posterior tongue Assess IX and X Test swallow and gag reflexes Assess symmetrical uvula and soft palate rise when saying "Ah" Test ability to speak clearly
X	Vagus	Medulla	Motor: Pharynx, larynx, and palate Sensory: Pharynx, larynx, and palate Parasympathetic fibers innervate abdominal and thoracic viscera	Assess with IX
XI	Spinal Accessory	Medulla	Motor: Sternocleidomastoid and trapezius muscles	Test ability of patient to shrug shoulders and turn head against resistance
XII	Hypoglossal	Medulla	Motor: Tongue	Note deviation of protruded tongue Test tongue strength

Physical Assessment—cont'd

Pupil shape	Oval or irregularly shaped pupil *due to increased ICP and early CN III compression from transtentorial herniation.* Irregularly shaped pupil *may also indicate orbital trauma, a nuclear midbrain lesion, or previous iridectomy.*[53]
Pupil size, equality, and reactivity to light	Pupil abnormalities can be associated with compression or damage to specific anatomical areas of the brain. (See Table 4-6.) *Abnormally small or large pupils may also be caused by orbital trauma or use of certain drugs.* Impaired direct and/or consensual pupil reaction to light *due to dysfunction of CNs II or III.* • *Loss of direct response is due to CN III lesion or CN II lesion resulting in blindness.* • *Loss of direct & consensual response, due to CN III damage.* • *Loss of direct response with the consensual response preserved due to blindness in that eye.* Sluggish pupil reaction to light *may signal impending loss of pupil reactivity to light.* Hippus (vacillating pupil constriction, and then dilatation in response to light) is normal if observing the pupil under high magnification; but if not, it may indicate CN III compression and impending transtentorial herniation.[53]
Corneal reflex (Eye should blink in response to touching the cornea with a wisp of cotton)	Absent *due to CN V or VII integrity, or dysfunction of the brainstem from where these CNs originate*
Doll's eyes (oculocephalic) reflex. Assessed ONLY after a cervical injury has been ruled out! (During brisk side to side rotation of the head, the eyes should conjugately deviate opposite the direction that the head is turned.)	Abnormal or absent *due to CN III, VI, or VIII dysfunction, or loss of brainstem integrity* Abnormal response if eye movement is asymmetrical Absent if there is no eye movement
Caloric (oculovestibular) reflex. This test should NOT be performed if the tympanic membrane is not intact. (With the head of the bed elevated 30 degrees, when iced saline is instilled into the patient's ear, conjugate eye deviation toward the irrigated ear should occur. If the cerebral cortex control is still intact, the eyes will then deviate rapidly back toward the opposite side.)	Abnormal or absent *due to CN III, VI, or VIII dysfunction, or loss of brainstem integrity* Abnormal if eyes move asymmetrically Absent if there is no eye movement
Respiratory rate and rhythm	Abnormal respiratory patterns *due to effect of brain injury on respiratory centers in the brain. Specific respiratory patterns have been correlated with various locations of brain injury. (Table 4-7.) Although the effect of brain injury on respiration is variable, and multiple other factors are known to affect respiratory rate and rhythm.*

TABLE 4-6 Pupil Abnormalities Related to Specific Areas of Brain Dysfunction

Pupil findings	Related brain dysfunction
Fixed and dilated pupil	Ipsilateral third cranial nerve (oculomotor) compression or injury
Bilateral fixed and dilated pupils	Severe brain anoxia and ischemia; bilateral CN III compression
Pinpoint, nonreactive pupils	Interruption of sympathetic innervation due to pons damage
Small, equal, reactive pupils	Bilateral diencephalic damage affecting sympathetic innervation originating from the hypothalmus or metabolic dysfunction
Nonreactive, midpositioned pupils	Loss of sympathetic and parasympathetic innervation due to midbrain damage

Source: Hickey JV: *The clinical practice of neurological and neurosurgical nursing,* ed 3, Philadelphia, 1992, JB Lippincott.

TABLE 4-7 Respiratory Patterns Associated with Brain Dysfunction

Name	Description	Neuroanatomical brain lesions
Cheyne-Stokes respirations	Regular cycles of respirations that gradually increase in depth to hyperpnea and then decrease in depth to short periods of apnea	Usually bilateral lesions deep within the cerebral hemispheres, diencephelon or basal ganglia; occasionally metabolic lesions
Central neurogenic hyperventilation	Regular, deep, rapid respirations	Midbrain, upper pons
Apneustic respirations	Prolonged inspiration followed by an end-inspiratory pause of 2 to 3 seconds and end-expiratory pause	Pons; usually associated with basilar artery occlusion
Cluster respirations	Clusters of irregular breaths followed by apneic periods lasting varied amounts of time	Lower pons or upper medulla
Ataxic or biots respirations	Irregular, unpredictable pattern of shallow and deep respirations and pauses	Medulla

Sources: Hickey JV: *The clinical practice of neurological and neurosurgical nursing,* ed 3, Philadelphia, 1992, JB Lippincott; and Mitchell PH: *Central nervous system 1: closed head injuries.* In Cardona VD, et al, editors: *Trauma nursing from resuscitation through rehabilitation,* Philadelphia, 1994, WB Saunders, pp 383-434.

Physical Assessment—cont'd

Cardiac rhythm

Sinus tachycardia, sinus bradycardia, premature atrial and ventricular contractions, paroxysmal atrial tachycardia, atrial fibrillation, atrial flutter, ventricular tachycardia, and atrioventricular blocks may be seen. Also, multiple changes in the ECG configuration have been associated with brain injury, including ST segment elevation or depression, T wave changes, prolonged QT interval, and Q or U waves. *Often ECG abnormalities are associated with the presence of subarachnoid blood. Excessive catecholamine release and autonomic nervous system stimulation are hypothesized to be the primary causes for these neurogenic ECG changes.*[19,99]

Blood pressure (BP)

Rising systolic blood pressure, widening pulse pressure, and bradycardia make up a triad of symptoms known as Cushing's response, a late sign of increased ICP and brain herniation.

Hypotension is rarely due to intracranial injury, but may be seen in conjunction with tachycardia when death from increased ICP and brainstem compression is imminent.

Temperature

Hyperthermia *may result from injury to the hypothalamic temperature regulating center, blood in subarachnoid space, seizures, or later from intracranial infections. Extracranial sources for temperature elevation (e.g., infection) must be ruled out.*

Hypothermia *may occur with destructive lesions of the brainstem or hypothalamus.*[53]

Complaint of pain	If awake, the patient may complain of pain from associated injuries, and headache pain *due to head trauma and increasing ICP.*
Presence of seizure activity	Seizures may occur *due to irritation of the brain tissue.*
Presence of vomiting	Vomiting *due to vestibular nerve dysfunction or compression of the medullary vomiting center.*
ICP	Elevated: >15 mm Hg *due to increased intracranial volume from cerebral edema, hyperemia, intracranial hemorrhage, and/or post-traumatic hydrocephalus. Possible ICP waveform changes associated with increased ICP and poor brain compliance are discussed in Guideline 12 on ICP monitoring.*
Cerebral perfusion pressure (equal to the mean arterial blood pressure minus the ICP)	May be decreased: <70 mm Hg *due to high ICP or systemic hypotension.* Increased: >100 mm Hg *due to excessive systemic hypertension.*

Laboratory Data

ABG	PaO_2 decreased: <60 mm Hg in approximately one third of patients on admission.[19] Often associated with hyperventilation and hypocapnea. *Exact mechanism for this early hypoxemia is unknown. Possible mechanisms include ventilation perfusion mismatch, abnormal respirations, pulmonary microemboli, atelectasis, aspiration, lung injury, and increased oxygen consumption.*[28] Hypocapnea and respiratory alkalosis will be present if the patient hyperventilates, whereas hypercapnea and respiratory acidosis will accompany depressed respirations. Metabolic acidosis may be present if systemic hypotension or hypoxia exists.
Glucose	Hyperglycemia >105 mg/dl (>5.8 mOsm/L) is common after severe head injury *in response to increased catecholamines.*[64,135] It is important to rule out hypoglycemia, which can adversely affect neurologic status
Electrolytes and Osmolarity	Electrolyte and fluid imbalance (excess, deficit, or combinations) may be present (e.g., sodium imbalance, hypokalemia) *due to hormonal stress response, treatment (e.g., diuretics) or onset of complications (e.g., diabetes insipidus or syndrome of inappropriate antidiuretic hormone).*
Coagulation profile	FDP >10 μg/ml PT >12.5 sec APTT >40 sec *Increased values are common due to endothelial disruption and thromboplastin release associated with brain injury.*[20]
Hgb and Hct	May not be affected by brain injury but assessed to ensure adequate oxygen-carrying capacity
WBC count with differential, sedimentation rate	Monitored for evidence of infection
Toxicology screen	Detects if the patient ingested drugs, which may skew neurologic assessment findings

Diagnostic Tests

Skull x-rays	Bony anomalies (i.e., skull fractures) and presence of metallic objects are detected. Shift of the calcified pineal gland *due to hematoma or edema* may be apparent.
Cervical spine x-ray	Rules out or confirms associated cervical spine injury.
Computerized tomography (CT)	The presence, extent, and location of hemorrhage or hematomas, edema, and contusions are identified. Complications, including brain herniation, hydrocephalus, and infarct, can be detected. Serial scans show the progression of brain injury.[53,56]

Magnetic resonance imaging (MRI)	The presence, extent, and location of ischemia, contusion, edema, hemorrhage or hematomas, and nonhemorrhagic lesions (i.e., axonal shear injury) can be detected in the brain, including the hard-to-visualize brainstem and basilar skull areas.[37,38,113]
Cerebral angiography	Identifies vascular injuries and presence of vasospasms.
Cerebral blood flow	Regional cerebral blood flow alterations are identified.
Positron emission transaxial tomography (PETT)	Used primarily for research, this test detects alterations in the brain's physiologic function, including abnormalities in brain metabolism caused by injury.[82]
Single-photon-emission computed tomography (SPECT)	Areas of brain dysfunction are detected by assessing regional cerebral blood flow to estimate metabolic activity.[89]
Transcranial Doppler ultrasound	Altered flow velocity through cerebral vessels may be detected. Examples: decreased flow velocity with drop in CPP below 60 mm Hg; increased flow velocity with vasospasms.[79]
Electroencephalogram (EEG)	Abnormal cerebral function and seizure activity can be detected.
Evoked potentials	Abnormal evoked potential response *due to dysfunction or disruption of pathways that carry specific sensory stimuli. Visual, somatosensory, and auditory pathways can be evaluated to provide information about lesion location and patient prognosis.*[59,82]
Neuropsychological testing	Mild to severe behavioral and cognitive deficits may be detected.

PLAN OF CARE

INTENSIVE PHASE

Traumatic brain injury is often a lifetime injury. The following section describes the intensive phase of care, detailing current therapeutics. Although the goals are constant, different settings may emphasize different interventions. When there is controversy or an alternative approach, this is indicated, along with the rationale that will promote the best possible outcome for the patient with traumatic brain injury.

PATIENT CARE PRIORITIES	EXPECTED PATIENT OUTCOMES
Ineffective airway clearance *r/t* *Decreased LOC with upper airway relaxation* *Absent or weak gag or cough reflexes* *Aspiration* *Secretion retention* *Associated injuries compromising the airway*	Patent airway maintained Breath sounds normal throughout lung fields Clear chest x-ray Airway secretions removed
Ineffective breathing pattern *r/t* *Injury to areas of the brain controlling respirations* *Associated injuries affecting respirations* *Metabolic imbalance*	Effective ventilation established and maintained ABG normal or within desired range Breath sounds normal throughout lung fields
Impaired gas exchange *r/t* *Airway obstruction* *Ineffective breathing patterns* *Onset of pulmonary complications (See 1)*	Airway patency maintained Effective ventilation established and maintained Chest x-ray and breath sounds clear ABG: WNL or within desired range: $Pa{O_2}$ >70 mm Hg $Pa{CO_2}$: WNL or reduced to desired range
Impaired cerebral tissue perfusion *r/t* *Brain tissue injury* *Increased ICP* *Hypotension* *Onset of neurologic complications*	ICP <20 mm Hg Cerebral perfusion pressure always greater than 50 mm Hg and maintained when possible over 70 mm Hg and less than 130 mm Hg Neurologic function maintained or improved

Plan of Care (cont'd)

High risk for fluid volume deficit *r/t*
Fluid loss; i.e., diuresis, vomiting, associated hemorrhage
Brain injury induced hormone imbalances; e.g., antidiuretic hormone (ADH) deficiency causes diabetes insipidus
Diuretic therapy
Inadequate fluid intake
Hemorrhage exacerbated by onset of coagulopathy

Serum and urine electrolytes normal
Serum osmolality within desired range
Blood pressure stable and sufficient to maintain adequate CPP
Urine output ≥30 cc but <200 cc/hr
Hemodynamic parameters (i.e., CVP, PCWP, and PA pressures) normal
Coagulation parameters normal
Control of any hemorrhage
Adequate hemoglobin for oxygen transport
Resolution of complications that alter fluid or electrolyte balance

High risk for decreased cardiac output *r/t*
Dysrhythmias
Hypotension

Cardiac output normal
Dysrhythmias controlled
Blood pressure adequate to maintain adequate CPP

High risk for fluid volume excess *r/t*
Brain injury induced hormone imbalance (e.g., syndrome of inappropriate ADH)

Serum and urine electrolytes normal
Serum osmolality within desired range
Urine output at least 30 cc/hr
Hemodynamic parameters (i.e., BP, CVP, PCWP, PA pressures) normal
ICP maintained <20 mm Hg
Resolution of complications that alter fluid and electrolyte balance

Alteration in comfort *r/t*
Headache
Traumatic injury
Invasive procedures

Pain is relieved
ICP maintained <20 mm Hg

Ineffective thermoregulation *r/t*
Injury to thermoregulatory centers

Normothermia maintained

High risk for infection *r/t*
Immunocompromise
Aspiration
Traumatic interruption of the skin and/or dura
Invasive procedures

Free of infection
Resolution of any infection

Inadequate nutrition *r/t*
Hypermetabolic and hypercatabolic state
Inadequate intake due to dysphagia, inability to feed self, vomiting, decreased level of consciousness

Caloric intake meets metabolic need
Maintain an equal or positive nitrogen balance
Normal metabolic parameters
Blood glucose within normal range
Minimal weight loss during hospitalization

Impaired physical mobility *r/t*
Injury to areas of the brain enabling movement
Decreased level of consciousness
Spasticity
Abnormal posturing
Sedation or paralytics
Bed rest

No evidence of complications related to immobility, including:
- Absence of venous thrombosis
- Absence of contractures
- Clear chest x-ray
- No skin breakdown
- No constipation
- No corneal abrasions

Potential for injury *r/t*
Neurological deficit
Altered level of consciousness
Sedation/analgesia
Onset of seizures

No further injury occurs
Seizures controlled

Plan of Care (cont'd)

Potential for impaired gastric tissue integrity *r/t* *Intracranial pathology* *Stress*	No evidence of a gastrointestinal bleed
Altered thought processes *r/t* *Neurologic impairment* *Perceptual or cognitive deficits*	Maintain or improve awareness and ability to interact with the environment appropriately Regain optimal level of cognitive function
Impaired family coping *r/t* *Traumatic event* *Sudden disability of family member or significant other* *Sudden role changes*	Family/significant other will: Verbalize an accurate understanding of patient injuries, condition, and treatment Express concerns Uses effective coping mechanisms and support systems to deal with the situation appropriately

INTERVENTIONS

Establish and maintain a patent airway.

Provide supplemental oxygen *to ensure adequate cerebral oxygen availability.*

Use mechanical ventilation, as necessary, *to facilitate effective lung ventilation and, if desired, to hyperventilate the patient.*

Provide pulmonary toilet *to keep airway patent and facilitate adequate gas exchange.*

Suction the airway only when necessary, passing the suction catheter as few times as possible (one or two) for no longer than 10 seconds each pass[61,107] *to avoid hypoxia, hypercapnea, and detrimental alterations in cerebrovascular parameters during suctioning.*

Hyperoxygenate the patient for 20 to 30 seconds or three to four lung volumes prior to and after each passage of the suction catheter[25,61] *to avoid hypoxia, hypercapnea, and detrimental alterations in cerebrovascular parameters during suctioning.*

Hyperventilate the patient for at least 20 to 30 seconds prior to and after each passage of the catheter, using caution in the already hypocapnic patient *to avoid reducing* $Paco_2$ *below 25 mm Hg.*[61]

Unless otherwise contraindicated, provide prescribed chest physiotherapy (including postural drainage) as tolerated *to facilitate secretion removal.*[77]

Monitor respiratory status, including frequent evaluation of ABGs, pulse oximetry, and capnography.

Administer fluids and use vasoactive and inotropic agents as appropriate *to maintain adequate BP and cardiac output necessary for sufficient brain perfusion.*

Monitor hemodynamic status.

Perform and document serial neurological assessments, ensuring physician notification when deterioration in neurological status is noted.

Rule out other physiologic causes (i.e., hypoxia, hypoglycemia, drug ingestion) that may also be contributing to alterations in neurologic status.

If present, maintain ICP monitoring device and monitor ICP, ICP waveform, and calculated CPP.

If an intraventricular catheter is in place, drain cerebrospinal fluid as prescribed, noting the character and amount of drainage.

Note the effect that specific interventions have on ICP and CPP, as well as other monitored parameters reflecting the brain's status. Space interventions as necessary *to avoid cumulative rises in ICP.*

Allow ICP and CPP to return to acceptable baseline levels before initiating additional interventions.

Maintain head and neck alignment, avoiding neck flexion and head rotation, *to promote cerebrovenous outflow and minimize ICP.*[10,84,93,132]

Position the head of the bed at the prescribed level (usually a 30° to 45° elevation). *The head-of-bed position selected ideally should be whatever level optimizes the patient's CPP.*[82]

Administer prescribed diuretics *to reduce cerebral edema and ICP.*

Plan of Care (cont'd)

Reduce cerebral stimulation and metabolic demand *to decrease ICP.*

Administer prescribed sedatives *to reduce cerebral stimulation and metabolic demand, thereby lowering ICP.*

Provide sedation with caution, preferably using small, frequent doses and administering the drug(s) slowly *to avoid systemic hypotension, which can compromise CPP.*

Institute comfort measures and administer prescribed analgesics as necessary *to control pain, which increases metabolic demand and ICP.*

Administer prescribed sedatives, analgesics, or lidocaine prophylactically prior to interventions known to raise ICP (e.g., respiratory care procedures) *to minimize ICP elevation.*

Prevent shivering and excessive muscle activity, *which increases cerebral metabolic demand and raises ICP.*

Administer any prescribed paralytic agents *to alleviate excessive muscle activity (i.e., abnormal posturing) or to control patient asynchrony with the ventilator.*

Maintain normothermia *to avoid elevations in cerebral oxygen consumption and ICP typically associated with hyperthermia.*

Avoid rapid cooling of the hyperthermic patient or prolonged hypothermia blanket use *to reduce the risk of shivering onset.*

Minimize unnecessary noxious stimuli, *which raises ICP.*[57]

Prevent the patient from performing the Valsalva maneuver, *which elevates ICP.*

Decompress the bowel until the gastrointestinal tract is functional *to reduce intra-abdominal pressure, which can elevate ICP, and to prevent possible aspiration.*

Avoid placement of tubes through the nasopharynx if a basilar skull fracture is suspected *to avoid intracranial intubation.*

Monitor electrocardiogram for the potential presence of cardiac arrhythmias. If present, treat appropriately and rule out other physiologic causes for these abnormalities.

Administer prescribed blood and/or blood products *to correct anemia or coagulopathy.*

Monitor clinical and laboratory data for evidence of coagulopathy.

Monitor fluid and electrolyte balance, including assessment of intake/output, urine specific gravity, and serum and urine electrolytes and osmolality, *to evaluate for potential imbalances caused by stress response, diuretic therapy, or onset of syndrome of inappropriate antidiuretic hormone or diabetes insipidus.*

Unless otherwise contraindicated, insert a bladder catheter *to facilitate accurate assessment of urine output and character.*

Institute seizure precautions and administer prescribed anticonvulsants.

Monitor therapeutic drug levels (e.g., barbiturate, phenytoin) as indicated.

If CSF drainage from the ear or nose is present or suspected, do not place anything into the leaking orifice. Instead, place a drip pad loosely outside the nose or ear to collect the drainage. If rhinorrhea is present, do not allow the patient to blow his or her nose.

Monitor for evidence of infection. Use aseptic technique when performing care to wounds, incision lines, or invasive devices *to prevent infection.*

Use hand mittens and protective restraints as ordered *to protect the agitated or localizing patient from self-harm.*

Collaborate with the nutritionist and physician to determine a diet that meets the patient's caloric and metabolic needs.

Administer nutritional support as prescribed, taking precautions to prevent aspiration with enteral feedings and to avoid hyperglycemia.

Administer prescribed antacids or Sucralfate (Carafate) *to avoid gastric ulceration.*

Assess gastric aspirate and stool for presence of blood *to evaluate for presence of gastrointestinal bleeding.*

Secure any drains coming from an operative site or head wound. Note drainage amount and character.

Provide eye care and apply eye lubricant q2h to q4h for the patient with absent corneal reflexes *to prevent corneal abrasions.*

Turn patient at least q2h as tolerated *to prevent complications associated with immobility.*

Provide meticulous skin care.

Plan of Care (cont'd)

Institute a bowel regimen *to establish a regular pattern of bowel elimination.*

Use pneumatic compression devices as prescribed *to decrease peripheral venous stasis and deep-vein thrombosis.*

Provide range of motion at least q8h *to prevent contractures caused by immobility and spasticity.*

Collaborate with physical therapy to develop a plan that optimizes pulmonary toilet and helps preserve functional mobility.

Communicate with the patient, even if unresponsive, to describe interventions and reorient frequently.

Collaborate with speech therapy to develop a plan for cognitive rehabilitation that can be instituted once the patient's condition has stabilized.

Provide the family with clear and concise information about the patient's condition and plan of care. Occasional mutlidisciplinary family conferences provide an excellent forum for sharing information and clarifying misperceptions.

Assess available family support systems and effective coping strategies and encourage the family to make use of these.

Teach family members how they can interact with the patient.

INTERMEDIATE PHASE

Nursing care in the intermediate phase focuses on continued stabilization of body systems, surveillance for onset of potential complications, developing the patient's adaptive processes for self-care, and ongoing preparation for discharge. Nursing care priorities in the intermediate phase can vary depending on the type and severity of neurologic deficits and multisystem complications present.

PATIENT CARE PRIORITIES	EXPECTED PATIENT OUTCOMES
Maintain effective gas exchange	Airway patency maintained Effective ventilation maintained Chest x-ray and breath sounds clear ABG within acceptable range
Alteration in comfort *r/t* *Headache* *Traumatic injury*	Pain relief
Potential for injury *r/t* *Altered LOC* *Agitation* *Impulsiveness* *Neurological deficit* *Onset of seizures*	No further injury occurs Seizures remain controlled
Maintain fluid and electrolyte balance	Urine and serum electrolytes remain normal
High risk for infection *r/t* *Invasive devices still in place* *Aspiration* *Inability to clear secretions*	Remain free of infection Resolution of any infection
Maintain adequate nutrition	Caloric intake meets metabolic need Maintains a positive or equal nitrogen balance Normal metabolic parameters
Impaired physical mobility *r/t* *Injury to areas of the brain enabling movement* *Decreased LOC* *Spasticity* *Abnormal posturing*	No evidence of complications related to immobility

Plan of Care (cont'd)

Alteration in pattern of urinary elimination *r/t* *Injury to areas of the brain that affect bladder emptying* *Altered LOC* *Cognitive impairment*	Regular bladder emptying Absence of bladder distension Incontinence contained
Altered sensory perception *r/t* *Injury to afferent pathways or to areas of the brain perceiving or interpreting sensory stimuli*	No injury results Establish strategies to compensate for sensory/perception deficits and to optimize perceived sensory input
Altered thought processes *r/t* *Neurologic impairment* *Persistent perceptual or cognitive deficits* *Memory and/or attention-span deficits*	Awareness of orientation to the environment improves Interacts with the environment appropriately, as able Regains optimal cognitive function
Self-care deficits in feeding, bathing/hygiene, toileting *r/t* *Impaired cognition, sensory perception, and/or mobility*	Feed, bathe, and perform hygiene and toileting measures as able Establish and utilize strategies that optimize self-care capabilities
Impaired verbal communication *r/t* *Tracheal intubation* *Neurologic impairment causing dysphasia or dysarthria*	Develop an effective method for communication Utilize established methods to communicate Participate in therapy to improve ability to communicate
Impaired individual coping *r/t* *Traumatic event* *Disability* *Personal vulnerability* *Role changes* *Loss of control*	Uses effective coping and support systems to deal with the situation appropriately Participates, as able, in planning and making decisions about care Participates in own care Acknowledges neurologic deficits Ventilates feelings
Altered self-concept *r/t* *Neurologic deficit*	Participates in therapies aimed at optimizing functional outcome Accepts positive reinforcement
Impaired family coping *r/t* *Traumatic event* *Disability of family member or significant other* *Role changes*	The family or significant other will: Continue to verbalize an understanding of the patient's condition and treatment plan Ventilate feelings about situation Use effective coping strategies and available support system to deal with the situation appropriately

INTERVENTIONS

Provide pulmonary toilet, including suctioning and chest physiotherapy, as needed *to facilitate secretion removal and maintain airway patency.*

Ensure the gag and swallow are intact prior to initiating oral feedings; elevate the head of the bed and monitor gastric residuals when administering enteral tube feedings *to prevent aspiration.*

Monitor respiratory status.

Perform and document neurological assessments.

Administer prescribed analgesics as necessary, taking caution to avoid obscuring the neurologic exam or causing respiratory depression.

Monitor fluid and electrolyte balance.

Use prescribed hand mittens and protective restraints as needed *to protect the patient from self-harm.*

Administer medications as prescribed to control severe agitation.

Plan of Care (cont'd)

Maintain seizure precautions and take appropriate action should a seizure occur.

Continue to monitor for infection and maintain aseptic technique as appropriate.

Collaborate with physical and occupational therapy *to determine how to best preserve and improve the functional mobility of the patient.*

Advance patient activity as prescribed and tolerated by the patient.

Position patient to ensure airway patency, body alignment, and patient comfort utilizing head and body supports and securing devices as necessary.

Elevate and support flaccid extremities. Do not to place a flaccid arm over the thorax *to prevent reduction in lung expansion.*

Reposition patient at least once q2h *to prevent complications associated with immobility.*

Achieve transition from passive to active range of motion as able.

Maintain extremity splints or casts applied *to prevent spasticity-induced joint deformities.*

Administer prescribed diet, ensuring that patient's metabolic requirements are met and that aspiration is prevented.

Consult speech therapy to evaluate patient's swallowing ability prior to starting oral feedings.

Supervise patient's initial feedings *to observe for choking or aspiration. Pureed foods or thick liquids, rather than thin liquids or regular foods, are usually preferred in the patient with chewing or swallowing difficulties.*

Remove indwelling urinary catheter as soon as possible *to prevent urinary tract infection.*

Monitor patient for adequate bladder elimination and use incontinence aids (e.g., male condom catheter, female incontinence pouch) as necessary. When patient is sufficiently aware, a bladder retraining program should be initiated.

Continue bowel regimen *to ensure regular bowel evacuation.*

Provide skin care including areas beneath braces and splints.

Collaborate with the physician and consulting services (e.g., speech therapy, audiology, opthamology) to determine the type and severity of sensory perception impairments that may be present and to develop an effective plan of care that considers these deficits. For example:

- If the patient has hemianopsia, approach and interact with the patient on the unaffected side. Place objects in view of the unaffected side.
- If visual acuity is impaired, use large-print reading materials and describe surrounding activities and location of necessities.
- If hearing is impaired, use assistive hearing aids, speak loud and clear, and use gestures and writing to communicate.
- If superficial sensation is impaired, protect that area from exposure to extremes in temperature and other sources of injury. Visually inspect this area frequently for evidence of injury.
- If agnosia is present, repeatedly reinforce the meaning of unrecognized but familiar objects.
- Encourage the use of intact senses to receive and/or recognize environmental input.[53]

Collaborate with physical and occupational therapy to devise alternative methods for the patient with neurologic deficits to perform activities of daily living, and to retrain the patient in self-care activities.

Maintain a quiet, calm environment that limits unnecessary stimuli *due to patient difficulty deciphering stimuli.*

Continue to reorient the patient frequently and explain interventions, even if the patient is unresponsive.

Use aids such as calendars, clocks, and posted schedules *to assist patient with memory and reorientation.*

Collaborate with speech and occupational therapy to implement a cognitive rehabilitation plan.

Plan of Care (cont'd)

- For the comatose patient, provide time-limited (15 to 30 minutes) directed stimulation to each of the senses (beginning with the tactile sense) *to develop environmental awareness and activate behavioral responses*. Use a stimulus familiar to the patient and stimulate only one sense at a time.[12]
- Maintain an organized, structured environment that provides consistency and repetition *to optimize the patient's cognitive processing*.[82]
- Incorporate rest periods into the established daily schedule.[12]

Remove aggravating stimuli and distract the confused and agitated patient who becomes upset or disruptive.[82]

Collaborate with speech therapy to determine the type of communication deficit that exists and formulate an appropriate plan of care. Examples of interventions that typically are part of such a plan include the following:

- Identify alternative methods for patient communication and encourage their use.
- Use nonverbal forms of communication and speak slowly to the patient in short, simple terms that may require repetition *to improve patient assimilation and understanding of the message*.
- Allow sufficient time for the patient to process and organize a response. Encourage the patient to take plenty of time when communicating.[53]
- Provide rest periods when communicating *to prevent patient fatigue and frustration*.
- When the patient has difficulty with expression, ask simple questions that enable the patient to provide one-word responses.

If the patient has dysarthria, encourage the patient to speak slowly, overarticulating each word. Have the patient perform prescribed oral facial exercises.

Educate the patient and family about the patient's condition, neurologic deficits that exist, and the treatment plan.

Include the patient, when possible, and the family in planning the patient's care and discharge.

Encourage the patient to participate in therapies aimed at improving and maximizing function.

Encourage the patient, when possible, and family to ventilate feelings about the injury and resulting deficits.

Suggest a neuropsychiatric consultation to assist the patient in dealing with post-traumatic anxiety and to help evaluate for cognitive and behavioral deficits.

Educate the family about how to interact and communicate with the patient and involve the family in the patient's care.

Explain to the family the need to foster independence in the patient by allowing the patient to perform activities as able.

Explain to the family that inappropriate or aggressive behavior may be out of the patient's control.

Provide referrals for family support services and head-injury support groups.

TRANSITION TO DISCHARGE

The severity of neurologic dysfunction and associated disabilities that persist as the patient's condition stabilizes will determine the most appropriate place for patient disposition. Patients with neurological disabilities that prohibit their participation in the rehabilitation process (i.e., persistent vegetative state) will require disposition to a long-term care facility or coma management program. Other patients with neurologic deficits may have good rehabilitation potential and require disposition to an inpatient rehabilitation program. In some cases, outpatient rehabilitation services may be sufficient. Others may benefit most from a specialized program that facilitates reentry into the community, or that offers vocational retraining.[82] Patients who have sustained mild brain injury are typically discharged home, but prior to discharge will require careful evaluation to ensure they can function safely and have adequate support systems in the home environment. The patient being discharged home also must be educated about postconcussive syndrome and other follow-up care. During the transition to discharge, priorities continue to focus on working in collaboration other health care team members to assist the patient in developing adaptive mechanisms to compensate for neurologic disabilities and to promote self-care.

REFERENCES

1. Adams JH, et al: Diffuse axonal injury in head injury: definition, diagosis, and grading, *Histopathology* 15:49-59, 1989.
2. Albrecht RJ, Miletich DJ, Ruttle M: Cerebral effects of extended hyperventilation in unanesthetized goats, *Stroke* 18:647-655, 1987.
3. American Association of Critical-Care Nurses: *Outcome Standards for Nursing Care of the Critically Ill,* Laguna Niguel, Calif, 1990, AACN.
4. Ammons AM: Cerebral injuries and intracranial hemorrhages as a result of trauma, *Nurs Clin North Am* 25:23-33, 1990.
5. Batjer HH, et al: Intracranial and cervical vascular injuries. In Cooper PR, editor: *Head injury,* ed 3, Baltimore, 1993, Williams & Wilkins, pp 373-403.
6. Battistella FD, Wisner DH: Combined hemorrhagic shock and head injury: effects of hypertonic saline (7.5%) resuscitation, *J Trauma* 31:182-188, 1991.
7. Becker DP: Common themes in head injury. In Becker DP, Gudeman SK, editors: *Textbook of head injury,* Philadelphia, 1989, WB Saunders, pp 1-22.
8. Bedford RF, et al: Lidocaine or thiopental for rapid control of intracranial hypertension? *Anesth Analg* 59:435-437, 1980.
9. Bloomfield EL: Extracerebral complications of head injury, *Crit Care Clin* 5:881-892, 1989.
10. Boortz-Marx R: Factors affecting intracranial pressure: a descriptive study, *J Neurosci Nurs* 17:89-94, 1985.
11. Borel C, et al: Intensive management of severe head injury, *Chest* 98:180-189, 1990.
12. Boss BJ: Cognitive systems: nursing assessment and management in the critical care environment, *AACN Clin Iss Crit Care Nurs* 2:685-698, 1991.
13. Braughler JM, Hall ED: Involvement of lipid peroxidation in CNS injury, *J Neurotrauma* 9(suppl 1):S1-S7, 1992.
14. Brawley BW, Kelley WA: Treatment of basal skull fractures with and without cerebralspinal fluid fistulae, *J Neurosurg* 26:57-61, 1967.
15. Braakman R, et al: Megadose steroid in severe head injury—results of a prospective double-blind clinical trial, *J Neurosurg* 58:326-330, 1983.
16. Brucia JJ, Owen DC, Rudy EB: The effects of lidocaine on intracranial hypertension, *J Neurosci Nurs* 24:205-214, 1992.
17. Bullock R, Fujisawa H: The role of glutamate antagonists for the treatment of CNS injury, *J Neurotrauma* 9(suppl 2):S443-S462, 1992.
18. Changaris DG, McGraw CP, Greenberg RA: Optimal cerebral perfusion pressure in head injury. In Hoff JT, Betz AL, editors: *Intracranial pressure VII,* Berlin, 1989, Springer-Verlag, pp 640-643.
19. Chesnut RM: Medical complications of the head-injured patient. In Cooper PR, editor: *Head injury,* ed 3, Baltimore, 1993, Williams & Wilkins, pp 459-501.
20. Chesnut RM, Marshall LF, Marshall SB: Medical management of intracranial pressure. In Cooper PR, editor: *Head injury,* ed 3, Baltimore, 1993, Williams & Wilkins, pp 225-246.
21. Cold GE: Does acute hyperventilation provoke cerebral oligaemia in comatose patients after acute head injury? *ACTA Neurochir (Wien)* 96:100-106, 1989.
22. Cook RJ, et al: Outcome prediction in extradural hematomas, *ACTA Neurochir (Wien)* 95:90-94, 1988.
23. Cooper PR: Post-traumatic intracranial mass lesions. In Cooper PR, editor: *Head injury,* ed 3, Baltimore, 1993, Williams & Wilkins, pp 275-329.
24. Cooper PR, et al: Dexamethasone and severe head injury—a prospective double-blind study, *J Neurosurg* 51:307-316, 1979.
25. Crosby LJ, Parsons LC: Cerebrovascular response of closed head injured patients to a standardized endotracheal tube suctioning and manual hyperventilation procedure, *J Neurosci Nurs* 24:40-49, 1992.
26. Cruz J, et al: Continuous monitoring of cerebral oxygenation in acute brain injury: injection of mannitol during hyperventilation, *J Neurosurg* 73:725-730, 1990.
27. Dearden NM, et al: Effect of high-dose dexamethasone on outcome from severe head injury, *J Neurosurg* 64:81-88, 1986.
28. Demling R, Riessen R: Pulmonary dysfunction after cerebral injury, *Crit Care Med* 18:768-773, 1990.
29. Department of Health and Human Services, National Institutes of Health, National Institute of Neurological Disorders and Stroke: *Interagency Head Injury Task Force Report,* Bethesda, Md., February 1989, National Institutes of Health.
30. Dickman CA, et al: Continuous regional cerebral blood flow monitoring in acute craniocerebral trauma, *Neurosurg* 28:467-472, 1991.
31. Donegan MF, Bedford RF: Intravenously administered lidocaine prevents intracranial hypertension during endotracheal suctioning, *Anesthesiology* 52:516-518, 1980.
32. Ducey JP, et al: A comparison of the cerebral and cardiovascular effects of complete resuscitation with isotonic and hypertonic saline, hetastarch, and whole blood following hemorrhage, *J Trauma* 29:1510-1518, 1989.
33. Durward QJ, et al: Cerebral and cardiovascular reponses to changes in head elevation in patients with intracranial hypertension, *J Neurosurg* 59:938-944, 1983.
34. Faden AI, Salzman S: Pharmacological strategies in CNS trauma, *Trends Pharmacol Sci* 13:29-35, 1992.
35. Feldman Z, et al: Effect of head elevation on intracranial pressure, cerebral perfusion pressure, and cerebral blood flow in head-injured patients, *J Neurosurg* 76:207-211, 1992.
36. Gennarelli TA: Cerebral concussion and diffuse brain injuries. In Cooper PR, editor: *Head injury,* ed 3, Baltimore, 1993, Williams & Wilkins, pp 137-158.
37. Gentry LR, et al: Prospective comparative study of intermediate field MR and CT in the evaluation of closed-head trauma. *AJR Am J Roentgenol* 150:673-682, 1988.
38. Gentry LR, Godersky JC, Thompson BH: Traumatic brainstem injury: MR imaging, *Radiology* 17:177-187, 1989.
39. Giannotta SL, et al: High-dose glucocorticoids in the management of severe head injury, *Neurosurg* 15, 497-501, 1984.
40. Gobiet W, et al: Treatment of acute cerebral edema with high-dose dexamethasone. In Beks JWF, Bosch DA, Brock M, editors: *Intracranial pressure III,* Berlin, 1976, Springer-Verlag, pp 232-235.
41. Graham DI, Adams JH, Gennarelli TA: Pathology of brain damage in head injury. In Cooper PR, editor: *Head injury,* ed 3, Baltimore, 1993, Williams & Wilkins, pp 91-113.
42. Gualtieri T, Cox DR: The delayed neurobehavioral sequelae of traumatic brain injury, *Brain Injury* 5:219-232, 1991.
43. Gudeman SK, Miller JD, Becker DP: Failure of high-dose steroid therapy to influence intracranial pressure in patients with severe head injury, *J Neurosurg* 51:301-306, 1979.

44. Gudeman SK, et al: Indications for operative treatment and operative technique in closed head injury. In Becker DP, Gudeman SK, editors: *Textbook of head injury,* Philadelphia, 1989, WB Saunders, pp 138-181.
45. Gunnar W, et al: Head injury and hemorrhagic shock: studies of the blood-brain barrier and intracranial pressure after resuscitation with normal saline solution, 3% saline solution, and dextran-40, *Surgery* 103:398-407, 1988.
46. Hall ED: Free radicals and CNS injury, *Crit Care Clin* 5:793-805, 1989.
47. Hall ED: Inhibition of lipid peroxidation in CNS trauma, *J Neurotrauma* 9(suppl 1):S31-S41, 1991.
48. Havill JH: Prolonged hyperventilation and intracranial pressure, *Crit Care Med* 12:72-74, 1984.
49. Hayes RL, Jenkins LW, Lyeth BG: Neurotransmitter-mediated mechanisms of traumatic brain injury: acetylcholine and excitatory amino acids, *J Neurotrauma* 9(suppl 1):S173-S187, 1992.
50. Heikkinen ER, et al: Development of post-traumatic epilepsy, *Stereotact Funct Neurosurg* 54 + 55:25-33, 1990.
51. Helling TS, et al: Infectious complications in patients with severe head injury, *J Trauma* 28:1575-1577, 1988.
52. Hendrickson SL: Intracranial pressure changes and family presence, *J Neurosci Nurs* 19:14-17, 1987.
53. Hickey JV: *The clinical practice of neurological and neurosurgical Nursing,* ed 3, Philadelphia, 1992, JB Lippincott.
54. Hovda DA, Becker DP, Katayama Y: Secondary injury and acidosis, *J Neurotrauma* 9(suppl 1):S47-S60, 1992.
55. Ignelzi RJ, VanderArk GD: Analysis of the treatment of basilar skull fractures with and without antibiotics, *J Neurosurg* 43:721-726, 1975.
56. Johnson MH, Lee SH: Computed tomography of acute cerebral trauma, *Radiol Clin North Am* 30:325-352, 1992.
57. Johnson SM, Omery A, Nikas D: Effects of conversation on intracranial pressure in comatose patients, *Heart Lung* 18:56-63, 1989.
58. Jones GA: Alcohol abuse and traumatic brain injury, *Alcohol Health & Research World* 13:105-109, 1989.
59. Judson JA, Cant BR, Shaw NA: Early prediction of outcome from cerebral trauma by somatosensory evoked potentials, *Crit Care Med* 18:363-368, 1990.
60. Kenning JA, Tautant SM, Saunders RL: Upright patient positioning in the management of intracranial hypertension, *Surg Neurol* 15:148-152, 1980.
61. Kerr ME, et al: Head-injured adults: recommendations for endotracheal suctioning, *J Neurosci Nurs* 25:86-91, 1993.
62. Kirsch JR, et al: Evidence for free radical mechanisms of brain injury resulting from ischemia/reperfusion-induced events, *J Neurotrauma* 9(suppl 1):S157-S163, 1992.
63. Kraus J: Epidemiology of head injury. In Cooper PR, editor: *Head injury,* ed 3, Baltimore, 1993, Williams & Wilkins, pp 1-25.
64. Lam AM, et al: Hyperglycemia and neurological outcome in patients with head injury, *J Neurosurg* 75:545-551, 1991.
65. Landesman S, Cooper PR: Infectious complications of head injury. In Cooper PR, editor, *Head injury,* ed 3, Baltimore, 1993, Williams & Wilkins, pp 503-523.
66. Lee S-T: Intracranial pressure changes during positioning of patients with severe head injury, *Heart Lung* 18:411-414, 1989.
67. Logan A: CNS growth factors, *Br J Hosp Med* 43:429-437, 1990.
68. Lyeth BG, Hayes RL: Cholinergic and opioid mediation of traumatic brain injury, *J Neurotrauma* 9(suppl 2): S463-S474, 1992.
69. MacKenzie EJ, Edelstein SL, Flynn JP: Hospitalized head-injured patient in Maryland: incidence and severity of injuries, *Md Med J* 38:725-732, 1989.
70. March K, et al: Effect of backrest position on intracranial and cerebral perfusion pressures, *J Neurosci Nurs* 22:375-381, 1990.
71. Marmarou A: Intracellular acidosis in human and experimental brain injury, *J Neurotrauma* 9(suppl 2):S551-S562, 1992.
72. Marmarou A, et al: Impact of ICP instability and hypotension on outcome in patients with severe head trauma, *J Neurosurg* 75:S59-S66, 1991.
73. Marshall SB, et al: *Neuroscience critical care pathophysiology and patient management,* Philadelphia, 1990, WB Saunders.
74. McBurney RN, et al: New CNS-specific calcium antagonists, *J Neurotrauma* 9(suppl 2):S531-S543, 1992.
75. McCormick PW, et al: Noninvasive cerebral optical spectroscopy for monitoring cerebral oxygen delivery and hemodynamics, *Crit Care Med* 19:89-97, 1991.
76. McIntosh TK: Pharmacologic strategies in the treatment of experimental brain injury, *J Neurotrauma* 9(suppl 1):S201-S209, 1992.
77. McQuillan KA: The effects of the Trendelenburg position for postural drainage on cerebrovascular status in head-injured patients, *Heart Lung* (abstract) 16:327, 1987.
78. Meyerson BA, et al: Bedside monitoring of regional cortical blood flow in comatose patients using laser Doppler flowmetry, *Neurosurg* 29:750-755, 1991.
79. Miller JD: Changing patterns in acute management of head injury, *J Neurol Sci* 103:S33-S37, 1991.
80. Miller JD, Becker DP: Secondary insults to the injured brain, *J R Coll Surg Edin* 27:292-298, 1982.
81. Mirvis SE, et al: Post-traumatic cerebral infarction diagnosed by CT: prevalence, origin, and outcome, *Am J Neuroradiol* 11:355-360, 1990.
82. Mitchell PH: Central nervous system 1: closed head injuries. In Cardona VD, et al, editors: *Trauma nursing from resuscitation through rehabilitation,* Philadelphia, 1994, WB Saunders, pp 383-434.
83. Mitchell PH, Mauss NK: Relationship of patient-nurse activity to intracranial pressure variations: a pilot study, *Nurs Res* 27:4-10, 1978.
84. Mitchell PH, Ozuna J, Lipe HP: Moving the patient in bed: effects on intracranial pressure, *Nurs Res* 30:212-218, 1981.
85. Muelleman RL, Mlinek EJ, Collicott PE: Motorcycle crash injuries and costs: effect of reenacted comprehensive helmet use law, *Ann Emerg Med* 21:266-272, 1992.
86. Muizelaar JP, et al: Adverse effects of prolonged hyperventilation in patients with severe head injury: a randomized clinical trial, *J Neurosurg* 75:731-739, 1991.
87. Muizelaar JP, van der Poel HG: Cerebral vasoconstriction is not maintained with prolonged hyperventilation. In Hoff JT, Betz AL, editors: *Intracranial pressure VII,* Berlin, 1989, Springer-Verlag.
88. Narayan RK: Emergency room management of the head-injured patient. In Becker DP, Gudeman SK, editors: *Textbook of head injury,* Philadelphia, 1989, WB Saunders, pp 23-66.
89. Newton MR, et al: A study comparing SPECT with CT and MRI after closed head injury, *J Neurol Neurosurg Psychiatry* 55:92-94, 1992.
90. Obrist WD, et al: Cerebral blood flow and metabolism in comatose patients with acute head injury—relationship to intracranial hypertension, *J Neurosurg* 61:241-253, 1984.
91. Offner PJ, Rivara FP, Maier RV: The impact of motorcycle helmet use, *J Trauma* 32:636-642, 1992.
92. Pappius HM: Brain injury: new insights into neurotransmitter and receptor mechanisms, *Neurochem Res* 16:941-949, 1991.
93. Parsons LC, Shogun JSO: The effects of the endotracheal tube suctioning/manual hyperventilation procedure on patients with severe closed head injuries, *Heart Lung* 13:372-380, 1984a.
94. Parsons LC, Smith Peard AL, Page MC: The effects of hygiene interventions on the cerebrovascular status of severe closed head injured persons, *Res Nurs Health* 8:173-181, 1985.
95. Parsons LC, Wilson MM: Cerebrovascular status of severe closed head injured patients following passive position changes, *Nurs Res* 33:68-75, 1984b.
96. Pollay M, et al: Effects of mannitol and furosemide on blood-brain osmotic gradients and intracranial pressure, *J Neurosurg* 59:945-950, 1983.

97. Povlishock JT, Erb DE, Astruc J: Axonal response to traumatic brain injury: reactive axonal change, deafferentation, and neuroplasticity, *J Neurotrauma* 9(suppl 1):S189-S200, 1992.
98. Quattrocchi KB, et al: Severe head injury: effect upon cellular immune function, *Neurol Res* 13:13-20, 1991.
99. Rea JB, Dunbar SB: Neurogenic electrocardiographic abnormalities in subarachnoid hemorrhage, *Focus Crit Care* 19:50-54, 1992.
100. Ribas GC, Jane JA: Traumatic contusions and intracerebral hematomas, *J Neurotrauma* 9(suppl 1):S265-S278, 1992.
101. Robertson CS, Goodman JC, Grossman RG: Blood flow and metabolic therapy in CNS injury, *J Neurotrauma* 9(suppl 2):S579-S594, 1992.
102. Ropper AH, O'Rourke D, Kennedy SK: Head position, intracranial pressure, and compliance, *Neurology* 32:1288-1291, 1982.
103. Rosenblum WI: Pathology of human head injury. In Becker DP, Gudeman SK, editors: *Textbook of head injury,* Philadelphia, 1989, WB Saunders, pp 525-537.
104. Rosenwasser RH, Andrews DW, Jimenez DF: Penetrating craniocerebral trauma, *Surg Clin North Am* 71:305-316, 1991.
105. Rosner MJ, Coley IB: Cerebral perfusion pressure, intracranial pressure, and head elevation, *J Neurosurg* 65:636-641, 1986.
106. Rosner MJ, Daughton S: Cerebral perfusion pressure management in head injury, *J Trauma* 30:933-940, 1990.
107. Rudy EB, et al: Endotracheal suctioning in adults with head injury, *Heart Lung* 20:667-674, 1991.
108. Schwab ME: Regeneration of lesioned CNS axons by neutralization of neurite growth inhibitors: a short review, *J Neurotrauma* 9(suppl 1):S219-S221, 1992.
109. Seelig JM, et al: Traumatic acute subdural hematoma: major mortality reduction in comatose patients treated within four hours, *N Eng J Med* 304:1511-1518, 1981.
110. Siegal JH, et al: Effect of associated injuries and blood volume replacement on death, rehabilitation needs, and disability in blunt traumatic brain injury, *Crit Care Med* 19:1252-1265, 1991.
111. Sheinberg M, et al: Continuous monitoring of jugular venous oxygen saturation in head-injured patients, *J Neurosurg* 76:212-217, 1992.
112. Skaper SD, Leon A: Monosialogangliosides, neuroprotection, and neuronal repair process, *J Neurotrauma* 9(suppl 2):S507-S516, 1992.
113. Sklar EML, et al: Magnetic resonance applications in cerebral injury, *Radiol Clin North Am* 30:353-366, 1992.
114. Snyder M: Relation of nursing activities to increases in intracranial pressure, *J Adv Nurs* 8:273-279, 1983.
115. Sosin DM, Sacks JJ, Holmgreen P: Head injury—associated deaths from motorcycle crashes, relationship to helmet-use laws, *JAMA* 264:2395-2399, 1990.
116. Sosin DM, Sacks JJ, Smith SM: Head-injury-associated deaths in the United States from 1979 to 1986, *JAMA* 262:2251-2255, 1989.
117. Sparadeo FR, Gill D: Effects of prior alcohol use on head injury recovery, *J Head Trauma Rehabil* 4:75-82, 1989.
117a. *St Anthony's DRG guidebook 1995,* Reston, Va, 1994, St Anthony.
118. Steward O, Jane JA: Repair and reorganization of neuronal connections following CNS trauma. In Becker DP, Gudeman SK, editors: *Textbook of head injury,* Philadelphia, 1989, WB Saunders, pp 466-506.
119. Sutin KM, Ruskin KJ, Kaufman BS: Intravenous fluid therapy in neurologic injury, *Crit Care Clin* 8:367-408, 1992.
120. Teasdale G: The treatment of head trauma: implications for the future, *J Neurotrauma* 8(suppl 1):S53-S58, 1991.
121. Teasdale G, Jennett B: Assessment of coma and impaired consciousness: a practical scale, *Lancet* 2:81-84, 1974.
122. Temkin NR, et al: A randomized, double-blind study of phenytoin for the prevention of post-traumatic seizures, *New Engl J Med* 323:497-502, 1990.
123. Testani-Dufour L, Chappel-Aiken L, Gueldner S: Traumatic brain injury: a family experience, *J Neurosci Nurs* 24:317-323, 1992.
124. Thompson RS, Rivara FP, Thompson DC: A case-control study of the effectiveness of bicycle safety helmets, *New Eng J Med* 320:1361-1367, 1989.
125. Treloar DM, et al: The effect of familiar and unfamiliar voice treatments on intracranial pressure in head-injured patients, *J Neurosci Nurs* 23:295-299, 1991.
126. Tsementzis SA, Harris P, Loizou LA: The effect of routine nursing care procedures on the ICP in severe head injuries, *ACTA Neurochir (Wien)* 65:153-166, 1982.
127. Vollmer DG: Prognosis and outcome of severe head injury. In Cooper PR, editor: *Head injury,* ed 3, Baltimore, 1993, Williams & Wilkins, pp 553-581.
128. Vollmer DG, et al: Age and outcome following traumatic coma: Why do older patients fare worse? *J Neurosurg* 75:S37-S49, 1991.
129. Walleck CA: Controversies in the management of the head-injured patient, *Crit Care Nurse Clin North Am* 1:67-74, 1989.
130. Walleck CA: Preventing secondary brain injury, *AACN Clin Issues* 3:19-28, 1992.
131. Wilkinson HA, Rosenfeld S: Furosemide and mannitol in the treatment of acute experimental intracranial hypertension, *Neurosurg* 12:405-410, 1983.
132. Williams A, Coyne SM: Effects of neck position on intracranial pressure, *Am J Crit Care* 2:68-71, 1993.
133. Yoshida K, Marmarou A: Effects of tromethamine and hyperventilation on brain injury in the cat, *J Neurosurg* 74:87-96, 1991.
134. Yoneda S, et al: Continuous measurement of intracranial pressure with SFT: clinical experience, *Surg Neurol* 4:289-295, 1975.
135. Young B, et al: Nutrition and brain injury, *J Neurotrauma* 9(suppl 1):S375-S383, 1992.
136. Young B, et al: Failure of prophylactically administered phenytoin to prevent late post-traumatic seizures, *J Neurosurg* 58:236-241, 1983.
137. Young W: Role of calcium in central nervous system injuries, *J Neurotrauma* 9(suppl 1),S9-S25, 1992.

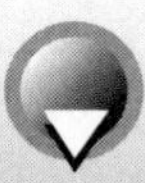

CLINICAL GUIDELINE

5

Supratentorial Craniotomy

Kathy A. Coburn, RN

DESCRIPTION

A craniotomy is a surgical opening through the scalp, muscle, and bone to allow access to the brain. Approximately two-thirds of all craniotomies performed are supratentorial; that is, above the tentorium cerebelli. The tentorium cerebelli (tentorium) is the double layer of dura mater that separates the cerebrum from the cerebellum and brainstem (Figure 5-1). Supratentorial craniotomies allow the surgeon access to lesions of the frontal, temporal, parietal, and occipital lobes of the brain. In clinical practice, a craniotomy is usually described by the site of the surgery, the region of the brain, and the indication for surgery (e.g., right frontal meningioma). It is not common for critical care staff to identify craniotomies as either supratentorial or infratentorial. However, there are characteristics associated with the nursing care of patients following surgical intervention, whether above or beneath the tentorium, that facilitate discussion using that division. Infratentorial craniotomies involving the brainstem or cerebellum are discussed in more detail in the following guideline.

PATHOPHYSIOLOGY

Regardless of the pathology indicating the need for surgery, a craniotomy is performed to repair damage or contain the progression of cerebral dysfunction. Surgical intervention, however, cannot reverse cerebral damage that has already occurred. Supratentorial craniotomies are indicated to remove space-occupying lesions (tumors, hematomas, abscesses) and to correct vascular abnormalities (arteriovenous malformations or aneurysms).

The surgeon determines the patient's need for a craniotomy after careful evaluation to determine the location of the lesion and its most likely composition.[5] For elective procedures, this evaluation may include laboratory, radiology, neurodiagnostic, and electrocardiogram studies, in addition to the physical examination and history. Understanding of the intraoperative events serves as a basis for evaluating postoperative physiological changes that signal potential complications. In addition, anesthetics have effects and side effects that impact cerebral blood flow, intracranial pressure, cerebral metabolism, and vasomotor tone. Patients are positioned intraoperatively to facilitate optimal visualization of the surgical field. Wilkins and Odom[10] describe several basic incisions which are modified by the neurosurgeon to provide maximum access to the lesion and in response to the medical and physiological status of the patient. Patient positioning is key to minimizing tissue injury caused by pressure and immobility. Pin fixation is used to immobilize the head during the operative procedure; postoperative care of pin sites may be indicated.

Postoperative Complications

General postoperative complications following surgical procedures include bleeding, infection, pain, and the complications of immobility (pneumonia, atelectasis, urinary retention, deep-vein thrombosis). Specific postoperative complications following craniotomy include increased intracranial pressure resulting from brain edema, accumulation of a blood clot (extradural hematoma), obstruction of CSF flow, and/or absorption of CSF.

Postoperative brain edema, or an increase in the volume of water in brain tissues, is more likely following lengthy surgery or procedures that require extensive retraction of cerebral tissue for optimal surgical exposure. The symptoms of postoperative brain edema include deterioration in levels of consciousness (LOC) and worsening of any neurological deficits. It is important not to discount even the most subtle

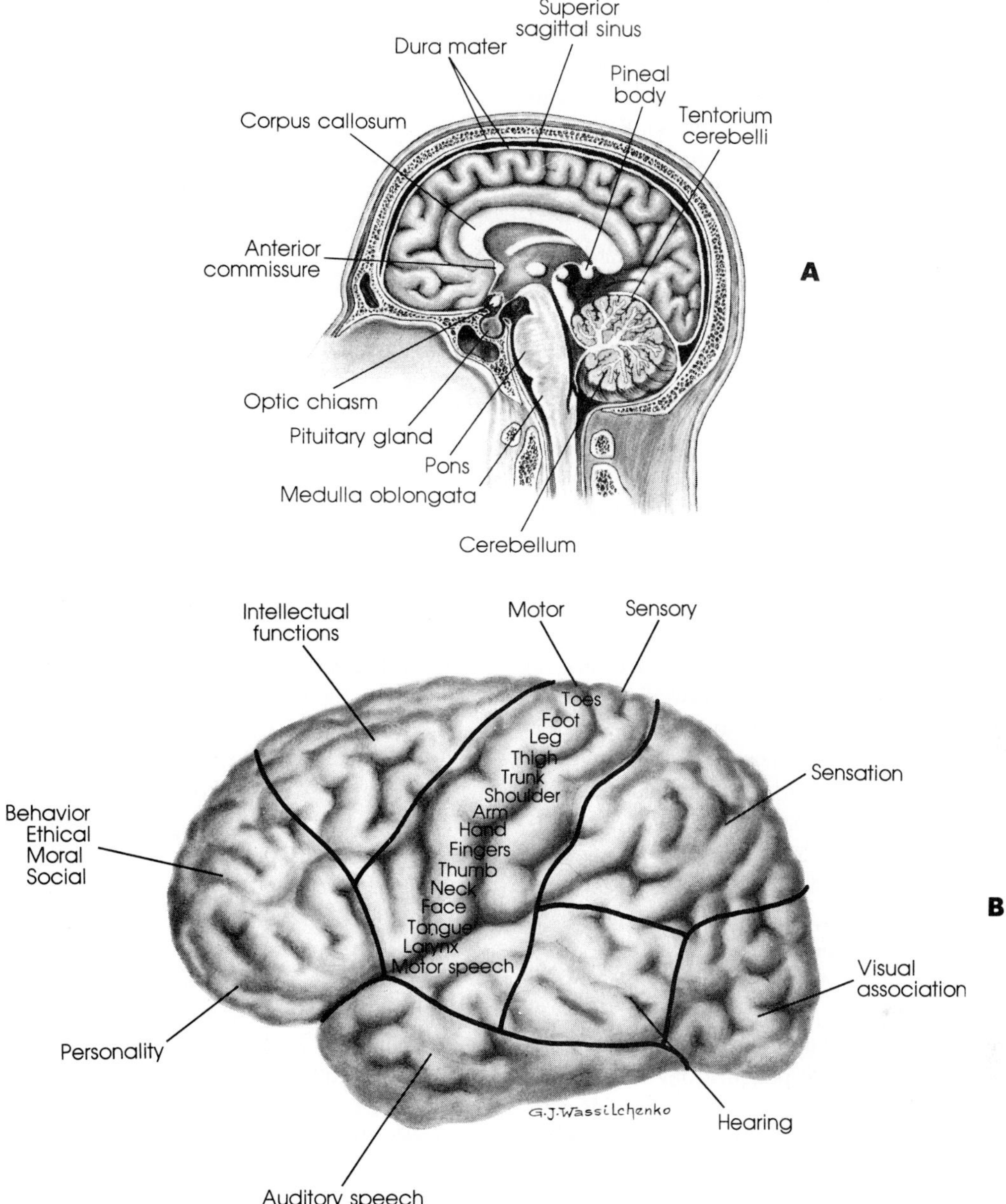

Figure 5-1 A. Sagittal view. **B.** Lateral view of cerebral hemisphere, cerebellum, pons, and medulla. (From Rudy EB: *Advanced neurological and neurosurgical nursing,* St Louis, 1984, Mosby–Year Book.)

changes in LOC following surgery. The treatment of choice for brain edema is mannitol, although Lasix is also used in some institutions.[6] Although not seen as frequently, an intracranial hematoma may develop following tumor surgery. Bleeding may occur as a result of vessels once compressed by the swollen brain losing the effect of the compression as the edema subsides. Bleeding also may occur in the tumor bed. Symptoms include complaints of a headache, the development of new focal signs, and a deterioration in LOC.

Postoperative hydrocephalus may develop as a result of bleeding. Blood acts to plug the arachnoid villi and prevents the normal reabsorption of CSF, enlarging the ventricles and producing a communicating hydrocephalus which is best treated with surgical shunting.

Monitoring of continuous EEG (CEEG) is neuro-intensive care units has demonstrated that seizure activity among acute brain injuries is more common than previously thought.[4] Seizure activity, including nonconvulsive seizures, serves to increase ICP, cerebral blood flow, and oxygen utilization.[8] Although CEEG is not commonly monitored in all critical care units, nurses should be aware of the potential for seizure activity and the signs of nonconvulsive seizures. Abnormal eye movements, limb posturing, periodic aphasia, or mental dullness may indicate a need for a bedside EEG to rule out nonconvulsive seizure activity.

LENGTH OF STAY/ANTICIPATED COURSE

It is not unusual for patients to be discharged from the hospital in less than one week following surgery. The wide range of indications for surgery and underlying medical status of the patient ultimately determine the length of hospital stay for a given individual patient. The average length of stay for a DRG diagnosis of craniotomy is approximately 13.9 days based on DRGs 1 and 2: Craniotomy greater than age 17 with or without trauma.[9]

MANAGEMENT TRENDS AND CONTROVERSIES

The introduction of the surgical microscope made a dramatic impact on intracranial surgery. Today, incisions are smaller and less brain retraction is necessary because of improvements in surgical instruments and lighting. Developments in operative technique also have improved craniotomy patient outcomes.[6] Prior to the increased use of ventriculostomies and improved medical intervention for increased ICP, the bone flap was not replaced at the end of the surgical procedures to allow for postoperative brain swelling. Today, craniectomies are seen less frequently and are usually performed only if an infectious or tumorous process involves the skull, or for decompression when cerebral edema cannot be controlled by medical intervention.

There has been an increased awareness of the benefit of intraoperative evoked potential and/or electroencephalographic (EEG) monitoring when the operative site is near cranial nerves or the sensory or motor strips. Additionally, many neuro-intensive care units are performing continuous EEG (CEEG) monitoring postoperatively to monitor seizure activity and to evaluate ICP and perfusion pressure treatment modalities. Current data indicate patients may require systolic blood pressures nearing 200 mm Hg to provide adequate cerebral perfusion and prevent ischemia in the postoperative period. Lowering a patients' blood pressure, when autoregulation is intact, has been shown to significantly increase ICP.[2]

The transphenoidal approach to pituitary tumors has dramatically improved patients' postoperative course and decreased their hospital stay. Using this approach, the surgeon accesses the tumor via an incision in the upper submucosa gum and resection of the floors of the sphenoid sinus and sella turcica. This approach avoids the potential complications associated with extensive brain retraction.[3]

Stereotactic surgery allows for precise biopsy and treatment of lesions based on three-dimensional coordinates provided by CT or MRI. Once the target has been identified, a probe is passed through a burr-hole incision. Patients are frequently observed overnight in the intensive care unit, receive a follow-up CT scan, and are discharged the following day. Indications for stereotaxis have expanded dramatically since its development in the 1940s. Currently stereotaxis neurosurgery is indicated for implantation of radioactive seeds into brain tumors (brachytherapy), aspiration of intracerebral hematomas, localization of seizure foci, drainage of intracranial abscesses, removal of thrombosed arteriovenous malformations (AVMs), thalamotomy for intractable cancer pain or tremor, and tumor biopsy.[1,3]

The gamma knife has made intervention possible for many nonsurgical candidates by providing a closed, bloodless operation that used high-dose radiation to obliterate an AVM or stop tumor growth. The gamma knife was designed as an adjunct to other neurosurgical and neuroradiological procedures. Patients have the stereotactic frame applied and undergo a CT scan. Using the coordinates obtained from the scan, the physicist and radiosurgeon calculate the total dose and treatment time for the patient. Under local anesthesia, the patient is placed in the unit and the treatment initiated. In general, treatments last less than one hour. The frame is removed, the patient is returned to the nursing unit, and preparations are initiated for discharge the following day.[7]

ASSESSMENT

Table 5-1 provides a list of signs of specific cerebral lobe dysfunction. However, the central nervous system is very complex. Comprehension and expression of information frequently require an integrated response from several areas of the brain, confounding the assessment.[6]

PARAMETER	ANTICIPATED ALTERATION
Neurological Status	
LOC	Difficult to arouse Disorientation to time, place, or person Behavior/personality changes Communication skill deterioration (aphasia or dysphasia)

TABLE 5-1 Assessment of Specific Focal Signs of Frontal, Temporal, Parietal, and Occipital Lobes[3,6]

Involved lobe of the brain	Common focal signs observed
Frontal lobe: *Controls affect and personality*	Changes in personality Impairment of memory Difficulty following instructions Mood changes, emotional Apathy Contralateral (opposite side from lesion) motor weakness or paralysis Sucking and/or grasping reflexes Expressive (Broca) aphasia if dominant hemisphere is involved. *Patient is able to comprehend language, but lacks the motor ability for expression.* Motor seizures Agraphia (inability to express thoughts in writing) Cranial nerve mediation dysfunction Apraxia (loss of the ability to perform familiar, purposeful movements in the absence of paralysis) Changes in extra-ocular movements Urinary incontinence
Temporal lobe: *Reception and interpretation of auditory information*	If lesion is in the dominant hemisphere, difficulty interpreting auditory information ranging from difficulty with repetition and comprehension to fluent, meaningless speech *(Wernicke's area is in the dominant hemisphere)* Memory impairment. *The hippocampus, in the medial temporal lobe, is responsible for recent memory and transfer of short-term to long-term memory.* Visual field defect of upper contralateral quadrant Auditory illusions and hallucinations Personality changes—psychotic behavior. *Connections of the temporal lobe, the hypothalamus and cingulate gyrus, form the limbic system and are involved in the expression of emotion and in autonomic function.* Complex partial seizures *are difficult to diagnose secondary to unusual manifestations characterized by purposeful, inappropriate actions. For example:* • *lip smacking or masticatory movements, abnormal speech* • *hallucinations (feelings of deja vu, depersonalization, changes in size perception, or dream state)* • *autonomic experiences such as hypertension or tachycardia*
Parietal lobe: *Ability to delineate sensations—pain, vibration, pressure, touch, and position—and awareness of spatial orientation*	Sensory disturbances including: • Loss of two-point discrimination • Loss of ability of judge size and shape of objects • Contralateral hypoesthesia/paresthesia • Impairment or loss of position sense Defects in the inferior aspect of contralateral visual field *(Parietal lobe contains visual radiations to the occipital lobe)* If dominant-lobe involvement, difficulty comprehending symbols required in writing or math If nondominant hemisphere involvement, there is an inability to understand spatial relationships. Patients will frequently neglect one half of their body.
Occipital lobe: *Reception, interpretation, and integration of visual information*	Contralateral homonymous hemianopsia Visual illusions and hallucinations Cortical blindness Inability to name or identify the use of objects Loss of color perception

Visual acuity	Diplopia or double vision
Ocular movements	Loss of ocular movement through any of the cardinal fields Ptosis or drooping of the eyelid Dysconjugate, nonparallel eye movement Gaze toward the side of the lesion Nsytagmus
Pupil signs	Unequal pupils: The larger pupil will not readily react to light, while the normal-sized pupil continues to react normally. *If a new finding, it should be reported immediately, since it represents downward pressure from the lesion or edema on the brain, causing compression of the oculomotor nerve between the uncus of the temporal lobe and the tentorium. The lesion will be on the same side as the dilated pupil.* Small, equal, reactive pupils *due to bilateral damage to sympathetic pathway in thalamus and hypothalamus or metabolic coma. If a new finding, report immediately. Review blood electrolyte and glucose levels, which may reveal metabolic process.* Bilateral, fixed, dilated pupils *due to terminal state and also from atropine-like drugs. If a new finding, emergency action is required if the process is to be reversed. Immediately evaluate airway and administer oxygen to prevent/reverse cerebral ischemia.*
Sensory function	Changes in perception of touch, pain, heat, cold, vibration, pressure, position
Motor function	Changes in muscle tone (flaccidity spasticity, rigidity) Changes in muscle strength Asymmetrical response
CT or MRI scans	Hemorrhage, edema, shifting of brain structures, hydrocephalus, and postsurgical changes

Vital Signs

Temperature	Elevated *due to infection, subarachnoid hemorrhage, hypothalamic lesion*
RR	Tachypnea Irregular or ineffective breathing patterns Cheyne-Stokes: waxing and waning in depth of respirations followed by a period of apnea *due to lesion located deep in the cerebral hemispheres and basal ganglia, with damage to thalamus and/or hypothalamus. May be normal in those <1 year or >70 years old.*
HR	Bradycardia Tachycardia *due to decreased vascular volume resulting from hemorrhage or dehydration*
BP	Hypertension >180 mm Hg systolic Hypotension <90 mm Hg systolic
ICP	Normal: 0 to 10 mm Hg. Increased: ≥15 mm Hg *due to brain edema or obstruction of CSF flow*
CPP	Normal: 70 to 100 mm Hg, with range from 60 to 150 mm Hg. *Calculated value = mean arterial pressure − intracranial pressure. CPP must be >60 mm Hg to prevent ischemia. CPP <30 mm Hg is not compatible with life.*
UO	Polyuria *due to diabetes insipidus (DI) which is suspected when urine output is >200 cc/hr, urine specific gravity is <1.005, serum sodium is >145, serum osmolarity is >295 mOsm/L, and urine osmolarity is <300 mOsm/L.*

Laboratory Data

Hgb and Hct	Serum: WNL CSF: absent

Na^{++}	Serum and CSF: WNL at 135 to 145 mEq/L
K^{++}	Serum: WNL at 3.5 to 5 mEq/L CSF: WNL at 2.8 mEq/L
Cl^{+}	Serum: WNL at 99 to 102 mEq/L CSF: WNL at 113 to 119 mEq/L or 700 to 750 mg/dl
Glucose	Serum: WNL at 70 to 110 mg/dl CSF: WNL at 50 to 75 mg/dl or 60 to 80% of serum glucose level
Ca^{++}	Serum: WNL at 8.5 to 10.5 mg/dl CSF: WNL at 2.1 to 4.6 mg/dl
Protein	Serum: WNL at 6800 to 7000 mg/dl CSF: WNL at 15 to 45 mg/dl and up to 70 mg/dl in elderly or children
pH	Serum: WNL at 7.40 CSF: WNL at 7.33
BUN and creatinine	Serum: WNL

PLAN OF CARE

INTENSIVE PHASE

Not all patients with craniotomy will require hospitalization in an intensive care unit. However, when the surgery is extensive, the risk of post-operative complications is high, or the patient's neurological status requires intense support, an intensive phase is indicated.

PATIENT CARE PRIORITIES	EXPECTED PATIENT OUTCOMES
High risk for increased ICP *r/t pathology and procedure*	Maintain normal ICP
Ineffective airway clearance *r/t* *Intubation* *Decreased LOC*	Clear lungs Patent airway Adequate management of secretions
High risk for cerebral edema *r/t pathology and procedures*	ICP: WNL
High risk for seizures *r/t pathology and procedures*	No seizures
High risk of infection and/or meningitis *r/t invasive procedures and monitoring*	No infection
High risk of thrombophlebitis *r/t impaired mobility*	No deep-vein thrombosis or pulmonary emboli
Impaired communication *r/t* *Decreased LOC* *Focal injury* *Intubation*	Adequately communicate needs
High risk for inadequate nutrition *r/t* *Decreased LOC* *Focal injury* *Intubation*	Nutritional needs met Maintain anabolic state
Pain/discomfort *r/t* *Bed rest* *Periorbital edema* *Intubation*	Report pain relief

INTERVENTIONS

Assess breath sounds and note respiratory pattern and rate *to assure patency of airway and effective air exchange.*

Plan of Care (cont'd)

Keep head in neutral position *to facilitate venous drainage and prevent increases in ICP.*

Assess patient for changes in LOC or increases in ICP *to identify symptoms of postoperative brain edema or obstruction of CSF flow.*

Monitor and report seizure activity (seizure activity may be as subtle as limb posturing, abnormal eye movements, aphasia, or mental dullness) *to prevent major increases in cerebral blood flow and metabolism.*

Monitor anticonvulsant levels *to minimize seizure risk.*

Maintain incision dressing clean, dry, and intact.

Elevate head of bed (HOB) as ordered. Assess patient to identify response of ICP and CPP to HOB elevation.

Perform frequent neurological assessment. Note and report deterioration of LOC, pupil reactions, eye movements, sensation, and motor ability.

Do not cluster nursing activities. Avoid activities known to increase patient's ICP (e.g., Valsalva, frequent suctioning, sensory stimulation).

Pre-medicate patient prior to unavoidable activities that are known to increase ICP *to enable activity without cerebral insult.*

Turn immobile patients at least q2h *to provide adequate drainage of oral secretions, assist with the mobilization of pulmonary secretions, and prevent complications of immobility.*

Monitor intake, urine output, urine specific gravity, blood and urine osmolarity and electrolytes closely. Daily weights. *Following surgery near the sella turcica or pituitary gland, there is a risk of diabetes insipidus.*

Monitor serum electrolytes *to assess for potential postoperative electrolyte imbalance.*

Maintain bed in low position with side rails up, and restrain patient as needed *to prevent potential injury related to altered LOC.*

INTERMEDIATE PHASE

Continued involvement of the entire health care team is required during the intermediate phase to optimize the patient's rehabilitation. Focus of care in this phase centers on preparation of the patient to return to independent function.

PATIENT CARE PRIORITIES	EXPECTED PATIENT OUTCOMES
High risk for ineffective airway management *r/t potential neurologic deficits*	Patent airway Clear breath sounds Able to clear secretions
High risk for immobility *r/t potential neurologic deficits*	No complications of immmobility Improved motor function Able to peform ADL and ambulate within capabilities Improved feeling of well-being
High risk for confusion or disorientation *r/t residual neurologic deficit*	Alert and oriented Aware of environment
High risk for injury *r/t potential seizure activity*	Free from seizure activity Side effects from anticonvulsant absent or controlled Protected from injury during seizure events
Self-care deficit *r/t inadequate knowledge of care requirements and rehabiltation needs*	Able to perform ADL within capabilities Patient/family able to verbalize care regime Patient/family able to identify appropriate discharge plan to home or rehabilitation facility

INTERVENTIONS

Collaborate with physical, occupational, and/or speech therapist in organizing acute rehabilitation care *to provide adequate therapy without tiring.*

Initiate discharge planning with social services, medical staff, family, and third-party payor *to insure patient needs will be met once discharged from hospital.*

Plan of Care (cont'd)

Advance diet as tolerated *to facilitate recovery, and increased strength and endurance.*

Maintain incision dressing clean, dry and intact.

Provide for time out of bed and turn immobilized patients frequently *to prevent complications of immobility.*

Monitor closely for any sign of seizure activity *to protect the patient from injury and to evaluate anticonvulsant effectiveness.*

Administer anticonvulsant medication as prescribed and observe for side effects *to maintain therapeutic blood levels and to enhance patient compliance post discharge.*

Monitor electrolytes, blood counts, and anticonvulsant levels *to ensure therapeutic blood levels of medication and to detect some drug side effects.*

Instruct patient/family regarding importance of medication regime, S/S to report to the physician, and safety strategies *to protect the patient from/during seizure activity.*

Encourage the patient/family to verbalize concerns regarding potential ADL limitations (e.g., ambulation, self-care, work, driving) and identify adaptive compensatory strategies *to facilitate coping and general well-being.*

TRANSITION TO DISCHARGE

The focus of nursing care as the patient nears discharge is to assist the patient and family in developing confidence in their ability to continue the recovery process once the patient is discharged from the hospital. Often patients will require inpatient acute rehabilitation, and they and their families need to be prepared for the change in nursing focus they will experience in that setting. In a rehabilitation setting, the patient will be guided to develop skills to compensate for neurological deficits. If the patient is being discharged home, the patient and family should practice aspects of the patient's care they will be expected to continue after discharge.

REFERENCES

1. Arbour RB: Stereotactic localization and resection of intracranial tumors, *J Neurosci Nurs* 25(1):14-21, 1993.
2. Bouma GJ, et al: Blood pressure and intracranial pressure-volume dynamics in severe head injury: relationship with cerebral blood flow, *J Neurosurg* 77:15-19, 1992.
3. Hickey JV: *The clinical practice of neurological and neurosurgical nursing,* ed 3, Philadelphia, 1992, WB Saunders.
4. Jordan KG: Nonconvulsive-status epilepticus in the neuro-ICU detected by continuous EEG monitoring, *Neurology* 42(suppl 1):194, 1992.
5. Litel GR: *Neurosurgery and the clinical team,* New York, 1980, Springer.
6. Marshall SB, et al: *Neuroscience critical care: pathophysiology and patient management,* Philadelphia, 1990, WB Saunders.
7. Neatherlin JS, Brent VS: The gamma knife: implications for nursing practice and patient education, *J Neurosci Nurs* 23(1):71-74, 1991.
8. Nevander G, et al: Status epilepticus in well-oxygenated rats causes neuronal necrosis, *Ann Neurol* 18:281-290, 1985.
9. *St Anthony's DRG guidebook 1995,* Reston, Va, 1994, St Anthony.
10. Wilkins RH, Odom GL: General operative technique. In Youmans, JR, editor: *Neurologic surgery,* vol 2, Philadelphia, 1982, WB Saunders, pp 1160-1193.

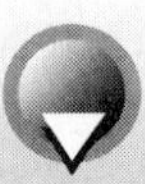

C L I N I C A L G U I D E L I N E

6

Infratentorial Craniotomy

Kathy A. Coburn, RN

DESCRIPTION

An infratentorial craniotomy allows surgical access to the portion of the brain positioned beneath the tentorium cerebelli. The tentorium cerebelli (tentorium) is the double layer of dura mater that separates the cerebrum from the cerebellum and brainstem (Figure 5-1). The infratentorial approach provides access to lesions of the cerebellum, midbrain, pons, medulla, fourth ventricle, and the cerebellar pontine angle.[6] Generally, critical care staff do not identify craniotomies as either supratentorial or infratentorial. However, there are characteristics associated with the nursing care of patients following surgical intervention, whether above or beneath the tentorium, that facilitate discussion using that division.[3] The nursing care of patients following supratentorial craniotomies, involving the cerebral lobes of the brain above the tentorium, are discussed in more detail in the previous guideline.

PATHOPHYSIOLOGY

There are several differences between infratentorial and supratentorial surgeries. Intraoperative infratentorial procedures tend to be technically more difficult because of the close proximity of the lesion to areas of the brain that control respiratory effort and wakefulness. Generally, patients have longer recovery periods following infratentorial craniotomies. The signs and symptoms common to patients with lesions in the infratentorial space vary more dramatically than the symptoms noted in patients with supratentorial lesions. This variability in symptoms is attributed to variations in extent and location of the lesion, rate at which it has grown, effectiveness of the brain to compensate, degree of compression on other brain structures, and effect on cerebrospinal fluid (CSF) flow.[4] Infratentorial lesions are of major clinical concern because of their potential to cause damage to the reticular activating system.

LENGTH OF STAY/ANTICIPATED COURSE

A 13.5-day hospital stay is typical for the patient undergoing an infratentorial craniotomy, as listed under DRG 1: Craniotomy, age greater than 17 except for trauma. DRG 2 includes trauma with essentially the same LOS.[11] This stay usually includes several days in the intensive care unit.

MANAGEMENT TRENDS AND CONTROVERSIES

A trend specific to infratentorial craniotomies is the increased utilization of neurodiagnostic intraoperative monitoring. Brainstem surgery is associated with significant morbidity. Methods to monitor the integrity of both motor and sensory cranial nerves intraoperatively have been developed over the past decade. Brainstem auditory evoked potentials (BAEPs) have been shown to reduce the incidence of permanent neurological deficits.[7] Intraoperative facial nerve monitoring aids the surgeon in preserving facial nerve function by providing early recognition of surgical trauma to the facial nerve.[9] Routine intraoperative monitoring of the facial nerve is recommended in all acoustic neuroma surgeries by the National Institutes of Health (NIH) Consensus Development Conference.[8] Although postoperative hearing cannot always be predicted from the findings obtained at the end of acoustic neuroma surgery,[5] utilization of intraoperative BAEPs has demonstrated a significant decrease in operative auditory morbidity.[10]

TABLE 6-1 Common Symptoms of Brainstem, Cerebellum, and Cerebellar Pontine Angle Lesions

Location of lesion	Common symptoms
Cerebellum	Lesions produce ipsilateral symptoms Uncoordination Impaired balance Disorders of equilibrium and gait Hypotonia Muscles tire easily Impaired ability to perform alternating repetitive movements rapidly Tremor *(usually intention tremor)* Inability to stop motor activity at desired point *(over- and/or underreaching)* Ataxia Scanning speech Nystagmus
Midbrain	Weber syndrome: Ipsilateral ptosis, diplopia, external strabismus, dilated pupil, inability to gaze up or down; *following damage to oculomotor (CN III) nerve* Dilated ipsilateral pupil, *following damage to oculomotor (CN III) nerve* Contralateral cerebellar signs; *following damage to red nucleus and fibers of superior cerebellar peduncle* Contralateral loss of senses of pain and temperature, and discriminative senses; *following damage to spinothalamic tract and medial lemniscus* Contralateral lower facial expression weakness, *following corticobulbar and corticoreticular fiber damage*
Pons	Inability to abduct eye to same side as lesion, and horizontal diplopia that worsens when patient attempts to gaze toward the side of lesion; *following damage to abducens (CN VI) nerve* Contralateral loss of discriminative (position, muscle and joint, vibration) senses, *following damage to corticospinal fibers and medial lemniscus* Disturbance of conjugate horizontal eye movements (abduction and adduction), *following damage to medial longitudinal fasciculus* Ipsilateral loss of sensation on face, forehead, nasal, and oral cavities; absence of corneal sensation and reflex; paralysis of muscles of mastication with chin deviating to lesion side when mouth is opened; *following damage to trigeminal (CN V) nerve* Diminished contralateral hearing, *following damage to lateral lemniscus* Ipsilateral cerebellar signs, *following interruption of pontocerebellar fibers*
Medulla	Hypoglossal nerve (CN XII) damage; initially fasciculation of tongue may occur followed by atrophy Tongue deviates to paralyzed side during protrusion Loss of position, muscle, and joint sense, impaired tactile discrimination; loss of vibration sense on contralateral side of body; *following damage to corticospinal tract (motor) and medial lemniscus (discriminative general senses)* Contralateral loss of senses of pain and temperature, *following spinothalamic tract damage* Ipsilateral loss of senses of pain and temperature of face and in nasal and oral cavities, *following damage to spinal trigeminal tract and nucleus* Ipsilateral dysphagia, hoarseness, and loss of gag reflex, *following damage of vagal (CN X), hypopharyngeal (CN XII), and spinal accessory (CN XI) nerves*
Cerebellopontine angle	Ipsilateral paralysis of muscles of facial expression (Bell's palsy), and loss of taste on anterior two thirds of tongue; *following damage to facial (CN VII) nerve* Tinnitus, followed by progressive ipsilateral deafness, tilting and rotating of head with chin pointing to lesion side; *following acoustic (CN VIII) nerve damage* Ipsilateral coarse intention tremor, ataxic gait, and under- or overreaching; *following cerebellar peduncle damage* Ipsilateral loss of senses of pain and temperature on face, and oral and nasal cavity; *following damage to spinal trigeminal tract* Contralateral loss of pain and temperature sensation, *following spinothalamic tract damage*

Continued.

TABLE 6-1 Common Symptoms of Brainstem, Cerebellum, and Cerebellar Pontine Angle Lesions—cont'd

Location of lesion	Common symptoms
Fourth ventricle	Hydrocephalus Increased intracranial pressure (ICP) which may result in additional damage by displacement and compression of brain tissue Herniation syndromes, both upward through the tentorial notch and downward through the foramen magnum Accumulation of cerebrospinal fluid (CSF) resulting from overproduction or interference with normal reabsorption and circulation that may result in increased ICP. *Initial treatment is the insertion of a catheter (ventriculostomy) into a lateral ventricle to provide a mechanism for CSF drainage and monitoring of ICP. This external drainage system may be left in place for several days. If hydrocephalus continues, an internalized shunting mechanism will usually be inserted.*

Stereotactic surgery allows for precise biopsy and treatment of lesions based on three-dimensional coordinates provided by CT or MRI scanner software. Advances in scanning ability and surgical technique now allow not only stereotactic biopsy, but stereotactic resection of tumors in the pons and thalamus.[2] Previously, open craniotomy approaches to the pons and thalamus were associated with high (60%) mortality rates.[1]

The common symptoms associated with lesions of the brainstem, cerebellum, fourth ventricle, and cerebellar pontine angle are outlined in Table 6-1. It is important to remember that lesions in an adjacent area may cause compression or displacement, obscuring the original site of the pathological condition.[4] Key signs and symptoms indicating an infratentorial lesion include cranial nerve palsies, abnormal oculovestibular (cold caloric reflex) response, disconjugate gaze, increased intracranial pressure (ICP), abnormal respiratory patterns, and unstable heart rate and blood pressure.[3]

ASSESSMENT

PARAMETER	ANTICIPATED ALTERATION
Neurological Status	
LOC	Decreased LOC Unresponsive
Focal neurological signs	Cranial nerve dysfunction Balance disturbances Uncoordination Headache Nausea and vomiting Papilledema Impaired extraocular movements Diplopia Blurred vision Nystagmus Visual field deficits Diminished or loss of hearing Tinnitus Vertigo
Pupil response	Midposition, nonreactive pupils. *If pupils are round and regular, may be caused by a lesion in the dorsal portion of the midbrain; if the pupils are irregular and unequal, indicates a nuclear midbrain lesion.* Small, bilateral, nonreactive pupils (pinpoint). *May result from a pontine hemorrhage.*

Sensory	Hearing loss Loss of sense of taste Loss of temperature, pain, position, vibration senses Impaired tactile discrimination Loss of corneal reflex Loss of facial sensation Loss of gag, cough reflex
Motor	Incoordination Hypotonia Tremor Ataxia Nystagmus Deviation of tongue Ptosis Facial weakness Paresis or paralysis of extremities Disturbance of ocular movements

Vital Signs

Temperature	Elevated *due to infection, brainstem hemorrhage* Subnormal *due to brainstem lesion*
RR	Changes in respiratory rate and pattern as follows: Central neurogenic hyperventilation. *Regular, rapid, continuous respirations. The lesion is in the reticular formation and may include a midbrain or pontine infarction or ischemia, anoxia, or tumor of midbrain.* Apneustic breathing. *Prolonged inspiration followed by a pause prior to expiration, alternated with expiratory pause. Seen with lesions of the pons such as infarction or severe meningitis.* Cluster breathing. *Irregular clusters of breaths with irregular periods of apnea. Lesion is usually a tumor or infarction in the upper medulla.* Ataxic breathing. *Completely irregular, unpredictable pattern. Lesion involves the medulla and may include cerebellar bleeding, pontine bleeding, compressing supratentorial tumors, or severe meningitis.*
HR	Bradycardia: <60 bpm *due to increased ICP* Tachycardia: >100 bpm *due to hypoxia, hypoxemia, bleeding*
BP	Hypotension with MAP <70 mm Hg will lead to inadequate cerebral perfusion pressure (CPP), *seen in terminal states* Hypertension with MAP >100 mm Hg *due to increased intracranial pressure*

PLAN OF CARE

INTENSIVE PHASE

Not all patients with craniotomy will require intensive monitoring. However, when the surgery is extensive, the risk of postoperative complications is high, or the patients' neurological status requires intense support, an intensive phase is indicated.

PATIENT CARE PRIORITIES	EXPECTED PATIENT OUTCOMES
Potential for secondary brain injury *r/t increased ICP*	ICP: WNL
Ineffective airway clearance *r/t* *Intubation* *Mechanical ventilation* *Decreased LOC* *Damage to CN I, X, or XII*	Clear lungs ABG: WNL Secretions removed/managed

Plan of Care (cont'd)

High risk for inadequate nutrition *r/t*
Intubation
Nausea and vomiting
Decreased LOC
Increased metabolic need

Adequate intake/output
Lab values WNL, especially albumen, nitrogen balance
Maintain weight
Maintain anabolic state

Impaired skin integrity *r/t surgical incisions and drainage devices*

No signs/symptoms of infection
Skin intact

High risk of visual impairment *r/t damage to CN II, III, IV, and VI*

Vision within patient norms
Extraocular movements intact

Impaired communication *r/t*
Decreased LOC
Focal injury
Intubation

Able to communicate

INTERVENTIONS

Assess breath sounds and note respiratory pattern and rate *to assure patency of airway and effective air exchange.*

Keep head in neutral position *to facilitate venous drainage.*

Assess patient for changes in LOC or increases in ICP.

Monitor and report seizure activity (seizure activity may be as subtle as limb posturing, abnormal eye movements, aphasia, or mental dullness) *to prevent major increases in cerebral blood flow and metabolism.*

Monitor anticonvulsant levels *to minimize seizure risk.*

Maintain incision dressing clean, dry, and intact.

Elevate head of bed (HOB) as ordered. Assess patient to identify individual response to ICP and CPP to HOB elevation.

Perform frequent neurological assesssment. Note and report deterioration of LOC, pupil reactions, eye movements, sensation, and motor ability.

Do not cluster nursing activities.

Avoid activities known to increase patient's ICP (e.g., Valsalva, frequent suctioning, sensory stimulation) *to prevent elevations in ICP.*

Pre-medicate patient prior to unavoidable activities that are known to increase ICP.

Turn immobile patients at least q2h *to provide adequate drainage of oral secretions, assist with the mobilization of pulmonary secretions, and prevent complications of immobility.*

Assess quality of breath sounds, sputum production and characteristics, and ABG *to reduce the development of nosocomial pneumonia and/or atelectasis.*

Maintain bed in low position with side rails up, restrain patient as needed *to prevent potential injury.*

INTERMEDIATE PHASE

The intermediate phase requires continued involvement of the entire health team to maximize patient outcome. Focus of care centers upon preparation for discharge and optimizing the patient's independent function. Patients transferred out of the ICU with no expectation of returning to routine activities enjoyed prior to hospitalization provide a difficult challenge to the health care team and the family.

PATIENT CARE PRIORITIES

High risk for ineffective airway management *r/t potential neurologic deficits.*

EXPECTED PATIENT OUTCOMES

Patent airway
Clear breath sounds
Able to clear secretions

Plan of Care (cont'd)

High risk for immobility *r/t potential neurologic deficits*	No complications of immobility Improved motor function Able to perform ADL and ambulate within capabilities Improved feeling of well-being
High risk for confusion or disorientation *r/t residual neurologic deficit*	Alert and oriented Aware of environment
Self-care deficit *r/t inadequate knowledge of care requirements and rehabilitation needs*	Able to perform ADL within capabilities Patient/family able to verbalize care regime Patient/family able to identify appropriate discharge plan to home or rehabilitation facility

INTERVENTIONS

Collaborate with physical, occupational, and/or speech therapist in organizing acute rehabilitation care *to provide adequate therapy without tiring patient.*

Initiate discharge planning with social services, medical staff, family, and third-party payor *to insure patient's needs will be met once patient is discharged from the hospital.*

Provide for time out of bed and turn immobilized patients frequently *to prevent complications of immobility.*

Monitor neurological status. Note and report changes.

Monitor lab values for changes in electrolyte and blood count.

TRANSITION TO DISCHARGE

The focus of nursing care, as the patient nears discharge, is to assist the patient and family in developing confidence in their ability to continue the recovery process once the patient is discharged from the hospital. Often patients will require inpatient acute rehabilitation, and they and their families need to be prepared for the change in nursing focus they will experience in that setting. In a rehabilitation setting, the patient will be guided to develop skills to compensate for neurological deficits. If the patient is being discharged home, allow the patient and family to practice aspects of the patient's care they will be expected to continue after discharge.

REFERENCES

1. Abernathy CD, Camacho A, Kelly P: Stereotaxic suboccipital transcerebellar biopsy of pontine mass lesions, *J Neurosurg* 70:195-200, 1989.
2. Baron MC: Advances in the care of children with brain tumors, *J Neurosci Nurs* 23(1):39-43, 1991.
3. Hickey JV: *The clinical practice of neurological and neurosurgical nursing,* ed 3, Philadelphia, 1992, WB Saunders.
4. Johanson BC, et al: *Standards for Critical Care,* ed 3, St Louis, 1988, Mosby–Year Book.
5. Kanzaki J, et al: Hearing preservation in acoustic neuroma surgery and postoperative audiological finding, *Acta Otolaryngol Stockh* 107(5-6):474-478, 1989.
6. Marshall SB, et al: *Neuroscience critical care: pathophysiology and patient management,* Philadelphia, 1990, WB Saunders.
7. Moller AR: Neuromonitoring in operations in the skull base, *Keio J Med* 40(3):151-159, 1991.
8. National Institutes of Health Consensus Development Conference on Acoustic Neuromas: Acoustic neuroma, *Consens Statement* 9(4):1-24, Dec 11-13, 1991.
9. Niparko JK, et al: Neurophysiologic intraoperative monitoring: II. facial nerve monitoring, *Am J Otol* 10(1):55-61, 1989.
10. Radtke RA, Erwin CW, Wilkins RH: Intraoperative brainstem auditory evoked potentials: significant decrease in postoperative morbidity, *Neurology* 39(2):187-191, 1989.
11. *St Anthony's DRG guidebook, 1995,* Reston, Va, 1994, St Anthony.

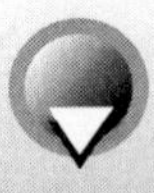

C L I N I C A L G U I D E L I N E

7

Cerebrovascular Accident

Patricia A. Blissitt, MSN, RN, CCRN, CNRN

DESCRIPTION

Cerebrovascular accident is one of the more commonly encountered neurological afflictions in critical care. The term cerebrovascular accident (CVA) is used interchangeably with the term stroke.[9,9a,16a,29] More current terms are brain attack or cerebral ischemia (CI). Cerebrovascular accident or brain attack is broadly defined as an interruption of cerebral blood flow with resultant death of cerebral tissue.[31] Another definition of brain attack is "a sudden, nonconvulsive, focal neurological deficit" that is correlated with a known vascular territory and lasts for 24 hours or more.[2] The clinical presentation may range from mild motor or sensory deficit to coma. However, CVA is not a single entity. Cerebral ischema has multiple pathophysiological and clinical presentations that are dynamic over time.[45] In fact, the term *stroke syndrome* has been adopted to emphasize the multiplicity and diversity of CVA.[23,31]

Statistically, the incidence and mortality of CVA is on the decline[3,20] due to improvements in medical management and risk-factor reduction.[23] However, CVA remains the third leading cause of death in the United States.[20,23,32] Each year approximately 400,000 to 750,000 individuals are afflicted with cerebral ischema[3,5] and approximately 150,000 die annually from CVA.[5,20] Furthermore, CVA remains the leading cause of adult disability in the United States.[27] Fourteen billion dollars was spent on CVA care in 1987.[19] This figure does not include the loss of money from the decreased earning capacity of the CVA patient, or the emotional cost of a brain attack. Those who have sustained a CVA and their families typically experience a gamut of emotions, including depression, fear, inability to cope, grief, anxiety, altered self-concept, feelings of powerlessness, and social isolation.[23]

PATHOPHYSIOLOGY

Brain attacks can be categorized as ischemic or hemorrhagic.[17] Ischemic CVAs account for approximately 80% to 85% of all strokes.[3,23] In ischemic or occlusive CVA, the brain injury occurs when the cerebral vessel is occluded and cells die. Subtypes of ischemic CVA include atherothrombotic, lacunar, and cardioembolic.[23]

Atherothrombotic brain attacks account for about 40% to 53% of all CVAs. In atherothrombotic attacks, damage to the endothelium of the cerebral blood vessels has occurred, primarily due to atherosclerosis. Ulcerations and an irregular surface on the atheroma may contribute to the buildup of clot on the vessels. Atheroma or clots adhering to the atheroma may embolize to occlude more distal vessels.[9] Atherothrombotic strokes tend to occur during inactivity.[5] They are typically associated with transient ischemic attacks (TIAs) and may progress slowly.[23]

A specific type of atherothrombotic attack, lacunar, is associated with long-standing hypertension and diabetes mellitus; it is also referred to as small-vessel stroke. Lacunar stroke occurs as a result of lipohyalinosis. In lipohyalinosis, a hyaline lipid material lines the small penetrating cerebral vessels, narrowing the lumen. Clots form and obstruct cerebral blood flow, typically in the basal ganglia, thalamus, or brainstem.[23,45]

Atherothrombotic brain attacks are frequently linked with terms that explain their associated pathophysiological process over time. The temporal profile of the atherothrombotic accident includes all of the following: asymptomatic phase, transient ischemic attack, reversible ischemic neurological deficit, stroke-in-evolution (progressing stroke), and completed stroke. Asymptomatic phase refers to the time period during which atherosclerotic damage to the

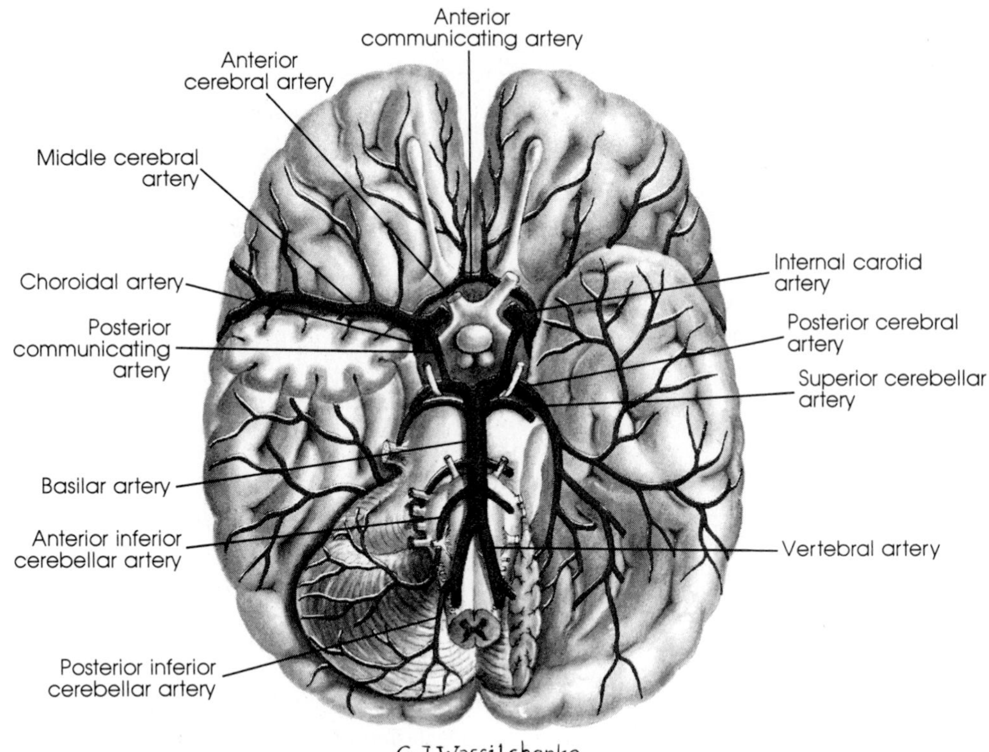

Figure 7-1 Blood supply of the brain, basilar view. (From Rudy EB: *Advanced neurological and neuroscience nursing,* St Louis, 1984, Mosby–Year Book.)

blood vessel and stenosis occur without symptomatology.[45] Transient ischemic attack (TIA) refers to the onset of a neurological deficit correlating with specific cerebral vasculature but lasting less than 24 hours. TIAs typically last less than 15 minutes[5] and are frequent precursors to stroke.[32] Following a TIA, the individual returns to a pre-TIA neurological status. In contrast, reversible ischemic neurological deficit (RIND) refers to the onset of a neurological deficit associated with a specific cerebrovascular territory, lasting longer than 24 hours but less than 3 weeks. Minimal to no residual neurological deficit results.[32] With a stroke-in-evolution, the person may experience a gradual worsening of neurological deficits as the thrombus enlarges to create more occlusion.[5] Finally, with the completed stroke, the neurological deficit has stabilized. However, not all atherothrombotic CVAs are associated with TIAs, RINDs, or strokes-in-evolution.

The other subtype of ischemic brain attack is the cardioembolic cerebrovascular accident. Cardioembolic stroke accounts for 15% to 31% of all CVAs.[5,30] As the name implies, a clot originating in the heart is released into the cerebral circulation, lodges in a blood vessel too small for its passage, occludes the vessel, and infarcts the tissue supplied by that blood vessel.[9] Predisposing cardiac conditions include: nonvalvular atrial fibrillation; valvular disease; ischemic heart disease, including myocardial infarction with mural thrombi; cardiomyopathy; and rheumatic heart disease.[4,5,27,32] Nonvalvular atrial fibrillation alone increases a person's risk of cardioembolic stroke five to six times.[27,32] Cardioembolic strokes typically are maximal at onset.

The other major category of CVA, hemorrhagic stroke, accounts for the remaining 20% of all CVAs and is subdivided into intracerebral hemorrhage and subarachnoid hemorrhage at an incidence of 14% and 6% respectively.[23,27] Intracerebral hemorrhage results from the rupture of small blood vessels, most commonly in the presence of hypertension. Clots are formed within the brain parenchyma and the blood may extend into the ventricles.[9] These cerebrovascular accidents typically occur while a person is active, and symptoms have an abrupt onset. Subarachnoid hemorrhage usually occurs with the rupture of a vascular anomaly such as a cerebral aneurysm or arteriovenous malformation. Both intracerebral hemorrhage and subarachnoid hemorrhage may occur as a result of trauma. However, this discussion is limited to nontraumatic intracerebral hemorrhage; traumatic brain injury and subarachnoid hemorrhage are discussed in other guidelines. Other mechanisms underlying stroke include blood dyscrasias, vasculitis, fibromuscular dysplasia, dissections, and substance abuse.[9,23]

Another approach to the pathophysiology of CVA is anatomical correlation with clinical presentation. Regardless of the exact mechanism—atherothrombosis or cardioembolism—occlusion of a blood vessel supplying a specific region of the brain results in distinct clinical syndromes (see Figure 7-1 and the following Box). In addition, hemorrhage

Symptoms Related to Cerebrovasculature Disease

Carotid region

Internal carotid artery syndrome

Symptoms of the typical ICA syndrome include the following:

- Paralysis of the contralateral face, arm, and leg
- Sensory deficits of the contralateral face, arm, and leg
- Aphasia, if the dominant hemisphere is involved
- Apraxia, agnosia, and unilateral neglect, if the nondominant hemisphere is involved
- Homonymous hemianopia

Middle cerebral artery syndrome

MCA syndrome is by far the most common of all cerebral occlusions. If the main stem of the MCA is occluded, a massive infarction of most of the hemisphere results. Initially, there may be vomiting and a rapid onset of coma, which may last a few weeks. Cerebral edema is extensive.

Symptoms of MCA syndrome include:

- Hemiplegia (involving the face and arm on the contralateral side; the leg is spared or has less deficits than the arm)
- Sensory impairment (same area as hemiplegia)
- Aphasia (global aphasia if the dominant hemisphere is involved)
- Homonymous hemianopia

Anterior cerebral artery syndrome

The ACA is least often occluded. If the occlusion occurs proximal to a patent anterior communicating artery, the blood supply will not be compromised. If the occlusion is distal, or if the communicating artery is inadequate, there will be infarction of the medial aspect of one frontal lobe. Bilateral medial frontal lobe infarction occurs if one ACA is occluded and the other artery is small and dependent on blood flow.

Symptoms of ACA syndrome include the following (note that aphasia and hemianopia are not part of the profile):

- Paralysis of the contralateral foot and leg (footdrop is a consistent finding)
- Impaired gait
- Sensory loss over the toes, foot, and leg
- Abulia (inability to perform acts voluntarily or make decisions)
- Flat affect, lack of spontaneity, slowness, distractibility, and lack of interest in surroundings
- Mental impairment, such as perseveration and amnesia
- Urinary incontinence (usually lasts for weeks)

Vertebrobasilar region

Occlusion of the vessels within the vertebrobasilar system produces unique syndromes. The vertebral and basilar arteries and their branches supply the brain stem and cerebellum. The posterior cerebral arteries are the terminal branches of the basilar artery and supply the medial temporal and occipital lobes, as well as part of the corpus callosum.

Vertebral artery syndrome

The following signs and symptoms are characteristic of VA occlusion:

- Wallenberg's syndrome (lateral medullary syndrome)
- Pain in face, nose, or eye
- Ipsilateral numbness and weakness of face
- Dizziness
- Staggering gait and ataxia
- Nystagmus
- Clumsiness
- Dysphagia and dysarthria

Basilar artery syndrome

The following signs and symptoms are characteristic of basilar artery occlusion:

- Quadriplegia
- Weakness of facial, tongue, and pharyngeal muscles
- Possibly, the "locked-in" syndrome

Anterior inferior cerebellar artery syndrome

Occlusion of the anterior inferior cerebellar artery is also known as the lateral inferior pontine syndrome.

Symptoms of the anterior inferior cerebellar artery syndrome include vertigo, nausea, vomiting, tinnitus, and nystagmus. Other symptoms include:

- Ipsilateral paresis of lateral conjugate gaze
- Ipsilateral Horner's syndrome
- Ipsilateral cerebellar signs (ataxia, nystagmus)
- Contralateral impaired pain and temperature sensation in the trunk and limbs (may also involve face)

Posterior inferior cerebellar artery syndrome (Wallenberg's syndrome)

Posterior inferior cerebellar artery syndrome involves the lateral portion of the medulla as a result of the occlusion of the posterior inferior cerebellar artery.

Symptoms include:

- Nausea and vomiting
- Dysphagia and dysarthria
- Loss of pain and temperature sensation on the contralateral side of the trunk and limbs
- Horizontal nystagmus
- Ipsilateral Horner's syndrome
- Cerebellar signs (ataxia and vertigo)

Symptoms Related to Cerebrovasculature Disease—cont'd

Posterior cerebral artery syndrome

Few strokes involve the PCA. The usual consequence of the superficial occlusion (peripheral areas) of a PCA is contralateral homonymous hemianopia. If the penetrating branches (central areas) are occluded, the cerebral peduncle, thalamus, and upper brain stem are involved. There is wide variation in the manifestations of the syndrome.

Symptoms of PCA syndrome include:

Peripheral area

- Homonymous hemianopia
- Several visual deficits, such as color blindness, lack of depth perception, failure to see objects not centrally located, visual hallucinations, and so forth
- Memory deficits
- Perseveration

Central area

- If the thalamus is involved, there is sensory loss of all modalities, spontaneous pain, intentional tremors, and mild hemiparesis.
- If the cerebral peduncle is involved, Weber's syndrome (oculomotor nerve palsy with contralateral hemiplegia) occurs.
- If the brain stem is involved, there are deficits involving conjugate gaze, nystagmus, and pupillary abnormalities, with the other possible symptoms of ataxia and postural tremors.

Deep cortical syndromes

Four syndromes are associated with intracerebral hemorrhagic stroke. In addition to an altered level of consciousness (confusion to coma), headache, nausea, vomiting, nuchal rigidity, hypertension, and bradycardia related to increased ICP, each syndrome has its own distinguishing characteristics.

Putaminal hemorrhage

This type of hemorrhage often involves the internal capsule.

- Contralateral hemiplegia
- Contralateral hemisensory deficits
- Hemianopia
- Slurred speech
- Ocular/deviation/away from paretic side (occurs in first 30 min)

Thalamic hemorrhage

- Contralateral hemiplegia
- Contralateral hemisensory deficits
- Deficits of vertical and lateral gaze

Pontine hemorrhage

- "Locked-in" syndrome (paralysis of all four extremities)
- Deficits in lateral eye movement

Cerebellar hemorrhage

- Occipital headache
- Dizziness
- Inability to sit or walk

Used with permission from Hickey JV: Stroke. In *The clinical practice of neurological and neuroscience nursing,* 3e, Philadelphia, 1992, JB Lippincott, pp 527-528.

from a cerebral vessel can result in clinical presentations specific to the location of the hemorrhage.

LENGTH OF STAY/ANTICIPATED COURSE

According to the federal government's prospective payment system, the average length of stay for a patient with a cerebrovascular accident is 8.7 days in acute care (DRG 14).[9,39,43] However, in reality the length of stay is frequently significantly longer due either to the CVA itself or complications associated with CVA including: increased intracranial pressure; atelectasis and pneumonia; adult respiratory distress syndrome (ARDS); neurogenic pulmonary edema; pulmonary emboli; syndrome of inappropriate antidiuretic hormone (SIADH); diabetes insipidus (DI); hyperthermia; infection; cardiac arrhythmias and heart disease; stress ulcer; fluid and electrolyte imbalance; nutritional compromise; bowel and bladder impairment; seizures; and impaired mobility. Cerebrovascular accidents do not typically exist in isolation from other systemic diseases. Pre-existing cardiovascular disease, diabetes mellitus, renal disease, and hypertension may contribute to the prolonged length of stay. Hemorrhagic stroke also may result in a longer length of stay related to rebleeding or greater potential for increased intracranial pressure resulting in herniation.[29,31]

Only a small percentage of patients with atherothrombotic or cardioembolic stroke are admitted to intensive care. Those who are admitted to ICU with occlusive stroke are patients who present with a decreased level of consciousness, decreased respiratory effort, and/or life-threatening arrhythmias.[32] However, a significant number of occlusive strokes are admitted to cardiac telemetry. In addition, many units specially designed as acute stroke units possess cardiac monitoring capability. Recent research has shown that stroke patients may benefit from admission to a designated stroke unit.[20,29] The prognosis for stroke is extremely variable. Depending on the patient's progress during acute care, functional ability, rehabilitation potential, physical stamina, social support, and fiscal resources, the patient may be discharged to a rehabilitation center, skilled nursing facility, home with home health, and/or outpatient therapies.[20]

MANAGEMENT TRENDS AND CONTROVERSIES

Numerous controversies exist regarding the management of cerebrovascular accidents.[12,15,42] The multitude of stroke studies provide incomplete data because of flaws in methodology.[7,32] In the management of stroke due to carotid artery disease, surgical versus nonsurgical intervention continues to be debated.[13,25,37] In carotid endarterectomy, the carotid artery is opened and the atherothrombotic plaque is excised.[9] In TIAs and CVAs resulting from either stenosis or ulceration, the question arises as to whether the benefit of surgery outweighs the risk.[10] In addition, even the asymptomatic patient with a normal ECG and no symptoms of heart disease is at significant risk for myocardial infarction within 5 years. Furthermore, no conclusive evidence exists that the carotid will remain free of disease or that a daily aspirin will maintain patency.[11,22]

A second surgical approach is extracranial-intracranial bypass, in which a scalp vessel is anastomosed to the occluded cerebral vessel to restore blood flow distal to the blockage.[9] Even though the negative findings of a large multicenter study on extracranial-intracranial bypass was widely accepted, bypass procedures are still performed on selected individuals with TIAs and completed strokes.[40] Again, the risk-benefit ratio must be considered. Complications of extracranial-intracranial bypass include occlusion of the graft, hematoma, scalp necrosis, and systemic complications.[9]

Similarly, there are no conclusive data about the benefits of pharmacological agents commonly prescribed for atherothrombotic stroke. The efficacy of antiplatelet agents versus anticoagulants and/or combination therapy is debatable.[16,21,28,35] Furthermore, optimal dosing of aspirin, the efficacy of aspirin in males versus females, the advantage of ticlopidine over aspirin in females, and the efficacy of combining dipyridamole with any other agent have not been clearly established.[8,14,18,21,26] In regard to heparin therapy, use of intravenous heparin for stroke-in-evolution and completed stroke is controversial, as is the optimal Activated Partial Thromboplastin Time (APTT). The long-term risk-benefit ratio of coumadin administration is also questionable.[14,24]

The use of anticoagulants in the treatment of cardioembolic stroke is also under scrutiny.[16] While heparin and coumadin decrease the risk of additional emboli, their administration may result in hemorrhagic transformation of the cardioembolic stroke. Intracranial hemorrhage may occur once the clot fragments and migrates to smaller cerebral vessels distally. Furthermore, when anticoagulation is delayed to minimize risk of hemorrhage, the optimal time to begin heparinization with or without consideration for the size of the infarct has not been established definitively.[38,41] The optimal APTT in heparin therapy, or the Prothrombin Time (PT) and International Normalized Ratio (INR) in coumadin therapy, may depend on the type of cardiac disease.[4,24,41]

Other modalities used to limit additional damage once the stroke has occurred include calcium channel blockers and hemodilutional hyperperfusion, which are used in atherothrombotic stroke to limit infarct size by vasodilating cerebral vessels and diluting plasma to increase cerebral perfusion. Hemodilutional hyperperfusion may increase blood pressure and intracranial pressure dangerously, and/or result in pulmonary edema.[9,44] Calcium channel blockers, such as nimodipine, may cause cardiac arrhythmias or hypotension.[36,46]

Surgical clot evacuation versus nonsurgical management with intracerebral hemorrhage is controversial in certain instances. Some physicians feel that the outcome is directly related to the patient's level of consciousness immediately after the hemorrhage. Therefore, they may choose nonsurgical supportive care over surgical evacuation of the clot.[32]

Investigational procedures used by interventional neuroradiologists may aid in the treatment of atherothrombotic stroke. Cerebral angioplasty and intravascular thrombolysis have been tried. In cerebral angioplasty, the plaque is compressed against the vessel wall to widen the lumen. However, plaque and clots may embolize during this procedure. In intravascular thrombolysis, agents such as urokinase and tissue plasminogen activator (tPA) may result in hemorrhage.[34] There are data suggesting that patients who receive thrombolytics within 6 hours of experiencing initial symptoms of atherothrombotic or embolic brain attacks experience improved neurological outcomes compared to patients who do not receive this therapy. Thrombolytics are contraindicated for patients with hemorrhagic stroke.

A number of multicenter studies are underway to determine optimal treatment for carotid stenosis. They include the Asymptomatic Carotid Atherosclerosis Study (ACAS); Carotid Artery Stenosis with Asymptomatic Narrowing: Operation Versus Aspirin (CASNOVA); and the North American Symptomatic Carotid Endarterectomy Trial (NASCET).[25] In addition, a regional study is being conducted to determine racial predilection in stroke—the Southeastern Consortium on Racial Differences in Stroke (SECORDS). A number of pharmacological agents are being studied as well, including intravenous tissue plasminogen activator (tPA) and low molecular weight heparinoids (ORG 10172). Tissue plasminogen activator lyses the clot at the onset of an atherothrombotic stroke. However, tPA may result in intracranial hemorrhage.[14] Low-molecular-weight heparinoids may lessen the risk of intracerebral hemorrhage when compared with heparin.[33]

ASSESSMENT

PARAMETER	ANTICIPATED ALTERATION
Neurological Status	
LOC	Decreased (lethargic to comatose); disoriented; impaired cognition; seizures
Pupils	Unequal; sluggishly reactive to nonreactive; pinpoint to fully dilated
Motor	Weakness to total paralysis of extremities; flaccid then spastic tone; abnormal reflexes; posturing; positive Babinski; negative Doll's eyes (in coma); abnormal or no response to Cold Caloric testing (in coma); ataxia; nuchal rigidity (with hemorrhage)
Cranial nerves	Ptosis; dysconjugate gaze; gaze preference; diplopia; visual field cut; facial asymmetry/motor weakness/numbness; inability to handle oral secretions; uvula/tongue deviation
Sensation	Numbness/paresthesias of extremities; headache
Speech	Dysarthria; expressive/receptive/global aphasia
Vital signs	Increased temperature Increased blood pressure Increased, decreased, and/or irregular heart rate Increased, decreased, and/or irregular respirations Carotid bruit
Perceptual deficits	Neglect; right-left disorientation; apraxia
Bowel and bladder	Incontinence; retention; constipation
Behavioral style	Right hemisphere CVA: spatial-perceptual deficits; denial of deficits; impulsive; poor judgment; left visual field deficit; easily distractable Left hemisphere CVA: aphasia; slow and cautious; right visual field deficit; more likely to have speech problems
Respiratory	Crackles; rhonchi; wheezes; increased or decreased rate; irregular *due to decreased LOC, neuronal damage, or impaired mobility*
Cardiac	Increased or decreased pulse rate; systemic hypertension; widened pulse pressure *(with increased intracranial pressure);* arrhythmias
Renal	Increased or decreased urine output *in the presence of renal failure; syndrome of inappropriate antidiuretic hormone (SIADH); or diabetes insipidus*
Diagnostic Tests	
CT of head	With infarct, may be normal first few days, then infarct visualized; blood immediately seen if hemorrhage present; *MRI may demonstrate brainstem lesions better.*
Cerebral arteriogram/digital subtraction	Thrombosis, narrowing or emboli in cerebral blood vessel. Also, aneurysm or leakage may be seen.
Angiography	May show occlusion, plaque ulceration in carotids, dissection, recanalization; may demonstrate an aneurysm or AVM. *75% level is significant for carotid artery stenosis.*
Magnetic resonance arteriogram (MRA)	Same as cerebral arteriogram
Duplex carotid ultrasound	Carotid artery stenosis; ulceration
ICP	Increased: >15 mm Hg
EEG	Rule out seizure activity; focal slowing, diffuse slowing, or no activity (brain death, barbiturates)

Lumbar puncture	Opening pressure >200 cm H_2O. *(In the presence of increased intracranial pressure, a lumbar puncture is contraindicated due to risk of herniation.)* If hemorrhage, CSF positive for blood.
Cerebral perfusion pressure (MAP − ICP = CPP)	Decreased: <60 mm Hg represents significant ischemia
12-lead ECG	Arrhythmias, especially atrial fibrillation
Heart disease	History of myocardial infarction
Echocardiogram, transesophageal echocardiogram	Cardiac embolus: valvular disease, patent foramen ovale, left atrial and atrial appendage abnormalities
24-hour Holter monitor	Dysrhythmias
Chest x-ray	Pulmonary edema; pneumonia/infiltrate related to aspiration
PAP/PCWP/CVP	Increased *due to concurrent heart disease or cardiac depressant factors released with brain injury*
CO/CI	Decreased with CO <4 L/min and CI <2.5 L/min/m^2 *due to cardiac suppression*
ABG	Hypoxemia, hypercapnea *due to depressed respiratory system*
CBC	Polycythemia
Platelets	Decreased: <150,000/mm^3 *due to hemorrhage* Increased: >400,000/mm^3 *due to presence of cerebral thrombus*
WBC count	Elevated: >10,000/mm^3 *due to possible septic emboli*
Lipid profile	Total cholesterol, triglycerides, and LDL all elevated, and HDL decreased *due to possible atherosclerotic cerebral vascular disease*
APTT/PT	Prolonged with APPT >40 sec and PT >12.5 sec *r/t hemorrhage*
Antiphospholipid antibody (+APA)	Positive *in the presence of thrombosis*
Circulating lupus anticoagulant (+CLA)	Positive *in the presence of thrombosis*
Antithrombin III	Increased *in the presence of thrombosis*
Protein C and protein S	Decreased *in the presence of thrombosis*
Clotting factor assays	Increased *r/t thrombosis* Decreased *r/t hemorrhage*
Hemoglobin electrophoresis	Positive *r/t sickle cell disease*
Blood cultures	Positive *in presence of septic emboli*

PLAN OF CARE

INTENSIVE PHASE

Few patients with an acute CVA will require intensive monitoring and care. However, CVA is a frequent complication of other diseases, and surgical interventions and care of this patient population are an important component of the critical care nurse's repertoire of skills. Those patients with an acute CVA requiring intensive level care generally have difficulty with airway management, breathing/gas exchange, or circulatory instability.

PATIENT CARE PRIORITIES	EXPECTED PATIENT OUTCOMES
Decreased cerebral tissue perfusion *r/t occlusion of cerebral vasculature and/or disruption of cerebral vasculature, increased ICP*	Regain or maintain optimal neurological status in regard to LOC; cognition; pupils, vision; EOMs; movement; sensation; speech; cranial nerves; vital signs; and absence of headaches, seizures, and nausea and vomiting ICP maintained <15 mm Hg

Plan of Care (cont'd)

Ineffective breathing pattern *r/t decreased LOC; neurological impairment; decreased mobility*	Regain or maintain optimal respiratory status in regard to rate, depth, and pattern of respirations; breath sounds; ABG; oxygen saturation; chest x-ray; pulmonary function studies; ventilation perfusion lung scans; sputum cultures
Impaired swallowing *r/t neuronal damage and/or decreased LOC; presence of artificial airway*	Regain or maintain optimal swallowing ability in regard to absence of aspiration of food or liquids while eating Optimal respiratory status Adequate oral intake
Impaired physical mobility *r/t neuronal damage to motor tracts; decreased LOC; activity restrictions necessary to control ICP; restrictions of movement due to placement of invasive devices*	Intact skin and mucous membranes Absence of deep-vein thrombosis and pulmonary embolus Absence of contractures; subluxation of joints Optimal range of motion of joints
High risk for fluid volume excess *r/t syndrome of inappropriate antidiuretic hormone (SIADH); hemodilutional hyperperfusion; decreased cardiac output*	Regain or maintain fluid balance: balanced intake and output Daily weights within 5% of baseline CO: WNL
Alteration in bowel and bladder elimination *r/t neuronal injury; decreased LOC; impaired mobility; restriction of movement due to placement of invasive devices; preexisting GI or GU disease or autonomic neuropathy; prolonged NPO status or diet inadequate in fluid/fiber; constipation related to meds; diarrhea*	Regain or maintain optimal bowel and bladder elimination as evidenced by completely emptying the bladder with or without catheterization; absence of urinary tract infection; soft-formed bowel movements with or without bowel training
Impaired verbal communication *r/t neuronal injury; cranial nerve involvement; presence of artificial airway; impaired hearing and vision; extremity weakness, flaccidity, or spasticity*	Regain or maintain effective communication with family and health care team members
Anxiety *r/t neuronal injury; knowledge deficit; sleep deprivation; alteration in LOC*	Patient/family able to demonstrate basic understanding of disease process and treatment as evidenced by cooperation with therapeutic regimen and verbal feedback as condition permits

INTERVENTIONS

Monitor neurological status q1h to q2h and prn *to detect neurological deterioration immediately and coordinate care with medical staff.*

Monitor ICP and CCP q1h to q2h and prn if ICP monitoring device present.

Provide rest periods between individual nursing interventions *to minimize increased ICP. Clustering activities may contribute to increased ICP.*

Elevate head of bed 30° to 45° *unless CPP is inadequate due to blood pressure decrease with head elevation.*

Maintain head in neutral position neither tilted to one side nor extended or flexed *to minimize ICP.*

Monitor respiratory function.

Administer oxygen therapy and/or ventilatory support as prescribed.

Suction orally or per artificial airway as needed. *Preoxygenate and hyperventilate to minimize ICP increases.*

Monitor response to IV fluids, vasoactive agents, and/or antihypertensives as prescribed to maintain BP, RAP, PAP, PCWP, CO, and CI within established parameters.

Avoid wide fluctuations in BP *to minimize risk of additional cerebral ischemia, infarction, and/or hemorrhage.*

For occlusive CVAs/TIAs, administer heparin at prescribed dose and rate. Monitor APTT. Observe for signs and symptoms of hemorrhage.

Plan of Care (cont'd)

Monitor heart rate and rhythm and administer antiarrhythmics as prescribed.

Administer pharamacological agents (e.g., loop diuretics) for treatment of cerebral edema or other fluid overload as prescribed.

Monitor intake and output and fluid status. *Avoid hypotonic IV solutions, which increase cerebral edema.*

Avoid Valsalva, including hip flexion, straining at stool, rectal temperatures, sustained cough, or isometric muscle contraction. *Valsalva increases ICP.*

Monitor frequency and character of stools, discourage straining, and administer stool softeners as prescribed *to minimize increased ICP and risks of hemorrhagic stroke.*

Monitor urine output, avoid bladder distension, and maintain patency of indwelling catheter (if present) or perform intermittent catheterization as needed *to minimize increased ICP.*

Administer medications as prescribed to minimize coughing, sneezing, vomiting, seizure activity, and/or pain *to minimize increased ICP.*

Monitor for signs and symptoms of pulmonary edema, aspiration pneumonia, deep-vein thrombosis, and/or pulmonary emboli.

If nasogastric tube is present, maintain patency and low intermittent suction (as ordered) *to minimize risk of aspiration.*

Check feeding tube residuals q4h and hold tube feeding if residuals exceed prescribed parameters *to prevent aspiration.*

Assess swallowing reflex prior to feeding by observing ability to handle oral secretions, ice chips, and/or water *to prevent aspiration.*

Note absence or presence of cough. *(Aspiration may be silent.)*

Note any pocketing of food in cheeks, if eating. If swallowing is impaired, hold diet, and notify physician.

Assist patient to keep head up when eating. Remind patient to take small bites and chew thoroughly. Minimize distractions during feeding. Unless ordered otherwise, keep tracheostomy tube cuff inflated during feeding.

Monitor for signs and symptoms of aspiration.

Monitor nutritional status.

Monitor blood glucose and administer insulin as prescribed. *Hyperglycemia can contribute to neuronal injury and infarct in the presence of ischemia.*

Monitor for signs and symptoms of seizures.

Monitor and report electrolytes, anticonvulsant levels, and other medication levels. Administer anticonvulsants as prescribed.

During seizure activity, protect from injury.

Assess ability to hear, read, express thought, and comprehend verbal and written language. Consider speech therapy consult.

Use alternate forms of communication as needed and instruct family and health care team members accordingly.

INTERMEDIATE PHASE

Once the patient's neurological, cardiovascular, and pulmonary systems have stabilized, emphasis will be placed on rehabilitation in acute care. During this phase, the patient will be transferred to a neurological unit, stroke unit, and/or unit with telemetry with the following goals as priorities: (1) increase physical endurance; (2) increase rehabilitation in acute care; (3) increase rehabilitation efforts based on the patient's response to the various therapies. An interdisciplinary approach is essential.

PATIENT CARE PRIORITIES	EXPECTED PATIENT OUTCOMES
Impaired neurological status *r/t CVA*	Maintain or improve neurological status, recovery of functional capability
High risk for impaired gas exchange *r/t residual effects of CVA*	Regain or maintain optimal respiratory status

Plan of Care (cont'd)

High risk for ineffective breathing pattern *r/t residual effects of CVA*	Regain or maintain optimal respiratory status
High risk for impaired swallowing *r/t residual effects of CVA*	Regain or maintain optimal swallowing ability. No evidence of aspiration complications
Impaired physical mobility *r/t residual effects of CVA*	Intact skin and mucous membranes Absence of deep-vein thrombosis, contractures, and subluxation Optimal range of motion
High risk for inadequate nutrition *r/t swallowing deficits, depression*	Regain or maintain optimal nutritional status
High risk for alteration in bowel and bladder elimination pattern *r/t residual effects of CVA*	Regain or maintain optimal bowel and bladder elimination
High risk for alteration in thought processes *r/t residual effects of CVA*	Regain or maintain thought processes
High risk for impaired verbal communication *r/t potential aphasia or inability to vocalize*	Regain or maintain effective communication
High risk for alteration in sensory perception *r/t residual effects of CVA*	Regain or maintain optimal sensory perception
High risk for unilateral neglect *r/t potential hemiparesis*	Experience improvement in and/or adaptation to unilateral neglect
Self-care deficit *r/t inadequate knowledge about disease, recovery process, and adaptive devices and activities*	Patient/family indicate basic understanding of disease process and treatment regimens Patient/family demonstrate adaptive coping behaviors

INTERVENTIONS

Monitor neurological status q4h to q8h and prn *to detect deterioration and intervene immediately.*

Administer antiplatelet, anticoagulant agents as prescribed. Monitor APTT and PT/INR as needed. Observe for any signs or symptoms of bleeding.

Assess swallow reflex. Collaborate with other health care team members as needed (speech therapy, dietitian).

Monitor for signs and symptoms of aspiration.

Monitor for and prevent consequences of immobility.

Assess for signs and symptoms of fluid and electrolyte imbalance.

Monitor nutritional status. Assist with meals/enteral feeding/parenteral nutrition.

Monitor for seizures. Administer anticonvulsants as prescribed. Monitor anticonvulsant levels.

At appropriate level of consciousness, attempt bladder and bowel retraining by offering urinal, bedpan, or bedside commode q2h to q4h during waking hours and if restlessness is noted at night.

Assess thought processes: LOC, orientation, appropriateness of response, affect, short- and long-term memory, ability to concentrate, judgment, and emotion.

Evaluate all medications for effect on cognitive function.

Reorient and talk with patient each time the room is entered. Explain procedures and note response.

Encourage participation in repetition of tasks and assimilation of new tasks.

Allow choices and some control.

Provide consistency in approach.

Interrupt inappropriate behavior and promote self-care behavior. Give immediate feedback on inappropriate behavior.

Continue to assess ability to communicate. Develop and implement alternate forms of communication.

Plan of Care (cont'd)

Assess alterations in sensory perception. Incorporate intact sensory perception in prompting completion of activities.

Assess for signs and symptoms of unilateral neglect. Implement compensatory measures *to protect patient from potential injury.*

Collaborate with other health care members on a daily basis. Consider weekly patient care conferences *to maximize coordination of services and shared goals.*

Educate patient and family regarding disease process and treatment regimens.

TRANSITION TO DISCHARGE

In preparing the stroke patient for discharge, the interdisciplinary team approach is essential to maximize the patient's potential in acute rehabilitation. Team members consulted in the acute care of the stroke patient may include physical therapist, occupational therapist, speech therapist, dietitian, psychologist, orthotist, chaplain, psychiatrist, social worker, respiratory therapist, and the clinical nurse specialist. Also essential to maximizing potential in acute care and preparing for rehabilitation is patient and family education. However, the patient and family must be ready to learn and receive educational information appropriate to their level of learning and learning style. Items to be included in the education of the patient or family may include basic disease process, risk-factor modification, medications, medical and surgical intervention, and the rehabilitation process. In addition, depending on the severity of the stroke, the patient and family may need to acquire a number of skills, including feeding tube care, rehabilitation techniques, and range of motion. Future success with stroke rehabilitation begins with emphasis on initiating CVA rehabilitation in acute care once the patient's condition has stabilized.

REFERENCES

1. AACN, *Outcome standards for nursing care of the critically ill,* Laguna Niguel, Calif, 1990, AACN.
2. Adams RD, Victor M: Cerebrovascular disease. In *Principles of neurology,* New York, 1989, McGraw-Hill, pp 617-692.
3. Alberts MJ: Diagnosis of acute stroke, *Postgrad Med* 86(8):95-102, 1989.
4. Asinger RW, et al: Cardiogenic brain embolism, *Arch Neurol* 46:727-743, 1989.
5. Barnaby W: Stroke intervention, *Emerg Med Clin North Am* 8(2):267-280, 1990.
6. Barnett HJM: The contribution of multicenter trials to stroke prevention and treatment, *Arch Neurol* 47:441-443, 1990.
7. Barnett HJM: Symptomatic carotid endarterectomy trials, *Stroke* 21(11):III 2-5, 1990.
8. Blissitt PA: Ticlopidine hydrochloride, *J Neurosci Nurs* 24(5):296-300, 1992.
9. Bronstein KS, Popovich JM, Stewart-Amidei C: *Promoting stroke recovery,* St Louis, 1991, Mosby–Year Book.

9a. Brott TG, et al: Urgent therapy for stroke, *Stroke* 23:633-639, 1992.

10. Callow AD, Mackey WC: Optimum results of the surgical treatment of carotid territory ischemia, *Circulation* 83(2):1190-1195, 1991.
11. Cebul RD, Whisnant JP: Indications for carotid endarterectomy, *Ann Intern Med* 3(8):675-677, 1989.
12. Charness ME: Controversies in the medical management of stroke, *West J Med* 142:74-78, 1985.
13. Crowell RM: Surgical management of cerebrovascular disease, *Nurs Clin North Am* 21(2):297-308, 1986.
14. Dutka AJ, Hallenbeck JM: Pharmacologic therapy for ischemic cerebrovascular disease, *Neurol Clin North Am* 8(1):161-176, 1990.
15. Dyken ML: Controversies in stroke: past and present, *Stroke* 24(8):1251-1258, 1993.
16. Estol CJ, Pessin MS: Anticoagulation in treatment of atherothrombotic stroke, *Stroke* 21(5):820-824, 1990.

16a. Fagan SC, Zorowitz BJ, Robert S: Brain attack: an indication for thrombosis? *Ann Pharmacother* 23:633-639, 1992.

17. Feldmann E: Intracerebral hemorrhage, *Stroke* 22(5):684-691, 1991.
18. Fitzgerald GA: Dipyridamole, *New Engl J Med* 316(20):1247-1257, 1987.
19. Gorelick PB: Treatment of ischemic stroke, *Postgrad Med* 86(8):107-118, 1989.
20. Grotta JC: Acute stroke management, *Stroke Clinical Updates* 3(5):17-20, 1993.
21. Hass W: Ticlopidine: an antiplatelet drug useful in stroke prevention, *Stroke Clinical Updates* 2(6):21-24, 1992.
22. Healy DA, et al: Immediate and long-term result of carotid endarterectomy, *Stroke* 20(9):1138-1142, 1989.
23. Hickey JV: Stroke. In *The clinical practice of neurological and neurosurgical nursing,* Philadelphia, 1992, Lippincott, pp 519-540.
24. Hirsh J, et al: Oral anticoagulation: mechanism of action, clinical effectiveness, and optimal therapeutic range, *Chest* 102(4):312S-326S, 1992.
25. Howard VJ, et al.: Comparison of multicenter designs for investigation of carotid endartectomy efficacy, *Stroke* 23(4):583-593, 1992.
26. Jonas S: The physician's health study, *Arch Neurol* 47:1352-1353 1990.
27. Kelly RE: Cerebrovascular disease. In *Neurology of the non-neurologist,* Philadelphia, 1989, Lippincott, pp 52-66.
28. Kushner M, Simonian N: Lupus anticoagulants, anticardiolipin antibodies, and cerebral ischemia, *Stroke* 20(2):225-229, 1989.
29. Leahy NM: Complications in the acute stages of stroke, *Nurs Clin North Am* 26(4):971-983, 1991.
30. Leonard AD, Newburg S: Cardioembolic stroke, *J Neurosci Nurs* 24(2):69-78, 1992.
31. Licata-Gehr EE: Etiology of stroke subtypes, *Nurs Clin North Am* 26(4):943-956, 1991.

32. Marshall SB, et al: Cerebrovascular disease. In *Neuroscience critical care,* Philadelphia, 1990, WB Saunders, pp 215-248.
33. Massey EW, et al: Large-dose infusions of heparinoid ORG 10172 in ischemic stroke, *Stroke* 21(9):1289-1292, 1990.
34. McDowell FH, et al: Stroke: the first six hours, *Stroke Clinical Updates* 4(1):1-12, 1993.
35. Miller A, Lees RS: Simultaneous therapy with antiplatelet and anticoagulant drugs in symptomatic cardiovascular disease, *Stroke* 16(4):668-675, 1985.
36. Mohr JP: Clinical trial of nimodipine in acute ischemic stroke, *Stroke* 23(1):3-8, 1992.
37. Neville RF, Hobson RW: Indications for carotid endarterectomy: an update, *Stroke Clinical Updates* 2(2):5-8, 1991.
38. Okada Y, et al: Hemorrhagic transformation in cerebral embolism, *Stroke* 20(5):598-603, 1989.
39. Phipps MA: Assessment of neurological deficits in stroke, *Nurs Clin North Am* (26)4:957-970, 1991.
40. Relman AS: The extracranial-intracranial bypass study: what have we learned? *New Engl J Med* 316(13):809-810, 1987.
41. Rothrock JF, Dittrich HC, McAllen S: Acute anticoagulation following cardioembolic stroke, *Stroke* 20(6):730-734, 1989.
42. Scheinburg P: Controversies in the management of cerebrovascular disease, *Neurology* 38(1):1609-1615, 1988.
43. *St Anthony's DRG guidebook 1995,* Reston, Va, 1994, St Anthony.
44. Stewart-Amidei C: Hypervolemic hemodilution: a new approach to subarachnoid hemorrhage, *Heart Lung* 18(6):590-598, 1989.
45. Whisnant JP, et al: Classification of cerebrovascular diseases III, *Stroke* 21(4):637-676, 1990.
46. Wong MCW, Haley EC: Calcium antagonists: stroke therapy coming of age, *Stroke* 21(3):494-501, 1990.

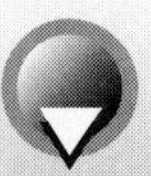

CLINICAL GUIDELINE

8

Seizures

Kara Lee Rusy, MSN, RN, CCRN

DESCRIPTION

A seizure can be described as involuntary behavioral manifestations secondary to abnormal cortical electrical activity. This finite event, for reasons not fully understood, occurs when certain nerve cells fire together in a sudden, paroxysmal burst, resulting in electrical disturbances and disruption of the brain's normal activity. The outward manifestations, or abnormal neurological functions, that subsequently occur are related to the region(s) of cerebral cortex involved and may consist of transient alterations in level of consciousness; impairment of mentation; disturbances of sensorimotor, autonomic, or psychic function, or varied combinations of symptoms.[1,3,5,12] Most authorities propose that an isolated seizure is a symptom of an underlying pathological condition, and they suggest that the term "epilepsy" be restricted to describing a group of syndromes that share a tendency to produce repeated seizures. Subdivisions of epilepsy include "primary" or recurrent seizures of unknown cause (formally called "idiopathic"), thought to result from a genetic predisposition; or "secondary" seizures resulting from a known disease process or pathological lesion.[10,12,13]

It has been estimated that the prevalence of epilepsy is from 0.5% to 2.0% of the United States' population, making it second only to cerebral vascular accident as the leading neurological disorder.[3,15] Eighty percent occur before the age of 20, and more than one quarter of all patients with epilepsy are refractant to medical therapy.[3] Secondary social and economic costs are staggering, along with the biological and psychological effects each individual suffers.[11]

PATHOPHYSIOLOGY

Seizures may be caused by a variety of pathological conditions that alter the neuron's cellular environment. The mechanism remains elusive but is thought to involve an autonomous paroxysmal discharge of electrical activity, and depolarization of the involved neuron's membrane potential, called the paroxysmal depolarization shift (PDS). This is the site of the epileptogenic focus. An accumulation of intracellular sodium and calcium along with extracellular potassium occurs, causing a continuous hyperexcited state and repeated generation of action potentials. A deficiency in the inhibitory neurotransmitter gamma aminobutyric acid (GABA) is also thought to contribute to the abnormal discharges. The wave of hyperexcitability may spread from the epileptogenic focus to other parts of the brain. Cessation of the seizure occurs when there is a reversal of cellular polarity.[5,11]

Many of the patients seen in the critical care setting are at risk for developing seizures because of the multiple etiologies or precipitating events that can induce seizure activity (See Box, Etiologies and Precipitating Events for Seizures.) The most common types of intracranial disorders causing seizures are vascular lesions, tumors, craniocerebral trauma, and infectious diseases.[12] From 5% to 50% of patients who suffer head trauma develop posttraumatic seizures, as well as 10% to 20% of patients who have suffered a CVA.[11] Factors that may precipitate seizure activity include various metabolic and electrolyte disturbances, toxic processes, hyperthermia, and extreme physical or emotional fatigue. Some environmental stimuli may also precipitate seizures, such as blinking lights or loud noises.[1,2,6,12]

Seizures have been classified in various ways according to site, electroencephalogram (EEG) correlates, symptomatology, therapy responses, and others. The classification system most frequently cited is the International Classification of Epileptic Seizures. (See Box, International Classification of Epileptic Seizures, on p. 80.) A partial or focal seizure involves abnormal electrical discharges from a lo-

Etiologies and Precipitating Events for Seizures

Idiopathic
Congenital anomalies (e.g., tuberous sclerosis, Tay-Sachs disease)
Perinatal trauma or injury
Postnatal trauma or injury
Cerebral tumors
Cerebral aneurysm or subarachnoid hemorrhage
Cerebrovascular disease (e.g., embolic or hemorrhagic stroke, arteriovenous malformations)
Craniocerebral trauma (e.g., contusion, epidural hematoma)
Infectious process (e.g., meningitis or encephalitis, cerebral abscess)
Degenerative disorders (e.g., multiple sclerosis, Alzheimer's disease)
Metabolic disorders (e.g., acidosis, hypoxemia, hypoglycemia)
Electrolyte disturbances (e.g., hypocalcemia)
Toxic processes (e.g., drug or alcohol overdose or withdrawal)
Uremic encephalopathy
Hyperpyrexia in children
Emotional or physical fatigue or stress
Sleep deprivation
Flashing lights, loud noises
Menstruation
Noncompliance with prescribed anticonvulsant therapy

calized region of the cerebral cortex. Clinical manifestations are related to the site of origin and localized area(s) affected by the seizure activity. Partial seizures are further divided into two main groups—simple and complex. Simple partial seizures have no impairment of consciousness. A jacksonian seizure is an example of a simple partial seizure that originates in the motor strip area of the frontal lobe and is characterized by focal twitching of a finger or toe that spreads sequentially in a stepwise fashion to various parts of the body. The patient, however, remains alert. Other examples include somatosensory simple partial seizures that arise from the sensory strip of the parietal lobe (postcentral gyros) and may manifest in a tingling or "pins and needles" sensation. Visual seizures arising from the occipital lobe may present as unformed visual hallucinations. Autonomic changes such as sweating, epigastric sensations, flushing, or pallor characterize autonomic seizures.[7,11,12] These signs and symptoms, referred to as "auras," often become warning signs to patients of further seizure activity.

Complex partial seizures also involve abnormal electrical discharges from a localized region but are accompanied by some impairment of consciousness. They most often originate from the temporal lobe.[12,15] Symptoms may include cognitive disruptions (e.g., deja vu), affective symptoms (e.g., fear, increased anxiety), and "autonomatisms," or repetitive, involuntary activity such as lipsmacking, chewing, mumbling, repetitive speech, or walking around inappropriately. The patient usually has no recall of the behavior displayed. The complex partial seizure eventually may spread to the opposite cerebral cortex, called "secondary generalization."

A generalized seizure involves abnormal electrical discharges from both cerebral hemispheres with no local onset and is characterized by a sudden loss of consciousness and immediate symmetrical abnormal motor activity.[5,7,11] There are many different types of generalized seizures. Absence seizures, previously referred to as petit mal, are most commonly seen in children ages 5 to 12 and involve a sudden onset and cessation of loss of consciousness without violent muscular activity. They can be induced by hyperventilation. Tonic-clonic seizures, previously referred to as grand mal, can be the most frightening type of generalized seizure because they are characterized by loss of consciousness, violent stiffening and jerking of the extremities, incontinence of stool or urine, tongue-biting and foaming at the mouth, and fatigue and confusion in the post-ictal (post-seizure) stage.

Status epilepticus is a state of recurrent, successive, and/or prolonged seizure activity (greater than 30 minutes) without intervening periods of physiologic recovery. Roughly 100,000 cases occur per year with morbidity and mortality rates as high as 10% to 12%, related to the duration of status and irreversible neuronal death that occurs from repetitive electric discharges.[7,19] Experimental and clinical research indicates that prolonged seizure activity for longer than 60 to 90 minutes may result in irreversible brain damage.[19] This condition is a life-threatening emergency because of the potential for developing cardiac dysrhythmias, metabolic acidosis, respiratory depression, laryngospasm, cerebral anoxia, and irreversible brain death.[5,19] Cerebral metabolic rate, oxygen and glucose use, and glycolysis increase two to three times above normal, and cerebral blood flow may increase to five times normal.[1] The most common cause is subtherapeutic antiepileptic drug levels in a patient with a known seizure disorder due to intercurrent infection or noncompliance. Time is of the essence in treatment of status epilepticus.

LENGTH OF STAY/ANTICIPATED COURSE

The length of stay for patients with seizures depends heavily on the etiology or precipitating event, timing of the diagnosis, and subsequent treatment. The ultimate outcome depends on removal of epileptogenic source, control of seizure activity, degree of cerebal injury, and control of complicating physiological and psychological factors. DRGs related to seizure disorders include DRGs 24 and 25. Both of these DRGs address seizure and headache in adults. DRG 24 includes an adjustment for complications with an average LOS of 6.6 days.[18] DRG 25 refers to seizure and headache without complications with an average LOS of 4.1 days.[18]

International Classification of Epileptic Seizures

Partial (focal) seizures

Abnormal discharge involving limited part(s) of one cerebral hemisphere

Types

Simple partial

No loss of consciousness
"Aura" (local cortical discharge)
Symptoms r/t area involved—may be motor, visual, auditory, olfactory, or gustatory (i.e., clonic hand movement, tongue tingling, epigastric sensation, vocalizations, hallucinations, pallor)

Complex partial

Impairment of consciousness/alteration in awareness
May begin as simple partial or impairment of consciousness at onset
"Automatisms" (involuntary repetitive movements) such as lipsmacking, repetitive mumbled speech, walking in circles
May be post-ictal afterwards (confusion, fatigue, etc.)
Todd's paralysis possible (temporary hemiparesis)
May generalize to tonic-clonic seizure

Primary generalized seizures

Abnormal discharge involving widespread areas of both cerebral hemispheres

Types

Absence (traditionally called "petit mal")

Sudden onset and cessation of loss of consciousness, "starting spells"
Usually begins at ages 5-12
Induced by hyperventilation

Myoclonic

Repetitive jerky movements, brief sudden muscle contractions

Clonic

Sudden hypotonia of muscle followed by bilateral jerks

Tonic

Sudden increase in muscle tone

Tonic-clonic (traditionally called "grand mal")

Begins suddenly with loss of consciousness; ends gradually
Quick, severe tonic-clonic movements
Stretorous respirations
Autonomic Sx (dilated pupils, HTN, tachycardia)
Possible loss of bowel and bladder function
Post-ictal period (muscle flaccidity, amnesia, fatigue and confusion)
Bilateral Babinski signs

Atonic (akinetic)

"Drop attacks"
Sudden loss of axial muscle tone
Patient may fall to ground
Seen as "head nodding" in infants

MANAGEMENT TRENDS AND CONTROVERSIES

The goals for management of a patient with seizures are aimed at determination and removal of the cause if possible, prevention of precipitating factors by effective anticonvulsant drug control (either short-term or long-term), and promotion and regulation of physical and mental hygiene. An array of diagnostic procedures are implemented to determine if there is an underlying pathological cause. In some cases, the cause of the seizure symptomatology may be surgically removed, such as with vascular lesion or tumor. Other pathological conditions causing seizures, such as metabolic or electrolyte disturbances or renal dysfunction, may be managed with medical therapy. Approximately 70% to 80% of patients may benefit from anticonvulsants to control their seizures. Many different antiepileptic medications are available, each with a selective efficacy for one or more seizure types; therefore, seizure classification is essential. The therapeutic goal is eradication of seizure activity without producing intolerable drug side effects, and control of precipitating events. Because of their superior efficacy and relative safety, phenytoin, carbamazepine, valproic acid, and phenobarbital are preferred medications. Monotherapy, whenever possible, has been shown to minimize toxicity with adequate seizure control.[11] Because different patients metabolize, absorb, and eliminate drugs at different rates, dosage and serum levels need to be individualized and monitored closely. Long-term follow-up helps prevent untoward drug side effects that may involve decreased mental abilities and difficulties in psychosocial functions.

Advances in the neurosciences have made temporal lobectomy, or surgical excision of an epileptogenic focus via craniotomy, an option for patients with complex partial seizures refractant to medical management.[15,17] Presurgical evaluation may be lengthy, involving multiple diagnostic procedures to localize the origin of seizure activity, but 60% to 90% of surgical candidates achieve an excellent outcome, demonstrated by a 95% decrease in seizure frequency one year after surgery.[15,16] Corpus callosotomy, or surgical resection of the corpus callosum to prevent hemispheric spread of the seizure activity, may be used as a last resort in patients with generalized atonic or "drop" seizures.[3]

Management of status epilepticus usually requires admission to the intensive care setting because major concerns are respiratory depression, laryngospasm, and cardiac dysrhythmias. After airway stabilization and cardiovascular management are established, the pharmacologic agent of choice for short-term control of seizures is diazepam (Valium). However, lorazepam (Ativan) has been shown to be as or more effective in suppressing the spread of abnormal cerebral electrical activity; it also has less respiratory suppression and hypotension associated with intravenous administration, as well as a longer duration of action.[4] For those patients who do not respond to Valium or Ativan, who have a limited pulmonary reserve, or in whom consciousness depression is undesirable, lidocaine appears to be a rapid-acting, short-term anticonvulsant in the management of status epilepticus.[14] Phenytoin and phenobarbital are also administered to control seizures. Paraldehyde may be administered, particularly in patients suffering from prolonged seizure activity due to alcohol withdrawal. If the above regimens do not stop the status epilepticus, general anesthesia, such as the inhalation agent isoflurane, may be employed. However, general anethesia needs to be regulated by an anesthesiologist and requires diagnostic follow-up to ensure cessation of abnormal electrical brain activity.[4,5,9,19]

A patient with seizures is often followed for years, requiring regular clinic visits to monitor progress. Living with seizures can lead to emotional and psychosocial complications. Because of the social stigma often associated with seizures, many patients and their families require psychological, educational, and vocational counseling. Often the seizure disorder becomes the central focus of the patient's life, significantly affecting self-concept, which in turn influences social relationships and choices or options of education or employment. Patient care requires a joint effort of multiple members of the interdisciplinary team, including the nurse, neuropsychologist, social worker, neurologist, speech and physical therapists, and others.

The focus on current and future research on seizures relates primarily to classification, diagnostic procedures, and appropriate management. New methods of EEG analysis and more selective electrical stimulations of the brain may help further classify seizure origin and type. New anticonvulsants are being investigated as well as various drugs to treat status epilepticus. Creative methods of imaging the brain structurally and metobolically with positive emission tomography (PET) and magnetic resonance imaging (MRI) scanning may provide better direction for medical and surgical management.[16]

ASSESSMENT

PARAMETER	ANTICIPATED ALTERATION
Specific description of previous seizure activity	Time of first occurrence Frequency of seizures Onset, duration, progression, type Occurrence of an aura or specific types of abnormal neurological activity Changes or fluctuation in LOC Abnormal eye/head movements or deviations Abnormal pupillary function Incontinence of bowel/bladder Tongue biting, mouth frothing, chewing/sucking Apnea/cyanosis Behavioral changes Post-ictal status (i.e., lethargy, confusion, headache, Todd's paralysis, aphasia, amnesia) Presence of any precipitating factors such as fever, hypoglycemia, emotional/physical stress If multiple seizures, any variation in activity or similarity of episodes Longest seizure-free period
Other neurological symptoms	Onset, duration, and progression Association to seizure activity Cerebrovascular accident Head trauma Space-occupying lesion

Patient history	Associated congenital anomalies Presence of cardiovascular or endocrine disease Previous exposure to toxins Previous infectious processes such as meningitis Previous drug or alcohol withdrawal Poor patient anticonvulsant compliance Acidosis/hypoxia
Metabolic nutritional habits	Inadequate nutrition Allergic reaction to foods Electrolyte imbalance Hypo- or hyperglycemia Fat/amino acid metabolism disorder
Presence and degree of physical, emotional, and psychological stress	High fever Physical exhaustion Sleep deprivation Family/environmental stresses
Patient's perceptions/reactions to diagnosis, treatment modalities; level of anxiety related to hospitalization	Denial Depression Anxiety Altered coping responses
Level of patient/family knowledge of seizure disorder, treatments, medication regimens, precipitating factors etc.	Incomplete knowledge Inadequate knowledge for informed consent or active participation
Alterations in function and image	Altered body image Fears of permanent disability or deficit, altered role in family, normal occupational performance, performance of activities of daily living, restrictions caused by disorder stigma reactions
Laboratory results	Potential for abnormal serum electrolyte levels, clotting profile, hypoxemia, hypercarbia, acid-base imbalance, drug toxicity, therapeutic anticonvulsant drug level, liver and renal function (to clear prescribed medications)
EEG • Routine hard-wire scalp electrodes • Nasopharyngeal or sphenoidal electrodes • Cortical strip electrodes/depth electrodes • Sleep-deprived	Abnormal frequency or amplitude of brain waves
Computed tomography (CT)	Visualization of neoplasm, infarction, cerebral hemorrhage, or abnormal vasculature may indicate etiology of seizures
Cerebral angiography	Cerebral blood flow is evaluated to detect presence of ischemic-induced seizures
Skull radiographs	Detects unilateral space occupying lesions, which may be source of seizure
Lumbar punctures	Abnormalities/infections of cerebrospinal fluid may contribute to seizures Glucose $<60\%$ of serum value Chloride <700 mg/dl LDH >7.2 U/ml of blood Presence of tumor cells Positive culture Protein >45 mg/dl

Magnetic resonance imaging (MRI)	Abnormal tissue in the intracranial vault
Psychological testing	Used to determine predisposing factors and coping
Electrocardiography (ECG)	Cardiovascular disorders may contribute to seizures

PLAN OF CARE

INTENSIVE PHASE

Seizures can occur in any setting. The section below describes the care of the patient with seizures in an ICU setting. However, unless the patient is in status epilepticus, it is unlikely that seizure is the primary admitting diagnosis for ICU hospitalization. Regardless of patient location, a siezuring patient requires an intensive level of care and monitoring until their condition stabilizes.

PATIENT CARE PRIORITIES	EXPECTED PATIENT OUTCOMES
Ineffective airway clearance *r/t* *Seizure activity* *Decreased LOC* *Retained secretions*	Patent airway Secretions managed/removed Improved ABG Adequate alveolar ventilation No evidence of cerebral damage secondary to ineffective oxygenation
High risk for injury *r/t* *Seizure activity* *Decreased LOC* *Aspiration*	Patient is protected from injury Optimal seizure control and safety maintenance
High risk for status epilepticus	Absence of complications Resolution or control of status epilepticus Adequate alveolar ventilation and perfusion Fluid and electrolyte balance within normal range
High risk for cardiovascular alterations *r/t* *Seizure activity* *Hypoxemia* *Anticonvulsant administration*	Normal cardiovascular function
Anxiety *r/t* *Seizure activity* *Hospitalization* *Threat of seizure* *Lack of knowledge, misconceptions* *Disturbances in self-concept*	Patient/family verbalizes concerns Patient/family demonstrates or verbalizes required knowledge and skills
High risk for impaired communication *r/t* *Intubation* *Seizure activity in post-ictal state*	Means for effective communication provided
High risk for impaired mobility *r/t status epilepticus*	Maintained, increased mobility Skin intact

INTERVENTIONS

Implement care for underlying disease process that causes seizures, if determined.

Loosen constricting clothing *to facilitate breathing*.

Support the head in a manner that allows secretions to drain out of the mouth *to avoid aspiration*.

Plan of Care (cont'd)

Observe for signs of airway obstruction.

Do not try to force objects/fingers into patient's mouth or restrain patient during seizure activity. *It is a myth that a patient may "swallow" the tongue.*

Insert airway if needed and teeth are not clenched.

Provide oropharyngeal suctioning *to maintain patent airway.*

Administer oxygen as needed.

Be prepared to assist with endotracheal intubation and emergency measures *if respiratory distress continues.*

Obtain arterial blood gases as needed. *ABG must be used to monitor acid-base balance in addition to oxygenation status.*

Bed is placed in low position and padded side rails are kept in up position *to provide seizure precaution.*

Call light within easy reach. *Patient may be able to call before onset of seizure activity.*

Keep drugs used for management of seizure activity immediately available.

Ongoing neurological assessment and observation.

Instruct patient to sit or lie in a safe place/position if a patient has an aura.

Protect head from injury during a seizure but do not restrain patient, *which may result in limb fractures or further injury.*

Do not leave patient during seizure but call for help *since further injury may occur.*

Observe seizure activity and document carefully. *Accurate description of seizure activity is vital in assisting with classification and management.*

Provide privacy if possible during the seizure.

Reorient following a seizure and provide slow, simple directions and commands. *The patient may be fatigued, frightened, and confused in the post-ictal phase.*

Monitor post-ictal state including LOC, vital signs, neurological status, patient discomfort, and adequate airway/ventilation.

Administer anticonvulsants as prescribed and monitor vital signs during and immediately after seizure. *Drugs given intravenously may have a hypotensive effect.*

Monitor anticonvulsant drug levels for therapeutic range maintenance *for adequate seizure control. Elevated levels of phenytoin (Dilantin) may induce serious cardiac dysrhythmias or neurological dysfunction; subtherapeutic levels may increase seizure activity.*

Prevent precipitating factors if possible, including hypoxia, hyperventilation, hypoglycemia, extreme fatigue, emotional stress.

Have emergency equipment and medications readily available if status epilepticus occurs.

Monitor vital signs, and respiratory, cardiovascular, and neurological status during status epilepticus q15min or as ordered.

Monitor ECG for any abnormalities during status epilepticus.

Provide analgesics and sedation with caution *to prevent masking neurological function, but as needed to maintain comfort.*

Administer prescribed anticonvulsants and monitor for effective seizure control and side effects.

Monitor I/O, weight, and serum electrolytes including calcium, glucose, phosphorus. *Disorders may potentiate or prolong status epilepticus occurrence.*

Monitor temperature q2h or prn for elevations and institute measures to maintain normothermia *since fever may potentiate seizures.*

Monitor urine for red or cola color *due to muscle cell breakdown and myoglobin in the bloodstream during or after status epilepticus, which may cause renal dysfunction.*

Administer diuretics and volume replacement as ordered.

Monitor for signs of dehydration or overhydration.

Enhance communication through alternative mechanism if intubated (e.g., writing board, letter board, or gesture messages).

Consider pressure-reducing mattress *to prevent skin breakdown secondary to immobilization if status epilepticus occurs.*

Plan of Care (cont'd)

Provide ongoing assessments of patient/family's level of anxiety.
Collaborate with physician in providing realistic information and assurance based on expected prognosis.
Assess and monitor level of understanding of seizure disorder and needed information and skills (i.e., seizure recognition, emergency management).
Explain pathophysiology, reasons for medications and treatments, anticipated course, and prognosis.
Interact with patient *to maintain orientation and instill hope.*
Assist with activities of daily living as necessary after a seizure.

INTERMEDIATE PHASE

Recovery will depend on the precipitating event of seizure activity. Once the diagnosis is made and the seizure activity is controlled, discharge planning and nursing care with interventions to achieve maximal independent function are implemented.

PATIENT CARE PRIORITIES	EXPECTED PATIENT OUTCOMES
Maintain effective airway (ongoing)	Patent airway
High risk for injury *r/t possible breakthrough seizure activity*	Patient is protected from injury Control of seizure activity is achieved Anticonvulsant serum levels are therapeutic without undue side effects
Anxiety *r/t* *Threat of future seizure activity* *Knowledge deficit* *Social stigma associated with seizures* *Altered life-style and restrictions*	Patient/family verbalizes concerns Patient/family demonstrates or verbalizes required knowledge and skills Patient/family describes means to achieve maximal independence in ADL, promote safety, and prevent complications

INTERVENTIONS

Monitor for seizure activity ongoing *to detect possible breakthrough seizure activity.*
Monitor anticonvulsant drug levels for therapeutic range, maintenance, and potential intolerable side effects.
Prevent precipitating factors of seizure activity.
Encourage verbalizations of fears, concerns, anger related to potential continuation of seizure disorder and management.
Encourage patient/family verbalization and questions regarding restrictions imposed by threat of potential seizure and effects on life-style. *Restrictions of prior activities or job responsibilities may include revocation of driver's license, a symbol of adult independence; constant supervision for certain activities; restrictions on operating dangerous equipment at work or home.*
Explore ways patient/family can cope with condition, and capabilities to maximize potential for independent functioning within confines of necessary safety precautions.
Explore patient's self-concept and its effect on interpersonal relationships.
Promote collaboration of patient/family and health team in achieving maximal control, independence, positive attitude, and as normal a life-style as possible.
Provide facts and realistic information to correct fallacies and misconceptions including dealing with "stigma" misperceptions.
Obtain orders for appropriate referrals such as social services, vocational training, National Epilepsy Foundation, community resources. *Underemployment/unemployment and isolation are often major problems for patients with seizures due to public misconceptions and fears.*

Plan of Care (cont'd)

Instruct, demonstrate, and evaluate patient's/family's knowledge acquisition and performance of needed information/skills such as:
- Knowledge of seizure disorder
- Patient's own specific seizure manifestations
- Identification and control of precipitating factors including excessive fatigue, poor nutrition, electrolyte imbalance, fever, emotional stress
- Necessary interventions if seizure occurs
- Restrictions necessitated by seizure disorder including dietary, activity, alcohol intake, seizure precautions
- Obtaining identification tag/bracelet and wallet card to alert others to needs
- Driving laws in the state of residence
- Pregnancy and parenting issues

Describe medication regimen and include information on:
- Name, purpose
- Route, dosage, frequency, times
- Side effects
- Special precautions necessary including drugs, foods, alcohol contraindicated or quantity regulated, factors potentiating/decreasing effects safety measures
- Blood testing required
- Scheduling of regimen to enhance compliance. A major reason for breakthrough seizure activity is lack of patient compliance.

Describe proper observations and method for recording if seizure occurs to monitor for increased activity and possible required medication adjustment.

Describe plan for follow-up care including purpose of appointments, when and where to go, who to see, specimens to bring, record of seizure activity to bring.

Describe signs/symptoms of seizure disorder requiring immediate medical attention.

TRANSITION TO DISCHARGE

As the patient moves from the intermediate phase and out of the critical care setting, the focus is to prepare the patient for discharge and return to a lifestyle as normal and functional as possible. This preparation builds on the care provided in the intermediate phase and involves further assistance to the patient to establish self-care regimes, adaptive techniques to live with potential for seizure activity, vocational productivity, and emotional and psychosocial adjustment. Social isolation is a problem that may be imposed internally or externally on a person with a seizure disorder. Long-term care involves efforts to encourage the patient and family to live as normal a life as possible despite the "invisible" disability.

REFERENCES

1. Alspach J: *Core curriculum for critical care nursing,* Philadelphia, 1991, WB Saunders, pp. 427-437.
2. Beare PG, Myers JL: *Principles and practice of adult health nursing,* St Louis, 1990 Mosby–Year Book.
3. Cammermeyer M, Ozuna J: Seizure disorders *AANN Core Curriculum,* ed 3, Ig1-Ig3, 1990.
4. Couldwell W, Weiss M: Critical care of the neurosurgical patient. In Berk J, Sampliner J, editors, *Handbook of critical care,* ed 3, Boston, 1990, Little, Brown, pp. 455-486.
5. Dolan JT: *Critical care nursing: clinical management through the nursing process,* Philadelphia, 1991, Davis.
6. Gauntlett P, Myers J: *Principles and practice of adult health nursing,* St Louis, 1990, Mosby–Year Book.
7. Greenberg MS: *Handbook of neurosurgery,* ed 2, Lakeland, Fla, 1991, Greenberg Graphics.
8. Gress D: Stopping seizures, *Emergency Medicine,* Jan, 1990.
9. Hilz MJ, et al: Isoflurane anesthesia in the treatment of convulsive status epilepticus, *J Neurol,* 239(3):135-137, 1992.
10. Marshall S, et al: *Neuroscience critical care pathophysiology and patient management,* Philadelphia, 1990, WB Saunders.
11. Mitchell M: *Neuroscience nursing—a nursing diagnosis approach,* Baltimore, 1989, Williams & Wilkins.
12. Netter F: *The CIBA collection of medical illustrations—nervous system, neurologic and neuromuscular disorders,* Summit, NJ, 1986, CIBA Pharmaceutical Co.
13. Niedermeyer E: *The epilepsies: diagnosis and management,* Baltimore, 1990, Urbain and Schwargenberg.
14. Pascual J, Cindad J, Berciano J: Role of lidocaine in managing status epilepticus, *J Neurol Neurosurg Psychiatry* 55(1):49-51, 1992.
15. Rusy K: Temporal lobectomy: a promising alternative, *J Neurosci Nurs* 23(5):48-52, 1991.
16. Rutecki P, Grossman R: Evaluation and surgical treatment of patients with complex partial seizures. In Appel S, editor, *Current neurology,* vol 10, Chicago, 1990, Year Book Medical Publishers.
17. Santilli N, Sierzant T: Advances in the treatment of epilepsy, *J Neurosci Nurs* 19(3):141-152, 1987.
18. *St Anthony's DRG Guidebook 1995,* Reston, Va, 1994, St Anthony.
19. Watson C: Status epilepticus—clincial features, pathophysiology, and treatment, *West J Med* 155(6):626-631, 1991.

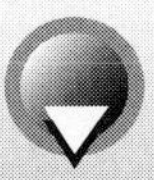

CLINICAL GUIDELINE

9

Meningitis/Encephalitis

Noreen Mocsny, MEd, RN

DESCRIPTION

Meningitis and encephalitis are common infectious processes of the central nervous system (CNS) that may occur as primary diseases, or as secondary complications of neurosurgery, certain diagnostic procedures, trauma, ear/sinus infections, systemic infections, and even certain drugs.[13]

Approximately 20,000 to 25,000 cases of bacterial meningitis occur annually in the United States.[13] About 70% of all cases occur in children under the age of 5.[1,5] More than 2000 deaths due to bacterial meningitis are reported in the United States every year.[10]

The mortality of fulminant meningococcal meningitis remains high primarily because patients are often in irreversible shock when treatment is instituted.[5] Most deaths occur within 24 to 48 hours of admission.[9,10]

A multitude of bacteria are capable of producing a suppurative meningitis. The most common forms of meningitis are Haemophilus, meningococcal, and pneumococcal.[4] Meningococcal meningitis frequently occurs in epidemic form and causes from 10% to 35% of cases in adults, and from 25% to 40% in children up to age 15.[5] Haemophilus influenzae, type B, is responsible for 40% to 60% of cases in children, but only 1% to 3% in adults and virtually none in infants.[5] Twelve thousand cases of H. influenzae meningitis are reported annually.[8] Pneumococcal meningitis predominates in adults.[4] Death rates associated with these three major meningeal pathogens have not changed over the past 30 years.[11]

A polysaccharide vaccine for one organism, groups A, C, Y, and W-B5 meningococci, has reduced the incidence of meningococcal infection among military recruits.[10] A vaccine for Haemophilus meningitis is licensed in the United States and recommended for routine use for all children at 18 months of age.[1]

Encephalitis is an inflammation of the tissues of the brain and spinal cord, resulting in altered function of various portions of these tissues.[4] It is usually caused by a viral infection, but the infectious agent may also be bacteria, fungi or parasites.[6]

Viral encephalitis is found worldwide and may be epidemic or sporadic and is usually associated with other viral diseases. Mosquito-borne encephalitides (equine and St. Louis encephalitis) are found in summer and early fall when mosquitoes are most plentiful, and in warm, moist climates. Amebic meningoencephalitis is found worldwide but is rare, and greatest occurrence is in previously healthy nonimmunocompromised children or young adults in warm climates and during summer.[2]

Few statistics are available regarding the overall incidence of encephalitis. Mortality rates for herpes simplex virus I can be 40% to 50%, whereas for other types it is much lower.[7] Neurological deficits occur in about one fifth of patients. Permanent neurologic sequelae are more common in herpes infections.[4] In mosquito-borne viral encephalitis, motor and mental disabilities (e.g., seizures, hydrocephalus, and mental retardation) are more likely to occur in infants and children.[4] In amebic meningoencephalitis, severe and rapidly fatal fulminating pyogenic cases may occur.[4] In encephalitis, death is most apt to occur in the first 72 hours when the cerebral edema is most pronounced, and in those who have progressed to the comatose state.[6]

PATHOPHYSIOLOGY

Meningitis

Meningitis is an inflammation of the arachnoid, the pia mater, and the intervening cerebrospinal fluid.[13] Since the subarachnoid space is continuous around the brain, spinal cord, and optic nerves, an infective agent gaining entry to any one part of the CNS may extend immediately to all of it, even its most remote recesses; therefore, meningitis is always cerebrospinal.[5] There is no direct invasion of cerebral tissue, but the subjacent brain becomes congested and edematous. The effectiveness of the pial barrier accounts for the fact that cerebral abscess does not complicate bacterial meningitis.[13]

The three most common bacteria causing meningitis (meningococcus, Haemophilus, and pneumococcus) are inhaled in mucous droplets from infected persons or carriers. These droplets invade the respiratory passages and are disseminated by way of the blood to meninges of the brain and spinal cord.[4] Direct routes to the CNS might include trauma or surgery. The infective agent or its toxin injures those structures that lie within the subarachnoid space (cranial and spinal roots) or ventricles (choroid plexuses) and adjacent to it (pial arteries and veins, peripheral fibers of optic nerves, subpial white matter of the spinal cord).[5]

Bacteria in the meninges elicit an inflammatory response and the production of an exudate consisting of leukocytes, fibrin, and bacteria in the subarachnoid space. With progress of the infection, the pia-arachnoid becomes thickened and adhesions may form. Adhesions at the base may interfere with the flow of CSF from the fourth ventricle and may produce hydrocephalus.[7]

Aseptic meningitis is a term used to describe a clinical symptomatology entity that can be produced by a variety of infective agents, the majority of which are viral. The common viruses involved are enteroviruses, paramyxovirus, and herpes simplex virus. Many times the specific virus cannot be isolated. Data that may assist in the differential diagnosis of viral meningitis include recent immunizations, past infectious diseases, animal bites, recent travel, epidemic outbreaks of meningitis, and seasonal/geographical distributions.

Encephalitis

Encephalitis is a syndrome characterized by an acute febrile stage; signs of meningeal involvement; and signs/symptoms of dysfunction of the cerebrum, brainstem, or cerebellum. Similar to meningitis, encephalitis may result from at least four causes: (1) a toxemia accompanying an infectious disease, (2) an allergic response to microbial antigens, (3) direct invasion by pathogens as a primary focal infection, or (4) direct invasion secondary to hematogenous dissemination from a primary focal infection elsewhere in the body.[4] The onset of neurological signs is commonly preceded by a prodromal illness of a few days duration with fever, headache, malaise, aches, sore throat, nausea, and vomiting resulting from organism invasion. The resultant pathological condition may include destruction of neurons, demyelination, diffuse edema, hemorrhage, and necrosis.

The list of signs and symptoms of viral encephalitis is long and varies depending on the particular invading organisms and the area of the brain involved.[6] The basic syndrome of viral encephalitis is characterized by an acute febrile stage; signs of meningeal involvement; and signs/symptoms of dysfunction of the cerebrum, brainstem, or cerebellum. The neurological dysfunctions may include weakness, aphasia, ataxia, involuntary movements, myoclonic jerks, ocular palsies, nystagmus, facial weakness, and coma.

When viruses attack the brain, they have a particular propensity for the frontal and temporal lobes. The brain becomes edematous, and necrotic areas with or without hemorrhage develop. Once the cerebral edema develops, it is pronounced, and abruptly increased intracranial pressure can result in temporal and/or brainstem herniation with coma, and changes in vital signs and respiratory patterns.[6]

Patients with herpes simplex encephalitis may also exhibit bizarre behavior, olfactory/gustatory hallucinations, temporal lobe seizures and anosmia. The frontal and temporal lobes are commonly affected. Herpes zoster (shingles) encephalitis produces an acute inflammatory reaction in spinal or cranial sensory ganglia, the posterior gray matter of the spinal cord, and adjacent meninges. Clinical signs include rash, pain, palsies, itching, and burning or tingling sensations.

LENGTH OF STAY/ANTICIPATED COURSE

The length of stay for a patient with bacterial meningitis or encephalitis averages 11.7 days in accord with DRG 20: Nervous system infection except viral meningitis.[12] The average length of stay for a patient with viral meningitis is 8.6 days, classified as DRG 21: Viral meningitis.[12] For those patients who survive the acute episode, neurological deficits are common and may include cognitive deficits (e.g., memory, reasoning), personality changes with dementia, seizure disorders, motor deficits, and dysphagia.[6] On the other hand, many recover completely. Minor disabilities may not require any special intervention because they will reverse themselves with time. Others require an aggressive rehabilitation plan.[6]

MANAGEMENT TRENDS AND CONTROVERSIES

Speed is of the essence, especially in acutely ill patients. Delays in diagnosis and therapy increase the likelihood of poor outcome. Drugs commonly administered for encephalitis include dexamethasone in tapering doses to reduce cerebral edema, histamine blockers to decrease gastric secretion and prevent development of gastric hemorrhage associated with the use of steroids, furosemide or mannitol for diuresis, phenytoin to prevent or control seizures, acetaminophen to control hyperthermia and headache.[6]

ASSESSMENT

PARAMETER	ANTICIPATED ALTERATION
Cerebral spinal fluid (CSF)	Varies with infectious agent. May be thick or thin and have plaquelike accumulations. Lymphocytes >5/mm^3 with largest percentage as neutrophils.[4]
Neurological status	Headache Nuchal rigidity Seizures
LOC	Anxious Communication impaired Restless Confusion Coma
Neurological Tests	
EEG	May show abnormalities such as slowing
CT scan	May show cerebral edema
Brain biopsy	May reveal causal agent
Meningeal signs	Stiff neck Positive Kernig sign *(resistance or pain while extending the knee after flexing the upper leg at the hip)* Positive Brudzinski sign *(when both the upper legs at the hips and the lower legs at the knees are flexed in response to passive flexion of the neck and head on the chest)*[6] Photophobia
Motor/sensory function	Opisthotonia *(marked retroflexion of the head, stiffness of the neck, and extension of the arms and legs)*
Cranial nerves	Ocular palsies (CN III, IV, VI) Facial paresis (CN VII) Decreased visual abilities (CN II) Deafness and vertigo (CN VIII) Pupils unequal, sluggish (CN III) Ptosis and diplopia (CN III)
Systemic	Vomiting, tachycardia, respiratory difficulties, dysrhythmia *related to medullary involvement*
Skin	Purpuric lesions/petechial rash
Cardiovascular Status	
HR	Bradycardia <60 bpm
Hematology	
• WBC	Elevated: >10,000/mm^3
• Erythrocyte sedimentation rate (ESR)	Increased: >15 to 20 mm/hr
• Antibody detection	Diagnostic for organism
• Toxin screens	May be elevated
Culture and sensitivity including blood, sputum, urine, nasal secretions, wound/sinus drainage, CSF	Diagnostic for specific organism

PLAN OF CARE

INTENSIVE PHASE

Meningitis/encephalitis is uncommon. Patients with this diagnosis may develop needs that can be cared for only in an ICU. Some patients in an ICU may experience this as a secondary ICU diagnosis, perhaps as a complication of open traumatic brain injury. The section below describes the intensive care of the patient even if not admitted to an ICU.

PATIENT CARE PRIORITIES	EXPECTED PATIENT OUTCOMES
Increased ICP *r/t infectious or viral process*	ICP: WNL HR: WNL Absence of nausea, vomiting
Decline in neurological status *r/t* *Acute infection-swelling* *Inflammatory process/hydrocephalus*	Maximal neurological functioning
High risk for infection progression *r/t underlying pathology or difficulty matching therapy to cause*	Resolution of infection
High risk for injury *r/t* *Altered neurological status* *Depressed/altered LOC* *Restlessness, agitation, irritability* *Seizures*	Safe environment Absence of injuries Absence or control of seizures
Ineffective breathing pattern *r/t CNS dysfunction*	Patent airway Alveolar ventilation and perfusion WNL RR: WNL

INTERVENTIONS

Contact the hospital infection control department for information on the possible need for isolation *since precautions to prevent the spreading of the disease depend on the type of invading organism and the stage of illness.*

Prevent hypoxia, hypercapnia, fever, Valsalva maneuver, *which increase intracranial pressure.*

Maintain patent airway *to prevent hypoxia with resultant increased ICP.*

Monitor neurological status continuously *to detect deterioration and prevent complications.*

Monitor for bradycardia and assess for any correlation with neurological deterioration *as clinical signs of increased ICP.*

Maintain temperature within normal range *to avoid increased cerebral metabolism associated with hyperthermia.*

Monitor ventricular drainage system *to maintain patency/sterility of system.*

Maintain continuous ICP monitoring *to detect change due to treatment and interventions.*

Administer antibiotics as ordered *to prevent complications/mortality.*

INTERMEDIATE PHASE

As the patient stabilizes and no longer requires continuous monitoring, transfer to an intermediate or general unit may occur. Regular assessment will continue to be required. In addition, reconditioning and possible rehabilitation will be required, especially if neurological complications have occurred.

PATIENT CARE PRIORITIES	EXPECTED PATIENT OUTCOMES
High risk for GI complications *r/t CNS factors, stress, steroid administration*	Absence or resolution of GI bleeding, stress ulceration, S/S of stress Able to tolerate oral intake

Plan of Care (cont'd)

High risk for neurological deficit *r/t infectious/viral trauma*	Maximal neurological functioning
Fears, anxiety, or anger *r/t neurological deficit and possible alterations in life-style*	Maximal independence in ADL within capabilities Patient/family able to verbalize concerns Patient/family demonstrate adaptive coping behavior

INTERVENTIONS

Collaborate with physical/occupational therapy *to increase strength and return to ADL.*
Ensure adequate sleep/rest periods *to promote physical healing and strength.*
Check stools for occult blood, *which would indicate gastrointestinal bleeding.*
Encourage patient/family to verbalize fears, questions, and concerns *to facilitate determination of effective coping strategies.*
Instruct patient/family in self-care ADL as indicated.
Explain all tests, procedures, and medications *to alleviate fears.*

TRANSITION TO DISCHARGE

The specific rehabilitative needs of a patient depend on the degree of disability resulting from the meningitis or encephalitis. With many, there is no residual effect, but sequelae of encephalitis may include mental deterioration, paralysis, and possible convulsive disorders. Postmeningitis sequelae may include visual impairment, optic neuritis, deafness, personality change, headache, seizure activity, paresis or paralysis, hydrocephalus, pneumonia and endocarditis.[4]

A team approach with team conferences including the patient/family is most effective in planning discharge. Nursing responsibilities may include patient/family teaching in ADL, medications, equipment or therapeutic devices, and reportable symptoms. In addition, teaching the need for periodic evaluation and long-term physical therapy and identifying potential coping resources are recommended.[4]

REFERENCES

1. Benenson AS, editor: *Control of communicable disease in man,* ed 15, New York, 1990, American Public Health Association, pp 154, 277-289.
2. Centers for Disease Control: Primary amebic meningoencephalitis—North Carolina, 1991, *Morb and Mortal Wkly Rep* 41(25):437-440, 1992.
3. Chaudhry HJ, Cunha BA: Drug-induced aseptic meningitis, *Postgrad Med* 90(7):65-70, 1991.
4. Grimes D: *Infectious diseases,* St Louis, 1991, Mosby–Year Book, pp. 52-65.
5. Harter DH, Petersdorf RG: Bacterial meningitis and brain abscess. In Wilson JD, et al, editors: *Harrison's principles of internal medicine,* ed 12, New York, 1991, McGraw-Hill, pp 2023-2027.
6. Hickey JV: *The clinical practice of neurological and neurosurgical nursing,* ed 3, Philadelphia, 1992, JB Lippincott, pp 605-618.
7. Ignatavicius D, Bayne MV: Interventions for clients with CNS disorders. In *Medical-surgical nursing,* Philadelphia, 1991, WB Saunders, pp 897-903.
8. Janai H, Stutman HR, Marks MI: Invasive Haemophilus influenzae type b infections: a continuing challenge, *Am J Infect Control* 18(3):160-166, 1990.
9. Kaiser AB, McGee AZ: Central nervous system infections. In Shoemaker WC, editor: *Textbook of critical care,* ed 2, Philadelphia, 1989, WB Saunders, pp 830-840.
10. Miller JR, Jubelt B: Infections of the nervous system: bacterial infections. In Rowland LP, editor: *Merritt's textbook of neurology,* ed 8, Philadelphia, 1989, Lea and Febiger, pp 63-68.
11. Scheld WM: New approach to lowering meningitis deaths uses steroids with antibiotics, *J Infect Dis* 3(1):3, 1992.
12. *St Anthony's DRG guidebook 1995,* Reston, Va, 1994, St Anthony.
13. Swartz MN: Bacterial meningitis. In Wyngaarden JB, Smith LH, Bennett JC, editors: *Cecil textbook of medicine,* ed 19, Philadelphia, 1992, WB Saunders, pp 1655-1667.

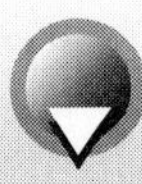

CLINICAL GUIDELINE

10

Spinal Cord Trauma

Teresa Heise Halloran, MSN, RN, CCRN

DESCRIPTION

Spinal cord trauma (SCT) is the result of a combination of vector forces (mechanism of injury) and the pathophysiological destruction of neuronal tissue within the spinal cord. The protective mechanisms of the vertebral column, spinous ligaments, meninges, and surrounding tissue are unable to absorb the magnitude of force and prevent SCT. The most frequent sites of SCT are the lower cervical region (C4 to C7 and T1) and the area of the thoracolumbar junction (T12, L1, and L2).[11] The majority of SCT patients admitted to critical care units are those with acute cervical injuries.

It is estimated that the prevalence of SCT is 12.4 to 53.4 per million population.[13] Approximately 30% of individuals with these injuries will die before reaching the hospital and another 10% will die during hospitalization. Three risk factors have been associated with this injury: age, sex, and alcohol/drug use. Males between the ages of 20 to 30 have a higher incidence of SCT than females. The average age at the time of injury ranges from 15 to 35 years. Causative factors include motor vehicle accidents, motorcycles, falls, sports injuries, diving accidents, and gunshot wounds.[15] Primary prevention strategies such as seat belt use, maintaining highway speed limits, motorcycle helmets, and educating the public of the consequences of drinking and driving are our only means to decrease the incidence of SCT. The socioeconomic impact of SCT is estimated at $2.4 billion per year. There is currently an expanding population of individuals with SCT who require life-long support and treatment, ranging from acute care management to rehabilitation. The cause of death in SCT, if not directly related to the level of spinal cord involvement at the time of injury, is generally due to pulmonary complications and infection.

PATHOPHYSIOLOGY

Clinically, the causative factor or force of cervical SCT can be inferred on the basis of historic, clinical, and radiologic evidence. A classification scheme for the mechanism of injury is outlined in the following Box. Flexion injuries are caused by forward rotation of a cervical vertebra. Clinically, the flexion teardrop fracture is the most devastating of all flexion injuries, as it is associated with the anterior cord syndrome. Simultaneous flexion and rotation is associated with the dislocation of a facet joint at one level on the side opposite that of the direction of rotation.

A second force-of-injury type is vertical compression, also known as axial loading. The force is usually transmitted to the spine from a blow to the top of the skull, as seen with a diving injury.

Hyperextension injuries, usually a result of a fall, are the opposite of flexion injuries. The head and cervical spine are propelled into hyperextension as a result of a direct posterior force on the face.[10]

The extent of injury to the spinal cord after trauma depends on the ability of the vertebral column to dissipate the energy generated by the mechanism of energy. The mechanism for diminished perfusion of the spinal cord after injury is still unclear. The final common pathway for necrosis of neurons within the spinal cord is hypoxia.[12] Microangiographic studies of experimental cord injury reveal necrosis of the central gray matter within 4 hours. Vasogenic edema spreads into the surrounding white matter. The microvasculature remains normal although neuronal and axonal degeneration is apparent by 8 hours.[5,8] Clinically, cord edema may change the baseline neurologic examination findings, especially within the first 4 hours after injury. Respiratory

Cervical Spine Injuries by Mechanism of Injury

I. Flexion
- Anterior subluxation (hyperflexion sprain)
- Bilateral interfacetal dislocation
- Simple wedge (compression) fracture
- Clay-shovelar fracture
- Flexion teardrop fracture

II. Flexion-rotation
- Unilateral interfacetal dislocation

III. Extension-rotation
- Pillar fracture

IV. Vertical compression
- Jefferson bursting fracture of atlas (C1)
- Burst fracture

V. Hyperextension
- Hyperextension dislocation
- Avulsion fracture of anterior arch of atlas
- Extension teardrop fracture of axis (C2)
- Fracture of posterior arch of atlas
- Laminar fracture
- Traumatic spondylolisthesis (hangman's fracture)
- Hyperextension fracture-dislocation

VI. Lateral flexion
- Uncinate process fracture

VII. Diverse or imprecisely understood mechanisms
- Atlanto-occipital disassociation (C1)
- Odontoid fractures (C2)

failure can result from ascending cord edema in the cervical region.

After spinal cord necrosis occurs, complete lesions or incomplete syndromes represent the clinical presentation. Complete cord lesions result in total loss of sensory and motor function below the level of the lesion. Incomplete lesions result in three syndromes: central cord, anterior cord, and Brown Sequard syndrome, described below. The first clinical sign of an incomplete lesion is often described as sacral sparing or sensation in the perineal area. Some neurologic function ultimately may return.

Central cord syndrome is characterized by microscopic hemorrhage and edema to the central cord. There is motor weakness in both the upper and lower extremities, but the weakness is much greater in the upper extremities. Sensory dysfunction varies, generally more pronounced in the upper extremities. Lower-extremity reflexes may be hyperactive. Bladder dysfunction is common.

Anterior cord syndrome is characterized by motor paralysis below the level of the injury. Sensory function of touch, position, and vibration remain intact if the posterior cord remains uninjured.

Brown Sequard syndrome occurs as a result of damage to one side of the spinal cord. The patient will have loss of voluntary motor function, and position and vibration sense on the same side (ipsilateral) of the injury, accompanied by loss of pain, temperature, and touch on the opposite side (contralateral) of injury.

Spinal Shock

Spinal shock is the manifestation of a complete lesion. With high cord injury level, there is a significant risk of cardiovascular instability. This is due to loss of sympathetic or vasomotor tone. Cervical spinal shock is characterized by hypotension because of a decrease in systemic vascular resistance and dilatation of capacitance vessels. Bradycardia results from loss of sympathetic innervation and cardioaccelerator reflexes. Depressed left ventricular function also occurs and is thought to be due to high levels of circulating beta-endorphins.[7] Other clinical signs and symptoms of spinal shock include flaccid paralysis; loss of sensory and spinal reflexes below the level of the lesion; bowel and bladder dysfunction; inability to perspire below level of injury, therefore leading to temperature instability and warm, dry extremities. The duration of spinal shock is variable, from a range of 2 days to several months. The return of reflex activity generally indicates resolution.

After resolution of spinal shock, high cord injuries are at risk for autonomic dysreflexia due to unchecked reflex sympathetic discharge. The clinical presentation includes a pounding headache, severe hypertension, reflex bradycardia, and vasodilation above the level of the lesion. The treatment of this life-threatening complication requires elimination of the cause of the sympathetic discharge. Common causes are a distended bladder or bowel, skin pressure from positioning, tight clothing and splints, or other GI stimuli such as enemas.[4]

LENGTH OF STAY / ANTICIPATED COURSE

Length of stay and the anticipated course of treatment are dependent on the level of injury, stabilization of the injury, degree of ventilatory compromise with need for mechanical ventilation, hemodynamic instability of spinal shock, and the development of complications. The risk of complications such as deep-vein thrombosis, pulmonary infections, and decubiti increases with the length of immobility. As a result, hospitalization may range from 1 week to 3 months with an average rehabilitation time of 2 months. The acute care phase of SCT averages 11 days for surgical cases as noted in DRG 4: Spinal procedures, and 8.8 days for medically managed cases as per DRG 9: Spinal disorders and injuries.[14] The increased life expectancy of SCT patients is a testimony to improved medical and nursing care.

MANAGEMENT TRENDS AND CONTROVERSIES

Initial medical management focuses on airway, breathing, and circulation. If required, intubation of the airway is managed with normal spinal alignment, rather than hyperextension. Next, stabilization of the spinal column can be considered. This can be achieved through the use of tongs or a halo device. The halo's advantage is that it allows early mobilization of the patient; tongs require bed rest. Surgical interventions for permanent stabilization can be considered once the risk of further cord injury or ischemia due to edema is past, usually 10 to 14 days postinjury.

Methylprednisolone for the treatment of acute spinal cord injury has been reevaluated by Bracken and coworkers.[3] When given within 8 hours after injury, methylprednisolone was found to be associated with an improved neurologic recovery in patients with complete and incomplete spinal cord injury. An initial bolus of 30 mg/kg is given over 15 minutes. A continuous infusion of 5.4 mg/kg × 23 hr is started within 45 minutes after completion of the bolus dose. A naloxone dose of 5.4 mg/kg and a maintenance dose of 4.0 mg/kg/hr was used as an additional treatment parameter. The naloxone results showed no improvement in neurologic recovery. The findings were considered significant by the National Institute of Neurologic Disorders and Stroke of the National Institutes of Health. The institutes notified physicians in an April 1990 clinical alert to expedite this important clinical information.

Further treatment for SCT is concerned with prevention of complications and maintenance of function. Potential complications pertinent to the acute injury and recovery periods include deep-vein thrombosis and pulmonary dysfunction and infection.

Deep-vein thrombosis (DVT) is a common complication of spinal cord injury. Nursing care plans frequently suggest the use of serial leg measurements to establish clinical diagnosis of DVT in spite of extensive studies showing that clinical signs and symptoms have a specificity and sensitivity hardly better than chance. Factors contributing to this difficulty include premorbid leg asymmetry, atrophy of the legs after spinal cord injury, true changes in circumference due to factors other than DVT, and lack of measurement reliability.[16] Primary prevention appears to be the best method to reduce incidence of this complication.

TABLE 10-1 Complete Cervical Cord Lesions According to Specific Vertebral Level

C1 to C4	Quadriplegia with total loss of respiratory function
C4 to C5	Quadriplegia with possible phrenic nerve involvement
C5 to C6	Quadriplegia with gross arm movements; sparing of diaphragm leads to diaphragmatic breathing
C6 to C7	Quadriplegia with biceps muscles intact; diaphragmatic breathing
C7 to C8	Quadriplegia with triceps and biceps intact, no function of intrinsic hand muscles; diaphragmatic breathing
T1 to L2	Paraplegia with loss of varying amounts of intercostal and abdominal muscle function
Below L2	Cauda equina injury; mixed picture of motor-sensory loss, bowel and bladder dysfunction

One recommendation for preventive measures of pulmonary complications is the use of a kinetic treatment table (KTT). One study compared the difference between the KTT and a wedge device. Results indicate that those clients treated with the KTT experienced a lower incidence of pulmonary infection and required less time on mechanical ventilation. Length of ICU stay and hospitalization were not significantly influenced.[2]

Microprocessor computer technology has contributed to improvement in prosthetic devices and potential implantation for innervated to paralyzed muscles. Although not curative, the future of this technology can improve the quality of life in the rehabilitation phase.

ASSESSMENT

PARAMETER	ANTICIPATED ALTERATION
Airway	Decreased cough effort and hypoventilation *due to level of injury*
Chest excursion, tidal volume	Loss of intercostal muscle function with cervical injury results in decreased spontaneous tidal volume Asymmetry secondary to incomplete lesions
ABG	Increased Pa_{CO_2}, decreased pH. Hypoxemia may result as hypoventilation worsens *secondary to decreased use of intercostal or diaphragmatic muscles r/t level of injury.*
Motor function	Complete injuries: loss of all movement below the level of cord injury. This includes loss of diaphragmatic effort with injuries at C5 or higher (Table 10-1). Incomplete injuries: varies, see text

Sensory function	Complete injuries: loss of all sensation (touch, proprioception, temperature, vibration, and pressure) below the level of cord injury Incomplete injuries: varies, see text
LOC	Normal, unless associated with decreased cerebral perfusion or head trauma
Pain	Usually at the level of the injury
BP	Hypotension *due to venous pooling and loss of vasoconstriction*
HR	Bradycardia *due to loss of sympathetic innervation*
Temperature	Hypothermia/hyperthermia *due to loss of neurogenic control of peripheral blood vessels*

PLAN OF CARE

INTENSIVE PHASE

Acute cervical spinal trauma nearly always requires an intensive care phase of hospitalization, usually within an ICU. Thoracic and lumbar injuries are less likely to require intensive level care; thus they are not described in this section.

PATIENT CARE PRIORITIES	EXPECTED PATIENT OUTCOMES
Neurologic dysfunction *r/t spinal instability*	Maintenance or improvement of neurologic function. Adequate relief of pain.
Impaired physical mobility *r/t loss of innervation*	Absence of contractures. Absence of deep-vein thrombosis, pulmonary emboli, pulmonary complications.
High risk for impairment of skin integrity *r/t loss of sensation*	Intact skin
Decreased tissue perfusion *r/t autonomic dysfunction*	Absence of orthostatic hypotension MAP ≥70 mm Hg HR ≥60 bpm UO ≥30 cc/min Immediate recognition/treatment of autonomic dysreflexia Maintenance of LOC
Ineffective airway clearance *r/t* *Intubation* *Mechanical ventilation* *Retained secretions* *Reduced muscular innervation*	Clear breath sounds Patent airway Optimal $Paco_2$ Adequate tidal volume, NIF Effective cough
Impaired gas exchange	Pao_2 ≥60 mm Hg on room air
Ventilation/perfusion mismatch *r/t intrapulmonary shunting and/or alveolar collapse*	Sao_2 greater than 92% Arterial/alveolar ratio ≥0.6 Breath sounds in all lung fields
Inadequate nutrition *r/t* *Intubation* *Decreased gastric motility* *Hypermetabolic state*	Adequate caloric/po intake per calorimetry Positive nitrogen balance: 1.5 to 2.5 gm/kg/day of protein
Alteration in bowel elimination *r/t paralytic ileus or altered bowel innervation*	Gastric motility Established bowel program Absence of impaction
Alteration in urinary elimination *r/t loss of innervation to bladder*	Bladder elimination program established Absence of incontinence and urinary tract infection

Plan of Care (cont'd)

Sexual dysfunction *r/t loss of innervation or autonomic function*	Access to information and resources to address concerns about sexual function
Grieving *r/t loss of function and resultant life-style changes*	Express grief Experience success with short-term goals
Alteration in family process *r/t crisis and potential role changes*	Family remain intact Reintegration of self within family structure
Disturbance in self-concept *r/t loss of function*	Begin to develop new plans and goals

INTERVENTIONS

Maintain patent airway

Assess motor and sensory function every hour. *Changes from admission assessment will assist to identify incomplete syndromes, ascending cord edema, and impending ventilatory failure.*

Maintain cervical alignment at all times with tongs/weights or halo vest. *Surgical intervention and decompression of the cord is indicated in partial cord injuries if there is spinal cord compression from bone, disk, or ligamentous tissue. Surgical stabilization is required for vertebral subluxation greater than 3.5 mm or angulation of a vertebra greater than 11 degrees.*

Measure respiratory parameters q2h prn: vital capacity, tidal volume, negative inspiratory force. *Alveolar ventilation may be affected by retained secretions, coexistent chest injuries, or paralytic ileus and gastric distention.*

Monitor ABG and correlate with pulse oximetry (SpO_2) or transcutaneous monitoring *to detect hypoventilation from inadequate innervation, due to level of injury or cord edema.*

Monitor patient's response to mechanical ventilation.

Suction as necessary per assessment. Preoxygenate before each suction pass and consider hyperinflation.

Monitor for vasovagal reflex, which may result in cardiac arrest *due to vagal stimulation and hypoxia.*

Stop any activity associated with >10% decrease in heart rate.

Teach quadriplegics assisted-coughing technique.

Administer chest physiotherapy.

Consider use of kinetic treatment table.

Monitor for hypotension and administer fluids or vasopressor therapy as ordered. *Loss of vasomotor tone and venous pooling will decrease venous return, potentially decreasing CO. Also, a lack of compensatory vasoconstriction compromises perfusion state.*

Monitor HR and institute measures to relieve bradycardia *resulting from loss of sympathetic innervation.*

Use gradual elevation of head of bed, abdominal binder, and pneumatic compression stockings *to avoid orthostatic hypotension with position changes. Abrupt changes in backrest position will further impede venous return.*

Administer deep-vein thrombosis prophylaxis; pneumatic compression stockings or anticoagulant therapy. Note sudden onset of dyspnea or respiratory failure.

Begin physical therapy program as soon as patient is hemodynamically stable and spinal stabilization is achieved.

Maintain body and environmental temperature. *Temperature regulation is altered due to lack of SNS innervation, resulting in loss of appropriate perspiration and shivering.*

Auscultate bowel sounds and monitor for abdominal distention.

Utilize NG decompression if absent bowel sounds. *Loss of peristalsis may lead to paralytic ileus.*

Evaluate gastric pH and presence of occult blood *due to prevalence of stress ulcers r/t steroid or anticoagulant therapy and hypersecretion of HCl and pepsin, which erodes the gastric mucosal barrier.*

Plan of Care (cont'd)

Initiate tube feedings with return of peristalsis. TPN may be initiated within 3 days postinjury if enteral feeding is contraindicated. *Trauma patients have a 25% to 40% increase in basal energy expenditure. Sepsis will further increase nutritional requirements.*

Check for presence of impaction.

Initiate bowel training program, stool softeners, or suppositories within first 72 hours of injury.

Palpate bladder for distention.

Institute intermittent catheterizations (when hemodynamically stable) q4h to q6h to maintain a bladder volume of 500 cc or less. *Intermittent catheterization lessens the risk of urinary tract infections and avoids bladder overdistention.*

Monitor I/O.

Monitor for signs and symptoms of infection: elevated temperature and leukocytosis; changes in color, odor, and character of urine.

Inspect all skin surfaces, including under Halo vest and back of head. Inspect tong sites every shift for redness and drainage, and clean with normal saline. *Changes in peripheral circulation, altered temperature regulation, and loss of sensation below level of injury contribute to risk of skin impairment.*

Protect pressure points.

Protect from injury; e.g., falls, positioning, and burns *due to sensory and motor deficits.*

Provide means to summon help, such as a special sensitivity call light to promote the patient's sense of control and reduce fear of being left alone. Enhance trust by answering promptly.

Allow expression of emotions, including loss, anger, despair, and rage.

Set limits on acting out or manipulative behavior when necessary, but in context with the importance of supporting expression of angry feelings.

Provide accurate information about treatment plan.

Encourage patient to take control when possible; i.e., diversional activities, diet choices, schedule of daily care routines.

Emphasize small victories and incremental progress.

Assess for extended denial or dysfunctional grieving; consult other resources for assistance. *Prolonged intubation after SCT may lead to depression and false perception of reality, as communication of thoughts and feelings is delayed.*

Help patient openly discuss what life was like before loss.

Determine the impact of the loss and of changes in bodily functions for the patient and family.

Provide touch where sensation is present.

Use prism glasses *to facilitate interaction with the environment and enhance sense of safety and control.*

Bolster the family's feelings of competence by early structured involvement in care activities. *Including the family at an early stage will help the family regain control and deal with the loss.*

Provide hope within the framework of injury and potential for rehabilitation.

Facilitate grieving. *The longer grieving is delayed, the more difficult the emotional work and the greater the depression.*

Validate coping strategies that benefited patient and family in the past and identify new coping behaviors.

INTERMEDIATE PHASE

Resolution of spinal shock is exhibited as the return of perianal reflexes, appearance of involuntary spastic movement, and return of deep-tendon reflexes. The cardiovascular status is increasingly stable. The patient with cervical injury is now at greater risk for autonomic

Plan of Care (cont'd)

dysreflexia. If pulmonary complications, such as aspiration pneumonitis, atelectasis, pneumonia, and/or sepsis, have been minimized, the patient may be transferred directly to a rehabilitation program. If the patient remains on a ventilator and long-term weaning is necessary, the patient may be transferred to an intermediate specialized care unit or remain in the ICU.

SCT patients experience a dramatic life-threatening event. It is not uncommon for the first stage of the grieving process, shock-denial, to be in process as the patient enters the intermediate phase. Crisis intervention is a useful model to provide emotional support for families. Crisis intervention focuses on short-term, immediate intervention with the intention of restoring the individual and/or family to their pre-crisis level of functioning or possibly even to a higher functional level.[6]

PATIENT CARE PRIORITIES	EXPECTED PATIENT OUTCOMES
Potential for autonomic hyperreflexia *r/t SCT*	Absence of elevated BP, HR
Potential for secondary complications *r/t immobility*	Intact skin Absence of pulmonary complications, UTIs Demonstrates ability to perform skin checks and weight shifts independently
Wean from mechanical ventilation	Maintain spontaneous ventilation
High risk for ineffective coping *r/t magnitude of physical changes and life-style changes needed*	Develop a sense of trust with health care team Move through the shock-denial stage of grieving Identify a plan for the future

INTERVENTIONS

Maintain intensive phase interventions for immobility. *Patient is still at risk for DVT, pulmonary complications, decubitus, and urinary tract infections.*
Monitor for clinical signs of hypertension: facial flushing, tachycardia.
Recognize and intervene for precipitating factors of autonomic dysreflexia.
Treat emergent hypertension per order and remove causative factors.
Coordinate care with multidisciplinary team.
Develop teaching plan for patient and family as a multidisciplinary effort. Include social services, psychiatric counselor, physical therapy, occupational therapy, and spiritual advisor.
Assess patient's ability to perform activities of daily living.
Assess family's requirements for assistance *to proactively plan for discharge.*
Allow independent decision-making/activity whenever possible *to facilitate coping and sense of control.*
Help patient/family redefine life goals. Realign roles according to abilities and interests.
Reinforce established/new coping behaviors.

TRANSITION TO DISCHARGE

The patient's level of injury and rehabilitation potential will greatly influence the teaching required prior to discharge. The primary goal of rehabilitation is to assist the patient and family to provide self-care at the maximal functional level. Over 89% of people with spinal cord injuries will return to their homes.[1]

This success is dependent on acquiring new knowledge and optimizing self-care activity. Teaching components may include, but are not limited to, skin care, fluid and diet management, bowel and bladder care, sexual functioning, home safety factors, and equipment.[9] The outcome is to enable the patient to live as satisfactory and fulfilling a life as possible. The critical care nurse is key to implementing the beginning plan of achieving success in short-term goals and integrating the patient, family, and significant others into the multidisciplinary health care team.[13]

REFERENCES

1. Belbrook G, Beer NI, McLaren RK: Preventive measures in the tertiary care of spinal cord-injured people, *Paraplegia* 23:69, 1985.
2. Borkowski C: A comparison of pulmonary complications in spinal cord-injured patients treated with two modes of spinal immobilization, *J Neurosci Nurs* 21:79, 1989.
3. Bracken MB, et al: A randomized, controlled trial of methylprednisolone or naloxone in the treatment of acute spinal-cord injury, *New Engl J Med* 322:1405-1411, 1990.
4. Erickson R: Autonomic hyperreflexia: pathophysiology and medical management, *Arch Phys Med Rehabil* 61:431, 1980.
5. Fairholm DJ, Turnbull IM: Microangiographic study of experimental spinal cord injuries, *J Neurosurg* 216:473, 1971.
6. Friedman-Campbell M, Hart CA: Theoretical strategies and nursing interventions to promote psychosocial adaptation to spinal cord injuries and disability, *J Neurosci Nurs* 16:335, 1984.
7. Gilbert J: Critical care management of the patient with acute spinal cord injury, *Crit Care Clin* 3:550, 1987.
8. Griffiths IR: Vasogenic edema following acute and chronic spinal cord compression in the dog, *J Neurosurg* 42:155, 1975.
9. Hamric A: A teaching tool for spinal cord injured patients, *J Neurosci Nurs* 13:234, 1981.
10. Harris J, Edeiken-Monroe E, Kopaniky D: A practical classification of acute cervical spine injuries, 17:15-38, *Orthop Clin North Am* 1986.
11. Hughes M: Critical care nursing for the patient with a spinal cord injury, *Critical Care Nursing Clinics of North America* 2:33-40, 1990.
12. Kelly DL, Lassister KRL, Calogero JA: Effects of local hypothermia and tissue oxygen studies in experimental paraplegia, *J Neurosurg* 33:554, 1970.
13. Richmond T: Spinal cord injury, *Nurs Clin North Am* 25:57, 1990.
14. *St Anthony's DRG guidebook 1995,* Reston, Va, 1994, St Anthony.
15. Stover SL, Find PR: *Spinal cord injury: the facts and figures,* Birmingham, Ala, 1986, University of Alabama.
16. Swarczinski C, Dijkers M: The value of serial leg measurements for monitoring deep-vein thrombosis in spinal cord injury, *J Neurosci Nurs* 23:306, 1991.
17. Young W, Bracken MB: The second national acute spinal cord injury study, *J Neurotrauma* 9(suppl 1):S 397-405, 1992.

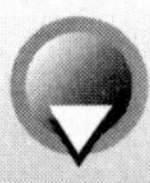

CLINICAL GUIDELINE

11

Cervical Spine Laminectomy

Peter A. Gonzalez, BSN, RN

DESCRIPTION

Laminectomy is the total or partial removal of the lamina, which is the posterior, protective element of the spine. This surgical technique is designed to limit disease processes, disability, and pain. The procedure allows decompression of the spinal cord from various pathological events. Decompression involves removal of pathology that acts to compress, invade, and infiltrate the nervous tissue, bone, and cartilage. Indications include traumatic injuries, disc herniation common to cervical and lumbar spine,[4] tumor excision, degenerative disc disease, and other stenotic conditions. Two major approaches are used: the standard posterior approach, and the anterior approach developed by Cloward and others in the early 1960s.[1] Figure 11-1 helps illustrate these approaches by describing anatomical landmarks in the vertebral column.

Posterior approach to the cervical spine involves a midline incision over the spinous process and dissection of tissue, bone, and cartilage, allowing visualization by way of the posterior spinal cord. Complications include bleeding, edema, and infection. Anterior approach involves entry to the cervical spine by way of dissection of tissue on either side of the neck. All or a portion of the vertebral body and cartilage of the spine are removed. This allows visualization of anterior structures. Since the lamina are not removed, this newer procedure does not constitute a laminectomy. The severity of complications arise from the proximity of the trachea, esophagus, vascular structures, and musculature of the neck to the surgical site. Diseased intervertebral discs, osteophytes, and anterior cord pathology can be appreciated from either approach.

Fusion of the cervical spine may or may not be performed with a laminectomy. Fusion involves use of autologous bone grafting, screws, plates and acrylic compounds as stabilizing elements. Stabilization prevents or minimizes rotation, flexion, extension, and lateral movement that is normal to the spine. Halo apparatus may be required in the postoperative phase for stabilization of the spine. Stabilization enhances mobility, safety, and patient recovery.

PATHOPHYSIOLOGY

The age range for patients undergoing cervical laminectomy varies with the underlying pathology. Degenerative conditions generally affect those 55 and older. Trauma impacts on those 15 to 30 years of age.[9]

The cervical spine is affected by encroachment from gradual deterioration, hypertrophy, and calcification of bone and cartilage or acutely, from trauma. The canal space becomes narrowed (Parke, 1988), resulting in impingement of nerve roots and pain, or impairment of impulse conduction and parasthesia or paralysis.

Another pathology associated with cervical laminectomy is the posterior herniation of a disc's nucleus pulposus. Such herniation may be caused by trauma, lifting, and strain injuries. Mechanisms of injury during trauma can produce hyperextension, hyperflexion, dislocation, and compression injuries to the vertebral elements. Traction is used initially to stabilize the spinal column. Surgical intervention is usually postponed until the edema resolves and the patient's condition permits. The result of these pathologies can be damage to nerves and nerve roots, illustrated in Figure 11-2.

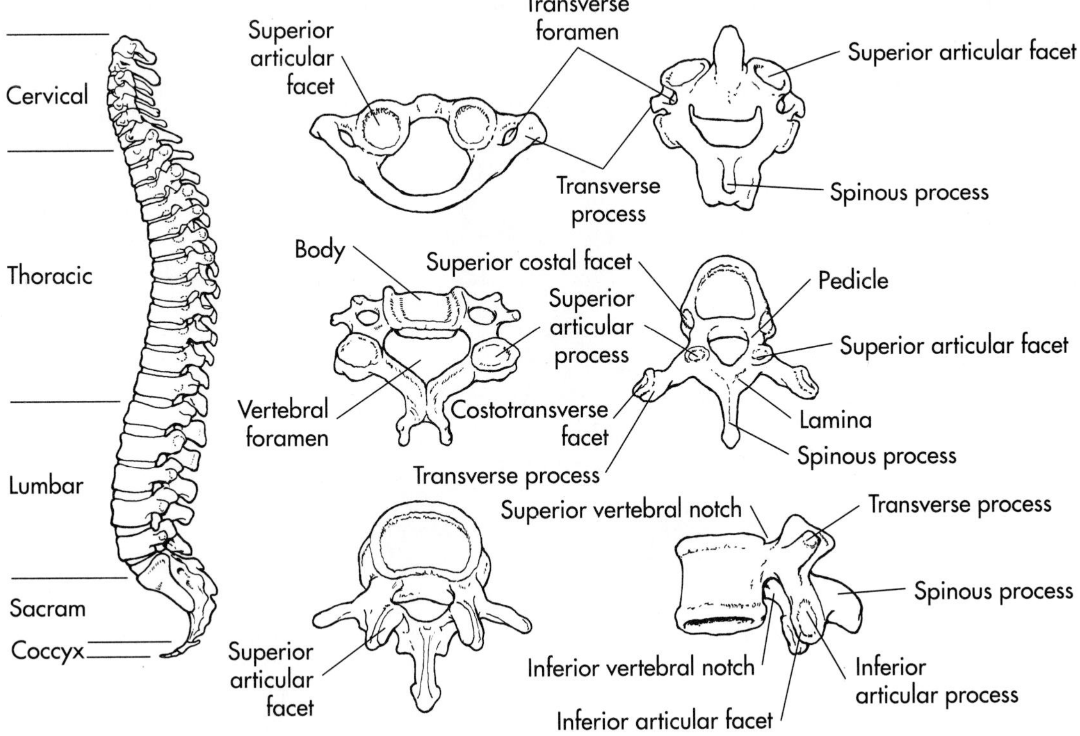

Figure 11-1 The vertebral column, with individual vertebrae: (A) atlas; (b) axis; (C) C4; (D) T6; (E) L3, superior view; (F) L3, lateral view. (Redrawn from DeCoursey RM, *The human organism,* ed 4, New York, 1974, McGraw-Hill.)

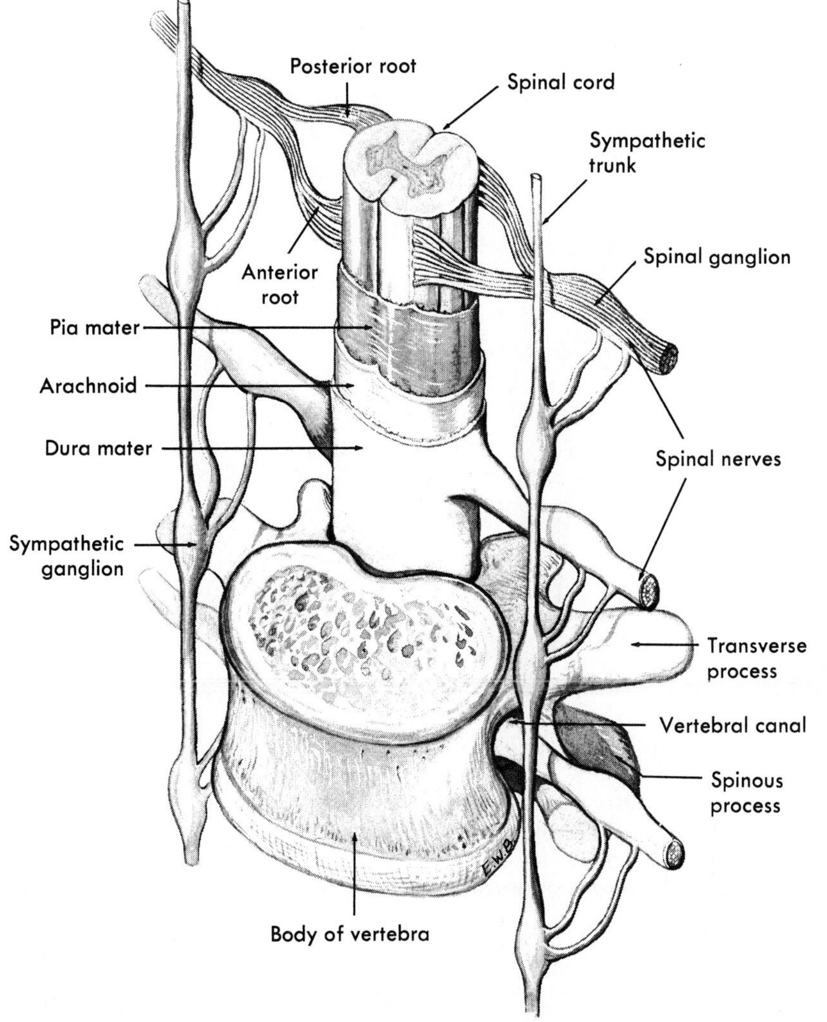

Figure 11-2 Spinal cord, showing meninges, formation of the spinal nerves, and relations to a vertebra and to the sympathetic trunk and ganglia. (From Anthony CP, Kolthoff NJ: *Textbook of anatomy and physiology,* ed 9, St Louis, 1975, Mosby–Year Book.)

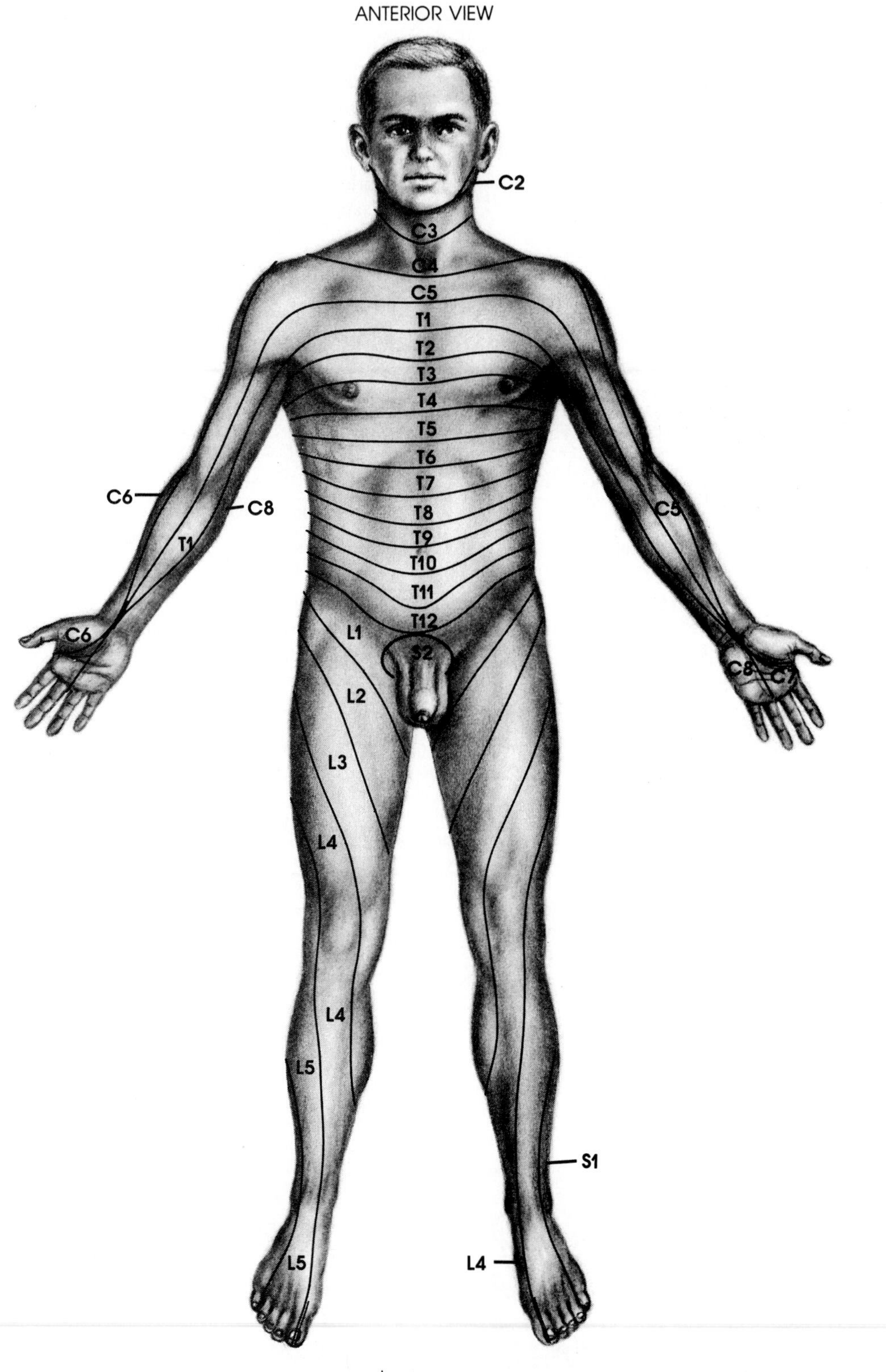

Figure 11-3 Dermatomes of the body. Each dorsal (sensory) spinal root innervates one dermatome. The first cervical nerve usually has no cutaneous distribution. (From Rudy EB: *Advanced Neurological and Neurosurgical Nursing*, St Louis, 1984, Mosby–Yearbook.)

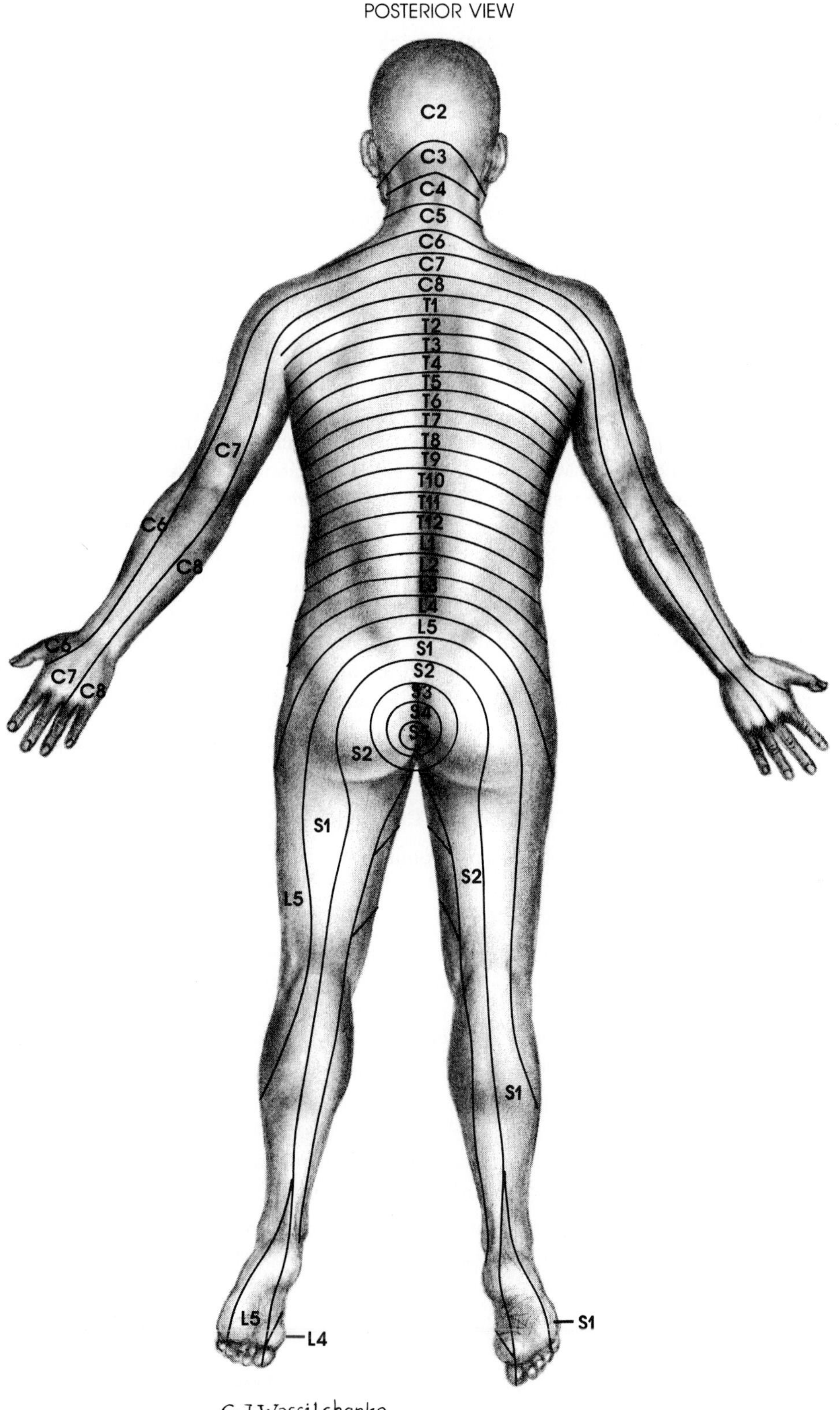

Figure 11-3, cont'd.

LENGTH OF STAY/ANTICIPATED COURSE

The average length of stay for uncomplicated spinal surgery is approximately 11 days in accord with DRG 4: Spinal procedures.[8] The length of stay in the ICU is usually less than 48 hours.

The predominant surgical goal of cervical spine laminectomy is to decompress, stabilize, and align the cervical spine.[2] Nursing goals focus on measures to prevent further complication and disease, and to enhance the reintegration of the individual into family and society via the rehabilitation process.

Motor Strength Scale

4+	Very brisk, hyperactive, may indicate disease
3+	More brisk than average, but may be normal
2+	Average or normal response
1+	Decreased response
0	No response

From Kinney MR, et al: *AACN's clinical reference for critical care nursing*, ed 3, St Louis, 1993, Mosby–Year Book.

MANAGEMENT TRENDS AND CONTROVERSIES

Diagnosis of the underlying pathology and the decision to operate are heavily dependent on technology. Magnetic resonance imaging (MRI) and computerized tomography (CT) scans are particularly useful in detecting underlying pathology and planning medical intervention. Myelography and conventional x-rays are still used.

Baseline data on the patient's function is important. Awareness of the patient's previous level of function alerts the nurse to ascending injury. Ascending injury occurs when edema causes spinal cord ischemia, injury, or infarct above the level of surgical intervention. This condition constitutes a medical emergency. Postoperative edema may be more catastrophic if the dura is violated. The dura surrounding the nervous tissue may require opening when tumors and vascular anomalies are present.

A dermatome chart must accompany the admission. The chart identifies the sensory regions that are innervated by the spinal nerves and serves as a guide for assessment. Usually an anterior and posterior view of the body is provided (see Figure 11-3 on pages 102-103). Familiarity with the anatomy and physiology of the spinal structure is necessary for accurate, consistent assessment. The medical team is notified when an abnormal result occurs.

ASSESSMENT

PARAMETER	ANTICIPATED ALTERATION
Respiratory	Decreased or compromised function *due to cervical spine ischemia, injury at C4 and higher, anesthetic agents or opiate sedation used during intra- or postoperative periods*
Cardiovascular	Potential bradycardia, hypotension, and shock *due to CNS injury with interruption of descending sympathetic pathways. These findings may signal neurogenic shock, which is a medical emergency. Symptoms also include orthostatic hypotension, loss of the ability to perspire below level of injury, and hypothermia from loss of innervation.*
Motor-sensory	Diminished motor-sensory function from the established baseline *via dermatome chart, which corresponds to the areas innervated by the spinal nerves. The motor system is best assessed by measuring strength in flexion, extension, and range of motion (see Box above).*
Pain	Physical pain may impair assessment and result in less than adequate performance *due to surgical incision, bone graft site, equipment in use after surgery, or intraoperative positioning of the patient's body.*
Surgical dressing	Presence of blood or serous fluid *due to arterial or venous bleeding. Presence of serous fluid is suspect for cerebrospinal fluid leakage. Serous fluid must be checked for glucose by use of dextrose measuring sticks or similar equipment. Glucose in CSF is usually 60% of serum or 20 to 30 mg/dl less than that of serum. CSF leakage leaves a characteristic "halo" on linen that surrounds a blood leak.*
Gastrointestinal	Potential stress ulcers, paralytic ileus, and hemorrhage *due to related drug therapy or temporary loss of reflex control below the level of injury*

Genitourinary	Predisposition to urinary tract infections, atonic bladder, or bladder rupture *due to loss of innervation*
Skin integrity	Potential pressure sores and reddened bony areas *due to loss of vasomotor tone and disuse of body*
Nutrition	Potential delayed healing of wound *due to low protein, iron, albumin, electrolytes, or absorptive difficulties in the gut from lack of innervation to GI tract*

INTENSIVE PHASE

Cervical laminectomy is a relatively safe procedure and one that does not absolutely require hospitalization in an ICU. However, frequent postoperative assessment and care needs may suggest a stay of 24 to 48 hours in an ICU to promote optimal patient outcomes.

PATIENT CARE PRIORITIES	EXPECTED PATIENT OUTCOMES
Ineffective airway clearance *r/t immobility and impaired neurological function*	Patent airway Sao_2 >96% Pao_2 >90 mm Hg
Sensory-perceptual alterations *r/t diminished tactile sensation secondary to inflammation of or injury to spinal nerves*	Maintenance of or improvement in baseline sensory-motor function
Immobility *r/t prolonged bed rest or disuse of extremities or muscle groups*	Return of mobility Skin intact
High risk for fluid deficit *r/t surgical intervention, possible hemorrhage, or diuresis from osmotic diuretics*	UO >30 cc and <200 cc per hour Minimal bleeding or wound drainage Electrolytes WNL
Pain *r/t surgical incision, edema of surrounding structures*	Patient achieves acceptable pain control within 30 minutes of intervention

INTERVENTIONS

Provide supplemental oxygen to maintain Sao_2 >96%.

Auscultate lungs q1h to q2h *to assess surgical recovery and prevent complications.*

Assist in cough effort by performing assisted-cough and chest percussion therapy.

Assist in secretion clearance as needed.

Monitor respiratory rate and effort *to detect ventilatory impairment.*

Encourage the use of an incentive spirometer *to prevent respiratory complications associated with decreased mobility.*

Collaborate with respiratory therapy in evaluating ABG and clinical responses to therapy.

Monitor sensory and motor functions of body q1h for the first 24 hours postoperatively for return or diminishment of sensations or motor functions, *to detect new motor or sensory losses early.*

Maintain body alignment at all times *to optimize return of full ROM and function.*

Turn by log-roll method q2h or as needed *to protect surgical site integrity.*

Assess skin on upper back, arms, and neck q8h to q10h and prn, especially when specialized beds, cervical collars, and halo head frames are used.

Begin ROM exercises 24 to 48 hours after surgery *to allow initial stabilization of surgical site.*

Use elastic and/or sequential compression hose *to prevent surgical complications such as DVT.*

Assess vital signs q15min times 4, then q30min times 2, then q1h times 8 hours. Advance to q2h if no abnormal signs are present after 24 hours.

Administer prescribed fluids. Monitor I/O and wound drainage *to prevent fluid excess/deficit.*

Monitor CBC and electrolyte results *to maintain normal values and aid healing.*

Inspect surgical site for drainage and bleeding, noting amount, color, and character *to detect signs of hemorrhage or infection. Report findings that may indicate CSF leak, such as fluid testing positive for glucose on dextrose stick, and appearance of halo effect on linen.*

Assess and document level, quality, and intensity of pain using a 0 to 10 rating scale. Report response to pain intervention(s).

Inspect surgical area for possible factors contributing to pain, such as position of head or body, edema, or wrinkles in linen.

Administer appropriate pain medication and reevaluate as indicated *to maintain comfort level and enhance patient participation in care.*

Implement alternative interventions, such as repositioning, distraction, and imagery, *to decrease pain response.*

INTERMEDIATE PHASE

The intermediate phase of care can be characterized by the patient's postoperative stability and return to neurologic assessment baseline. The focus turns to maintaining normal body functions and mental well-being that may otherwise impair the rehabilitation phase.

PATIENT CARE PRIORITIES	EXPECTED PATIENT OUTCOMES
Alteration in urinary elimination *r/t immobility or lack of spinal innervation to bladder*	*Bladder emptied adequately.* *Free of infection.*
Alteration in elimination *r/t* *Bed rest* *Immobility* *Anorexia* *Inadequate diet*	*Bowel regimen returns to baseline.* *Free from ileus and/or constipation.*
Neurological deficit *r/t precipitating pathology.*	*No further deterioration from baseline.* *Positive adaptation and adjustment to deficit.*

INTERVENTIONS

Monitor bladder for distension using a catheter only when necessary.

Assess color and odor of urine *for potential infection.*

Institute an intermittent catheterization program as soon as possible if patient is unable to void spontaneously, *to facilitate return of normal bladder function.*

Maintain NPO status until bowel sounds return, *to prevent aspiration and complications of ileus.*

Assess bowel sounds every shift or prn *to determine readiness for po intake.*

Begin feeding as soon as possible *to optimize nutrition.*

Maintain adequate hydration *to promote circulation and healing.*

Initiate bowel training including stool softeners *if patient is unable to defecate spontaneously by the third postoperative day.*

Assess motor and sensory systems *to determine impairment or improvement.*

Ensure appropriate health care team referrals *to meet patient's needs.*

Include patient and family in patient care conferences that focus on rehabilitation *to prepare for discharge.*

TRANSITION TO DISCHARGE

For those with neurological deficits, either new or long-standing, discharge to rehabilitative services may enhance the transition to independent living. Discharge instructions include (1) halo and brace care if the equipment is used, (2) activity restrictions and any other limitations imposed by the laminectomy, and (3) follow-up appointments and phone numbers of attending physicians.

REFERENCES

1. Cloward RB: The anterior surgical approach to the cervical spine: the Cloward procedure: past, present and future, *Spine* 13:823-827, 1988.
2. Hickey, JV: *The clinical practice of neurological and neurosurgical nursing,* ed 3, Philadelphia, 1992, Lippincott.
3. Kinney MD, et al: *AACN's clinical reference for critical care nursing,* ed 3, St Louis, 1993, Mosby–Year Book.
4. McCance KL, Huether SE: *Pathophysiology: the biological basis for disease in adults and children,* St Louis, 1990, Mosby–Year Book.
5. Parke WW: Correlative anatomy of cervical spondylotic myelopathy, *Spine* 13:831-837, 1988.
6. Rhodes MJ, Grendemann BJ, Ballinger WF: *Alexander's care of the patient in surgery,* St Louis, 1978, Mosby–Year Book.
7. Rudy, EB: *Advanced neurological and neurosurgical nursing,* St Louis, 1984, Mosby–Year Book.
8. *St Anthony's DRG guidebook 1995,* Reston, Va, 1994, St Anthony.
9. Stover SL, Kennedy EJ: *Spinal cord injury: the facts and figures,* Birmingham, 1986, University of Alabama at Birmingham.

DEVICE GUIDELINE

12

Intracranial Pressure Monitoring

Chris Winkelman, MSN, RN, CCRN

DESCRIPTION

Intracranial pressure (ICP) monitoring permits continuous, direct measurement of the pressure inside the skull. Monitoring ICP has become a standard and necessary part of the management of severely head-injured patients in most major institutions.[12] The normal ICP ranges from 0 to 10 mm Hg. The adverse effects of intracranial hypertension (i.e., pressures in excess of 15 to 20 mm Hg) during the acute stages of injury are well-documented.[6,17,23,26] Early diagnosis and rapid evaluation of treatment of elevated intracranial pressure can minimize morbidity and mortality.[8,12]

A variety of methods are available to monitor ICP: fiberoptic device, intraventricular catheter, subarachnoid or subdural bolt, and epidural sensor. The characteristics and potential complications associated with each method are compared in Table 1.[15] The clinical situation, patient's age, physician preference, and device availability and characteristics all influence the selection of the method used.[9] The devices are illustrated in Figures 12-1 through 12-4.

INDICATIONS

Any patient condition associated with actual or potential intracranial hypertension may indicate the need for ICP monitoring. Intracranial hypertension results from an increase in volume in the rigid skull. It is defined as a pressure in excess of 15 to 20 mm Hg.[1] A commonly used indicator for initiating ICP monitoring in many institutions is a finding of a severely depressed neurologic status, defined as a Glasgow coma score of 8 or less, in the presence of known neurologic injury.[2] Other patient conditions that indicate potential need for ICP monitoring include:

- Head injury
- Intracranial hemorrhage
- Subarachnoid hemorrhage
- Hydrocephalus
- Intracranial tumors/space-occupying lesions
- Cerebral edema
- Intracranial infection
- Ischemic/hypoxic brain injury
- Toxic or metabolic encephalopathies
- Use of paralytics, high-dose sedatives, or anesthetic agents in patients at high risk for intracranial hypertension
- The need for extensive surgical manipulation of brain tissue
- Initiation of a neurodiagnostic test demonstrating a high probability for ICP elevation

LIMITATIONS

Limitations, complications, and possible contraindications also guide the decision to initiate ICP monitoring. ICP monitoring has several limitations. It does not define the extent, location, or type of injury present. It does not determine the degree of neurological impairment. It is possible that pressure gradients could develop within the cranial vault, especially in the presence of a mass lesion.[21] These localized areas of high pressure may not be reflected by ICP monitoring. However, it is believed that pressure gradients are transient and of limited importance.[1] Lastly, the location of the brain lesion, the rate of intracranial volume expansion, and the presence of a cranial and dural defect or cerebrospinal fluid leak can limit the accuracy of monitoring values.[11]

POTENTIAL COMPLICATIONS

The three major complications associated with ICP monitoring are intracranial infection, brain injury, and CSF leak. Reported infection rates vary from 1% per device used to

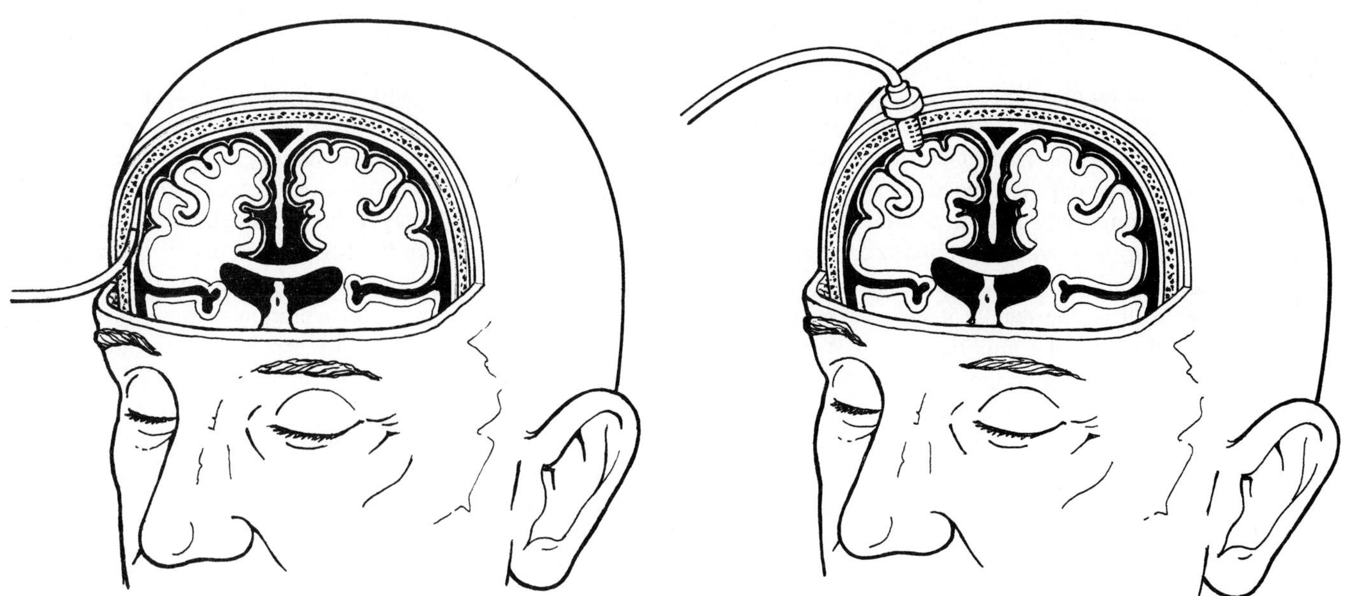

Figure 12-1 Epidural sensor. (Redrawn from McQuillan: Intracranial pressure monitoring: technical imperative, *AACN Clin Iss Crit Care Nurs,* 2:623-636, 1991.)

Figure 12-2 Subarachnoid screw. (Redrawn from McQuillan: Intracranial pressure monitoring: technical imperative, *AACN Clin Iss Crit Care Nurs,* 2:623-636, 1991.)

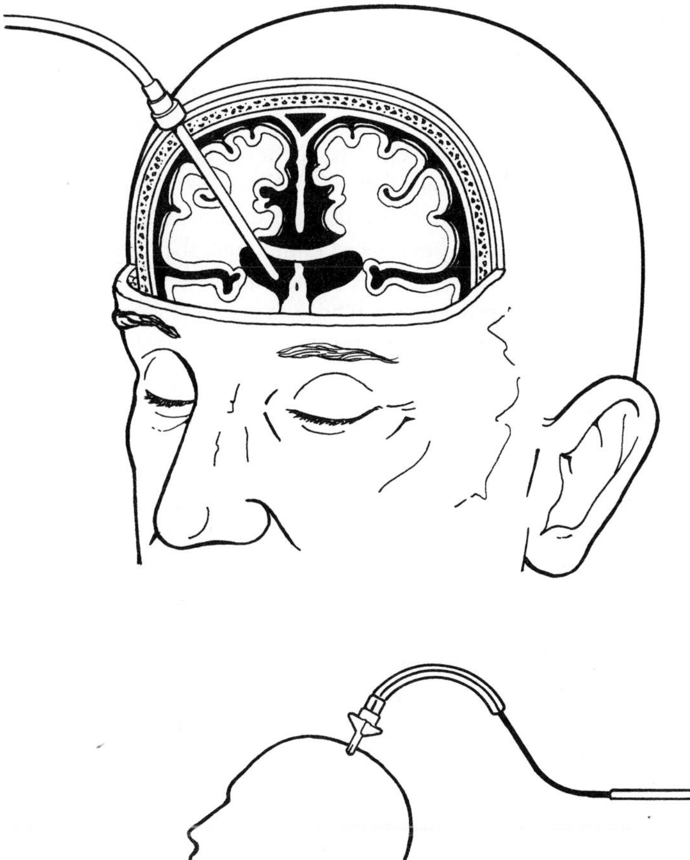

Figure 12-3 Intraventricular catheter. (Redrawn from McQuillan: Intracranial pressure monitoring: technical imperative, *AACN Clin Iss Crit Care Nurs,* 2:623-636, 1991.)

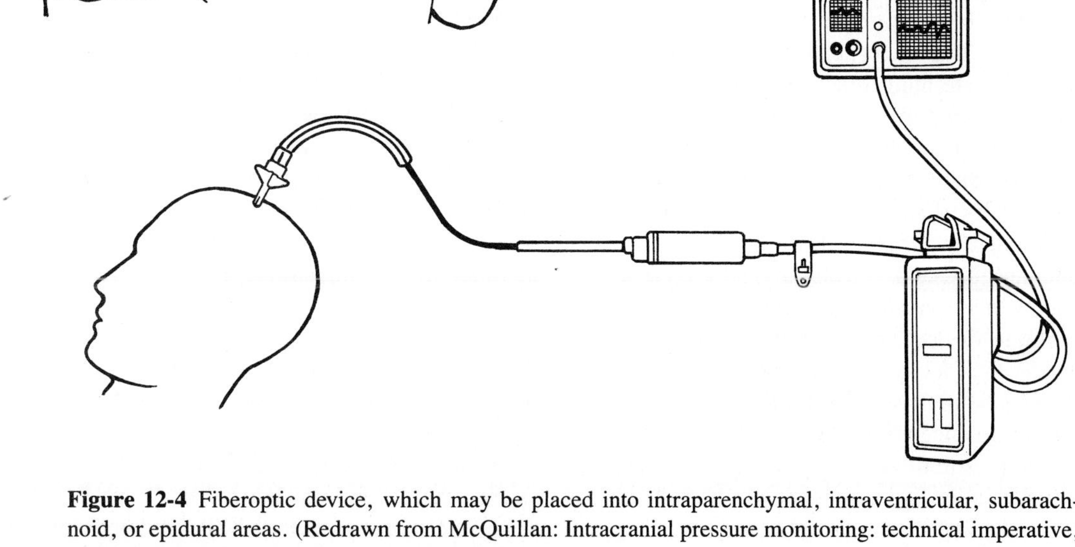

Figure 12-4 Fiberoptic device, which may be placed into intraparenchymal, intraventricular, subarachnoid, or epidural areas. (Redrawn from McQuillan: Intracranial pressure monitoring: technical imperative, *AACN Clin Iss Crit Care Nurs,* 2:623-636, 1991.)

10%.[7,13] This variation may be related to the type of device used (see Table 12-1) and the length of time the device is in place. Some physicians recommend rotation of the insertion site every three days to reduce the risk of infection.

Finally, ICP monitoring may be contraindicated in the presence of a scalp or cranial infection, coagulopathy, or lack of sufficient knowledge by the staff about the device and system as well as the data it supplies. Despite these limitations and the risk of complications, ICP monitoring is a valued and effective intervention in the evaluation and treatment of brain-injured patients. ICP monitoring is used to guide therapy, can detect changes in intracranial dynamics when other signs of neurological impairment are unreliable, and, when placed intraventricularly, can provide a method of CSF displacement and reduce ICP.

GENERAL NURSING INTERVENTIONS

Several nursing activities are essential to the effective use of any ICP monitoring device. These activities include assisting with ICP device insertion, maintaining an established ICP monitoring system, monitoring patient response to interventions, preventing complications, recording ICP pressure readings and analyzing waveforms, and monitoring cerebral perfusion pressure.[14] Each of these activities is described in detail below and summarized in Table 12-2.

Initiating Monitoring

Assisting with insertion of an ICP monitoring device varies with the device used and institutional resources. Some nursing responsibilities, however, can be anticipated. Typically, in obtaining informed consent prior to insertion, the physician provides initial information to the patient and family/significant others about the device and the rationale for its use. The nurse may reinforce this information and share data about trends and patient responses.

Insertion of any intracranial device must occur with attention to strict aseptic technique; vigilance is a shared physician and nursing concern. In addition, the critical care nurse may be responsible for irrigating flush systems prior to insertion, leveling the transducer, calibrating the system, and setting alarms. Irrigate fluid-filled systems using manufacturer's guidelines. Level the transducer to the foramen of Monro. Choose an anatomic point, such as the outer canthus of the eye, the tragus of the ear, or a point halfway between these landmarks as an external marker, indicating the level of the foramen of Monro.[24] More important than the anatomic landmark selected is using a single reference point consistently with all balancing.[15] Note that epidural sensors and fiberoptic devices do not need to be leveled because the transducer is located within the cranial vault; simply zero the device before insertion. Calibrate the system and set alarms in congruence with monitor/manufacturer's recommendations and institutional policy. In general, alarm limits include a range indicating disconnection (0 to 1 mm Hg) and a prescribed value that indicates a need for intervention (usually 20 or 25 mm Hg).

Recalibrate and zero any fluid-filled system with any change in patient ICP waveform or trends, after patient transport, after system manipulation (e.g., collection of cerebrospinal fluid for analysis), or apparent device malfunction. Routine frequency of zero and calibration varies from every 2 to 12 hours for fluid-filled systems[19,20,24] and depends on type of transducer and monitor used, the manufacturer's recommendations, and consideration of the risk in system violation. Fiberoptic systems can be zeroed only prior to insertion; calibration can be done as suggested by these guidelines to correlate values with the bedside monitor because the current manufacturer of ICP fiberoptic systems, Camino, does not provide alarms to indicate high/low pressure or disconnection.

Maintenance and Prevention of Complications

Once established, maintaining an intracranial monitoring device involves three areas of nursing responsibility: care of the insertion site; care of the transducer/drainage system; and prevention of complications, especially central nervous system infection. All insertion sites require a dry and intact occlusive dressing. No data exist to recommend frequency of dressing changes. Some institutions use the original dressing until the monitor is removed, recommending that nurses only reinforce nonocclusive dressings and assist the physician in replacing the dressing when it becomes soiled or wet. Another approach is to routinely change the dressing at day 3 to 5, using aseptic technique (including mask and sterile gloves). There are no data to recommend the definitive dressing. Despite these limitations, the nurse can evaluate the site with each ICP measurement for evidence of infection, cerebrospinal fluid leak, and/or hematoma formation near the occlusive dressing. Physician notification and evaluation is imperative should any of these conditions be discovered.

Maintaining the transducer and pressure tubing means avoiding dislodgment or breakage of the system. Affix the tubing to the patient/head dressing rather than the bed to avoid tension on the line. Fiberoptic cables are made of glass filaments; maintaining this system requires avoidance of tension and kinking in the line. Monitor fluid-filled pressure tubing for the presence of air bubbles; air in the line will dampen the waveform and give false values for ICP. Notify the physician if the device is loose within the skull. Typically, when devices are secure, no movement occurs in any direction; no rotational, lateral, or vertical displacement occurs when the device is minimally manipulated, such as manipulation during a dressing change. Changing the transducer and pressure tubing also varies with institutional practice and is without any researched base. Perhaps the critical determinants in changing the tubing are whether the device is changed at the recommended 3 to 5 day interval[13] and how often the system is entered.

In the presence of a cerebrospinal fluid (CSF) drainage system (e.g., an intraventricular device that also may be fiberoptic), ensure that the air-fluid interface in the drip chamber or collection bag is at the prescribed height, usually

TABLE 12-1 Comparison of ICP Monitoring Devices

Device	Characteristics	Potential complications
Epidural devices. Placed between the dura and skull. Fiberoptic.	Low risk for brain injury and/or infection because the dura remains intact Unable to drain CSF in presence of IICP or collect CSF for analysis No risk for CSF leakage Technically easy to insert	Questionable accuracy because it is placed above the dura with a possibility of drift as unable to rezero post-insertion.[4] Possible extradural infection
Subdural/subarachnoid devices. Inserted through a burr hole into the subarachnoid space. Used in patients whose ventricles cannot be cannulated (e.g., small ventricles due to cerebral edema).	Less infection risk than intraventricular catheter Requires intact skull and closure of fontenales Unable to drain or collect CSF	Risk for brain infection Risk for brain injury (i.e., hematoma, contusion) Protruding screw/bolt at risk for trauma and/or dislodgement Accuracy of the waveform and values is questionable in the patient who has increased pressure and in whom the brain substance impinges on the end of the screw[21] Questionable reliability in evaluating brain compliance Risk for CSF leakage at insertion site with subarachnoid placement
Intraventricular devices. Typically inserted in the frontal horn of the lateral ventricle of the nondominant hemisphere. A radiopaque catheter is threaded into the ventricle over a stylet through a burr hole.	Considered most accurate and reliable in determining ICP and brain compliance because it directly measures the pressure within the ventricular space Permits CSF sampling and drainage Allows ventricular instillation of medications and diagnostic material Most difficult of devices to place, especially when ventricles are distorted or collapsed	Highest risk of all devices for brain infection Risk for brain injury (i.e., intracerebral hemorrhage, cerebral edema around catheter) Excessive CSF removal can cause ventricular collapse Risk for CSF leakage at insertion site Risk for ventricular air entry with improper system maintenance System may become obstructed with tissue, blood, or bone, impairing ICP readings
Fiberoptic transducer-tipped device. Can be used for intraventricular, subarachnoid, epidural, and direct parenchyma measurement. Senses changes in the amount of light reflected from a pressure-sensitive diaphragm at the catheter tip.	Less artifact, usually clear, high-fidelity ICP wave Can be placed in brain parenchyma Transducer leveling not required To get accurate brain pressure, stopcock must be positioned to prohibit drainage.	Unable to rezero or balance after insertion Pressure drift may occur Can be easily damaged or dislodged—fragile glass filaments provide fiber optics Tissue can occlude the sensor tip, elevating ICP values or impairing waveform. Potential for CSF leak at insertion site Relationship between parenchymal and intraventricular pressures not yet known

CSF: cerebrospinal fluid; ICP: intracranial pressure; IICP: increased intracranial pressure

15 to 20 cm above the foramen of Monro. This step is known as setting the "pop off" value and ensures drainage when intracranial pressure exceeds the pop off value (10 to 15 mm Hg). Rebalance the interface after each patient position change. Evaluate and document the clarity, color, rate, and amount of CSF drainage whenever outflow occurs. Notify the physician of new onset of discolored CSF, bloody drainage, or suspected infection (cloudiness, odor, or sediment in CSF). Monitor the system for evidence of occlusion; cessation of CSF flow may indicate catheter dislodg-

TABLE 12-2 General Nursing Interventions Associated with ICP Monitoring

General considerations	Related nursing interventions
Initiation of monitoring	Reinforce information about the device for patient and family Share data about trends and patient responses to therapy Irrigate the flush system prior to insertion Level the transducer at the foramen of Monro Calibrate/recalibrate the system Set alarms
Maintenance and prevention of complications	Monitor/care for the insertion site Ensure accurate "pop-off" level Monitor the system for occlusion and malfunction Monitor alarm settings
Analysis of ICP waveforms	Analyze ICP waveform: clarity of P_1, P_2, and P_3 Determine presence of A, B, or C waves Evaluate ICP trend data Relate ICP waveforms to patient responses to interventions Communicate findings and abnormalities to physician
Calculation of cerebral perfusion pressure	Calculate the cerebral perfusion pressure (CPP) Relate CPP to patient responses to interventions

ment, blood or debris in the system, or a collapse of the ventricle so that CSF is no longer able to accumulate for drainage. Notify the physician of the presence of occlusion/CSF flow cessation in the presence of intracranial hypertension. Change the collection bag as needed using aseptic technique; occasionally CSF will cease to flow when the collection bag is only partly full.

Prevent infection by opening the system infrequently and only when necessary. Examples of necessary entry into the closed system include collection of CSF for analysis and irrigation to remove air or clots. In some institutions, these interventions may be nursing responsibilities; in other locations only physicians collect CSF and irrigate tubing. In either case, precepted experience is valuable in developing safe technique. Monitor serum white blood cell count, patient temperature, and results of CSF cultures to detect early signs of central nervous system infection. Check the patient for nuchal rigidity (e.g., inability to flex the neck, and/or neck flexion associated with sharp pain at neck, head, and jaw) with each neurological assessment, unless contraindicated by the patient's condition (such as a suspected or actual cervical injury). Keep all portals of entry covered with a deadender cap or a dry micron filter. Use sterile technique to interrupt the system, cleansing any connections thoroughly with a bacteriostatic solution prior to entry. Avoid placing solutions in the system with preservatives, alcohol, and heparin; such additives can damage brain tissue.[2]

Analyzing ICP Waveforms

Analyzing the ICP waveform and evaluating trend data has tremendous implications for nursing practice and patient outcome. A normal pulse waveform is characterized by low amplitude fluctuations of less then 15 mm Hg; this value is derived from the mean reading. Each individual waveform has at least three peaks (Figure 12-5). The first peak, or percussion wave, labeled P_1, is the tallest and has a relatively consistent amplitude. It is believed to originate from pulsations of the intracranial arteries. The second peak, P_2, or tidal wave, normally has a lower amplitude than P_1, although this amplitude is less consistent than P_1. The dicrotic wave, P_3, has the lowest peak; as this wave terminates, the waveform descends toward baseline. The second and third peaks of the ICP waveform are thought to originate from venous pulsations in the cranial vault. Smaller peaks, caused by retrograde venous pulsations, may follow this triad.[35]

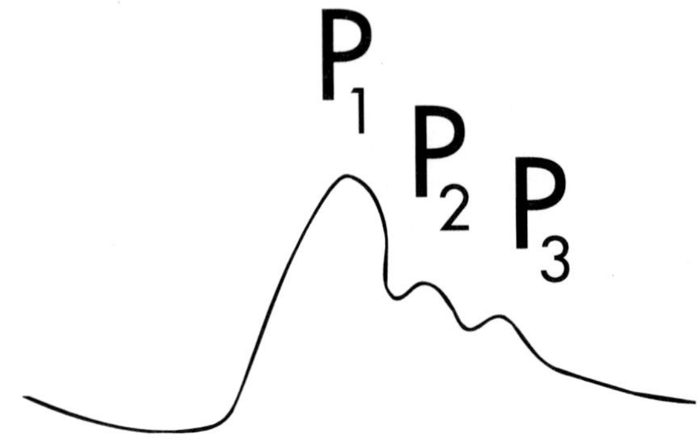

Figure 12-5 Normal intracranial pressure wave components. (Redrawn from McQuillan: Intracranial pressure monitoring: technical imperative, *AACN Clin Iss Crit Care Nurs,* 2:623-636, 1991.)

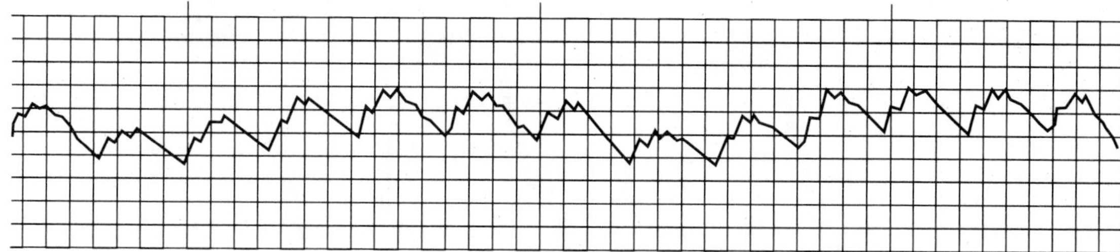

Figure 12-6 ICP waveform demonstrating P_2 elevation and rounding of waveform. (Redrawn from McQuillan: Intracranial pressure monitoring: technical imperative, *AACN Clin Iss Crit Care Nurs,* 2:623-636, 1991.)

Intracranial pressure waves correlate with cardiac systole and diastole. Respiratory fluctuation of the entire waveform also may occur.[16] Normal variations include transient increases in amplitude due to Valsalva, coughing, or suctioning, and during rapid eye movement (REM) sleep.[2]

Abnormal ICP waveforms can indicate a loss of intracranial compliance and an increase in elastance. Compliance describes the amount of compensation available before an increased volume causes a pathological increase in intracranial pressure. Compliance is defined as the change in volume per unit change in pressure.[1] Elastance is a reciprocal term and indicates brain stiffness. Elastance is defined as the pressure change per unit of volume change.[1] Greater detail about these terms can be found in the guidelines for increased intracranial pressure.

An abnormal trace waveform is characterized by an amplitude greater than 15 to 20 mm Hg. Also, a rounded upswing may appear on the abnormal waveform. Persistent elevations in ICP usually cause the P_2 wave to increase more than the P_1 or P_3 component as illustrated in Figure 12-6, contributing to the rounded appearance of an abnormal waveform. The P_2 wave amplitude may reflect the brain's compensatory capacity. When the P_2 wave amplitude is equivalent to or exceeds the height of the P_1 wave, the brain's compliance is believed to be poor.[3,5] Poor compliance means that, should additional volume be added to the intracranial vault, the brain's capacity to compensate is exhausted and significant ICP elevations could occur. Other techniques for directly assessing brain compliance are to add or remove ventricular fluid and observe ICP response. Usually done only by physicians, these techniques, known as the volume-pressure response and the volume-pressure index, are not without potential complication.[5,16] Most importantly, they may cause a pathological increase in intracranial pressure. No evidence supports routine irrigation of ICP monitoring systems as beneficial in maintaining patency. Additionally, because of the risk of serious complications such as pathologic ICP increases, and increased risk of infection, irrigation into the cranial vault should be done only when the patient's condition indicates a need for this highly invasive intervention. Indications for irrigation into a ventricle may include evaluating compliance and clearing the catheter of occlusion. Regardless, only an experienced operator should irrigate into the ventricle, a procedure likely to be limited to physician practice.

Another technique is being investigated to assist in describing or predicting intracranial compliance. Recently, researchers have demonstrated that a relationship exists between a computerized frequency analysis of the ICP waveform and intracranial compliance.[22] The accuracy and reliability of using the P_2 wave to assess the brain's compliance is not completely established. Nonetheless, in the presence of an elevated P_2 (possibly indicating decreased compliance and increased risk for elevated ICP) the nurse can focus interventions on improving compliance and on providing prophylactic measures prior to procedures known to increase ICP. Such interventions will not harm the patient and, in the absence of conclusive data, are reasonable.[2]

Abnormal Waveforms

A Waves

In addition to real-time waveform analysis, trend recordings of 5 to 10 minutes provide data key to patient assessment and outcomes. Three types of abnormal trend waveforms have been identified.[10,21] Of these three, the most pathological are A waves, also known as plateau waves (Figure 12-7). Characterized by sudden increases in pressure greater than 50 mm Hg, A waves last 2 to 20 minutes. They occur with an elevated ICP (20 to 40 mm Hg baseline can be expected) and recur with variable frequency. During this period of severe intracranial hypertension, neurologic deterioration and cerebral ischemia are likely, necessitating immediate intervention to reduce the ICP.[4,18]

B Waves

A second type of abnormal waveform that may occur over time is known as B waves (Figure 12-8). B waves occur in the presence of a normal baseline ICP (<20 mm Hg). They occur regularly, every 30 seconds to 2 minutes, and range in amplitude from 20 to 50 mm Hg. B waves often correspond to changes in respiration. For example, B-wave elevation may be seen during the apneic period of Cheyne-Stokes breathing patterns. Considered clinically significant, B waves may indicate a decline in intracranial compensation

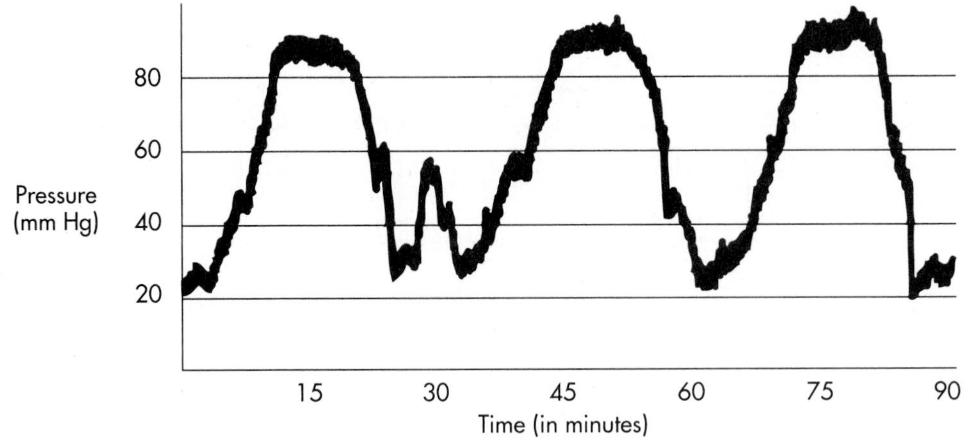

Figure 12-7 A (plateau) waves. (Redrawn from McQuillan: Intracranial pressure monitoring: technical imperative, *AACN Clin Iss Crit Care Nurs,* 2:623-636, 1991.)

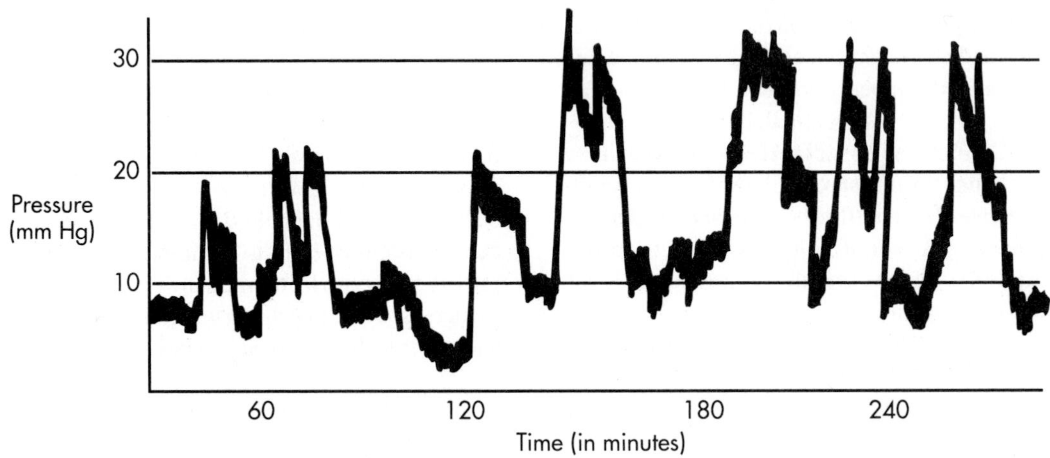

Figure 12-8 B waves. (Redrawn from McQuillan: Intracranial pressure monitoring: technical imperative, *AACN Clin Iss Crit Care Nurs,* 2:623-636, 1991.)

and their frequency may increase as compliance deteriorates.[2]

C Waves

C waves are the third abnormal trend that may be observed with ICP monitoring. These waves are low-amplitude (up to 20 mm Hg), rhythmic oscillations that usually occur at a rate of 4 to 8 per minute (Figure 12-9). Their clinical significance is not known.

Cerebral Perfusion Pressure

Intracranial hypertension is pathologic because of its compromising effects on cerebral blood flow. Under normal circumstances, cerebral blood flow remains constant despite a wide range of mean arterial blood pressures, and changes in arterial carbon dioxide ($PaCO_2$) or arterial oxygen tension (PaO_2). This stability in cerebral blood flow is known as autoregulation. Autoregulation may be lost with conditions such as head injury, subarachnoid hemorrhage, or craniotomy; the more severe the injury, the greater the degree of autoregulation loss. Since direct measurement of cerebral blood flow at the bedside is still in the future, the best indicator for perfusion to the brain is calculation of cerebral perfusion pressure. Cerebral perfusion pressure, not ICP, determines adequacy of cerebral blood flow. Calculating this pressure and initiating interventions in the presence of hyper-or hypoperfusion is a nursing responsibility.

Cerebral perfusion pressure (CPP) is the pressure at which cells of the brain are perfused. Its normal range in adults is 60 to 100 mm Hg. Hyperperfusion and increased intracranial pressure can occur when the CPP exceeds 100 mm Hg. Hypoperfusion and cerebral ischemia can result if the CPP decreases to less than 50 mm Hg.[19] Cerebral perfusion pressures less than 40 mm Hg in the adult are as-

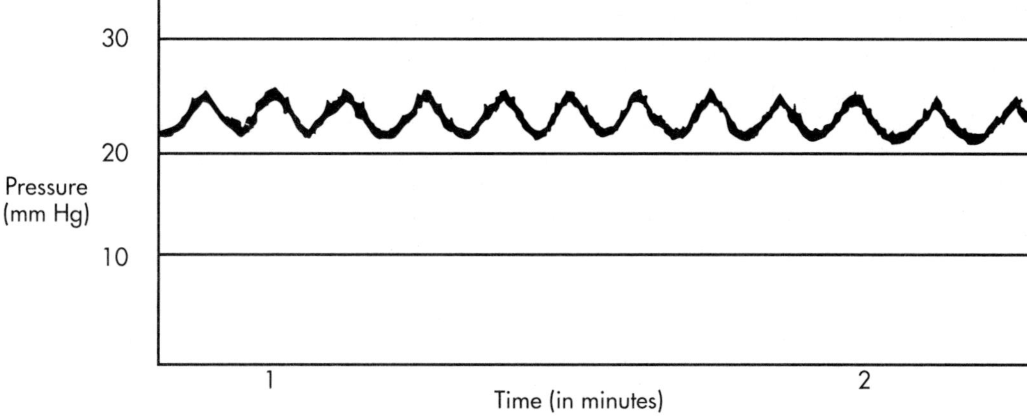

Figure 12-9 C waves. (Redrawn from McQuillan: Intracranial pressure monitoring: technical imperative, *AACN Clin Iss Crit Care Nurs,* 2:623-636, 1991.)

sociated with irreversible brain ischemia and infarction.[2] CPP can be calculated indirectly as the difference between the mean arterial pressure (MAP) and the ICP: CPP = MAP − ICP. Some clinicians advocate that MAP in this equation should be measured at the level of the fourth ventricle (rather than the left cardiac ventricle or phlebostatic axis).[2] The CPP must be considered in addition to the ICP when assessing the patient's cerebrovascular status and planning or evaluating therapeutic interventions.[15] Specifically, treatment focuses not only on maintaining normal intracranial pressures, but on maximizing CPP through manipulation of systemic blood pressure, $PaCO_2$, and PaO_2 to enhance cerebral perfusion and, indirectly, cerebral blood flow. The goal of therapeutic interventions is to maintain a CPP at levels greater than 60 mm Hg, although recent research indicates a goal of greater than 70 mm Hg or even 80 mm Hg is optimal.[25] Further discussion of CPP and related therapeutic interventions is found in the guidelines outlining the care of the patient with increased intracranial pressure.

TROUBLESHOOTING

A final consideration in the care of the patient with an ICP monitor is troubleshooting. Generally, there are two areas with problems to solve: a dampened or absent ICP waveform, and/or a false pressure reading.

Problem: Dampened/Absent Waveform

CAUSE	CORRECTIVE ACTION
Air between transducer and pressure source	Eliminate air bubbles with sterile preservative-free saline or Ringer's Lactate.
Occlusion of intracranial device with blood or debris, or of catheter tip by ventricular walls	Notify physician. Anticipate flushing intracranial catheter or screw with 0.25 cc preservative-free saline.
Transducer disconnected	Check all connections. Use Luer-Lok devices and/or tape slip-tip connections.
Incorrect gain setting for pressure	Generally, use 0 to 30 mm Hg scale. In the presence of A or B waves, adjust gain to permit higher readings (0 to 60 or 0 to 120 mm Hg scale).

Problem: False Pressure Value

CAUSE	CORRECTIVE ACTION
Transducer too low/too high	Evaluate position of transducer. *For every 1 inch displacement (above or below the foramen of Monro), anticipate >2 mm Hg change in value.*

Transducer incorrectly balanced	Reposition and rebalance transducer
Monitoring system incorrectly calibrated	Repeat calibration
Air or debris in pressure tubing	Remove air, clots, and debris from monitoring line through irrigation. *Air may attenuate or amplify pressure signal. Blood and debris may interfere with accurate signal reading.*

SUMMARY

Effective monitoring of intracranial pressure does not occur in isolation of the patient's condition or without considerable knowledge of the pathophysiology of increased intracranial pressure. These topics are covered in separate guidelines in this text. Additionally, ICP values and waveforms must be interpreted with the findings of neurologic examination, the results of neurodiagnostic testing, and multisystem assessment. The purpose of guidelines specific to ICP monitoring devices is to support the patient and extend the decision-making capabilities of the bedside nurse using a technology unique to critical care. The information provided by continuous ICP monitoring is extremely important in guiding interventions and improving patient outcome. It is also a fertile area for nursing research.[15] The benefit of ICP monitoring can be appreciated fully only when the critical care nurse is knowledgeable about the device, competent to properly care for the monitoring system, and able to correctly interpret and act on the data provided.[15]

REFERENCES

1. Barnet GH: Intracranial pressure monitoring devices: principles, insertion, and care. In Ropper A, editor: *Neurological and neurosurgical intensive care,* ed 3, New York, 1993, Raven Press.
2. Cammermeyer M, Appledorn C: *Core curriculum for neuroscience nursing,* ed 3, Chicago, 1990, American Association of Neuroscience Nurses.
3. Cardoso ER, Rowan JO, Galbraith S: Analysis of the cerebrospinal fluid pulse wave in intracranial monitor, *J Neurosurg* 59:817-821, 1983.
4. Crutchfield JS, et al: Evaluation of a fiberoptic intracranial monitor, *J Neurosurg* 72:482-487, 1990.
5. Germon K: Interpretation of ICP pulse waves to determine intracerebral compliance, *J Neurosci Nurs* 20:344-249, 1988.
6. Gilliam EE: Intracranial hypertension: advances in intracranial monitoring, *Advances in Neurologic Care,* vol 2:21-27, 1990.
7. Hickman KM, Mayer BL, Muwaswas M: Intracranial pressure monitoring: review of risk factors associated with infection, *Heart Lung* 19:84-91, 1990.
8. Klauber MR, Marshall LF, Toole BM: Cause of decline in head-injury mortality rate in San Diego County, *J Neurosurg* 62:528-531, 1985.
9. Lehman B: Intracranial pressure monitoring and treatment: a contemporary view, *Ann Emerg Med* 19:295-303, 1990.
10. Lundberg N: Continuous recording and control of ventricular fluid pressure in neurosurgical practice, *Acta Psychiatr Neurol Scand Suppl* 149:1-193, 1960.
11. Marmamou A, Tabaddor K: Intracranial pressure: physiology and pathophysiology. In Cooper PR, editor: *Head injury,* Baltimore, 1987, Williams & Wilkins, pp 159-176.
12. Marshall SB, et al: *Neuroscience critical care: pathophysiology and patient management,* Philadelphia, 1990, WB Saunders.
13. Mayhall CG, et al: Ventriculostomy-related infections—a prospective epidemiologic study, *N Engl J Med* 310:552-559, 1984.
14. McCloskey JC, Bulechek GM: *Iowa intervention project: nursing interventions classification,* St. Louis, 1992, Mosby–Year Book.
15. McQuillan KA: Intracranial monitoring: technical imperatives, *AACN Clin Iss Crit Care Nurs* 2:623-636, 1991.
16. Miller ER: Nursing care of the head-injured patient. In Becker DP, Gudeman SK, editors: *Textbook of head injury,* Philadelphia, 1989, WB Saunders.
17. Miller JD, Becker DP, Ward JD: Significance of intracranial hypertension in severe head injury, *J Neurosurg* 47:503-516, 1977.
18. Pacult A, Gudeman SK: Medical management of head injuries. In Becker DP, Gudeman SK, editors: *Textbook of head injury,* Philadelphia, 1989, WB Saunders, pp 192-220.
19. Pollock-Latham C: Intracranial pressure monitoring. Part I: Physiologic principles, *Crit Care Nurse* 7:40-51, 1987.
20. Pollock-Latham C: Intracranial pressure monitoring. Part II: Patient care, *Crit Care Nurse* 7:53-72, 1987.
21. Richmond TS: Intracranial pressure monitoring, *AACN Clin Iss Crit Care* 4:148-160, 1993.
22. Robertson CS, et al: Clinical experience with a continuous monitor of intracranial compliance, *J Neurosurg* 71:673-680, 1989.
23. Robertson CS, et al: Treatment of hypertension associated with head injury, *J Neurosurg* 59, 1983, pp 289-296.
24. Robinet K: Increased intracranial pressure: management with an intraventricular catheter, *J Neurosci Nurs* 17:95-104, 1985.
25. Rosner MJ, Daughton S: Cerebral perfusion pressure management in head injury, *J Trauma* 30:933-940, 1990.
26. Saul TG, Ducker TB: Effect of intracranial pressure monitoring and aggressive treatment on mortality in severe head injury, *J Neurosurg* 56:498-503, 1982.

UNIT

II

Cardiovascular System

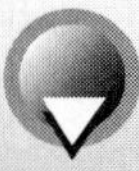

CLINICAL GUIDELINE

13

Angina

Debra Lynn-McHale, MSN, RN, CS, CCRN
Eileen M. Kelly, MSN, RN, CCRN

DESCRIPTION

Angina pectoris is a clinical syndrome resulting from transient myocardial ischemia.[8] Clinical manifestations of angina vary greatly from individual to individual. Commonly reported clinical manifestations of angina can be found in Table 13-1. Anginal symptoms may also vary significantly in severity. It is essential that patients are able to identify their anginal symptoms and initiate appropriate interventions for their symptoms as soon as they develop.

In 1989 over 69 million Americans were estimated to have one or more forms of cardiovascular disease.[1] Since angina is usually an early warning of cardiovascular disease and seldom causes death in itself, statistical evaluation is difficult.[5] Estimates are that over 3 million people in the United States have angina.[1]

There are two general types of angina: stable angina and unstable angina.

Stable Angina

Stable angina usually does not occur at rest. It usually occurs when additional demand is placed on the myocardium, such as during exercise or periods of high anxiety or stress. The additional demand causes an increase in heart rate (HR), blood pressure (BP), and myocardial wall tension, thus increasing myocardial oxygen consumption (MV_{O_2}).

The average annual mortality in patients with chronic stable angina is 4%.[12] Mortality is increased in male patients; in patients who have risk factors such as hypertension, previous MI, or abnormal ECGs; and in patients who have low exercise tolerance, exercise-induced ischemia, or a poor hemodynamic response to exercise.[12]

Patients with stable angina may not undergo cardiac catheterization. In those patients who do undergo cardiac catheterization, the most important determinant of survival is left ventricular function, followed by the number of diseased vessels.[12] The annual mortality rate is five times greater in those with three coronary arteries significantly diseased compared to those with disease in only one coronary artery.[17]

Unstable Angina

Unstable angina may occur at rest or when minimal exertion is required. According to Shah, patients are classified as having unstable angina if they meet any of the following criteria:[18]

1. Abrupt onset of ischemic symptoms at rest or precipitated by physical effort in a patient without history of coronary artery disease (CAD).
2. Intensification or a change in the pattern of ischemic symptoms in a patient with a history of CAD such as (a) an increase in frequency, severity, and duration of symptoms and increased ease of provocation; and (b) symptoms at rest or minimal effort.
3. Recurrences of ischemic symptoms soon after an acute myocardial infarction (usually within 4 weeks).

Prinzmetal's angina is a form of unstable angina, usually caused by coronary artery spasm, during which the 12-lead ECG may show significant signs of myocardial injury. The ECG returns to normal when the angina is relieved.

Unstable angina in medically treated patients is associated with a 3% to 5% hospital mortality and 7% to 8% mortality in the first year.[12] The rate of nonfatal myocardial infarction is approximately 8% to 10% in the first 2 weeks.[12]

TABLE 13-1 Clinical Manifestations of Angina

Substernal chest pain described as
- burning
- pressure
- heaviness
- aching
- crushing
- squeezing
- choking

Chest pain may radiate to the
- jaw
- teeth
- left arm or individual joints
- right arm or individual joints
- epigastric area

Discomfort may be accompanied by
- nausea
- vomiting
- diaphoresis
- shortness of breath
- dizziness

Mortality is increased in those with the presence of moderate or severe left ventricular dysfunction, left main coronary artery disease, and increased myocardium at risk from diseased vessels.[13]

PATHOPHYSIOLOGY

Stable Angina

Stable angina may be nonatheromatous or atheromatous in nature. Nonatheromatous stable angina occurs due to valvular heart disease, left ventricular failure, inappropriate coronary vasodilator reserve, or coronary artery spasm.[15] In general, angina develops when there is an imbalance between oxygen supply and demand. Increased myocardial oxygen demand under circumstances when oxygen supply is compromised or inadequate will result in ischemic cellular insult, which usually produces anginal discomfort as a warning sign.

Atheromatous stable angina pectoris usually occurs in patients with atherosclerotic lesions within one or more coronary arteries.[15] These lesions decrease the amount of coronary blood flow available to the myocardium.

Stable angina is more often associated with stable coronary artery stenosis characterized angiographically by smooth, usually concentric borders, and is not associated with plaque rupture, intramural hemorrhage, or thrombus.[15] Figure 13-1 depicts the various types of coronary artery lesions.

An important pathophysiologic mechanism for the production of ischemia in CAD may be the loss of normal endothelial vasodilator function as a result of atherosclerotic injury.[15] Another factor influencing coronary blood flow is transmural oxygen distribution from the epicardium to the endocardium. According to Lambert, the distribution of blood flow to the subendocardium is approximately 1.25 times greater than to the epicardium because of greater systolic compressive forces and resultant wall stress.[15] This preferential subendocardial flow is dependent upon vasodilation of vessels in this region. As a result, the subendocardium has less coronary flow reserve to respond to further stress. Therefore, factors such as decreased coronary perfusion pressure, elevation of left ventricular end diastolic pressure (LVEDP), and tachycardia all tend to make the subendocardium ischemic before affecting the epicardial layers.[15]

Adenosine will also influence coronary blood flow. When adenosine triphosphate (ATP) demand exceeds the capacity of myocardial cells to synthesize high-energy phosphate compounds, adenosine monophosphate is produced. Adenosine is a potent vasodilator and may be the primary physiologic modulator of coronary blood flow.[15]

During the first several minutes of ischemia, production of ATP and creatine phosphate declines and tissue stores are depleted.[15] When ATP levels are reduced to less than 20% of control values, cellular ability to balance intracellular volume, generate high-energy phosphates, and maintain ionic integrity is lost.[20] Cell swelling results in damage to the sarcolemma, which may herald calcium accumulation and irreversible cell death.[15]

Patients with stable angina usually have brief periods of reversible ischemia. According to Lambert, the earliest mechanical changes detectable are related to diastolic dysfunction, followed by systolic abnormalities that reflect dysfunctional contraction in the ischemic region.[15] This may be followed by ECG changes and symptomatic angina.

Approximately 20% of patients with stable angina are shown to have angiographically normal coronary arteries. Among patients with obstructive CAD, the incidence of one-, two-, and three-vessel disease is roughly evenly divided.[14] In addition, most patients with stable angina pectoris have fixed atherosclerotic narrowing in one or more major coronary arteries, with at least 50% diameter reduction. Lesser degrees of luminal reduction may be responsible when the obstruction stimulates vasospasm.[14]

Unstable Angina

Unstable angina results from an interplay between the fixed coronary stenosis due to atherosclerotic plaque and dynamic factors that contribute to intermittent coronary artery occlusion or near-occlusion.[18] The exact mechanisms involved in the progression from stable angina are not clearly understood.

Angiographic studies have shown that patients with stable and unstable angina do not differ from each other when traditional indices of the severity of CAD, such as the number of vessels with significant stenoses, the percent

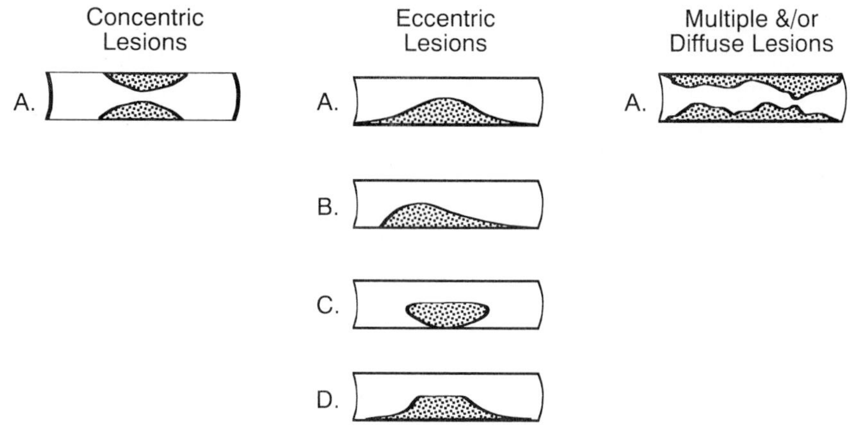

Figure 13-1 Types of coronary artery lesions. (Adapted from Ambrose JA, et al: Angiographic morphology and the pathogenesis of unstable angina pectoris, *J Am Coll Cardiol* 5:609, 1985.)

and length of stenosis, and the presence or absence of collateral vessels, are examined.[2,10,22] There are two differences that do exist. Seventy percent of patients with unstable angina demonstrate eccentric coronary stenosis (refer to Figure 13-1) with overhanging or irregular margins and filling defects.[3,16] In addition, atherosclerotic plaques in the coronary arteries of patients with unstable angina are complex, with fissures or cracks in the fibrous cap of the plaque.[6,7]

Ulceration or rupture of an atherosclerotic plaque is considered a major cause in the progression to unstable angina.[11] Changes in vascular tone, platelet aggregation, and platelet-fibrin thrombus formation are additional causes in the development of unstable angina.[18]

Atherosclerosis impairs the normal vasoactive responses of the vascular muscle.[18] The vasodilator effects of normal vascular endothelium are believed to be mediated by the release of substances such as endothelium-derived relaxation factor (EDRF). The ability of the coronary arteries to dilate, thus allowing increased blood flow, during times of increased oxygen demand is essential to prevent angina. The vascular smooth muscle cells in atherosclerosis may reflect endothelial dysfunction leading to deficient release of EDRF and excessive release of endothelin, which is a potent vasoconstrictor.[23] The resulting coronary artery spasm results in angina and may progress to myocardial infarction if not relieved. Local thrombin formation may also contribute to vasoconstriction in the presence of endothelial dysfunction.[18]

Studies have demonstrated evidence of platelet activation during unstable angina, creating microemboli in myocardial microvasculature distal to stenosis.[4,9] Plaque fissure also leads to platelet adhesion, aggregation, and subsequent fibrin-platelet thrombus formation.[18] When thrombus formation is associated with brief periods of coronary occlusion, the result is unstable angina. When the coronary occlusion is more prolonged, the result is acute myocardial infarction.[18]

LENGTH OF STAY / ANTICIPATED COURSE

Length of stay and anticipated course vary greatly depending upon patient condition. For the most part, patients with stable angina will be discharged much sooner than patients with unstable angina. Length of stay is also dependent on the diagnostic studies that may be prescribed. Noninvasive tests may be done on an outpatient basis. Invasive studies such as cardiac catheterization may require longer hospitalization, especially if aggressive or invasive intervention becomes necessary; for example, percutaneous transluminal coronary angioplasty (PTCA) or coronary artery bypass graft (CABG) surgery.

Patients who are admitted with a diagnosis of angina will usually be classified under DRG 140: Angina pectoris. The average LOS for this DRG is noted as 4 days, assuming that invasive testing such as cardiac catheterization or interventions such as PTCA or CABG surgery are not performed as part of the initial hospitalization.[19]

MANAGEMENT TRENDS AND CONTROVERSIES

The exact mechanism of angina remains unclear. Many investigations have established that most ischemic episodes in patients with stable angina are not accompanied by angina but are asymptomatic, or silent.[5,8,12,14,15] Subsequently, the mechanisms by which angina does or does not present as a symptom of ischemia have been the object of a great deal of investigation.[15] Many agents such as lactic acid, kinins, potassium, and hydrogen ions have been implicated as causing the actual anginal symptoms, but no single agent has been linked definitively to anginal pain.[15] Sympathetic nerve stimulation within the myocardium has also been postulated as a mechanism for the development of angina.[15]

Pharmacologic therapy may decrease the occurrence of anginal symptoms for many patients. Medications commonly prescribed for patients with stable and unstable angina include nitrates, beta-blockers, and calcium channel blockers. These medications improve myocardial oxygen supply by improving myocardial blood flow. Intermittent use of sublingual nitrates may be all that is necessary for patients with minimal symptoms.[21] Patients who have moderate symptoms may require a beta-blocker, a calcium-channel blocker, or long-acting nitrates. If symptoms do not improve despite therapy with adequate doses of a given class of drug, another class of agent should be substi-tuted. If some improvement occurs with one agent, but the patient still has symptoms, combination therapy with two different classes of agents should be considered.[21] Unless contraindicated, all patients with unstable angina should be treated with aspirin or full-dose heparin anticoagulation followed by long-term aspirin therapy.[11]

In addition to medical therapy, significant emphasis must be given to risk factor assessment and management. Patients should be given information about risk factors that contribute to coronary artery disease and how to manage them. Long-term follow-up and involvement of the patient's family have been suggested as the most effective methods to ensure necessary life-style modification.[21]

Patients who have left main coronary artery disease or three-vessel disease with diminished left ventricular function are candidates for CABG surgery. Other patients with one-, two-, and even three-vessel disease can be successfully managed medically, but PTCA and CABG surgery always are additional options.[21] PTCA is a viable option for most coronary artery disease. Treating left main coronary artery disease with PTCA or CABG surgery remains an active debate even though the current trend is to perform cardiac surgery.

Intra-aortic balloon counterpulsation is indicated for unstable angina refractory to medical management until emergency cardiac catheterization or CABG surgery is available. This treatment is important in patients with severe left main coronary disease since they are at high risk for myocardial infarction and sudden death.

Other therapies for patients with angina and unstable angina include atherectemy, stents, and laser ablation of plaque. Optimal therapy in treating patients with CAD and angina remains the subject of debate and development.

ASSESSMENT

PARAMETER	ANTICIPATED ALTERATION
Chest discomfort or pain and level of severity	See Table 13-1. Rating scale (0 to 10 or 0 to 5) useful in trending pain or evaluating intervention.
Associated Syptoms	See Table 13-1.
Duration of chest pain or discomfort	Seldom starts abruptly unless during coronary spasm. Usually has a crescendo-decrescendo quality and lasts 1 to 30 minutes.
Occurrence of symptoms	Increased frequency and/or severity is associated with disease progression that may warrant more aggressive intervention.
Activity	Symptoms with exertion or stress associated with stable angina. Symptoms at rest associated with unstable angina.
Relief of symptoms	Symptoms are relieved by nitroglycerin tablets within 1 to 2 minutes, or by increasing the dose of IV nitroglycerin.
Physical Assessment	
HR	May increase *due to pain, anxiety or decreased cardiac output.* May have bradycardia *due to vasovagal response.*
BP	May increase *due to sympathetic stimulation associated with pain or anxiety.* May decrease *if angina is associated with decreased ventricular function.*
RR	May increase *due to pain or anxiety.*
Pulse oximetry	May decrease *due to dyspnea or decreased cardiac output.*
Diagnostic Tests	
Cardiac enzymes	Nondiagnostic
12-lead ECG	Enlargement and inversion of T wave *due to ischemia.* ST segment changes above or below the isoelectric baseline greater than 1 mm *due to injury.*

ST-segment monitoring via bedside monitor, telemetry, or Holter monitor	ST segment deviates from baseline in the leads that reflect the ischemic area. ST-segment elevation or depression greater than 1 mm considered significant. May detect silent ischemia or ischemia of short duration
Exercise ECG	Responses considered predictive for severe multivessel and/or left main CAD: • ST-segment depression >2.5 mm • ST-segment downsloping or elevated >1 mm • Serious ventricular dysrhythmias at heart rates of 120 to 130 bpm • Ischemic ST-segment changes during the first 3 minutes of exercise • Ischemic changes >8 minutes in the postexercise recovery period • Heart rate does not increase >120 bpm with exercise • Decrease in systolic BP of 10 mm Hg in the absence of antihypertensive medication or hypovolemia • Increase in diastolic BP >110 to 120 mm Hg. Inability to exercise beyond 3 min
Thallium-201 imaging	Detects perfusion abnormalities associated with CAD
Dipyridamole thallium imaging	Indicated for patients unable to perform exercise stress test. Dipyridamole causes coronary vasodilation. Regional myocardial perfusion differences may be detected. Contraindicated in patients with severe bronchospastic pulmonary disease. Aminophylline antagonizes the effects of dipyridamole on vascular smoothness and may be used to reverse coronary ischemia induced by dipyridamole.
Exercise echocardiography	Detects regional wall-motion abnormalities
Radionuclide ventriculography	Evaluates ventricular function and wall motion at rest and exercise
Cardiac catheterization	Provides precise assessment of location and severity of CAD

PLAN OF CARE

INTERMEDIATE PHASE

Most patients with angina do not require an intensive phase of care unless their status is considered high risk for complications such as acute MI or sudden death. Typically the entire hospitalization of a patient with angina manifests at the intermediate level. Diagnostic tests such as exercise stress test and scans will be performed after the patient has stabilized or on an outpatient basis. All angina patients will require teaching with emphasis on education regarding self-care in order to slow CAD progression and prevent complications.

PATIENT CARE PRIORITIES	EXPECTED PATIENT OUTCOMES
Decreased myocardial tissue perfusion *r/t myocardial oxygen supply/demand imbalance*	ST-segment changes promptly return to baseline following intervention.
Chest pain or discomfort *r/t myocardial ischemia*	Relief from pain or discomfort. Episodes of angina minimized and controlled.
Dyspnea *r/t pain, anxiety, or decreased cardiac output*	Respiratory rate within normal limits. Pulse oximetry >90%.
Anxiety *r/t pain, decreased CO, lack of knowledge about diagnostic procedures and/or invasive interventions (PTCA or surgery)*	Demonstrates relaxed appearance and speech. Describes rationale for procedure. Verbalizes understanding of treatment and care associated with procedures. States acceptable level of comfort with information and readiness to proceed.
High risk for complications *r/t progression of the disease process:* *Acute MI* *Sudden death* *Arrhythmias*	Complications prevented or promptly noted and treated.

Plan of Care (cont'd)

Activity intolerance *r/t episodes of angina*	Performs ADL without angina. Avoids activities that trigger angina and/or takes preventive measures such as sublingual nitroglycerin prior to the activity. Alternates activity with rest. Recognizes timing of angina (i.e., morning) and plans medication schedule to prevent episodes.
Self-care deficit *r/t reducing risk for further CAD and managing angina episodes*	Verbalizes basic understanding of coronary artery disease. Describes symptoms of angina, appropriate actions to relieve symptoms, and appropriate actions if angina is not relieved. Verbalizes the name, action, dose, and side effects of medications. Identifies personal risk factors for CAD and plans to reduce or control them.

INTERVENTIONS

Continuous bedside ECG monitoring in leads that demonstrate ischemic changes on 12-lead ECG *to reveal ST-segment changes associated with silent ischemia or angina, and to detect dysrhythmias associated with ischemia.*

Administer oxygen *to increase myocardial oxygen supply.*

Administer nitroglycerine immediately with episodes of angina *to increase coronary blood supply and decrease myocardial workload by decreasing preload.*

Provide rest periods *to decrease myocardial oxygen demand.*

Administer narcotics *to relieve chest pain or discomfort not relieved by nitroglycerine.*

Administer anticoagulant *to prevent platelet aggregation, which may contribute to decreased myocardial blood supply or cause coronary thrombosis and resulting MI.*

Administer beta-blocking agents *to decrease heart rate, which increases myocardial oxygen consumption; to decrease myocardial contractility; and to decrease hypertension, which will decrease myocardial oxygen demand.*

Administer calcium channel blocking agent *to dilate the coronary arteries and the peripheral arteries, which decreases ventricular afterload and prevents coronary artery spasm.*

Administer sedation or tranquilizer *to decrease emotional responses, which may trigger angina.*

Monitor patient's response to medications.

Prepare patient for diagnostic or interventional procedures as indicated.

Teach basic pathophysiology associated with coronary artery disease, risk factors, signs and symptoms of angina, associated variables that may trigger angina, and medication information.

Assist in planning methods to reduce personal risk factors and modify associated triggers for angina.

Assist in identifying community sources for help with life-style modification.

Assist in obtaining information regarding access to emergency medical treatment in the community.

Provide information related to follow-up care, diagnostic procedures, or invasive interventions that may be scheduled on an elective basis.

TRANSITION TO DISCHARGE

As the patient progresses to discharge, the individual will need assistance in setting realistic goals to modify CAD risk factors and reduce the triggers associated with angina. Patients may experience anxiety or fear related to leaving the protection of the hospital. The nurse may need to provide emotional support so that the patient is able to remember the instructions provided. While hospitalized, linking the patient with community resources for ongoing support and education in heart-healthy living may be the most effective intervention to ensure long-term positive outcomes.

REFERENCES

1. AHA: *1992 Heart and Stroke Facts,* Houston, 1991, American Heart Association.
2. Alison HW, Russel RO, Mantle JA: Coronary anatomy and arteriography in patients with unstable angina pectoris, *Am J Cardiol* 41:204-209, 1978.
3. Ambrose JA, Winters SL, Stern A: Angiographic morphology and the pathogenesis of unstable angina pectoris, *J Am Coll Cardiol* 5:609-616, 1985.
4. Ashton JH, Taylor AL, Ogletree ML: Serotonin and thromboxan mechanisms are both important in mediating cyclic flow variation in severely narrowed canine coronary arteries, *Clin Res* 34:707A, 1986.
5. Burden LL: The person with angina pectoris. In Guzetta and Dossey, editors: *Cardiovascular Nursing Bodymind Tapestry,* St Louis, 1984, Mosby–Year Book.
6. Davies MJ, Thomas AC: Thrombosis and acute coronary artery lesions in sudden ischemic cardiac death, *N Engl J Med* 310:1137-1140, 1984.
7. Davies MJ, Thomas AC: Plaque fissuring: the cause of acute myocardial infarction, sudden ischemic death, and crescendo angina, *Br Heart J* 53:363-373, 1985.
8. Dehmer GJ: Angina pectoris: diagnosis, treatment, and prognosis, *Curr Prob Cardiol* 12(4):219-281, 1987.
9. Edit JF, Ashton J, Golino P: Treadmill exercise promotes cyclic alterations in coronary blood flow in dogs with coronary artery stenoses and endothelial injury, *J Clin Invest* 84:517-527, 1989.
10. Fuster V, Frye RL, Connolly DC: Arteriographic patterns early in the onset of coronary syndromes, *Br Heart J* 37:1250-1262, 1975.
11. Gottlieb SO, Flaherty JT: Medical therapy of unstable angina pectoris, *Cardiol Clin* 9(1):89-98, 1991.
12. Hilton TC, Chairman BR: The prognosis in stable and unstable angina, *Cardiol Clin* 9(1):27-38, 1991.
13. Keaney JF: Natural history and prognosis of unstable angina. In Rutherford, editor: *Unstable Angina,* New York, 1992, Marcel Deker.
14. Kulick DL: Coronary arteriography in the anginal syndromes, *Cardiol Clin* 9(1):63-71, 1991.
15. Lambert CR: Pathophysiology of stable angina pectoris, *Cardiol Clin* 9(1):1-10, 1991.
16. Levin DC, Fallon JT: Significance of angiographic morphology of localized coronary stenosis, *Circulation* 66:316-3, 1982.
17. Oliver MF: Epidemiology and prognosis of stable angina. In Julian, editor: *Angina Pectoris,* ed 2, New York, 1985, Churchill Livingstone.
18. Shah FK: Pathophysiology of unstable angina, *Cardiol Clin* 9(1):11-26, 1991.
19. *St Anthony's DRG guidebook 1995,* Reston, Va, 1994, St Anthony.
20. Steenberger C, Hill ML, Jennings RB: Volume regulation and plasma membrane injury in aerobic, anaerobic, and ischemic myocardium in vitro, *Circ Res* 57:864-886, 1985.
21. Thadani U: Medical therapy of stable angina pectoris, *Cardiol Clin* 9(1):73-87, 1991.
22. Wilson RF, Holida MD, White CS: Quantitative angiographic morphology of coronary stenosis leading to myocardial infarction or unstable angina, *Circulation* 73:286-292, 1986.
23. Yanagisawa M, Kurihara H, Kimura S: A novel potent vasoconstrictor peptide produced by vascular endothelial cells, *Nature* 332:411-415, 1988.

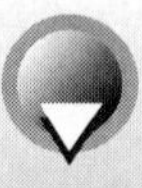

CLINICAL GUIDELINE

14

Cardiac Catheterization

Tamera Mahaffey, MSN, RN

DESCRIPTION

Cardiac catheterization is considered the gold standard for precise diagnosis of coronary artery disease (CAD) and cardiac function.[18]

Cardiac catheterization involves insertion of radiopaque catheters into a large artery and vein. The venous catheter is advanced to the right side of the heart to measure right heart and pulmonary pressures. The arterial catheter is advanced to the aortic root where the openings of the coronary arteries are located and into the left ventricle (LV). Pressure gradients within the left heart chambers and aorta are measured. Injection of contrast material into the coronary arteries assesses the absence or presence and severity of coronary artery disease. Injection of a bolus of contrast material (25 to 40 ml) into the LV enables assessment of LV wall motion and calculation of ejection fraction. All contrast injections of coronary arteries and LV are recorded on X-ray film (cineangiography) to permit further analysis.[12]

According to the American Heart Association, over one million heart catheterizations are performed in the United States each year. The risk of major complication from the procedure is 0.01% or less.[10,15] Emergency catheterizations or procedures performed on very sick patients (patients with pulmonary hypertension, dysrhythmias, renal failure, severe CAD, hypoxemia, or children with complex congenital heart disease) carry a somewhat higher risk. The risk of the procedure is small, especially when compared to the risk of making an incorrect or incomplete diagnosis.

The indications for cardiac catheterization are listed in Table 14-1. Information obtained from this procedure is also valuable in determining a patient's prognosis because of the correlation between subsequent mortality and LV dysfunction, severity of CAD, and/or significant valvular disease. Determination of the need for medical treatment or invasive intervention such as coronary artery bypass graft surgery (CABG), valvular surgery, percutaneous transluminal coronary angioplasty (PTCA), or directional coronary atherectomy (DCA) is made from the information obtained from cardiac catheterization. In spite of the very low risk associated with cardiac catheterization, there are a number of contraindications to the procedure, as listed in Table 14-2.

PATHOPHYSIOLOGY

Knowledge of cardiac anatomy is essential to understanding cardiac catheterization. Figure 14-1 demonstrates the flow of venous and arterial blood throughout the heart and vascular system. It is important to note that the left side of the heart functions under much higher pressure than the right side due to the difference in vascular resistance each side must overcome. In addition, it is important to recall that the four intracardiac valves should allow blood only to flow forward.

There are two coronary arteries, the right coronary artery (RCA) and the left coronary artery (LCA), which provide the myocardium with its blood supply (Figure 14-2). These arteries arise at the base of the aortic valvular ring behind the right and left aortic cusps. The RCA and its branches, referred to as marginals, supply the atria, the RV, and, in 70% of the population, the inferior wall of the LV. The major LCA branches are the left anterior descending (LAD) branch, with branches called diagonals; and the circumflex (Cx) branch, with branches called marginals. The branches of the LCA supply the interventricular septum, the anterior wall of the LV, and the posterior and lateral walls of the LV. Arterial branches from the epicardial vessels supply the

TABLE 14-1 Possible Indications for Cardiac Catheterization and Angiography[16]

Diagnosis of obscure or confusing cardiac problems
Chest pain of uncertain etiology
Young patients with stable angina pectoris
Patients of any age with unstable angina pectoris
Elderly patients with disabling stable angina pectoris
Patients with abnormal stress ECG or stress thallium tests
Post-MI treated with thrombolytic therapy
Post-MI angina
Patients with valvular heart disease
Patients undergoing major surgery who have abnormal thallium studies
Patients for whom corrective heart surgery is anticipated (congenital defects, valvular disease, etc.)

TABLE 14-2 Relative Contraindications for Cardiac Catheterization and Angiography

Elderly patients who are not candidates for invasive interventions (such as CABG, PTCA, etc.)
Patients with uncorrected electrolyte imbalance (especially hyper- or hypokalemia, hypomagnesemia, hypocalcemia, or hyponatremia)
Patients who are digitalis toxic
Patients with febrile illness or infection
Patients who are fully anticoagulated with warfarin (PT >18 sec)
Patients with uncorrected hypertension
Patients with severe renal insufficiency or renal failure (unless measures are taken to remove contrast material, such as dialysis, diuretics, or fluids)
Patients with known allergy to contrast material (unless the patient can be premedicated with antihistamines and anti-inflammatory medication)
Recent cerebrovascular accident (>1 month)
Pregnancy

epicardial layer of the myocardium. Vessels that plunge deep into the myocardium supply the endocardium. The myocardium is rich in capillaries. Blood passes through these capillaries into the venous collecting system and back into the RA through the coronary sinus.

During cardiac catheterization, a radiopaque catheter is inserted through an artery and vein and threaded to the heart. This process is guided by fluoroscopy. Percutaneous puncture of the femoral vessels, known as the Judkins technique, is the most common approach.[11,12] When the antecubital site is accessed via an incision, the technique is referred to as the Sones technique.[11,12] After vascular access is gained, the catheter is connected to a pressure transducer via a manifold

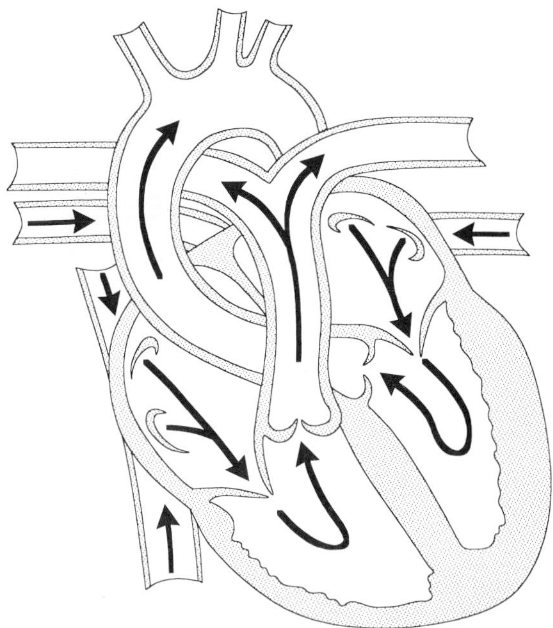

Figure 14-1 Intracardiac circulation.

system that permits pressure monitoring and catheter flushing with heparinized solution. The catheter is then advanced into the coronary arteries and LV. The venous catheter is advanced to the right atrium (RA), across the tricuspid valve into the right ventricle (RV), then across the pulmonary valve into the pulmonary artery. Pressures are measured in each of the chambers catheterized, as well as the pressure gradient across the valves. Pulmonary hypertension, elevated RV or RA pressure, blood oxygen content and tension in each chamber, and cardiac output (CO) can be assessed by this technique.

A transseptal approach may be used to catheterize the left atrium. In this procedure, the catheter is advanced across an atrial septal puncture site, and left atrial pressure measurements are obtained. Further advancement across the mitral valve into the left ventricle is used to assess left ventricular pressure. Left heart pressures and valve gradients are measured and evaluated. More commonly, left cardiac chamber pressures and valvular gradients are measured by retrograde insertion of a catheter from the aorta backward into the LV and LA.

Cineangiography involves injecting a radiopaque solution into cardiac chambers or vessels with cine x-ray film recording. Once the catheter is advanced through the aorta to the origin of the coronary arteries, the catheter is directed to either the right or left coronary artery, contrast material is injected, and cineangiograms obtained (Figure 14-3). Cineangiography provides an opportunity for diagnosis and quantification of CAD and coronary artery spasm. Coronary artery disease that may require intervention includes significant left main coronary artery stenosis, or significant stenosis in the LAD, Cx, RCA, or any of their branches

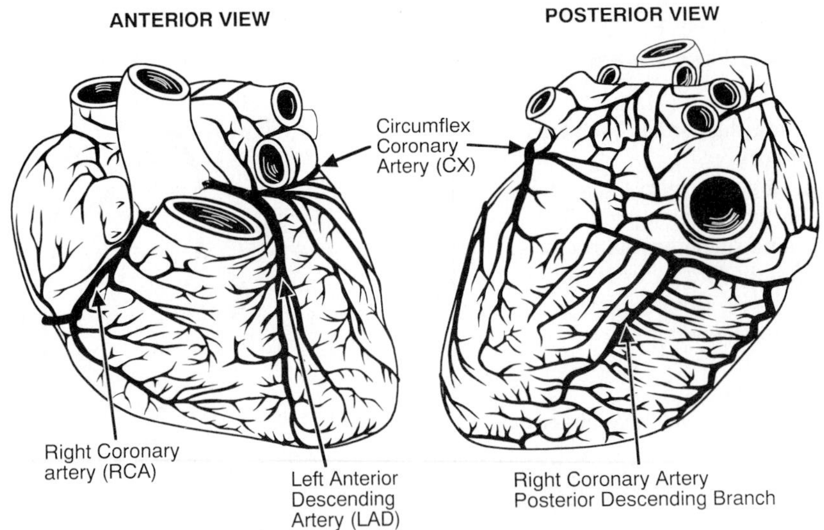

Figure 14-2 Anatomy of the coronary arteries.

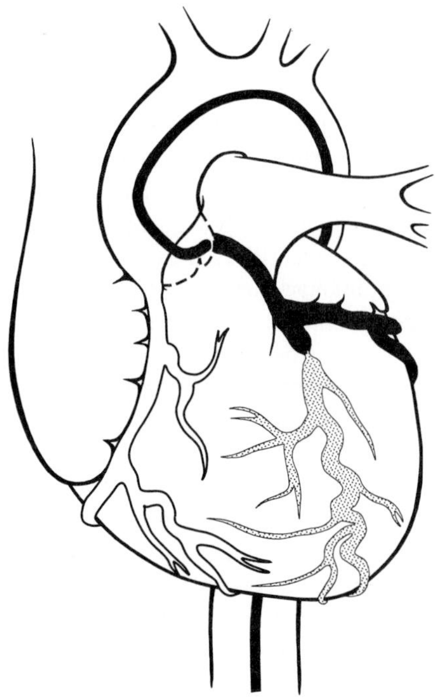

Figure 14-3 Catheter position for left coronary artery angiogram with stenosis in LAD.

with or without reported symptomatology. Left main stenosis is considered significant if greater than 50%; other coronary artery stenosis is judged significant if greater than 75%. Injection of contrast material into the left ventricle provides information about left ventricular size and function, presence of left ventricular aneurysm, mitral valve competence, or abnormalities such as ventricular septal defect or cardiomyopathy.

Additional procedures may be done in conjunction with the cardiac catheterization. These include PTCA, electrophysiologic studies, DCA, and direct laser ablation of intracoronary plaque.

Incidence of major complication from cardiac catheterization is 0.01% or less.[4] Complications include myocardial infarction (MI), cerebrovascular accidents (CVA), arterial thrombosis, vasovagal reactions, dysrhythmias, allergic reactions to the contrast material, and infection.[11,13] Premedication with antihistamines and steroids may be used to prevent allergic reactions to the contrast material. Anticoagulation with intravenous heparin during the procedure is common to prevent thrombolic complications. Cardiac catheterization is performed under sterile conditions to decrease the incidence of infection.[8]

LENGTH OF STAY/ANTICIPATED COURSE

Cardiac catheterization is commonly done as an outpatient procedure unless an interventional procedure is also planned, or the patient has been admitted with unstable angina, an acute MI, severe diabetes, or renal failure.[5,16] As a result, traditional DRG coding does not apply. Outpatient catheterization has proven to be safe, cost-effective, and less inconvenient to the patient and family; it promotes more efficient use of hospital beds and is offered by most facilities that provide cardiac services.[2,3] Outpatient cardiac catheterization labs are located in hospital facilities as well as in mobile catheterization laboratory units. While mobile cath labs provide improved patient access, a major impetus for their development has been marketing of services. It is recommended that catheterization labs be located in or in close proximity to institutions that have cardiovascular surgery programs, and that mobile cath labs be associated with transport services (helicopter or fixed wing) that can carry patients to institutions that provide surgery if necessary.[6,9]

The usual length of hospital stay for outpatient catheterization is 8 to 10 hours.[3] Most protocols require 4 to 6 hours of bed rest following the procedure.[2] Additional procedures such as PTCA or DCA require an average hospital stay of 1.5 to 3 days. Complications of cardiac catheterization, depending on the severity, may also prolong the length of stay.

MANAGEMENT TRENDS AND CONTROVERSIES

Nuclear procedures such as thallium stress tests may augment the data obtained from cardiac catheterization. These procedures may be used first to determine the need for cardiac catheterization, or following cardiac catheterization to determine if CAD diagnosed by catheterization is causing ischemia.[19] In addition, various techniques such as magnetic resonance imaging (MRI), positron emission tomography (PET), and digital subtraction angiography (DSA) may enhance the diagnostic information obtained by cardiac catheterization and, some day, may be developed to a point that they replace cardiac catheterization entirely.[7] New techniques such as intravascular ultrasound and fiberoptic angioscopy have the capability of allowing visualization of a vessel lumen to assess the structure of the arterial wall, extent of atherosclerosis, and lesion characteristics.[14] These techniques may also complement coronary arteriography.

ASSESSMENT

PARAMETER	ANTICIPATED ALTERATION
BP	Potential hypotension: MAP <70 mm Hg *due to hypovolemia from contrast-induced diuresis* Potential hypertension: MAP >90 mm Hg *due to the stress of the procedure*
Right heart pressures	Pulmonary hypertension: PAS >35 mm Hg, PAD >15 mm Hg RV hypertension: RVS >35 mm Hg, RVD >8 mm Hg RA hypertension: RAM >8 mm Hg *all due to potential cardiopulmonary disease*
CO/CI	May be decreased: CO <4 L/min, CI <2.5L/min *due to ischemic heart disease, structural defects, or valve defects*
Left heart pressures	LV hypertension: LVS >140 mm Hg, LVD >10 mm Hg LA hypertension: LAM >12 mm Hg *all due to potential cardiac disease*
Ventricular cineangiography	Valvular stenosis Valvular insufficiency Congenital heart disease Abnormal ventricular wall motion Decreased LV ejection fraction (<50%)
Coronary cineangiography	Coronary artery disease, anomalies, or spasm

Renal Function

UO	Decreased: <30 cc/hr
Creatinine	Elevated: >1.2 mg/dl
BUN	Elevated: >20 mg/dl
K^+	Elevated: >5.0 mEq/L *all due to reaction to contrast material*

PLAN OF CARE

INTERMEDIATE PHASE

Advancement in cardiac catheterization techniques, the trend toward outpatient catheterization, and the need for shortened hospital stays have essentially eliminated the intensive phase of care for the patient undergoing cardiac catheterization. The close monitoring of the postcardiac catheterization patient is reasonably managed in the outpatient or general unit setting.

Plan of Care (cont'd)

PATIENT CARE PRIORITIES	EXPECTED PATIENT OUTCOMES
Anxiety *r/t* *Cardiac disease* *Procedure* *Fear of complications*[1,17]	Decreased anxiety. Verbalize understanding of procedure and possible complications.[1,17]
Decreased cardiac output *r/t* *Cardiac disease* *Dysrhythmias* *Hemorrhage* *Cardiac perforation* *Reaction to contrast material* *Diuresis-induced hypovolemia*[2,3]	Stable BP and heart rhythm No bleeding at access site No angina Adequate UO
High risk for decreased tissue perfusion in cannulated extremity *r/t* *Indwelling invasive catheter* *Possible disruption in vascular plaque* *Vessel perforation*	Perfusion of extremity within precatheterization norms
Self-care deficit *r/t* *Care of insertion site* *Interventions for possible complications* *Follow-up care or interventions*	Verbalizes proper care of site, activity limits, s/s of complications such as hematoma or infection, and recommended follow-up care

INTERVENTIONS

Educate the patient and family regarding the procedure *to decrease anxiety and enable the patient to participate as needed during the procedure.*[1] Emphasize the following aspects:

- Length of the procedure
- Fast response to request to cough
- Hot flash sensation most pronounced in mouth, axilla, groin, and rectum during ventriculogram portion of study
- The need to maintain immobility post-procedure
- The need for increased fluids post-procedure
- Importance of splinting catheter site when coughing, sneezing, laughing, getting up, or having a bowel movement
- Relaxation and distraction techniques.

Premedicate the patient with antihistamine and/or anti-inflammatory drugs *to reduce the risk of allergic reactions.*

Monitor VS, ECG, and UO *to ensure adequate hydration and prevent complications.*

Observe catheter insertion site for bleeding, erythema, or hematoma *to prevent blood loss, perfusion deficit, and discomfort.*

Monitor extremity of insertion site for pulse, temperature, color, and sensory changes *to treat possible perfusion deficit.*

Observe for allergic reaction to contrast material such as hives (especially on abdomen and chest), itching, difficulty swallowing or breathing.

Administer fluids po or IV *to prevent dehydration and hypovolemia.*

Monitor body temperature, site drainage, and general perfusion *to assess for possible infection.*

Monitor neurological status *to assess for embolic complications.*

Reinforce explanation of results and options for future interventions *to assist patient in future care.*

TRANSITION TO DISCHARGE

With the trend toward outpatient catheterization procedures, it is especially important to provide the patient and family with adequate instruction about care at home following cardiac catheterization. Instructions should include care of the catheterization site, signs and symptoms of infection, activity restrictions, and when to follow up with the physician. Patient instruction about the treatment program, whether medical or interventional, should also be done prior to discharge. Patients with documented CAD should be referred to a cardiac rehabilitation program, if available, for risk-factor modification education, exercise programs, and stress management programs.

REFERENCES

1. Anderson KO, Masur FT: Psychologic preparation for cardiac catheterization, *Heart Lung* 18(2):154-163, 1989.
2. Clark DA, et al: Guidelines for the performance of outpatient catheterization and angiographic procedures, *Cathet Cardiovasc Diagn* 27:5-7, 1992.
3. Clements SD, Gatlin S: Outpatient cardiac catheterization, *Clin Cardiol* 14:477-480, 1991.
4. Dault LH, Groene J, Herick R: Helping your patient through cardiac catheterization, *Nursing* 22(2):52-5, 1992.
5. Fierens E: Outpatient coronary arteriography. A report on 12,719 studies, *Cathet Cardiovasc Diagn* 10:27, 1984.
6. Goss JE, Cameron A: Mobile cardiac catheterization laboratories, *Cathet Cardiovasc Diagn* 26:71-72, 1992.
7. Gould K: PET perfusion imaging and nuclear cardiology, *J Nucl Med* 32:579-606, 1991.
8. Heupler FA, et al: Infection prevention guidelines for cardiac catheterization laboratories, *Cathet Cardiovasc Diagn* 25:260-263, 1992.
9. Holmes DR: The mobile catheterization laboratory: should we pick it up and move? Editorial, *Cathet Cardiovasc Diagn* 26:69-70, 1992.
10. Hurst JW, et al: *Atlas of the Heart,* New York, 1988, Gower Medical Publishing.
11. Johnson LW, Krone R: Cardiac catheterization 1991: a report of the registry of the Society for Cardiac Angiography and Interventions, *Cathet Cardiovasc Diagn* 28:219-220, 1993.
12. Judkins MP: Selective coronary arteriography: a percutaneous transfemoral technique, *Radiology* 89:815, 1967.
13. Kennedy JW, et al: Complications associated with cardiac catheterization and angiography, *Cathet Cardiovasc Diagn* 8:5, 1982.
14. Liebson PR, Klein LW: Intravascular ultrasound in coronary atherosclerosis: a new approach to clinical assessment, *Am Heart J* 123(6):1643-1660, 1992.
15. O'Brien C, Recker D: How to remove a femoral sheath, *Am J Nurs* 10:34-37, 1992.
16. Pappenheim CL, Kirkpatrick B: Cardiac catheterization: performing the procedure in an outpatient setting . . . patient selection guidelines, *AORN J* 48(6):1130-2, 1134-7, 1988.
17. Peterson M: Patient anxiety before cardiac catheterization: an intervention study, *Heart Lung* 20(6):643-7, 1991.
18. Rossi L, Leary E: Evaluating the patient with coronary artery disease, *Nurs Clin North Am* 27(1):171-88, 1992.
19. Waller BF, et al: Anatomy, histology, and pathology of coronary arteries: a review relevant to new interventional and imaging techniques. Part II, *Clin Cardiol* 15:535-540, 1992.

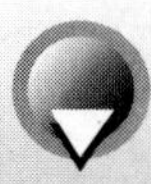

CLINICAL GUIDELINE

15

Percutaneous Transluminal Coronary Angioplasty

Patricia Swanson VerMass, MSN, RN

DESCRIPTION

Percutaneous transluminal coronary angioplasty (PTCA) is a widely accepted procedure for the treatment of occlusive coronary artery disease. PTCA involves the use of a double-lumen balloon catheter inserted into the coronary artery and across an atherosclerotic lesion, where repeated balloon inflations increase the lumen size and subsequently improve distal blood flow. The use of balloon angioplasty on occlusive peripheral arteries was first reported in 1964.[14] Gruentzig performed the first coronary angioplasty in a human in 1977. In 1980, the Food and Drug Administration (FDA) approved its use in the United States. Since its inception, the PTCA procedure has proven to be a desirable and successful nonsurgical alternative to coronary artery bypass graft surgery (CABG).

The prevalence of this procedure has grown rapidly, from a reported 39,000 procedures performed in 1983[17] to 100,000 in 1985 and 300,000 in 1989.[6] It is estimated that nearly half of all patients considered for myocardial revascularization are initially managed with PTCA.[31] Initially, the selection criteria allowed only stable patients with good ventricular function and single-vessel disease involving a proximal, discrete, and readily accessible lesion. With the advancement of catheter technology as well as improved operator technique, the selection criteria have been expanded to include patients with multivessel disease, poor ventricular function, and unstable cardiac status such as acute myocardial infarction (MI) and cardiogenic shock.[27] The type of lesion acceptable for angioplasty has also broadened to include more complex, moderately calcified, and distal lesions.

Angioplasty is the treatment of choice for the majority of patients with single-vessel disease and in many patients with multivessel disease.[27] Positive outcomes have been achieved in patients with unstable angina and in providing emergent revascularization during an evolving MI, especially when thrombolytic therapy is contraindicated or in the presence of cardiogenic shock, where time is critical. Indications for PTCA are not standardized, and vary with center and physician. The American Heart Association/American College of Cardiology Task Force on Assessment of Diagnostic and Therapeutic Cardiovascular Procedures has reported guidelines for patient selection for PTCA using a classification system based on patient characteristics and lesion morphology, and favorable outcome for the procedure.[1,36] Best results are still found with discrete, concentric, noncalcified, smooth lesions. However, increased success rates have been seen with tubular, eccentric, and moderately calcified lesions.[27] PTCA, initially reserved for only single-vessel lesions, has been increasingly performed with success in patients with double- and triple-vessel disease. Patients with multiple noncomplex lesions are usually at no higher risk than those who undergo single-vessel angioplasty.[21] Ongoing clinical trials such EAST, ERACI, GABI, BARI, and RITA are examining the outcome of PTCA in multivessel disease involving complex lesions as compared with CABG as the initial intervention.[20,35] The largest of these, the Randomised Intervention Treatment of Angina (RITA) trial, compares the long-term effects of PTCA and CABG in patients with one- to three-vessel disease with its primary objective being to compare the combined 5-year incidence of death and MI in the two groups.[35] Interim findings at 2.5

years into the trial have reported no significant difference in mortality or MI in the two groups.[35] However, the PTCA group had a greater incidence of revascularization and primary event (including further PTCA, CABG, MI, or death): 38% of the PTCA patients compared with 11% of CABG patients. In addition, angina was more prevalent in PTCA: 32% versus 11% at 6 months, and 31% versus 22% at 2 years.[35] Further findings reported CABG patients to have a longer hospitalization and recovery but in the long term have fewer subsequent events. Reports on treatment costs and resource allocation and continued follow-up will be forthcoming as the RITA trial continues for at least 5 years.

Chronic total occlusions, highly calcified lesions, and vein graft narrowing do not fare as well with PTCA. There continue to be low success rates in opening these types of lesions, although promising advances are continually being made. Left main disease is the one remaining contraindication for PTCA. PTCA of the left main coronary artery carries high mortality, high restenosis rates, and poor late survival.[27] In addition, the presence of thrombus or ulceration at the lesion site, the amount of myocardium that is in jeopardy, and the patient's ability to withstand an ischemic insult must be considered in selecting suitable PTCA candidates.

Initial success rates of 69% to 76% have improved to as high as 91% to 95% with the development of catheters that can be more easily directed into hard-to-reach vessels along with improved operator technique.[27] These numbers are quite impressive considering the expansion of selection criteria to include patients with multivessel and unstable disease. Abrupt occlusion of the involved coronary artery produces the majority of complications seen during or soon after the angioplasty procedure and occurs at a rate of 1.7% to 8.0%.[27,36] Coronary artery dissection, with or without thrombus, is the major cause of abrupt artery occlusion, with coronary spasm and hypotension being contributing factors.[36] Even with the availability of emergent repeat PTCA or bypass surgery, the mortality rate from acute closure is significant at 4.0% to 10.0%.[36]

Despite the advances in PTCA success rate, restenosis of the previously dilated arteries remains the major limitation of the PTCA procedure. The incidence of restenosis remains unchanged since the early years of this procedure in the 1970s.[17,36]

Even with the relatively high rate of restenosis, PTCA remains a widely accepted treatment for coronary disease. With successful PTCA the patient is dismissed from the hospital within 24 to 48 hours and is able to return to work within a week. This results in substantial savings in both health care and patient costs compared with coronary artery bypass graft (CABG) surgery.

PATHOPHYSIOLOGY

Procedure

Ideally, PTCA is not performed at the same time as the diagnostic coronary angiogram. This allows time for patient education and preparation, in addition to decreasing the exposure to contrast material during a single procedure. In emergent situations, when time is critical, PTCA may be performed immediately following the angiogram. Patient education is carried out before and during the procedure. The use of contrast material is kept to a minimum. A surgery suite and staff should be readily available during the PTCA procedures to allow for emergent CABG if complications occur. As a result, the American College of Cardiology recommends that PTCA patients must be reasonable candidates for CABG, and PTCA should be performed only in hospitals with cardiac surgical facilities readily available.[36]

Before the procedure, the patient is given aspirin (325 milligrams) for its antiplatelet properties. The patient may also receive a calcium antagonist, such as nifedipine, to prevent coronary artery spasm during and after PTCA.

The PTCA procedure is performed in the cardiac catherization lab using local anesthesia with arterial access performed in the same manner as the coronary angiogram (see Guideline 14). The patient is attached to a monitor using standard limb and chest leads to allow continuous ECG monitoring during the procedure. A temporary pacing electrode may be inserted through the femoral vein before the procedure. This is usually done when dilating the right coronary artery or circumflex artery as a prophylactic measure to compensate for potential bradycardia. Femoral artery access is obtained, and under continuous angiographic visualization, the guiding catheter is advanced to the origin of the coronary ostium. A 5000 to 10,000 U bolus of intravenous (IV) heparin is administered to prevent thrombus formation. An additional bolus of heparin may be administered every hour. More commonly, the patient is started on a continuous heparin IV infusion to maintain the partial thromboplastin time at 2 to 2½ times the normal or the activated clotting time (ACT) at greater than 300 seconds. In addition, 200 μg of intracoronary nitroglycerin may be administered to prevent coronary spasm and to aid in dilatation of the stenotic artery just before insertion of the balloon catheter.

Selection of the balloon catheter is dependent on coronary artery size, lesion characteristics, and physician preference. Inflated diameter size of PTCA balloons ranges from 1.5 mm to 4.0 mm; balloons are 20 mm in length, although there are shorter or longer balloons available, depending on the patient's needs.[27] In general, balloon size should approximate the size of the normal artery segment adjacent to the stenosis.[27] There are many PTCA balloon catheters to select from, and they are continually being improved in an attempt to optimize success and prevent complications of the procedure.

Once the appropriate catheters are selected, the guide wire and balloon catheter are passed through the guiding catheter and advanced 1 to 2 cm beyond its distal tip. The guide wire is passed independently to the correct vessel and advanced through the lesion (see Figure 15-1). Contrast material injections through the guide catheter are done in-

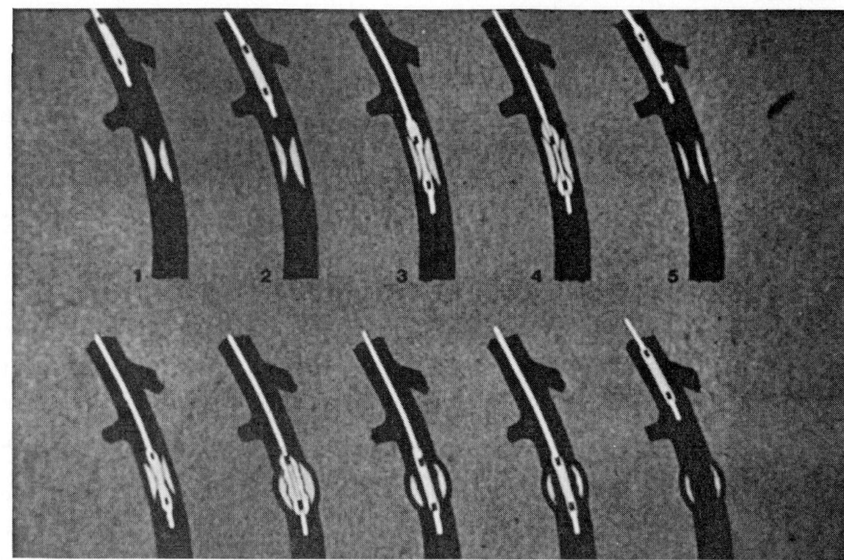

Figure 15-1 Insertion of PTCA balloon catheter across atherosclerotic lesion with repeat balloon inflations and catheter withdrawal. (From Andreoli KG, et al: *Comprehensive cardiac care,* ed 6, St Louis, 1987, CV Mosby.)

termittently to ensure correct position. Once the guide wire has crossed the lesion, it is advanced to a distal point in the coronary artery. The dilatation catheter is then carefully advanced into the lesion, making sure that it is fully engaged across the entire length of the lesion before it is inflated. The balloon is inflated under pressure with a mixture of saline and contrast material to a point at which a sausagelike balloon shape appears. The optimal inflation pressure is dependent on several factors: size of balloon catheter, size of artery dilated, type of lesion, and the presence of myocardial ischemia during dilatation. Overinflation of the balloon with the use of higher pressures can result in arterial trauma. Inflation duration is usually 30 to 60 seconds with repeat inflations until desired results are obtained. Longer inflation times may be needed to achieve plaque molding or to enhance adherence of a dissection. Careful assessment and monitoring for myocardial ischemia occurs throughout the PTCA procedure.

Patients frequently experience angina with ST-T changes during balloon inflation. These symptoms are usually tolerated for a brief period of time and should be promptly relieved with deflation. Sublingual nitroglycerin or nifedipine may be administered to relieve angina pain. In addition, continuous IV infusions of nitroglycerine may be used, especially when the PTCA procedure stimulates coronary spasm. If necessary, small increments of IV morphine may be titrated slowly to relieve persistent discomfort. Perfusion balloon catheters that allow continued coronary blood flow during inflation can be used on those patients who do not tolerate brief periods of balloon inflation or when longer inflation times are needed. The occurrence of refractory chest pain, prolonged ventricular ectopy, or hemodynamic deterioration would indicate more severe ischemia and demand abrupt deflation of the balloon. On occasion, further supportive measures, such as intraaortic balloon pump insertion, are needed.

Repeat angiography is performed after each inflation/deflation cycle to assess patency of the vessel. Translesional pressure gradients, the difference in the intracoronary pressure proximal to the lesion and that distal to the lesion, may also be obtained to assess improvement in coronary blood flow. A gradient of less than 15 to 20 mm Hg is considered an indicator of successful dilatation.[27] In addition, successful PTCA is defined as (1) less than 50% residual stenosis (in a lesion that was initially greater than 50%); (2) 20% or greater increase in arterial lumen diameter; and (3) the absence of major complications defined as death, acute MI, or need for emergent CABG.[36]

Mechanism of Action

Since its inception, several theories have been proposed for the mechanism of balloon angioplasty. Initially, many believed that dilatation of the balloon caused compression of liquid elements from the atheromatous plaque, resulting in flattening of the plaque with resultant reduction in obstruction. Further research found this mechanism to be a minor contributor to increased lumen size and identified a multitude of other factors that resulted in successful dilatation. Although the exact mechanism of PTCA effectiveness remains unknown, current studies have revealed that plaque splitting and stretching of the medial layer of the vessel are most likely the major mechanisms of successful angioplasty.[33] Balloon inflation results in splitting or fracturing of the atheromatous plaque. In addition, inflation causes stretching of the media and destruction of its elasticity, resulting in increased arterial lumen.[27] Plaque compression

TABLE 15-1 Factors Associated with Acute Vessel Closure

Multivessel disease
Female sex
Eccentric, heavily calcified and/or long lesions
Lesions with irregular edges
Lesions with thrombus present
Translesional gradient >20 mm Hg after PTCA
Presence of arterial dissection following PTCA

Adapted from Kulick DL, Kawanishi DT: Percutaneous transluminal coronary angioplasty. In Goldberg S, editor: *Techniques and applications in interventional cardiology*, St Louis, 1991, Mosby–Year Book.

and endothelial denudation are also contributing factors to the remodeling of the arterial lumen. Braden et al. used intracoronary ultrasound before, during, and after the PTCA procedure to examine the coronary vessel wall at the stenosis site and concluded that lumen enlargement was predominantly the result of vessel stretching, with reduction in plaque being a contributing factor.[5] The resulting vascular injury initiates a cascade of events that results in vessel remodeling and repair.[33] The final outcome of long-term lumen patency versus the occurrence of acute vessel closure or restenosis depends on the individual's response to this injury.

Once desired results have been achieved, a pressure dressing may be applied to the vascular access site. The leg is kept extended until the heparin infusion is discontinued and an appropriate interval of time has passed following discontinuation of the heparin to allow for safe removal of the arterial sheath. Hemostasis is again established with manual pressure and 4 to 8 hours of additional immobility to ensure clot stabilization at the sheath sites.

Complications

Despite technical advances and improved physician skill, acute vessel closure and restenosis remain the major complications of PTCA. In general, acute vessel closure is defined as abrupt occlusion or narrowing of the affected coronary artery with clinical or ECG evidence of myocardial ischemia during or within 24 hours of PTCA; restenosis is narrowing of the affected coronary artery of greater than 50% diameter within 6 months post-PTCA.[11,36]

Three major acute complications are associated with PTCA: acute MI, 2.4% to 4.7%; emergent CABG surgery, 1.8% to 3.5%; and death, 0.1% to 1.0%.[27] The majority of acute complications are due to acute occlusion of the coronary artery during or within 24 hours after the angioplasty procedure. The majority of abrupt occlusions are the result of arterial dissection during the angioplasty procedure, with elastic recoil of the vessel wall, vasoconstriction, and coronary spasm being contributing factors.[11] Extensive dissection with a large intraluminal flap or deep medial injury may result in occlusive thrombus formation.[11] The use of aspirin, heparin, and vasodilating agents has reduced the incidence of acute closure caused by coronary spasm or thrombosis. The incidence for acute vessel closure is reported at 1.7% to 8.0%, with the majority occurring before the patient leaves the cath lab.[12,24,36] Factors associated with increased risk of acute vessel closure are listed in Table 15-1. Acute vessel closure may result in acute MI (9.0%) or the need for emergent CABG surgery (20% to 30%) and is associated with a significant mortality rate (4% to 10%), especially if a large area of myocardium is jeopardized.[36] Patient complaints of chest pain, especially associated with ECG changes, should be immediately reported so that repeat PTCA or emergent CABG may be done as needed. Repeat PTCA, often successful in "tacking down" an overly dissected plaque, should be performed with the use of a perfusion balloon catheter that will allow continued coronary blood flow during prolonged inflation. When repeat PTCA fails to reopen the occluded vessel, emergent CABG surgery is the only option unless only a small portion of myocardium is at stake, with less risk associated with the small MI versus the CABG surgery. Newer devices, specifically directional coronary atherectomy and intracoronary stents, have been successful in the management of acute dissection associated with PTCA. However, prolonged interventions should not be deployed if they delay surgery and risk even greater loss of myocardium.[36]

Additional complications associated with PTCA include refractory chest pain; bradycardia; arrhythmias; hypotension; and hematoma, bleeding, arterial thrombosis, and false aneurysms at the sheath site. The need for nitrates, analgesics, and atropine along with other antidysrhythmic and inotropic agents should be anticipated and readily on hand. Possible insertion of an intra-aortic balloon pump is associated with refractory chest pain or hemodynamic compromise or can be used to help maintain vessel patency. Close monitoring of the arterial site and peripheral pulses is mandatory. Loss of peripheral pulses should be immediately reported and the patient prepared for possible emergent embolectomy.

Since 1980, when PTCA became a therapeutic option for revascularization, the incidence of restenosis has remained unchanged and continues to be the major complication of PTCA. Restenosis is the result of the pathophysiological mechanisms involved in vascular injury as a result of balloon inflation. Disruption of the endothelium, itself a very important regulator of normal blood flow, by balloon inflation results in adherence of platelets and fibrin at the injured site. Thrombus formation, associated with endothelial damage and deep vessel injury, stimulates further platelet accumulation. In addition, elastic recoil of the vessel and vasoconstriction may contribute to thrombus formation. Platelet aggregation results in the release of platelet-derived growth factor and other vasoactive, mitogenic, and chemoactive substances.[27] The release of platelet-derived growth factor and other substances stimulates the migration

TABLE 15-2 Risk Factors for Restenosis
Unstable or variant angina
Diabetes mellitus
Hypercholesterolemia
Cigarette smoking
Total and/or high grade occlusions
LAD lesions
Proximal-bifurcation lesions
Heavily calcified and eccentric lesions
Diffuse disease
Saphenous vein graphs (especially old graphs)
Translesional gradient after PTCA >15–20 mm Hg

Adapted from Fanelli C, Aronoff R: Restenosis following coronary angioplasty, *Am Heart J*, 119:357-365, 1990.

of smooth muscle cells from the media to the intima with subsequent proliferation and the end result of intimal hyperplasia and restenosis. Macrophages, endothelial cells, and smooth muscle cells themselves may also play a part in releasing harmful substances.[27] Analysis of tissue obtained in atherectomy procedures has revealed the restenotic plaque to consist primarily of smooth muscle cell hyperplasia.[27] The fibroproliferative process described is the normal response to PTCA; it results in needed vessel remodeling. When the fibroproliferative response becomes excessive, restenosis and subsequent myocardial ischemia result.[33]

The incidence of restenosis is highest in the first 3 to 4 months after PTCA, with greater than 90% developing within 6 months.[27] Restenosis occurring 6 months after PTCA is rare. The majority of patients will have anginal characteristics similar to symptoms prior to their original PTCA. However, some may experience silent restenosis with signs of myocardial ischemia noted during a follow-up exercise stress test. A number of factors related to patient, lesion morphology, and procedure have been identified as risk factors for restenosis and are outlined in Table 15-2. Severe or recent onset of anginal symptoms and diabetes mellitus are the most frequent patient-related risk factors cited. Treatment of restenosis involves repeat PTCA, CABG, or medical management. Repeat PTCA has been reported to be highly successful at rates of 92% to 98%.[27] Restenosis rates after the second PTCA are similar to those with the initial procedure. Patients who present with symptoms less than 3 months after PTCA are at greater risk for restenosis with the second procedure. Patients who tolerated the initial procedure poorly or in which the procedure was technically difficult would be better candidates for medical or surgical intervention.

LENGTH OF STAY/ANTICIPATED COURSE

DRG 112: Percutaneous Cardiovascular Procedures is associated with PTCA.[37] The documented average length of stay is 5.3 days but may be prolonged if complications occur. The expected length of stay includes use of atherectomy and laser adjuncts to PCTA.

Patients undergoing stent placement routinely remain hospitalized 4 to 5 days. Patients are usually kept on bed rest for the first 12 to 24 hours with their activity slowly increased 6 to 12 hours after the sheath is removed. Patients are kept on intravenous heparin while oral anticoagulation with warfarin is initiated. Patients are closely monitored for signs of bleeding and are discharged from the hospital once a safe, therapeutic prothrombin time of 17 to 21 seconds (or INR of 3 to 4) has been reached.

MANAGEMENT TRENDS AND CONTROVERSIES

Abrupt closure and long-term restenosis continue to be the major complications associated with PTCA as well as with the newer interventional devices.

Pharmacologic Intervention

Adjunctive pharmacologic therapy has been employed to decrease thrombus formation, prevent coronary spasm, and decrease the rate of restenosis. Antiplatelet agents, specifically aspirin and dipyridamole, have been effective in decreasing thrombin formation and platelet aggregation and thus preventing abrupt closure following PTCA.[3] Ticlopidine, a newer antiplatelet agent, has been shown to be effective in preventing acute closure, although its use is somewhat limited due to delay (24 to 48 hours) in therapeutic effects from time of ingestion.[2] Although these antiplatelet agents have been effective in preventing acute closure, their role in preventing restenosis has been less successful.[33] Other antiplatelet agents, such as the monoclonal antibody fragment 7E3 F(ab)2, are currently being investigated for their effectiveness in reducing acute closure and restenosis.[9] Studies with omega-3 fatty acids (fish oil), effective as an antiplatelet and possible growth factor inhibitor, have reported conflicting results but may be promising in preventing restenosis.[17]

The use of systemic heparin during the angioplasty procedure has long been established as an adjunct for preventing thrombi from forming on the catheter and the balloon-injured site. Heparin is frequently continued post-procedure for 12 to 24 hours, especially in the event of dissection, to prevent thrombus formation and abrupt vessel closure. It is believed that the groundwork for restenosis, that is, smooth muscle cell proliferation and release of platelet-derived growth factor, begins within minutes of balloon dilatation.[16] Heparin, an effective anticoagulant and inhibitor of smooth muscle cell proliferation, should theoretically be effective in retarding the process of restenosis. Studies thus far have not proven this to be true, although several clinical trials are under way to determine the correct heparin dosage and duration of administration post-procedure as related to its efficacy in preventing long-term restenosis.

Hirulog (BG867), a synthetic thrombin inhibitor, is currently being compared with heparin in clinical trials for its effectiveness and safety in reducing acute complications and restenosis. Preliminary results of the use of recombinant hirudin, CGP 39 393, a derivative of hirulog and also a potent inhibitor of thrombin, have reported its safe and effective use compared with heparin in patients with stable angina undergoing PTCA.[38]

Warfarin is frequently used for long-term anticoagulation following PTCA augmented by stent placement. However, routine PTCA patients are managed with heparin initially and aspirin and dipyridamole long term. Although effective in preventing acute thrombus formation, Warfarin does not prevent restenosis. As with other anticoagulants, the risk of bleeding needs to be thoroughly investigated. Thrombolytic agents such as urokinase have been used successfully in emergent PTCA with thrombus formation.[11]

The use of calcium channel blockers such as diltiazem and nifedipine is common practice for preventing coronary vasospasm associated with balloon-induced injury. Intracoronary nitroglycerin is also routinely used for reducing coronary vasoconstriction during the procedure. Although effective adjuncts in reducing ischemia and preventing acute closure during the angioplasty procedure, these agents have not proven to be effective in preventing long-term restenosis.[33] Clinical trials are under way with other agents that reduce coronary vasoconstriction and inhibit vascular response to injury, including prostocyclin and ciprostene, a prostocyclin analogue.

With increasing knowledge of the fibroproliferative response and factors involved in the restenotic process, many pharmacologic agents are being investigated as adjuncts to modify or inhibit these responses to vascular injury. Corticosteroids have been studied for their ability to decrease tissue inflammation and cell proliferation following vascular injury. However, trials thus far have not shown any effect on preventing restenosis.[17] Other studies have aimed at agents that inhibit growth factors, such as triazolopyrimidine and eicosopentanoic acid, and antiproliferative agents, such as cilazapril (an angiotensin-converting enzyme inhibitor), mevinolin, colchicine, cyclophosphamide, and methotrexate.[33]

An effective method of preventing long-term restenosis following coronary angioplasty has not yet been found. Continued refinement of mechanical interventions along with ongoing investigation of pharmacologic adjuncts will hopefully yield a solution to this major complication.

Catheter Design and Support Therapy

During the early years of PTCA, patient selection was restricted to relatively healthy individuals with good left ventricular function. As catheter technology and operator technique improved, the criteria broadened. Although still at high risk, patients with poor left ventricular function or with a large amount of myocardium in jeopardy are considered candidates for PTCA. The development of perfusion balloon catheters has made it possible to continue coronary blood flow through a stenotic vessel during balloon inflation, thus preserving myocardial perfusion. Autoperfusion balloon catheters allow for prolonged inflation (up to 30 minutes) to tack down an intimal flap in the event of dissection.[11] In the event of a failed procedure, autoperfusion catheters can be placed across the stenosis to reduce ischemia and stabilize the patient until emergency surgery can be performed.

Cardiopulmonary bypass is now being employed in the catheterization lab as a support device for high-risk patients. Femfemoral bypass was first used in emergent cases involving abrupt closure or cardiac arrest. The femfemoral approach has been replaced in most centers by percutaneous cardiopulmonary bypass. This technique eliminates the need for cutdowns and has reported a lower in-hospital mortality for both emergent and elective cases.[39] The use of prophylactic cardiopulmonary bypass during PTCA has shown favorable results, especially in patients with reduced left ventricular ejection fractions.[40]

The intra-aortic balloon pump (IABP) as a support device to augment coronary perfusion and reduce left ventricular workload has been effectively used in high-risk patients undergoing PTCA.[24,26] In patients with acute myocardial infarction, after undergoing successful PTCA, the IABP proved effective in preventing reinfarction.[22]

Adjunctive Interventions

The need for new technology to overcome the limitations of PTCA was first identified in the late 1970s and early 1980s. New mechanical interventional cardiac devices were developed in an attempt to overcome acute vessel closure and restenosis rates associated with PTCA, and to treat more complex lesions in which PTCA has thus far failed, such as total occlusions, elastic lesions, and rigid lesions.[32] Coronary athrectomy, coronary laser angioplasty, and intracoronary stents have recently been employed as alternatives or adjuncts to PTCA. These procedures are increasingly being used in the clinical setting, and trials are ongoing in establishing short- and long-term efficacy.

Coronary atherectomy is the selective excision of atherosclerotic material from the coronary artery. The advantages of atherectomy over PTCA are a more stable lumen after atherectomy with actual debulking of the vessel, a decrease in elastic recoil of the vessel, and a smoother surface post-procedure resulting in less accumulation of platelets and fibrin.[32] In theory, the mechanisms of atherectomy, such as a smoother vessel surface and less tissue damage, should result in reduced restenosis rates. However, thus far, atherectomy has not been shown to be superior to PTCA, with complication and long-term restenosis rates similar for both procedures.[7,8,15]

Three types of atherectomy devices have been identified. The **directional coronary atherectomy (DCA),** developed by Simpson and colleagues in California in 1984 and approved by the Food and Drug Administration for coronary revascularization in September 1990, has been increasingly used, with 17,000 reported cases in 1991 and an estimated 33,000 procedures in 1992.[8] It consists of a distal cylindrical

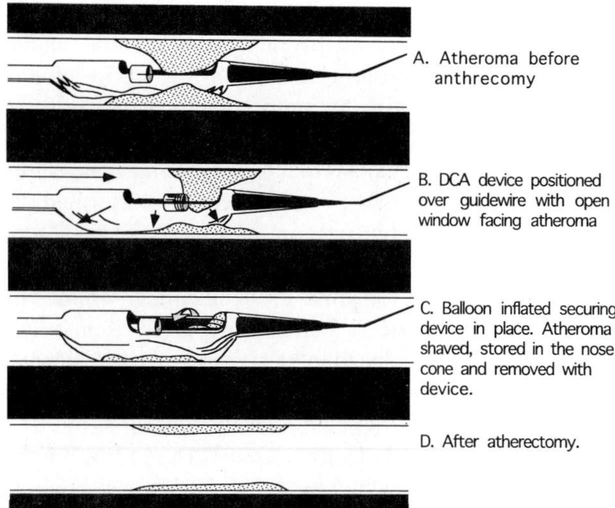
A. Atheroma before anthrecomy
B. DCA device positioned over guidewire with open window facing atheroma
C. Balloon inflated securing device in place. Atheroma shaved, stored in the nose cone and removed with device.
D. After atherectomy.

Figure 15-2 Use of the DCA device. **A,** Atheroma before atherectomy. **B,** DCA device positioned over guide wire with open window facing atheroma. **C,** Balloon inflated to secure DCA firmly against atheroma. Shaved portions of atheroma stored in the nose of the device and removed along with the catheter. **D,** Atheroma following atherectomy.

metal housing with an open window on one side and a balloon on the other (see Figure 15-2). A rotating cutting blade, located within the housing and powered by a handheld, battery-operated device, revolves at 2000 rpm. The metal housing is placed across the lesion with the open window pressed against the plaque. Stabilized by balloon inflation, the blade shaves off atherosclerotic material, which is collected in the housing unit and removed when the catheter is withdrawn. Immediate success rates for the DCA have been reported at 85% to 96% in both native arteries and vein grafts.[8,28] Incidence of acute closure is 1% to 4%, with restenosis rates reported at 30% to 50%, reflecting no improvement over PTCA.[8,28] Further improvement in catheter technology, along with greater lesion selectivity, is needed to improve on these complication rates. At present, DCA has demonstrated the greatest success in large vessels (i.e., proximal left anterior descending) with noncalcified, focal de novo lesions; ulcerated and eccentric lesions; and in failed PTCA lesions, especially if they contain thrombus.[19,28] A lower success rate is associated with lesions greater than 1 cm in length, vessels with less than 3 mm diameter, highly calcified and angulated lesions, and post-PTCA lesions of native and saphenous vein grafts with subintimal dissection.[19,28,32] Although theorized to create less vascular injury, intimal hyperplasia from proliferation of smooth muscle cells is also seen after DCA as in PTCA. One of the major advantages of DCA may be its ability to obtain a larger post-procedural arterial lumen by removing the atherosclerotic plaque, although further refinement of DCA technique and methods for treating the fibroproliferative response to vascular injury are needed.[8]

A second type of atherectomy device is the **mechanical rotational atherectomy.** This high-speed rotational atheroablation device was developed by Auth and associates and first used on human coronary arteries in 1988.[28,32] The rotational atherectomy device consists of a brass burr, available in varied sizes, with a diamond-chip-coated tip. It is driven by a compressed air turbine at speeds of 160,000 to 190,000 rpm. The rotating burr cuts away at the hard plaque, resulting in distal embolization of microparticles. The resultant microparticles are reported to be smaller than red blood cells and thus cause no obstruction to distal blood flow.[32] However, studies have reported that a small percentage of microparticles, especially with the use of large burrs, may be large enough to cause myocardial microinfarcts.[28] The initial success rate for the rotational atherectomy is 90% to 95%.[15,28] Acute complications, reported at an overall rate of approximately 5.0% to 8.9%, are primarily the result of distal embolization of microparticulate debris or perhaps bubbles produced by the burring turbulence which result in slow or no reflow of the affected coronary vessel.[15,28] Acute MI, acute vessel closure, and slow reflow without infarction are the most frequent ischemic complications seen, with coronary perforation, emergent CABG surgery, and death occurring rarely.[15] Restenosis rates range from 30% to 50%, showing no advantage over either DCA or PTCA.[28] Rotational atherectomy is probably most effective in heavily calcified lesions where other techniques have failed to reach the reported success rate of 91%.[15] Rotational atherectomy may also be indicated for ostial, moderately angulated (less than 60 degrees), and restenotic lesions, although other techniques have reported similar success rates. Increased complications have been associated with longer and more angulated (greater than 60 degrees) lesions and right coronary artery stenosis.[15] Technical disadvantages of the rotational atherecotmy apparatus have been identified and need further refinement. At present, further clinical investigation of the rotational atherectomy procedure is needed to better determine its effectiveness in treating coronary artery disease.

The third type of atherectomy device, the **transluminal extraction-endarterectomy catheter (TEC),** has not been as extensively researched as either DCA or rotational atherectomy. The TEC consists of a distal rotary cutting device that rotates at speeds of 750 rpm. It is powered by a handheld device that also controls suction used to aspirate debris from the artery and remove it through the central lumen of the catheter. In the majority of cases, a large residual stenosis remains and PTCA is required to obtain desirable results. The success rate for TEC, used in conjunction with balloon angioplasty, is reported at greater than 90% for both native and saphenous vein graft lesion.[28] The overall complication rate is 3% to 5% with long-term restenosis rates at 40% to 45%.[28] More extensive clinical trials are needed to determine the efficacy of TEC. At present it appears to demonstrate the greatest success in large, bulky lesions containing thrombus and in diffuse disease in both native and vein grafts.

Several **laser systems** used for coronary angioplasty are undergoing clinical trials. The two most widely studied are the excimer coronary laser angioplasty (ECLA) and laser balloon angioplasty (LBA).

The **excimer laser,** first used clinically in 1988, delivers pulsed ultraviolet energy through a fiberoptic catheter directly to the lesion. Plaque ablation occurs as a result of disruption of molecular bonds, with plaque being removed by laser vaporization. Because the excimer laser delivers a very rapid, localized heat, little if any thermal injury occurs.[41] The major disadvantage of the excimer laser is the lack of adequate delivery systems that are small and flexible enough to cannulate the coronary artery and reach the lesion.

The procedure is the same as PTCA except the laser catheter is passed over a guide wire to the lesion site and advanced through the lesion while delivering 10- to 30-second bursts of laser energy. As the catheter is slowly withdrawn the lesion is again lased. The procedure may be repeated until successful angiographic results are obtained. In many cases balloon angioplasty is also required to achieve satisfactory results. Multicenter trials have reported success rates for the excimer laser at 84% to 90%, with the majority of cases requiring additional balloon dilatation.[42] Acute occlusion occurs at a rate of 6.5%, with a restenosis rate of 45%.[29] A higher restenosis rate has been found in patients requiring both laser and balloon angioplasty.[25] Additional complications for excimer laser angioplasty include perforation, dissection, and coronary spasm. Lesions most suitable for ECLA include those that are greater than 20 mm in length, heavily calcified and diffuse; total occlusions; saphenous vein graft lesions; and those unsuccessfully treated by PTCA alone.

Laser balloon angioplasty (LBA), first used in humans in the late 1980s, uses laser energy to heat the arterial walls during balloon angioplasty. The plaque is heated to subvaporization temperatures, which molds the arterial segments, decreases elasticity to prevent recoil, and seals arterial dissections. In addition, the heat produced by laser energy smooths the luminal surfaces and dehydrates thrombi, leaving a larger, potentially less thrombogenic vessel.[23] The LBA uses continuous-wave neodymium: yttrium-aluminum-garnet (Nd:YAG) laser energy delivered through a fiberoptic lumen with a diffusing tip located within a conventional angioplasty balloon (Spears catheter). The laser energy diffuses circumferentially along the length of the balloon. The procedure is performed as a routine balloon angioplasty with repeated balloon inflations until the most optimal angiographic appearance is obtained. At this point, during the final inflation, laser energy is delivered for 20 seconds, diffusing to the arterial walls in contact with the inflated balloon. After laser exposure the balloon is left inflated for 30 seconds to allow the tissue to cool.

Clinical trials with the LBA are ongoing. Preliminary data thus far report the LBA useful for treating failed angioplasty involving thrombus, dissection, or spasm.[23] One clinical trial reported a 95% success rate in patients who had LBA following abrupt closure with PTCA.[34] Severe pain during laser energy delivery is one of the main complications associated with the procedure, although the occurrence of this has lessened with the use of lower-energy doses. Additional complications include acute MI in patients requiring emergent CABG surgery after unsuccessful laser balloon angioplasty for treatment of failed conventional angioplasty, femoral artery pseudoaneurysm, and progressive thrombus formation.[34] Preliminary data reveal LBA to be a safe procedure for treating abrupt closure following PTCA. Restenosis rates reported in small clinical trials have been high at 51% and 56%.[34,42] More recent studies have shown no long-term benefit of the LBA over conventional PTCA, and many centers have stopped using it.

Intracoronary stents, used in humans in the late 1980s, were designed to treat abrupt closures following PTCA and possibly to prevent long-term restenosis. Placed in the coronary artery, stents reduce lumen obstruction by displacing plaque and stretching vessel walls. They also serve as a scaffolding within the lumen to tack up dissected intimal plaque flaps. Once in place, the stent is covered by a neointimal layer, creating a smoother surface that results in less turbulent blood flow and less exposure to platelets. Stents are categorized as self-expanding or balloon expanding, and by the type of material they are made of. The majority of stents are made of surgical stainless steel, although other materials being investigated include tantalum, nitonol, and various polymers. All stainless steel stents have the disadvantage of minimal radiopacity and increased tendency for thrombosis. Use of anticoagulant agents pre- and post-procedure is essential to prevent thrombosis. Two stents currently available for use are the Palmaz-Schatz stent and the Gianturco-Roubin flex stent.[10] Both are balloon-expandable stents made of stainless steel. The Palmaz-Schatz stent is a tubular mesh with eight rows of offset slots (see Figure 15-3). the Gianturco-Roubin stent is arranged in a zigzag pattern similar to a coil (see Figure 15-4). Other stents currently being investigated include the Wall stent, a multifilament, woven stainless steel self-expanding stent; and the Wiktor and Zigzag stents,both of which are balloon expandable and made of tantalum.

The procedure for placement of a balloon-expandable stent begins with balloon dilatation of the lesion. Once satisfactory results are obtained (or if abrupt closure occurs), the stent, placed over a balloon catheter, is delivered to the site. The balloon is then inflated and the stent expands against the arterial wall. In some cases the stent is dilated after placement to ensure contact with the vessel wall. With a self-expanded stent, predilatation is not required. The stent is advanced to the lesion site by a delivery catheter and begins to expand against the arterial wall as it is released from the catheter. Before stent placement, patients receive aspirin and dipyridamole, with low-molecular-weight dextran given just before placement, during the procedure, and post-procedure. Intravenous heparin is given following stent placement, and warfarin is initiated to maintain a prothrom-

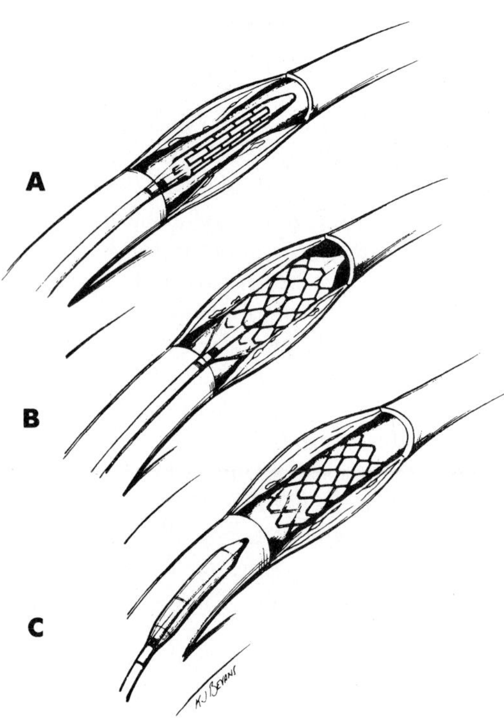

A. Stent is crimped onto balloon catheter for placement.
B. Stent is expanded against vessel wall.
C. Stent is supporting the vessel wall. Balloon catheter is withdrawn from coronary artery.

Figure 15-3 The Palmaz-Schatz stent available as a single or articulated multiple segments to improve stent flexibility. (From Thelan, et al: *Critical care nursing,* ed 2, St Louis, 1993, Mosby–Year Book.)

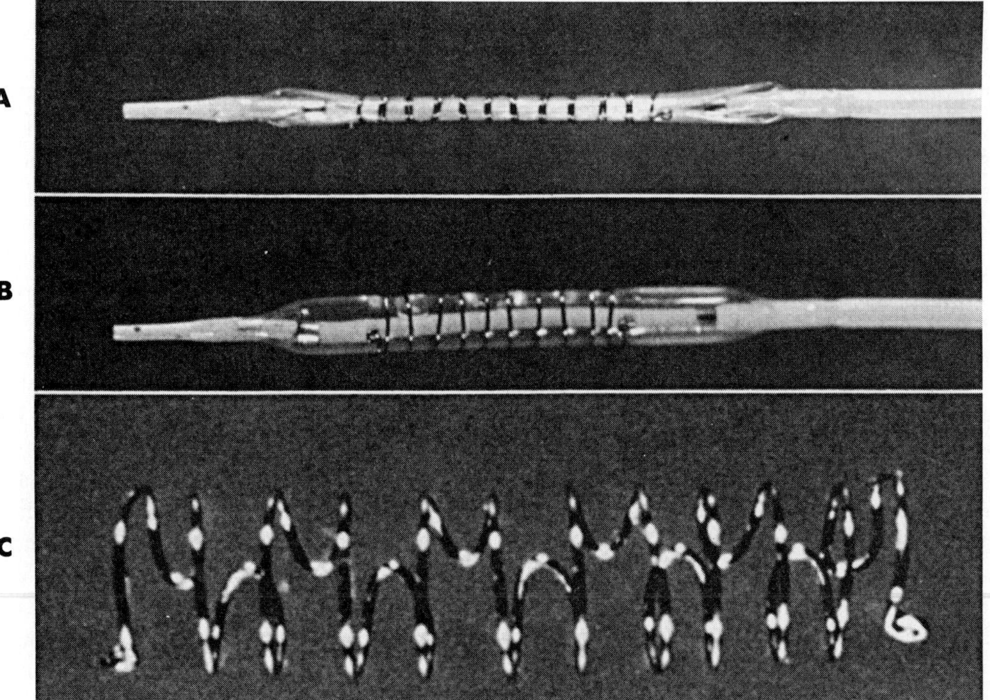

Figure 15-4 The Gianturco-Roubin stent. **A,** Deflated balloon delivery system with coil stent wrapped tightly around deflated balloon. **B,** Inflated balloon showing deployment of the stent. **C,** Enlarged photograph of the expanded coil stent showing the reversing interdigitating coils. (From Vogel, King: *Interventional cardiology: future directions,* St Louis, 1989, Mosby–Year Book.)

bin time (PT) of 17 to 21 seconds or an International Normalized Ratio (INR) of 3.0 to 4.0. Hospital stay may be lengthened in order to achieve therapeutic PT/INR levels. Patients receive warfarin and dipyridamole for approximately 2 to 3 months and aspirin indefinitely. Prophylactic antibiotics may also be recommended post–stent placement and especially during other invasive procedures. The meshwork of the stent remains at risk for bacterial seeding until it is completely endothelialized.

Success and complication rates vary according to the device used. Success rates for the Palmaz-Schatz and Gianturco-Roubin stents have been reported at greater than 90%.[10] The major complications reported are thrombus formation and bleeding from excessive anticoagulation. Preliminary trials of stent use report reocclusion rates of 20% to 40%.[10] Stents used for failed angioplasty versus elective stenting reportedly have greater thrombosis and restenosis rates.[18] The major limitations cited for the use of intracoronary stents are thrombus formation and the need for anticoagulation, restenosis, and failure to deliver to the appropriate site. Ongoing investigation of stents made with tantalum and other materials, along with improved technology, may bring a reduction in these limitations.

Current health care reform warrants the evaluation of the economic impact of the newer mechanical devices for coronary revascularization. Previous studies have demonstrated the cost savings with PTCA as compared with coronary bypass surgery. A group at Emory reported the average cost of multivessel PTCA to be approximately 40% of the cost for CABG even with repeat PTCA.[4] Few studies thus far have examined the cost/benefit ratio of the newer mechanical devices such as DCA, lasers, and stents. Dick et al. reported an in-hospital cost analysis comparing PTCA, coronary atherectomy, and intracoronary stent placement.[13] In-hospital charges were 102% higher for intracoronary stent placement and 34% higher for atherectomy patients as compared with PTCA.[13] The increased cost associated with stent placement was due to prolonged hospital stay to regulate anticoagulation with warfarin or bleeding complications. Although refinement of these techniques is ongoing, atherectomy, laser, and intracoronary stent devices have not produced lower restenotic rates than PTCA.[30] In addition, the majority of procedures require balloon dilatation in conjunction with the newer techniques. Further development of mechanical and pharmacologic interventions needs to be evaluated not only for safety and efficacy but also for cost/benefit ratio.

ASSESSMENT

PARAMETER	ANTICIPATED ALTERATION
Cardiovascular	
HR	Tachycardia: HR >100 bpm
Rhythm	Bradycardia: HR <60 bpm *may occur while pulling sheath secondary to vasovagal response.* Ventricular ectopy *due to reperfusion or may be a sign of myocardial ischemia.*
BP	Hypertension: SBP >150 mm Hg Hypotension: SBP <100 mm Hg *Due to contrast material reaction or bleeding at sheath site*
12-lead ECG	ST segment changes consistent with ischemia *due to underlying CAD, balloon inflation or post-PTCA coronary thrombosis, dissection or coronary spasm*
Chest pain	Angina *due to CAD, PTCA procedure or post-PTCA complications*
Vascular integrity	Change in color, pulses, temperature, capillary refill, or sensation of affected extremity *due to presence of sheath, thrombosis, hemorrhage, or hematoma*
Sheath site	Excessive bleeding at sheath/puncture site Development of hematoma or retroperitoneal bleed
Laboratory Findings	
Hgb/Hct	Abnormal drop in hemoglobin and/or hematocrit compared with preprocedure values *due to potential bleeding at site*
UO	Excessive UO *due to osmotic diuresis from contrast material* Decreased: <30 cc per hour *due to renal insufficiency from contrast material*
Creatinine	Elevated: >1.5 mg/100 ml *due to renal insufficiency from contrast material*
Partial thromboplastin time (PTT)	PTT within therapeutic range as defined by the physician *for patients receiving IV heparin.*

Prothrombin time (PT) International normalized ratio (INR)	PT therapeutic at 18 to 20 seconds INR at 3 to 4 *Only in patients receiving oral anticoagulant.* *The therapeutic prothrombin time is expressed as an INR value, a standardized level of anticoagulation that takes into account the differences in reagents used in measuring the PT.*
CPK	Increased: >10 mg/ml with positive MB index *in the event of myocardial damage*
K^+	Decreased: <4.0 mEq/L *due to excessive urine output*

PLAN OF CARE

INTERMEDIATE PHASE

Unless a complication evolves such as refractory angina or AMI, the majority of patients undergoing PTCA with or without an adjunctive procedure will be placed on a telemetry unit. ICU admission may be warranted for the intense PTT and PT monitoring needed for intracoronary stent patients. In general, however, PTCA patients may be adequately monitored and cared for outside the ICU environment.

PATIENT CARE PRIORITIES	EXPECTED PATIENT OUTCOMES
High risk for decreased cardiac output *r/t* *Dysrhthmias* *Acute vessel closure* *Coronary artery spasm* *Acute MI*	Normal sinus rhythm BP within patient norms Absence of angina Stable ECG Normal CK
High risk for decreased extremity tissue perfusion *r/t* *Cannulization of artery* *Excessive bleeding* *Hematoma formation*	Palpable peripheral pulses Extremity appearance within patient norms Absence of bleeding or hematoma at sheath site
Fluid volume and electrolyte imbalance *r/t osmotic diuresis associated with use of contrast material or renal insufficiency*	Stable vital signs Adequate hydration Serum potassium and creatinine: WNL UO: WNL
Back, joint, and leg pain/discomfort *r/t* *Prolonged extension of extremity* *Strict bed rest* *Generally immobilized state*	Comfort within acceptable patient-determined range Able to rest and sleep
Self-care deficit *r/t lack of knowledge about procedure, medications, follow-up care*	Verbalizes knowledge of procedure, medications, when to contact physician, life-style modification strategies

INTERVENTIONS

Monitor rhythm and ECG, compare with pre-procedure ECG. *Be alert for ventricular ectopy and/or ST segment changes signifying ischemia.*

Monitor for presence of angina. Encourage patient to report onset of chest discomfort immediately: note onset, location, severity. Be familiar with character of preprocedure angina.

Obtain stat ECG and notify physician for anginal episodes.

Anticipate the need for emergent repeat PTCA if angina occurs.

Administer antianginal medications (nitroglycerin, calcium blockers) as directed.

Monitor blood pressure. *Elevated BP may increase bleeding at puncture site. Decreased BP will decrease coronary artery perfusion precipitating myocardial ischemia and possible coronary artery closure at PTCA site(s).*

Monitor creatinine phosphokinase levels *to determine presence/absence of myocardial damage.*

Plan of Care (cont'd)

Maintain strict bed rest while sheath in place *to prevent increased vascular trauma at sheath site.*

Turn patient from side to side without allowing hip flexion.

Immobilize affected leg following sheath removal *to prevent arterial bleed.*

Head of bed elevated no more than 30°, especially following sheath removal.

May place a pillow under unaffected leg/knee *to decrease strain on lower back and enhance comfort while on bed rest.*

Maintain bed rest until 6 to 8 hours after sheath removal. *Patients with intracoronary stents will be on total bed rest for 24 hours after sheath removal with activity slowly advanced.*

Frequently check sheath/puncture site dressing for bleeding, hematoma, or expanding ecchymosis.

Instruct patient to report feelings of warmth or wetness at puncture site and the presence of numbness or tingling of the affected extremity.

Instruct patient to splint sheath site when laughing, coughing, sneezing, or having a bowel movement *to prevent disruption of clot at sheath site.*

Apply direct pressure to site if excessive bleeding occurs. Maintain pressure until new clot forms at site. Redress with pressure dressing.

Frequently assess appearance and pulses of affected extremity for adequate tissue perfusion.

Monitor urine output *to assess for decreased renal perfusion and/or excessive diuresis.*

Avoid venipunctures and intramuscular injections unless absolutely necessary, *especially with patients who received thrombolytic therapy or those on extended anticoagulation therapy such as intracoronary stent patients.*

Administer sedation/analgesics as needed prior to sheath removal *to maximize patient comfort and reduce risk of vasovagal reaction.*

Monitor Hgb and Hct, comparing to pre-procedure values *to assist in monitoring for potential retroperitoneal bleeding.*

Monitor serum K^+ *especially if excessive urine output secondary to diuretic effect of contrast material to prevent ventricular dysrhythmias.*

Maintain adequate fluid replacement through IV infusion and/or oral intake *to maintain adequate cardiac output.*

Closely monitor heparin infusion and PTT values *to ensure therapeutic anticoagulation and prevent bleeding complications in the acute post-procedure period. This is a critical intervention for stent patients.*

Remove sheath as directed once PTT within a safe range, being alert for bradydysrhythmias *which may occur as result of vagal stimulation.*

Closely monitor the administration of warfarin as related to daily PTs *to ensure adequate long-term anticoagulation, especially in patients with intracoronary stents.*

Administer analgesic/antianxiety agents *to maintain immobility of extremity, reduce anxiety, and promote comfort.*

Instruct patient in the importance of any new medications, especially antiplatelet medications, calcium antagonists, and, when necessary, anticoagulants *to maximize the potential for long-term success of the procedure.*

Instruct patient to notify their physician for episodes of anginal chest pain, change in color or sensation of affected extremity, additional or new swelling, or expansion of hematoma at sheath site.

Instruct stent patients in the need for prophylactic antibiotic therapy for dental work or any invasive procedures *to prevent stent infection.*

Instruct patient in strategies to modify personal risk factors for coronary artery disease.

TRANSITION TO DISCHARGE

With a hospital stay of 24 hours to 2 days, patients are usually discharged from the telemetry unit. This may differ for those patients receiving intracoronary stents whose hospitalization is longer due to regulation of anticoagulation therapy. In both cases, the short LOS mandates a highly organized process of care with discharge planning from the moment of admission. Discharge instructions must focus on the following points:

- Care of puncture site
- Signs of infection
- Activity limitations
- Medications
- Readily reporting return of angina
- Alterations in risk factors

Most patients will also need follow-up stress testing to evaluate their progress and detect early signs of restenosis. In addition, participation in a phase II cardiac rehabilitation program is strongly encouraged with emphasis on alteration of risk factors and routine exercise.

REFERENCES

1. ACC/AHA Subcommittee on Percutaneous Transluminal Coronary Angioplasty: Guidelines for percutaneous transluminal coronary angioplasty, ACC/AHA Task Force Report, *J Am Coll Cardiol* 12:529-545, 1988.
2. Barnathan ES, Hershfeld JW: Adjunctive pharmacologic treatment. In Goldberg S, editor: *Coronary angioplasty,* Philadelphia, 1988, FA Davis, pp 41-78.
3. Barnathan ES, et al: Aspirin and dipyridamole in the prevention of acute coronary thrombosis complicating coronary angioplasty, *Circulation* 76(1):125-134, 1987.
4. Black, AJ, et al: Comparative costs of percutaneous coronary angioplasty and coronary artery bypass grafting in multivessel coronary artery disease, *Am J Cardiol* 62:809-811, 1988.
5. Braden GA, et al: Qualitative and quantitative contrasts in the mechanisms of lumen enlargement by coronary balloon angioplasty and directional coronary atherectomy, *J Am Coll Cardiol* 23(1):40-48, 1994.
6. Califf RM, et al: Restenosis after coronary angioplasty: an overview. *JACC* 17(6):2B-13B, 1991.
7. Carrozza JP, Baim DS: Complications of directional coronary atherectomy: incidence, causes, and management, *Am J Cardiol* 72:47E-54E, 1993.
8. CAVEAT Study Group: A comparison of directional atherectomy with coronary angioplasty in Patients with coronary artery disease, *N Engl J Med* 329(4):221-227, 1993.
9. Cheseboro JH, Badimon L, Fuster V: Importance of antithrombin therapy during coronary angioplasty, *J Am Coll Cardiol* 17(6):96B-100B, 1991.
10. Dean LS, Roubin GS: Use of intracoronary stents for arterial stenosis or occlusion. In Kulick DL, Rahimtoola SH, editors: *Techniques and applications in interventional cardiology,* St Louis, 1991, Mosby–Year Book, pp 215-229.
11. de Feyter PJ, et al: Abrupt coronary artery occlusion during percutaneous transluminal coronary angioplasty, *Am Heart J* 123(6):1633-1642, 1992.
12. Detre KM, et al: Incidence and consequences of periprocedural occlusion, *Circulation* 82(3):739-750, 1990.
13. Dick RJ, et al: In-hospital costs associated with new percutaneous coronary devices, *Am J Cardiol* 68:879-885, 1991.
14. Dotter CT, Judkins MP: Transluminal treatment of arteriosclerotic obstruction, *Circulation* 30:654-670, 1964.
15. Ellis SG, et al: Relation of clinical presentation, stenosis morphology, and operator technique to the procedural results of rotational atherectomy and rotational atherectomy-facilitated angioplasty, *Circulation* 89(2):882-892, 1994.
16. Ellis SG, et al: Effect of 18- to 24-hour heparin administration for prevention of restenosis after uncomplicated coronary angioplasty, *Am Heart J* 117:777-782, 1989.
17. Fanelli C, Aronoff R: Restenosis following coronary angioplasty, *Am Heart J* 119:357-365, 1990.
18. Foley JB, Brown RI, Penn IM: Thrombosis and restenosis after stenting in failed angioplasty: comparison with elective stenting. *Am Heart J* 128(1):12-20, 1994.
19. Garratt KN, Holmes DR. Directional coronary atherectomy, *Cardio Intervention* 12-22, October 1991.
20. Hamm CW, et al: Angioplasty vs bypass-surgery in patients with multivessel disease: in-hospital outcome in the G.A.B.I. trial, *Circulation* 86(4) (suppl I): I-374, 1992 (abstract).
21. Hartzler GO, et al: What to expect from PTCA today, *Patient Care* 36-67, Feb. 15, 1992.
22. Ishihara M, et al: Intraaortic balloon pumping as the post angioplasty strategy in acute myocardial infarction, *Am Heart J* 122(2):385-389, 1991.
23. Jenkins RD, Spears JR: Laser balloon angioplasty, *Circulation* 81(suppl IV):IV-101-IV-108, 1990.
24. Kahn JK, et al: Support "high risk" coronary angioplasty using intraaortic balloon pump counterpulsation, *J Am Coll Cardiol* 15:1151-1155,1990.
25. Karsch KR, et al: Percutaneous coronary excimer laser angioplasty in patients with stable and unstable angina pectoris, *Circulation* 81:1849-1859, 1990.
26. Kern MJ, et al: Augmentation of coronary blood flow by intra-aortic balloon pumping in patients after coronary angioplasty, *Circulation* 87(2):500-511, 1993.
27. Kulick DL, Kawanishi DT: Percutaneous transluminal coronary angioplasty. In Golberg S, editor: *Techniques and applications in interventional cardiology,* St Louis, 1991, Mosby–Year Book, pp 43-119.
28. Lau KW, Sigwart U: Novel coronary interventional devices: an update, *Am Heart J* 123(2):497-506, 1992.
29. Lee G, Mason DT: Excimer coronary laser angioplasty: it's time for a critical evaluation, *Am J Cardiol* 69:1640-1643, 1992.
30. Muller DWM, et al: Quantitative angiographic comparison of the immediate success of coronary angioplasty, coronary atherectomy and endoluminal stenting, *Am J Cardiol* 66:938-942, 1990.
31. Myler RK: Coronary angioplasty: baloons and new devices, *J Invasive Cardiol* 5(2):74-78, 1993.
32. O'Neill WW: Mechanical rotational atherectomy, *Am J Cardiol* 69:12F-18F, 1992.
33. Popma JJ, Topol EJ: Factors influencing restenosis after coronary angioplasty, *Am J Med* 88:1-16N-1-23N, 1990.
34. Reis GJ, et al: Laser balloon angioplasty: clinical, angiographic and histologic results, *J Am Coll Cardiol* 18:193-202, 1991.
35. RITA Trail Participants: Coronary angioplasty versus coronary artery bypass surgery: the Randomised Intervention Treatment of Angina (RITA) trial, *Lancet* 341:573-580, 1993.
36. Ryan TJ, et al: Guidelines for percutaneous transluminal coronary angioplasty: a report of the AHA/ACC Task Force on assessment of

diagnostic and therapeutic cardiovascular procedures, *Circulation* 88(6):2987-3007, 1993.

37. *St Anthony's DRG Guidebook 1995,* Reston, Va, 1994, St Anthony.
38. van den Bos AA, et al: Safety and efficacy of recombinant hirudin (CGP 39 393) versus heparin in patients with stable angina undergoing coronary angioplasty, *Circulation* 88(5):2058-2066, 1993.
39. Vogal RA, Tommaso CL: Myocardial and systemic circulatory protection during coronary angioplasty. In Golberg S, editor: *Techniques and applications in interventional cardiology,* St Louis, 1991, Mosby–Year Book, pp 269-281.
40. Vogel RA: Elective supported angioplasty registry: benefit of prophylactic cardiopulmonary bypass support in low ejection fraction patients, *Circulation* 86:(suppl I)I-374, 1992 (abstract).
41. Waller BF: "Crackers, breakers, stretchers, drillers, scrapers, shavers, burners, welders and melters"—the future of atherosclerotic coronary artery disease? A clinical-morphologic assessment, *J Am Coll Cardiol* 13:969-987, 1989.
42. White CJ, Ramee SR: Laser angioplasty in peripheral and coronary artery disease. In Golberg S, editor: *Techniques and applications in interventional cardiology,* St Louis, 1991, Mosby–Year Book, pp 230-268.

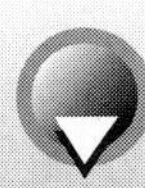

CLINICAL GUIDELINE

16

Acute Myocardial Infarction

Susan G. Osguthorpe, MS, RN, CNA

DESCRIPTION

Acute myocardial infarction (AMI) is the death or necrosis of myocardial tissue due to inadequate tissue perfusion. Inadequate tissue perfusion occurs when there is an imbalance of the cardiac oxygen supply relative to demand. Myocardial infarction (MI) is a dynamic process that takes place over several hours. An *evolving* myocardial infarction is present when the patient has chest discomfort or other symptoms, due to myocardial ischemia, usually lasting longer than 20 minutes but less than 4 to 6 hours; however, chest discomfort or other symptoms lasting longer than 4 to 6 hours are classified as a *completed* myocardial infarction.[27]

Dead cardiac tissue is unevenly surrounded by severely ischemic tissue that may recover or die over time.[27] In the *evolving* myocardial infarction, this cellular death progresses from the endocardium out toward the epicardium. The concept of myocardial salvage presumes that interventions to improve myocardial perfusion can be used to limit infarct size and return ischemic cells to normal. As a result, there has been increased emphasis on interventions that increase myocardial oxygen supply rather than those that alter the myocardial oxygen demand.[19,27]

Heart disease is the leading cause of death in the United States, and it is responsible for more years of potential life lost before age 65 than any other illness, regardless of gender or race.[43] At least 7 million Americans have diagnosed coronary artery disease, with mortality of more than 514,000 people each year.[43]

Significant coronary artery syndromes include sudden cardiac death (SCD), angina, and MI. More than 350,000 people die from SCD annually.[43] Approximately two thirds of sudden deaths due to coronary disease take place outside the hospital and usually occur within 2 hours of the onset of symptoms.[13] About 1.5 million MIs occur each year in the United States, with an approximate mortality of 25%, more than half of which occur in the prehospitalization phase.[31]

Although adjusted death rates for MI have declined dramatically from more than 300 per 100,000 population in 1950 to slightly less than 200, the total number of deaths due to MI has not declined due to population growth.[43] The decrease in age-adjusted death rates from MI over the past 25 years is estimated to be as high as 47%, and it is attributed to several factors identified in the Box on p. 147.[13,43]

MI is one of the most common diagnoses occurring in hospitalized patients in Western countries, with approximately 750,000 hospital admissions annually in the United States alone.[31,43] Patients who recover from MI are at risk for recurrent nonfatal MI, with 5% to 10% dying in the first year following MI.[31]

PATHOPHYSIOLOGY

MI is an end-point clinical presentation of myocardial ischemia resulting from coronary atherosclerosis, thrombus formation, and/or dynamic coronary artery changes such as coronary spasm, intimal injury, and trauma.[33,49] Environmental factors, associated illness, vasoconstricting drugs, and abrupt withdrawal of antianginal drugs have also been implicated as aggravating factors in AMI.[33]

Thrombotic occlusion of a coronary vessel caused by exposure of a thrombogenic lipid-rich plaque core is responsible for 80% to 90% of AMIs.[15] Therefore, initial mangement of AMI is based on thrombolytic reperfusion therapy. Less than 10% of MIs are due to other causes such as coronary emboli, thrombotic coronary artery disease, coronary vasculitis, infiltrative and degenerative coronary vascular disease, coronary ostial occlusion, trauma, or aug-

Factors Influencing Decreased Cardiovascular Death Rates[13]

Improved approaches to cardiovascular disease diagnosis and therapy
Use of drugs with cardioprotective effect on high-risk persons
Improved revascularization/reperfusion techniques
- Thrombolytic agents
- Percutaneous transluminal coronary angioplasty
- Coronary artery bypass grafting

Improved emergency cardiac care
- Early access
- Early cardiopulmonary resuscitation
- Early defibrillation
- Early advanced cardiac life support

Modification of cardiovascular risk factors
- Smoking cessation
- Control of hypertension
- Low-cholesterol diet
  - decreased low-density lipoprotein cholesterol
  - decreased serum triglycerides
- Physical fitness
- Weight control
- Stress management
- Control of diabetes

mented myocardial oxygen requirements that exceed oxygen delivery capacity.[15,43] Primary management of the underlying condition is essential for successful patient outcomes in patients with AMI due to these various causes.

The diagnosis of AMI is based on characteristic clinical history, electrocardiogram (ECG) changes, and cardiac enzyme elevations. The characteristic clinical history of chest pain occurs when myocardial oxygen demand is not met by oxygen supply. This symptom must be differentiated from other cardiac and noncardiac conditions. A description of differential analysis of chest pain is found in Table 16-1.

The ECG is an important diagnostic tool in AMI. The indicative ECG changes over the area of ischemia, injury, and infarction as well as the reciprocal ECG changes seen on the opposite side of the infarct are depicted in Figure 16-1. However, Morris has summarized the limitations of electrocardiography in the diagnosis of AMI as follows:

- Delayed appearance of ECG changes
- Cancellation of new infarction ECG changes by a diametrically opposed previous infarction
- Frequent absence of QRS complex changes of AMI in isolated posterolateral and apical regions
- Inability to diagnosis AMI in the presence of left bundle branch block[27]

The terms Q-wave and non–Q-wave infarction have recently been used instead of transmural and subendocardial infarction.[31] *Q-wave infarction* has replaced the term *transmural infarction* because morphologic studies have demonstrated a lack of specificity of Q waves as a marker for infarction involving all layers of the myocardium.[31,33,43] *Non–Q-wave* infarction has replaced the term *subendocardial infarction* because of a lack of morphologic limitations to this region and correlates with transient ST-segment and sustained T-wave changes.[31,33] Patients with non–Q-wave infarctions have smaller infarctions and reduced mortality compared to patients with Q-wave infarctions. However, they have a higher incidence of early reinfarctions.[33]

During a myocardial infarction, cardiac enzymes are released into the blood. Currently, creatine phosphokinase (CPK or CK) and lactic dehydrogenase (LDH) are used in the diagnosis of AMI. The MB isoenzyme of CK is preferred because it is not found in significant concentration in noncardiac tissue. Therefore, elevations are specific for cardiac damage. A summary of cardiac enzyme changes is found in Table 16-2.

Radionuclear imaging techniques may be used to diagnose MI, but they are of limited use in facilitating reperfusion therapy decision making. Radionuclear imaging techniques to establish myocardial infarction include identification of a "cold spot" (the ischemic necrotic tissue fails to pick up the thallium) on a resting and redistribution thallium-201 scan, or a "hot spot" (the necrotic tissue only avidly picks up the technetium pyrophosphate) on a technetium-99m stannous pyrophosphate scan.[15,27] These techniques are of little value in the acute phase of a myocardial infarction because the thallium-201 scan does not differentiate between new and old myocardial infarction, and the technetium pyrophosphate scan is not very sensitive until the AMI is 24 hours old.[27]

LENGTH OF STAY/ANTICIPATED COURSE

The length of stay (LOS) and anticipated course for patients with AMI depend upon the size of the infarction, the extent of ventricular dysfunction, and preexisting conditions that may complicate recovery.[33,49] In patients with successful early reperfusion, the degree of myocardial necrosis is significantly decreased.

Patients with a completed MI may have an uncomplicated course without experiencing shock, heart failure, cardiac arrhythmias, recurrent angina, or unusual psychologic distress.[27] The diagnosis of uncomplicated MI is made on the third or fourth day following initial chest pain and in the absence of complications.[27] The average LOS for a patient with an uncomplicated MI based on DRG 122: Circulatory disorders with AMI without complications average 6 days but may be as long as 10 to 14 days.[44] The last three days of the hospitalization period are used for diagnostic testing to determine residual ventricular function, the presence or absence of ventricular ectopy, the adequacy of coronary circulation, and education in risk-factor modification. It is important to note that complete healing or absence of necrotic fibers usually requires 35 days.[16]

TABLE 16-1 Analyzing Subjective Characteristics of Chest Pain[42]

Subjective characteristics	Angina	Myocardial infarction	Pericarditis	Pleuropulmonary disorders	Gastric disorders
Onset	Gradual or sudden	Sudden	Sudden	Gradual or sudden	Gradual or sudden
Precipitating factors	May be nothing specific; can occur at rest or after physical exertion, emotional stress, eating, exposure to cold or hot, humid weather, or during micturition or defecation	May be nothing specific; can occur at rest or after physical exertion or emotional stress	Not induced by activity but related to respiratory movement; increases with coughing	Pneumonia or other respiratory infection	Esophagitis and gastritis often occur after eating or taking medication or when person leans over
Location	Substernal, anterior chest (not sharply localized)	Substernal, anterior chest, or midline	Substernal (to left of midline) or precordial only	Over lung fields to side and back; substernal or retrosternal	Epigastric, slightly to left of midline
Radiation	To back, neck, arms, or jaw; occasionally to upper abdomen or fingers	Down one or both arms; to jaw, neck, or back	To back or left supraclavicular area	To anterior chest, shoulder, or neck; none with some disorders	Under sternum or to back of neck, left shoulder, or lower thoracic spine
Quality	Deep, squeezing, or tight sensation; feeling of heavy pressure	Deep, burning, stabbing, choking, squeezing, or viselike sensation; feeling of heavy pressure	Sharp, stabbing, deep, or superficial sensation	Sharp, burning, stabbing, shooting, deep, crushing, or tearing sensation	Gnawing, burning, or aching (sharp or dull) sensation; feeling of bloating or pressure
Intensity	Mild to moderate; tends to build in intensity (crescendo pattern)	Asymptomatic to severe	Moderate to severe pain or only an ache	Sharp ache (mild to severe)	Mild to severe

Duration	Usually less than 15 minutes (rarely more than 30 minutes); average duration is about 3 minutes	Often 30 minutes, but usually 1-2 hours; residual soreness lasts 1-3 days	Continuous (may last for days); residual soreness	Intermittent (may last for hours, days, or weeks)	Varies (may be intermittent or continuous, lasting seconds, minutes, or hours)
Relieving factors	Rest, nitroglycerin	Rest (but only temporarily)	Shallow breathing, sitting up, leaning forward	Warm, moist air; rest; splinting; heat; sitting up	Food, antacid, standing upright, belching
Aggravating factors	Physical or emotional stress, cold weather	Physical or emotional stress	Lying down, leaning forward, muscle movement, inspiration, laughter, coughing, or left lateral position	Cold air or dry environment, high altitude, hypoxia, carbon monoxide, coughing, exertion, immobility	Emotional stress; caffeine, protein, and some spices; constipation; heavy meal (or lying down after meal); carbonated beverage; cold liquids; exercise; aspirin; smoking
Associated symptoms	Indigestion, dizziness, urge to void, belching	Dizziness, nausea, fatigue	Air hunger, tachypnea, dizziness, restlessness	Air hunger, dyspnea, restlessness, splinting	Nausea, vomiting, dysphagia, restlessness, diaphoresis, foul breath, bad taste in mouth
Emotional response	Anxiety, fear	Anxiety, fear, feeling of impending doom	Anxiety, fear	Anxiety, anger (over shortness of breath)	Anxiety, withdrawal

Used with permission from Smith CE: Assessing chest pain, *Nursing* 88:56-57, May, 1988.

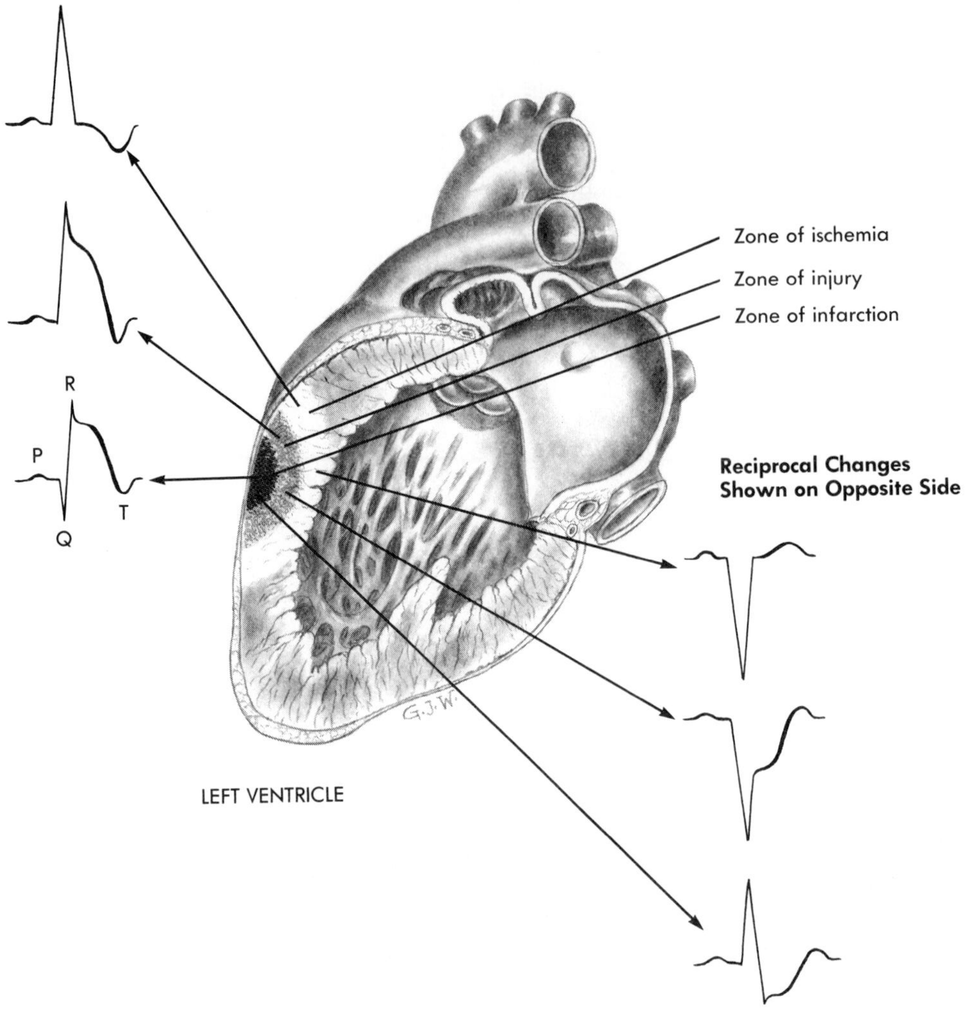

Figure 16-1 Zone of ischemia, zone of injury, and zone of infarction, showing ECG waveforms and reciprocal waveforms corresponding to each zone. (From Thelan, et al: *Critical Care Nursing Process and Application,* ed 2, St Louis, 1993, Mosby–Year Book.)

TABLE 16-2 Enzyme Changes in Acute Myocardial Infarction

Cardiac enzymes	Elevation (hours)	Peak (hours)	Duration (days)
Creatine phosphokinase (CPK)	4-8	12-24	3-4
Creatine phosphokinase-MB (CPK-MB)	4-8	12-20	2-3
Lactate dehydrogenase (LDH)	12-48	72-144	8-14
$LDH_1:LDH_2$*	12-14	72-144	14

*LDH_1: LDH_2 ratio is normally ≤1. Ratio >1 highly indicative of myocardial infarction.

Other patients may suffer MI complicated by cardiac arrhythmias, recurrent pain, ventricular dysfunction, hypotensive states, cardiogenic shock, nonarrhythmic cardiac arrest, pericarditis, venous thrombosis and embolism, systemic arterial embolism, ventricular septal rupture, papillary muscle rupture, external cardial rupture, or unusual psychologic distress.[27] Complications are termed early or late as they may occur in the prehospitalization period, the hospitalization period, or following discharge.[27] A summary of the diagnosis and treatment of several more common complications in AMI is found in Table 16-3. LOS for these patients would depend upon the type of complications and

TABLE 16-3 Common Complications of Myocardial Infarction (MI)

Complication	Diagnosis	Treatment
Arrhythmias	In inferior-wall MI, ECG shows bradycardia and junctional rhythms or atrioventricular (AV) block. In anterior-wall MI, tachycardia or heart block. In all MIs, premature ventricular contractions, ventricular tachycardia, or ventricular fibrillation.	Antiarrhythmics, pacemaker, cardioversion, and defibrillation
Congestive heart failure	Auscultation reveals rates at the base of the lungs, muffled or abnormal heart sounds, S_3 gallop, and possible systolic ejection murmur. Chest x-rays show pulmonary venous congestion and cardiomegaly. Catheterization shows increased pulmonary artery, pulmonary capillary wedge, and left ventricular end-diastolic pressures and central venous pressure.	Diuretics, vasodilators, inotropics, cardiac glycosides
Cardiogenic shock	Catheterization shows decreased cardiac output, and increased pulmonary artery and pulmonary capillary wedge pressures. Other signs include hypotension, tachycardia, decreased level of consciousness, decreased urinary output, neck vein distension, cool, pale, moist skin, and S_3/S_4 summation gallop.	IV fluids, vasodilators, cardiotonics, cardiac glycosides, intra-aortic balloon pump (IABP), and beta-adrenergic stimulants
Mitral regurgitation	Auscultation reveals rales and apical holosystolic murmur. Catheterization shows increased pulmonary artery and pulmonary capillary wedge pressures. Dyspnea is prominent.	Nitroglycerin, nitroprusside, IABP, and surgical replacement of the mitral valve and concomitant myocardial revascularization (may be postponed 7-14 days if possible)
Ventricular septal rupture	In left-to-right shunt, auscultation reveals a harsh holosystolic murmur and thrill at LLSB. Catheterization shows increased pulmonary artery and pulmonary capillary wedge pressures. Confirmation by increased oxygen saturation of right ventricle and pulmonary artery, SVo_2 >75%.	Surgical correction (may be postponed several weeks), IABP, nitroglycerin, or nitroprusside
Pericarditis	Auscultation reveals a friction rub. Chest pain is relieved by sitting up or increased by deep inspiration.	Anti-inflammatory and analgesic drugs
Ventricular aneurysm	Auscultation reveals S_3 gallop, and palpation reveals paradoxical heave at the apex. Chest x-rays may show cardiomegaly or ballooning of the aneurysm. Left ventriculography shows altered left ventricular motion (akinesis) or paradoxical motion (dyskinesis). Complications include congestive heart failure, arrhythmias, and systemic embolization.	Cardioversion, antiarrhythmics, vasodilators, anticoagulants, cardiotonic glycosides (digitalis), and diuretics. If nonoperative treatment fails to control complications, surgical resection is necessary.
Dressler's syndrome (postmyocardial infarction syndrome)	Auscultation reveals a friction rub. Chest x-rays may show pleural effusion.	Anti-inflammatory drugs and analgesics

Adapted from Nurses Reference Library, vol *Diseases,* Springhouse, Pa, 1981, Intermed Communications.

early or late occurrence in the recovery period. DRG 121, which denotes AMI with complications, notes an average LOS of 8.6 days.[44]

Prognostic indicators after AMI include the size and location of the infarction, residual ventricular function, other coronary artery obstruction, recurrent myocardial ischemia (either silent or symptomatic), ECG changes (Q waves, intraventricular conduction disturbances, or late potentials), dysrhythmias (including ventricular tachycardia/fibrillation, PVCs, supraventricular dysrhythmias, or heart block), and risk factors such as hypertension, cigarette smoking, hyperlipidemia, or diabetes mellitus.[48] Presence of one or more of these indicators increases the risk of subsequent myocardial infarction.

MANAGEMENT TRENDS AND CONTROVERSIES

The goals of medical management of AMI are to

- restore coronary blood flow and minimize the infarct size
- provide adequate tissue oxygenation
- improve ventricular performance
- detect and treat complications early
- stratify AMI and ischemic risk and treatment

Although the emphasis has shifted from interventions that alter myocardial oxygen demand to those that affect myocardial oxygen supply, both are important aspects of care for the patient with AMI. Therapies to improve oxygen supply include oxygen administration, pain relief, thrombolytic drugs, and procedures such as percutaneous transluminal coronary angioplasty (PTCA) and coronary artery bypass grafting (CABG). Therapies to decrease myocardial oxygen demand and thereby limit infarction size include use of calcium channel blockers, beta-blockers, nitrates, angiotensin-converting enzyme (ACE) inhibitors, and aspirin.

Restoration of Coronary Blood Flow and Minimization of Infarct Size

Research indicates that patients with an evolving AMI who receive thrombolytic therapy within the first 4 to 6 hours demonstrate reduced in-hospital and 1-year mortality rates.[3,23,38,47] Furthermore, improved residual left ventricular function due to preservation of ischemic myocardium has been demonstrated in patients who receive thrombolytic treatment in the first few hours.[47,51]

Studies also show that patients with acute transmural or Q-wave MI and with new bundle-branch block who are treated within 6 hours of symptom onset unequivocally benefit from thrombolytic therapy, although thrombolytic therapy in patients with non–Q-wave MI or those seen more than 6 hours after the onset of symptoms is controversial.[35,38]

Data presented at the 14th Annual Congress of the European Society of Cardiology in Barcelona, Spain, demonstrate reduced mortality in patients treated with thrombolytics up to 12 hours after the onset of symptoms.[14] Therefore, the American Heart Association recommendations for early treatment of patients with chest pain and possible AMI (Figure 16-2) emphasize the roles of the community, emergency medical system (EMS), and emergency department in the early screening and diagnosis of AMI to facilitate initiation of early thrombolytic therapy for all patients with symptoms and ECG findings of AMI.[14] A 30 to 60 minute "door to drug" interval has been recommended as the standard of care.[14]

Currently available thrombolytic agents include APSAC, streptokinase, t-PA, and urokinase. A comparison of these agents is found in Table 16-4.[15] Despite the potential benefits of these agents, the possible risks of thrombolytic therapy include varying degrees of systemic fibrinogen depletion, systemic bleeding, and intracranial hemorrhage.[14] Furthermore, streptokinase and APSAC are derived from group C beta-hemolytic streptococci and, therefore, may elicit an allergic response in some patients.[12,18]

Anticoagulation in conjunction with thrombolytic therapy has been an area of concern due to potential bleeding complications. Studies support the use of intravenous heparin therapy in conjunction with t-PA and streptokinase to maintain vessel patency.[5,24] However, heparin is contraindicated with APSAC thrombolytic therapy due to increased risk of bleeding complications.[30] Aspirin 150 to 325 mg po as soon as possible (within 24 hours of chest pain) should be used in conjunction with thrombolytic therapy in all patients to reduce mortality and reinfarction.[38,52]

Early intravenous beta-blockade has been shown to limit infarct size, reduce the risk of reinfarction, reduce the risk of intracranial bleeding following thrombolysis, and decrease mortality and morbidity.[21,47] Long-term beta-blocker therapy for 1 to 2 years following AMI has demonstrated a 39% reduction in mortality when used in adequate doses to achieve a resting heart rate of less than 60 beats per minute and an exercise heart rate of less than 90 beats per minute.[26] Intravenous nitroglycerin has also been shown to be beneficial in limiting infarct size.[26]

The role of calcium channel blockers in limiting infarct size has yet to be demonstrated despite rigorous investigation. Studies have shown that nifedipine is ineffective in reducing infarct size or altering mortality in AMI.[28,39] Studies also have failed to demonstrate the efficacy of verapamil.[11] On the other hand, diltiazem has been shown to reduce the risk of reinfarction in non–Q-wave AMI and improve long-term survival.[20,29] Diltiazem is not beneficial for patients with Q-wave infarction and significant left ventricular dysfunction.[29]

An important indication for use of calcium channel blockers is in providing myocardial protection from *stunned myocardium*. Clinical evidence of stunned myocardium includes:

- slow return of regional function after thrombolytic therapy for AMI
- prolonged left ventricular abnormalities of regional wall motion in patients with unstable angina

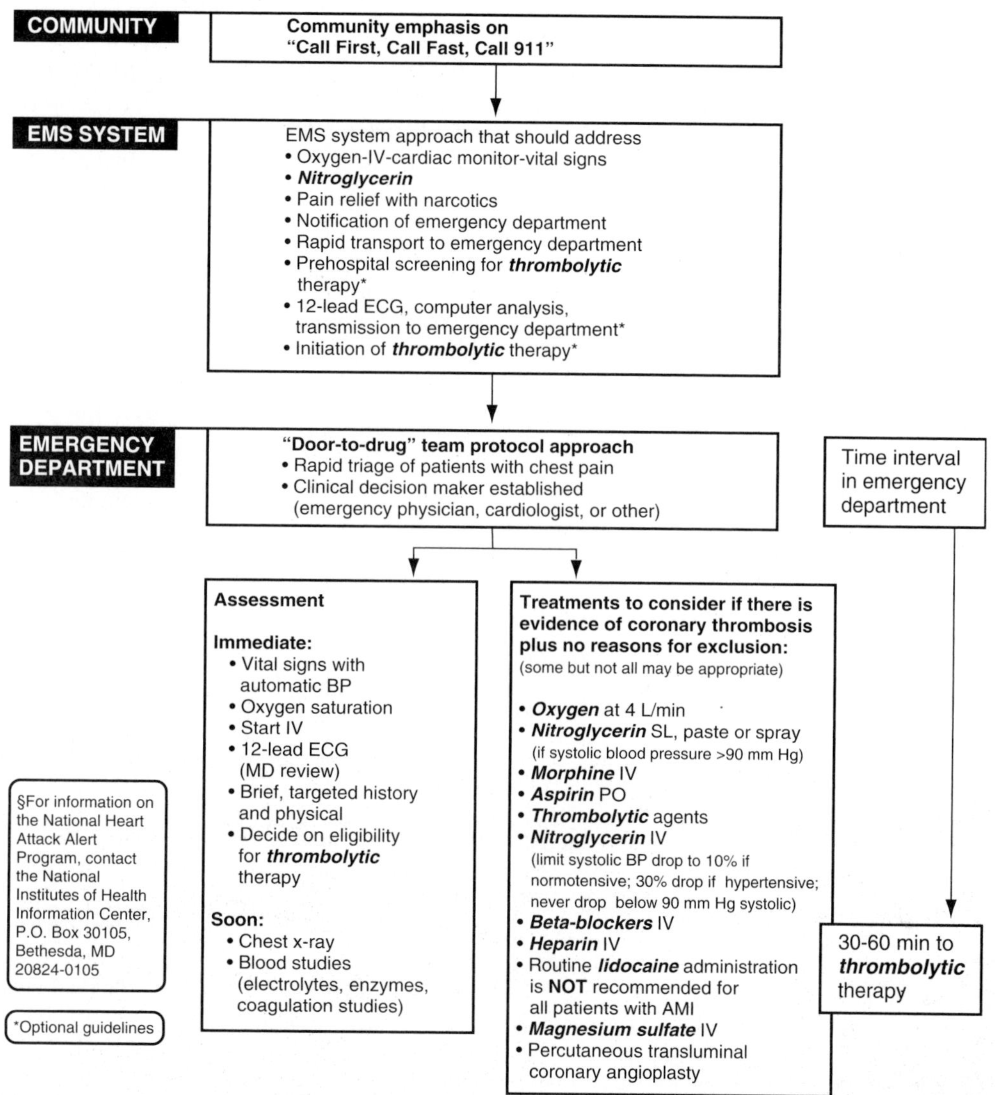

Acute Myocardial Infarction Algorithm
Recommendations for early management of patients with chest pain and possible AMI§
COMMUNITY
Community emphasis on "Call First, Call Fast, Call 911"
EMS SYSTEM
EMS system approach that should address
• Oxygen-IV-cardiac monitor-vital signs
• Nitroglycerin
• Pain relief with narcotics
• Notification of emergency department
• Rapid transport to emergency department
• Prehospital screening for thrombolytic therapy*
• 12-lead ECG, computer analysis, transmission to emergency department*
• Initiation of thrombolytic therapy*
EMERGENCY DEPARTMENT
"Door-to-drug" team protocol approach
• Rapid triage of patients with chest pain
• Clinical decision maker established (emergency physician, cardiologist, or other)
Time interval in emergency department
Assessment
Immediate:
• Vital signs with automatic BP
• Oxygen saturation
• Start IV
• 12-lead ECG (MD review)
• Brief, targeted history and physical
• Decide on eligibility for thrombolytic therapy
Soon:
• Chest x-ray
• Blood studies (electrolytes, enzymes, coagulation studies)
Treatments to consider if there is evidence of coronary thrombosis plus no reasons for exclusion:
(some but not all may be appropriate)
• Oxygen at 4 L/min
• Nitroglycerin SL, paste or spray (if systolic blood pressure >90 mm Hg)
• Morphine IV
• Aspirin PO
• Thrombolytic agents
• Nitroglycerin IV (limit systolic BP drop to 10% if normotensive; 30% drop if hypertensive; never drop below 90 mm Hg systolic)
• Beta-blockers IV
• Heparin IV
• Routine lidocaine administration is NOT recommended for all patients with AMI
• Magnesium sulfate IV
• Percutaneous transluminal coronary angioplasty
30-60 min to thrombolytic therapy
§For information on the National Heart Attack Alert Program, contact the National Institutes of Health Information Center, P.O. Box 30105, Bethesda, MD 20824-0105
*Optional guidelines

Figure 16-2 Acute myocardial infarction algorithm—recommendations for early management of patients with chest pain and possible AMI. (From Newman MM, editor: The algorithm approach to emergency cardiac care, *Currents in Emergency Cardiac Care* 3(4):19, 1992.)

- persistent left ventricular abnormalities of regional wall motion after exercise-induced ischemia
- diastolic abnormalities after coronary angioplasty procedures
- prolonged but reversible left ventricular dysfunction after cardiac surgery[36]

Braunwald proposed that repeated, brief episodes of ischemia may lead to myocardial stunning.[7] In the context of AMI, stunned myocardium can be defined as "prolonged but transient abnormality in contractile function and high-energy metabolism of viable myocardium salvaged by timely reperfusion."[36]

Theories of causation of stunned myocardium include reduction of ATP levels, regional microvascular ischemia, cytotoxic oxygen-derived free radicals, and abnormalities of calcium flux during reperfusion.[22] Stunned myocardium will have either no contractile function (akinesis) or depressed contractile function (hypokinesis) resulting in mild to severe heart failure.[22] The following effects of calcium channel blockers have been associated with reducing the degree of stunned myocardium: direct cardioprotective effects, prevention of calcium accumulation in the mitochondria of ischemic cells, reduction in oxygen consumption, reduction of coronary artery spasm, prevention of ischemia-induced arrhythmias, and increased coronary blood flow to ischemic tissue directly or through enhanced collateral flow.[25]

TABLE 16-4 Thrombolytic Agents

Agent	Fibrin selectivity	Systemic lytic effect	Dosage	Half-life (min)	Adverse effects/comments
Streptokinase (SK)	0	+ + + +	IC: 2000-4000 U/min for 60 min up to 250,000 U (a bolus of 20,000 U may be given) IV: 1.5 million U over 1 hr	23	Bleeding, allergic reactions, hypotension, fever Inexpensive ($200/1.5 million U)
Recombinant tissue plasminogen activator (rt-PA), single chain	+ + + +	+	IV: 6-mg bolus, 54 mg over 1st hour, 20 mg over 2nd hour, 20 mg over 3rd hour IV: entire dose over 90 min	5	Bleeding Expensive ($2200/100 mg)
Anisoylated plasminogen streptokinase activator complex (APSAC)	+	+ + + +	IV: 30 U over 2-5 min	90	Side-effect profile similar to SK No maintenance infusion necessary ? Lower incidence of reocclusion ($1500/30 U)
Single chain urokinase plasminogen activator (scu-PA, pro-urokinase)	+ + + +	+	Optimal dose, either alone or in combination with rt-PA, not known	7	May be best used in synergistic combination with rt-PA Expensive
Urokinase (UK)	0	+ + +	IC: 4000-6000 U/min for 2 hr, average total dose 500,000 U IV: 1.5-million U bolus, then 1.5 million U over 90 min or ? 2.0 million U over 5-15 min†	16	Optimal IV dose has not been established Not antigenic Expensive ($2200/3 million U)

0 = none: + + + + = highest; IC = Intercoronary artery; IV = Intravenous.
*Adapted from Marder VJ, Sherry S: Thrombolytic therapy: Current Status.
†Exceeds dosage recommended by the manufacturer.
Used with permission from Rakel RE, editor: *Cohn's current therapy, 1992,* Philadelphia, 1992, WB Saunders.

TABLE 16-5 Hemodynamic Classification of Forrester and Associates[17]

Subgroup	Clinical findings	Hemodynamic	Interventions
I	No pulmonary congestion or peripheral hypoperfusion	PCWP <18 mm Hg CI >2.2 L/min/m^2	Beta-blockade, if no contraindications
II	Isolated pulmonary congestion	PCWP >18 mm Hg CI >2.2 L/min/m^2	Diuretics, correct hypoxia
III	Isolated peripheral hypoperfusion	PCWP <18 mm Hg CI <2.2 L/min/m^2	Volume replacement
IV	Pulmonary congestion and peripheral hypoperfusion	PCWP >18 mm Hg CI <2.2 L/min/m^2	Diuretics vasodilators, positive inotropes, IABP

PCWP = pulmonary capillary wedge pressure, CI = cardiac index, IABP = intra-aortic balloon pump
Reprinted by permission of the New England Journal of Medicine, 295:1360, 1976.

TABLE 16-6 Diagnosis and Treatment of Shock Following Acute Myocardial Infarction

Pathophysiology abnormality	Diagnostic evaluation: *Clinical*	*Hemodynamic*	*Noninvasive*	Guides to management	Prognosis
Hypovolemia	Clear lungs on chest film	BP <100 mm Hg PCWP <18 mm Hg CI <2.2 L/min/m^2	Vigorous left ventricular function	Rapid but cautious volume expansion until PCWP = 15-18 mm Hg	Very good
Right ventricular infarction	Inferior MI on ECG, JVP elevation, minimal LV failure, Kussmaul's sign	BP <100 mm Hg RA pressure ≥PCWP, reduced PA and RV pulse pressure, CI <2.2 L/min/m^2	Dilated RV with RVEF ≤.30%, LVEF generally <45%, inferior and/or posterior LV dysfunction	Volume expansion if PCWP <15 mm Hg, inotropic support, maintain atrial transport	Good unless severe LV dysfunction coexists
Cardiogenic shock	Pulmonary rales, S_3 gallop, pulmonary congestion on CXR	BP <90 mm Hg PCWP ≥18 mm Hg CI <2.2 L/min/m^2 Elevated SVR	LVEF ≤.40%, marked regional LV wall motion abnormalities	Inotropes and/or vasopressors to maintain BP <90 mm Hg and CI approx 2 L/min/m^2, vasodilators & diuretics to keep PCWP <18 mm Hg IABP support	Poor, mortality 80%; early reperfusion (PTCA, rt-PA) may improve outlook
Acute mitral regurgitation	Holosystolic murmur at apex, pulmonary rales, S_3 gallop, pulmonary congestion on chest film	PCWP ≥18 mm Hg with large V waves. CI <2.2 L/min/m^2, SVR elevated, BP <90 mm Hg	LVEF may be high, normal, or depressed, depending on extent of infarction	Vasodilators and inotropes, IABP, prompt MVR	Surgical mortality 30-40%, medical mortality 80%
Acute ventricular septal rupture	Shock syndrome, rales, S_3, holosystolic murmur at LLSB, thrill in 50% of patients	BP <90 mm Hg O_2 "step-up" from RA to RV or PA	L to R shunts; by first-pass RVG, LVEF, and RVEF are variable. 2D echocardiography should visualize defect; Doppler confirms shunt.	Vasodilators & inotropes, IABP Early VSD closure	Surgical mortality 40-50%, medical mortality 80-85%, outlook better with anterior MI

PCW = pulmonary capillary wedge pressure; CI = cardiac index (L/min/m^2); SVR = systemic vascular resistance; BP = blood pressure, LVEF = left ventricular ejection fraction; RVEF = right ventricular ejection fraction; LV = left ventricle; RV = right ventricle; RA = right atrium; IABP = intra-aortic balloon pump; PA = pulmonary artery; JVP = jugular venous pressure; PTCA = percutaneous transluminal coronary angioplasty; rt-PA = tissue plasminogen activator; VSD = ventricular septal defect; MVR = mitral valve replacement; LLSB = lower left sternal border; RVG = radionuclide ventriculography; CXR = chest X-ray.

*Used with permission from Rakel RE, editor: *Cohn's Current Therapy, 1992,* Philadelphia, 1992, WB Saunders.

Adequate Tissue Oxygenation

Supplemental oxygen is recommended in AMI.[43] Nitrates also improve cardiac and systemic tissue oxygenation. The hemodynamic effects of nitrates include relaxation of conduit arteries, increased arterial compliance, dilation of collateral vessels in the myocardium, and, possibly, increased myocardial compliance.[10] However, the nonhemodynamic effects of nitrates are also significant and include inhibition of vascular smooth muscle growth, myocyte hypertrophy, and ventricular remodeling.[10] Ventricular remodeling following AMI is due to the loss of contractile function of the necrotic tissue, expansion of the infarct, and compensatory dilation of the nonischemic myocardium.[4,6,34,40,50]

ACE inhibiting drugs are another important drug therapy for AMI. The early treatment of AMI patients with ACE inhibiting drugs has been shown to optimize the oxygen supply–demand ratio in evolving AMI; decrease myocardial infarct size by reducing regional wall stress; decrease ventricular dilation and remodeling by reducing ventricular wall stress and hypertrophy; and decrease ischemia, arrhythmias, and risk of recurrent infarction by optimizing the oxygen supply–demand ratio.[40]

Magnesium sulfate is another relatively new drug treatment used in the management of AMI. It has been shown to lower mortality by up to 50% and decrease arrhythmias.* Magnesium sulphate is a physiologic calcium antagonist with actions that include coronary and systemic vasodilatation, platelet inhibition, and antidysrhythmic effects.[54]

Improvement of Ventricular Performance

Many patients with AMI have an uncomplicated course; however, others require extensive medical management to maintain adequate ventricular performance. In patients with a complicated AMI, hemodynamic monitoring is often used to provide information for clinical decision making. A hemodynamic classification and intervention system developed by Forrester and modified by Farmer and Young uses cardiac index (CI) and pulmonary capillary wedge pressure (PCWP) to classify AMI patients into four subgroups.[15,17] Each group has distinct clinical findings, mortality, and recommended interventions as presented in Table 16-5.[15,17]

Patients with right ventricular failure due to right ventricular infarction fall into subset III. These patients require augmentation of vascular volume to maintain left ventricular preload, as well as positive inotropes to maintain right ventricular contractility.[15,17,43]

*References 2, 8, 37, 41, 46, 53, 54.

Early Detection and Treatment of Complications

The complications from AMI fall into four primary groups:

1. Electrical failure—arrhythmias, heart blocks, and asystole
2. Pump failure—right or left congestive heart failure and cardiogenic shock
3. Mechanical disruption—papillary muscle dysfunction or rupture that causes mitral valve regurgitation, ventricular septal rupture, or ventricular aneurysm
4. Inflammatory syndromes—pericarditis or Dressler's syndrome

Diagnosis and treatment of these complications are summarized in Table 16-3. The pathophysiology, diagnostic evaluation, management, and prognosis for the five principal causes of shock following AMI are summarized in Table 16-6.[15]

AMI and Ischemic Risk Stratification and Treatment

It is useful to stratify patients presenting with AMI to determine appropriate and timely medical management and interventions. The emergent interventions for patients with AMI with hemodynamic instability, contraindications for thrombolysis, diffuse ST-segment depression, recurrent pain, and high-risk predischarge ischemia include revascularization by PTCA, atherectomy, or CABG.[32] Other revascularization procedures such as coronary laser angioplasty are promising but need continued research and development.[32]

There are several important differences reported concerning women in the treatment and management of AMI. Although risk factors for CAD in women parallel men, diabetic women have the same or greater risk for CAD than nondiabetic men. Reduced ECG and ETT sensitivity and lower cardiac enzyme levels seen in women may affect accurate diagnosis of AMI in women. Women experience higher mortality with traditional treatment modalities such as PTCA and CABG. Finally, women experience a higher rate of early in-hospital reinfarction, increased incidence of CHF, and a higher rate of stroke. Despite experiencing a lower incidence of sudden cardiac death, women have a higher overall mortality.[9] Accurate nursing assessment of the AMI patient is essential and should consider these important differences.

ASSESSMENT

PARAMETER	ANTICIPATED ALTERATION
History of coronary risk factors, CAD, angina, MI, cardiac failure, cardiac surgery, or cardiac medications	Presence of one or more of these conditions increases likelihood of AMI.

General appearance and level of distress	Awake, alert, and oriented unless CO significantly decreased. Restlessness and anxiety *due to circulating catecholamines from fear and pain*

Noninvasive Cardiac Tests

Chest x-ray	WNL or cardiomegaly, vascular engorgement or pulmonary infiltrates
Multiple-gated acquisition (MUGA) scan	May reveal decreased LVEF <50%, decreased wall motion (hypokinesis), systolic bulging (dyskinesis), or absent wall motion (akinesis)
Radionuclear imaging with technetium-99	May reveal "hot spots" where infarcted areas show increased levels of uptake
Radionuclear imaging with thallium-201	May reveal ischemic areas that show normal uptake at rest and decreased uptake or "cold spots" on exercise. No uptake will occur in areas of infarction appearing as dark or "cold" areas on scan.
Echocardiography	May reveal abnormal cardiac chamber size, intracardiac shunts, valvular heart disease, cardiomyopathy, pericardial effusion, pericardial tamponade, or papillary muscle dysfunction
ECG	May reveal rhythm or conduction abnormalities. Signs of ischemia, injury, and infarction will be seen in leads corresponding to the area of insult: • Septal wall—V_{1-2} • Anterior wall—V_{2-4} • Lateral wall—I, aVL, V_{5-6} • Inferior wall—II, III, aVF • Posterior wall—reciprocal changes in V_{1-2}
Signal-averaged ECG	May reveal evidence of late potentials, identifying patients at risk for life-threatening arrhythmias who may need follow-up electrophysiology testing
Exercise tolerance test (ETT)	May reveal ST-segment depression>1 mm during exercise with or without hypotension, chest pain, or ventricular dysrhythmias

Invasive Cardiac Tests

Cardiac catheterization	May reveal lesions of arteries or valves, abnormalities of ventricular function, elevated cardiac pressures, or decreased CO <4 L/min
Chest pain evaluation that includes onset, precipitating factors, location, radiation, quality, intensity, duration, relieving factors, aggravating factors, associated systems, and emotional response	See Table 16-1 for differentiation of chest pain

Hemodynamic Status

BP	WNL, or hypotension with SBP <90 mm Hg *due to decreased CO.* Hypertension with SBP > patient norm *due to anxiety and/or chest pain*
HR	HR <60 bpm *due to bradydysrhythmia or heart blocks associated with inferior wall MI (especially first degree type I heart block)* HR >100 bpm *due to CHF more often seen in anterior wall MI or tachydysrhythmias.* Irregularities *due to PACs or atrial fibrillation seen in CHF or atrial infarction, and PVCs seen in all types of AMI.*
Jugular veins	JVD with HOB >30° *due to backward failure*
Heart sounds	S_3 *due to LV failure.* S_4 *due to decreased ventricular compliance.* Pericardial friction rub, or valvular murmurs.

Breath sounds	WNL unless CHF present. Crackles (rales), wheezes, or gurgles (rhonchi) *due to CHF if present.*
Abdomen	Nausea and vomiting are frequently associated with AMI. There may also be liver engorgement and distension *due to backward failure of the right heart.*
Genitourinary	UO <30 cc/hr *due to decreased CO*
Peripheral perfusion	Extremities may be cool, pale, and diaphoretic with weak or thready pulses *due to decreased CO and resulting compensatory catecholamines.* Mottling in the lower extremities is often seen in cardiogenic shock *due to severely decreased CO and failure to oxygenate tissues.*
Invasive hemodynamic monitoring	Significant hemodynamic changes seen in AMI are presented in Table 16-6.
Temperature	Elevations ≥38.3° C *due to inflammatory response to myocardial tissue injury in the first 48 to 72 hours. Continued or higher temperature elevation may be due to pericarditis or infection.*

Laboratory Findings

Serial cardiac enzymes	See Table 16-2.
Electrolyte values	Usually WNL

PLAN OF CARE

INTENSIVE PHASE

The medical goals in the intensive phase of care include restoration of blood flow to minimize infarct size and improve ventricular performance, and to provide adequate tissue oxygenation. The detection and treatment of complications in the intensive phase focuses on arrhythmias and pump failure. Nursing care priorities include management of pain, anxiety, and fear of death; management of decreased CO and/or tissue perfusion; and facilitating appropriate patient coping mechanisms.[1,45]

PATIENT CARE PRIORITIES	EXPECTED PATIENT OUTCOMES
Anxiety *r/t pain and fear of death*	Demonstrates decreased anxiety. Able to rest, sleep, and engage in other care-related activities.
Pain/discomfort *r/t cardiac ischemia, decreased CO, or pericarditis*	Absence of chest pain, discomfort, and associated symptoms. Notifies staff immediately if pain/discomfort occur. Demonstrates knowledge of activities to decrease oxygen consumption.
Decreased CO *r/t dysrhythmias, ventricular dysfunction, or complications*	CO: WNL CI: WNL UO ≥30 cc/hr Absence of dysrhythmias other than patient norms BP and pulse within patient norms Absence of S_3, S_4 Clear lungs Absence of peripheral edema Normal mentation
High risk for decreased tissue perfusion *r/t deep-vein thrombosis or embolization of mural thrombi from infarcted myocardium*	Absence of venous thrombosis, pulmonary embolism/infarction, or systemic embolism, especially to the bowel
High risk for ineffective patient coping *r/t anxiety, depression, or denial*	Demonstrates usual coping responses without denial or depression hindering recovery

Plan of Care (cont'd)

INTERVENTIONS

Create a calm, quiet environment and provide information regarding procedures, medications, and treatment *to decrease anxiety, promote patient comfort, decrease catecholamine release, and minimize oxygen demand.*

Treat chest pain promptly with IV narcotics, oxygen, sedation as needed, and reassurance *to decrease pain, reduce anxiety, and minimize infarct size.*

Assess and document full description of chest pain using a scale of 0 to 10 *to assist with appropriate evaluation and management of pain.*

Assess and document hemodynamic status before, during, and after chest pain and medications *to evaluate effect of therapies to relieve chest pain.*

Assist patient in the use of imagery, breathing techniques, and relaxation exercises *to maximize response to pain-relieving medications and decrease oxygen demand.*

Instruct patient how and when to notify staff of chest pain, discomfort, or associated symptoms *to provide timely pain management.*

Obtain 12-lead ECG with episodes of chest pain following initial diagnosis of AMI *to promptly identify potential extension of MI.*

Differentiate pericarditis as source of pain and treat pain with anti-inflammatory agents *to decrease inflammatory response.* If patient is anticoagulated, check with the physician regarding anti-inflammatory therapy *due to the risk of cardiac tamponade.*

Monitor and assess for abnormalities or changes in cardiac rhythm, rate, and dysrhythmias. Observe for reperfusion dysrhythmias associated with successful thrombolysis or sustained/recurrent ST- or T-wave changes associated with unsuccessful thrombolysis or reocclusion *to monitor effectiveness of thrombolytic therapy.*

Complete and document cardiovascular assessment q4h and prn *to detect significant changes in cardiovascular status or complications.*

Administer IV fluids, diuretics, nitrates, inotropes, vasodilators, beta-blockers, calcium channel blockers, and magnesium sulfate as order *to maximize CO and to protect and preserve viable myocardium.*

Be prepared for possible emergent interventions *to manage catastrophic complications, including administration of emergency medications, insertion of intra-aortic balloon pump, pericardiocentesis, or insertion of pacemaker.*

Monitor and record accurate I/O and obtain daily weight *to evaluate fluid balance and potential CHF.*

Limit meals and/or meal size *to decrease oxygen demand and minimize pain.*

Instruct patient regarding activity limitation and expected activity progression *to increase patient knowledge of and compliance with activity restrictions to decrease oxygen demand.*

Assist patient with leg exercises while in bed and instruct not to cross ankles *to increase muscle movement and venous return.*

Ambulate patient once pain-free ≥24 hours and apply appropriately sized elastic support stockings *to enhance venous circulation and psychoemotional well-being.*

Provide rest periods before and after spaced activities and meals *to decrease oxygen demand.*

Administer anticoagulants as ordered *to decrease thrombogenicity.*

Assess, report, and document any signs of venous thrombosis such as positive Homan's sign; any changes in the color, girth, or temperature of extremities; and the presence of tenderness and/or cords in lower extremities *to insure early recognition and intervention for DVT.*

Assess, report, and document any signs of pulmonary embolism *to insure early recognition and intervention.*

Assess, report, and document any signs of systemic embolism such as the color, girth, temperature, or decreased/absent pulses in an extremity, or abdominal distension and tenderness *to insure early recognition and intervention.*

Explain what AMI is and the healing process *to help patient and/or family cope with diagnosis.*

Plan of Care (cont'd)

Openly acknowledge coping behavior *to assist patient to explore feelings; work through denial and depression and engage patient and family in cardiac rehabilitation activities.*

INTERMEDIATE PHASE

The patient with AMI is usually transferred to a telemetry or intermediate care unit as soon as the cardiac enzymes begin to fall and in the absence of complications. Intermediate phase goals include progressive cardiac rehabilitation, including patient and family teaching, and early detection and management of late complications of AMI.

PATIENT CARE PRIORITIES	EXPECTED PATIENT OUTCOMES
Self-care deficit *r/t AMI, discharge regimen, and lifestyle modification*	Verbalize basic knowledge of CAD and AMI. Identify personal risk factors and how they can be modified. Demonstrate home exercise program and describe work simplification techniques. Describe symptoms requiring immediate medical attention and verbalize how and when to activate the emergency medical system in their area. Verbalize knowledge of discharge medications. Verbalize knowledge of diet regimen. Discuss the future realistically.
Pain and discomfort *r/t Dressler's syndrome*	Absence of pain and associated complications

INTERVENTIONS

Collaborate with the cardiac rehabilitation staff to provide information about illness and discharge regimen, including:

- Nature and significance of AMI and healing process
- Risk factors, modification, and sources of support
- Nature and significance of angina
- Factors that commonly precipitate angina, with emphasis on specific factors that the patient identifies:
  - -Activity
  - -Cold
  - -Emotional stress
  - -Ingestion of heavy meal
- Progressive exercise program with continued activity progression after discharge
- Diet regimen low in saturated fats, cholesterol, and sodium, with calorie control in overweight patients
- Resumption of work and sexual activity

Obtain appropriate consultations from other health care providers such as dietician, physical therapist, occupational therapist, social worker, or psychologist *to address individual patient concerns and education.*

Discuss symptoms requiring immediate medical attention *to assure early recognition and treatment, including:*

- An increase in frequency or duration of angina
- Additional symptoms associated with angina, such as shortness of breath, diaphoresis, change in quality or duration of pain
- Recurrent angina previously controlled by medications
- Heart palpitations or fainting
- Side effects or difficulty in maintaining medication regimen

Instruct patient and/or family how and when to activate the emergency medical system (EMS) *to insure early intervention prn.*

Plan of Care (cont'd)

Provide teaching and written discharge information on medication regimen including name, purpose, dosage, frequency, prophylactic use, side effects, and storage.

Provide opportunities for patient and families to attend group support classes *to improve ability to cope with illness and treatment.*

Provide private and separate opportunities for patient and family to ask questions.

Assess patient's potential for compliance with medical treatment regimen and implement appropriate interventions or referrals as needed.

Determine if there is a recent history of AMI *to differentiate potential Dressler's syndrome, which is related to a hypersensitivity reaction to the necrotic cardiac muscle that develops within a few weeks to months after AMI.*

Assess for and document presence of pericardial-type pain, pericardial friction rub, and prolonged fever *due to immune response.*

Assess for and document signs and symptoms of pericardial effusion or tamponade such as decreased pulse pressure, muffled heart tones, rising and equalizing right and left atrial pressures, and decreased CO.

Assess for and document signs and symptoms of pleuritis or pneumonitis, *which is sometimes associated with Dressler's syndrome.*

Administer aspirin, indomethacin, or corticosteroids as ordered *to decrease immune response.*

TRANSITION TO DISCHARGE

As patients with AMI and their families approach discharge, the health care team should assure that the discharge plan for resuming activities of daily living, diet, progressive exercise including sexual relations, medications, and return to work are clear. Information including medical appointments, future invasive or noninvasive tests, and additional interventional procedures should be provided to assist the patient and family in anticipating plans for continued medical evaluation and follow-up. Patients and families should be made aware that periods of depression and fatigue are not uncommon, particularly during the first few weeks at home.

After the patient and family return home, fear of the future can seriously impact cardiac rehabilitation and quality of life. Providing reality-based information reinforced by an outpatient cardiac rehabilitation program will enhance the ability of AMI patients and their families to return to an optimal level of function and enjoyment of life.

REFERENCES

1. Alspach JG: *Core curriculum for critical care nursing,* ed 4, Philadelphia, 1991, WB Saunders.
2. Abraham AS, et al: Magnesium in the prevention of lethal arrhythmias in acute myocardial infarction, *Arch Intern Med* 147:753-755, 1987.
3. AIMS Trial Study Group: Effect of intravenous APSAC on mortality after acute myocardial infarction: preliminary report of a placebo-controlled clinical trial, *Lancet* 2:545-549, 1988.
4. Anversa P, Olivetti G, Capasso JM: Cellular basis of ventricular remodeling after myocardial infarction, *Am J Cardiol* 68:7D-16D, 1991.
5. Bleich SD, et al: Effect of heparin on coronary arterial patency after thrombolysis with tissue plasminogen activator in acute myocardial infarction, *Am J Cardiol* 56:1412-1417, 1990.
6. Braunwald E, Pfeffer MA: Ventricular enlargement and remodeling following acute myocardial infarction: mechanisms and management, *Am J Cardiol* 68:1D-6D, 1991.
7. Braunwald E, Kloner RA: The stunned myocardium: prolonged, postischemic ventricular dysfunction, *Circulation* 66:1146-1149, 1982.
8. Ceremuzynski L, et al: Threatening arrhythmias in acute myocardial infarction are prevented by intravenous magnesium sulphate, *Am Heart J* 118:1333-1334, 1989.
9. Cochrane B: Acute myocardial infarction in women, *Crit Care Nurs Clin North Am* 4(2):279-289, 1992.
10. Cohn PF: Mechanism of myocardial ischemia, *Am J Cardiol* 70:14G-18G, 1992.
11. Danish Study Group on Verapamil in Myocardial Infarction: Verapamil in acute myocardial infarction, *Eur Heart J* 5:518-528, 1984.
12. Elliott JM, et al: Streptokinase titers 1 to 4 years after intravenous streptokinase, *Circulation* 84(suppl II):110-116 (abstract).
13. Emergency Cardiac Care Committee and Subcommittees, American Heart Association: Guidelines for cardiopulmonary resuscitation and emergency cardiac care. I: Introduction, *JAMA* 268:2172-2183, 1992.
14. Emergency Cardiac Care Committee and Subcommittees, American Heart Association: Guidelines for cardiopulmonary resuscitation and emergency cardiac care. III: Adult advanced cardiac life support, *JAMA* 268:2199-2242, 1992.
15. Farmer JA, Young JB: Acute myocardial infarction. In Rakel RE, editor: *Cohn's Current Therapy, 1992,* Philadelphia, 1992, WB Saunders.

16. Fishbein MC, Maclean D, Maroko PR: The histopathologic evolution of myocardial infarction, *Chest* 73:843-849, 1978.
17. Forrester JS, et al: Medical therapy of acute myocardial infarction by application of hemodynamic subsets. Part one, *N Engl J Med* 295:1356-1362, 1976.
18. Gardiner-Caldwell SynerMed: *Nursing management in thrombolytic therapy: a slide/lecture guide,* 1989, Genentech, Inc.
19. Gawlinski AG: Opening remarks, *Heart Lung* 16(6):739-740, 1987.
20. Gibson RS, et al: Diltiazem and reinfarction in patients with non-Q-wave myocardial infarction, *N Engl J Med* 315:423-429, 1986.
21. Gore JM, et al: Intracerebral hemorrhage, cerebral infarction, and subdural hematoma after acute myocardial infarction and thrombolytic therapy in the Thrombolysis in Myocardial Infarction Study: Thrombolysis in Myocardial Infarction, phase II, Pilot and Clinical Trial, *Circulation* 83:448-459, 1991.
22. Griego LC: The phenomenon of "stunned" myocardium: implications for coronary care nurses, *Prog in Cardiovasc Nurs* 5(4):126-131, 1990.
23. Gruppo Italiano Per lo Studio della Streptochinasi nell'Infarto Miocardico (GISSI): Effectiveness of intravenous thrombolytic treatment in acute myocardial infarction, *Lancet* 1:397-402, 1986.
24. Hsia J, et al: A comparison between heparin and low-dose aspirin as adjunctive therapy with tissue plasminogen activator for acute myocardial infarction, *N Engl J Med* 323:1433-1437, 1990.
25. Kern MJ: Perspective, the cellular influences of calcium antagonists on systemic and coronary hemodynamics, *Am J Cardiol* 69:3B-7B, 1992.
26. May GS: A review of long-term beta-blocker trials in survivors of myocardial infarction, *Circulation* 67(suppl I):46-49, 1983.
27. Morris DC, Walter PF, Hurst JW: The recognition and treatment of myocardial infarction and its complications. In Hurst JW, et al, editors: *The heart arteries and veins,* ed 7, New York, 1990, McGraw-Hill.
28. Muller JE, et al: Nifedipine therapy for patients with threatened and acute myocardial infarction: a randomized, double-blind, placebo-controlled comparison, *Circulation* 69:740-747, 1984.
29. Multicenter Diltiazem Postinfarction Trial Research Group: The effect of diltiazem on mortality and reinfarction after myocardial infarction, *N Engl J Med* 319:385-392, 1988.
30. O'Connor CM, et al: A randomized trial of heparin in conjunction with anistreplase (APSAC) in acute myocardial infarction, *J Am Coll Cardiol,* 23(1):11-18, 1994.
31. Pasternak RC, Braunwald E: Acute myocardial infarction. In Wilson JD, et al, editors: *Harrison's principles of internal medicine,* ed 12, New York, 1991, McGraw-Hill.
32. Pepine CJ, Kern MJ, Boden WE: Advisory group reports on silent myocardial ischemia, acute intervention after myocardial infarction, and postinfarction management, *Am J Cardiol* 69:41B-46B, 1992.
33. Pepine CJ: New concepts in the pathophysiology of acute myocardial infarction, *Am J Cardiol* 64:2B-8B, 1989.
34. Pfeffer MA: Ventricular enlargement following infarction is a modifiable process, *Am J Cardiol* 68:127D-131D, 1991.
35. Piegas LS, et al: Arterial patency and ejection fraction after late thrombolysis with streptokinase: results from EMERAS, *Eur Heart J* 12:97, 1991 (abstract #598).
36. Przyklenk K, Kloner RA: What factors predict recovery of contractile function in the canine model of the stunned myocardium? *Am J Cardiol* 64:18F-26F, 1989.
37. Rasmussen HS, et al: Magnesium infusion reduces the incidence of arrhythmias in acute myocardial infarction. A double-blind placebo-controlled study, *Clin Cardiol* 10:351-356, 1987.
38. Second International Study of Infarct Survival (ISIS-2) Collaborative Group: Randomized trial of intravenous streptokinase, oral aspirin, both, or neither among 17,187 cases of suspected acute myocardial infarction: ISIS-2, *Lancet* 2:349-360, 1988.
39. Secondary Prevention Reinfarction Nifedipine Trial (SPRINT): A randomized intervention trial of nifedipine in patients with acute myocardial infarction, *Eur Heart J* 9:354-364, 1988.
40. Sharpe N: Early preventive treatment of left ventricular dysfunction following myocardial infarction: optimal timing and patient selection, *Am J Cardiol* 68:64D-69D, 1991.
41. Shechter M, et al: Beneficial effect of magnesium sulfate in acute myocardial infarction, *Am J Cardiol* 66:271-274, 1990.
42. Smith CE: Assessing chest pain, *Nursing* 88:56-57, May 1988.
43. Sobel BE: Acute myocardial infarction. In Wyngaarden JB, et al, editors: *Volume 1: Cecil textbook of medicine,* ed 19, Philadelphia, 1992, WB Saunders.
44. *St Anthony's DRG guidebook 1995,* Reston, Va, 1994, St Anthony.
45. Tachibana C: Care of the patient with myocardial infarction. In Reiner A, editor: *Manual of patient care standards,* Gaithersburg, Md, 1990, Aspen Publishers.
46. Teo KK, et al: Effects of intravenous magnesium in suspected acute myocardial infarction: overview of randomized trials, *Br Med J* 303:1499-1503, 1991.
47. TIMI Study Group: Comparison of invasive and conservative strategies after treatment with intravenous tissue plasminogen activator in acute myocardial infarction: results of the Thrombolysis in Myocardial Infarction (TIMI) Phase II Trial, *N Engl J Med* 320:618-627, 1989.
48. Vander Wall EE, Cats VM, Bruschke AVG: Silent ischemia after acute myocardial infarction, *Am J Cardiol* 69:19B-24B, 1992.
49. Vetrovec GW: Changing concepts in the pathophysiology of myocardial ischemia, *Am J Cardiol* 64:3F-9F, 1989.
50. Weiss JL, Marina PN, Shapiro EP: Myocardial infarct expansion: recognition significance and pathology, *Am J Cardiol* 68:35D-40D, 1991.
51. White HD, et al: Effect of intravenous streptokinase on left ventricular function and early survival after acute myocardial infarction, *N Engl J Med* 317:850-855, 1987.
52. Wilcox RG, et al: Trial of tissue plasminogen activator for mortality reduction in acute myocardial infarction: Anglo-Scandinavian Study of Early Thrombolysis (ASSET), *Lancet* 2:525-530, 1988.
53. Woods KL, et al: Intravenous magnesium sulphate in suspected acute myocardial infarction: results of the second Leicester Intravenous Magnesium Intervention Trial (LIMIT-2), *Lancet* 339:1553-1558, 1992.
54. Woods KL, Fletcher S, Smith LFP: Intravenous magnesium in suspected acute myocardial infarction, *Br Med J* 304:119, 1992.

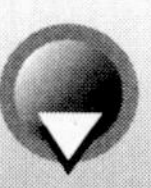

C L I N I C A L   G U I D E L I N E

17

Congestive Heart Failure

Mary G. Schigoda, MSN, RN, CCRN

DESCRIPTION

Congestive heart failure (CHF) is a primary complication of almost all forms of heart disease. It is defined as the pathophysiological state in which an abnormality of cardiac function results in failure of the heart to pump blood at a rate commensurate with the requirements of metabolizing tissues and/or the ability to do so only from an elevated filling pressure.[4] An alternative definition focuses on the clinical consequences of heart failure and identifies CHF as a complex clinical syndrome characterized by abnormalities of left ventricular function and neurohumoral regulation accompanied by activity intolerance, fluid retention, and reduced survival.[22] Both definitions represent a broad spectrum of impaired myocardial function ranging from the mildest, which is clinically manifested only under marked stress, to the most advanced, in which the heart requires mechanical support to sustain life.

Heart failure results from any condition that decreases the heart's ability to pump. (See Table 17-1.) The inability to maintain adequate cardiac output (CO) results in diminished forward flow and pooling of blood behind the right and/or left ventricle. These two mechanisms form the basis for the forward-backward theories of heart failure. The backward failure hypothesis, first introduced in 1832 by James Hope, postulates that when ventricular emptying is incomplete, blood accumulates and pressure rises in the atrium and venous system emptying into it. There is substantial physiological evidence in favor of this theory.[4] Eighty years after publication of Hope's work, Mackenzie proposed the forward failure theory, which attributes the clinical manifestations of heart failure to inadequate delivery of blood to the arterial system. Although seemingly opposite, it is evident now that both mechanisms are operant in chronic heart failure. Exceptions do occur and are most notable in acute cardiac decompensation, where relatively pure forms of backward failure have been reported, such as in ruptured papillary muscle with resultant acute mitral/tricuspid valve insufficiency.[4]

Implied in the backward theory of failure is the idea that fluid accumulates behind the specific chamber that is initially affected. Thus, symptoms of pulmonary congestion predominate with left ventricular dysfunction and symptoms of systemic congestion tend to originate with right ventricular dysfunction. Ultimately, left or right ventricular failure will lead to global CHF if uncorrected because both ventricles share a common intraventricular septum with continuous muscle bundles. Unilateral CHF, however, is 30 times more prevalent in the left ventricle than in the right.[15] Clinical manifestations for left versus right heart failure are listed in Table 17-2.

The clinical manifestations of heart failure are dependent on the rate at which the syndrome develops and whether sufficient time has lapsed for compensatory mechanisms to engage. The most common cause of acute CHF is myocardial infarction (MI). Loss of contractility is due to intracellular acidosis and the accumulation of intracellular phosphates following the MI.[27] Ischemic heart disease and dilated cardiomyopathy are the most frequent causes of chronic CHF. The mechanisms responsible for chronic CHF are as yet unclear.[27]

Low CO is the most common characteristic of heart failure. High CO also may lead to heart failure in select situations in which unusually extreme metabolic demand exceeds the ability of an otherwise normal heart. These include thyrotoxicosis, arteriovenous fistulas, beriberi, Paget's disease, anemia, and pregnancy.[4,27,40] Clinical manifestations

TABLE 17-1 Causes of CHF

Cause	Examples
Primary muscle disease	Cardiomyopathy Myocarditis
Secondary myocardial dysfunction	Coronary artery disease with ischemia/infarction Biochemical alterations, such as low calcium or magnesium
Congenital, rheumatic, or acquired valvular disease	Aortic, mitral, pulmonic, or tricuspid insufficiency or stenosis
Congenital anomalies	Atrial/ventricular septal defect Patent ductus arteriosus Arteriovenous fistula
Obstructive disorders	Hypertension Coarctation of the aorta Hypertrophic disorders, such as idiopathic hypertrophic subaortic stenosis (IHSS)
Restrictive disorders	Cardiac tamponade Restrictive pericarditis
Endocrine/metabolic disorders	Thyrotoxicosis Anemia Fever Pregnancy Systemic infection Beriberi Paget's disease

From Wright SM: Pathophysiology of congestive heart failure, *Cardiovasc Nurs,* 4(3):7, 1990.

of low CO failure include impairment of peripheral circulation with systemic vasoconstriction and pale, cool, and sometimes cyanotic extremities. As heart failure progresses, pulse pressure may begin to narrow. In contrast, high CO failure usually demonstrates warm and flushed extremities with widened or normal pulse pressure.[4,27]

Based on the physiological definition of heart failure, a defect in systolic function (inability to move blood out of the ventricle) or in diastolic function (impaired ventricular filling) are primary causes.[1,3,4] Systolic heart failure is the more familiar, classic heart failure caused by impaired contractility. Diastolic heart failure, less familiar but equally important, is caused by impaired ability of the ventricle to accept blood. Heart failure is most commonly caused by coronary atherosclerosis and is an example of combined systolic and diastolic failure. Systolic failure is caused by chronic loss of contracting myocardium due to infarction and acute loss from transient ischemia. Diastolic failure is due to the ventricle's decreased compliance secondary to development of scar tissue, which neither contracts nor expands in the area of the infarct.

TABLE 17-2 Clinical Manifestations of Right and Left Heart Failure

Left heart failure	Right heart failure
Breathlessness Exertional dyspnea Orthopnea Paroxysmal nocturnal dyspnea Dyspnea at rest Fatigue and weakness Decreased urine output Nocturia Cough Crackles, wheezes, or pleural fluid Hemoptysis Cyanosis Palpitations Tachycardia Dysrhythmias Elevated PCWP Gallop rhythm (S_3)	Jugular venous distension Elevated CVP Splenomegaly Hepatomegaly Hepatojugular reflex Abdominal distension Anorexia Nausea/vomiting Ascites Peripheral edema Weight gain

An estimated 3 million people in the United States and 15 million people worldwide are afflicted with CHF.[29] Unlike other cardiovascular disorders, which have decreased over the past 10 years, CHF has increased at an alarming rate. Approximately 400,000 people in the United States develop CHF each year.[17] This number is likely to increase as more people survive myocardial infarction, but with compromised ventricular function. Hospitalizations for CHF have increased threefold over the past 15 years, with CHF now representing the most common medical discharge diagnosis for those over the age of 65 years.[24] As a result of extensive research, advances in the understanding of CHF and cardiogenic shock have occurred. Initial studies of myocardial mechanics clarified the influence of preload on myocardial fiber shortening.[5] Further studies suggested that such hemodynamic alterations could be improved with pharmacologic intervention.[6] Regional blood flow measurements confirmed reduced blood flow to vital organs, especially the kidneys.[21] More recent studies have focused on delineating many of the neurohormonal abnormalities associated with CHF.[20] Based on this research, a variety of treatment options are now available to enhance the functional capacity of the CHF patient, such as the use of home inotropic therapy.[2,34]

Despite all this, CHF remains a progressive, debilitating syndrome that ultimately results in death for all but those few who are candidates for cardiac transplantation.

PATHOPHYSIOLOGY

CHF is a complex syndrome in which CO is inadequate for the metabolic demands of the body, resulting in poor tissue perfusion.[40] As a result, treatment is directed to optimize oxygen delivery (DO_2) to the vital organs and peripheral tissues. Assuming adequate hemoglobin concentrations and arterial saturation, CO becomes the critical determinant of survival in these patients.

CO is the quantity of blood pumped by the heart into the aorta each minute. Cardiac index (CI), an indicator derived from the CO, is a more specific indicator of the adequacy of CO for a specific individual as it reflects body surface area (BSA). Cardiac output is derived from the product of heart rate (HR) and stroke volume (SV).[3,15,16]

Stroke volume is the amount of blood ejected from the ventricle during each systolic contraction. Three factors contribute to the regulation of SV: preload, afterload, and contractility.[15]

Preload is the length to which myocardial muscle is stretched at the end of diastole. A relationship between fiber length and force of contraction was first identified in 1895 when Frank demonstrated that the tension generated by a muscle fiber was proportional to the initial fiber length at end-diastole.[13] Starling confirmed that the force of contraction is determined by end-diastolic fiber length, also adding that it is related to the diastolic filling pressure or volume in the ventricle.[26] Because myocardial muscle is usually compliant or distensible, the end-diastolic volume results in maximum stretching of the myocardial muscle fibers. Within physiological limits, the left ventricle will eject the volume of blood returning to the right atrium without buildup or back pressure. Thus, according to Starling's law of the heart, CO equals venous return. This allows for alteration in CO in response to changing demand. In the normal heart, greater end-diastolic pressure or volume will increase the force of contraction, resulting in an increase in CO up to the physiologic limit of the heart.

Preload volume cannot be measured directly in the intact heart. However, pulmonary capillary wedge pressure (PCWP) and left ventricular end-diastolic pressure (LVEDP) are related to left ventricular end-diastolic volume (LVEDV) and can be determined with a pulmonary artery (PA) catheter. Central venous pressure (CVP), right atrial mean pressure (RAMP), and right ventricular end-diastolic pressure (RVEDP), reflective of right ventricular end-diastolic volume (RVEDV), also may be measured using the proximal lumen of a PA catheter or an independent central line.

Afterload is the resistance against which the ventricle must pump, which impacts the tension in the ventricular wall at the onset of muscle fiber shortening.[15] The law of Laplace ($T = Pr/2h$) states that myocardial wall tension (T) is directly dependent on intraventricular pressure (P) and the internal radius of the ventricle (r), and inversely on the ventricular wall thickness (h).[15] Thus, wall tension in an enlarged heart must be greater than in a normal heart resulting in hypertrophy over time. As wall tension increases, myocardial oxygen consumption greatly increases. The other major component of afterload is aortic impedance, which is primarily influenced by systemic vascular resistance (SVR) and blood viscosity.

Contractility refers to the ability of cardiac muscle to alter its force of contraction independent of influences such as myocardial fiber length. This ability is primarily mediated by the sympathetic nervous system. Catecholamines activated by sympathetic stimulation and positive inotropic agents facilitate exchange of calcium across the cell membrane, which enhances contractility and increases CO. Conversely, negative inotropic agents, acidosis, and hypoxemia inhibit catecholamine release and suppress contractility.[3]

Heart rate is the other major determinant of CO, in addition to SV. It is primarily regulated through the pressure receptors in the carotid sinus and aortic arch. Tachycardia is an extremely important compensatory mechanism in CHF due to the heart's limited ability to augment SV. However, extremely fast heart rates reduce diastolic filling, which limits coronary artery perfusion, increases myocardial oxygen consumption, and may negatively impact CO. In the absence of other causative factors (drugs, fever, anemia, etc.), sinus tachycardia in CHF is generally compensatory in nature and should not be suppressed unless it results in myocardial ischemia.[25]

Several compensatory mechanisms are activated in response to reduction in CO and tissue perfusion. These include the Frank-Starling mechanism, activation of the autonomic nervous system, fluid retention by the kidneys, cardiac hypertrophy, and increased extraction of oxygen, all of which are intended to increase contractility and blood volume to return CO to normal levels.[3,27,40] The sympathetic nervous system (SNS) is activated within 30 seconds of the onset of decreased CO.[16] This momentary drop in CO triggers the pressure receptor and chemoreceptor feedback mechanisms, stimulating the release of norepinephrine by the adrenal medulla, heart, and peripheral blood vessels. In turn, the parasympathetic nervous system (PNS) is inhibited.

Stimulation of the SNS augments CO by (1) increasing heart rate and contractility; (2) constricting the venous beds, which enhances venous return and augments contractility via the Frank-Starling mechanism; (3) constricting the arterial beds, which improves blood pressure and redistributes blood flow from the periphery to the vital organs; and (4) constricting the renal arteries, which stimulates reabsorption of sodium and water by the kidneys to increase blood volume.

Myocardial hypertrophy, another compensatory mechanism, occurs in response to sustained increased hemodynamic workload. However, the hypertrophied cells require more energy due to the increase in mass, result in less contractile force, and ultimately worsen the failure state.[3,15]

Two distinct patterns of hypertrophy have been identified: concentric hypertrophy, most often associated with increased afterload, and eccentric hypertrophy, usually resulting from chronic volume overload.[3,15]

As blood flow to the tissues decreases in heart failure, the affinity of hemoglobin for oxygen declines. An increase in 2,3,diphosphoglycerate shifts the oxyhemoglobin curve to the right, facilitating the release of oxygen to the underperfused tissues. An increase in tissue extraction of oxygen also occurs, resulting in decreased venous oxygen saturation (SVO_2) and increased arteriovenous oxygen (AVO_2) difference. Increased oxygen extraction by the myocardium also occurs due to the increase in oxygen consumption by the failing heart.[3,16,40]

LENGTH OF STAY/ANTICIPATED COURSE

The average hospital length of stay for CHF is reported by Sorrentino at 8 days with a mean charge of $6,022.00 and a mean reimbursement of $3,330.00.[32] This information is consistent with HCFA data for DRG 127: Heart Failure and Shock, which reports an average LOS of 7.1 days.[33,40] Combined with a high rate of hospital readmission, the economic implications of CHF for the health care community are tremendous.

MANAGEMENT TRENDS AND CONTROVERSIES

The two primary treatment goals for patients with heart failure are to improve the quality of life and enhance survival. Three general approaches are used to achieve these goals: (1) removal of the underlying cause(s); (2) removal of the precipitating cause(s); and (3) control of congestive symptoms.

The most desirable approach in treating heart failure is to remove the underlying cause. This usually involves surgical correction of structural abnormalities such as congenital anomalies, acquired valvular lesions, and ventricular aneurysms or effective medical management of conditions such as hypertension and infective endocarditis. If heart failure is due to an impairment in diastolic relaxation rather than systolic contraction, specific measures to reduce ventricular hypertrophy or myocardial ischemia are employed.

Early recognition, prompt intervention, and, whenever possible, prevention of the specific precipitating causes are critical to successful management of CHF. Examples of precipitating factors of heart failure include dysrhythmias, infection, and pulmonary embolism.

The control of congestive symptoms is accomplished through three therapeutic approaches. First, *reduction of myocardial workload,* which involves reducing the demand on the heart to pump blood and/or to generate pressure. Second, *improvement in myocardial pumping performance,* which consists of efforts to restore the heart's contractile abilities. Third, *control of excessive sodium and water retention,* or extracellular fluid volume, which is the primary cause of most congestive symptoms such as dyspnea and edema.[30]

Management of Congestive Symptoms in Heart Failure

Reducing myocardial workload

Activity restriction
Optimizing weight
Vasodilator therapy
Assisted circulation

Improving pump performance

Digitalis glycosides
Sympathomimetic amines
Other positive inotropic agents

Controlling water and sodium retention

Low-sodium diet
Diuretic therapy
Mechanical fluid removal

Within each of these approaches, a number of therapeutic interventions exist depending on the severity of the heart failure (see Box). Severity of heart failure has been categorized by the New York Heart Association (NYHA) into four classes based on functional capacity.[30] Table 17-3 correlates progressively increasing one-year mortality rates with functional class.[19]

Reduction of myocardial workload is achieved through the use of various vasodilating agents including angiotensin-converting enzyme (ACE) inhibitors, nitrates, and hydralazine. Vasodilators promote arterial and venous vasodilation, resulting in the reduction of preload, afterload, or both. Vasodilators do not directly increase contractility. The ability of these drugs to improve CO depends on the degree of reduction in preload and afterload.

Optimal vasodilator therapy continues to be the only therapeutic intervention for CHF proven to reduce mortality. The first Veterans Affairs Cooperative Vasodilator–Heart Failure Trial (VHeFT-I) compared placebo, hydralazine plus isosorbide, and prazosin in patients with mild to moderate heart failure.[7,8] The study reported a 36% reduction in mortality in patients receiving the hydralazine/isosorbide combination as compared to the placebo or prazosin groups. LV ejection fraction also increased in the nitrate/hydralazine group.

The CONSENSUS Trial Study Group evaluated enalapril versus placebo and found that enalapril reduced mortality by 27% in patients with severe, NYHA Class IV heart fail-

TABLE 17-3 New York Heart Association Functional Classification Correlated with 1-Year Mortality

Functional class	Definition	Manifestation	1-year mortality
I	Patients with cardiac disease but without resulting limitations of physical activity	Ordinary activity does not cause undue fatigue, palpitations, dyspnea, or angina	0%-5%
II	Patients with cardiac disease resulting in slight limitation of physical activity, but comfortable at rest	Ordinary physical activity results in fatigue, palpitations, dyspnea, or angina	10%-20%
III	Patients with cardiac disease resulting in marked limitation of physical activity but comfortable at rest	Less than ordinary physical activity results in fatigue, palpitations, dyspnea, or angina	35%-45%
IV	Patients with cardiac disease resulting in an inability to carry out any physical activity without discomfort	Symptoms of cardiac insufficiency or of angina may be present even at rest	85%-95%

Used with permission from the New York Heart Association.

ure.[12] There was no reduction in the incidence of sudden death.

The second Veterans Trial (VHeFT-II) found the ACE inhibitor enalapril superior to hydralazine plus isosorbide in reducing mortality in patients with stable CHF.[10] Annual mortality in the enalapril group was 11.4% versus 14% in the vasodilator combination group. However, in looking at the 20% mortality in the placebo group from the first trial it can be inferred that both treatment groups in VHeFT-II favorably reduced mortality.

The SOLVD trial compared enalapril to standard treatment and placebo in patients with moderate to moderately severe NYHA Class II-IV heart failure and an LV ejection fraction of <35%.[31] A significant reduction in mortality of 16% was reported for the enalapril group.

Treatment with vasodilators of asymptomatic patients or those with only minimal symptoms remains controversial. Whether vasodilators can alter the natural history of the syndrome in patients with left ventricular dysfunction is currently under intense investigation. The various vasodilators currently used to treat CHF are outlined in Table 17-4.

Improvement of the heart's pumping performance is accomplished through the use of a variety of inotropic agents including the digitalis glycosides, sympathomimetic amines, and phosphodiesterase inhibitors. Inotropic usefulness is based on the theory that there is significant residual myocardial function able to be elicited from the failing heart. Inotropes act by increasing the amount of calcium available for contraction. It should be noted that they do not alter the underlying cause of poor contractility and are only a palliative measure in the treatment of CHF. It has been theorized that long-term use of these agents may actually damage the heart by further increasing its workload.[18] The various inotropes used to treat CHF are outlined in Table 17-5.

Elimination of sodium and water by the kidney is enhanced through the use of diuretics, which ultimately decreases left ventricular filling pressure or preload. Diuretic therapy subjectively decreases dyspnea and objectively increases urine output, decreasing weight, edema, JVD, S_3, and pulmonary crackles. Hemodynamically, diuretic therapy reduces pulmonary capillary wedge pressure (PCWP) by 12% to 32% and mean pulmonary artery pressures (PAM) by 0% to 35%.[15] A notable limitation of diuretic therapy is its failure to produce predictable improvement in CO.[15,22] Diuretics provide symptom relief but have no direct effect on the failing heart. Improvement in SV and CO is directly related to the reflex decrease in SVR.[22] The various diuretic agents are outlined in Table 17-6.

A growing body of research indicates that combination drug therapy for both acute and chronic CHF results in improved management of congestive symptoms and increased survival.[9,11,12,14,23,28] Some individuals who are refractory to standard therapy with vasodilators, inotropes, and diuretics have responded to more intensive pharmacological approaches tailored to specific hemodynamic goals in advanced heart failure.[35,36]

Although many treatment options exist for the CHF patient, severe heart failure progressing to cardiogenic shock may not respond to conventional or investigational pharmacologic interventions. Cardiogenic shock treated with pharmacologic agents has a mortality of 90% or greater.[40] This has led to the evolution of a variety of mechanical devices to assist the failing heart, including the intra-aortic balloon pump (IABP), ventricular assist devices (VADs), and total artificial hearts (TAHs).

Cardiac transplantation has become a treatment option for many with advanced heart failure as advances in operative technique and immunosuppression therapy increase

TABLE 17-4 Vasodilators Used to Manage CHF

Drug	Usual dose	Mechanism of action	Venous dilating effect (preload reduction)	Arterial dilating effect (afterload reduction)	Comments
Nitroglycerin	10-100 μg/min IV 5-20 mg transdermal qd 0.4-0.6 mg sl prn	Direct action on smooth muscle of arteries and veins	+ + +	+	Headache, flushing, dizziness, hypotension Give nitrate-free interval—determined by type and route of administration—controversial Acetaminophen for headache If hypotensive, remove patch or wipe off ointment
Isosorbide	5-40 mg q6h po Sustained release: 40-80 mg q8-12h po	Direct arterial vasodilation	+ + +	+	Similar to nitroglycerin
Captopril Enalapril Lisinopril	6.25-25 mg q6h po 2.5-10 mg q12h po 0.625-2.5 mg q6h IV 10-40 mg daily po	ACE inhibition	+ + +	+ +	Hypotension, headache, dizziness, dysgeusia Decrease dose according to renal function Watch for hyperkalemia!! Rash—esp with captopril—change to another ACE-I Cough—change class of vasodilator only if cough is bothersome to patient
Hydralazine	10-75 mg q6h po/IV	Direct arterial vasodilation		+ + +	Nausea, vomiting, headache, flushing, palpitations, angina, MI, drug-induced systemic lupus erythematosus (at high doses) Tolerance occurs in 30% of patients Must be titrated carefully, esp in volume depleted and elderly
Prazosin Terazosin Doxazosin	1-5 mg q6h po 1-5 mg po 1-16 mg po	α-adrenergic blockade	+ + +	+ +	First dose syncope—give first dose at HS Postural hypotension, drowsiness, headache, dizziness, palpitations
Nitroprusside	0.3-10 μg/kg/min IV	Direct effect on arterial and venous smooth muscle	+ + +	+ + +	Marked hypotension—discontinue drug Need invasive monitoring Light sensitive Caution—thiocyanate toxicity—usually seen in high doses for long periods of time or in hepatic or renal dysfunction (more than 500 μg/kg total at a rate >2 μg/kg/min)

TABLE 17-5 Inotropes Used to Manage CHF

Drug	Dose	Mechanism of action	Hemodynamic effects	Side effects	Comments
Digoxin	Load: 0.25 mg slow IV 0.25 mg q6h × 3 (varies) Maintainance: 0.125-0.25 mg po	↑ Force of contraction Prolongs conduction through AV node	↓ HR ↑ CO	Nausea, vomiting, diarrhea, bradycardia, arrhythmias Toxicity: Nausea, vomiting, anorexia, diarrhea, yellow or blurred vision, premature beats, heart blocks, tachy/bradycardias	4 reasons to check a digoxin level: • Verify compliance of medication • At point of conversion or control of A.Fib. • Changing renal function • Suspect toxicity Drug interactions: Quinidine, Amiodarone, Verapamil—↑ digoxin levels Questran, antacids—↓ digoxin levels
Dopamine	1-4 μg/kg/min IV 5-10 μg/kg/min IV 10-20 μg/kg/min IV	Dopaminergic receptor stimulant: dilates mesenteric and renal arteries β-stimulant: + inotrope α-stimulant: ↑ SVR	↑ RBF and U/O ↑ RBF, MAP, PCWP—↑ CO ↑↓ RBF, ↑ MAP, PCWP, CO, SVR CHF patients need doses < 10 μg/kg/min	Angina, headaches, nausea, tachydysrhythmias, ectopic beats, hypotension ↓ Peripheral perfusion Fever	Must be diluted Incompatible with bicarbonate—degrades dopamine Painful extravasation—requires phentolamine and/or steroid injections Isolated cases of gangrene in low dose recipients with occlusive vascular disease Ideal patient = ↓ CO and BP due to ↓ SVR
Dobutamine	2.5-5 μg/kg/min IV titrated for effect Intermittent infusion: 1.5-15 μg/kg/min IV over 4 to 72 hours weekly	Selective β-stimulant: ↑ Contractility	↑ CO, RBF ↓ PCWP Reflex ↓ SVR may ↑ HR	Tachycardia, hypertension, ectopic beats, phlebitis at injection site, nausea, headache, angina, SOB	Improves LV contractility without ↑ O_2 demand unlike dopamine No dose-dependent functions Usually preferred over dopamine Ideal patient = ↓ CO, ↑ PCWP and SVR, normal BP
Amrinone	Load: 0.75 mg/kg IV over 2 min Maintainance: 5-10 μg/kg/min IV May re-bolus in 30 min No more than 10 mg/kg/day	+ Inotrope Vasodilating activity Actual mechanism unknown	↑ CO, RBF ↓ PCWP, SVR ↑↓ HR ↓ MAP	Hypotension, Thrombocytopenia Hepatotoxicity Hypersensitivity in therapy >2 weeks duration	Long half-life—titrate in increments of 1 μg/kg/min Dilute in NORMAL SALINE Many side effects are dose related
Milrinone	Load: 50 μg/kg IV over 10 min Maintainance: 0.375-0.75 μg/kg/min IV	Inotrope with arterial vasodilating activity	↑ CO ↓ PCWP, SVR	Ventricular arrhythmias (more than amrinone) Thrombocytopenia (less than amrinone) Hypotension (more than amrinone)	Monitor BP and HR frequently ↓ Dose for hypotension and renal dysfunction May use D5W OR SALINE as diluent

RBF: renal blood flow.

TABLE 17-6 Diuretics Used to Manage CHF

Drug	Usual dose (mg/day)	Site of action	Effect on serum electrolytes	Extrarenal effects	Side effects
Thiazides					
Chlorothiazide Hydrochlorothiazide Metolazone	500-1000 25-100 5-10	Early distal tubule Proximal—added effects on NaCl and K excretion with loops	↓ Na, Cl, Mg ↑ HCO_3, Ca	↑ Blood glucose ↑ LDL, TG ↑ ↑ Serum uric acid	Dizziness, hypotension, headache, syncope, drowsiness, frequent urination, muscle cramps, acute gouty attacks, hypokalemia, hypercalcemia, hyponatremia Only useful if creatinine clearance >30 ml/min
Loops					
Furosemide Bumetanide	20-400 0.5-2.0	Thick ascending loop of Henle—inhibition of Na/K/Cl transport	↑ HCO_3 ↓ K, Na, Cl, Mg, PO_4 ↑ Uric acid	↓ Preload ↑ Venous capacitance ↑ SVR	Useful to creatinine clearance of 10 ml/min Side effects similar to those of thiazides but also pancreatitis, thrombocytopenia, and blood dyscrasias Irreversible ototoxicity greater with furosemide than bumetanide Metabolic alkalosis
K-sparing					
Spironolactone Triamterene Amiloride	25-100 50-300 5-20	Late distal tubule Aldosterone antagonist Inhibits Na transport	↑ K, ↓ Na, ↓ HCO_3	↓ ADH release	Gynecomastia Side effects similar to thiazides Hyperkalemia!! Watch out for ACE inhibitors and potassium supplements!!
Acetazolamide	250-500	Proximal tubule carbonic anhydrase inhibition	↓ HCO_3, Na, K	↑ Ventilatory drive	Metabolic acidosis May be used to correct alkalosis caused by other diuretics Side effects similar to other diuretics plus: sulfonamide hypersensitivity reactions may occur, melena, bone marrow depression, blood dyscrasias, nervousness, depression, flaccid paralysis, paresthesias of the extremities, convulsions If nausea occurs, give with food, watch for sore throat, fever, or unusual bleeding—notify MD
Mannitol	50-200 GM/day	Proximal tubule	↓ Na, Cl	↑ H_2O elimination ↓ Intracranial pressure	May enhance loop diuresis by maintaining GFR May cause edema, pulmonary congestion, thrombophlebitis, hypotension, hypertension, tachycardia, angina-like chest pain, fluid and electrolyte imbalances, acidosis, dehydration

survival.[40] However, the limited supply of donor hearts has made this option available to only a small percentage of those who might potentially benefit. Because of this, other surgical treatment options are being explored. Dynamic cardiomyoplasty is a surgical option currently being investigated. In this procedure, skeletal muscle, usually the latissimus dorsi, is wrapped around the weakened heart and is paced in synchrony with ventricular systole to augment ventricular function.[37,39] The first successful attempt at this procedure occurred in 1985. Since then, more than 200 patients have undergone this procedure worldwide.[39] If trials continue to produce positive outcomes, this procedure may become an important bridge to transplant. Considering the scarcity of donor hearts, dynamic cardiomyoplasty may also be a promising long-term alternative to cardiac transplantation.

The prevalence and complexity of this syndrome make CHF one of the most important public health concerns in the United States today. Continued research and innovative interventions based on sound scientific principles are needed to assist the growing number of individuals afflicted with CHF.

ASSESSMENT

PARAMETER	ANTICIPATED ALTERATION
Cardiovascular Status	
HR	Tachycardia: resting HR >100 bpm
Rhythm	Dysrhythmias
MAP	Decreased: <70 mm Hg
CI	Decreased: <2.0 L/min/mm^2 *due to decreased contractility, especially in cardiogenic shock*
SVR	Increased: >1200 to 1500 dynes/sec/cm^{-5} *due to compensatory mechanisms, especially in cardiogenic shock*
SVRI	Increased: >2390 dyne · sec/cm^{-5} · −m^2
PVR	Increased: >97 dynes/sec/cm^{-5} *due to pulmonary congestion and hypoxia*
PVRI	Increased: >285 dyne · sec/cm^{-5} · −m^2
Neck veins	JVD present with HOB >30°
Peripheral perfusion	CRT >3 sec; pale, cool extremities; cyanosis
Pulmonary Status	
RR	Tachypnea: >30/min Dyspnea
PAP (S/D/M)	Elevated: >35/15/20 mm Hg *due to pulmonary congestion and LV dysfunction*
FiO_2	Increased percentage needed to maintain adequate oxygenation
DO_2	Decreased: <900 ml/min at rest
VO_2	Increased: >275 ml/min at rest
Breath sounds	Crackles, decreased in bases
Neurological Status	
LOC	Anxious, restless, confused
Noninvasive Tests	
12-lead ECG	Atrial/ventricular ectopy Atrial/ventricular enlargement Aneurysm formation Ischemia/infarction

Echocardiography	Concentric vs. eccentric ventricular hypertrophy Septal hypertrophy Atrial enlargement Valvular insufficiency/stenosis Septal and ventricular wall motion abnormalities (akinesis, hypokinesis, dyskinesis) Decreased ventricular ejection fraction: LVEF <60% RVEF <45% *due to decreased contractility*
Chest x-ray	Cardiomegaly Pulmonary vascular congestion Alveolar and/or interstitial edema Pleural effusions
MUGA scan	Decreased ventricular ejection fraction: LVEF <60% RVEF <45% Wall motion abnormalities

Laboratory Findings

Na^+	Hyponatremia: Na^+ <136 mEq/L *dilutional or due to diuretics*
K^+	Hyperkalemia: K^+ >5.0 mEq/L *due to renal insufficiency* Hypokalemia: K^+ <3.5 mEq/L *due to diuretics*
Cl^-	Hypochloremia: Cl^- <96 mEq/L *due to diuretics*
BUN	Elevated: >20 mg/dl *due to renal impairment*
Creatinine	Elevated: >1.2 mg/dl *due to renal impairment*
SGOT	Elevated: >40 IU/L *due to hepatic involvement*
LDH	Elevated: >225 IU/L *due to hepatic involvement*
UA	Proteinuria (1 to 2 g/dl) Elevated specific gravity >1.030
Creatinine clearance	Decreased: <88 ml/min
PT	Prolonged: >12.5 sec *due to hepatic compromise*
RBC	Polycythemia: RBC >6.1 million/mm^3 *due to renal impairment and compensatory response to decreased tissue perfusion*
Hgb	Anemia: Hgb <8.6 mmol/L
WBC	Leukocytosis: WBC >10,000/mm^3
ABG	Metabolic acidosis *due to decreased tissue perfusion* • pH <7.35 • Pao_2 <80 mm Hg • $Paco_2$ <35 mm Hg • Hco_3 <21 mEq/L Respiratory alkalosis *due to hyperventilation* • pH >7.45 • $Paco_2$ <35 mm Hg Respiratory acidosis *due to pulmonary edema and hypoventilation* • pH <7.35 • Pao_2 <80 mm Hg • $Paco_2$ >45 mm Hg

PLAN OF CARE

INTENSIVE PHASE

The intensive phase of care for heart failure patients is clearly focused on hemodynamic stabilization and adequate oxygenation to preserve organ and tissue integrity. Acute CHF, especially when it manifests as fulminating pulmonary edema or cardiogenic shock, is typically managed in the ICU where full hemodynamic monitoring, aggressive vasoactive and cardiotonic support, and possible mechanical support for both circulation and ventilation may be employed. Chronic CHF presenting with exacerbation of failure symptoms requiring inotropic "rescue" intervention may be managed in the intermediate care unit setting depending on its severity and in the absence of invasive hemodynamic monitoring. Initially, both types of heart failure patients require intensive nursing care, monitoring, and intervention regardless of the unit they are admitted to.

PATIENT CARE PRIORITIES	EXPECTED PATIENT OUTCOMES
Decreased CO/CI *r/t diminished ventricular function*	Hemodynamic stability (see Appendix A) Normal fluid and electrolyte balance Peripheral perfusion WNL Alert and oriented
Impaired gas exchange *r/t pulmonary vascular congestion*	Absence of dyspnea, orthopnea, paroxysmal nocturnal dyspnea, frothy sputum, tachypnea, tachycardia, restlessness Breath sounds clear ABG: WNL
Fatigue *r/t limited cardiac reserve*	Able to perform ADLs
Decreased physical mobility *r/t decreased cardiac output*	Absence of skin breakdown, pneumonia, PE, constipation, thromboembolism/phlebitis
Decreased nutrition *r/t dyspnea, fatigue, anorexia, impaired absorption*	Positive nitrogen balance and weight within optimal range
Anxiety/fear *r/t acute/chronic illness, dyspnea, fear of dying*	Verbalizes feelings of anxiety/fear Uses effective coping strategies throughout the course of the illness Demonstrates beneficial use of relaxation techniques

INTERVENTIONS

Monitor hemodynamic parameters.

Administer diuretics as prescribed *to increase the elimination of sodium and water by the kidneys, resulting in a decrease in both vascular volume and left ventricular filling pressure (preload).*

Administer vasodilators as prescribed *to decrease vasoconstriction, resulting in reduction of preload and afterload.*

Administer inotropic agents as prescribed *to increase contractility, resulting in increased cardiac output.*

Monitor intake and output, *especially in the stabilization of acute CHF.*

Monitor daily weight, *especially in the ongoing management of chronic CHF.*

Monitor for ongoing signs/symptoms of pulmonary congestion and impaired gas exchange.

Provide supplemental oxygen *to improve oxygen supply.*

Position in high Fowler's with legs dependent *to lower diaphragm, increase lung expansion, and dilate peripheral arteries and veins, resulting in peripheral pooling, decreased venous return to the heart, and reduction in preload.*

Administer morphine sulfate as prescribed *to reduce anxiety, decrease tachypnea, and cause peripheral pooling of blood, resulting in decreased preload and afterload.*

Plan of Care (cont'd)

Space activities *to prevent fatigue and further decompensation.*

Monitor for complications of physical immobility.

Offer high-calorie, high-protein, low-volume supplements between meals *to maintain adequate caloric intake and positive nitrogen balance.*

Organize care to allow for 1-hour periods of rest before and after meals *to conserve energy for eating and enhance nutrient absorption.*

Offer small, frequent meals *to decrease the amount of blood needed for digestion, which helps maintain the blood supply to other vital organs.*

Encourage use of previously successful coping strategies *to focus patient on strengths and abilities.*

Teach relaxation strategies *to increase sense of control.*

Encourage active participation in planning care *to increase sense of control and reestablish confidence in decision-making abilities.*

Provide realistic reassurance.

Control and manage the environment *to ensure safety and comfort.*

INTERMEDIATE PHASE

If the patient survives the intensive phase, recovery will depend on the precipitating event. Nursing care will focus on reducing myocardial workload and assisting the patient in adapting to physical and life-style changes resulting from the acute illness and the chronic nature of the disease process.

PATIENT CARE PRIORITIES	EXPECTED PATIENT OUTCOMES
High risk for ineffective gas exchange *r/t chronic degenerative disease process with probable future exacerbation of symptoms*	Demonstrate absence of dyspnea and adequate tissue perfusion
High risk for ongoing activity intolerance *r/t chronic, degenerative disease process.*	Adjust activity level to avoid fatigue Demonstrate increased energy levels and ability to perform ADLs Participate in a supervised cardiac rehabilitation program
Self-care deficit *r/t complexity of CHF and treatment/care requirements*	Verbalizes signs/symptoms of heart failure, risk factor modification, medication regime, diet, activity, pulse counting, daily weight, when to call the physician, and when to return for follow-up

INTERVENTIONS

Teach patient to count pulse before and after activities and record *to identify activities that place high demands on the heart.*

Space activities known to increase fatigue. New activities should not be initiated until heart rate returns to preactivity level *to ensure adequate tissue perfusion and minimize symptoms.*

Ensure adequate sleep/rest periods *to promote physical healing and strength.*

Teach patient to obtain daily weight at approximately the same time each day on the same scale and to contact their physician for a weight gain of >2 lb within 24 hours or >5 lb within one week *to optimize potential modification of medications or other interventions without acute exacerbation of CHF and need for readmission. Monitoring daily weight has been found to be a highly effective indicator of the status of chronic CHF, although its value in the evaluation of acute pulmonary edema has been disputed.*

Teach patient/family regarding medications, activity plan, general indicators of worsening CHF, diet prescription (especially the need to avoid sodium), and follow-up care requirements *to ensure optimal self-care after discharge and to decrease the frequency of readmission.*

TRANSITION TO DISCHARGE

As the patient moves from the intensive phase to the intermediate phase, the focus of nursing care is to prepare the patient for discharge. For most patients with CHF, the cause of this complex syndrome is not correctable. Thus, nursing care during the transition phase must focus on enhancing the quality of the patient's life through symptom control. This involves assisting the patient in the development of a self-care regime using adaptive techniques that reduce myocardial workload, maintain the heart's pumping performance, and control sodium and fluid retention.

REFERENCES

1. Applegate RJ, Little WC: Systolic and diastolic dysfunction in congestive heart failure, *Cardiology* 8(6):57, 1991.
2. Bousquet GL: Congestive heart failure: a review of nonpharmacologic therapies, *J Cardiovasc Nurs* 4(3):35-46, 1990.
3. Braunwald E: Pathophysioloy of heart failure. In Braunwald E, editor: *Heart disease—a textbook of cardiovascular medicine,* vol I, Philadelphia, 1992, WB Saunders.
4. Braunwald E, Grossman W: Clinical aspects of heart failure. In Braunwald E, editor: *Heart disease—a textbook of cardiovascular medicine,* vol I, Philadelphia, 1992, WB Saunders.
5. Braunwald E, Ross J, Sonneblick EJ: *Mechanisms of contraction of the normal and failing heart,* ed 7, Boston, 1976, Little, Brown.
6. Chatterjee L, Rosenweig J: The role of vasodilator therapy in heart failure, *Cardiovasc Dis* 19:301, 1977.
7. Cohn JN, et al: Veterans administration cooperative study on vasodilator therapy in heart failure: influence of prerandomization variables on the reduction of mortality by treatment with hydralazine and isosorbide dinitrate, *Circulation* 75(suppl IV):49-54, 1987.
8. Cohn JN, et al: Effect of vasodilator therapy on mortality in chronic congestive heart failure, *N Engl J Med* 314:1547-1552, 1986.
9. Cohn JN, Francisosa JA: Selection of vasodilator, inotropic or combined therapy for the management of heart failure, *Am J Med* 65:181, 1978.
10. Cohn JN, et al: A comparison of enalapril with hydralazine-isosorbide dinitrate in the treatment of chronic congestive heart failure, *N Engl J Med* 325:303, 1991.
11. Cohn JN, Rector TS: Prognosis of congestive heart failure and predictors of mortality, *Am J Cardiol* 62:25A, 1988.
12. CONSENSUS Trial Study Group: Effects of enalapril on mortality in severe congestive heart failure, *N Engl J Med* 316:1429-1435, 1987.
13. Frank O, Chapman CB, Wasserman E, trans: On the dynamics of cardiac muscle, *Am Heart J* 58:282-467, 1959.
14. Gheorghiade M, et al: Comparative hemodynamic and neurohormonal effects of intravenous captopril and digoxin, and their combination in patients with severe heart failure, *J Am Coll Cardiol* 13:134-143, 1989.
15. Guyton AC: *Textbook of medical physiology,* Philadelphia, 1986, WB Saunders.
16. Hurst J, et al: *The heart,* New York, 1990, McGraw-Hill.
17. Kannel WB: Epidemiologic aspects of heart failure. In Wever KT, editor: *Heart failure: current concepts and management,* 1989.
18. Katz A: Cellular mechanisms in congestive heart failure, *Am J Cardiol* 62:3A-8A, 1988.
19. Killip T: Epidemiology of congestive heart failure, *Am J Cardiol* 56:2A-7A, 1985.
20. Kubo S: Neurohormonal activity in congestive heart failure, *Crit Care Med* 18:39, 1990.
21. Leithe ME, et al: Relationship between central hemodynamics and regional blood flow in normal subjects and in patients with congestive heart failure, *Circulation* 69:57, 1984.
22. Packer M: Survival in patients with chronic heart failure and its potential modifications by drug therapy. In Cohn JH, editor: *Drug treatment of heart failure,* 1988.
23. Packer M: Physiological determinants of survival in congestive heart failure, *Circulation* 75(suppl. 4):1-3, 1987.
24. Packer M: Prolonging life in patients with congestive heart failure: the next frontier, *Circulation* 75(suppl. 4):1-111, 1987.
25. Passmore JM, Goldstein RA: Acute recognition and management of congestive heart failure, *Crit Care Clin* 5(3):497-532, 1989.
26. Patterson S, Piper H, Starling E: The regulation of the heart beat, *J Physiol* 48:465-513, 1914.
27. Quaal SJ: The person with heart failure and cardiogenic shock. In Guzzetta C, Dossey BM, editors: *Cardiovascular nursing: holistic practice,* Chicago, 1992, Mosby–Year Book.
28. Ribner HS, et al: Vasodilators as first-line therapy for congestive heart failure: a comparative hemodynamic study of hydralazine, digoxin, and their combination, *Am Heart J* 114:91, 1987.
29. Schwartz DW, Piano MR: New inotropic drugs for treatment of congestive heart failure, *Cardiovascular Nurs* 26(2):7, 1990.
30. Smith TW, Braunwald E, Kelly RA: The management of heart failure. In Braunwald E, editor: *Heart disease—a textbook of cardiovascular medicine,* vol I, Philadelphia, 1992, WB Saunders, pp 464-519.
31. SOLVD investigators: Effect of angiotensin converting enzyme inhibitor enalapril on survival in patients with reduced left ventricular ejection fraction and congestive heart failure, *N Engl J Med* 325:293, 1991.
32. Sorrentino E: Hospitals vary by length of stay, changes, reimbursements, and death rates, *Nurs Management* 20:54-60, 1989.
33. *St Anthony's DRG Guidebook 1995,* Reston, Va, 1994, St Anthony.
34. Stanley R: Drug therapy of heart failure, *J Cardiovasc Nurs* 4(3):17-34, 1990.
35. Stevenson LW: Tailored therapy before transplantation for treatment of advanced heart failure: effective use of vasodilators and diuretics, *J Heart Lung Transplant* 10:468-476, 1991.
36. Stevenson LW, Dracup KA, Tillisch JH: Congestive heart failure: efficacy of medical therapy tailored for severe congestive heart failure in patients transferred for urgent cardiac transplantation, *Am J Cardiol* 63:461-464, 1989.
37. Stewart JV, et al: Cardiomyoplasty: treatment of the failing heart using the skeletal muscle wrap, *J Cardiovasc Nurs* 7(2):23-31, 1993.
38. The Criteria Committee of the New York Heart Association: *Nomenclature and criteria for diagnosis of diseases of the heart and great vessels,* New York, 1979, Little, Brown.
39. Vargo R, Dimengo JM: Surgical alternatives for patients with heart failure, *AACN Clin Issues Crit Care Nurs* 4(2):244-259, 1993.
40. Wright SM: Pathophysiology of congestive heart failure, *J Cardiovasc Nurs* 4(3):1-16, 1990.

Lisa Pauley, Pharm. D., Clinical ICU Pharmacist, and Dennis Brierton, Pharm. D., Clinical Coordinator, St. Luke's Medical Center, Milwaukee, WI, are thanked for their assistance in developing and editing the tables on diuretics, vasodilators, and inotropic agents.

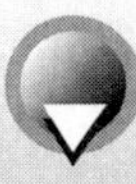

CLINICAL GUIDELINE

18

Dysrhythmias

Siobhan Bremner, BSN, MPH, RN
Kelly Scholz, BSN, RN

DESCRIPTION

Dysrhythmias are disturbances of impulse formation and/or conduction within the heart that occur as a result of structural or functional abnormalities of the conduction system. They may be broadly categorized as ectopy, tachycardias, and bradycardias. An ectopic beat, often referred to as a premature beat or escape beat, is an impulse that interrupts the normal sinus cycle. Tachycardias, by definition, include rapid rhythms with atrial or ventricular rates exceeding 100 beats per minute (bpm). Bradycardias, on the other hand, include rhythms with atrial or ventricular rates below 60 bpm. Dysrhythmias that are common and have the greatest impact on mortality and quality of life include ventricular tachycardia (VT), supraventricular tachycardia (SVT), and bradycardias. In addition, neurocardiogenic syncope (NCS) has been identified as a significant clinical presentation associated with bradycardia and hypotension.

Ventricular tachycardia includes ventricular rhythms greater than 100 bpm that originate from impulses generated in the right or left ventricle. Ventricular rhythms with rates between 60 and 100 bpm are termed accelerated idioventricular rhythm and are usually benign. However, VT has a significant likelihood of becoming lethal. Its severity is related to dissociation of AV contraction, decreased diastolic filling time, and potential degeneration into ventricular fibrillation. As a result, identification and treatment of persons with VT is critical

The variety of VT mechanisms and associated structural heart disease make it difficult to measure incidence rates accurately. Adequate ECG documentation is not possible with every case. However, of the 300,000 annual victims of sudden cardiac death (SCD), more than 70% have associated ventricular dysrhythmias.[4] Unfortunately, SCD is often the first indication of heart disease and/or VT.[17]

Supraventricular tachycardia, as the name implies, originates above the ventricle in either the atrium or the AV junction. There are three types of tachycardia that originate in the atrium: atrial fibrillation (>350 bpm), atrial flutter (250 to 350 bpm), and atrial tachycardia (160 to 250 bpm). AV junctional SVT includes AV nodal reentry tachycardia and accessory pathway mediated tachycardia. Though accessory pathway mediated tachycardia may be lethal in rare cases, SVT typically causes nonlethal symptoms ranging from palpitations to syncope. In addition to tachycardic-specific symptoms, patients with underlying heart disease may experience exacerbation of heart failure or ischemia with rapid ventricular response to SVT.

Though the frequency of each type of SVT is not clear, the incidence of AF/AFL is significant in the general population. Rates increase with age: 2 to 3 per 1000 for ages 25 to 35 years, and 30 to 40 per 1000 for ages 55 to 64 years.[16] SVT originating in the AV junction is clearly prevalent in the general population and accounts for the "garden variety" of SVT (sometimes termed PAT).

Bradycardia refers to a mixture of dysrhythmias that cause abnormally slow heart rates (below 60 bpm). Though rates closer to 60 bpm may not produce symptoms, the combination of bradycardia at any rate with hemodynamic compromise requires immediate attention. Syncope, dizziness, or fatigue are often the symptoms that prompt individuals to seek treatment. The incidence rate of bradycardia is unclear. However, the tremendous volume of artificial pacemakers implanted in the United States each year (more than 90,000) is one indicator of the problem's magnitude.[4]

Neurocardiogenic syncope is a manifestation of an abnormal reflex involving both neurologic and cardiovascular responses. Up to 30% of the general adult population in the United States will experience some form of syncope at least once in their lives.[3] In fact, as many as 3% of all emergency room visits are for episodes of syncope.[3] While often due to the dysrhythmias just reviewed, the complex combination of responses known as NCS is increasingly being recognized as a cause of previously unexplained syncope (e.g., the common faint or vasovagal syncope) especially in young individuals without structural heart disease.

PATHOPHYSIOLOGY

The two primary electrophysiologic mechanisms of ectopy and tachycardia are enhanced automaticity and reentry. **Enhanced automaticity** may occur due to the rapid depolarization rate of a cell or group of cells in response to physiologic stimuli or functional abnormalities. The enhanced automatic site causes cardiac depolarization at a rate rapid enough to usurp the sinoatrial node. Potential predisposing factors include increased catecholamines, hypoxia, electrolyte and acid base disturbances, ischemia, and hypertrophy. This dysrhythmic mechanism may develop in the normal conduction system or the myocardium. Specific sites include the atria, the atrioventricular (AV) junction, the His-Purkinje system, or the ventricles. A ventricular origin generally implies a more ominous consequence.

Reentry is an electrophysiologic phenomenon resulting from impulse transmission around a circuit (loop) within or outside the normal conduction system (Figure 18-1). The impulse travels at a tachycardic rate, depolarizes cardiac tissue, and thus usurps the sinus and AV nodes. The genesis of reentry requires at least two anatomically or functionally distinct conductive pathways (limbs that complete the circuit) and unidirectional block.[27] Reentry tachycardia is usually initiated by a premature impulse that reaches the normal conduction pathway when it is still refractory from the previous impulse (unidirectional block). As a result, the premature impulse propagates through the alternate (second) limb of the circuit. Once it has reached the end of the alternate limb, the impulse turns around and finds the previously refractory tissue of the primary limb recovered. Propagation through the primary limb at this point completes the reentrant circuit. This process, if aborted, results in a single premature reentrant beat; if persistent, it leads to tachycardia.[27] Reentrant circuits may be near the SA node, within the atria, within the AV node, between the AV node and an accessory pathway, or within the ventricles.

Ventricular tachycardia is due to either abnormal automaticity or reentry and is categorized as monomorphic or polymorphic. Monomorphic VT manifests identical QRS complexes in several ECG leads, whereas changing QRS morphology implies polymorphic VT (Figure 18-2). Generally speaking, monomorphic VT is more common and is seen in the presence of a prior myocardial infarction or fibrosis associated with dilated cardiomyopathy. In the majority of cases, this tachycardia is associated with a microreentrant circuit located near the fibrotic or scar tissues.[2] The occurrence of VT in these individuals is due to a complex interaction between the diseased tissue and a variety of triggers such as ischemia, electrolyte imbalance, antidysrhythmic drugs, or hypoxia.

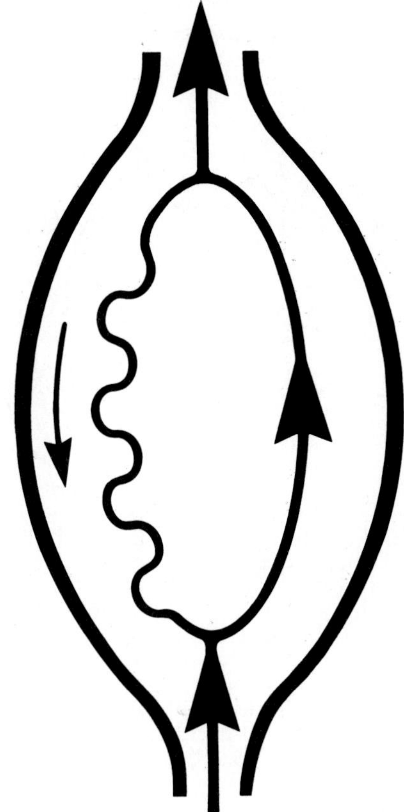

Figure 18-1 Schematic representation of a reentrant circuit depicting two limbs with varying conduction times (straight line vs. curly line). The tachycardic impulse travels around this circuit, and as it reaches the common end(s), travels to the myocardium which then depolarizes. A similar reentrant circuit can be located around the sinus node, within the atrial or ventricular myocardium, within the AV node, or between the AV node and an accessory pathway.

Although infrequent, monomorphic VT may occur in persons with seemingly normal hearts. The exact mechanism is unclear: there is limited evidence of reentry and automaticity. It typically occurs in young persons, produces symptoms that are not malignant (e.g., palpitations), and may be mistaken for SVT.[2]

The etiology and management of polymorphic VT will vary according to the presence or absence of a prolonged QT interval prior to its onset. Torsade de pointes (TDP) is the most common form of polymorphic VT and is associated

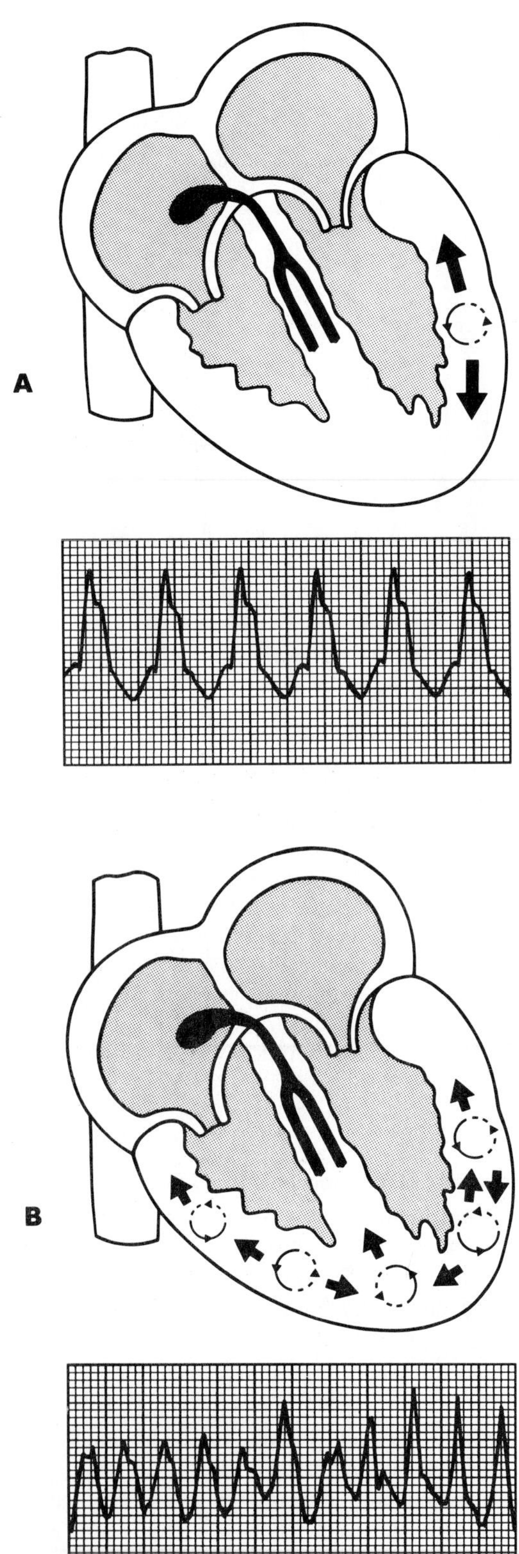

Figure 18-2 Ventricular tachycardia (VT). Panel **A** depicts VT where each QRS complex is identical, also known as monomorphic VT (see ECG) due to a micro-reentrant circuit (see heart figure). Panel **B** depicts polymorphic VT where QRS complexes vary from beat to beat (see ECG) due to either enhanced automaticity or reentry (see heart figure).

with prolonged QT interval.[14] TDP gets its name from the fact that, in some cases, the polymorphic QRS complexes appear to twist around the ECG baseline. Although its exact mechanism is unclear, it may be either acquired (from the effects of drugs such as class IA or III antidysrhythmics, diet, hypokalemia, hypomagnesemia, or bradycardia) or congenital. The most distinguishing factor of TDP is not necessarily a prolonged QT interval during normal sinus rhythm, but a prolonged QT interval with bizarre T- and U-wave morphologies apparent just prior to the onset of tachycardia. While the onset of acquired TDP is typically post-pause (after a PVC or during bradycardia), congenital TDP is triggered by an adrenergic surge such as that which occurs with excitement or exercise. Because both forms of TDP may result in sudden cardiac death and treatment is unique, initial identification of TDP is crucial.[14] Antidysrhythmic drugs that prolong QT interval are absolutely contraindicated.

Polymorphic VT that is not associated with a prolonged QT frequently develops in the presence of myocardial ischemia but can also be seen with advanced cardiomyopathies.[12] Its ECG will not reveal QT prolongation, but there will be beat-to-beat differences in QRS morphology during tachycardia, as depicted in Figure 18-2. In contrast to TDP, it may be successfully treated with antidysrhythmic drugs or revascularization.[12]

Identification of VT in the clinical setting, even with telemetry, may be challenging. The most distinguishing criteria are wide QRS intervals (greater than 160 milliseconds) and AV dissociation.[12] These factors may not be evident on one or two leads as seen with most monitoring systems. Therefore, a 12-lead ECG is often helpful. SVT with intraventricular conduction delay due to either bundle-branch block or antegrade conduction over an accessory pathway may also produce a wide QRS complex. On occasion, differentiation of wide-QRS complex tachycardias is very difficult to make without an intracardiac electrogram.

Supraventricular tachycardias originating in the atrium may be associated with coronary artery disease, hypertension, valvular disease, cardiomyopathy, pericarditis, post-cardiac surgery, or drug toxicity. However, a significant proportion of these patients have otherwise normal hearts. AF is characterized as a rapid disorganized atrial rhythm with a variable ventricular response depending on the conduction ability of the AV node (Figure 18-3, panel *D*).[21] Both AF and AFL are considered to be reentrant in nature. Atrial tachycardia is due to reentry or abnormal automaticity and originates in either the right or left atrium (Figure 18-3, panel *C*).[22] Whether SVT that originates in the atrium is paroxysmal (comes and goes abruptly) or chronic, it is challenging to manage medically.

SVT that originates in the AV junction is due to enhanced automaticity or reentry and reaches rates of up to 250 bpm. Automatic AV junctional tachycardias are usually seen in acutely ill patients in association with ischemia, infarction, metabolic disturbances, or drug toxicity. Correction of the

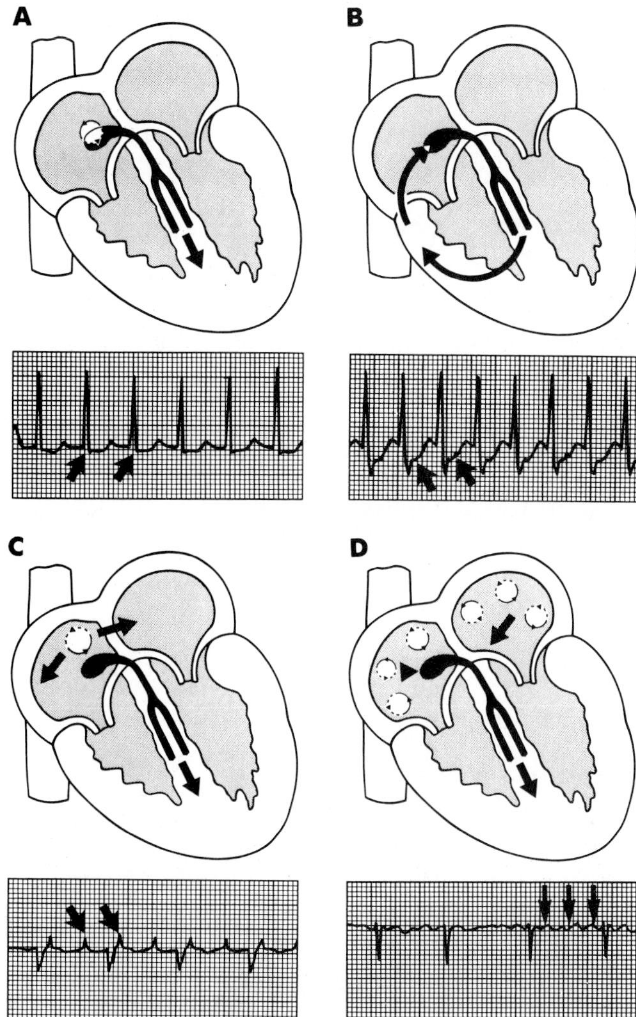

Figure 18-3 Representations of reentrant supraventricular tachycardias (SVT). Panel **A** portrays AV nodal reentry: reentrant circuit is around the AV node; tachycardia is regular with a narrow QRS complex; and p wave, depicted by the arrow, is usually hidden within the QRS. Panel **B** portrays orthodromic supraventricular tachycardia utilizing a right-sided accessory pathway whose ECG reveals a rapid rate and regular rhythm, with a p wave in the ST segment. Panel **C** represents atrial tachycardia originating in the right atrium. The ECG shows a 3:2 p:QRS relationship due to AV block. Panel **D** represents atrial fibrillation due to multiple reentrant circuits within the atria. The corresponding ECG shows the resulting fibrillatory p waves with variable ventricular response.

etiology usually terminates the tachycardia. Reentrant mechanisms, on the other hand, are not related to structural heart disease but are due to preexisting reentrant circuits that are present from the time of birth. These tachycardias manifest at any age, usually in persons without structural heart disease, and are largely paroxysmal in nature.

The most common type of AV junctional SVT is due to a second conductive pathway within the AV node and is referred to as AV nodal reentry.[22] The impulse circulates around the atrioventricular node at a rapid rate, simultaneously activating the atria and ventricle (Figure 18-3, panel *A*). Electrocardiograms during sinus rhythm do not normally reveal clues about the potential for AV nodal reentry tachycardia, such as the existence of two conductive pathways in the AV node.

Potential for AV junctional SVT in the form of accessory pathway mediated tachycardia is electrocardiographically apparent during sinus rhythm in approximately one half the population of patients with accessory pathways. Wolf-Parkinson-White (WPW) syndrome is an example of an accessory pathway (a muscular fiber with electrical properties that bridges the atrium and ventricle) that propagates an impulse from the atria to the ventricle (antegrade) instead of or in addition to the AV node. This pre-excites the ventricle, making a "delta" wave (slurred upstroke on the QRS) appear on the surface ECG. In actuality, little more than one half of identified accessory pathways have antegrade conduction capabilities. The others can conduct only retrograde and, therefore, are not apparent on a surface ECG.[10] The latter are called concealed accessory pathways. Due to the varying conduction properties of accessory pathways, there is a family of accessory pathway mediated tachycardias.

The most common SVT involving an accessory pathway is called orthodromic reentrant tachycardia. Its circuit incorporates the AV node and the accessory pathway. Essentially, the impulse travels antegrade through the AV node, the His-Purkinje system, the ventricle, and then up (retrograde) the accessory pathway and through the atria at a rate of up to 250 bpm (Figure 18-3, panel *B*). If the accessory pathway has antegrade conduction properties, it has the potential to propagate reentrant tachycardia in the opposite direction just described, and SVT originating in the atrium. Atrial fibrillation that conducts antegrade through a rapidly conducting accessory pathway has the potential to cause ventricular fibrillation. Thus there is a small incidence of SCD associated with WPW.[20]

Bradycardia is caused by either SA node dysfunction or AV block as depicted in Figure 18-4.[19] Sinus bradycardia may be physiologic or pathologic. Physiologic sinus bradycardia is most evident in well-conditioned athletes who may have rates well below 60 bpm without symptoms. Pathologic states leading to sinus bradycardia include drug-induced suppression of the SA node (usually calcium channel blockers or beta-blockers), or intrinsic disease of the SA node, commonly referred to as sick sinus syndrome.[6]

Bradycardia resulting from AV block despite normal SA node function may be congenital but most often is due to damaged conductive tissues above (AV node), within, or below the His bundle; it causes the sinus impulse to be either slowed or completely blocked at the AV junction. Acquired damage may be due to myocardial infarction (especially anteroseptal), myocardial ischemia, idiopathic fibrosis, cardiomyopathy, cardiac surgery, or ablation of the conduction system whether purposeful or unintentional.[6] Electrolyte imbalance and drug toxicity may also cause tran-

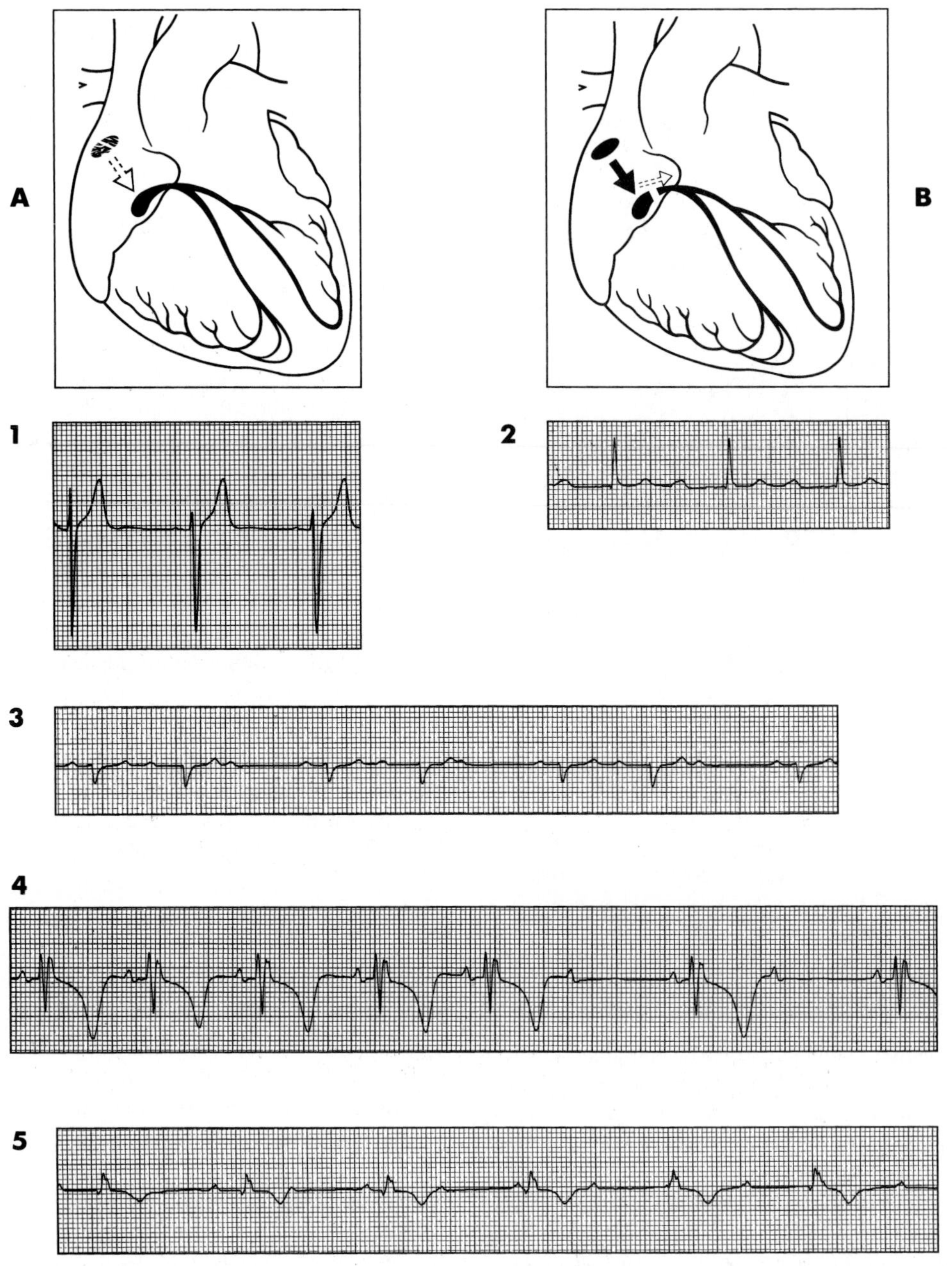

Figure 18-4 Bradycardias due to disturbance of impulse formation in the sinus node **(A),** or impulse conduction through the AV node or His bundle **(B).** ECG manifestations include panels **(1)** sinus bradycardia (due to sinus node dysfunction), **(2)** first-degree AV block usually due to block within the AV node, **(3)** second-degree AV heart block (Mobitz type I or Wenckebach) usually due to block within the AV node, **(4)** second-degree AV heart block (Mobitz type II) usually due to block within the His-Purkinje system, **(5)** third-degree AV heart block (complete heart block) usually due to block within or below the His bundle. The latter two usually require permanent pacing.

sient heart block. Figure 18-4 illustrates ECG indications of benign and significant AV blocks. The former category usually includes first- and second-degree (type I) heart block while the latter includes second-degree type II and third-degree AV heart block.

Finally, **neurocardiogenic syncope** is thought to involve a combination of abnormal neurologic and cardiovascular responses. The usual trigger is reduction in venous return, often precipitated by prolonged standing or extreme emotion. Normally decreased venous return leads to sinus tachycardia and hypercontractility of the ventricles: compensatory mechanisms to maintain blood pressure and cardiac output. The compensatory mechanism in patients with NCS becomes abnormal when hypercontractile ventricles stimulate vagal nerve endings within the myocardium, affecting the vagal and sympathetic centers in the brainstem.[3] Vagal overstimulation leads to bradycardia, while sympathetic dysfunction causes vasodilatation. The two responses in combination lead to presyncope or syncope.[3,23]

LENGTH OF STAY / ANTICIPATED COURSE

Hospitalization will vary for dysrhythmia patients depending on the type of dysrhythmia, the etiology of the condition, potential complications, and preferred intervention. In general, primary diagnoses of dysrhythmia fall under DRGs 138 and 139: Cardiac dysrhythmia and conduction disorders with or without cardiac catheterization. In either case, the average length of stay (LOS) is noted as 3.3 to 5.2 days.[25] In the event that an artificial pacemaker is implanted, the average length of stay increases to almost 6.5 days as listed under DRG 116: Other permanent cardiac pacemaker implant or AICD lead or generator procedure.[25]

Dysrhythmias such as VT may involve repeated electrophysiology studies (EPS), cardiac surgery, or extensive medical management yielding lengths of stay up to 60 days in extreme cases. SVT, on the other hand, may be resolved with interventions such as ablation or pacemaker with a 3- or 6-day LOS respectively. NCS may require up to a 5-day LOS for initial evaluation and treatment with follow-up studies conducted on an outpatient basis.

MANAGEMENT TRENDS AND CONTROVERSIES

Patients with dysrhythmias may have nonlethal symptoms such as palpitations, near-syncope, shortness of breath, and atypical chest pain. Serious symptoms such as syncope or SCD also occur. History and physical examination alone are not likely to uncover the origin and cause of dysrhythmia. Thus, after patients are stabilized and underlying problems are addressed, patients are assessed for the presence of primary electrophysiologic abnormalities, which involves the use of one or more diagnostic procedures. Several diagnostic modalities may be used to isolate the type and source of dysrhythmia present. Summarized in Table 18-1, the tests range from a simple 12-lead ECG to full electrophysiology studies (EPS). Prior to EPS, noninvasive tests including signal-averaged ECG (SAECG), Holter monitoring (HM), transtelephonic monitoring (TTM), and/or stress testing (ST) facilitate diagnosis of structural heart disease and mechanism of dysrhythmia.[13,15] The decision to proceed with EPS, an invasive procedure, should be individualized after careful consideration of the risk-benefit ratio.

Once diagnosed, management of dysrhythmia may be categorized into two basic approaches: acute intervention and long-term treatment. Considering dysrhythmias have the potential to be life-threatening, acute intervention may involve activation of the emergency medical system (EMS) and advanced cardiac life support (ACLS) protocols.

Ventricular tachycardia requires perhaps the most dramatic acute intervention. Symptoms of VT vary depending on factors such as underlying heart disease, ventricular function, rate and duration of the VT, and condition of the patient during VT. If the patient is unconscious and has monomorphic VT, polymorphic VT, or VF, the first line of treatment is defibrillation with 200 joules.[5] If the patient is conscious with an unstable blood pressure, the first line of treatment is cardioversion (50 to 100 joules) following sedation.[5] If the patient is conscious with a stable blood pressure and the VT is monomorphic, the first line of treatment is lidocaine.[5] If there is doubt whether a wide-QRS complex tachycardia is ventricular or supraventricular, adenosine may be given. If this is ineffective, treatment should proceed with the assumption that the tachycardia is VT. In addition to electrical or pharmacologic treatment, a 12-lead ECG and lab values such as electrolytes and cardiac enzymes are obtained so that underlying disease or precipitating factors can be identified and treated.

Patients who are conscious and have TDP are not given antiarrhythmic medication due to the risk of further prolonging the QT interval. Instead, removal of the offending agent and administration of magnesium sulfate or potassium may be helpful.[5] Artificial pacing or adrenergic-stimulating drugs such as isuprel may be used when TDP is related to rhythm pauses or bradycardia (acquired TDP). Beta-blockade is recommended in cases of congenital TDP. In all cases, full resuscitation may be required prior to any emergent drug therapy.

Long-term treatment of VT includes determination of the risk of recurrent VT followed by prescription and evaluation of treatment (Figure 18-5). Patients with ischemia, infarction, or electrolyte imbalance should be diagnosed and treated prior to any further testing or treatment. Once a diagnosis of recurrent VT is determined, the patient's risk is ranked or stratified.

Patients identified to be at risk of recurrent, sustained (>30 seconds) monomorphic VT and or SCD are treated with either antiarrhythmic drugs, surgical aneurysmectomy, ablation, or, more commonly, the implantable cardiovertor defibrillator (ICD). Empiric treatment of ventricular ectopy or VT with antiarrhythmic drugs is no longer considered acceptable based on the Cardiac Arrhythmia Suppression Trial (CAST), which demonstrated that patients randomized to receive class I antiarrhythmic drugs for suppression of PVCs had a higher incidence of death than those randomized to placebo.[8] Instead of empirically treating VT, use of antiarrhythmic drugs is evaluated for effectiveness by EPS.

EPS-guided suppression of recurrent VT with antidysrhythmic drugs is challenging because of the following factors: (1) the initial inducibility of tachyrhythmia varies, (2) the efficacy of antidysrhythmic drugs is variable, (3) a variety of events and conditions may trigger VT that drugs cannot prevent, and (4) these drugs often have side effects that may not be tolerated by patients.[27] Although antidysrhythmic drugs are not ideal for primary treatment of most VT, they are commonly used to partially suppress VT or

TABLE 18-1 Diagnostic Tests Used for Evaluation of Dysrhythmias

Test	Description	Indication	Technique	Risk
Electrocardiogram (ECG)	Simultaneous recording of 12 ECG leads (I, II, III AVR, AVL, AVF, V1-6)	Differentiate wide complex QRS tachycardias Diagnose myocardial infarction or ischemia Identify hypertrophy Evaluate intraventricular conduction delay	Application of 12 electrodes in standardized position	None to patient
Signal-Averaged ECG (SAECG)	Recording process that averages several QRS complexes in order to produce a "clean" signal Amplification of terminal portion of the averaged QRS	Determine presence of late electrical activity (late potentials) that can predispose one to VT Ancillary test for VT/VF risk stratification and medical management	Acquisition of ECG using a variety of lead configurations Requires electrically noise-free environment and relaxed patient	None to patient Limitation: inaccurate in patients with atrial fibrillation or bundle-branch block
Holter Monitor (HM)	24-48 hour magnetic tape recording of 1-2 ECG leads	Diagnoses of paroxysmal dysrhythmias in patients who report symptoms suggestive of nonlethal dysrhythmias (palpitations, dizziness, near syncope)	Application of 5 electrodes Small recorder is attached to leads for ambulatory patients (newer hospital telemetry units have Holter capability Diary of symptoms and activity is kept by patient	None to patient Limitation: may not capture a dysrhythmia that occurs less than every 24-48 hours
Transtelephonic Monitor (TTM)	Ambulatory patient records ECG at time of symptoms and plays it back over the phone	Alternative to Holter monitor (patients can keep recorder for a month or more) Diagnose dysrhythmia for patients with suggestive nonlethal symptoms	Instruct patient in application of leads (usually chest or wrist) and use of recording equipment Trained personnel available 24 hours for ECG evaluation, patient instruction	None to patient Limitation: may be difficult for some patients to use effectively

Stress Test (ST)	Monitored, controlled treadmill to determine: • presence of underlying coronary artery disease • presence of exercise-induced dysrhythmias (AV block, VT) • maximal sinus rate achieved with exercise	Nonspecific symptoms suggestive of myocardial ischemia (in conjunction with other diagnostic tests) Paroxysmal symptoms of dysrhythmias that are associated with exercise Active patients with ICDs	Patient instruction Application of 12-lead set-up and B/P monitoring equipment Use one of many treadmill exercise protocols Environment with life-support facility available	Development of life-threatening ischemia, dysrhythmia
Electrophysiologic Studies (EPS)	An accurate test for reproduction of reentrant tachycardias and AV block 1-4 multi-electrode catheters placed near critical areas of normal conduction system (high right atrium, His bundle, right ventricle) Recording/pacing from electrodes allows measurement of conduction/refractory characteristics and induction/differentiation of dysrhythmia	Patients with symptoms suggestive of dysrhythmia: • sustained palpitations • near syncope • syncope • SCD Patients with documented dysrhythmias (to determine the mechanism and site of origin) Follow-up evaluation of anti-dysrhythmic drug, ICD, and ablation effectiveness	Patient instruction Catheters positioned in right heart via femoral, brachial, or jugular vein using aseptic technique and fluoroscopic guidance Patient's heart rhythm, blood pressure, and O_2 sat monitored continuously Patient positioned for safety Emergency equipment readily available Medications commonly used: • heparin • versed • adenosine • atropine • isuprel • procainamide	Morbidity (<2%) • cardiac tamponade • embolic events • thrombosis • bleed • infection Mortality (<.1%)
Tilt Table Test (TTT)	A procedure carried out in EP lab which is accurate for the reproduction of presyncope and syncope due to an abnormal neurocardiogenic reflex. The reflex leads to vasodilation and bradycardia in situations when just the opposite is needed (e.g., venous pooling).	Unexplained syncope or near syncope Follow-up for persons with positive TTTs and on drug therapy (e.g., oral beta-blockers, ephedrine)	Patient secured on fluoroscopy table with tilt capabilities ECG monitor/O_2 monitor BP monitor via cuff (q 1-2 min) or arterial line Head-up tilt 70-90 degrees for 20 minutes Medications commonly used: • isuprel • esmolol	None to patient Development of symptoms may cause discomfort

ICD: implantable cardiovertor defibrillator, SCD: sudden cardiac death, VT: ventricular tachycardia.

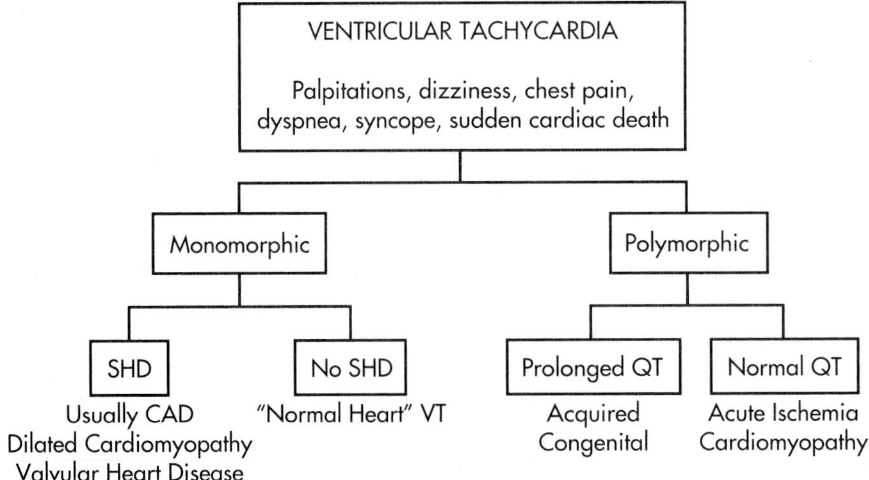

Figure 18-5 Classifying ventricular tachycardia into monomorphic (MVT) and polymorphic (PMVT) is critical for long-term management. MVT is usually associated with structural heart disease (SHD), but in rare cases can occur in persons with normal hearts. PMVT is subclassified based on the presence of a prolonged QT interval prior to onset. Symptoms of MVT and PMVT (regardless of type or associated heart disease) range from palpitations to sudden cardiac death.

atrial dysrhythmia in patients with ICDs.[7] Table 18-2 summarizes common antidysrhythmic drugs used for patients with dysrhythmias.

Whereas antidysrhythmic drugs are targeted to suppress a specific VT induced in EPS, **ICDs** serve as a broad-spectrum treatment for any ventricular tachydysrhythmia. That is, regardless of the cause or type of VT/VF, each occurrence will be treated with either antitachycardia pacing, cardioversion, or defibrillation. It is now standard practice to implant ICDs in patients with clinical VT that is reproducible in the electrophysiologic laboratory and refractory to antidysrhythmic drugs, or in patients who have been fortunate enough to be resuscitated from SCD.[1] Implantation of leads is accomplished in the operating room using one of many approaches: left thoracotomy, mid-sternotomy, sub-xiphoid, and the newest nonthoracotomy/transvenous approach. The leads are attached to one of many ICD generators available. While simpler ICDs are capable of sensing VT/VF and delivering a shock when the rhythm reaches a preprogrammed heart rate, newer ICDs incorporate low-energy shocks and antitachycardia and bradycardia pacing. In addition, these newer devices have sophisticated detection algorithms that diminish the likelihood of a patient receiving inappropriate shocks (e.g., during sinus tachycardia or AF). The increasing detail of stored information surrounding each shock delivered enhances the evaluation of events (e.g., electrograms, shock information) so that appropriate ICD or antiarrhythmic drug adjustments are made when necessary.

The newer transvenous approach to lead implantation eliminates the morbidity and mortality associated with open chest surgery, shortens surgical recovery time, and shortens LOS. It has thus become the preferred approach if concomitant surgery (e.g., revascularization) is not required. Other ICD developments being researched include increasing the efficiency of ICD system, decreasing generator size, prolonged battery life, and automatic capacitor reformation. Research and development is essentially aimed at increasing patient acceptability of ICDs.

Despite the rapid evolution of ICD technology, patients with ICDs require close follow-up. They are routinely seen in the clinic every two or three months for evaluation of ICD battery and function. Depending on the patient's condition and use of antidysrhythmic drugs, follow-up EPS may be necessary. In addition, ICD generators are replaced every 3 to 5 years.

Surgical ablation of VT is possible for a selected group of patients and is limited by a significant operative risk of 8% to 16% and VT recurrence of up to 15%.[9] Catheter ablation for ventricular tachycardia is similarly useful in a select group of patients. In both instances, technical expertise and experience influence outcome. Regardless of the treatment chosen, follow-up EPS are required to ensure patient safety.

Supraventricular tachycardias that require acute intervention are those that present with sustained palpitations, near syncope, syncope, or SCD. Acute treatment of AF/AFL includes control of the ventricular response with IV drugs such as diltiazem, verapamil, and beta-blockers. Synchronized cardioversion in the acute setting is reserved for patients who are hemodynamically unstable. Assessment of predisposing factors, such as underlying heart disease, and dysrhythmia triggers, such as exercise, emotion, and alcohol, is also carried out.

Long-term treatment of AF/AFL includes cardioversion to sinus rhythm and subsequent maintenance with antidysrhythmic drugs (class Ia or III), or merely ventricular rate control (digoxin, calcium channel blockers, beta-blockers)

TABLE 18-2 Classification of Commonly Used Antidysrhythmic Drugs

Vaughn Williams class	Drug name (tradename)	Usual dose	Dysrhythmic indications	Side effects
IA	Procainamide (Pronestyl)	IV: 20-50 mg/min (10-15 mg/kg) po: 250-1000 mg q4-6h	SVT VT	Prodysrhythmia Hypotension Heart failure Lupus-like syndrome (procainamide) CNS disturbance (class IB/IC) GI disturbance Rash Blood dyscrasias
	Quinidine	po: 200-400 mg q6h		
IB	Lidocaine	IV *loading:* 1-1.5 mg/kg *maintenance:* 1-4 mg/min	VT	
	Mexiletine (Mexitil)	po: 150-300 mg q8h		
IC	Flecainide (Tambocor)	po: 100-300 mg q12h	Life-threatening VT without SHD	
	Encainide (Enkaid)	po: 25-50 mg q12h		
II Beta-blockers (cardioselective)	Atenolol (Tenormin)	po: 50-100 mg q24h	SVT	Prodysrhythmia (especially bradycardia) Hypotension Heart failure Asthma Fatigue Blunted hypoglycemic response
	Metoprolol (Lopressor)	po: 50-100 mg q12h	VT	
	Esmolol (Brevibloc)	IV *loading:* 500 mg/kg/min *maintenance:* titratable		
Beta-blockers (noncardioselective)	Propranolol (Inderal)	po: 10-80 mg q8h	SVT VT	
III	Amiodarone (Cordarone)	po: *loading:* 800-2400 mg/day (1-2 weeks) *maintenance:* 100-600 mg/day	VT	Prodysrhythmia Pulmonary fibrosis Skin discoloration GI disturbance Thyroid dysfunction Neurologic disturbance
	Sotalol (Betapace)	po: 80-240 mg q12h	VT	Prodysrhythmia Heart failure Hypotension
	Bretylium	IV *loading:* 5 mg/kg *maintenance:* 1 mg/min	VT	Hypotension Prodysrhythmia Headache

All antidysrhythmic drugs have the potential of being "prodysrhythmic": making the existing dysrhythmia worse or predisposing the patient to a new dysrhythmia.
SVT: supraventricular tachycardia; VT: ventricular tachycardia.

and prevention of thromboembolism.[18] Cardioversion of stable patients may be attempted after considering the risk of embolism. If AF/AFL is present for more than three days, anticoagulation is recommended for 3 weeks prior to and 2 to 4 weeks following cardioversion.[21,24] Conversion to sinus rhythm is then accomplished by either pharmacologic or electrical therapy. Unfortunately, successful cardioversion does not assure long-term maintenance, especially without concomitant drug therapy. In cases where AF/AFL is persistent and problematic despite drug therapy, AV nodal ablation may be performed followed by the insertion of a permanent pacemaker.

Acute treatment of reentrant AV junctional SVT is similar in that it is predicated upon the presence of symptoms such as palpitations, shortness of breath, atypical chest pain, near syncope, syncope, and, rarely, SCD. Immediate conversion is ideally accomplished with vagal maneuvers or administration of adenosine.[5] Alternatively, calcium channel or beta-blockers may be used for narrow-QRS complex tachycardias. If the patient is hemodynamically unstable, cardioversion is performed following sedation. Since reentrant AV junctional SVT is usually paroxysmal, it may spontaneously convert to sinus rhythm before the patient is medically evaluated.

Whereas reentrant AV junctional tachycardia typically reoccurs in an unpredictable manner, automatic AV junctional tachycardia is limited by its concomitant illness. As mentioned previously, automatic AV junctional tachycardia occurs in the setting of myocardial ischemia, infarction, metabolic abnormalities, or drug toxicity. If the offending illness is corrected, tachycardia terminates and long-term treatment becomes irrelevant.

Symptoms of reentrant AV junctional tachycardia are bothersome at least, and at worst interfere with activities and life-style. Long-term treatment is dependent upon verification of the SVT through diagnostic tests such as HM, TTM, or EPS. Once validated, SVT is treated with oral antidysrhythmic drugs such as digoxin, beta-blockers, verapamil, and class I drugs in an attempt to suppress reoccurrence. In cases where several drug regimens have been unsuccessful, have caused intolerable side effects, or result in noncompliance due to activities, sports, or the desire to have a child, ablation is an option. In fact, transcatheter ablation of the source of the SVT has emerged as a safe and effective cure at specialized centers.[10]

Where available, *radiofrequency catheter ablation* has become the treatment of choice for permanently terminating recurrent AV junctional SVT. The procedure involves applying radiofrequency energy through electrode catheter to a critical portion of a reentrant circuit. The initial phase of the procedure is similar to an EPS in that catheters are positioned in the high right atrium, near the His bundle, in the right ventricle, and often in the coronary sinus vein. Electrophysiologic measurements (conduction and refractory properties) are obtained, and tachycardia is induced so that its characteristics and origin can be studied. Following localization of the tachycardia reentrant circuit, a deflectable, large-tipped (4-mm) electrode catheter is positioned using intracardiac recordings and fluoroscopic guidance. Radiofrequency energy is directed through the catheter tip, which produces heat and a small homogeneous lesion. An effective lesion interrupts the circuit permanently so that it is no longer able to participate in reentry tachycardia. The success of the procedure is evaluated immediately and sometimes 1 day and 2 months after the procedure. The majority of cases take between 2 and 6 hours to complete.[9,10] This, coupled with the fact that most patients are sedated or given general anesthesia, necessitates that patients are properly positioned, have adequate skin protection, and are continuously monitored throughout the procedure.

Ablation sites vary according to the SVT origin. Ablation of atrial tachycardia, AF, and AFL remains challenging due to difficulty in localizing the tachycardic site, existence of multiple sites, and difficulty in maintaining adequate catheter placement. When ablation of SVT that originates in the atrium is not possible and medical treatment is inadequate, complete AV node ablation may be chosen in combination with a pacemaker.

AV junctional tachycardias have discrete reentrant circuits that are amenable to catheter ablation. In the case of AV nodal reentry, the AV node is "modified"—that is, one of the functioning pathways in the AV node (slow pathway) is ablated, leaving the other intact so that normal conduction is maintained.

In the case of accessory pathway mediated tachycardia, the accessory pathway is ablated wherever it crosses the mitral or tricuspid annuli. Accessory pathways may be on the right or, more commonly, left side of the heart and are located using EPS mapping techniques. The ablation catheter is placed on either the atrial or ventricular side of the valvular annuli near the accessory pathway, and radiofrequency energy is applied. This obliterates the accessory pathway so that it can no longer conduct, making reentrant tachycardia impossible.[9]

Bradycardias may be treated acutely with transcutaneous pacing or drugs such as atropine.[5] Since transcutaneous pacing will require sedation due to its associated discomfort, transvenous pacing should be initiated as soon as possible. Isuprel, due to its positive inotropic effects, is no longer used as a first-line drug for patients with symptomatic bradycardia.

Once the patient is stabilized, the need for a permanent pacemaker is addressed. If AV block intermittently produces symptoms, documentation may be accomplished with ST, HM, or TTM. Occasionally, EPS is required to determine the exact location of the block (above, within, or just below the His bundle).[5] High-degree AV blocks signify tissue damage within or below the His bundle and thus require permanent pacing.

There are many types of pacemakers available with varying features. For active patients, a pacemaker incorporating a sensor that triggers an increase in rate with exercise and increased metabolism has made a positive impact on quality of life. However, standard VVI pacing may still be used for less-active individuals (see Guideline 31 for more information regarding pacemakers).

Neurocardiogenic syncope rarely requires acute intervention other than care for witnessed syncopal events. Once NCS is verified by TTT, drug therapy is prescribed for prevention of future syncopal episodes due to the abnormal reflex. Beta-blockers, theophylline, ephedrine, diisopyramide, or scopolamine may be used alone or in combination.[23] Artificial pacing alone for the bradycardia associated with NCS is insufficient since vasodilation is a significant factor in this syndrome.[24] As a result, drug therapy remains the preferred current mode of therapy.

ASSESSMENT

PARAMETER	ANTICIPATED ALTERATION
History and physical	Common symptoms include palpitations, atypical chest pain, shortness of breath, near syncope, syncope, or SCD. Determining the frequency, duration, associated activities, and relief may be helpful in identifying dysrhythmia and NCS.

Previous treatments, other medical diagnoses (e.g., coronary artery disease, cardiomyopathy) and family history will contribute to diagnosis and long-term plan of action.

BP

Decreased: <100 mm Hg systolic

Diminished tissue perfusion may be present *due to dysrhythmia that is not tolerated, or NCS.*

ECG

Abnormal heart rate and rhythm *due to dysrhythmias such as SVT, VT, sinus bradycardia, or AV block.*

Intraventricular conduction delays, ischemic changes, presence of old myocardial infarction *due to concomitant structural heart disease.*

Laboratory tests

Abnormal electrolytes or cardiac enzymes *due to ongoing ischemia*

Signal averaged ECG

May have evidence of "late potentials" *due to delayed depolarization in fibrotic tissue*

Holster monitor

May document dysrhythmia on ECG with associated symptoms/activity recorded in diary

Transtelophonic monitor

Evidence of dysrhythmia at time of symptoms

Stress test

Evidence of dysrhythmia *due to exercise*

Presence of ischemia *due to underlying coronary artery disease.*

Determination of exercise tolerance and maximum heart rate *in order to optimize treatment (e.g., rate cut-off criteria for ICDs)*

Electrophysiologic studies

Determine mechanism and origin of dysrhythmia and effectiveness of treatment with antidysrhythmic drugs, ICDs, or ablation

Tilt table test

Detect abnormal reflex manifested by syncope/presyncope *due to hypotension and bradycardia without discomfort related to reproduction of symptoms*

Treatments

Antidysrhythmic drugs

Suppression of dysrhythmia without side effects. Risk for intolerance *due to major side effects of hypotension and prodysrhythmia.*

Catheter ablation

Effective cure of tachydysrhythmia with risk for complications *due to complex procedure using up to five electrode catheters.*

Recurrence of tachycardia or new dysrhythmia.

ICD implantation

Effective treatment/interruption of each episode of VT/VF.

Absence of ICD generator or lead malfunction *due to faulty battery, interrupted lead integrity, or lead migration.*

PLAN OF CARE

INTERMEDIATE PHASE

Patients with dysrhythmias are routinely managed on intermediate or telemetry units. The ICU environment is necessary only in the event of SCD with life-threatening complications. Unless the dysrhythmias are both life-threatening and intractable, a monitored, non-ICU environment supports the goals of care for dysrhythmia patients: (1) localize the type and source of the dysrhythmia, (2) select and evaluate the effectiveness of intervention(s), and (3) provide the patient/family with support and information to optimize self-care after discharge.

PATIENT CARE PRIORITIES	EXPECTED PATIENT OUTCOMES
Decreased cardiac output *r/t dysrhythmia, NCS*	Maintain LOC and mentation within patient norms Free of angina, heart failure, AMI
Anxiety *r/t fear of recurrent dysrhythmia, inadequate knowledge, multiple procedures*	Patient/family verbalize concerns and demonstrate decreased anxiety

Plan of Care (cont'd)

High risk for inadequate cardiopulmonary tissue perfusion *r/t complications from EPS or surgery such as tamponade, embolic event, pneumothorax, bleeding*	BP and heart rhythm stable following procedures Free of complications If complications occur, they are detected, reported and treated quickly
Self-care deficit *r/t inadequate knowledge of dysrhythmia, diagnostic procedures, treatment regimen*	Patient and family verbalize knowledge of dysrhythmia, diagnostic tests, treatments, and follow-up requirements

INTERVENTIONS

Continuously monitor ECG *to detect dysrhythmia characteristics: onset, rate, morphology, and duration.*

Use V_1 or MCL_1 for continuous monitoring *to detect morphological cues for differentiation of VT from SVT.*[11]

Obtain 12-lead ECG as ordered and with dysrhythmia *to determine baseline abnormalities, characteristics of dysrhythmia (rate, mechanism), and to differentiate wide-QRS complex tachycardias.*

Monitor VS with and without dysrhythmia to *determine baseline and tolerance of dysrhythmia.*

Implement ACLS as needed *to protect patient from life-threatening dysrhythmia.*

Administer antidysrhythmic drugs as ordered and monitor for tolerance and effectiveness. *Class I and III drugs may alter ECG intervals, especially lengthening QT interval, which may result in TDP. Most antidysrhythmic medications may compromise hemodynamic stability and/or prodysrhythmia.*

Measure HR, pr interval, QRS duration, and QT interval routinely *to detect potential dysrhythmias and expected or adverse drug effects.*

Assess as appropriate to site of catheter ablation and monitor for success and development of complications. *Site of ablation varies with tachycardic mechanisms. Complications (e.g., tamponade, AV block) may manifest after procedure.*[9]

Assess and document the following ICD parameters: (1) model, (2) HR above which ICD will deliver antitachycardia pacing, (3) HR above which ICD will deliver shocks, and (4) bradycardia pacing rate *to ensure optimal dysrhythmia and ICD management.*

Obtain and evaluate electrolytes and cardiac enzymes *to detect possible underlying causes of the dysrhythmia.*

Monitor neurologic, respiratory, renal, and circulatory status *to detect possible complications from dysrhythmia or interventions.*

Prepare for diagnostic procedures *to ensure special preparation needed for some tests (EPS, TTT, SAECG, radiofrequency ablation).*

Provide emotional support to patient and family *to decrease anxiety and enable learning.*

Instruct patient/family about dysrhythmia, its origin, and associated diagnostic tests and treatments *to decrease anxiety.*

Instruct patient/family regarding self-care concerns such as drug regimes, recurrent symptoms and when to report them, and pacemaker and ICD follow-up *to ensure patient safety and optimize self-care.*

TRANSITION TO DISCHARGE

Patients and their families must be well-informed of all medications, follow-up care, and an emergency plan prior to discharge. Depending on the type of dysrhythmia and intervention, life-style modification and/or role changes may require community-based suport for implementation and to facilitate coping.

REFERENCES

1. Akhtar M, Jazayeri MR, Sra JS: Implantable cardioverter-defibrillator therapy for prevention of sudden cardiac death, *Cardiol Clin* 11(1):97-105, 1993.
2. Akhtar M: Clinical spectrum of ventricular tachycardia, *Circulation* 82(5):1561-1573, 1990.
3. Akhtar M, Jazayeri M, Sra J: Cardiovascular causes of syncope: identifying controlling trigger mechanisms, *Postgrad Med* 90(2):87-94, 1991.
4. American Heart Association: *Heart and Stroke Facts Statistics,* Dallas, 1993.
5. American Heart Association: Guidelines for cardiopulmonary resuscitation and emergency cardiac care recommendations of the 1992 National Conference, *JAMA* 268(16):2171-2302, 1992.
6. Braunwald E: *Heart disease: a textbook of cardiovascular medicine,* ed 3, Philadelphia, 1988, WB Saunders, pp 383-742.
7. Bremner SM, McCauley KM, Axtell KA: A follow-up study of patients with implantable cardioverter defibrillators, *J Cardiovasc Nurs* 7(3):40-51, 1993.
8. CAST Investigators: Mortality and morbidity in patients receiving encainide, flecainide, or placebo: the Cardiac Suppression Trial, *N Engl J Med* 324(12):781-787, 1991.
9. Craney JM: Radiofrequency catheter ablation of supraventricular tachycardias: clinical consideration and nursing care, *J Cardiovasc Nurs* 7(3):26-39, 1993.
10. Deshpande S, et al: Control of supraventricular tachycardia with transcatheter ablative technique using radiofrequency as the energy source, *Wis Med J,* 92(9):507-516, 1993.
11. Drew BJ: Bedside electrocardiogram monitoring, *AACN Clin Iss Crit Care Nurs* 4(1):25-33, 1993.
12. Harlan RG, Scheinman M: Evaluation and management of patients with polymorphic ventricular tachycardia, *Cardiol Clin* 11(1):39-55, 1993.
13. Hsia HH, Buxton AE: Work-up and management of patients with sustained and nonsustained monomorphic ventricular tachycardias, *Cardiol Clin* 11:21-38, 1993.
14. Jackman WM, Friday JL, Anderson EM: The long QT syndromes: a critical review, new clinical observations and a unifying hypothesis, *Prog Cardiovasc Dis* 31:115-172, 1988.
15. Josephson ME: *Clinical cardiac electrophysiology,* ed 2, Philadelphia/London, 1993, Lea and Febiger, pp 1-70.
16. Kannel WB, et al: Epidemiologic features of chronic atrial fibrillation: the Framingham Study, *N Engl J Med* 306:1018-1022, 1982.
17. Kannel WB, Schatzkin A: Sudden death: lessons from subsets in population studies, *J Am Coll Cardiol* 5(6):141B-149B, 1985.
18. Pritchett ELC: Management of atrial fibrillation, *N Engl J Med,* 326(19):1264-1271, 1992.
19. Rosenthal JE. In Zipes, Jalife, editors: *Cardiac electrophysiology from cell to bedside,* ed 1, Philadelphia, 1990, WB Saunders, pp 409-417.
20. Sheinman MM: Radiofrequency catheter ablation for patients with supraventricular tachycardia, *Pace* 16:671-679, 1993.
21. Stanton MS, Miles WM, Zipes DP: *Cardiac electrophysiology from cell to bedside,* ed 1, Philadelphia, 1990, WB Saunders, pp 735-740.
22. Swerdlow CD, Liem LB. In Zipes, Jalife, editors: *Cardiac electrophysiology from cell to bedside,* ed 1, Philadelphia, 1990, WB Saunders, pp 742-756.
23. Sra JS, et al: Unexplained syncope evaluated by electrophysiologic studies and head-up tilt testing, *Ann Intern Med* 114:1013-1019, 1991.
24. Sra JS, et al: Comparison of cardiac pacing with drug therapy in the treatment of neurocardiogenic (vasovagal) syncope with bradycardia or asystole, *N Engl J Med* 328:1085-1090, 1993.
25. *St Anthony's DRG guidebook 1995,* Reston, Va, 1994, St Anthony.
26. Wit AL, Dillon SM. In Zipes, Jalife, editors: *Cardiac electrophysiology from cell to bedside,* ed 1, Philadelphia, 1990, WB Saunders, pp 353-363.
27. Wyse GD: Pharmacologic therapy in patients with ventricular tachyarrhythmias, *Cardiol Clin* 11(1):65-85, 1993.

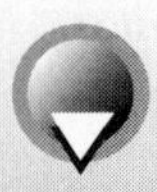

CLINICAL GUIDELINE

19

Inflammatory Heart Disease

Marguerite Scaduto-Philips, MA, RN

DESCRIPTION

Inflammatory heart disease is a term that refers to inflammation of any or all layers of the heart with potential inclusion of the valvular structures. As a result, endocarditis, pericarditis, and myocarditis are all forms of inflammatory heart disease.

Endocarditis is an inflammation of the endothelium and/or the valves of the heart.[9] As early as 1885, Osler noted that infective endocarditis was a difficult disease to diagnose and treat. Modern medicine has not altered this situation.[4] Endocarditis may be infective or noninfective. The vegetative lesion is sterile in the noninfective processes. Actually, endocarditis presents as a thrombolytic process more often than as an inflammatory condition.

In addition, the population at risk has changed since the introduction of antibiotics and cardiac surgery. Endocarditis was previously associated with rheumatic heart disease. Currently, it is seen more often as a complication of cardiac valve surgery, especially aortic valve replacement. Patients with aortic valve disease, mitral insufficiency, and congenital defects are among the high-risk group for infective endocarditis.[17]

Endocarditis occurs more frequently in older males, median age of 50, with approximately one fourth of all patients over the age of 60. Acute cases are seen more frequently than chronic cases due to an increased number of intravenous drug abusers. Before the era of antibiotics, infective endocarditis was usually fatal. With the advent of penicillin therapy, the prognosis has changed dramatically with mortality rates now 20% to 40%.[14] Infective endocarditis occurs after invasive dental and surgical procedures in approximately 20% of all patients with this condition.[2]

Infective endocarditis may also be subacute or acute. The subacute form has a longer clinical course with insidious onset and less toxicity. The causative organism is usually of low virulence (most often *Streptococcus viridans*). In contrast, the acute form has a shorter course with rapid onset, increased toxicity, and a more pathogenic causative organism (usually *Staphylococcus aureus*).[4]

Pericarditis is a syndrome caused by inflammation of the pericardial sac. Acute pericarditis in adults is often idiopathic. A variety of viral causes may be suspected but a proven etiology is rarely demonstrated. When a viral agent is identified, *Coxsackie B* group is the most common cause. Other causes of pericarditis are listed in the Box, Causes of Pericarditis.

Postcardiotomy (postpericardiotomy) syndrome is another form of pericarditis that occurs after cardiac surgery in which the pericardium has been opened. This syndrome was first recognized in patients after mitral commissurotomy for rheumatic heart disease. It was realized that the syndrome could occur following cardiac operations in patients without rheumatic heart disease. The common denominator appeared to be a wide incision and manipulation of the pericardium. An identical clinical syndrome has been reported following any form of cardiac perforation and its causes are listed in the Box, Procedures or Injuries Resulting in Postpericardiotomy-like Syndrome. The incidence of postpericardiotomy syndrome following cardiac surgery ranges from 10% to 40% in adults.[15] Pericarditis is also common with connective tissue disorders, such as systemic lupus erythmatosus.[17]

Myocarditis is inflammation of the heart muscle itself. The inflammation may be focal or diffuse. Patients may experience severe heart failure with myocarditis. The various causes of myocarditis are listed in the Box, Causes of Myocarditis. *Coxsackie B* virus appears to be the chief causative agent.[6] In addition, patients with immune deficiency

Causes of Pericarditis
• Viral infection • Bacterial infection • Uremia • Acute MI • Cardiac surgery • Systemic lupus erythematosus

Procedures or Injuries Resulting in Postpericardiotomy-like Syndrome
• Insertion of a transvenous pacemaker • Blunt chest trauma • Percutaneous diagnostic left ventricular puncture • Epicardial pacemaker implantation

Causes of Myocarditis
• Bacteria • Viral rickettsia • Mycotic, helminthic, or parasitic organisms • Alcoholism • Malnutrition • Poor sanitation • Fulminating systemic sclerosis

disorders, who are malnourished, who have a history of alcoholism, or who live in areas where there is poor sanitation are at high risk. Myocarditis has been reported in patients with progressive systemic sclerosis. These patients have favorable therapeutic responses to intravenous methylprednisone. Patients with scleroderma and new onset heart failure may have acute myocarditis.[5]

PATHOPHYSIOLOGY

Inflammatory heart disease is the direct result of an agent affecting one or all parts of the heart. **Acute endocarditis** occurs when the body is invaded by a substantial number of organisms to create an infectious process in the endothelium. It may occur in patients without valvular disease. Vegetations grow and colonize the valve leaflets. The vegetations have irregular edges and may dislodge, causing systemic embolization. Patients who receive antimicrobial therapy may still experience progressive valvular infection. This may occur due to metabolic activity of deeply imbedded microorganisms that have slow metabolism and high density. This may reduce the effect of antimicrobial agents.[3]

TABLE 19-1 Unique Signs and Symptoms of Endocarditis

Term	Description
Osler nodes	Cutaneous nodules that vary in size from 1 mm-10 mm. Reddish, tender lesions with a white center located on the pads of the distal finger or toes, sides of the fingers, palms, or thighs.
Janeway lesions	Nontender, hemorrhagic, erythematous lesions found on the palms, soles, arms, and legs. 1 mm-5 mm in diameter, they are accentuated when the extremity is elevated.
Roth's spots	Boat-shaped retinal hemorrhages 3 mm-10 mm, pale or white center, located near the optic nerve disk.

Patients with endocarditis may develop unique signs and symptoms. These signs and symptoms are described in Table 19-1. In addition, low-grade fever, diaphoresis and/or chills (most common at night), anorexia, weight loss, malaise, and arthralgias are common cues associated with endocarditis.[9]

Subacute bacterial endocarditis is an indolent but progressive process of damaged valves caused by organisms with low virulence such as *Streptococcus viridans* and bacteria commonly found in the oral cavity. The process evolves over several weeks or months and is characterized by remittent fever, weight loss, and other chronic symptoms. It may mimic many systemic diseases.[14] The mitral valve is most commonly involved, followed by the aortic, tricuspid, and pulmonic valves. Cardiac failure may develop or be aggravated by perforation of a cusp.[9] Patients who have undergone valve replacement surgery may develop an infection of the artificial valve as well. The infection is most likely to develop within the first 60 days after surgery.[17]

Pericarditis develops when pericardial tissue is damaged or inflamed by bacteria or other substances. Chemical mediators associated with inflammation are released into the pericardial tissue in response to the causative agent, starting the inflammatory process. The inflamed pericardial surfaces rub against each other, producing a pericardial friction rub. As the inflammatory process progresses, exudate begins to form. This exudate (purulent or serous) may cause cardiac tamponade in severe cases. In addition, fibrosis and scar tissue form. Scarring, which can be extensive, may cause heart failure due to its restrictive impact on cardiac function.[1]

Pericarditis may be classified as acute or chronic. Patients with acute pericarditis develop sharp chest pain, dyspnea, and a pericardial friction rub. The pain is usually located over the left precordium but may radiate to the trapezius ridge or the neck. The pain is often more intense when the patient is lying down. Initially, the pain of acute pericarditis may be mistaken for an acute MI. The landmark sign of acute pericarditis is the pericardial friction rub. This may or may not accompany the symptom of pain. Pericardial friction rubs are best heard during inspiration with the diaphragm of a stethoscope. Friction rubs have been described as grating, scraping, squeaking, superficial, leathery, crunching, or scratchy.[15]

The two most serious complications of acute pericarditis are pericardial effusion and cardiac tamponade. Pericardial effusion is the accumulation of fluids in the pericardial sac. A pear-shaped silhouette may be noted on the chest x-ray of a patient with pericardial effusion. Echocardiography is also used to confirm the presence and extent of effusion. When fluid accumulates rapidly and/or extensively, the heart cannot compensate and cardiac tamponade occurs. The patient with cardiac tamponade may appear confused, agitated, and restless. In addition, neck veins become distended, color becomes dusky to cyanotic, and pulsus paradoxus is present.[14]

Patients with **constrictive pericarditis** begin with acute pericarditis. Fibrin deposits are found in the pericardial sac with the accumulation of fluid. As the fluid is reabsorbed, scarring and thickening of the pericardium occurs. The resulting restriction of cardiac function may mimic CHF. A pericardial knock is often heard when assessing the patient. Resection of the pericardium, known as pericardiectomy, may be required for patients with extensive scarring, fibrosis, and signs and symptoms that are unresponsive to medical management.

Postpericardiotomy syndrome appears within 1 to 3 weeks after cardiac surgery. It is believed that this syndrome is autoimmune in nature. The autoimmune reaction is due to damaged autologous tissue in the pericardial cavity. The autoimmune theory of etiology is based on the presence of heart-reactive antibodies that appear in significant titers in the majority of patients undergoing cardiac surgery. However, the titer is higher in patients with this syndrome a few weeks to months after surgery. This syndrome may reoccur with reoperation.[12] Presentation of this syndrome includes persistent chest pain, an intermittent pericardial friction rub, pleurisy, fever, tachycardia, dyspnea, and leukocytosis. The appearance of pericardial effusion and friction rub is considered diagnostic of this syndrome.[7]

Myocarditis may be focal or diffuse in nature. The clinical findings depend on the location and extent of the disease. Viral myocarditis can progress from severe to lethal.[17] There are three mechanisms that cause myocardial damage in myocarditis: (1) invasion of the myocardium by an echovirus (2) production of myocardial toxins, and (3) autoimmunity reaction.[16] A clear understanding of the pathophysiology of myocarditis is lacking. As a result, this diagnosis is often made on autopsy.

LENGTH OF STAY/ANTICIPATED COURSE

The length of stay and anticipated course for patients with inflammatory heart disease vary according to the specific diagnosis and its severity. Patients with endocarditis are often classified under DRG 126: Acute and Subacute Endocarditis with an average length of stay of 18.4 days.[19] However, these patients may need intravenous antibiotic therapy for from 4 to 6 weeks. These patients are often able to complete their therapy at home or as an outpatient. DRG 124: Circulatory Disorders except acute myocardial infarction with complex diagnoses carries an average length of stay of 5.5 days. DRG 125 refers to the same diagnosis without complex diagnoses and averages 3.2 days LOS. Pericarditis and myocarditis are among the diagnoses often classified by either of these DRGs. Extended length of stay is seen with more severe forms of these inflammatory cardiac conditions, including postpericardiotomy syndrome. Following cardiac surgery, severe, complicated acute phases of any form of inflammatory heart disease may require admission to an intensive care unit. On the other hand, some patients with myocarditis can be treated on an outpatient basis.

MANAGEMENT TRENDS AND CONTROVERSIES

The care of patients with inflammatory heart disease is directed at identifying the source of the condition. Symptom management is implemented until a specific diagnosis can be made. It is imperative that cardiac output be maintained.

Cheitlan and associates noted that the prevention of infective endocarditis involves early treatment of bacteremia, social and educational programs for control of "mainline" drug abuse, and early recognition of systemic infections in the compromised host.[4] The American Heart Association has recommended chemoprophylaxis when bacteremia is likely. The cure for infective endocarditis is sterilization of the vegetation. In order to achieve this, bacteriocidal rather than bacteriostatic agents have been recommended for use in high concentrations.[3] High doses are required because of the organism's high density. With the advent of prospective payment for hospitalization, home therapy for endocarditis has become more common. Home therapy should be used only after response to treatment (i.e., afebrile with negative blood cultures) has been ensured and in patients who will receive follow-up daily. The preferred method of antibiotic therapy is IV or IM. Although oral therapy has been used, the risks of failure are clearly higher than with parenteral therapy.[13]

Pericarditis and myocarditis are inflammatory diseases that are often initiated by common viruses. Pericarditis rarely causes serious long-term disability, whereas myocarditis may lead to chronic congestive cardiomyopathy and permanent disability.[11] Topaz and Mackall observed patients with angina, myocardial ischemia, and myocardial infarction. In two of the cases the patients had constrictive pericarditis; however, imaging modalities were not useful in establishing the diagnoses. Topaz and Mackall concluded that accurate hemodynamic measurements play a key role in diagnosis.[21]

In a study by Hehrlein and associates, 72 patients with constrictive pericarditis were found to get the best hemodynamic results with total immobilization of the pericardium.[10] Among the population they observed, only two patients required the heart-lung machine. They suggest using this therapy only when the patient has critical myocardial dysfunction or with patients who have compounding additional diseases.

The treatment of pericarditis depends on the symptoms. If the symptoms do not resolve, steroid therapy is usually initiated. However, there is no conclusive evidence that steroids are effective.[4]

Myocarditis remains a mystery. According to Maisch and associates, the controversy regarding the benefits of immunosuppressive treatment in myocarditis will continue long after the trials are completed.[16] In viral heart disease, immunosuppressive drugs should be avoided. Immunomodulating factors (e.g., immunostimulatory or antiviral substances like ribavirin, the interleukins, and the interferons) have demonstrated some effect in animals. Zhang and associates established a model to test the effects of cyclosporine, prednisolone, and aspirin on rats. They found that autoimmune myocarditis is preventable by cyclosporine but not by prednisolone or aspirin.[22]

There are clinical situations in which conventional methods are not effective. Grundl found the use of ECHMO helpful in the case of a 13-month-old boy with viral myocarditis.[8] Important factors to consider before using ECHMO are reversibility of the primary disease process, inability to use conventional treatment, and the ability to provide life support while awaiting a heart transplant. Myocardial rest provided by ECHMO permitted the patient to resolve what most likely would have been lethal cardiac infection, injury, and dysfunction.[8] In patients with acute myocarditis, ventricular assist devices can be used to provide support for a failing myocardium.[20]

In some instances the diagnosis of myocarditis may be overlooked because the patient appears to have a myocardial infarction. Once the presence of normal coronary arteries is confirmed, an antimyosin scan has been recommended to provide information regarding a myopathic process rather than an ischemic one.[18]

ASSESSMENT

PARAMETER	ANTICIPATED ALTERATION
History and physical exam	Patient may have had an invasive procedure, infection, or virus recently
Chest pain	Precordial pain may be burning, sharp, stabbing, dull, or constant ache
LOC	Anxious, restless *due to pain, fear of AMI, cardiac tamponade*
Heart sounds	Pericardial friction rub *due to inflammatory process* Muffled heart tones *due to tamponade*
ECG	Diffuse ST segment elevation with or without T wave inversion ST segments appear slightly concave or flat and horizontal *due to typical patterns of pericarditis* ST segments return to baseline with T wave flattening several days after onset of treatment T waves return to normal weeks or months later Dysrhythmias (especially atrial) *due to cardiac inflammation*
BP	WNL or slightly hypertensive *due to pain* Hypotensive *due to decreased CO* Paradoxical BP *due to cardiac tamponade*
Neck veins	WNL or distended *due to cardiac tamponade*
RR	Dyspnea and splinting *due to pericardial and/or pleuritic chest pain that worsens with deep inspiration*
Chest x-ray	Presence of CHF *due to endocarditis* Pear-shaped cardiac silhouette *due to cardiac effusion* Widened mediasternum *due to cardiac tamponade*
Temperature	Low-grade fever
Blood cultures	Causative agent in bacterial endocarditis

Pericardiocentesis	Serous or purulent exudate *due to tissue responses to inflammatory process*
Endomyocardial biopsy	Confirmation of myocarditis Must be done during the first 6 weeks of acute illness Inflammatory infiltrate, usually lymphocytic necrosis or degeneration of adjacent myocytes *due to myocarditis*

PLAN OF CARE

INTENSIVE PHASE

Patients with the diagnosis of inflammatory heart disease usually do not require intensive care. However, if cardiac function is compromised severely, as in acute myocarditis, intensive care is necessary.

PATIENT CARE PRIORITIES	EXPECTED PATIENT OUTCOMES
Pain *r/t* *Inflammation of the myocardium or pericardium* *Local or systemic infection* *Ischemia of the myocardium*	Absence of pain Able to sleep, rest, and engage in ADLs Requires decreasing amounts of pain medication
High risk for decreased CO *r/t* *Increased fluid in the pericardial sac* *Valvular stenosis/insufficiency* *Restriction of cardiac filling and ventricular contraction* *Possible dysrhythmias*	VS stable ECG rhythm stable Chest x-ray clear
High risk for infection *r/t possible causative organism*	Temperature: WNL WBCs: WNL Blood cultures negative
Activity intolerance *r/t* *Impaired oxygenation with shallow, splinted respirations* *Possible decreased CO or valvular dysfunction*	Verbalize less fatigue and weakness Participate in self-care activities
High risk for inadequate nutrition *r/t lack of appetite*	Maintain weight and nutritional intake Positive nitrogen balance
Anxiety *r/t* *Pain* *Fear of death* *Possible permanent cardiac damage*	Verbalize decreased anxiety Demonstrate relaxation techniques

INTERVENTIONS

Assess for the presence of pain noting onset, intensity, quality, severity, site, radiation, and influence of movement and deep inspiration.

Monitor heart rate and cardiac rhythm *to detect potential dysrhythmias.*

Auscultate heart sounds *to provide early detection of developing complications (e.g, CHF, cardiac tamponade).*

Investigate rapid pulse, hypotension, narrow pulse pressure, pulsus paradoxus, elevated CVP/jugular venous distention, changes in heart tones, diminishing levels of consciousness *as clinical manifestations of cardiac tamponade.*

Evaluate complaints of fatigue, dyspnea, palpitations, continuous chest discomfort *as clinical manifestations of CHF that may accompany endocarditis or myocarditis.*

Evaluate mental status *to detect any changes associated with decreased CO. Note any weakness in the extremities due to septic embolization of the brain.*

Check fingernails for splinter hemorrhages *due to endocarditis.*

Inspect fingers, toes, palms, and soles of feet for nodes *due to endocarditis.*

Plan of Care (cont'd)

Monitor vital signs *to detect decreased CO, cardiac tamponade.*
Monitor blood cultures *to assist in determination of causative agents and evaluate response to therapy.*
Monitor WBC *to detect evidence of infection.*
Assess patient's response to activity *as an indication of cardiac status.*
Observe for verbal and physiological signs of anxiety.
Assess and provide sleep aids as needed.
Weigh patient every day *to detect possible CHF.*
Assess nitrogen balance *to monitor nutritional status.*
Position patient in high Fowler's leaning forward *to decrease pain and enhance breathing for patient with pericarditis.*
Administer diuretics and inotrophic agents *to increase myocardial contractility and reduce the cardiac work load in the presence of CHF associated with myocarditis.*
Administer supplemental oxygen prn *to reduce cardiac work load and support other comfort measures.*
Administer analgesics as ordered *to relieve pain.*
Administer antiinflammatory agents *to relieve pain and decrease inflammatory response.*
Administer antipyretics *to decrease fever and relieve pain.*
Administer antibiotics *to treat identified causative agents and prevent further damage.*
Administer fluids *to maintain hydration and cardiac output.*
Administer anticoagulants as ordered *except when pericarditis and cardiac tamponade are suspected.*
Provide caloric intake as ordered *to meet body requirements.*
Encourage bed rest in semi-Fowler's position *to reduce cardiac work load and enhance comfort.*
Provide a quiet environment and comfort measures *to increase effectiveness of pain-relieving medication.*
Teach patient relaxation techniques and guided imagery *to enhance other comfort interventions.*
Allow for verbalization of fears regarding illness.
Assist with emergency pericardiocentesis *to reduce fluid pressure around the heart in the event of cardiac tamponade.*
Prepare patient for surgery, if indicated. *Valve replacement may be necessary for endocarditis. Pericardiotomy may be necessary for constrictive pericarditis.*

INTERMEDIATE PHASE

As the patient progresses from the intensive phase to the intermediate phase, complete recovery will depend on the patient's and family's knowledge of the illness and the plan of continued care. The focus of care during the intermediate phase is to prevent relapses, plan for discharge, and arrange for continued care as needed.

PATIENT CARE PRIORITIES	EXPECTED PATIENT OUTCOMES
Self-care deficit *r/t lack of knowledge about disease process, prevention, long-term therapy and follow-up*	Verbalize understanding of disease process and long-term therapy Identifies life-style changes Verbalizes protective actions needed prior to dental work and other procedures
Diversional activity deficit *r/t restricted mobility, long-term hospitalization, or homebound convalescence*	Engage in diversional activities based on restrictions

INTERVENTIONS

Explain the effect of inflammation on the heart *to help patient understand and comply with follow-up care.*
Instruct patient and family regarding drug therapy *to ensure optimal administration.*

Plan of Care (cont'd)

Discuss prophylactic use of antibiotics prior to dental work or other invasive procedures *to prevent reinfection.*

Identify risk factors such as drug use or extreme physical exertion for patient to control.

Identify diversional activities based on patient interest *to minimize boredom and enhance patient coping.*

Encourage visitors *to supplement diversional activities.*

Identify resources and support systems *to ensure adequate long-term care and life-style modification.*

Stress importance of follow-up care *to prevent reoccurrence and minimize risk of structural complications.*

TRANSITION TO DISCHARGE

As the patient progresses to discharge, the patient and family must be prepared for ongoing care requirements. The plan of care will differ depending on the site of heart muscle affected. Patients with endocarditis may need intravenous antibiotic therapy for 4 to 8 weeks. Because relapses may occur from 4 to 6 weeks following antibiotic therapy, weekly cultures during this extended time are advised. As a result, home care services or scheduled outpatient care will need to be arranged prior to patient discharge.[17]

Activity should be restricted for at least 1 month with avoidance of strenuous exercise or heavy work.[17] Since relapses may occur, the patient and family need to be able to recognize signs and symptoms. The patient must also be advised to adhere to the medical regime and follow-up care to prevent relapses and minimize the structural complications possible with pericarditis.

Patients with myocarditis may be treated on an outpatient basis and may resume normal activities as symptoms subside. Adequate rest and nutrition are essential to increase long-term resistance against infection.

REFERENCES

1. Bass L: Close up on pericarditis, *Nursing* 23(7):32H, 32J, 1993.
2. Bisno AL: Antimicrobial prophylaxis for infective endocarditis, *Hosp Prac (Off Ed)* 24:43, 46, 48, 52, 1989.
3. Boyer AS, Cromwell D, Nast C: Intravegetation antimicrobial distribution in aortic endocarditis analyzed by a computer generated model, *Chest* 97:611, 1990.
4. Cheitlan M, Sokolow M, McIllroy MB: *Clinical cardiology,* ed 6, Norwalk, Conn, 1993, Appleton & Lange.
5. Clemson BS, et al: Acute myocarditis in fulminant systemic sclerosis, *Chest* 101:872-874, 1992.
6. Friman G, Fohlman J: The epidemiology of viral heart disease, *Scand J Infect Dis* 88:7-10, 1993.
7. Fruth RM: Differential diagnosis of chest pain, *Crit Care Clin North Am* 3(1):59-67, 1991.
8. Grundl PD, et al: Successful treatment of acute myocarditis using extracorporeal membrane oxygenation, *Crit Care Med* 21(2):302-304, 1993.
9. Guzzetta CE: Infective endocarditis. In Dossey BM, Guzzetta CE, Kenner CV, editors: *Critical care nursing: mind-body-spirit,* Philadelphia, 1992, JB Lippincott, pp 515-534.
10. Hehrelein FW, Stertman WA, Roth M: Constrictive pericarditis with or without heart-lung machine? *Langenbecks Arch* Supplement:488-493, 1992.
11. Houghton JL: Pericarditis and myocarditis. Which is benign and which isn't? *Postgrad Med* 91(2):273-278, 281-282, 1992.
12. Kirklin JW, Barrett-Boyes B: *Cardiac surgery.* New York, 1986, John Wiley & Sons.
13. Korzenowksi OM, Kaye D: Infective endocarditis. In Braunwald E, editor: *Heart Disease: a textbook of cardiovascular medicine,* ed 4, Philadelphia, 1992, WB Saunders.
14. Kupper NS, Duke ES: Nursing role in management: inflammatory and valvular heart disease. In Lewis SM, editor: *Medical surgical nursing.* St Louis, 1992, Mosby–Year Book.
15. Lorrell B: Pericarditis. In Braunwald E, editor: *Heart disease: a textbook of cardiovascular medicine,* ed 4, Philadelphia, 1992, WB Saunders.
16. Maisch B, Herzum M, Schonian U: Immunomodulating factors and immunosuppressive drugs in the therapy of myocarditis, *Scand J Int Med* 88:149-162, 1993.
17. Monnig RL, Streit L: Nursing management of adults with disorders of cardiac structures and having heart surgery. In Burrell L, editor: *Adult nursing in hospital and community setting,* Engelwood Cliffs, NJ, 1991, Prentice Hall, pp 436-462.
18. Narula J, et al: Recognition of acute myocarditis masquerading as acute MI, *N Engl J Med* 328(2):100-104, 1993.
19. *St Anthony's DRG Guidebook 1995,* Reston, Va, 1994, St Anthony.
20. Starling RC, et al: Successful management of acute myocarditis with biventricular assist devices and cardiac transplantation, *Am J Cardiol* 62:341, 1988.
21. Topaz O, Mackall JA: Observations of angina and myocardial infarction in constrictive pericarditis, *Int J Cardiol* 39(2):121-129, 1993.
22. Zhang S, et al: Effects of cyclosporine, prednisolone, and aspirin on rat autoimmune giant cell myocarditis, *J Am Coll Cardiol* 21(5):1254-1260, 1993.

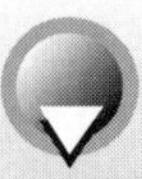

CLINICAL GUIDELINE

20

Coronary Artery Bypass Grafting

Catherine Ryan, MS, RN, CCRN

DESCRIPTION

Coronary artery bypass graft (CABG) surgery was first introduced in 1969 by Garrett and colleagues.[13] Since that time, the surgical procedure has been refined, myocardial protection techniques have improved, and there have been major changes in the profile of patients who undergo CABG. The result is a dramatic increase in the prevalence of the operation. CABG surgery is a technique used to shunt blood around stenotic portions of major coronary arteries. The procedure involves constructing conduits between the aorta (or other major artery) and segments of the coronary arteries beyond obstructing lesions. These conduits bring blood flow to areas of the myocardium that have become ischemic, or have the potential to become ischemic, related to these lesions.[13]

Because the overall goals of CABG surgery are to relieve symptoms, prolong survival, and improve quality of life through revascularization, the criteria for selection for CABG surgery remain controversial.[36] Generally accepted indications for CABG surgery are listed in the following Box.

Conduits most commonly used are the internal mammary arteries (IMA) and reversed segments of autologous saphenous veins (SVG). Superior patency rates of internal mammary grafts over saphenous vein grafts have been demonstrated in short- and long-term follow-up comparisons.[13,23,36] The IMA is also superior because it can constrict and dilate to provide blood flow according to myocardial demands, and it eliminates the necessity of leg incisions, thus facilitating early ambulation. IMA graft procedures, however, can be used only as bypasses for the anterior surface of the heart; are technically more difficult to perform and result in increased blood loss and longer operative and cardiopulmonary bypass times;[39,42] and account for more postoperative chest wall pain.[20] A combination of internal mammary and saphenous vein grafts are often used for patients requiring multiple bypasses. Figures 20-1 and 20-2 demonstrate various positions for IMA and SVG conduit combinations. Other conduits less commonly used include cephalic veins, segments of the radial artery, allograft arteries and veins, right gastroepiploic artery (as a free or in situ graft), inferior mesenteric artery, and inferior epigastric artery.[13,36] Long-term patency from these alternative grafts has been disappointing.[28] The necessity for alternative conduits is increasing as the population of patients requiring re-operation increases. As a result, researchers continue to search for new conduits to use for bypass grafts. Coronary endarterectomy is another alternative and may be performed in conjunction with CABG in select patients with diffuse multivessel disease.

It is estimated that 353,000 CABG procedures are done annually in the United States.[2] The Coronary Artery Surgery Study (CASS) showed that CABG surgery increases survival in patients with chronic, unstable angina; left main coronary artery disease; and patients with triple vessel disease combined with decreased left ventricular function.[10]

PATHOPHYSIOLOGY

Procedure

The CABG procedure is most commonly performed using a median sternotomy approach. The ribs are separated with a retractor and the pericardium is opened. Patients often complain of constant aching pain or soreness in the shoulders, upper back, ribs, and neck postoperatively as a result of retraction of the ribs and intraoperative positioning.[20] If

Indications for CABG Surgery

Symptomatic angina unresponsive to medical therapy[13,31,36]
Chronic, stable angina with >70% narrowing of the left main CA[31]
Multivessel disease with LV dysfunction[31,41]
Acute MI with residual high-grade CA stenosis postemergent intervention (thrombolytic therapy and/or PTCA)[41]
Acute MI with hemodynamic decompensation[41]
Severe triple vessel disease[41]
Persistent, recurrent, or post-infarction angina[1]
Severe left main CA stenosis >50%[42]

an IMA graft is used, it is dissected from the chest wall. After opening the pericardium, the end of the IMA is anastomosed to the coronary artery, distal to the blockage (Figure 20-1). If saphenous vein grafts are performed, the saphenous vein is removed from the leg and prepared. The vein graft is reversed to assure that venous valves do not interrupt blood flow. One end of the vein graft is anastomosed end-to-side to an opening in the coronary artery, distal to the obstructing lesion, and the other end is sutured into a small punch opening on the ascending aorta (Figure 20-2). Most surgeries involve a combination of these two procedures.

A number of techniques are employed to protect the patient from the complications of CABG surgery. The cardiopulmonary bypass pump (CPBP) provides the surgeon with a bloodless, motionless surgical field while the patient's blood is oxygenated and circulated to the other body organs. The goal of CPBP is to provide nearly normal cardiac output (CO) and metabolic conditions. Because the body's metabolic demands are reduced by hypothermia, a CI of 2.0 to 2.4 L/min/m^2 is considered acceptable.[42] Higher flow rates have been associated with cerebral bleeding.[42] CPBP is accomplished by cannulating the right atrium or inferior and superior vena cava to divert venous blood away from the surgical field to a mechanical pump and gas exchange system (Figure 20-3). Oxygenated blood is returned to the patient via a cannula in the ascending aorta. Blood from the right heart is drained by gravity and collected in a venous reservoir that contains a heat exchanger used to produce systemic hypothermia and warm the patient's blood. In addition, there is a cardiotomy suction reservoir where blood suctioned from the operative field is collected to be filtered and reinfused into the patient. A cardioplegia reservoir keeps cold cardioplegia solution readily available. Roller pumps producing a non-pulsatile flow pattern are most commonly used to propel blood through CPBP systems. These pumps have a number of disadvantages, including destruction of red blood cells and platelets, decreased phagocytic activity of WBCs, platelet dysfunction, and increased vascular resistance; however, they are easy to use and well-tolerated by patients undergoing CABG procedures. Because CPBP results in production of particulate matter and fat and gas emboli, blood filters play an important role in the system. It is especially important to filter cardiotomy blood because it has been shown to contain calcium fragments, suture fragments, fat, fibrin, and other debris.[7,42] Blood is also filtered and passes through a bubble detector before it is returned to the patient.

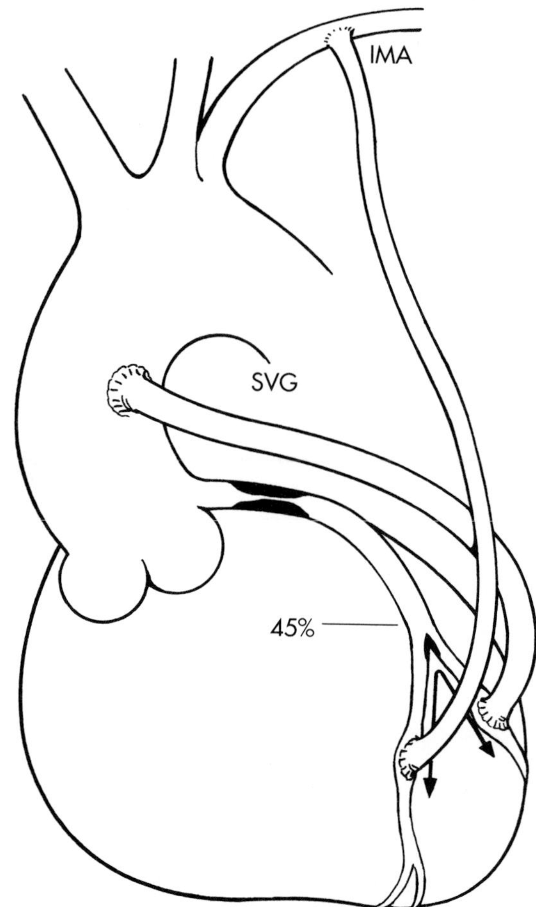

Figure 20-1 Internal mammary artery graft (IMA) remains attached to subclavian and is anastomosed end-to-side to a coronary artery, distal to an obstructing lesion. Saphenous vein free graft (SVG) is used to bypass an obstructing lesion. (From Mills NL: Physiologic and technical aspects of the internal mammary artery-coronary artery bypass graft. In *Modern techniques in surgery,* Mount Kisco, NY, 1982, Futura Publishing Company.)

There are two types of oxygenators that may be used to oxygenate the venous blood that has entered the CPBP system. Bubble oxygenators bubble an oxygen and CO_2 mixture through a vertical column of blood, allowing for direct contact of the blood with the gas. Oxygen and carbon dioxide diffuse between the bubbles and the blood due to concentration gradients. This system results in increased trauma to and destruction of blood cells and may contribute to formation of microemboli.[4] However, it is considered a safe choice if used for less than 3 hours.[7,42] In membrane oxy-

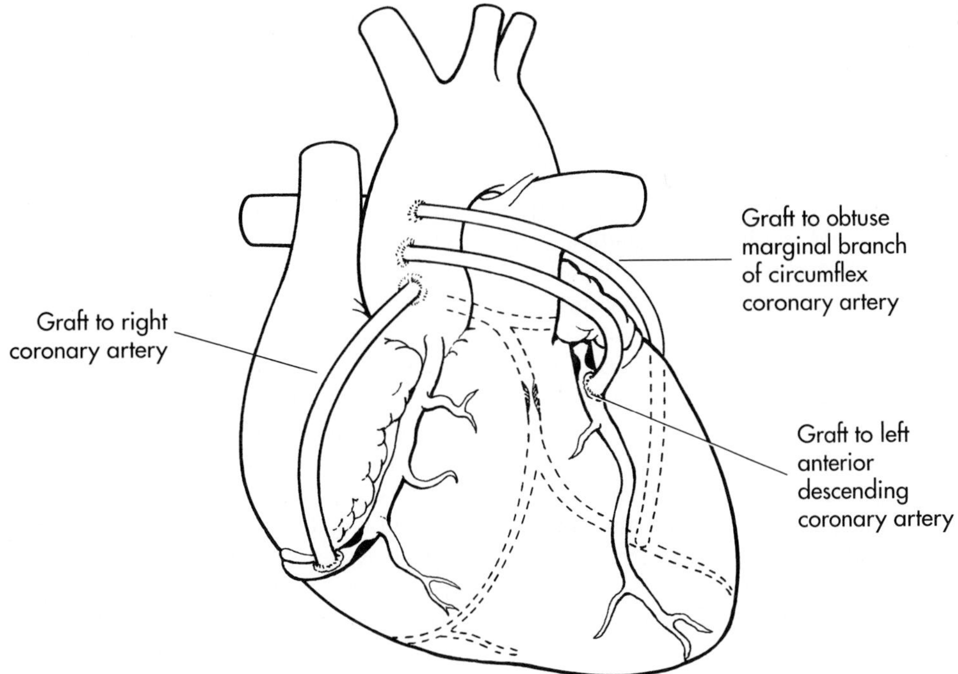

Figure 20-2 Graft to right coronary artery; graft to left anterior descending coronary artery; graft to obtuse marginal branch of circumflex artery. (From Monro JL, Shore G: *Color atlas of cardiac surgery: acquired disease,* London, 1982, Appleton-Century-Crofts/Wolfe Medical Publications, Ltd. By permission of Wolfe Medical Publications, Ltd.)

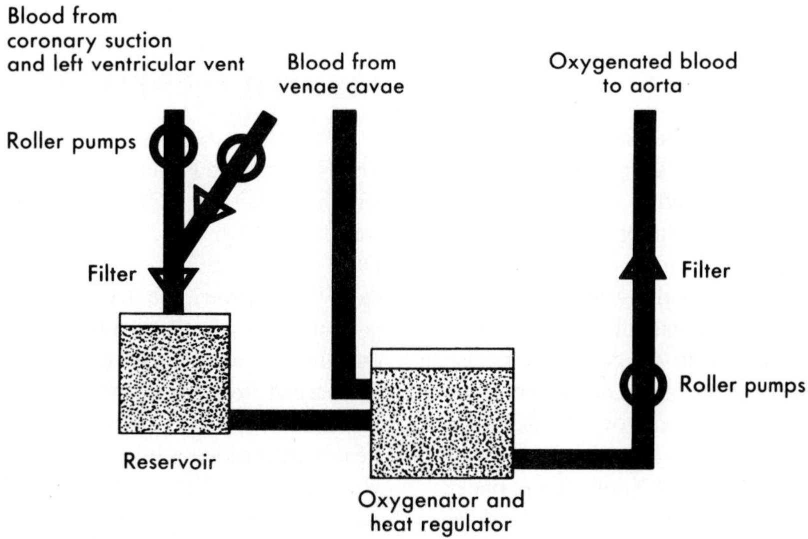

Figure 20-3 Basic components required for CPBP. (From Kinney M, et al: *Comprehensive cardiac care,* ed 7, St Louis, 1991, Mosby–Year Book.)

genators, gas exchange occurs through diffusion of gas across a semipermeable membrane that separates the circulating blood from the gas. This system closely parallels human alveoli and causes less blood cell trauma but is more difficult to use. Membrane oxygenators are the device of choice for CPBP runs greater than 3 hours. After the CPBP, hypothermia, and cardiac arrest are established, the distal grafts are completed. It is important to note that while the patient is on CPBP, the lungs are partially deflated and the ventilator is turned off. Oxygenation and circulation of blood as well as delivery of additional anesthetic agents are carried out through the CPBP.

During use of the CPBP, the heart is not included in the circulation, thus creating a bloodless surgical field. Interventions are initiated to protect myocardial tissue during the procedure. Cardioplegia solution with high concentrations of potassium, magnesium, or procaine are infused at low temperatures (4 to 8° C) into the coronary arteries at the aortic root to produce a rapid chemical arrest.[29] Aortic root cross-clamping ensures that the cardioplegia solution remains in the heart. The cold temperature of the solution lowers myocardial temperature to 5 to 15° C, protecting the myocardium against ischemia. Addition of the patient's own blood, glucose, buffers, calcium, and steroids assure a homeostatic solution. Cold saline or iced saline slush may also be instilled into the pericardial cavity to further assist in uniformly cooling the heart. However, this technique must be used cautiously because it may cause phrenic nerve damage or paralysis.[4,34] Hypothermia is maintained throughout the procedure by periodic addition of cold cardioplegia solution. When the intracardiac portion of the procedure is completed, warmed fluid or pump blood is infused to stimulate the heart to begin beating. In rare instances, internal defibrillation is necessary to stimulate the heart to beat independently. The patient is then weaned from the CPBP, atrial and ventricular pacemaker wires are placed on the pericardium, and pleural and mediastinal chest tubes are inserted. The pericardium may be partially closed with suture. The sternum is closed and stabilized with stainless steel wire. Patients complain of less postoperative chest pain than might otherwise be expected if the sternum is stabilized in this fashion.

Associated Interventions

Interventions that are related to initiation and use of CPBP play an important part in the patient's postoperative care and outcomes. Currently, CPBP systems are primed with pH-corrected colloid or crystalloid solutions (usually 1800 to 2000 ml).[7] Therefore, at the beginning of CPBP, the patient is maximally hemodiluted, resulting in a hematocrit of 25% to 30%. Hemodilution has a number of implications to the patient, including reduction in oxygen-carrying capacity due to decreased hemoglobin concentration, decrease in colloid osmotic pressure, and promotion of interstitial edema.[4,41] It also lowers blood viscosity and vascular resistance, improves capillary flow, reduces hemolysis and platelet aggregation, reduces the incidence of postoperative renal and pulmonary dysfunction, decreases postoperative bleeding, and decreases the use of banked blood.[42] Overall, the benefits outweigh the risk.

Anticoagulation is also required during CPBP to decrease the incidence of abnormal coagulation rates caused by blood contact with the nonbiological surfaces of the CPBP machine and air, and vascular occlusion during the procedure. Heparin 300 to 400 U/kg at the onset of bypass and every ½ to 1 hour is used to suspend clotting mechanisms during CPBP. The dosage is monitored by measurement of ACT during bypass. Because of the massive heparinization required, early recognition of heparin-sensitive patients and intervention to remove additional contact with heparin is essential to reduce morbidity and mortality. The heparin is reversed with a slow infusion of protamine sulfate administered over 10 to 15 minutes when CPBP is terminated.

Because the CPBP does not exactly reproduce heart and lung functions, other techniques must be employed to protect the patient from complications. The metabolic demands of other organs are decreased with the use of systemic hypothermia. Studies reveal that metabolic rate is decreased by approximately 7% for each 1° C the body temperature is lowered.[7,42] Body temperature is reduced to 28° to 32° C via the heat exchanger on the bypass pump. This results in core cooling, which provides better protection of key organs than surface cooling. A number of complications have been related to systemic hypothermia, including increased blood viscosity, sluggish capillary and organ flow, tighter oxygen binding to hemoglobin, and difficulties with rewarming.[6,16] Due to these complications, a number of centers are advocating normothermic cardiopulmonary bypass in an effort to decrease complications and length of hospitalization.[8,26]

Unfortunately, the ideal CPBP system does not exist. CPBP produces blood-cell trauma and has the potential to adversely affect nearly all body systems. For this reason, the majority of the nursing interventions performed in the first 24 hours postoperatively are geared to reversing the trauma of the very interventions that are used to enable patients to survive the surgical procedure.

LENGTH OF STAY/ANTICIPATED COURSE

The Health Care Financing Administration (HCFA) average length of stay for DRG 106: CABG with cardiac catheterization, is 13.6 days. The HCFA mean length of stay for DRG 107: CABG without cardiac catheterization, is 10.4 days.[19] However, the length of stay varies based on the patient's preoperative condition and comorbidities. It is not unusual for an otherwise healthy, younger patient to be discharged from the hospital within 5 days when provisions are made for close home surveillance.[8,13] An innovative treatment protocol called Fast Track is currently being investigated at a limited number of centers.[8] This protocol includes a combination of preoperative education; drug administration before, during, and after surgery; and accelerated physical activity. It attempts to identify the normal consequences of cardiac surgery and treat them in an anticipatory fashion. Thus far, the protocol has shown a decrease in the length of stay by 2.5 days.[8]

Care of the CABG patient can be divided into four phases. The preoperative phase, including cardiac catheterization and other diagnostic evaluation, is often performed on an outpatient basis. The intensive phase includes the operative day and approximately 24 hours after surgery. The intermediate phase lasts 3 to 5 days including transition to discharge. Cardiac rehabilitation, which begins while the patient is an inpatient, continues for several months.

MANAGEMENT TRENDS AND CONTROVERSIES

The highly competitive environment of modern health care has resulted in a proliferation of CABG programs. The Inter-Society Commission for Heart Disease Resources recommended as early as 1972 that a minimum of 200 to 300 procedures should be performed annually by institutions providing CABG services to assure quality and competence.[49] As hospitals consider initiating CABG programs, this recommendation remains the standard. While high volume does not always assure quality, ongoing scrutiny of low-volume programs must be a consideration.

As CABG surgery has become more prevalent, a trend has developed toward surgery in older patients. Over one half of the open-heart surgery procedures in 1989 were performed on people 65 years of age or older.[3] While it might be assumed that the postoperative care of an older patient would be more complicated, many consider the postoperative nursing care and recovery of elderly cardiac surgery patients to be similar to that of younger patients; the greatest age-related difference in nursing care is that the pace of recovery tends to be slower.[12,16,25] However, in spite of improved survival rates, elderly cardiac surgery patients demonstrate higher morbidity and mortality rates than younger patients.[12,16] This may be due in part to increased primary cardiac risk and chronic medical conditions in older patients.[14,33,36] The number of CABG re-operations has also increased, becoming the second most common cardiac surgery. These surgeries carry an exponential increase in risk of mortality, especially in females and the elderly.[18,36]

Another trend in recent years is admission of low-risk preoperative patients early on the morning of surgery. Certainly the trend relates to cost containment and use of hospital resources. While carefully planned and executed same-day admission programs have demonstrated a small cost saving combined with patient satisfaction, more research is needed to prove that this strategy is truly advantageous to the patient and the institution.[6,13]

Controversies abound related to optimal postoperative management of the CABG patient. Early ambulation of the CABG patient is encouraged to prevent complications of bedrest and help counteract the trauma caused by CPB. However, the optimal time to initiate ambulation and the amount of ambulation remain controversial. Current guidelines at some hospitals recommend that patients dangle immediately after extubation on the operative day and begin ambulation on the first postoperative day.[58]

The preoperative use of antiplatelet agents has shown promise in preventing saphenous vein graft occlusion. Aspirin and dipyridamole are commonly used alone or in combination.[15] Studies are underway to identify optimal timing and dosing for this therapy.[15,39,44] The CABADAS study on prevention of coronary artery bypass graft occlusion by aspirin, dipyridamole, and acenocoumarol/phenoprocoumon showed acceptable vein graft patency 1 year postoperatively when as little as 50 mg of aspirin per day was taken by the patient.[44] This compared to results obtained from higher doses of aspirin in previous studies. The study also demonstrated additional benefit when dipyridamole was added.[44]

Preoperative aspirin and dipyridamole therapy has also been shown to decrease postoperative morbidity and mortality associated with heparin-induced thrombocytopenia. CABG patients are at particular risk for this potentially devastating complication since most have been exposed to heparin preoperatively during diagnostic or interventional procedures such as PTCA. In addition, low-dose heparin therapy to reduce the incidence of stroke post-AMI is still practiced in many centers. Once sensitized, heparin antiplatelet antibodies (HAAB) may remain in the system for up to 2 years.[46] Subsequent massive heparin exposure to prevent clotting while on the CPBP may trigger a dangerous cycle of microembolization and bleeding in HAAB-positive patients. Continued postoperative exposure to heparin, as may occur from heparinized flush solution in arterial monitoring lines, will continue to feed this damaging reaction.

Elimination of even the most minute heparin exposure postoperatively has also been shown to significantly reduce the risk of morbidity and mortality from heparin-induced thrombocytopenia in heparin-sensitive patients.[45,46,47] As a result, rather than routinely screening patients for the presence of HAAB prior to surgery (a time-consuming and expensive process), many surgeons routinely prescribe aspirin and dipyridamole for all of their patients preoperatively. The increased risk of slightly greater postoperative bleeding in patients who receive preoperative aspirin is considered to be less than the risk of heparin-induced thrombocytopenia in heparin-sensitive patients.[46]

Other areas of research and controversy related to postoperative management of CABG patients include crystalloid versus colloid therapy,[15,27] management of supraventricular dysrhythmias,[15] types of preoperative skin preparation,[38] and optimal methods for rewarming after cardiac surgery.[21,22]

Nursing research is aimed at investigating nursing responsibilities and clarifying and validating nursing interventions. Nursing research has identified improved methods for predicting shivering, a dangerous postoperative complication, by monitoring the bladder-to-core temperature ratio.[9] A ratio of <1.0 was noted to significantly correlate with shivering, while a ratio of ≥ 1.0 was associated with no incidences of shivering.[36]

Techniques related to chest tube stripping, a common nursing practice, have also been investigated. Recent nursing research reinforces that stripping and milking chest tubes generates high negative pressure and creates potential lung injury without scientific evidence of any value in maintaining chest tube patency.[32,43]

There have also been studies that address the sleep disturbance problems that are so prevalent in CABG patients. For example, a study by Williamson demonstrated a significant improvement in amount and quality of sleep during the night by using recorded ocean sounds as a sleep-enhancing intervention.[48]

A number of studies have focused on outcomes and quality of life issues for CABG patients. Studies agree that long-term survival and activity tolerance are increased and angina is decreased in patients who undergo CABG surgery.[1] There are varying reports of return to work, recreational status, sexual functioning, and general functional status in this patient population.[1,35] Other studies indicate that there are a number of nonsurgical factors that influence recovery, such as perception of tension and anxiety[37] and degree of life satisfaction.[24] Because adjustment after CABG is a multidimensional phenomenon, information gained from these and other studies will prove to be valuable for discharge planning and counseling for CABG patients and their families.

The entire realm of post-CABG care offers fertile ground for ongoing medical and nursing research and innovations in practice.

ASSESSMENT

PARAMETER	ANTICIPATED ALTERATION
History of previous cardiac events: AMI, PTCA, or cardiac surgery	Most CABG candidates will have previous hospitalization experiences. *Previous CABG surgery significantly increases surgical morbidity and mortality.*
Risk factor assessment: • Hypertension • Diabetes • Hyperlipidemia • Cigarette smoking • Obesity • Sedentary life-style • Response to stress • Sex • Age • Family history	CABG candidates generally have several risk factors. *Preoperative risk-factor assessment enables more efficient focus for postoperative education.*
Comorbid conditions	Renal insufficiency, diabetes, past stroke, thrombophlebitis, pulmonary disease, dental caries. *Presence of any of these increases risk of morbidity or mortality and/or may prolong hospitalization.*
Preoperative autologous Blood	Donation of one unit every 2 to 3 weeks with 3 weeks between last donation and surgery to allow for recovery of hematocrit
Medication history	Antianginals: continue until surgery Diuretics: stop 1 to 2 days preoperatively *to allow for* K^+ *repletion* ASA and dipyridamole preoperatively with ASA continuing postoperatively once hemostasis is re-established.

Cardio-pulmonary Assessment

HR and rhythm	Regular, NSR
Heart tones	May have an S_4 *due to previous MI or CAD*
BP	BP within patient norms preoperatively and within 12 to 24 hours postoperatively. Hypertension immediately postoperatively with systolic BP >150 mm Hg; diastolic BP >100 mm Hg *due to hypothermia, sympathetic stress response, and fluid shift during surgery.*
Peripheral circulation	Presence of poor peripheral perfusion (decreased pulses, stasis ulcers) or varicosities or history of vein stripping *will have implications for graft site selection.*
Rate, rhythm and quality of respirations	Effortless respirations <20/min preoperatively and within 48 hours postoperatively.
Breath sounds	Clear breath sounds preoperative and at discharge postoperative.
Pulmonary screening	Ventilatory volumes and capacities WNL. *Decreased values are associated with increased pulmonary risk postoperatively.*

Chest x-ray (PA and lateral)	Chest x-ray clear and heart size WNL preoperative. *Fluid shifts may cause right or left heart failure.* Atalectasis common postoperative with slight degree of mediastinal widening *due to surgical effects.* Pleural effusion possible postoperative
Neurological Assessment	
Carotid bruits	Appropriate cerebral circulation is essential *to decrease the possibility of stroke during aortic clamping while on bypass.*
Mentation/LOC	Awake, alert, oriented
Carotid Doppler studies	WNL. Abnormalities are associated with higher risk.
Hematologic Assessment	
Recent ASA or antiplatelet drug use	Platelet count and bleeding times WNL. *Recent ASA, thrombolitic, antiplatelet, and ETOH use may increase bleeding potential postoperatively.*
History of ETOH use and abuse	
Recent thrombolytics	
Laboratory Findings	
Cardiac enzymes	WNL
Blood chemistries	WNL
Electrolytes	WNL
BUN	WNL
Creatinine	WNL
Blood sugar	WNL or slightly elevated postoperative *due to stress response*
Liver function tests	WNL or slightly elevated *due to stress response*
Activated clotting time (ACT)	May be prolonged (>180 sec) *if heparin is not fully reversed postoperatively*
Urinalysis	WNL. *Preoperative urinary tract infection may lead to postoperative sepsis.*
Psychosocial Assessment	
Anxiety level	Anxiety is expected in patients and families. Adequate coping mechanisms should be in evidence.
Knowledge of procedure	Verbalize basic knowledge of procedure and expected course.
Life-style assessment	Potential risk factors for CAD that will require modification.
Coping mechanisms	In evidence

PLAN OF CARE

INTENSIVE PHASE

The intensive phase of care for CABG patients lasts through the first 24 to 36 hours postsurgery in most patients. The majority of monitoring and interventions provided during this phase are focused on supporting patient recovery from anesthesia; the hematologic and organ trauma associated with the CPBP; and subsequent autonomic, immune, and stress responses that place the patient at high risk for serious complications. Many patients receive full hemodynamic monitoring while other, low-risk patients may be monitored with only a CVP and arterial line. Weaning for ventilatory support with subsequent extubation is typically ac-

Plan of Care (cont'd)

complished within 8 to 24 hours from the time of arrival in the ICU. Without the occurrence of significant complications, the current trend in CABG surgery is to transfer the patient from the ICU to an intermediate or general unit on the first postoperative day.

PATIENT CARE PRIORITIES	EXPECTED PATIENT OUTCOMES
High risk for confusion/complications *r/t emergence from anesthesia*	Awaken neurologically intact
Decreased cardiac output *r/t myocardial depression from* *Ischemia and reperfusion* *Hypothermia* *Anesthesia* *Hypoxia* *Cardiopulmonary bypass pump* *Vasoactive drugs* *Sympathetic stimulation* *Cellular metabolic abnormalities* *Hypovolemia* *Decreased contractility*	BP and HR: WNL CO and hemodynamic profile WNL or within prescribed ranges Normovolemic Absence of myocardial ischemia Absence of dysrhythmias Sao_2 >90% UO >30 cc/hr
Hypothermia *r/t the surgical procedure*	SVR, MAP, and Sao_2 within normal limits Absence of shivering Extremities pink and warm with strong pulses
Impaired gas exchange *r/t pulmonary trauma during surgery with resultant atelectasis and interstitial edema*	ABG: WNL Sao_2 >90% Respirations unlabored Breath sounds clear Absence of pulmonary embolism, pulmonary edema, pleural effusion, pneumothorax, hemothorax, CHF, ARDS
Decreased tissue perfusion *r/t* *Hypothermia* *Sympathetic stimulation* *Dysrhythmias* *Decreased CO* *Increased SVR*	Extremities pink, warm, and pulses present Absence of deep-vein thrombosis Absence of dysrhythmias BP and SVR within acceptable limits
Bleeding *r/t high risk for* *Heparin rebound* *Platelet dysfunction* *Thrombocytopenia* *Depletion of coagulation factors* *Tissue dissection during IMA graft dissection* *Inadequate hemostasis* *Preop antiplatelet agents* *Cardiopulmonary bypass pump* *Potential graft rupture*	Hemostasis Chest x-ray shows mediastinal width within preoperative norms Chest tube drainage non-pulsatile and within prescribed norms Hct and Hgb within acceptable parameters HR and BP: WNL ACT, PT/PTT within acceptable limits Absence of bleeding from incision, venipuncture sites, or invasive drains
Dysrhythmias *r/t ischemia, electrolyte abnormalities, pacemaker wire placement*	NSR or rhythm within patient norms
Alteration in fluid and electrolyte balance *r/t fluid shifts from* *Anesthesia* *Diuretic use* *Deep hypothermia and rewarming* *K^+ shifts with acidosis/alkalosis*	Urine output >.5 ml/kg/hr, or 30 cc/hr Potassium >4.0 mEq/L BP within patient norms PCWP 14 to 16 mm Hg Chest tube drainage <200 cc/hr the first hour and <100 cc/hr thereafter

Plan of Care (cont'd)

Hypoperfusion of the kidney *Blood loss* *Increase in capillary permeability/fluid shifts* *Dilution from pump solution*	Electrolytes: WNL
Alterations in acid-base balance *r/t CPBP trauma of* *Tissue hypoxemia* *Minimal perfusion* *Increased lactic acid production* *Postoperative interventions of diuretic use, high doses of vasopressors*	pH: WNL ABG consistent with preoperative baseline
Decreased renal perfusion *r/t decreased CO*	Urine output >.5 ml/kg/hr or 30 cc/hr Urine specific gravity 1.015 to 1.020
High risk for infection *r/t* *Sternal incision* *Multiple invasive lines* *Immunosuppression associated with cardiopulmonary bypass pump* *Mechanical ventilation* *Urethral catheter* *Possible inadequate preoperative nutrition*	Absence of infection: WBC: WNL Afebrile
High risk for decreased cerebral perfusion *r/t* *Cerebral hypoperfusion* *Particulate embolization* *Air embolism*	Awakens from anesthesia Oriented to time and place Pupil response within patient norms Absence of paralysis, seizures, numbness, confusion, disorientation, hallucinations, or psychosis
Pain and general discomfort *r/t* *Incisions* *Intubation* *Chest tubes* *Decreased mobility* *Rib retraction during surgery*	Able to sleep, eat, ambulate, and complete respiratory exercises States feeling of reasonable comfort as defined by the patient
Patient/family anxiety *r/t* *Fear of outcome* *Knowledge deficit* *Dependence on medical team*	Patient/significant others verbalize effective ways to deal with anxiety Patient/significant others state decreased anxiety Patient will sleep

INTERVENTIONS

Prepare the family for the patient's appearance after surgery (tubes, lines, monitoring equipment, generalized edema, cool skin, etc. Prepare the patient for awakening in the ICU *to decrease anxiety and facilitate coping.*

Monitor vital signs, hemodynamic profile, and peripheral perfusion q½h to q1h until stable correlating with clinical observations. *Studies indicate that 90% of CABG patients experience decreased LVEF and CI and transient LV dysfunctions postoperatively due to preoperative cardiac dysfunction, the stress of the procedure (anesthesia, bypass and surgical trauma), uncorrected physiology, or release of myocardial depressant factor (MDF).*[42]

Administer volume replacement therapy to keep MAP/BP within prescribed limits and optimize preload. *MAP <60 mm Hg can result in low flow through coronary grafts and early graft collapse.*[32] *Hypovolemia may be masked by vasoconstriction and increased SVR prior to rewarming.*

Administer vasodilators and/or antihypertensives *to stabilize immediate postoperative hypertension, decrease SVR, prevent graft rupture, and optimize O_2 supply.*

Administer positive inotropic agents as ordered *to increase CO and CI in the event that the myocardium is sluggish in its recovery.*

Plan of Care (cont'd)

Initiate rewarming techniques (radiant heat, warm blankets, warming mattress) as needed.

Monitor temperature continuously using core PA temperature and/or urinary bladder temperature.

Monitor PA: bladder temperature ratio *to predict and prevent shivering.*

Discontinue rewarming when patient temperature nears 37° C *to avoid elevated temperature, which increases O_2 demands. PA temperatures with the Swan Ganz catheter reflecting mixing of blood from all regions of the body, and urinary bladder temperatures are preferred sites over rectal temperatures, which are slow to stabilize.*[30] *Rapid rewarming can potentiate hypotension through vasodilation.*

During warming, administer fluids and colloids *in anticipation of a falling SVR.*

Position for optimal hemodynamic function and ventilation *but keep patient supine until hemodynamically stable.*

When hemodynamically stable, turn q1h to q2h and elevate the head of the bed *to promote diaphragmatic excursion, gas exchange, and chest tube drainage.*

Chest physiotherapy q1h to q2h with turning *to facilitate chest drainage.*

Continuously monitor ECG for dysrhythmias, and P-, ST-, or T-wave changes; or bundle-branch block *to detect presence of ischemia, infarction, abrupt graft closure, and electrolyte abnormalities.*

Promptly initiate antidysrhythmic therapy as indicated. *Supraventricular tachydysrhythmias, which may potentiate CHF, angina, myocardial ischemia, or mural thrombus formation, occur in as many as 30% of all patients undergoing CABG.*[15] *Postoperative atrial fibrillation may delay patient recovery.*[5]

Attach atrial and ventricular pacemaker wires to pulse generator and set at prescribed rate *to ensure prompt support in the event of bradycardia or heart block.*

Provide mechanical ventilation with oxygen therapy until respiratory depression from anesthesia has resolved.

Auscultate breath sounds q1h until stable.

Suction only as needed *to maintain patent airways and facilitate gas exchange.*

Monitor ventilator settings and parameters *to identify readiness for weaning including rate, volumes, oxygen, pressures, ABG, NIF, level of consciousness, presence of spontaneous respirations.*

Monitor for signs and symptoms of hypoxemia (tachycardia, use of accessory muscles, tachypnea, restlessness, confusion, decreased SaO_2). *Hypoxemia may increase blood pressure and SVR and decrease contractility.*

Monitor chest x-ray for atelectasis, pleural effusion, pulmonary interstitial edema, position of all tubes and lines, hemo- or pneumothorax, and width of mediastinum *to identify potential complications promptly and facilitate weaning process.*

Provide sedation *if patient inability to synchronize breathing with ventilator is not due to readiness for extubation or patient is shivering.*

Administer pain medications *to facilitate comfort, coughing, ventilator weaning, ambulation and rest. Patients undergoing IMA grafting may require more pain medication due to more extensive surgical dissection of the chest wall. Pain and anxiety may also cause postoperative hypertension.*

Monitor for bleeding: Hgb, Hct, chest drainage, preload indicators, bleeding times, and especially ACT *due to its greater specificity for heparin effect.* Notify physician as indicated.

Autotransfuse blood lost during the first 12 to 24 hours as indicated. Routinely return all cell saver blood from OR if not infused prior to arrival in ICU. *Returning patient's own blood decreases need for banked blood with its risks of infectious disease and calcium depletion and helps maintain blood volume and tissue oxygenation. Platelets are destroyed by the CPBP and counts will remain low for 3 to 5 days postsurgery.*[4]

Monitor UO every hour and correlate with hemodynamic profile *to ensure adequate renal perfusion and function.*

Monitor BUN and creatinine *as indicators of renal function.*

Plan of Care (cont'd)

Monitor for shivering and initiate treatment (Valium, MS, neuromuscular blockade) as necessary. *Shivering will increase SVR, BP, and O_2* consumption, and decrease CO.[9,21,34]

Administer diuretics cautiously *to balance fluid overload from third spacing associated with CPBP, blood loss, and the vasodilation of warming.*

Administer electrolyte solutions IV *to keep serum electrolytes within prescribed limits, facilitate cellular function, and prevent myocardial depression.*

Administer prophylactic antibiotics for 24 to 48 hours as prescribed.

Assess neurological function with each set of vital signs. *Failure to awaken from anesthesia or change in neuro functioning may indicate a perfusion deficit or cerebral embolic event. Subtle changes in cognitive function and psychological state related to the CPBP have been described by some authors and are transient.*[40]

Assure that chest tubes are patent *since occluded chest tubes can cause cardiac tamponade. However, excessive manipulation and negative pressure with stripping may promote bleeding.*[17] *Gently milk chest tubes that contain clots.*

Assure that chest tubes are connected to underwater seal drainage *to assure that there is lung reexpansion, to avoid pneumothorax, and to determine the presence of any air leak.*

Monitor chest tube bleeding per prescribed ranges. *Patients who have had reoperations and those who have had IMA grafts will have greater amounts of chest tube bleeding.*[32]

Monitor for bowel recovery and maintain NG tube if prescribed to *prevent gastric distension, diaphragmatic elevation, emesis, and potential aspiration.*

Monitor chest sounds including breath sounds, adventitious sounds, pleural or cardiac rub.

Monitor chest movements, especially noting asymmetrical movements, *which could indicate a damaged phrenic nerve resulting in diaphragmatic paralysis.*[40]

Monitor extremities and peripheral pulses *for signs and symptoms of peripheral emboli.*

Initiate antiplatelet or anticoagulant therapy as prescribed *to promote graft patency and minimize graft occlusion.*[15,39]

Apply antithromboembolism stockings, Ace wraps, or sequential compression boots as prescribed. Perform passive range of motion exercises to legs. Teach and encourage active leg exercises *to prevent formation of deep-vein thrombosis.*

Monitor blood sugar and administer insulin as indicated. *Stress-related hyperglycemia is common with blood sugars 250 to 500 in normal patients and higher in diabetics.*

Provide support and encouragement for patient/significant others. Teach and reinforce education as needed *to decrease anxiety levels.*

INTERMEDIATE PHASE

Monitoring of all body systems continues in the intermediate care phase where the goals of care relate to continued recovery toward discharge. The patient will be extubated and chest tubes will be removed unless an air leak persists. The patient is feeling better and progress toward recovery is seen by patient and family. In this phase, many patients express that they are thankful to be alive and may be quite emotional related to their condition.

PATIENT CARE PRIORITIES	EXPECTED PATIENT OUTCOMES
High risk for ineffective breathing pattern *r/t incisional pain*	Participate in coughing and deep-breathing exercises and incentive spirometry every 2 hours while awake, progressing to qid by discharge.
Pain *r/t* *Surgical incisions (chest and legs)* *Chest tubes* *Early mobility attempts*	Demonstrate comfort to enable coughing, moving, ambulating, eating, and sleep/rest.
High risk for infection *r/t* *Incisions*	WBC: WNL Afebrile

Plan of Care (cont'd)

Immunosuppression associated with CPBP *Potential pulmonary complications* *Inadequate nutrition* *Inadequate sleep*	Evidence of incisional healing
Activity intolerance *r/t* *Pain* *Anemia*	Participate in activity progression prescription Balance rest and activity periods
Decreased nutrition *r/t* *NPO status* *GI response to anesthesia* *Loss of appetite* *Pain* *Stress response* *Stress associated with procedure*	NG tube removed Diet progression to low salt, low cholesterol general diet with sufficient calories to promote wound healing and general recovery
High risk of ineffective sleep/rest pattern *r/t* *Hospital environment/routine* *Medications*	Patient will have at least 6 hours of uninterrupted sleep per night by postoperative day 2
High risk for patient/family anxiety *r/t uncertainty about caring for patient at home, fear of self-care*	Express fears related to recovery and self-care State decreased anxiety level Patient will sleep Family will leave hospital at appropriate times
Self-care deficit *r/t lack of knowlege about discharge regimen*	Verbalize dietary management Describe activity progression Perform physical care procedures within limitations of energy level Verbalize signs and symptoms of delayed complications and appropriate interventions Describe follow-up care

INTERVENTIONS

Perform incentive spirometry q2h while awake initially, progressing to qid by discharge *to promote lung expansion and combat atelectasis. Atelectasis and pleural effusions are more common in patients who have had IMA grafts.*

Instruct and assist in the use of a blanket or pillow to splint surgical incisions or use a sternal support/splint device *to decrease pain and promote lung expansion.*

Position patient in semi-Fowler's position *to promote chest expansion.*

Assist patient to chair prior to chest tube removal *to facilitate chest cavity drainage.*

Apply and maintain an occlusive dressing to the chest tube site(s) for 24 to 48 hours postremoval *to prevent pneumothorax or tension pneuomothorax.*

Facilitate early removal of invasive monitoring lines and urethral catheter *to prevent secondary infection.*

Assess GI system and advance diet as tolerated *to ensure adequate nutrition needed for wound healing and general recovery.*

Assist with ambulation at least 4 times per day progressing to independent ambulation 4 to 6 times per day in collaboration with cardiac rehabilitation staff.

Assist patient to chair and reinforce teaching related to elevation of lower extremities *to prevent deep-vein thrombosis and leg edema.*

Monitor neurologic function. *Transient confusion, behavioral changes, and depression are most common in patients with advanced age, severe preoperative cardiac dysfunction, history of psychiatric illness, sleep deprivation, or prolonged ICU stays.*[42] *Transient brachial plexus injury may be caused by sternal retraction.*

Provide for rest periods and 6 hours of uninterrupted sleep at night by postoperative day 2 *to enable wound healing, minimize infection risk, prevent post-pericardiotomy delirium, and promote general recovery.*

Plan of Care (cont'd)

Assess pain carefully, including the nature, location, intensity, and response to intervention. *Change in the nature, severity, or location of pain, or failure to respond to intervention, could signal a complication such as graft occlusion, myocardial ischemia, pulmonary emboli, post-pericardiotomy syndrome (PPS), or sternal wound infection.*[9]

Observe for signs and symptoms of PPS: persistent low-grade temperature, pericardial friction rub, persistent nonspecific chest discomfort, slightly elevated WBC, nonspecific ECG changes of ST-T-wave abnormalities, elevated sedimentation rate. *PPS occurs in 10% to 50% of patients and has been postulated to be an autoimmune response to blood remaining in the pericardial or pleural cavity.*[40]

Continue to carefully monitor I/O as well as weight *as an indicator of renal function and fluid volume status. The patient should return to preoperative weight in 3 to 5 days.*

Monitor for CHF, *which may occur 2 to 5 days postoperatively due to increased circulating volume from fluid shifts and poor cardiac reserve.*

Begin patient/family instruction regarding wound care, continued respiratory care, ambulation/activity regime, dietary requirements to promote recovery, and life-style modification requirements specific to the patient *to optimize patient and family potential for adequate self-care post-discharge.*

Begin patient/family instruction regarding follow-up care requirements, the importance of outpatient cardiac rehabilitation, and S/S to notify the physician for events such as fever, indicators of incision infection, palpitations, regression in activity tolerance, shortness of breath, increased chest or incisional discomfort, return of preoperative angina, or fluid retention *to ensure continued, safe surgical recovery following discharge.*

TRANSITION TO DISCHARGE

The patient who has had an uneventful postoperative course will make the transition to discharge on approximately postoperative day 4 or 5. An assessment of the patient's learning capabilities and motivation for life-style modification made preoperatively will be valuable to the nurse at this time to guide in the patient teaching process. Patients will need to learn specific techniques for self-care, specifically life-style modification to reduce cardiac risk factors, signs and symptoms of surgical complications, and plans for follow-up care. Patients and their families are anxious about discharge and must have all of their questions and concerns related to postoperative care answered openly and honestly. The family's involvement is essential at this time, as they will become the primary caretakers following patient discharge. Therefore, nursing priorities in the transition to discharge phase relate to patient/family education, continually improving activity tolerance, and promoting wound healing and general recovery.

REFERENCES

1. Allen JK: Physical and psychosocial outcomes after coronary artery bypass graft surgery: review of the literature, *Heart Lung* 19(1):49-54, 1990.
2. American Heart Association: *1991 heart and stroke facts,* Dallas, 1991, The American Heart Association.
3. American Heart Association: *1992 heart and stroke facts,* Dallas, 1992, The American Heart Association.
4. Bell PE, Diffe GT: Cardiopulmonary bypass: principles, nursing implications, *AORN J* 53(6):1479-1504, 1991.
5. Cardiology Preeminence Roundtable: *Aggressive bypass surgery recovery (decreasing postoperative LOS),* Washington, DC, 1993, The Advisory Board Co.
6. Cella AS, Bush CA, Codignotto B: Same-day admission for cardiac surgery: a benefit to patient, family, and institution, *J Cardiovasc Nurs* 7(4):14-29, 1993.
7. Coleman B, Lavieri MC, Gross S: Patients undergoing cardiac surgery. In Clochesy JM, et al, editors: *Critical care nursing,* Philadelphia, 1993, WB Saunders, pp 385-436.
8. Deaton DW, Engleman R: Fast-track treatment protocol speeds recovery of cardiopulmonary bypass patients. News release from the American College of Surgeons, October 11, 1993.
9. Earp JK, Finlayson DC: Urinary bladder/pulmonary artery temperature ratio of less than 1 and shivering in cardiac surgical patients, *Am J Crit Care* 1(2):43-52, 1992.
10. Evans SA: The economics of cardiac surgery, *AACN Clin Iss Crit Care Nurs* 4(2):340-348, 1993.
11. Feng WC, et al: Perioperative paraplegia and multi-organ failure from heparin-induced thrombocytopenia, *Ann Thorac Surg* 55(6):1555-1557, 1993.
12. Finkelmeier BA, et al: Influence of age on postoperative course in coronary artery bypass patients, *J Cardiovasc Nurs* 7(4):38-46, 1993.
13. Fisch C, et al: ACC/AHA guidelines and indications for coronary artery bypass graft surgery, *Circulation* 83(3):1125-1173, 1991.

14. Geraci JM, et al: Predicting the occurrence of adverse events after coronary artery bypass surgery, *Ann Intern Med* 118(1):18-24, 1993.
15. Gilski DJ: Controversies in patient management after cardiac surgery, *J Cardiovasc Nurs* 7(4):1-13, 1993.
16. Gortner SR, Dirks J, Wolfe MM: The road to recovery: elders after CABG, *Am J Nurs,* pp 44-49, Aug. 1992.
17. Gross SB: Current challenges, concepts, and controversies in chest tube management, *AACN Clin Iss Crit Care Nurs* 4(2):260-275, 1993.
18. Halfman-Franey M, Gabel K, Berg DE: Re-operation: cardiac surgery. *AACN Clin Iss Crit Care Nurs* 1(1):72-78, 1990.
19. Reference deleted in proofs.
20. Heye ML: Pain and discomfort after coronary artery bypass surgery, *J Cardiovasc Nurs* 27(4):19-24, 1991.
21. Howell RD, et al: Effects of two types of head coverings in the rewarming of patients after coronary artery bypass graft surgery, *Heart Lung* 21:1-5, 1992.
22. Howie JN: Hypothermia and rewarming after cardiac operation, *Focus Crit Care* 18(5):414-418, 1991.
23. Jansen KJ, McFadden PM: Postoperative nursing management of patients undergoing myocardial revascularization with the internal mammary artery bypass, *Heart Lung* 15(1):48-54, 1986.
24. King K, et al: Patient perceptions of quality of life after coronary artery surgery: was it worth it? *Res Nurs Health* 15(5):327-334, 1992.
25. King KB, et al: Coronary artery bypass graft surgery in older women and men, *Am J Crit Care* 1(2):28-35, 1992.
26. Ley SJ: Myocardial depression after cardiac surgery: pharmacologic and mechanical support, *AACN Clin Iss Crit Care Nurs* 4(2):293-308, 1993.
27. Ley SJ, et al: Crystalloid versus colloid therapy after cardiac surgery, *Heart Lung* 19(1):31-40, 1990.
28. Lytle BW: Conduit options for coronary artery bypass surgery. In Grillo, et al, editors: *Current therapy in cardiothoracic surgery,* Toronto, 1989, BC Decker.
29. Monsein S, Constancia P: Retrograde coronary sinus perfusion: a new approach to cardioplegia delivery, *AACN Clin Iss Crit Care Nurs* 1(1):59-64, 1990.
30. Mravinac CM, Dracup K, Clochesy J: Urinary bladder and rectal temperature monitoring during clinical hypothermia, *Nurs Res* 38(2):73-76, 1989.
31. Nair R, Thames MD: When to consider angioplasty or CABG in ischemic syndromes, *Consultant,* pp 62-75, May 1992.
32. Norris SO: Managing low cardiac output states: maintaining volume after cardiac surgery, *AACN Clin Iss Crit Care Nurs* 4(2):309-319, 1993.
33. Naunheim KS, et al: Coronary artery bypass surgery in patients aged 80 years or older, *Am J Cardiol* 59:804-807, 1987.
34. Osguthorpe SG: Hypothermia and rewarming after cardiac surgery, *AACN Clin Iss Crit Care Nurs* 4(2):276-292, 1993.
35. Rogers WJ, et al: Ten-year follow-up of quality of life in patients randomized to receive medical therapy or coronary artery bypass graft surgery—the coronary artery surgery study (CASS), *Circulation* 82:1647-1658, 1990.
36. Rosborough D: Surgical myocardial revascularization in the 1990s, *AACN Clin Iss Crit Care Nurs* 4(2):219-227, 1993.
37. Ruiz B, et al: Predictors of general activity 8 weeks after cardiac surgery, *Appl Nurs Res* 5(2):59-65, 1992.
37a. *St Anthony's DRG guidebook 1995,* Reston, Va, 1994, St Anthony.
38. Sellick JA, Stelmach M, Mylotte JM: Surveillance of surgical wound infections following open heart surgery, *Infect Control Hosp Epidemiol* 12:591-596, 1991.
39. Sethi GK, et al: Implications of preoperative administration of aspirin in patients undergoing coronary artery bypass grafting, *J Am Coll Cardiol* 15(1):15-20, 1990.
40. Shafer JA, Schulkers N, Wexler L: Ambulatory postoperative care of patients following coronary artery bypass and valve replacement surgery: discussion and algorithms, *Prog Cardiovasc Nurs* 6(1):3-12, 1991.
41. Shinn JA: Management of a patient undergoing myocardial revascularization: coronary artery bypass graft surgery, *Nurs Clin North Am* 27(1):243-256, 1992.
42. Stewart SL, et al: Cardiac surgery. In Kinney MR, Packa DR, Dunbar SB, editors: *AACN's clinical reference for critical care nursing,* ed 3, St Louis, 1993, Mosby–Year Book, pp 635-657.
43. Teplitz L: Update: are milking and stripping chest tubes necessary? *Focus on Critical Care* 18(6):506-511, 1991.
44. Van der Meer J, et al: Prevention of one-year-graft occlusion after aortocoronary-bypass surgery: a comparison of low-dose aspirin, low-dose aspirin plus dipyridamole, and oral anticoagulants, *Lancet* 342:257-264, 1993.
45. Walls JT, et al: Heparin-induced thrombocytopenia in patients undergoing intra-aortic balloon pumping after open heart surgery, *ASAIO Journal* 38(3):M574-M576, 1992.
46. Walls JT, et al: Heparin-induced thrombocytopenia in patients who undergo open heart surgery, *Surgery* 108(4):686-692, 1990.
47. Walls JT, et al: Heparin-induced thrombocytopenia in open heart surgery patients: sequelae of late recognition, *Ann Thorac Surg* 53(5):787-791, 1992.
48. Williamson JW: The effects of ocean sounds on sleep after coronary artery bypass graft surgery, *Am J Crit Care* 1(1):91-97, 1992.
49. Wright JS, Fredrickson DT, editors: Cardiovascular disease: guidelines for prevention and care: reports of the Inter-Society Commission for Heart Disease Resources, Washington DC, 1972, U.S. Government Printing Office.

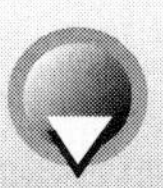

CLINICAL GUIDELINE

21

Cardiac Trauma

Kimberly Woods-McCormick, BSN, RN, CCRN

DESCRIPTION

Trauma is the leading cause of death in children and adults under the age of 44.[4] In fact, a manifestation of cardiac concussion known as commotio cordis is the single most common cause of traumatic death associated with youth sports.[1] Trauma of the heart and aorta that results in rupture or tamponade has the highest mortality. As many as 80% of cardiovascular trauma victims die before reaching the hospital.[17,19] Survival is dependent on the extent of the injury, time elapsed before treatment, and the speed of the health care team. In the event that only a superficial myocardial contusion occurred, mortality is rare and patients may be safely discharged within days.

Because there is a limited window of opportunity to intervene with cardiovascular trauma victims, rapid, aggressive intervention is essential. Assessment of the mechanism of injury must be carefully completed. An index of suspicion based on history helps in the prediction of serious complications. Rapid identification of all possible injuries must be a priority. Life-threatening injuries must be stabilized rapidly. Any delay in the assessment and intervention process significantly increases the risk of death. Persistent assessment is necessary because physiologic compensation responses may mask complications.

Trauma to the cardiovascular system is caused by two primary types of injuries: blunt and penetrating trauma. Blunt, or nonpenetrating, trauma is the result of an external force against the chest that results in injury to the chest wall and the heart itself. The majority of blunt trauma is caused by motor vehicle accidents in which the chest strikes the steering wheel, dashboard, or other passengers.[7]

Most penetrating trauma is associated with violent crime. Penetrating trauma is the result of an object or missile propelled through the chest wall into the heart, creating an opening to the outside. Stabbings and gunshot wounds to the heart are the most lethal of traumatic injuries, resulting in rapid deterioration of cardiac function. Although stabbings are the most frequent injuries seen, the number of gunshot wounds to the chest is increasing as violent crime increases in society. Increased mortality is associated with penetrating trauma that demonstrates the characteristics listed in the following Box.[4]

Historically, traumatic injuries to the heart have been beyond clinical intervention. The recent development of sophisticated trauma systems has increased effective resuscitation in the field, enabling more patients to reach the hospital alive. Once they arrive at a reasonably well-equipped emergency room, patient prognosis is much improved.

PATHOPHYSIOLOGY

Blunt Trauma

There is a broad spectrum of injury seen in blunt trauma, including myocardial contusion, concussion, cardiac chamber rupture, aortic rupture, and myocardial tamponade. Most blunt trauma occurs with motor vehicle accidents; other mechanisms include falls, crush injuries, sporting accidents, and acts of violence. The mechanism of injury in blunt trauma includes acceleration, deceleration, shearing, and compression.[5] Acceleration is an increase in the rate of velocity or speed of a moving object. Deceleration is a decrease in the velocity of a moving object. The rapid deceleration in motor vehicle accidents (MVA) can cause major vessels to stretch and bow.[5] Shearing is produced when stretching forces are applied at a 90-degree angle and exceed

Characteristics of Penetrating Cardiac Trauma Associated with Increased Mortality

Large, open wound
Wound created by a gunshot
Lacerated coronary arteries or aorta
Multiple cardiac chambers or left ventricle involved
Delayed diagnosis or treatment

the elasticity of vessels. Shearing damage causes the vessels to tear, dissect, rupture, or form aneurysms. Shearing damage occurs in the vessels as they decelerate at a different speed from the areas they perfuse. The most common horizontal deceleration pattern of injury seen with MVA results in torn, crushed, ruptured, lacerated, or concussed heart and great vessels.[16] When compressive forces are applied to vessels or tissues, the surface may remain unchanged while underlying structures sustain spasm, thrombus, and tissue failure.

Compressive force is a factor in contusion injuries.[5] Myocardial contusion is one of the most common injuries seen in blunt trauma. Contusion is the result of a direct blow to the chest. The heart's right ventricle is the most vulnerable to anterior trauma. The aortic and mitral valves are highly susceptible to injuries due to the increased pressure in the left side of the heart compounded by the force of the trauma and the resulting instability of the aorta. Contusions are caused by red blood cells extravasating around injured myocardial fibers.[6] Cellular rupture is thought to result in systemic increases in creatine kinase MB (CK-MB). Contusions are well-circumscribed lesions at both gross and microscopic levels and resolve as the hemorrhage is reabsorbed and fibrotic healing occurs.[6]

A predictable pattern of rhythm disturbances has been associated with cardiac contusion that includes cardiac arrest immediately after impact.[3] Additional dysrhythmias include AV blocks and bradycardias. ST segment changes are not attributed to myocardial contusion but to previously existing coronary artery disease. Myocardial dysfunction has been related to transient reduction in coronary blood flow resulting in global ischemia, electrical instability, and direct myocyte damage. Of all dysrhythmias requiring treatment, 80% are usually seen in the emergency department.[6] Dysrhythmias from myocardial contusion are rare to nonexistent after 24 hours.[7,8] Dysrhythmias seen after 24 hours are generally associated with preexisting cardiac disease or myocardial infarction. The spectrum of injury in myocardial contusion is related to the size and forces involved in the injury. If the injury is localized, the potential for complications remains small. When the injury is large, myocardial tearing, tamponade, and rupture may occur.

Aortic Disruption

Traumatic aortic rupture is considered the most severe of all traumatic cardiovascular injuries with less than 10% survival.[9] Acute traumatic aortic transection is described as dehiscence of all or part of the aortic wall.[20] The transection may be complete, involving the aortic adventitia and mediastinal pleura. Death occurs instantly from rupture that causes profound hemorrhage. If the tear involves all the layers of the aortic wall with the exception of the mediastinal pleura, blood may escape into the retropleural tissues with obvious signs of hemorrhagic shock. Victims of aortic rupture who arrive at the hospital alive do so because the aortic adventitia balloons out with the resulting aortic tamponade serving to compress the intimal tear. This false aneurysm prevents immediate exsanguination.[13] Pseudoaneurysm or partial circumferential hematoma formation will prolong the patient's life, but is clearly a time-limited effect.[5] The descending portion of the thoracic aorta is most often damaged because it is partially fixed posteriorly at the ligamentum arteriosum. This point of attachment takes the brunt of traumatic tensile forces, making it the most vulnerable to rupture. Shearing and tearing result when one area of the aorta moves while the isthmus remains immobile. Another reason for arterial layers to shear and tear is because the layers themselves vary in tensile strength. The adventitia has greater strength than the medial layer, causing shearing within the aorta itself.[15] Tears vary in size from millimeters to several centimeters.

Penetrating Trauma

The pathophysiology of penetrating cardiac injuries correlates with the penetrating object's size, the mode of entry, and the site of the injury. Knives, bullets, and other penetrating objects may lodge in the pericardium and ventricular wall. The chest wall offers little protection against such traumatic injuries. If ribs are fractured, they may become penetrating objects. Extensive damage from the forces created by the kinetic energy of the penetrating object and subsequent destruction of cells is compounded by contaminated materials that may be carried into the wound with the projectile. In addition, the presence of acidosis and shock have been suggested to correlate with reduced survival more than the actual site of the cardiac injury.[19] In stabbings, 90% present with tamponade and may deceivingly appear relatively stable.[19] Tamponade offers a protective effect by delaying exsanguination. Gunshot wounds, however, present with profound hemorrhage, shock, and exsanguination. In addition, penetrating injuries are often associated with other injuries of the abdomen and thorax that compound hypovolemic shock and tamponade.[19]

Cardiac Tamponade

Cardiac tamponade is another life-threatening complication of cardiac trauma. In acute cardiac trauma, blood rapidly accumulates in the pericardium. The pericardium can normally hold 25 cc of fluid.[5] In tamponade, blood enters the pericardial space and exerts pressure within the relatively nonelastic pericardial sac. This rapid accumulation of blood causes pressure that inhibits the ventricles from filling. Endocardial ischemia also occurs and progresses rapidly to cardiac failure. When tamponade occurs, compensatory mechanisms may initially maintain an adequate cardiac output. These include tachycardia, vasoconstriction, and increased venous return to the heart. However, as intrapericardial and ventricular end-diastolic pressures rise, stroke volume falls to a point where compensatory mechanisms can no longer maintain the cardiac output. The resulting severe reduction in cardiac output causes hypotension shock, and total circulatory collapse.[11]

Traumatic tamponade may differ from the classic presentation of tamponade. Beck's triad of systemic hypotension, muffled heart tones, and elevated venous pressure is the classic presentation of tamponade. However, elevated venous pressure may be obscured by hypovolemia in traumatic tamponade. Muffled heart tones and a paradoxical pulse may be impossible to assess. Hypotension that is unresponsive to volume infusion or vasopressors, or is out of proportion to the observed degree of blood loss, may be the best indication of tamponade.[19] In addition, blood that accumulates in the pericardium from trauma comes from the ventricle. As a result, it will clot almost immediately. Blood that does not accumulate rapidly will be affected by the motion of the heart and will not clot. Pericardiocentesis may relieve the pressure of tamponade in the classic presentation of this syndrome but may not be successful in traumatic injuries without repair of the injury first.

Coexistent Injuries

Identifying other coexisting injuries is a challenge for care givers of the victim with cardiac trauma. Injuries to the brain, spine, and abdomen may cloud the presentation of tamponade or contusion. Substance abuse is also a consideration in all types of myocardial trauma. Alcohol may decrease myocardial performance and potentiate dysrhythmias. Drug abuse may increase the risk for endocarditis, mycotic aneurysm, and vascular complications.[19] The use of cocaine prior to the injury may precipitate dysrhythmias or a myocardial infarction in an already gravely traumatized heart.

LENGTH OF STAY/ANTICIPATED COURSE

If the patient is alive upon admission to the emergency department, he or she is in extremis and requires full trauma resuscitation. Presentation with a systolic blood pressure over 90 mm Hg is associated with survival of 90% or greater.[14] In all cases, the anticipated course of the patient is dependent on the extent of the cardiac injuries and other concomitant traumatic injuries. DRG 487: Other Multiple Significant Trauma, with an average LOS of 10.2 days, is the most likely DRG assignment for patients with cardiac trauma who are not dead on arrival (DOA).[18]

Patients who have sustained a myocardial contusion that is uncomplicated and who are without risk factors for coronary artery disease no longer require observation in the intensive care setting. Observation on a telemetry unit is sufficient to rule out and treat dysrhythmias and pain. In contrast, the patient who has sustained a gunshot wound to the chest may spend weeks in the intensive care unit due to complications that may include heart failure, myocardial infarction, pericarditis, sepsis, and ineffective wound closure. In addition, over 50% of trauma patients may develop postpericodotomy syndrome, which may prolong the intermediate phase of care.[19]

MANAGEMENT TRENDS AND CONTROVERSIES

Changes in the care of the cardiac trauma patient have been precipitated by more effective resuscitation at the scene of the injury. More patients are surviving what was once certain death, even though the use of lifesaving devices such as pneumatic antishock garments (PASG) has been challenged. Although many prehospital protocols recommend their use, several sources cite concern that PASG may accelerate exsanguination by forcing more blood into the chest and injured heart.[10] Agreement does exist, however, that PASGs are useful in stabilizing pelvic fractures, abdominal bleeding, and femur fractures.

Traumatic cardiac injuries require a broad range of therapy. This may include such heroic measures as emergency thoracotomy in the emergency department as well as simple monitoring of heart rhythm. The medical-nursing team in the emergency department will begin resuscitative care as soon as the patient is received. Resuscitative care may include assessment of hemorrhage and life-threatening dysrhythmias, control of hemorrhage, and rapid administration of crystalloids and colloids for fluid resuscitation. Pleural chest tube insertion with autotransfusion or pericardiocentesis may be necessary as well.

The patient who is dying from penetrating chest injuries requires immediate surgical intervention. Available resources will dictate whether this is performed in the emergency department or the operating room. The surgical incision of choice is dependent on the stability of the patient. In the emergency room, a patient who cannot be stabilized will require a left anterior thoracotomy to decrease time and surgical resources. A patient who is stable enough to be transported to the operating room will undergo median sternotomy to allow optimal visualization of wound.[14] Once the chest is opened, immediate assessment of bleeding and/or tamponade is initiated. Digital pressure will be applied to bleeding sites initially followed by vascular clamps. Tamponade may be relieved by pericardial incision and evacuation of blood. A pericardial window may be created and drained via a closed chest drainage system. Wound closure must be done cautiously to avoid damaging coronary arteries or creating tears in the ventricles. Horizontal mattress sutures may be strengthened with Teflon felt pledgets or strips of pericardium to prevent sutures from tearing through damaged heart tissue. If damage is extensive, cardiopulmonary bypass may be used but with extreme caution because of the increased risk of bleeding for the traumatized patient.

Missiles may be difficult to remove immediately due to cardiovascular instability but may require surgery later to prevent migration. Valvular injuries may require immediate replacement if regurgitation and heart failure are present. Septal injury repair may be postponed for up to 3 months to allow for fibrosis and better wound closure.[19] Aortic tears will be repaired using Dacron grafts with aortic cross-clamping or shunt bypass techniques.[5]

In contrast to penetrating trauma, blunt cardiac trauma is managed medically with close observation for complications. Research regarding assessment of cardiac injuries from blunt trauma reveals considerable differences. The use of expensive diagnostic aids such as echocardiography and radionuclide studies may not be warranted in the initial diagnosis but are considered valuable in the diagnosis of hidden defects or myocardial decompensation later on.[6,7] Serum myocardial enzymes have been reported by some to be the most reliable indicator of injury whereas others consider them to be a poor predictor of pump failure or dysrhythmias.[2,6,7] More research is needed to determine the efficacy of CK-MB as a guide to the management of cardiac contusion.

An ECG is important in determining the presence of myocardial contusion. However, confusion exists regarding which dysrhythmias are most closely associated with contusion versus infarction. As a result, monitoring for ST segment changes and continuous ECG monitoring over 24 hours has been suggested to be unnecessary by some investigators but essential for up to 72 hours by others.[2,3,7] The cost of monitoring patients with cardiac contusion could be significantly reduced if a method could be found to differentiate the population at greatest risk for infarction following trauma so that only they would be monitored.

The age of the patient is another factor in the assessment and management of cardiac trauma. Patients over 60 years of age may not demonstrate the widened mediastinum typically seen on chest x-ray with tamponade or aortic injuries.[15] As a result, the elderly must be monitored clinically with even greater vigilance. Children and adolescents are more likely to present with cardiac contusion as a result of a sports injury. The associated activity serves as a useful adjunct in swift diagnosis and intervention. Unfortunately, cardiac concussion appears to have more immediate direct dire consequences than contusion for young adolescent victims. Commotio cordis often results in ventricular dysrhythmias and cardiac standstill that are resistant to resuscitative therapy.[12] The pathophysiologic reasons for this grim outcome are unclear.[1] More research is needed in this area to prevent children from dying secondary to blows to the chest by baseballs and hockey pucks, and other sports-related injuries.

A major trend in trauma care is rapid transport, assessment, and management. To change mortality statistics, the victim must receive rapid operative therapy. Trauma alert and "on-call" systems must be organized so that initiation of trauma surgery may be immediate. Such systems are costly, and the population that they serve is small. As a result, sophisticated trauma system have become very controversial outside large metropolitan trauma centers.

On a final note, the violence too often associated with cardiac trauma is finding its way into the once-safe confines of the hospital. Family and gang members are bringing weapons with them when they visit victims. The safety of both victims and health care workers is an escalating issue for all hospitals.

ASSESSMENT

PARAMETER	ANTICIPATED ALTERATION
Cardiac Tamponade	
HR	Tachycardia: HR >120 bpm
BP	Narrowed pulse pressure *due to impaired ventricular filling* Paradoxical pulse >10 mm Hg *due to increased effect of intrathoracic pressure changes associated with respiration on the compressed heart* Hypotension: SBP <90 mm Hg and often <70 mm Hg *due to blood loss and shock*
Heart sounds	Muffled, S3, murmurs *due to blood trapped in the pericardial sac*
Rhythm	Electrical alternans, pulseless electrical activity (PEA), ventricular dysrhythmias
CI	Decreased: <2.5 L/min/m^2 *due to frank cardiac failure*
CVP, PAD, PCWP	CVP increased: >12 mm Hg with equalization of pressure CVP = PAD = PCWP *due to external compression on entire heart*
Chest x-ray	Widended mediastinum *unless patient is over 60 or very hypovolemic*
ABGs	Respiratory/metabolic acidosis *due to respiratory failure and decreased CO*

RR	Tachypnea: RR >26, labored
LOC	Anxious, restless, confusion progressing to unresponsiveness
Physical findings	Skin cool, diaphoretic prolonged capillary refill >3 seconds, UO <30 cc/hr

Aortic Rupture

HR	Tachycardia: HR >110 bpm
BP	Initial hypertension until rupture, then profound hypotension with SBP <70 mm Hg *due to sympathetic response of stretched baroreceptors followed by rapid loss of circulating volume and failure of compensatory mechanisms*[17] In pseudocoarctation, BP may be elevated in upper extremities and decreased in lower extremities *due to the decrease in size of aortic lumen resulting from the hematoma*[17]
Rhythm	PEA, ventricular dysrhythmias
Chest wall	Ecchymosis, rib and sternal fractures *due to direct trauma of the chest and thorax*
Chest x-ray	Widened mediastinum Tracheal deviation
Chest pain	Searing, unrelenting deep pain that radiates to the back *due to tearing or dissecting of the aorta*
Aortograms/transesophageal echocardiography	Tears or aneurysms in compensating patients

Cardiac Contusion

Rhythm	Ventricular tachycardia, asytole, AV block, prolonged QT intervals *due to cellular action potential changes that occur with the myocardial injury, seen upon admission in 80% of cases*
Chest pain	Dull, intensity ranges from extreme to vague
BP	Variable: hypertension may be seen *due to catecholamine release, otherwise BP is related to rhythm*
CK-MB	Elevated >5% *due to cellular rupture in response to the force of injury*
CI	May be decreased: <2.5 L/min/m^2 *due to larger contusions causing decreased contractility*
Echocardiogram	May show wall motion abnormalities *due to the presence of hematoma*

PLAN OF CARE

INTENSIVE PHASE

The intensive care phase of care is characterized by uniting the routine care typical for cardiac surgery patients in the event surgical intervention was required with the potential for complications that characterizes the care of multiple-trauma patients. Cardiothoracic trauma patients have greater potential for developing DIC, systemic inflammatory response syndrome (SIRS), multiple organ dysfunction syndrome (MODS), and myocardial rupture than other critically ill cardiac patients.[8] The goal of therapy in this phase is rapid assessment and intervention for potentially catastrophic complications with or without surgical intervention.

PATIENT CARE PRIORITIES	EXPECTED PATIENT OUTCOMES
Decreased cardiac output *r/t tamponade, shock*	MAP: WNL CI: WNL
Fluid volume deficit *r/t hemorrhage*	VS stable CVP and PCWP: WNL Chest tube drainage within ordered parameters

Plan of Care (cont'd)

High risk for impaired gas exchange *r/t decreased CO, oxygen delivery, respiratory failure*	ABG: within patient norms SVO_2: WNL
Pain *r/t injury and/or surgical intervention*	Patient indicates pain is controlled Is able to engage in activity, rest, and sleep.
High risk for infection *r/t probable wound contamination*	Temperature: WNL Wounds clean, dry and intact WBCs: WNL Skin intact
Impaired mobility *r/t possibility of other injuries and initial care requirements*	Skin intact Joints remain supple Minimal loss of strength

INTERVENTIONS

Maintain a high level of suspicion when history may indicate covert injuries.
Maintain patent airway *to ensure optimal oxygenation.*
Monitor cardiac rhythm continuously *to promptly detect and treat the likely dysrhythmias.*
Monitor continuously for signs of tamponade, especially hypotension and equalization of CVP, PAD, and PCWP *to ensure rapid intervention.*
Monitor pulse oximetry *to ensure adequate oxygenation and oxygen delivery.*
Administer fluids *to maintain cardiac output.*
Monitor chest tube drainage, maintain water seal system, and use autotransfusion techniques *to prevent pneumothorax, tamponade, and anemia.*
Administer analgesics on a routine schedule with sedation as needed *to maintain reasonable patient comfort and ensure patient participation in care as needed.*
Turn patient and increase activity daily in collaboration with PT *to prevent complications of immobility.*
Monitor intake and output *to assess adequacy of cardiac output and renal function.*
Assess temperature, WBCs, and all wound and incision sites regularly *to detect potential infection as early as possible.*

INTERMEDIATE PHASE

Patients who have sustained blunt cardiac injury may be adequately managed within the context of an intermediate level of care from the time of admission. Patients who required surgical intervention will receive their initial care within the ICU environment and once stabilized, will move on to an intermediate care environment for continued care. The intermediate phase of care continues to focus on close and careful assessment for potential complications while gradually increasing patient strength, mobility, and general recovery.

PATIENT CARE PRIORITIES	EXPECTED PATIENT OUTCOMES
High risk for decreased CO *r/t late occurring dysrhythmias*	ECG within patient norms VS stable
Pain *r/t injury and/or possible surgical intervention*	Patient states pain is controlled and is able to engage in self-care activities, rest, and sleep.
Impaired activity/rest pattern *r/t injuries and initial care requirements*	Activity progresses daily Sleep/activity schedule is reestablished
Self care deficit *r/t knowledge of wound care s/s of infection, physical rehabilitation*	Verbalizes knowledge of all necessary care requirements, exercise program, and when to notify the physician.
High risk for ineffective coping *r/t psychological distress associated with the trauma*	Patient able to express fears and concerns openly and in realistic context.

Plan of Care (cont'd)

INTERVENTIONS

Monitor cardiac rhythm and treat any late occurring dysrhythmias *to ensure adequate CO.*

Monitor need for IV narcotics, weaning to oral analgesics within approximately 72 hours or as indicated *to ensure adequate pain control necessary for general recovery.*

Establish activity/sleep/exercise regime with patient and other members of the health care team *to optimize physical recovery and prevent powerlessness.*

Instruct patient/family regarding wound care regime and s/s of infection *to ensure uncomplicated recovery and appropriate notification of physician if necessary.*

Evaluate activity progression *to determine need for ongoing rehabilitation after discharge.*

Evaluate patient and family coping *to assess psychological recovery and identify potential need for follow-up counseling.*

TRANSITION TO DISCHARGE

The prognosis for the patient who has survived both the resuscitative and intensive phases of care is excellent. Psychological recovery from surviving a violent, near-death experience may present the greatest obstacle to full recovery. Flashbacks, nightmares, or feelings of unresolved anger may occur for an extended period of time. Physical care such as wound management and signs of infection are essential patient education priorities; however, the patient and family may not feel as comfortable with the need for psychological care. Survivors of severe traumatic injury have been shown to benefit from outpatient cardiac rehabilitation and psychotherapy. Both should be considered for the patient who may be faced with changed body image and cardiac sequelae upon discharge. Careful assessment of patient or family need for psychological counseling after discharge may be as important to the ultimate outcome as physical rehabilitation.

REFERENCES

1. Abrunzo TJ: Commotio cordis: the single most common cause of traumatic death in youth baseball, *Am J Dis Child* 45(11):1279-1282, 1991.
2. Bartlett R: Myocardial contusion using the index of suspicion of assessing blunt chest trauma, *DCCN* 10(3):133-139, 1991.
3. Baxter TB, et al: A plea for sensible management of myocardial contusion, *Am J Surg* 158:557-562, 1989.
4. Beaver BM: Care of the multiple trauma victim: the first hour, *Nurs Clin North Am* 25(1):11-21, 1990.
5. Cardona VD, et al: *Trauma nursing from resuscitation through rehabilitation,* ed 2, Philadelphia, 1994, WB Saunders.
6. Christensen MA, Sutton KR: Myocardial contusion: new concepts in diagnosis and management, *Am J Crit Care* 2(1):28-33, 1993.
7. Fabian TC, et al: Myocardial contusion in blunt trauma, *J Trauma* 28(1):50-57, 1988.
8. Fontaine DK: The cutting edge in trauma, *Crit Care Nurs* 13(suppl):14-15, 1993.
9. Hammond SG: Chest injuries in the trauma patient, *Nurs Clin North Am* 25(1):35-43, 1990.
10. Honigman B, et al: The role of the pneumatic antishock garment in penetrating cardiac wounds, *JAMA* 266(17):2398-2340, 1991.
11. Horvath PT: *Care of the adult cardiac surgery patient,* New York, 1984, John Wiley & Sons.
12. Kaplan JA, Korofsy PS, Volturo GA: Commotio cordis in two amateur ice hockey players despite the use of commercial chest protectors, *J Trauma* 34(1):151-153, 1993.
13. Kite JH: Cardiac and great vessel trauma assessment, pathophysiology, and intervention, *J Emerg Nurs* 13(6):346-351, 1987.
14. Mitchell ME, et al: Surgical approach of choice for penetrating cardiac wounds, *J Trauma* 34(1):17-20, 1993.
15. Moore EE: Blunt injury to the thoracic aorta. Presented at the Emergency Medicine and Nursing Symposium, Aspen, Colo, January 17-21, 1993.
16. Rea R, editor: *Trauma nursing core course,* ed 3, Chicago, 1991, ENA.
17. Rosen P, et al: *Emergency medicine concepts and clinical practice,* ed 3, St Louis, 1992, Mosby–Year Book.
18. *St Anthony's DRG guidebook 1995,* Reston, Va, 1994, St Anthony.
19. Smith A, Fitzpatrick E: Penetrating cardiac trauma: surgical and nursing management, *J Card Nurs* 7(2):52-70, 1993.
20. Turner JT: Cardiovascular trauma, *Nurs Clin North Am* 25(1):119-130, 1990.

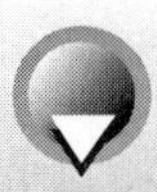

CLINICAL GUIDELINE

22

Percutaneous Transluminal Valvuloplasty

Nancie Urban, MSN, RN, CCRN

DESCRIPTION

Percutaneous transluminal valvuloplasty (PTV) is a nonsurgical method to improve blood flow through stenotic valves. The technique involves inflating one or more large balloons, inserted percutaneously, inside a stenotic valve to force the leaflets or cusps open. The resulting decrease in valvular gradient, or resistance, results in increased antegrade/forward flow through the valve, improved hemodynamics, and decreased signs and symptoms of the congestive heart failure that compromises quality of life for patients with valve stenosis.

Used primarily in the treatment of stenotic mitral or aortic valves, PTV has been used successfully with stenotic pulmonic valves as well.[27] First performed on a newborn in 1979, and then on an 8-year-old in 1982, pulmonic valve PTV established an ongoing outcome of success without mortality and with minimal morbidity in patients of all ages.[18,25,26,36]

Aortic valve PTV was first performed in 1984 in children, but immediate and long-term results were disappointing.[22,23,24] Aortic valvuloplasty has demonstrated the greatest success in adults, especially the elderly who could not withstand surgical aortic valve replacement.[35]

Since it was first attempted in 1984, mitral valve stenosis has been the most frequent target for PTV.[12] Mitral PTV continues to be safely performed with excellent outcomes in patients of all ages even though it is more difficult technically than PTV of other valves.[8] This is especially true in Third World countries where rheumatic heart disease remains endemic and the availability of valve replacement surgery is very limited.[41] In addition, mitral PTV compares favorably to the more traditional mitral commissurotomy procedure, with a double balloon technique producing larger post-PTV valve diameter than single balloon techniques.[37] Significant improvement in both left ventricular ejection fraction and reduction in pulmonary hypertension have been reported following mitral PTV.[2,10,31]

The lower pressure dynamics on the right side of the heart make the risk of performing PTV on the tricuspid valve greater than the problems typically associated with tricuspid stenosis. However, PTV can be performed on the tricuspid valve with results comparable to other valves.

The impact of PTV is related to its palliative intent. PTV results in decreased symptoms of stenosis but does not alter the disease process. PTV is considered a success with almost any reduction of valvular gradient, especially when coupled with reduction of heart failure symptoms in patients. In addition, improvement in quality of life has been reported by patients following PTV.[15] PTV may also have a beneficial effect on platelet activation. Kataoka demonstrated that platelet activation was favorably decreased in patients who experienced optimal dilation of their mitral valves.[19] This effect may have implications for reducing the thromboembolic risk of patients with mitral stenosis even though mitral PTV is not a curative procedure.

Restenosis rates vary based on the degree of calcification of the valves and range from 40% to 66%.[41] The return of severe symptoms of heart failure has also been related to the degree of valve calcification at the time of PTV, ranging from 5% to 7% for noncalcified valves to 30% to 40% for highly calcified valves.[1,30] A more recent study of 5-year survival following mitral PTV in 146 patients has demonstrated 76% overall survival.[8] Considering that 1 to 2 year mortality rates for valve replacement surgery in elderly patients has been quoted as high as 57%, the 95% procedural success rates of PTV coupled with reasonable improvement in symptoms make this procedure a viable option for patients who may not be good surgical candidates.[41] As a result, the very young and the very old benefit the most from PTV.

The impact of PTV on adults who are good candidates for surgical valve replacement remains disputed, with continued preference for surgery. In fact, the use of aortic PTV in the elderly has recently been disputed as no more effective in the long run than valve replacement surgery, despite the surgical risk in this patient population.[5] However, another study demonstrated that aortic PTV could be used to stabilize the hemodynamic and organ status of critically ill patients with aortic stenosis, resulting in a decreased risk profile for follow-up aortic valve replacement.[38] An agreed-upon exception to the use of PTV in the very young and very old is pregnant women with valve stenosis. Without PTV, these women would be unable to safely deliver full-term babies. Valve replacement, especially with a mechanical valve, would make pregnancy a contraindication due to the anticoagulation therapy required. Recent literature consistently reports success in using mitral PTV in pregnant women, enabling successful and safe delivery of healthy infants.[4,11]

PATHOPHYSIOLOGY

PTV is a clinically challenging procedure. While inflated, the balloon occludes the valve, totally obstructing antegrate blood flow through the heart. Balloon inflation is limited to only several seconds up to a maximum of 1 minute as a result. Even so, severe hypotension and dysrhythmias such as bradycardia, complete heart block, and PVCs are common during balloon inflation.[27,40] Vital signs are permitted to return to baseline prior to balloon reinflation that may be necessary for optimal outcomes.

The mechanisms by which PTV improve valvular performance are not clearly understood. At the very least, fused commissures of the mitral valve are stretched or separated.[44] The result is improved blood flow from the left atrium with associated decrease in left atrial pressure and improved left ventricular filling. Piercing the atrial septum with the Mullins catheter during mitral PTV does not result in significant atrial septal defect post-PTV.

In the case of aortic PTV, the noncalcified portions of the valve are thought to be stretched while calcified nodules are fractured.[16] Cardiac output increases as the aortic valve opening is increased. Left ventricular wall tension, afterload, and myocardial oxygen consumption all decrease as well. In all forms of PTV, the sudden improvement in cardiac hemodynamics typically produces a significant decrease in preload. The diuretic effects of contrast material, and diuresis due to the secretion of atrial naturetic hormone stimulated by the brief but significant increases in atrial pressure during balloon inflation, contribute to preload reduction as well. While a positive outcome in the long run, preload reduction may occur faster than the chronically overloaded cardiovascular system can compensate for. The result is often a hypovolemic-like shock pattern, with hypotension and renal impairment occurring within several hours of the procedure unless fluids are carefully managed throughout the procedure and recovery phase.

Considering the rather traumatic nature of the PTV procedure, mortality is surprisingly rare and complications relatively mild. The common complications of PTV are summarized in Table 22-1. Unusual complications of mitral PTV include rupturing of the posterior valve leaflet, rupturing of the chordae tendineae of the anterior leaflet, and tearing of the anterior leaflet, all of which produce mitral regurgitation but without significant clinical symptomatology, and with eventual nonsurgical recovery of all patients.[29]

LENGTH OF STAY/ANTICIPATED COURSE

Patients admitted for PTV require thorough preassessment of their valve disease and hemodynamic status. The sudden improvement in cardiac hemodynamics as a result of the procedure necessitates adequate time to allow hemodynamic stabilization. Most PTV patients also require considerable reevaluation of their medication regimes. As a result, total lengths of stay may range from 4 days to a week, including up to 24 hours in an ICU immediately post-procedure for invasive monitoring and preload management. Elective PTV is grouped under DRG 112: Percutaneous cardiovascular procedures, with an average LOS of 5.3 days.[39]

MANAGEMENT TRENDS AND CONTROVERSIES

PTV is performed in the cardiac catheterization laboratory and includes full hemodynamic monitoring and measurement of valvular gradients. In addition, full heparinization is required to protect the patient from thrombosis and embolization associated with the extensive cannulation and catheter manipulation required with PTV. Once vascular access has been achieved, 5000 to 10,000 units of heparin are administered as a loading dose, with maintenance doses of 2000 to 3000 units administered every 30 minutes during the procedure.[9]

The femoral vein is cannulated for pulmonic and mitral PTV and, occasionally, for aortic PTV as well. Using guide wires, the balloon catheters are maneuvered into position. In the case of pulmonic PTV, the balloon catheter(s) is threaded through the right side of the heart and positioned across the valve orifice. Aortic PTV is typically accomplished via femoral arterial cannulation. The balloon catheter(s) is threaded into the aortic valve in retrograde fashion from the aorta, pointing down into the left ventricle. The

TABLE 22-1 Complications of Percutaneous Transluminal Valvuloplasty

Complication	Cause	Comments
Embolization of calcium deposits	Fracture of calcified nodules within stenotic valves	Rare due to containment of calcification within the endothelium of the valve leaflets or cusps
Embolization of atrial thrombus	Extreme blood flow fluctuations due to balloon inflation that disrupts mural thrombi	Rare, as pre-PTV identification of atrial thrombus is a contraindication for PTV
Embolization of clot formed during the procedure	Presence and manipulation of guide wires, catheters, and balloons within diseased valves	Rare due to full heparinization during PTV procedure
Ventricular dysrhythmias and heart block	Mechanical irritation of myocardium and conduction system by guide wires, catheters, and balloons	Common but transient; resolves with balloon deflation and/or removal of the catheters and guide wires
Bradycardia or asystole	Obstruction of CO during balloon inflation and dramatic fluctuation in intercardiac pressures during procedure	Common but transient; resolves with balloon deflation and/or coughing by patient
Vascular thrombosis or hematoma at femoral cannulation site(s) with potential peripheral perfusion deficit	Large sheaths needed to hold large or multiple balloon catheters, frequent manipulation of catheters, heparinization	Seen in 5% to 20% of patients More common in elderly with tortuous or fragile vessels
Acute MI or death	Lack of coronary artery perfusion during balloon inflation, and potential, prolonged hypotension post-balloon deflation	Seen in 4% to 5% of patients
Hypovolemia with hypotension and renal failure	Sudden increase in antegrade blood flow in a dilated heart, diuresis from contrast material and atrial naturetic hormone released during balloon inflation, potential hemorrhage from femoral cannulation sites	May be prevented by prophylactic administration of fluids, and close monitoring of CVP and PCWP, H&H, APPT, ACT, and VS
Stroke, pulmonary embolus, mesenteric embolus	Embolization of unknown mural thrombus, plaque or valve fragment, inadequate heparinization	Very rare; more likely in debilitated elderly patients with severe valve stenosis
Severe valvular regurgitation	Tearing of the leaflets or cusps of friable valves	Seen in 5% to 6% of patients Usually older patients with less pliable valves
Pulmonary edema	Insufficiently dilated valve, or excess fluid or contrast material administration	Uncommon, but more likely early in the recovery period and in patients with renal insufficiency
Infection with sepsis or endocarditis	Highly invasive procedure; diseased valves are more prone to infection than healthy valves	Strict aseptic technique during procedure and during initial care of sheath sites
Restenosis	Ongoing process of valvular stenosis	Occurs eventually in all PTV patients since PTV is only palliative, not curative

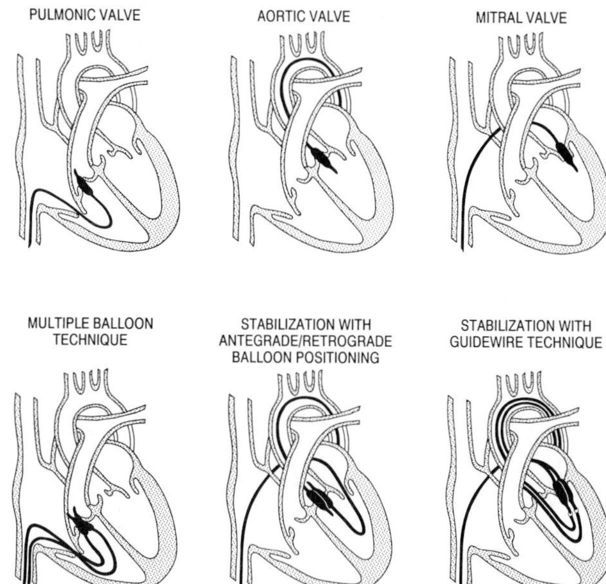

Figure 22-1 Positions of balloons for PTV of pulmonic, aortic, and mitral valves, and examples of multiple balloon and balloon stabilization techniques.

mitral valve is the most difficult to reach. The balloon catheter(s) may be threaded arterially through the left ventricle and positioned in retrograde direction across the mitral valve, pointing into the left atrium. The alternative is to use a Mullins introducer to pierce the atrial septum and provide a conduit through which a balloon catheter may be passed from the right side of the heart into the left atrium and across the mitral valve in antegrade position, pointing down into the left ventricle. Figure 22-1 summarizes the balloon positions for PTV of the various valves.

Due to the tendency of balloons to slip out of position when inflated, they may be placed in both antegrade and retrograde position in either the aortic or mitral valves. The friction between the balloons helps secure their positions during inflation and increases the potential for a successful outcome. As a result, many patients experience both venous and arterial cannulation with large introducers (12 to 14 fr) to accommodate multiple balloon catheters.

Traditional PTV catheters are large (8 to 12 fr) to accommodate the large balloons that vary in size from 5 to 20 mm in length and 8 to 25 mm in diameter. Initially, using a balloon equal to the size of the valve annulus was recommended. Soon thereafter, studies demonstrated that using balloons 20% to 30% larger than the valve annulus produces better results.[33] In the event that a 25-mm balloon is not large enough, several balloons may be used in combination. The alternative is to use an Inoue balloon, which has demonstrated considerable success in dilating even severely stenosed mitral valves with its single-balloon technique.[13,32] The Inoue balloon has also compared favorably to other single- and double-balloon techniques in the dilation of pulmonic valve stenosis.[6,24] Initial concerns regarding a slightly increased risk of mitral regurgitation with the Inoue balloon have been addressed by follow-up studies that demonstrated that the degree of post-PTV regurgitation is as likely due to the degree of valve calcification as to the catheter.[7,14]

The balloon(s) is inflated with a saline/contrast material mixture under variable amounts of pressure up to 4 to 5 atmospheres. Fluoroscopic observation of the inflated balloon(s) typically reveals a "waist," or pinched segment, where the balloon makes contact with the stenotic valve leaflets. The balloon(s) may be inflated repeatedly until the waist disappears, signaling the opening of the valve orifice, or until the balloon ruptures. More recently, transesophageal echocardiography has been used instead of fluoroscopy during PTV. This approach is beneficial when performing PTV on pregnant women so that exposure to fluoroscopy can be avoided.[21] Transesophageal echocardiography has also been shown to assist in catheter placement so that the risk of left atrial thrombus is reduced.[17]

Nursing care of PTV patients presents multiple challenges. Since PTV is most commonly performed on children or the elderly, age-related attention to coping capability as well as physiologic response may be integrated into routine care. Pregnant women require additional reassurance in light of the potential ramifications for the fetus as well as the patient.

The extreme changes in hemodynamics produced by PTV often warrant full hemodynamic monitoring in the ICU setting for a minimum of 24 hours post-procedure.[3,9,28] Preload status is most vulnerable to dramatic reduction due to sudden improvement in cardiac output, diuresis, and potential bleeding from the cannulation sites. As a result, both CVP and PCWP must be monitored closely in addition to vital signs. Early experience with PTV often resulted in the need for fluid resuscitation in response to the sudden decline in preload that routinely occurs within several hours of the procedure. Fluid administration, if begun early, maintains preload status and ensures adequate cardiac output and renal perfusion during the stabilization phase.

Clotting times must also be monitored carefully immediately following PTV to protect the patient from hemorrhage prior to the clearance of heparin from the system. APTT has traditionally been the lab value of choice in monitoring the effects of heparin. Activated clotting time (ACT) has recently been shown to be a more precise indicator of heparin effect and may be tested at the bedside with results available within seconds.[43] Arterial and venous sheath may be left in place until clotting times are within normal ranges. Since femoral placement of the sheaths requires strict activity limitation, sheath removal as soon as possible is advisable.

Additional standard PTV management includes frequent assessment of peripheral perfusion, especially in the cannulated extremities, as well as careful assessment for evidence of heart failure. Considerable readjustment of cardiac medications may be needed in light of the improved hemodynamics and cardiac performance associated with PTV.

Long-term assessment of the efficacy of aortic PTV in the elderly has been recommended, using a functional status questionnaire more accurate than the New York Heart Association classification.[42]

ASSESSMENT

Clinical Assessment

Vital signs	BP may be WNL or slightly decreased pre-PTV *due to CHF.* Hypotension (BP <90 mm Hg systolic) may be seen during balloon inflation and immediately post-PTV *due to interrupted blood flow with inflation and decreased preload following PTV.* HR may be increased: >100 bpm *due to CHF pre-PTV, and hypovolemia post-PTV* RR may be increased: >20/min at rest *due to CHF pre-PTV*
Heart tones	Regular in absence of dysrhythmias S_3 gallop *due to CHF and a dilated ventricle* S_4 with summation gallop *due to noncompliant ventricles, CHF, and tachycardia.* Ejection murmurs in accord with the affected valves *due to valve stenosis* Murmurs of valve regurgitation in accord with the affected valves may be present *due to severe stenosis pre-PTV, and due to reopening of stiff valve leaflets or cusps post-PTV.*
Breath sounds	Decreased breath sounds and/or crackles *due to CHF pre-PTV* Clear breath sounds within 24 to 48 hours post-PTV

Diagnostic Tests

Chest x-ray	Interstitial edema and cardiac enlargement *due to chronic CHF with atrial and ventricular dilatation*
ECG	P wave and/or QRS enlargement with ST-segment elevation *due to atrial and ventricular enlargement with possible ventricular strain pattern associated with chronic CHF* NSR or atrial dysrhythmias (PACs, atrial flutter, atrial fibrillation) with or without PVCs and ventricular tachycardia *due to elevated cardiac pressures and hypoxemia with CHF*
Echocardiography	Decreased ventricular ejection fractions, evidence of valve stenosis and regurgitation, dilated cardiac chambers, and potential wall motion abnormalities *due to valve disease and chronic CHF*
Transesophageal echocardiography	Similar to standard echo but more sensitive for identification of atrial thrombi *due to chronic atrial dilation associated with valve stenosis*[20]
Hemodynamic profile	Elevated preload status pre-PTV *due to valve stenosis and CHF* CVP >8 mm Hg and PCWP >16 mm Hg Decreased preload status post-PTV *due to sudden improvement in antegrade blood flow, diuresis, and possible hemorrhage* CVP <2 mm Hg and PCWP <14 mm Hg CO decreased: <4 L/min, and CI decreased: <2.5 L/min/m^2, pre-PTV *due to chronic CHF.* CO and CI: WNL post-PTV. Elevated afterload status pre- and post-PTV *due to compensatory sympathetic response to decreased CO of valve disease and preload alterations* • PVR >97 dynes/sec/cm^{-5} • PVRI >285 dyne · sec/m^2 · cm^{-5} • SVR >1200 dynes/sec/cm^{-5} • SVRI >2390 dyne · sec/m^2 · cm^{-5}

Cardiac catheterization	Increased pressure gradients across affected valves *due to resistance to blood flow caused by valve stenosis (normal valve gradient = 0%)* Reduction in valve gradient post-PTV

PLAN OF CARE

INTENSIVE PHASE

The initial 24 hours following PTV require vigilant monitoring of the hemodynamic status of patients. The sudden improvement in antegrade flow through the treated valve, in addition to the diuresis associated with the procedure, may result in significant hemodynamic compromise in patients who have long been compensating for an overload state. As a result, many facilities choose to recover PTV patients in the ICU during this phase of care, especially when full invasive hemodynamic monitoring is required.

PATIENT CARE PRIORITIES	EXPECTED PATIENT OUTCOMES
Fluid volume deficit *r/t decreased preload, diuresis, and potential hemorrhage*	BP, HR, CVP, and PCWP: WNL UO >30 cc/hr H&H, APTT, and ACT: WNL
High risk for decreased CO *r/t atrial or ventricular dysrhythmias or heart block during or immediately post-PTV*	NSR or rhythm within patient norms
High risk for peripheral perfusion deficit *r/t thrombosis or hematoma at femoral cannulation sites*	Pulses: WNL Extremities pink, warm CRT <3 sec
General discomfort *r/t strict bed rest and hemodynamic monitoring post-PTV*	Verbalizes comfort Able to rest and sleep

INTERVENTIONS

Monitor ECG continuously *to detect and treat serious dysrhythmias promptly.*

Monitor VS continuously until stable, then q1h to q4h and prn.

Assess CVP and PCWP (may substitute PAD if correlates well with PCWP) q30min to q1h until stable, then q4h and prn for a minimum of 24 hours post-PTV.

Administer fluids prophylactically as ordered *to prevent sudden preload losses, hypotension, and renal impairment.*

Assess femoral cannulation sites q15min initially, then q1h to q4h and prn *to prevent potential hemorrhage, hematoma, and peripheral perfusion deficit.*

Monitor APTT or ACT *to ensure that femoral sheaths are not removed until the effects of heparin have diminished and to prevent associated hemorrhage.*

Monitor heart and breath sounds q4h and prn *to evaluate stabilization of CHF and hemodynamic status.*

Administer analgesics, muscle relaxants, and back rubs with appropriate body positioning *to facilitate general comfort, rest, and sleep during post-PTV bed-rest requirement.*

INTERMEDIATE PHASE

The hemodynamic status of PTV patients usually stabilizes within 24 to 48 hours, eliminating the need for invasive hemodynamic monitoring. Transfer of patients to an intermediate care environment is appropriate at this time. Emphasis is placed on readjusting cardiac medications and preparing the patient for self-care post-discharge in this phase of care.

PATIENT CARE PRIORITIES	EXPECTED PATIENT OUTCOMES
High risk for self-care deficit *r/t changes in cardiac medication*	Patient/family verbalize knowledge of post-PTV medication regime

Plan of Care (cont'd)

Self-care deficit *r/t lack of knowledge about monitoring status of valve disease over time post-PTV*

Patient/family verbalize signs/symptoms of return of valve stenosis, CHF, actions to protect valves, and when to contact the physician

INTERVENTIONS

Instruct patient/family in new cardiac medication regime *to ensure that patients do not overmedicate following PTV.*

Reinforce prior learning about monitoring weight, exercise tolerance, and patient-specific indicators of returning CHF *to ensure that patients seek medical attention in a timely fashion when restenosis of their valves occurs.*

Instruct patient to contact physician prior to any procedure that might permit introduction of bacteria into the bloodstream and result in bacterial endocarditis (e.g., dental work or a proctoscope) *to determine if prophylactic antibiotics are needed since diseased valves are more vulnerable to infection than healthy valves.*

TRANSITION TO DISCHARGE

The relatively short LOS for elective PTV patients compresses the discharge preparation of these patients into the intermediate phase of care. Emphasis is placed on evaluating the ability of the individual to return to maximal independence in ADL. The importance of close follow-up with the patient's cardiologist is also stressed. In select cases, Phase II cardiac rehabilitation may be indicated to ensure maximum increase in exercise tolerance and quality of life post-PTV.

REFERENCES

1. Abscal VM, et al: Echocardiographic evaluation of mitral valve structure and function in patients followed for at least 6 months after percutaneous balloon mitral valvuloplasty, *J Am Coll Cardiol* 12:606-615, 1988.
2. Alfonso F, et al: Percutaneous mitral valvuloplasty with severe pulmonary artery hypertension, *Am J Cardiol,* 72:325-330, 1993.
3. Barden C, et al: Balloon aortic valvuloplasty: nursing care implications, *Crit Care Nurs* 10:22-29, 1990.
4. Ben Farhat M, et al: Percutaneous balloon mitral valvuloplasty in eight pregnant women with severe mitral stenosis, *Eur Heart J* 13:1658-1664, 1992.
5. Bernard Y, et al: Long-term results of percutaneous aortic valvuloplasty compared with aortic valve replacement in patients more than 75 years old, *J Am Coll Cardiol* 20:796-801, 1992.
6. Chen CR, et al: Long-term results of percutaneous mitral valvuloplasty with the Inoue balloon catheter, *Am J Cardiol* 70:1445-1448, 1992.
7. Chen CH, et al: Mitral regurgitation after double balloon or Inoue balloon mitral valvuloplasty, *Chin Med J* 51:176-182, 1993.
8. Cohen DJ, et al: Predictors of long-term outcome after percutaneous balloon mitral valvuloplasty, *N Engl J Med* 327:1329-1335, 1992.
9. Daily EK: Percutaneous balloon valvuloplasty in adult patients with valvular heart disease, *Crit Care Nurs Clin North Am* 1:339-357, 1989.
10. Georgeson S, et al: Effect of percutaneous balloon valvuloplasty on pulmonary hypertension in mitral stenosis, *Am Heart J* 125:1374-1379, 1993.
11. Glantz JC, et al: Percutaneous balloon valvuloplasty for severe mitral stenosis during pregnancy: a review of the therapeutic options, *Obstet Gynecol Surv* 48:503-508, 1993.
12. Glazier JJ, et al: The role of percutaneous transvenous balloon mitral valvuloplasty in the treatment of patients with symptomatic mitral stenosis, *Acta Clin Belg* 47:256-263, 1992.
13. Herrmann HC, et al: Comparison of results of percutaneous balloon valvuloplasty in patients with mild and moderate mitral stenosis to those with severe mitral stenosis, *Am J Cardiol* 71:1300-1303, 1993.
14. Herrmann HC, et al: Mechanisms and outcome of severe mitral regurgitation after Inoue balloon valvuloplasty, *J Am Coll Cardiol* 22:783-789, 1993.
15. Hixon M: Perceived quality of life before and after percutaneous balloon valvuloplasty, *Heart Lung* 21:290, 1990.
16. Isner JM, Samuels DA, Solvenkai GA: Mechanisms of aortic balloon valvuloplasty: fracture of valvular calcific deposits, *Ann Intern Med* 108:377, 1988.
17. Kamalesh M, Burger AJ, Shubrooks SJ: The use of transesophageal echocardiography to avoid left atrial thrombus during percutaneous mitral valvuloplasty, *Cathet Cardiovasc Diagn* 28:320-322, 1993.
18. Kan JS, et al: Percutaneous balloon valvuloplasty: a new method for treating congenital pulmonary valve stenosis, *N Engl J Med* 307:540-542, 1982.
19. Kataoka H, et al: Hemostatic changes induced by percutaneous mitral valvuloplasty, *Am Heart J* 125:777-782, 1993.
20. Kronzon I, et al: Transesophageal echocardiography to detect atrial clots in candidates for percutaneous transseptal mitral balloon valvuloplasty, *J Am Coll Cardiol* 16:1320-1322, 1990.
21. Kultursay H, et al: Mitral balloon valvuloplasty with transesophageal echocardiography without using fluoroscopy, *Cathet Cardiovasc Diagn* 27:317-321, 1992.
22. Lababidi Z, Weinhaus L: Successful balloon valvuloplasty for neonatal critical aortic stenosis, *Am Heart J* 112:913-916, 1986.
23. Lababidi Z, Wu JR, Walls JT: Percutaneous balloon aortic valvuloplasty: results in 23 patients, *Am J Cardiol* 53:194-197, 1984.
24. Lau KW, et al: Pulmonary valvuloplasty in adults using the Inoue balloon catheter, *Cathet Cardiovasc Diagn* 29:99-104, 1993.
25. Masura J, et al: Five-year follow-up after balloon pulmonary valvuloplasty, *J Am Coll Cardiol* 21:132-136, 1993.
26. Mullins CE, et al: Balloon valvuloplasty for pulmonic valve stenosis

two-year follow-up: hemodynamic and Doppler evaluation, *Cathet Cardiovasc Diagn* 14:76-81, 1988.

27. Nishimura RA, Holmes DR, Reeder GS: Percutaneous balloon valvuloplasty, *Mayo Clin Proc* 65:198-220, 1990.
28. Ohler L, Fleagle DJ, Lee BI: Aortic valvuloplasty: medical and critical care nursing perspectives, *Focus Crit Care* 16:275-287, 1989.
29. O'Shea JP, et al: Unusual sequelae after percutaneous mitral valvuloplasty: a Doppler echocardiographic study, *J Am Coll Cardiol* 19:186-191, 1992.
30. Palacios IF, et al: Follow-up of patients undergoing percutaneous mitral balloon valvuloplasty, *Circulation* 79:573-579, 1989.
31. Pan JP, et al: Response of left ventricular ejection performance following balloon valvuloplasty in patients with mitral stenosis, *Chin Med J* 49:303-312, 1992.
32. Park SJ, et al: Immediate and one-year results of percutaneous mitral balloon valvuloplasty using Inoue and double-balloon techniques, *Am J Cardiol* 71:938-943, 1993.
33. Radtke W, et al: Percutaneous balloon valvotomy of congenital pulmonary stenosis using oversized balloons, *J Am Coll Cardiol* 8:909-915, 1986.
34. Rupprath G, Neuhaus KL: Percutaneous balloon valvuloplasty for aortic valve stenosis in infancy, *Am J Cardiol* 55:1655-1656, 1985.
35. Saffian RD, et al: Balloon aortic valvuloplasty in 170 consecutive patients, *N Engl J Med* 319:125-130, 1988.
36. Semb BK, et al: Balloon valvulotomy of congenital pulmonary valve stenosis with tricuspid valve insufficiency, *Cardiovasc Radiol* 2:239-241, 1979.
37. Shrivastava S, et al: Comparison of immediate hemodynamic response to closed mitral commissurotomy, single-balloon and double-balloon mitral valvuloplasty in rheumatic mitral stenosis, *J Thorac Cardiovasc Surg* 104:1264-1267, 1992.
38. Smedira NG, et al: Balloon aortic valvuloplasty as a bridge to aortic valve replacement in critically ill patients. In *St Anthony's DRG guidebook 1995,* Reston, Va, 1994, St Anthony.
39. *St Anthony's DRG guidebook 1995,* Reston, Va, 1994, St Anthony.
40. Steinberg C, Levin AR, Engle MA: Transient complete heart block following percutaneous balloon pulmonary valvuloplasty, *Pediatr Cardiol* 13:181-183, 1992.
41. Straus B, Marquis JF: Percutaneous valvuloplasty as a treatment for aortic and mitral valve disease, *Am Heart J* 119:1184-1192, 1990.
42. Tedesco C, et al: Functional assessment of elderly patients after percutaneous aortic balloon valvuloplasty: New York Heart Association classification versus functional status questionnaire, *Heart Lung* 19:118-125, 1990.
43. Thomason T, et al: Clinical safety and cost of heparin titration using bedside activated clotting time, *Am J Crit Care* 2:81-87, 1993.
44. Vitello-Cicciu J: Aortic and mitral valvuloplasty, *J Cardiovasc Nurs* 1:70-78, 1987.

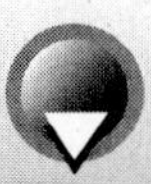

CLINICAL GUIDELINE

23

Valve Repair and Replacement

Gayle R. Whitman, MSN, RN, FAAN

DESCRIPTION

Valvular repair or replacement is primarily recommended for adults with acquired valve disease such as mitral stenosis or regurgitation and aortic stenosis or regurgitation. Presently, approximately 2 million people have an implanted mechanical or biologic valve.[20] Cumulative data on the number of valve repairs are not available but some institutions report that mitral valve commissurotomy and repair account for almost 50% of their mitral valve surgeries.[5] Valve repair techniques consist of commissurotomy, annuloplasty, resection and repair of valve cusps or leaflets, shortening of elongated chords, and chordal transposition.[14]

The valve repair technique of commissurotomy was commonly performed in the 1950s. With this procedure, an incision was made in the left atrium, and the mitral valve was blindly opened by a finger or a surgical dilator. If closed commissurotomy did not produce the desired outcome, the patient was placed on cardiopulmonary bypass and an open commissurotomy was performed. As improvement in cardiopulmonary bypass evolved, longer operative times became acceptable and valve repair decreased while valve replacement increased. Recently, however, there has been a resurgence in valve repair procedures especially of the mitral valve. Dilation of a regurgitant valve annulus can be corrected by an annuloplasty ring, which is a flexible oval ring sewn to the valve annulus. This reshapes the valve orifice so that the mitral leaflets or aortic cusps coapt. Elongated mitral chordae that result in regurgitation may be either surgically shortened, "pleated" upon themselves to shorten them, or have their bases transplanted to another section of the ventricle. Moving the chordae in this fashion prevents the leaflet from "flopping" upward into the atrium. Perforated or torn leaflets or cusps may be patched with pericardium. Studies demonstrate that 5- and 8-year survival rates are higher and complication rates are lower for patients undergoing mitral valve reconstruction techniques when compared to mitral valve replacement.[6,15,19,31] However, aortic valve repair techniques are still evolving, and aortic valve replacement remains the treatment of choice.[11]

Valve replacement consists of resection of the patient's native valve and insertion of either a mechanical, biologic, or allograft valve (Table 23-1). Although only a limited number of valves are currently available in the United States, many of the deleted models remain implanted in patients.[24] As a result, all of the valves will be included in this discussion. As Table 23-1 indicates, there are four types of mechanical valves: the caged ball, the caged disk, the tilting disk, and the bileaflet valve (Figure 23-1). The caged ball valve consists of a ball housed in a cage that is attached to a sewing ring. The ball rests on the sewing ring and moves forward in the cage when a pressure gradient develops. The Starr-Edwards valve still remains a popular valve for implantation, but a caged ball valve in the mitral position produces left ventricular outflow obstruction and ventricular septal irritation in some patients. For these patients a valve with a lower profile is desired. The caged disk valve was designed to meet this need for a lower-profile prosthesis. Caged disk valves have a disk that rests on a sewing ring that moves forward when a pressure gradient develops. Although this design does have a lower profile, it also produces high transvalvular pressure gradients due to the small clearance of the disk from the sewing ring. This also makes the valve more prone to thrombus formation. As can be seen from Table 23-1, none of these valves is currently in use. To counter the small orifice of the caged disk valve, the tilting disk valve was introduced. With a tilting disk valve,

TABLE 23-1 Types of Cardiac Prosthetic Valves

Mechanical	Biologic	Allografts
Caged ball	**Porcine**	
Starr-Edwards*	Hancock Modified Orifice*	CryoLife Allografts
Smeloff	Carpentier Edwards*	
Magovern-Cromie		
Caged disk	**Pericardial**	
Hufnagle-Conrad	Mitroflow†	
Cross-Jones	Carpentier Edwards*	
Kay-Suzuki	Ionescu-Shiley	
Kay Shiley		
Beall		
Tilting disk		
Lillehei-Kaster		
Wada-Cutter		
Bjork-Shiley Monostrut†		
Medtronic Hall*		
Omniscience*		
Omnicarbon†		
Bileaflet		
St. Jude*		
Gott-Daggert		
Kalke-Lillehei		
Duromedics†		
Carbomedics†		

*Indicates valves that currently remain available in the United States.
†Valves not available in the United States but currently in use internationally.[24]

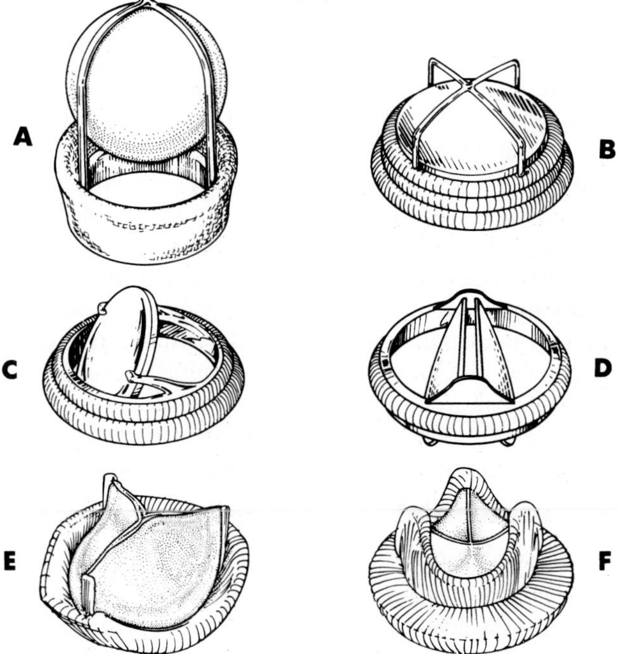

Figure 23-1 Schematic representations of various valves. **A,** Caged ball. **B,** Caged disk. **C,** Tilting disk. **D,** Bileaflet valve. **E,** Pericardial tissue valve. **F,** Porcine tissue valve.

a disk sets against the sewing ring when the valve is closed. The circular disk is held in place by hinges or struts that allow it to tilt forward when flow occurs through the valve orifice. The tilt occurs at an angle of up to 60 to 80 degrees, providing a significant valve orifice for blood flow. Most recently, bileaflet valves have been introduced. Bileaflet valves consist of two semicircular disks that, when open, pivot on hinges to allow centralized flow, and, when closed, occlude the valve orifice. These valves also provide a large orifice for blood flow.

There are currently two types of biologic or tissue valves being implanted: porcine and pericardial. Pericardial valves are made of bovine pericardium fashioned into valve leaflets. Porcine valves are constructed from porcine aortic valves that are mounted on stents and attached to a sewing ring.

Since the early 1960s, aortic hemografts (cadaver) have been used. Harvested within 24 hours of cardiac arrest, these cryopreserved valves have demonstrated a 92% actuarial freedom from moderate or severe incompetence at 10 years.[34] Fresh aortic homografts have also demonstrated superior hemodynamic function over bioprostheses. However, availability makes their use impractical based on the demand for valve surgery.[36]

Postoperative recovery patterns and complications for valve surgery patients are similar to those undergoing myocardial revascularization or other open cardiac procedures. However, there are unique complications associated with valve replacement surgery. These complications are structural and nonstructural valve dysfunction, thrombosis/thromboembolism, anticoagulant-related hemorrhage, and prosthetic valve endocarditis.

PATHOPHYSIOLOGY

The etiology of valvular heart disease has changed dramatically in the past few decades. Rheumatic heart disease, previously a major cause of valve disease, has all but disappeared in industrialized nations due to the effective prevention and control of group A streptococci infections. In contrast, the incidence and prevalence of rheumatic heart disease in developing countries has not improved.[12] Today, the major cause of valvular disease in the United States is nonrheumatic valvular heart disease, including mitral valve prolapse, congenital aortic disease, degenerative changes associated with aging, and mitral leaflet regurgitation from ischemia. Nonrheumatic valvular disease has replaced rheumatic valvular disease as a significant cause of mortality and morbidity in the United States. However, since the etiology of congenital and acquired nonrheumatic valve disease is poorly understood, primary prevention strategies are not available.[16]

Aortic Stenosis

Aortic stenosis may occur secondary to calcification of rheumatic inflammation. It may also be congenital in origin, producing a unicuspid, bicuspid, or multicuspid valve. Aortic stenosis is increasingly becoming a disease associated with the elderly. In patients 75 years of age or older, 40% demonstrate mild aortic calcification, 13% have severe calcification, and 2.9% demonstrate a critical level of aortic valve stenosis.[32] The normal aortic valve has a cross-sectional diameter of 2.5 to 3.5 cm^2.[37] Severe aortic stenosis results in an aortic valve diameter less than 0.7 cm^2. The resulting obstruction to left ventricular outflow causes persistent increase in left ventricular systolic pressure and cardiac workload leading to progressive ventricular hypertrophy and increased myocardial oxygen demand. Although a normal stroke volume (SV) and cardiac output (CO) may be maintained at rest, SV and CO fail to rise during exercise. Patients usually do not become symptomatic until their fifth or sixth decade because there is a relatively long latent period for the ventricular changes to occur. There are generally three hallmark signs of aortic stenosis: angina, syncope, or exertional dyspnea. Once these symptoms appear, the average life expectancy is 3 to 4 years. As the disease progresses, left ventricular failure develops and heralds mortality within 1 to 2 years. Severe reactive pulmonary artery hypertension may also develop.[41] Sudden cardiac death accounts for about 20% of the deaths associated with aortic stenosis.[37] Surgical correction is recommended once the patient becomes symptomatic and the aortic valve orifice demonstrates severe stenosis.[25]

Aortic Regurgitation

Aortic regurgitation is commonly caused by rheumatic fever, infective endocarditis, dissecting aortic aneurysm, and dilation of the aortic annulus. In patients over 50 years of age, 11% are reported to have aortic regurgitation.[27] In aortic regurgitation, blood is initially ejected out of the ventricle into the aorta. However, because the aortic valve does not completely close during diastole, blood flows back into the left ventricle. This increases left ventricular end-diastolic volume, and progressive ventricular dilation occurs. CO will be normal at rest but fail to rise with exercise. Left ventricular failure ensues. Angina and dysrhythmias may develop as CO and coronary artery perfusion pressure fall, failing to provide the dilated taxed left ventricle with oxygen. The majority of patients with asymptomatic chronic aortic regurgitation and normal left ventricular systolic function do well with medical management. However, once symptoms of syncope, angina, orthopnea, dyspnea at rest, and left ventricular systolic dysfunction (resting ejection fractions below normal) develop, surgical valve replacement is indicated.[2]

Mitral Stenosis

Mitral stenosis is generally caused by rheumatic fever and occurs most often in women. Exposed to rheumatic fever before their teenage years, women may be in their third decade before a murmur becomes present and in their fourth or fifth decade before cardiac symptoms develop.[38] Medically managed patients with mitral stenosis live to an average age of 48 years.[35] The normal mitral valve orifice is 5 cm^2. Once the orifice is half this size, significant symptoms appear. As the mitral valve stenoses, left atrial pressure rises, pulmonary vascular resistance (PVR) increases, and CO falls. As the pulmonary pressure rises, pulmonary edema develops, with the additional possibility of pulmonic and tricuspid regurgitation. Such pulmonary involvement may result in numerous episodes of respiratory problems prior to surgical repair and may lead to the development of pulmonary hypertension. Left atrial enlargement develops and thrombus formation may occur as blood sluggishly moves through the atrium. Embolization resulting in peripheral ischemia or neurologic deficit is sometimes the first indication that a patient has mitral stenosis. The CO remains normal at rest but cannot increase during exercise because blood volume is trapped in the left atrium.

Mitral Regurgitation

Unlike mitral stenosis, mitral regurgitation is seen more frequently in men than women. Linked to rheumatic and nonrheumatic causes, mitral regurgitation has been reported to occur in 48% of people over 50.[27] This age-related prevalance is believed to be associated with the increased thickness and sclerosis valves undergo as they age. It has also been reported that mitral regurgitation develops transiently in about 13% of patients during early myocardial infarction. Approximately 1% of these patients experience rupture of the papillary muscle and significant mitral regurgitation.[30] Additional causes of mitral regurgitation include mitral valve prolapse and endocarditis. Depending on the etiology, surgical correction will be recommended at different points in the disease. Fulminant pulmonary edema may develop following ischemic ruptures of the papillary muscle, requiring immediate surgery. However, rheumatic changes will occur more slowly, resulting in an insidious onset of symptoms. In mitral regurgitation, blood flows both through the aorta and back into the left atrium during systole. In order to maintain an effective CO with less blood flowing into the aorta, the ventricle attempts to compensate by emptying more completely. Ultimately, the ventricle dilates and left ventricular failure develops. Additionally, the regurgitant stream into the left atrium causes left atrial enlargement, resulting in increased pulmonary vascular resistance, pulmonary edema, and, eventually, right-sided heart failure. Thrombus formation in the left atrium is less likely than in mitral stenosis because there is constant movement of blood across the regurgitant valve.

LENGTH OF STAY/ANTICIPATED COURSE

Cardiac valve surgery and repair procedures fall into the Health Care Financing and Administration Diagnostic Related Grouping (DRG) under DRGs 104, 105, and 108. Patients receiving a valve replacement or aortic or mitral valvuloplasty with a cardiac catheterization within the same hospitalization fall into DRG 104, which is generally an 18-day length of stay.[42] If patients have had cardiac catheterization before admission for surgery, they are classified in DRG 105, which has an average length of stay of 13 days.[42] Finally, patients undergoing annuloplasty or repair of their papillary muscle or chordae are placed in DRG 108, which has a 14.7-day length of stay.[42] Generally, these lengths of stay are adequate for patients who do not develop major complications. In fact, uncomplicated cases may be discharged within 7 to 8 days after surgery. However, lengths of stay may become as long as several weeks to months if catastrophic complications such as severe strokes or acute renal failure develop.

MANAGEMENT TRENDS AND CONTROVERSIES

Postoperative management and care of cardiac valve patients is similar to that of patients undergoing myocardial revascularization or other cardiac procedures. The major tenets of management center on optimizing preload, enhancing contractility, and reducing afterload. In patients who have mixed lesions (i.e., stenosis and regurgitation of one or both valves), all three of these tenets are of equal importance because these patients are at risk for both right- and left-sided heart failure. However, in instances with an isolated lesion (such as singular mitral stenosis or singular aortic regurgitation), patients may be transiently at greater risk for one type of failure over another after cardiac surgical repair. For example, patients with chronic isolated mitral stenosis with a significant history of pulmonary hypertension and pulmonary congestion generally require more aggressive ventilatory management. The need for ventilatory support and the duration of that support may be significantly greater than for patients with other types of lesions. Additionally, filling pressures may need to be kept at the upper levels of normal or higher because these patients are accustomed to high left-atrial pressures. Positive inotropes may be required to assist both the left and right ventricle. Left ventricular failure may develop postoperatively because the left ventricle is receiving more blood than it previously had to contend with. During this transient period of adjustment, administration of inotropes or support with an intra-aortic balloon pump (IABP) may be required. The development of right heart failure is also a risk for mitral stenosis patients. In chronic mitral stenosis, the right ventricle hypertrophies in order to compensate for the resulting pulmonary hypertension. The transient operative insults of anesthesia, cardiopulmonary bypass, and volume overloading may be enough to push the right ventricle into a decompensated state and cause right-sided heart failure. Unloading the right ventricle with agents such as isoproterenol, sodium nitroprusside, nitroglycerin or, in severe instances, IABP of the pulmonary artery may be required.

The management of isolated mitral regurgitation may be somewhat different. If the patient had chronic mitral regurgitation, pulmonary problems from persistently elevated left atrial pressures may be present and require aggressive pulmonary support. Due to their history of elevated left atrial pressures, these patients may also require higher filling pressures to maintain CO. Patients with acute onset mitral regurgitation following rupture of a papillary muscle are not as likely to require such extensive ventilatory management or elevated filling pressures because their baseline respiratory and cardiac volume status are closer to normal levels. Because of the change in blood flow dynamics created by the replaced mitral valve, temporary inotropic support may be necessary. Such support may be needed because, previous to the mitral valve replacement, the left ventricle ejected blood out of two outflow tracts: the aortic valve into the aorta and the incompetent mitral valve into the left atrium. Although the route back into the left atrium was not beneficial, it did provide the left ventricle with a path of lesser resistance for ejection. With valve replacement, the left ventricle has only the aortic valve and aorta as an outflow tract. Adjusting to this workload may cause left ventricular failure unless inotropes or mechanical assistance are employed.

Mitral valve surgery patients may be plagued by pulmonary and biventricular heart failure, but patients following aortic valve replacement are generally spared such complications unless they have severe chronic aortic valve disease. Left ventricular failure becomes a greater problem in

TABLE 23-2 Complication Rates Associated with Prosthetic Valve Implantation[20] (% / Year)

Valve	Position	Leaks	Embolism	Thrombosis	Bleeding	Infection
Mechanical	Aortic	0-2.6	0-3.5	0-1.1	0-6.0	0.2-1.3
	Mitral	0-4.0	1-7.0	0-3.0	0-7.0	0-1.5
Biologic	Aortic	0-1.6	0-2.9	—	0-2.5	0.2-2.0
	Mitral	0.1-0.9	0.1-4.0	—	0-2.4	0.1-2.3

TABLE 23-3 Normal Sounds of Various Prosthetic Valves

	Aortic position	Mitral position
Caged ball	• Systolic opening click • Early systolic crescendo-decrescendo murmur Grade I-II/VI	• Systolic click of mitral valve closure • Click of mitral valve opening (after S_2)
Tilting disk	• Systolic opening click • Early systolic crescendo-decrescendo murmur Grade I-II/VI • Click from aortic valve closure (end systolic)	• Systolic click of mitral valve closure • Click of mitral valve opening (after S_2) • Rumbling mid-diastolic murmur
Bileaflet	• Systolic opening click • Early systolic crescendo-decrescendo murmur Grade I-II/VI • Click from aortic valve closure (end systolic)	• Systolic click of mitral valve closure • Click of mitral valve opening (after S_2) • Rumbling mid-diastolic murmur
Biologic	• Mid-systolic crescendo-decrescendo murmur Grade I-II/VI	• Diastolic rumble

these patients. In both aortic regurgitation and stenosis, the left ventricle dilates and hypertrophies to compensate for ejecting against a stenotic valve or dealing with the volume overload from regurgitation. The surgical experience itself, with hypothermia, surgical incisions, cardiac manipulation, anesthesia, cardiopulmonary bypass, and volume overload, can easily push ventricles into decompensated failure. Afterload reduction in the form of sodium nitroprusside, nitroglycerine, and the IABP may be required to manage a decompensated state. Once unloading has been optimized, inotropes may also be required. After 1 to 2 days, patients who have not developed complications are typically weaned from these supports and maintain stable hemodynamics on their own.

Although rarely a problem in the early recovery phase, nonstructural dysfunction and stuctural deterioration are problems that plague prosthetic valves. The incidence of paraprosthetic leaks is reported in Table 23-2. A paraprosthetic leak is an example of a nonstructural problem. Paraprosthetic leaks occur when there is abnormal retrograde flow of blood around the circumference of the prosthetic valve between the sewing ring and the annulus of the native valve. Such leaks are believed to be the result of tissue retraction during healing, using continuous rather than interrupted suture technique, heavily calcified annulus, or endocarditis following valve replacement. Auscultation for changes in prosthetic valve sounds are helpful in the diagnosis of paravalvular leaks. Normal prosthetic heart sounds are listed in Table 23-3. The normal murmurs from prosthetic valves result from turbulent flow that is present across all types of prosthetic valves. However, any prolonged diastolic mitral rumble is suggestive of prosthetic dysfunction.[17,29] Paraprosthetic leaks are not related to the type of valve used for replacement. However, valve design has been associated as a factor. The sutureless Magovern-Cromie valve, which has rows of interlocking pins holding it into the annulus rather than sutures, has been reported to have a leak rate of 2.6% to 15%, a rate higher than the other valves reported in the literature (Table 23-2).[33]

Valve failure from structural deterioration is a rare occurrence with mechanical valves, occurring at a rate of only 0.41% to 0.0001% per year.[20] However, the failure rate of biologic valves increases with time. Five-year failure rates are low. Ten-year failure rates are approximately 55% to 90% for aortic valves and 50% to 80% for mitral valves.[20] In biologic valves, structural deterioration occurs as the leaflets and cusps begin to tear away from the stents, or develop calcification or endocarditis. Phagocytosis has also recently been identified as playing a role in valve degeneration.[18] Failure is typically a slow process with gradual development of cardiac symptoms.[45] Failure of mechanical valves may be an insidious process, but may also be sudden, unexpected, and catastrophic. Structural deteriorations may develop as a ball or disk variance due to wear, strut or hinge fracture from stress, or disk or ball escape. As these structural problems develop, laminar blood flow is compromised

TABLE 23-4 Antithrombotic Therapy in Patients with Prosthetic Heart Valves*[43]

	Warfarin		Antiplatelet therapy†		
Clinical presentation	**Duration**	**International normalized ratio**	**Drug**	**Duration**	**Dose (daily)**
Biologic valve					
Mitral valve; normal sinus rhythm	3 months	2-3	Aspirin	Indefinite (optional as follow-up to warfarin therapy)	325 mg
Aortic valve; normal sinus rhythm	3 months (optional)	2-3	Aspirin	Indefinite (optional)	325 mg
Mitral or aortic valve; atrial fibrillation	Indefinite	2-3		No recommendation	
Mitral or aortic valve; left atrial thrombus	Uncertain	2-3		No recommendation	
Mitral or aortic valve; history of embolism	3-12 months	2-3		No recommendation	
Mechanical valve					
Mitral or aortic valve	Indefinite	2.5-3.5		No recommendation	
St. Jude aortic valve; normal sinus rhythm	Indefinite (optional)	2.5-3.5	Aspirin and dipyridamole	Indefinite (alternative to warfarin)	325 mg aspirin; 225 mg dipyridamole
Mitral or aortic valve; high-risk patient or patient with embolism on warfarin alone. Options‡	Indefinite	3-4.5	Aspirin	Indefinite (added to warfarin therapy)	160 mg
	Indefinite	3-4.5	Dipyridamole	Indefinite (added to warfarin therapy)	400 mg
	Indefinite	2-3	Aspirin and dipyridamole	Indefinite (added to warfarin therapy)	660 mg aspirin; 150 mg dipyridamole

*Recommendations based on the Third Consensus Conference of the Task Force on Antithrombotic Therapy of the American College of Chest Physicians (1992).

†Antiplatelet therapy may offer protection comparable to that of warfarin therapy.

‡Options may offer additional protection without increased risk of bleeding complications.

and thrombus begins to form. Thrombus may partially or completely immobilize the disk or ball in its cage, thereby creating a stenotic or regurgitant mechanical valve. Frequently, the symptoms from this type of stenosis or regurgitation or from an embolus lead to the diagnosis of structural deterioration. All artificial valves have some minor degree of regurgitation and the hemolysis created by this low-grade regurgitant flow is normally compensated for by erythropoiesis. However, severe hemolytic anemia develops when paravalvular leaks are significant or the poppet or disk is partially occluded or begins to wear.[13,39]

Thrombus formation is a major problem with mechanical valves even in the absence of structural deterioration. Despite the changes in design and materials that have occurred in valve construction, overall risk for thrombus formation is 1% to 3% per year (Table 23-2). In addition to the ability of thrombus to alter the valve's mechanical function, it may also lead to embolization. Thrombus formation and embolization are more likely to occur from valves in the mitral position than the aortic position. This is believed to be so because flow across and around the mitral valve is slower and the orifice is wider, thus allowing more turbulent flow and subsequent thrombus formation. The sequelae from embolization may range from transient peripheral embolization to catastrophic cerebral or myocardial embolism. Valve thrombosis is usually related to intervals of inadequate anticoagulation. In a report by Deviri and associates, 70% of patients who thrombosed appeared to be inadequately anticoagulated per laboratory tests.[10] Deviri is also quick to point out that using only one set of laboratory results to assess anticoagulation is inappropriate because values may change. Trending anticoagulant levels is suggested as more appropriate. Additionally, thrombus is not the only culprit in valve obstruction. Formation of pannus (vascular tissue growth) can also obstruct the valve mechanisms. Pannus formation may begin as early as within 1 month and may occlude a valve within 6 months.

Management of structural abnormalities may take a number of paths. If symptoms are minor, medical management is pursued. In the presence of cardiac decompensation, valve replacement is undertaken. Reoperation under these conditions may result in mortality rates as high as 33%.[22] Three options are available in the presence of thrombus: valve replacement, valve declotting and excision of pannus, and nonsurgical thrombolysis. The current standard is valve replacement. Pannus removal can be successfully performed 10% of the time.[22] Thrombolysis currently provides incomplete results and is associated with a 15% to 25% embolism rate.[19]

Prevention of thrombus has become a major goal of therapy after valve replacement. Anticoagulation is generally started within 48 hours after surgery unless the patient is still unstable, may require reoperation, or has significant oozing from the chest tubes. Warfarin is the drug of choice. However, antiplatelet therapy as an adjunct or alternative is also currently used (Table 23-4). The International Normalized Ratio (INR) has recently been suggested as more reliable than patient testing for anticoagulant control. An INR range of 3.0 to 4.5 (3.5 target) corresponds to a prothrombin activity of 25% to 30%.[28] Patients may be discharged from the hospital prior to reaching this level as long as they are followed as outpatients. Inadequate anticoagulation will lead to thrombus, but over-anticoagulation may cause internal and external bleeding, leading to death, stroke, hospitalization, reoperation, and transfusions. Rates of expected bleeding complications are listed in Table 23-2. The mortality rate is 5% in patients who develop this complication.

The incidence of prosthetic valve endocarditis (PVE) is reported in Table 23-2. Although the incidence is low, the mortality may be as high as 50%.[7] The risk of PVE is greatest in the first 6 to 12 months after valve surgery and decreases thereafter.[4] Causative agents are usually *coagulase-negative staphylococci* or diphtheroids. Gram-negative bacteria, streptococci, and fungi are less common. Recent evidence has shown that PVE caused by *coagulase-negative staphylococci* within 1 year after valve replacement was probably acquired at the time of surgery.[23] Thus, prevention

Standard Antibiotic Prophylaxis for Prosthetic Heart Valve and Other High-Risk Patients[8]

For dental/oral/upper respiratory procedures

- Amoxicillin 3 g orally 1 hour before procedure, then 1.5 g 6 hours after initial dose.
- For amoxicillin/penicillin allergic patients: erythromycin ethylaucinate 800 mg or erythromycin stearate 1.0 g orally 2 hours before a procedure, then one half the dose 6 hours after the initial administration; *or* clindomycin 300 mg orally 1 hour before a procedure and 150 mg 6 hours after initial dose.

Alternate prophylactic regimens for dental/oral/upper respiratory tract procedures in patients at risk

- For patients unable to take oral medications: Ampicillin 2.0 g IV (or IM) 30 minutes before procedure, then ampicillin 1.0 g IV (IM) *or* Amoxicillin 1.5 g orally 6 hours after initial dose.

OR

- For ampicillin/amoxicillin/penicillin allergic patients unable to take oral medications: clindamycin 300 mg IV 30 minutes before a procedure and 150 mg IV (or orally) 6 hours after intitial dose.
- For patients considered to be at high risk who are not candidates for the standard regimen: ampicillin 2.0 g IV (or IM) plus gentamicin 1.5 mg/kg IV (or IM) (not to exceed 80 mg) 30 minutes before procedure, followed by amoxicillin 1.5 g orally 6 hours after the initial dose. Alternatively, the parenteral regimen may be repeated 8 hours after the initial dose.
- For amoxicillin/ampicillin/penicillin-allergic patients considered to be at high risk: vancomycin 1.0 g IV administered over 1 hour, starting 1 hour before the procedure. No repeat dose is necessary.

For genitourinary/gastrointestinal procedures

- Standard regime: ampicillin 2.0 g IV (or IM) plus gentamicin 1.5 mg/kg IV (or IM) (not to exceed 80 mg) 30 minutes before procedure, followed by amoxicillin 1.5 g orally 6 hours after the initial dose. Alternatively, the parenteral regimen may be repeated once 8 hours after the initial dose.
- For amoxicillin/ampicillin/penicillin-allergic patients: vancomycin 1.0 g IV administered over 1 hour plus gentamicin 1.5 mg/kg/IV (IM) (not to exceed 80 mg) 1 hour before the procedure. May be repeated once 8 hours after initial dose.

and prophylaxis are essential. The current standard of practice is to administer antibiotics in the perioperative period to prevent the valve prosthesis from colonizing. After implantation, patients are on antibiotics whenever a bacteria-inducing oral, urogenital, or other invasive procedure is planned. Antibiotic coverage in these latter situations should follow American Heart Association guidelines (see Box). The American Heart Association recommends a cefazolin-based regimen of the initial cardiac surgical procedure. The duration of antibiotic administration should not exceed 24 hours into the postoperative period in order to avoid emergence of multiresistant organisms.[8] The specific cephalosporin chosen should be based on three criteria: susceptibility patterns within the hospital, patient-specific susceptibility, and costs. The risk for critical care units to develop a pattern of methicillin-resistant *Staphylococcus aureus* (MRSA), which may predispose future patients to PVE in that environment, is a problem associated with blanket administration of cephalosporin.[26] Although vancomycin is effective against MRSA, current American Heart Association recommendations suggest the use of vancomycin only in patients with allergy to cephalosporins or when endemic rates of MRSA become significant.[8]

ASSESSMENT

PARAMETER	PREOPERATIVE ANTICIPATED ALTERATION				POST-OPERATIVE ANTICIPATED ALTERATION
	Aortic Stenosis	*Aortic Regurgitation*	*Mitral Stenosis*	*Mitral Regurgitation*	
CO	WNL	WNL	WNL	WNL	WNL
CI	WNL Decreased: <2.2 l/min/m^2 in severe AS	WNL Decreased: <2.2 l/min/m^2 in severe AR	WNL	WNL	WNL
PAS	WNL Increased: >50 mm Hg in severe AS	WNL	Increased: >30 mm Hg	WNL	WNL or slightly increased *due to need for higher preload*
PAD	WNL Increased: >25 mm Hg in severe AS	WNL	Increased: >15 mm Hg	WNL	Increased at 15 to 18 mm Hg *due to need for higher preload*
PCWP	WNL Increased: >16 mm Hg in severe AS	WNL	Increased: >15 mm Hg	WNL	Increased at 12 to 16 mm Hg *due to need for higher preload*
CVP	WNL	WNL	WNL Increased: >12 mm Hg in severe MS with right-side failure	WNL	Increased at 8 to 12 mm Hg *due to need for higher preload*
SVR	WNL	WNL	WNL	WNL	Increased: >1200 dynes/sec/cm^{-5} *Decreases once rewarming and vasodilation occur*
PVR	WNL Increased: >200 to 480 dynes/sec/cm^{-5} in severe AS	WNL	Increased: >300 dynes/sec/cm^{-5}	WNL	WNL *May be higher if residual reactive pulmonary hypertension persists*

PARAMETER	PREOPERATIVE ANTICIPATED ALTERATION				POST-OPERATIVE ANTICIPATED ALTERATION
	Aortic Stenosis	***Aortic Regurgitation***	***Mitral Stenosis***	***Mitral Regurgitation***	
Arterial pressure wave	Delayed systolic peak Anacrotic notch	Widened pulse pressure with elevated BPS and decreased BPD *may even be heard when sphygmomanometer cuff is deflated* Corrigan's pulse (water hammer pulse) which quickly collapses during late systole *due to regurgitation*	Normal to diminished upstroke	Normal Sharp upstroke	WNL with a dicrotic notch
Heart sounds	Systolic crescendo-decrescendo murmur Low, harsh pitched, best heard at second intercostal space right of sternum Transmitted to neck and carotid vessels Begins shortly after first heart sound Systolic thrill at base of heart Paradoxical splitting of second heart sound (advanced stages) Atrial gallop (S4) Ventricular gallop (S3)	Three types of murmurs: Blowing high-pitched decrescendo diastolic murmur at third left intercostal space Systolic ejection murmur Austin flint murmur: low-pitched, soft diastolic murmur heard best at cardiac apex	Loud first heart sound Opening snap Diastolic murmur low pitched, rumbling best heard at apex with patient on left side Soft systolic murmur at apex Diastolic thrill at apex Right ventricular lift along left sternal border *Due to hypertrophied right ventricle*	Soft or absent first heart sound Normal second heart sound (widely split in severe regurgitation) Occasional atrial and ventricular gallop High-pitched blowing holosystolic murmur best heard at apex; radiates to axilla Short rumbling diastolic murmur Systolic thrill palpable at apex Rocking motion of chest *Due to left ventricular contraction and left atrial expansion during systole*	Normal prosthetic sounds (Table 23-3)
Jugular venous pulse	Normal	Normal	Abnormal prominent "a" wave *Due to powerful atrial systole* May be a singular pulsation cannon wave due to atrial fibrillation	Abnormal prominent "a" wave	WNL
Cardiac rhythm	NSR	NSR PVCs	NSR Atrial dysrhythmias common	NSR Atrial dysrhythmia common	NSR May require temporary or permanent pacing *due to edema and surgical disruption of conduction system*
Skin color	WNL	WNL	Peripheral cyanosis Flushed cheeks *Due to chronic low CO*	WNL	

	Aortic Stenosis	*Aortic Regurgitation*	*Mitral Stenosis*	*Mitral Regurgitation*	
Electrocardiogram	Left ventricular "strain" pattern if ST segment elevation, T wave inversion in leads I, AVL, V_5, V_6	Left ventricular hypertrophy "strain" pattern of ST segment elevation, T wave inversion in leads I, AVL, V_5, V_6	Atrial dysrhythmias (premature atrial contractions, paroxysmal atrial tachycardia, atrial fibrillation and flutter) Bifed P waves in leads I, II, and V_5 *Due to left atrial enlargement, right-axis deviation, and right ventricular hypertrophy*	Occasional atrial fibrillation with severe chronic mitral regurgitation	WNL *If perioperative myocardial infarction, ECG alterations will be consistent with typical myocardial infarction*
Pulses	WNL	DeMusset's sign (bobbing of head with systole) Duroziez's sign (to and fro murmur over femoral artery) Trabe's sign (pistol shot sound heard with bell of stethoscope over femoral arteries) Quincke's pulse (capillary pulsations demonstrated by applying pressure to tip of the nail and observing alternate blanching and flushing at nail bed root)	WNL	WNL	WNL *Diminished pulses present only in low-CO state or following embolization*
RR	Increased with exertion	Increased with exertion	Dyspnea *precipitated by excitement, exertion, fever, etc.* Hemoptysis not associated with pulmonary edema *due to ruptured alveoli from elevated pulmonary pressures* Orthopnea Paroxysmal nocturnal dyspnea Cough Decreased vital capacity and pulmonary compliance Hoarseness *due to compression of recurrent laryngeal nerve by enlarged left atrium*	WNL Increased *if left ventricular failure develops*	Per ventilator control to maintain ABGs Once extubated, WNL to slightly tachypneic *due to normal postoperative splinting*
Lung fields	Clear *until left ventricular failure*	Clear *until left ventricular failure*	Pulmonary congestion	Pulmonary congestion	Clear to auscultation *Pleural effusions may be present for first few days*

PARAMETER	PREOPERATIVE ANTICIPATED ALTERATION				POST-OPERATIVE ANTICIPATED ALTERATION
	Aortic Stenosis	*Aortic Regurgitation*	*Mitral Stenosis*	*Mitral Regurgitation*	
Chest x-ray	Enlarged left ventricle Congested (advanced stages)	Enlarged left ventricle Congested (advanced stages)	Dilated left atrium Calcified mitral valve	Enlarged left ventricle and left atrium	Heart size normalizing Pleural effusions possible
LOC	Syncope with exercise	WNL	Focal or global symptoms *due to left atrial embolization*	WNL	Awake, alert Orientation to person, place, time, and situation No motor deficits

PLAN OF CARE

INTENSIVE PHASE

Many care priorities for valve repair or replacement patients are similar to those for patients undergoing myocardial revascularization (see Guideline 20). The priorities addressed here are those that are unique to valve surgery patients. The primary goals of care focus on emergence from anesthesia, and normalization of hemodynamic, respiratory and thermoregulatory functions.

PATIENT CARE PRIORITIES	EXPECTED PATIENT OUTCOMES
Decreased cardiac output *r/t* *Right ventricular failure* *Left ventricular failure* *Biventricular failure* *Conduction defects*	CO: WNL CI: WNL Sufficient intrinsic or extrinsic temporary or permanent pacing to support adequate CO
Fluid volume excess *r/t* *Excess fluid administration during cardiopulmonary bypass* *Sodium and water retention from compensatory renin-angiotension aldosterone mechanism* *Peripheral vasoconstriction from intraoperative hypothermia and cardiopulmonary bypass*	BP: WNL CO: WNL CVP: WNL PAP: WNL
Fluid volume deficit *r/t* *Aggressive and rapid postoperative vasodilation* *Inability to maintain adequate preload* *Abnormal fluid losses from diuresis*	BP: WNL CO: WNL CVP: WNL PAP: WNL
Ineffective breathing pattern *r/t musculoskeletal impairment from cardiac cachexia*	Adequate ABGs Comfortable respiratory rate
High risk for impaired skin integrity *r/t* *Preoperative nutritional deficit* *Chronic low CO state* *Elderly* *Limited exercise capacity*	Intact skin Adequate nutritional intake Positive nitrogen balance
Impaired physical mobility *r/t preoperative deconditioning and prolonged preoperative bed rest*	Increased mobility Independent in ADLs Intact skin

Plan of Care (cont'd)

Altered tissue perfusion *r/t* *Decreased blood flow from intracardiac emboli to cerebral, coronary, renal, mesenteric, or peripheral beds* *Decreased blood flow from valvular dysfunction*	Adequate tissue and organ oxygenation to maintain function
High risk for infection *r/t* *Prosthetic valves* *Major operative procedure* *Numerous intravascular lines*	Temperature: WNL WBC: WNL Prosthetic valve sounds: WNL Negative blood cultures Clear, yellow urine Sputum production: WNL

INTERVENTIONS

Obtain hemodynamic parameters on admission and as often as necessary until stable.

Determine optimum right and left ventricular preload levels *to ensure adequate cardiac output.*

Administer appropriate volume (crystalloid, colloid, blood products, or autotransfusion) *to achieve optimum preload levels and adequate CO/CI.*

Administer pulmonary and/or systemic vasodilator agents *to bring SVR and/or PVR to normal levels and optimize CO/CI.*

Administer positive inotropes *to enhance contractility and achieve adequate CO/CI.*

Monitor heart rate and rhythm. Use temporary pacing if heart block occurs *due to edema of conduction system.*

Assess prosthetic valve sounds on admission and throughout hospitalization *to identify early postoperative paravalvular leaks.* Document to provide baseline for later postoperative follow-up.

Monitor chest tube, nasogastric, and urinary output, and replace volume as needed *to maintain adequate preload.*

Obtain daily weight *to assist in analysis of hemodynamic and nutritional status.*

Administer paralytic and sedation agents as needed *to maintain adequate ventilation until postoperative hemodynamic variables are stable and effects of preoperative valve disease are compensated.*

Wean patient from ventilator *ensuring maintenance of hemodynamic stability in context with both surgical recovery and hemodynamic adjustment after valve repair.*

Position patient *to prevent skin breakdown.*

Place patient on appropriate pressure-reducing mattress if not able to be mobilized out of bed within 24 hours *due to high-risk status of valve patients for skin breakdown.*

Assess neurologic status (pupillary response, monitor motor and cognitive function) as patient arouses from anesthesia *to determine possible intraoperative stroke.*

Obtain postoperative 12-lead ECG and cardiac enzymes *to determine if intraoperative myocardial infarction or embolization has occurred.*

Assess and record bowel sounds *to ensure absence of mesenteric emboli and recovery from anesthesia.*

Monitor temperature, WBC, valve sounds *to detect potential infection.*

Maintain aseptic techniques when working with invasive lines *to prevent surgical infection and protect the prosthestic valve from easily acquired infection.*

Administer antibiotics per protocols *to protect the prosthetic valve from initial colonization and prevent surgical infection.*

Remove invasive lines as soon as possible *to minimize the high risk for prosthetic valve infection.*

Obtain blood cultures per routine following a temperature elevation *to determine specific, optimum antibiotic therapy in the event of infection.*

Plan of Care (cont'd)

Observe for signs of valve failure and heart failure *to detect early valve dysfunction and hemodynamic recovery from preoperative cardiac impairment.*

INTERMEDIATE PHASE

Following recovery from anesthesia and development of hemodynamic stability, valve repair and replacement patients are discharged from the ICU. This will usually occur within 24 to 48 hours after surgery. Continued assessment and interventions to assist general surgical recovery will be necessary. The major intermediate recovery priority focuses on initiation of anticoagulation, and patient education related to antibiotic prophylaxis, anticoagulant regimes, and knowledge of symptoms of prosthetic valve failure and heart failure.

PATIENT CARE PRIORITIES

Self-care deficit *r/t complex medical regimes and discharge follow-up requirements*

EXPECTED PATIENT OUTCOMES

Verbalizes need for anticoagulation and follow-up patient testing

Demonstrates correct administration of anticoagulation

Describes symptoms of over-anticoagulation: bleeding gums, tarry stools, easy bruising

Verbalizes rationale for antibiotic prophylaxis and indications for initiation

Describes symptoms evidenced in valvular endocarditis: neurologic (stroke, visual changes, blindness, paralysis, severe headaches, aphasia, sensory loss, transient weakness); temperature elevation, shaking chills, night sweats, generalized fatigue, painful joints; and cardiac symptoms (shortness of breath, easy fatigue)

Describes, recognizes and knows to whom to report signs and symptoms of prosthetic valve and heart failure: weight gain, chest pain, dyspnea (sudden or insidious), paroxysmal nocturnal dyspnea, and cough

INTERVENTIONS

Emphasize the importance of anticoagulation and prophylactic antibiotics.

Collaborate with pharmacists in teaching patient/family about the anticoagulation regime prescribed *to increase potential compliance and avoid over- or undercoagulation.*

Instruct the patient/family regarding the types of procedures that necessitate prophylactic antibiotics (e.g., dental work, genitourinary exams, endoscopic exams, minor or major surgery) *to ensure adequate antibiotic protection of the artificial valves.*

Ensure patient/family has valve identification information *to facilitate adequate communication of valve status.*

Collaborate with dietician in teaching patient/family about dietary antagonists to warfarin *to ensure patient avoids these foods.*

Assist patient/family in completion of application for med-alert tags *to ensure that patient receives other medical care in context with protection of prosthetic valve or anticoagulant regime.*

Provide patient/family with verbal instructions and written patient education material on signs and symptoms of valve failure *to ensure prompt reporting of any symptoms.*

TRANSISTION TO DISCHARGE

Discharge will occur once the patient is hemodynamically stable, performs ADLs with minimal assistance, and demonstrates an initial understanding of discharge medical regimes. Follow-up reinforcement as an outpatient will be necessary. Early in-hospital mortality for valve surgery varies between 3% and 15% depending on the patient's preoperative condition.[1,3,21,44]

Within 10 years postoperatively, valve-related complications cause death or necessitate reoperation in 50% of patients.[40] However, as valve designs and management techniques improve, so will the survival statistics. In the meantime, valve repair and replacement procedures allow many patients to achieve a quality of life they have not experienced for years prior to their surgery.

REFERENCES

1. Bloomfield P, et al: Twelve year comparison of a Bjork-Shiley mechanical heart valve with porcine bioprosthesis, *N Engl J Med* 324:573-579, 1993.
2. Bonow RD, et al: Serial long-term assessment of the natural history of asymptomatic patients with chronic aortic regurgitation and normal left ventricular systolic function, *Circulation* 84:1625-1635, 1991.
3. Braile DM, et al: IMC Bovine pericardial valve: 11 years, *J Card Surg* 6:580-588, 1991.
4. Calderwood S, et al: Risk factors for the development of prosthetic valve endocarditis, *Circulation* 72:31-37, 1985.
5. Cosgrove DM, et al: Mitral valvuloplasty at the Cleveland Clinic Foundation, *Clev Clin J Med* 55:37-42, 1988.
6. Cosgrove DM, Stewart WM: Mitral valvuloplasty, *Curr Probl Cardiol* 14:355-415, 1989.
7. Counsell CE, de Belder MA, Oldershaw PJ: Prosthetic valve endocarditis, *Br J Hosp Med* 46:28-31, 1991.
8. Dajani AS, et al: Prevention of bacterial endocarditis: recommendations by the American Heart Association, *JAMA* 264:2919-2922, 1990.
9. Delocke A, Jebara VA, Relland JYM: Valve repair with Carpentier techniques: the second decade, *J Thorac Cardiovasc Surg* 99:990-1002, 1990.
10. Deviri E, et al: Obstruction of mechanical heart valve prosthesis: clinical aspects and surgical management, *J Am Coll Cardiol* 17:646-650, 1991.
11. Duran C, et al: Indications and limitations of aortic valve reconstruction, *Ann Thorac Surg* 52:447-454, 1991.
12. Eisenberg MJ: Rheumatic heart disease in the developing world: prevalence, prevention and control, *Eur Heart J* 14:122-128, 1993.
13. Flaschskampf FA, et al: Patterns of normal transvalvulor regurgitation in mechanical valve prostheses, *J Am Coll Cardiol* 18:1493-1498, 1991.
14. Galloway AC, Colvin SB, Baumann FG: Current concepts of mitral valve reconstruction for mitral insufficiency, *Circulation* 78:1087-1098, 1988.
15. Galloway AC, Colvin SB, Baumann FG: A comparison of mitral valve reconstruction with mitral valve replacement: intermediate results, *Ann Thorac Surg* 47:655-662, 1989.
16. Gillum RF: Nonrheumatic valvular heart disease in the United States, *Am Heart J* 125:915-918, 1993.
17. Gonzalez JF, Hummel BW, Rogers WJ: Prosthetic heart valves: an overview, *Hosp Med* 24:31-56, 1988.
18. Grabenwager M, et al: New aspects of the degeneration of bioprosthetic heart valves after long-term implantation, *J Thorac Cardiovasc Surg* 104:14-21, 1992.
19. Graver LM, Gelber PM, Tyras DH: The risks and benefits of thrombolytic therapy in acute aortic and mitral valve dysfunction: report of a case and review of the literature, *Ann Thorac Surg* 46:85-88, 1988.
20. Grunkemeier GL, Starr A, Rahimtoola SH: Prosthetic heart valve performance: long-term follow-up, *Curr Probl Cardiol* 17:329-406, 1992.
21. Hammermeister KE, et al: A comparison of outcomes in men 11 years after heart-valve replacement with a mechanical valve or bioprosthesis, *N Engl J Med* 328:1289-1296, 1993.
22. Jindani A, et al: Paraprosthetic leak: a complication of cardiac valve replacement, *J Cardiovasc Surg* 32:503-508, 1991.
23. Karchmer AW, Archer AL, Dismukes WE: Staphylococcus epidermidis causing prosthetic valve endocarditis: microbiologic and clinical observations as guides to therapy, *Ann Intern Med* 98:447-455, 1983.
24. Karp RB, Sand ME: Mechanical prosthesis: old and new, *Cardiovasc Clin* 23:235-253, 1993.
25. Kennedy KD, et al: Natural history of moderate aortic stenosis, *J Am Coll Cardiol* 17:313-319, 1991.
26. Kernodle DS, Barg NL, Kaiser AB: Low-level colonization of hospitalized patients with methicillen-resistant coagulase-negative staphylococci and emergence of the organisms during surgical antimicrobial prophylaxis, *Antimicrob Agents Chemother* 32:202-208, 1988.
27. Klein AL, et al: Age-related prevalence of valvular regurgitation in normal subjects: a comprehensive color flow examination of 118 volunteers, *J Am Soc Echocardiogr* 2:54-63, 1990.
28. Koepke JA: Coagulation testing systems. In Koepke JA, editor: *Laboratory hematology,* New York, 1984, Churchill Livingstone.
29. Kupari M, Harujula A, Mattila S: Auscultatory characteristics of a normally functioning Lillehei-Kaster, Bjork-Shiley and St. Jude heart valve prosthesis, *Br Heart J* 55:364-370, 1986.
30. Lehmann KG, et al: Mitral regurgitation in early myocardial infarction, *Ann Intern Med* 117:10-17, 1992.
31. Lessana A, Carbone C, Romano M: Mitral valve repair: results and the decision making process in reconstruction, *J Thorac Cardiovasc Surg* 99:622-630, 1990.
32. Lindroos M, et al: Prevalence of aortic valve abnormalities in the elderly: an echocardiographic study of a random population sample, *J Am Coll Cardiol* 21:1220-1225, 1993.
33. Magovern GJ, Liebler GA, Park SB: Twenty-five year review of the Magovern-Cromie sutureless aortic valve, *Ann Thorac Surg* 48(suppl):533, 1989.
34. O'Brien MF, Stafford EG, Gardner MAH: Cryopreserved viable allograft aortic valves. In Yankoah AC, et al, editors: *Cardiac valve allografts,* New York, 1988, Springer, pp 311-321.
35. Olesen KH: The natural history of 271 patients with mitral stenosis under medical treatment, *Br Heart J* 24:349-352, 1962.
36. Penta A, et al: Patient status 10 or more years after "fresh" homograft replacement of aortic valve, *Circulation* 70:182-186, 1984.
37. Rackley CE, Edwards JE, Wallace RB: Aortic valve disease. In Hurst JE, editor: *The heart,* ed 6, New York, 1986, McGraw-Hill.
38. Rackley CE, Edwards JE, Karp, RB: Mitral valve disease. In Hurst JE, editor: *The heart,* ed 6, New York, 1986, McGraw-Hill.
39. Saad RM, Wolf MW: Progressive hemolytic anemia due to a delayed recognition of a Beall mitral valve prosthesis, *Chest* 99:496-498, 1991.
40. Schoen FJ: The first step to understanding valve failure: an overview of pathology, *Eur J Cardiothorac Surg* 6:550-553, 1992.
41. Silver K, et al: Pulmonary artery hypertension in severe aortic stenosis: incidence and mechanism, *Am Heart J* 125:146-153, 1992.
42. *St Anthony's DRG Guidebook 1995,* Reston, Va, 1994, St Anthony.
43. Stein PD, et al: Antithrombotic therapy in patients with mechanical and biological prosthetic heart valves, *Chest* 102:445S-455S, 1992.
44. Teoh KH, et al: Survival and valve failure after aortic valve replacement, *Ann Thorac Surg* 32:270-275, 1991.
45. Walley VM, et al: Patterns of failure in Hancock pericardial bioprosthesis, *J Thorac Cardiovasc Surg* 102:187-194, 1991.

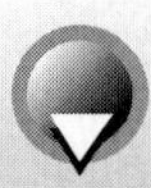

CLINICAL GUIDELINE

24

Sternal Wound Infection

Susan O'Brien Norris, MS, RN, CCRN

DESCRIPTION

Sternal wound infection, a potentially life-threatening complication of cardiac surgery, may result in increased mortality and morbidity and significant revenue loss. Poststernotomy wound infection has been categorized as a superficial presternal infection or deep retrosternal infection.[24] Superficial wound infection will be evident within the first week of surgery, probably caused by contamination, and is treated with local drainage and wound care. Deep retrosternal infection involves infection of the mediastinum and sternum. Mediastinitis requires re-operation for removal of mediastinal infection and necrosis and rewiring the sternum. Long-term parenteral antibiotic therapy and muscle flap reconstruction are usually required.

The incidence of sternal wound infection has been reported recently to range from 0.16% to 1.86%.[20,26,31,34] Stiegel et al. reported a 0.94% incidence of mediastinitis in a pediatric cardiac surgical population of 2242.[44] Mortality rates quoted in the literature vary widely and range from 52% to 70% due to mediastinitis, and 5.3% in patients with mediastinitis treated with muscle flap reconstruction.[8,30,39]

Early diagnosis and treatment of mediastinitis is critical in order to reduce morbidity, mortality, length of stay (LOS), and consumption of resources. Re-operation, long-term wound care, and extensive intravenous antibiotic therapy are often part of the extended care of patients with mediastinitis. This complication frequently occurs in the elderly. Cost was noted to increase by $8500 for an infection of a saphenous vein incision, $9000 for a deep subcutaneous incision infection, $40,000 for a sternal infection, and $73,000 for mediastinitis in one study alone.[23] Another study compared cardiac surgery patients who were without infection to patients who had sternal wound infections, leg incision infections, or prosthetic valve endocarditis. The infected group showed doubled hospital cost and an increase of 19 days in average LOS.[4]

Nurses caring for cardiac surgery patients must be expert in promotion of wound healing and early recognition of wound infection and sternal dehiscence. Timely, collaborative care will improve patient outcomes and, as a result, reduce cost. In the event that a sternal wound infection cannot be prevented, some have recommended less costly home care for patients who require extended parenteral antibiotics and wound care.[16]

PATHOPHYSIOLOGY

Median sternotomy is the most common approach used for patients requiring cardiac operations. It provides access to the heart and great vessels and has less respiratory complications and pain when compared to a thoracotomy incision. Mediastinitis is most likely to occur as a result of delayed wound healing and poor host defenses. Contamination of the mediastinum is less frequently the cause. Table 24-1 compares four studies that identified risk factors in the development of mediastinitis.

Advanced age, diabetes mellitus, impaired immunocompetence, inadequate perfusion, inadequate oxygenation, infection, malnutrition, obesity, and preoperative illness increase the risk of impaired wound healing.[33] Sternal wound infection rates in two studies of cardiac surgery patients 80 years or older were found to be 5% rather than the 1.86% seen in other adult cardiac surgery patients.[14,45]

Wound healing is impaired in diabetics because of deficits in wound perfusion and oxygenation caused by small-vessel disease and hyperglycemia. Diabetics who undergo cardiac

TABLE 24-1 Mediastinitis Risk Factors

Loop et al. n = 6504 1.1% developed mediastinitis or sternal dehiscence 1990	Ottino et al. n = 2579 1.86% developed mediastinitis 1987	Grossi et al. 0.97% developed mediastinitis 1985	Edwards and Baker Nine pediatric patients 1983
• Bilateral internal thoracic artery grafting in a diabetic • Obesity • Prolonged operating time • Blood transfusions	• Hospital environment (operating room had moved) • Preoperative length of stay • Reoperation • Blood transfusions • Early chest reexploration • Sternal rewiring	• Combined revascularization and valve replacement • Early reexploration for bleeding • Prolonged low cardiac output syndrome • Prolonged ventilatory support • Severe concomitant infection	• Bypass time of greater than 1 hour • Excessive postoperative bleeding • Low cardiac output for ≥24 hours postoperatively • Reexploration for bleeding • Inadequate antimicrobial prophylaxis

Adapted with permission from Norris, SO: Managing postoperative mediastinitis, *J Cardiovasc Nurs* 3(3):52-65, 1989.

surgery require careful assessment of serum glucose and continuous regulation of insulin to achieve control of hyperglycemia and minimize their added risk of sternal wound infection.

Immunosuppressed cardiac transplant patients have an increased incidence of mediastinitis of 1% to 10%.[17,22] One cardiac transplant study reported subclinical manifestation of fatal mediastinitis that demonstrated the role of immunosuppression in masking the true extent of the mediastinitis.[6]

Cardiopulmonary bypass temporarily causes vasoconstriction, anemia, and hypovolemia. Vasoconstriction directly reduces wound perfusion and the delivery of oxygen to the healing tissues.[47] Factors contributing to vasoconstriction include hypothermia, severed afferent nerves, hypovolemia, fear, pain, surgical stress, and sympathetic nervous system response.[47] Aggressive management of vasoconstriction and hypoxia reduce the risk of wound complications.

Excessive wound stress may cause wound dehiscence, herniation, and nonunion. Reduced tensile strength is seen in wounds of the obese. Sternal dehiscence risk factors include obesity, repeated sternotomy, bleeding or tamponade, debilitated patients, and osteoporosis.[32] Wound stress also may be caused by exaggerated coughing, vomiting, struggling with arm restraints, external cardiac massage, fighting the ventilator, or strenuous pulling or flexing activity of the upper extremities. Use of a circumferential ribcage splint increases patient comfort and decreases wound stress during coughing and deep breathing and movement in and out of bed (Figure 24-1). Large-breasted women should be encouraged to wear a supportive bra to minimize the weight of the breasts on the sternal incision. It is beneficial if the surgeon alerts the nursing staff of sternums that may be at risk due to poor bone quality.

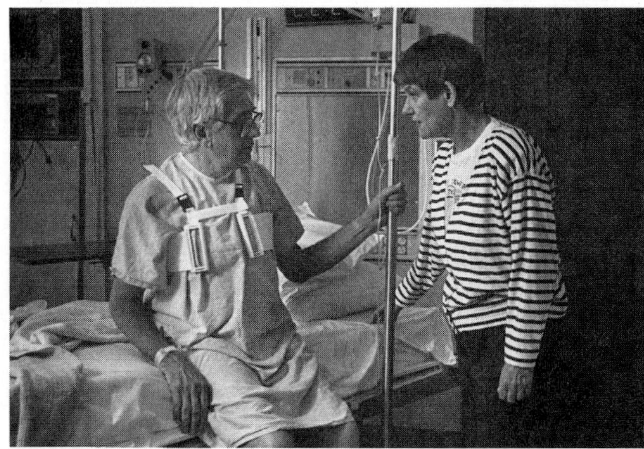

Figure 24-1 The *Heart Hugger* is a circumferential ribcage splint used to increase patient comfort while decreasing mechanical stress on the sternotomy. It is used during coughing and deep breathing, incentive spirometry, and moving in or out of bed or chair. The device's handles are positioned over the mid-sternal area a generous handwidth apart. When needed, the patient squeezes the handles together, thereby tightening ribcage support and lessening surgical incision stress. The *Heart Hugger* is applied early postoperatively and used for several weeks after hospital discharge. (Used with permission of General Cardiac Technology, Mountain View, California.)

The association between the internal mammary artery graft and the risk of sternal wound infection has been debated in the literature. An early study found a sternal wound infection rate of 1.1% to saphenous vein grafting, 2.3% for left internal mammary artery grafting, and 8.5% for bilateral internal mammary artery grafting.[12] However, diabetes mellitus and advanced age were the risk factors for sternal wound infection found in a study that employed multivariate logistic regression analysis to matched groups of patients receiving saphenous vein grafting, single internal mammary artery grafting, and bilateral internal mammary artery grafting.[10,21] In a comparison of saphenous vein grafts versus internal mammary artery grafts to the left anterior descending artery, no difference was seen in wound complication rates.[42] A fourth study demonstrated no statistical difference in sternal wound infection rates in nondiabetic patient groups receiving saphenous vein grafting, single internal thoracic artery grafting, or bilateral internal thoracic grafting.[26]

Delayed sternal wound closure due to myocardial edema or uncontrolled hemorrhage secondary to postcardiopulmonary bypass coagulopathy does not appear to be a risk factor for mediastinitis providing the mediastinum is isolated from the environment. In a study of 13 patients requiring delayed sternal wound closure until postoperative day 2 to 5, no sternal wound infection was seen.[29] In all patients, only the skin was closed and they were mechanically ventilated from the initial surgery to sternal wound closure.[29] No mediastinitis was found in a second study where the mediastinum was isolated from the environment by either skin approximation, patching a synthetic membrane to skin edges, or use of a plastic drape in situations where delayed sternal closure was necessitated by cardiac edema or uncontrolled hemorrhage.[27]

While not all factors that impair wound healing can be altered, early awareness of those risk factors and interventions to promote wound healing can reduce wound complications.

LENGTH OF STAY/ANTICIPATED COURSE

The usual LOS for uncomplicated myocardial revascularization or valve surgery is approximately 10 to 18 days according to HCFA data.[43] Some centers have demonstrated LOS as short as 4 to 5 days with a program built to support early transition to home. Some insurers have announced that a 5-day LOS for coronary artery bypass grafting will be the reimbursed standard.

The DRG system does not specify major complications to cardiac procedures. Additional payment is not automatically made if postoperative wound infections occur. While hospitals will seek a discharge diagnosis for patients that best matches the resources used to care for the patient, the original DRG for the cardiac surgery typically demonstrates a longer average LOS and commensurate reimbursement than the DRGs specific to the medical or surgical management of sternal wound infection.

Sternal wound infection results in longer LOS and increased costs as demonstrated in a study of patients experiencing sternal wound infection, saphenous vein donor site infection, or prosthetic valve endocarditis when compared with controls.[4] In the presence of one of these infections, LOS increased 18.5 days and cost doubled.[4] A mean increase of 43 days in LOS and a median cost increase of 2.8 times that of noninfected patients was determined in another study of patients with mediastinitis.[26]

The course of sternal wound infection includes diagnostic techniques, antibiotic therapy, debridement procedures, complex wound care, and muscle flap and/or skin grafting. LOS may be extended an average of 14 days to several months with systemic complications. Strategies to reduce LOS and costs include early diagnosis and treatment of the infection, early involvement of a plastic surgeon, and, if the wound is open and healing by secondary intent, discharge home once the wound is covered with a bed of granulation tissue.

MANAGEMENT TRENDS AND CONTROVERSIES

Early diagnosis and treatment of mediastinitis reduces mortality, complications, and costs. Infection involving the sternum or substernal space (mediastinal area) is required to make the diagnosis of mediastinitis.[11] The presentation of mediastinitis may be diverse: at times obvious, at times occult. Signs and symptoms of mediastinitis are listed in the following Box. Mediastinitis usually presents on the sixth to twenty-first postoperative day.[1] This has discharge teaching ramifications for all cardiac surgery patients, since they could develop mediastinitis after hospital discharge.

Signs and Symptoms of Sternal Wound Infection

Wound

Erythema
Edema
Warmth
Drainage, positive culture
Infected or necrotic tissue
Sternal instability or dehiscence
Tenderness
Atypical or excessive wound pain

Chest

Unilateral or bilateral pleural effusions
Pulmonary infiltrates
Pericardial effusion
Widened superior mediastinum
Crepitus of chest wall
Drainage from chest tube stab wounds or epicardial pacer wire site
Dyspnea or tachypnea

Systemic

Fever
Tachycardia
Elevated WBC count or differential
Elevated sedimentation rate
Weakness

Diagnostic Tests for Mediastinitis

White blood cell count and differential
Wound culture
Chest x-ray
Retrosternal aspirate culture
Computed tomography
Indium-111 leukocyte scan
Epicardial wire culture
Chest wall thermography
Plasma protein trends

In one study of 7949 cardiac surgery patients, temperature greater than 38.6° C, white blood cell count >12,000/mm^3, and drainage from the sternal wound or chest tube site correlated with mediastinitis.[20] Fever >38° C after the third postoperative day is abnormal and may signify respiratory or wound infection.[36] Wound drainage in combination with sternal instability is associated with advanced mediastinitis.[40] However, sternal drainage does not always indicate infection. Drainage may occur with hematoma or fat necrosis as well as mediastinitis or superficial tissue infection.[11] Sternal instability may also occur in the absence of infection.

Diagnostic tests may be used to confirm mediastinitis or if manifestations are unclear. The following Box describes the tests to diagnose mediastinitis. Negative wound or cardiac prosthesis cultures were found in 23% to 36% of patients with mediastinitis.[8,35] Staphylococcus was cultured in mediastinitis in 60% to 77% of patients in other studies.[9,20,30] *S. aureus* and *S. epidermidis* predominated in these studies, with gram negative pathogens occurring next in frequency. Survival has been shown to be enhanced when early antistaphylococcal and gram negative antibiotics are used.[38] However, more than half of patients with mediastinitis may be infected by the pathogens that are resistant to the prophylactic antibiotics most often used.[20]

Computed tomography (CT) scan provides a safe, rapid, noninvasive means to define mediastinitis, thereby expediting treatment. It accurately demonstrates sternal defects, fluid and gas collection, and abscesses of the presternal tissue, sternum, and retrosternal space.[5] Indium-111 leukocyte scan and epicardial pacer wire culture have also been identified to have diagnostic value in poststernotomy mediastinitis.[5]

Aspiration of retrosternal fluid in poststernotomy patients with suspected mediastinitis or evidence of infection of unknown etiology provides a mechanism of evaluation of mediastinal fluid. A technique of low-risk mediastinal tap in postcardiac surgical patients has been shown to document early mediastinitis in 9 of the 24 patients in a sample of 4000 cardiac surgery patients prior to the appearance of wound drainage or sternal instability.[40] The 15 remaining patients had a negative mediastinal culture and did not develop mediastinitis.[40]

TABLE 24-2 Flaps for Wound Closure in Postcardiotomy Mediastinitis*

Bypass conduit	Flap
Vein grafts or single internal mammary artery	Contralateral split pectoralis turnover Contralateral rectus abdominus Ipsilateral pectoralis rotation advancement
Bilateral internal mammary artery	Segmental pectoralis flap Pectoralis rotation advancement Bipedicled pectoralis-rectus flap Rectus abdominus (intercostal blood supply) Omentum Latissimus dorsi.

*Flaps are listed in order of preference.
Reprinted with permission. Craver JM, et al: Management of postcardiotomy mediastinitis. In Waldhausen JA, Orringer MB, editors: *Complications in cardiac surgery,* St Louis, 1991, Mosby–Year Book.

Chest radiography may be abnormal in mediastinitis and seen as a widened mediastinum, gas or fluid accumulation, or pulmonary changes.[7] However, chest x-ray changes may not occur until after clinical manifestations are apparent.

Changes in the skin temperature of patients with sternal wound infection have been detected noninvasively with thermography.[37] Plasma protein monitoring has also been investigated as an early indicator of mediastinitis in open-heart surgery patients. In a study of 188 poststernotomy patients, deviations in alpha$_1$-acid glycoprotein and C-reactive protein were highly predictive in the development of mediastinitis.[28] In another study, C-reactive protein increases occurring after the third day were found in all patients who developed mediastinitis.[46] Temperature elevation and white blood cell increase were seen in most but not all patients who developed mediastinitis.[46]

Mediastinitis is managed by eradicating the infection and healing the wound. Upon strong suspicion or confirmation of infection, incision and debridement are done to remove all infected or necrotic tissue and assess the extent of the infection. The entire wound is opened, sternal wires are removed, and infected or necrotic tissue is removed to the level of inducing bleeding in the tissue or bone.[1] The mediastinum is then irrigated with normal saline or an antimicrobial solution. Broad-spectrum intravenous antibiotics are begun until the drug sensitivities of the infecting organism are known. Incomplete debridement of infected tissue, bone, or rib cartilage often results in recurrent mediastinitis.[2,35] After debridement, the patient is closely monitored for evidence of infection. In one study, 25% of patients with mediastinitis required a second debriding.[20]

Wound management choices, following debridement, may be summarized as (1) muscle flap closure of the mediastinum, (2) closure of the mediastinum and continuous

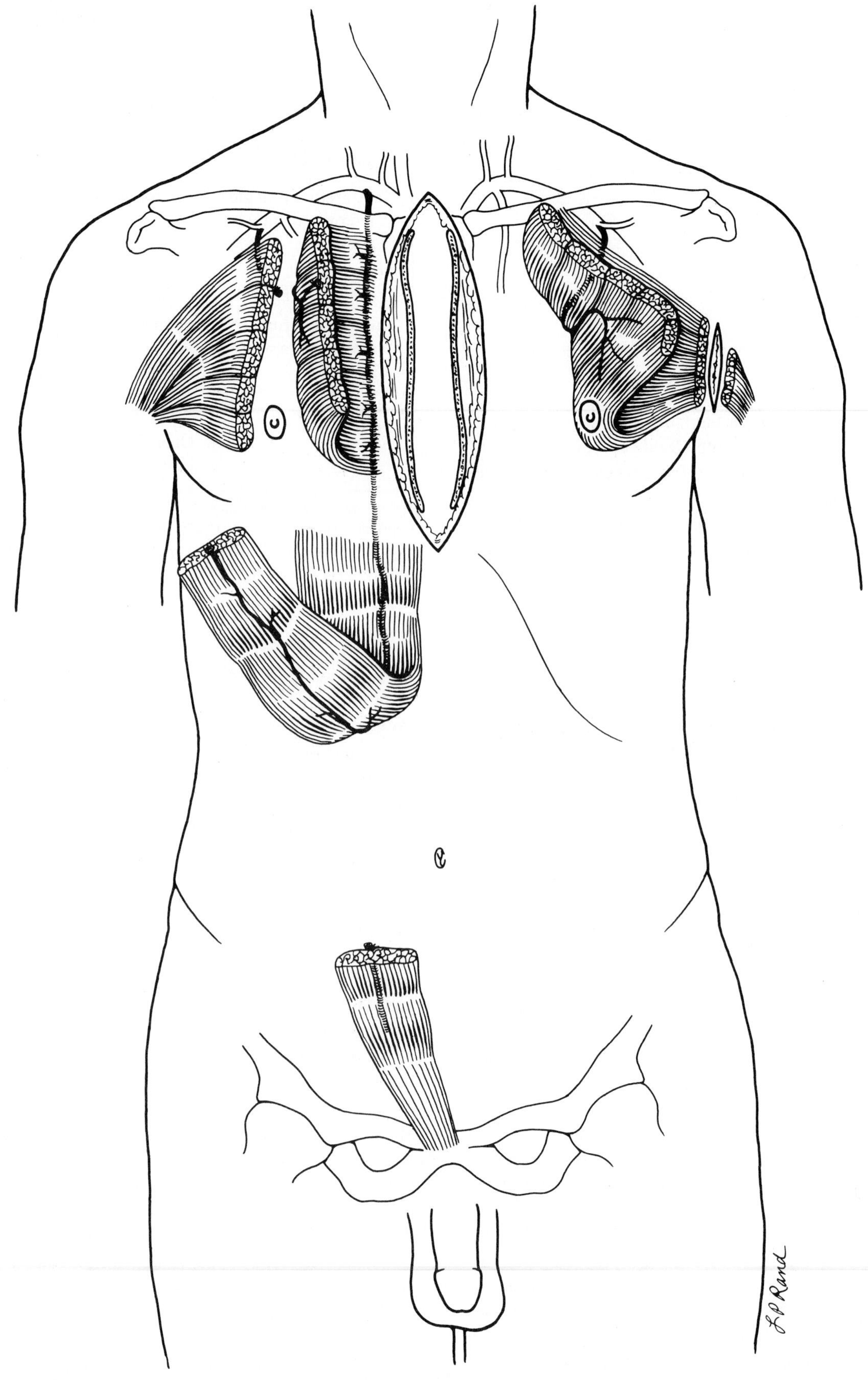

Figure 24-2 Examples of multiple muscle flaps: right pectoralis flap; left pectoralis rotation advancement flap; right rectus abdominus muscle flap. (Used with permission from Craver JM, et al: Management of postcardiotomy mediastinitis. In Waldhausen JA, Orringer ME, editors: *Complications in cardiothoracic surgery,* St Louis, 1991, Mosby.

mediastinal irrigation, or (3) wound care and monitoring with the mediastinum open.

Muscle flap reconstruction obliterates mediastinal dead space, speeds healing by providing well-vascularized tissue, reduces the risk of further infection, protects underlying tissue, and strengthens respiratory mechanics. Types of muscle flap procedures are listed in Table 24-2. Figure 24-2 illustrates muscle flap procedures.

In the early 1980s muscle flaps were used for refractory mediastinitis, extensive mediastinal defects, and sternal loss. However, recent research has demonstrated that muscle flap reconstruction results in significantly lower mortality, fewer complications, and shorter LOS, and should be the primary method of treatment for mediastinitis.[9,30,44] Using muscle flap reconstruction as the primary treatment of post-sternotomy mediastinitis, a fourfold decrease in mortality and decreased LOS were realized when compared to closed-chest irrigation or wound packing.[30] The use of muscle flap reconstruction rather than chest irrigation has been recommended in children with postoperative mediastinitis based on evidence that ventilator support could be shortened by up to 21 days, ICU stay could be reduced by 17 days, wound complications could be reduced, and emotional and physical trauma of otherwise extensive wound care in the child could be eliminated.[15,44] A comparative study showed 33% mortality in patients with mediastinitis treated with chest irrigation alone, while mortality was absent in the muscle flap reconstruction groups.[9] One group had wound closure after 3 to 5 days following debridement, while the other group had omentum reconstruction immediately after mediastinal debridement and sternal rewiring.[9]

Following muscle flap reconstruction, most patients are ready for hospital discharge within 2 weeks. No change in mobility of the shoulder girdle or torso, function, or final anesthetic outcome were found in a group of patients who received pectoralis major muscle flaps.[41]

Another treatment option, continuous mediastinal irrigation, is used to create a sterile wound and mediastinum. The sternum is rewired over a catheter placed in the chest used to infuse a broad-spectrum antimicrobial solution or an antibiotic specific to the cultured organism. Chest tubes are used to drain the solution. The chest drainage must be equal to the irrigation volume. The catheter is removed when the drainage is sterile and there is no evidence of infection.

Unfortunately, fatal iodine toxicity has been reported in a three-year old child with postoperative mediastinitis who was treated with povidone-iodine chest irrigation.[19] Povidone-iodine irrigation for mediastinitis caused significant metabolic complications in three other pediatric patients resulting in one death.[44] Systemic and local absorption of iodine manifested in part by severe chemical pericarditis was demonstrated in a canine model following povidone-iodine chest irrigation.[19] The study authors advise extreme caution in the use of povidone-iodine chest irrigation, a dilution of 1:1000, and frequent assessment of serum iodine levels.

When gentamycin is used in the irrigating solution, size-related outcomes of toxic levels of the antibiotic in small patients and subtherapeutic levels in large-sized patients have resulted in the recommendation to carefully monitor gentamycin blood levels during mediastinal irrigation.[25]

The third wound treatment option, open wound care, has the advantage of ongoing visualization of the wound and ability to readily debride nonviable tissues. The wound may be allowed to heal by secondary intent, or muscle flap reconstruction may be done once the infection is resolved. However, open management of the wound may result in impaired respiratory dynamics, contamination of the wound, or prolonged LOS. If the sternum is not intact, a decision must be made and communicated regarding the handling of cardiac massage in the event of cardiac arrest.

Wound dressings should provide a slightly moist environment within the wound and, upon removal, minimize injury to newly healing tissue.[13] Wet-to-damp dressings of normal saline are an example of this type of dressing. The dressing is wrung out and interfaced with all wound surfaces in a thin layer. This is then covered with a dry dressing and secured with Montgomery straps, paper tape, stretchy non-adherent tape, or a lightweight body stocking. The dressing will need tape across the top to hold it in place during ambulation. The wet-to-damp dressing must be moist when removed to avoid disruption of healing tissue. If the wound bleeds after dressing removal, healing tissue has been disturbed. If it is stuck to the wound, the dressing must be moistened with sterile saline as it is removed. Once the saturated dressing can be easily removed, it should be taken off.

Ongoing wound monitoring and documentation of wound appearance should include wound size; presence of necrosis, exudate, and granulation tissue; and new capillary development.

ASSESSMENT

PARAMETER	ANTICIPATED ALTERATION
Sternal wound appearance	Approximated versus separated wound edges Possible loss of wound tissue Wound may have evidence of normal, infected, and/or necrotic tissue. Skin around wound may be indurated, reddened, warm, or edematous. There may be pain, tenderness, or a change in sensation associated with the wound. Wound drainage may be malodorous, serous, serosanguineous, or purulent. The drainage may come from the wound, chest tube site, or epicardial pacer wire site.

Sternal integrity	Sternal instability or dehiscence evidenced by grating, clicking, or sternal separation with breathing or coughing. Patient may report chest "giving way." Patient may experience dyspnea. Sternal sucking or bubbling on deep breathing Palpation of a separated sternum Widened mediastinum may be seen on chest x-ray
Temperature	Elevated: >38° C after postoperative day 3
WBC	Elevated: >10,000/mm^3
Wound culture	Positive or negative wound culture
Chest x-ray	Sternal fragmentation, pleural effusion, or widened mediastinum

Cardiovascular Status

HR	Tachycardia: HR >100 bpm at rest
Rhythm	NSR, atrial dysrythmias
MAP	Decreased: <70 mm Hg *if septic syndrome accompanies mediastinitis*
SVR	Decreased: <800 dynes/sec/cm^{-5} *if septic syndrome accompanies mediastinitis*
Cardiac index (CI)	Elevated: >4 L/min/m^2 *if septic syndrome accompanies mediastinitis*
Pulmonary status	Hypoventilation and respiratory distress *if sternal dehiscence occurs*
RR and pattern	Tachypneic with change in respiratory pattern
ABG	Respiratory acidosis and hypoxia • pH: <7.35 • P_{CO_2}: >45 mm Hg • P_{O_2}: <80 mm Hg
LOC, behavior	May change *due to hypoventilation or sepsis*

Uncontrolled infection often results in sepsis, which may trigger hemodynamic deterioration, acute respiratory distress syndrome (ARDS), renal failure, and other system dysfunction. Sternal dehiscence may cause disrupted respiratory and cardiovascular dynamics.

PLAN OF CARE

INTENSIVE PHASE

The major goals for this phase include: limit the infectious process within the wound, promote wound healing, minimize anxiety in the patient and significant other, and manage pain. Most patients who remain in the ICU during this phase are there short-term following debridement or muscle flap grafting, or have significant multisystem compromise as a result of mediastinitis. Those patients with respiratory, cardiovascular, or multisystem sequelae of mediastinitis are at risk for suboptimal perfusion and oxygenation of the wound.

PATIENT CARE PRIORITIES	EXPECTED PATIENT OUTCOMES
High risk for infection *r/t* *Impaired tissue integrity* *Impaired wound healing* *Immunocompromise* *Wound stress*	Approximated wound edges or, if wound is open, evidence of granulation tissue No necrotic or infected tissue or wound drainage Intact sternum Adequate wound oxygenation and perfusion Controlled blood glucose if diabetic Adequate sleep Minimal wound stress Temperature: WNL Optimal nutrition

Plan of Care (cont'd)

Ineffective breathing pattern *r/t* *Dehised sternum* *Increased work of breathing* *Anxiety* *Pain*	WNL/improved respiratory pattern Intact sternum/chest stability Decreased anxiety Improved comfort Activity tolerance
Anxiety *r/t* *Unexpected, significant postoperative complication* *Fear of unknown*	Reduced anxiety Able to rest, sleep, maintain nutritional intake Demonstrates trust in caregivers
Pain *r/t wound infection and treatments*	Verbalizes adequate comfort Able to participate in ADL Able to rest, sleep

INTERVENTIONS

Ensure effective preoperative skin preparation prior to the initial surgery *to reduce the risk of postoperative wound infection.*[3]

Ensure optimal timing of preoperative and perioperative antibiotics at the time of the initial surgery *to reduce the risk of postoperative wound infection.*

Identify patients at risk for poor wound healing (e.g., immunocompromised, elderly, diabetic, malnourished, reexploration) and institute appropriate compensatory or protective measures.

Manage hypothermia, pain, hypovolemia, and vasoconstriction after initial surgery *to minimize wound hypoxia and promote wound healing and resistance to infection.*

Ensure adequate filling pressures, MAP, CI, and SaO_2 *to promote adequate wound oxygenation and perfusion.*

Do not remove original dressing for first 24 hours *to allow adequate time for skin edges to seal and thus reduce the risk of infection.*

Expose nondraining incisions to air after 24 hours *to promote wound healing.*

Practice meticulous handwashing and aseptic wound care *to reduce contamination.*

Splint the entire ribcage when suctioning or coughing *to minimize wound stress.*

Suppress exaggerated coughing, vomiting, struggling with arm restraints, or "bucking the ventilation" *to minimize wound stress.*

Recognize that exaggerated wound stress occurs in patients receiving external cardiac massage and patients who have repeat sternal opening in the immediate postoperative period.

Cover a newly dehised sternal wound with sterile towels moistened with sterile saline and immediately notify physician *to prevent wound contamination.*

Monitor the patient with new sternal wound dehiscence for potential respiratory and cardiovascular deterioration.

Cover sternal wounds that are not intact or are draining with a sterile dressing.

Monitor the color of the muscle flap reconstruction site for evidence of adequate oxygenation *to identify hypoperfused muscle flaps early.*

Protect all sternal wounds from respiratory secretions or drainage contamination by elevating head of bed and covering the chest with a waterproof drape when suctioning.

Assess and document the appearance of open wounds with each dressing change *to detect evidence of healing or infection. A healing wound is red or pink in color, is becoming smaller, or may have a healing ridge around the wound and/or granulation tissue in the wound. An infected wound may be yellow in color with purulent drainage and, over time, enlarge in size. A necrotic wound has a black eschar.*[13]

Apply a wet-to-damp dressing in a single layer on the wound *to avoid masceration of the skin.*

Use a net body stocking, Montgomery straps, or Co-ban nonstick tape *to avoid denuding the skin with repeated tape removal during dressing changes.*

Consult with a dietitian, pharmacist, and physician to develop an optimal nutritional plan *to provide wound healing substrates and promote immune function.*

Plan of Care (cont'd)

Monitor weight and intake of calories, protein, carbohydrates, fats, minerals, and vitamins.
Ensure adequate sleep *to improve immune function, tissue regeneration, and ability to cope.*
Maintain normal temperature.
Monitor for respiratory instability if sternum is not intact.
Encourage airway clearance by means of coughing and deep breathing, incentive spirometry, ambulation, repositioning, and postural drainage *to maximize oxygen delivery and exchange.*
Monitor pulse oximetry and pulmonary assessment *to detect changes in oxygenation.*
Ensure accurate perception of condition and plan of care *to reduce anxiety.*
Use the calming strategies of a consistent, supportive, caregiver using a reassuring manner, eye contact, touch, reality orientation, and simple, concrete commands *to reduce anxiety.*
Encourage the use of support, such as family/significant others and/or religion *to reduce anxiety and promote adaptive coping.*
Administer analgesics on a scheduled basis *to maintain adequate pain control and ensure patient cooperation with wound care and ADL.*
Use relaxation, distraction, imagery, and/or music *to enhance pain control and reduce anxiety.*

INTERMEDIATE PHASE

Once the infection is brought under control and potential sepsis-related complications are resolved or controlled, the priority of wound healing continues. In addition, the greater wound care involvement of the patient and/or family/significant other is emphasized to facilitate transition to discharge.

PATIENT CARE PRIORITIES	**EXPECTED PATIENT OUTCOMES**
High risk for impaired wound healing *r/t prolonged hospitalization and wound care process*	Free from infection Approximated wound skin edges or evidence of granulation tissue within wound Adequate wound perfusion and oxygenation Adequate nutrition Adequate sleep Blood glucose: WNL
High risk for ineffective coping *r/t* *Body image changes* *Dependency in self-care* *Loss of health*	Looks at wound and accurately discusses wound appearance Takes responsibility for wound care as appropriate Demonstrates activities to manage anxiety and cope with implications of illness Progresses activity to full ADL Resumes self-care Practices energy conservation
High risk for inadequate nutrition *r/t increased metabolic demands associated with wound healing*	Consumes adequate calories and protein

INTERVENTIONS

Ensure adequate MAP, SaO_2 *to maintain adequate wound perfusion and oxygenation.*
Ensure adequate nutrition *to provide additional substrate needed for tissue regeneration.*
Promote adequate sleep *to facilitate tissue regeneration, energy for ADL and coping.*
Assist patient and family/significant other in identifying issues related to body image changes and losses.
Discuss wound appearance and plan of wound management with patient and family/significant other.
Encourage the patient and family/significant other to view the wound to establish what the wound looks like *to ensure a realistic perception of the wound.*

Plan of Care (cont'd)

Point out evidence of healing within the wound.

Involve the patient and family/significant other in wound care and self-care.

Encourage the patient and family/significant other to examine the meaning of the losses they have experienced with this illness *to correct any misperceptions.*

Collaborate with cardiac rehabilitation and/or physical therapy *to progress strengthening exercises and ambulation.*

Use distraction techniques *to reduce the boredom and stress of prolonged hospitalization.*

Prior to hospital discharge, ensure that the patient and family/significant other have a clear understanding of activity progression, wound care, indicators of wound infection and healing, and nutrition.

TRANSITION TO DISCHARGE

Hospital discharge following mediastinitis occurs once there is significant wound healing and absence of infection. If the wound has been left open to heal by secondary intent, resistance to reinfection is greater when granulation tissue is present. Once the patient and/or family/significant other has demonstrated proper wound care and can verbalize the indicators of wound reinfection, activity restrictions, and the dosing and purpose of medications, discharge can occur. If sternal osteomyelitis has occurred, additional teaching and home care referral are necessary for at-home intravenous antibiotic administration, intravenous site evaluation and care, and drug and supply acquisition. Follow-up home care may provide important support, prevent reinfection, and ensure optimal, complete recovery in all patients discharged while previously infected sternal wounds are still in a healing phase.

REFERENCES

1. Acinapura AJ, et al: Surgical management of infected median sternotomy: closed irrigation vs. muscle flaps, *J Cardiovasc Surg* 26(5):443-446, 1985.
2. Arnold PG, Pairolero PC: Intrathoracic muscle flaps: a 10-year experience in the management of life-threatening infections, *Plast Reconstr Surg* 84(1):92-98, 1989.
3. Association of Operating Room Nurses: *1993 Standards and recommended practices,* Denver, 1993, AORN.
4. Boyce JM, Potter-Bynoe G, Dziobek L: Hospital reimbursement patterns among patients with surgical wound infections following open-heart surgery, *Infect Control Hosp Epidemiol* 11(2):89-93, 1990.
5. Browdie DA, et al: Diagnosis of poststernotomy infection: comparison of three means of assessment, *Ann Thorac Surg* 51(2):290-292, 1991.
6. Byl B, et al: Mediastinitis caused by *Aspergillus fumigatus* with a ruptured aortic pseudoaneurysm in a heart transplant recipient: case study, *Heart Lung* 22(2):145-147, 1993.
7. Carrol CL, et al: CT evaluation of mediastinal infections, *J Comput Assist Tomogr* 11(3):449-454, 1987.
8. Cheung EH, et al: Mediastinitis after cardiac valve operations, *J Thorac Cardiovasc Surg* 90(4):517-522, 1985.
9. Colen LB, Huntsman WT, Morain WD: The integrated approach to suppurative mediastinitis: rewiring the sternum over transposed omentum, *Plast Reconstr Surg* 84(6):936-941, 1989.
10. Cosgrove DM, et al: Does bilateral internal mammary artery grafting increase surgical risk? *J Thorac Cardiovasc Surg* 95(5):850-856, 1988.
11. Craver JM, et al: Management of postcardiotomy mediastinitis. In Waldhausen JA, Orringer MB, editors: *Complications in cardiothoracic surgery,* St Louis, 1991, Mosby–Year Book.
12. Culliford AT, et al: Sternal and costochondral infections following open-heart surgery: a review of 2594 cases, *J Thorac Cardiovasc Surg* 72(5):714-726, 1976.
13. Cuzzell JZ. Choosing a wound dressing: a systemic approach, *AACN Clin Iss Crit Care Nurs* 1(3):566-577, 1990.
14. Edmunds LH, et al: Open-heart surgery in octogenarians, *N Engl J Med* 319(3):131-136, 1988.
15. Edwards MS, Baker CJ: Median sternotomy wound infections in children, *Pediatr Infect Dis J* 2(2):105-109, 1983.
16. Fara AM, Wolff PH: Discharge planning for cardiothoracic patients requiring extensive wound care, *Crit Care Nurse* 7(2):103-108, 1987.
17. Gentry LO, Zeluff BJ: Nosocomial and other difficult infections in the immunocompromised cardiac transplant patient, *J Hosp Infect* 11(suppl A):21-28, 1988.
18. Glick PL, et al: Iodine toxicity in a patient treated with continuous povidone-iodine mediastinal irrigation, *Ann Thorac Surg* 39(5):478-480, 1985.
19. Glick PL, et al: Iodine toxicity secondary to continuous povidone-iodine mediastinal irrigation in dogs, *J Surg Res* 49(5):428-434, 1990.
20. Grossi EA, et al: A survey of 77 major infectious complications of median sternotomy: a review of 7949 consecutive operative procedures, *Ann Thorac Surg* 40(3):214-221, 1985.
21. Grossi EA, et al: Sternal wound infections and use of internal mammary artery grafts, *J Thorac Cardiovasc Surg* 102(3):342-347, 1991.
22. Hofflin JM, et al: Infectious complications in heart transplant recipients receiving cyclosporine and corticosteroids, *Ann Intern Med* 106(2):209-216, 1987.
23. Kaiser AB, et al: Efficacy of cefazolin, cefamandole, and gentamycin as prophylactic agents in cardiac surgery, *Ann Surg* 206(6):791-797, 1987.
24. Kay HR, et al: Use of computed tomography to assess mediastinal complications after median sternotomy, *Ann Thorac Surg* 36(6):706-714, 1983.
25. Kopel ME, et al: Gentamycin solution for mediastinal irrigation: sys-

temic absorption, bactericidal activity, and toxicity, *Ann Thorac Surg* 48(2):228-31, 1989.
26. Loop FD, et al: Sternal wound complications after isolated coronary artery bypass grafting: early and late mortality, morbidity, and cost of care, *Ann Thorac Surg* 49(2):179-187, 1990.
27. Mestres CA, et al: Delayed sternal closure for life-threatening complications in cardiac operations: an update, *Ann Thorac Surg* 51(5):773-776, 1991.
28. Miholic J, et al: Early prediction of deep sternal wound infection after heart operations by alpha$_1$-acid glycoprotein and C-reactive protein measurements, *Ann Thorac Surg* 42(4):429-433, 1986.
29. Milgater E, et al: Delayed sternal closure following cardiac operations, *J Cardiovasc Surg* 27(3):328-331, 1986.
30. Nahai F, et al: Primary treatment of the infected sternotomy wound with muscle flaps: a review of 211 consecutive cases, *Plast Reconstr Surg* 84(3):434-441, 1989.
31. Nishida H, et al: Discriminate use of electrocautery on the median sternotomy incision, *J Thorac Cardiovasc Surg* 101(3):488-494, 1991.
32. Norris SO: Managing postoperative mediastinitis, *J Cardiovasc Nurs* 3(3):52-65, 1989.
33. Norris SO, Provo B, Stotts NA: Physiology of wound healing and risk factors that impede the healing process, *AACN Clin Iss Crit Care Nurs* 1(3):545-552, 1990.
34. Ottino G, et al: Major sternal wound infection after open-heart surgery: a multivariate analysis of risk factors in 2579 consecutive operative procedures, *Ann Thorac Surg* 44(2):173-179, 1987.
35. Pairolero P, Arnold P: Management of recalcitrant median sternotomy wounds, *J Thorac Cardiovasc Surg* 88(2):357-364, 1984.
36. Pien F, Ho P, Fergusson D: Fever and infection after cardiac operation, *Ann Thorac Surg* 33(4):382-384, 1982.
37. Robicsek F, et al: The value of thermography in the early diagnosis of postoperative sternal wound infections, *Thorac Cardiovasc Surg* 32(4):260-265, 1984.
38. Rosenbaum GS, Klein NC, Cunha BA: Poststernotomy mediastinitis, *Heart Lung* 19(4):371-372, 1990.
39. Rutledge R, Applebaum RE, Kim BJ: Mediastinal infection after open-heart surgery, *Surgery* 97(1):88-92, 1985.
40. Sarr MG, Watkins L, Stewart JR: Mediastinal tap as useful method for the early diagnosis of mediastinal infection, *Surg Gynecol Obstet* 159(1):79-81, 1984.
41. Scully HE, et al: Comparison between antibiotic irrigation and mobilization of pectoral muscle flaps in treatment of deep sternal infections, *J Thorac Cardiovasc Surg* 90(4):523-531, 1985.
42. Sethi GK, et al: Comparison of postoperative complications between saphenous vein and IMA grafts to left anterior descending coronary artery, *Ann Thorac Surg* 51(5):733-738, 1991.
43. *St Anthony's DRG guidebook 1995*, Reston, Va, 1994, St Anthony.
44. Stiegel RM, et al: Management of postoperative mediastinitis in infants and children by muscle flap rotation, *Ann Thorac Surg* 46(1):45-46, 1988.
45. Tsai T, et al: Cardiac surgery in the octogenerian, *J Thorac Cardiovasc Surg* 91(6):924-928, 1986.
46. Verkkala K, et al: Fever, leukocytosis, and C-reactive protein after open-heart surgery and their value in the diagnosis of postoperative infections, *Thorac Cardiovasc Surg* 35(2):78-82, 1987.
47. West JM: Wound healing in the surgical patient: influence of the perioperative stress response on perfusion, *AACN Clin Iss Crit Care Nurs* 1(3):595-601, 1990.

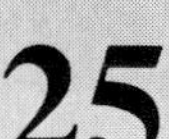

TRANSPLANT GUIDELINE

25

Cardiac Transplant

Nancy Abou-Awdi, MS, RN, CCRN, CCRC
Penny L. Powers, BSN, RN, CCTC

DESCRIPTION

Heart disease remains the number one cause of death in the United States. Estimates from the Centers for Disease Control are that 11.2 million people suffer from coronary artery disease alone. In addition, approximately 2.3 million people are in chronic heart failure, and 400,000 more people are diagnosed with this disease annually. Of those developing heart failure, 50% die within the first year.[5] Over the last three decades, cardiac transplantation has evolved into an accepted therapy for end-stage heart disease. Since the first heart transplant in 1967, more than 23,000 have been done worldwide.[9] Currently, there are 158 heart and 85 heart-lung transplant centers in the United States. Registry data reveals that 2173 heart and 48 heart-lung transplants were performed in 1992 in the United States alone.[11]

Progress in transplantation has been directly affected by advances in immunology and immunosuppression. In 1976, Jean Borel and other researchers in Switzerland revealed a major scientific breakthrough: the immunosuppressive properties of cyclosporine. This discovery was followed by animal studies showing improved graft survival, which led to clinical application in renal transplant recipients.[4] In 1983, the U.S. Food and Drug Administration approved cyclosporine (Sandimmune) for general use.

PATIENT SELECTION

Patients identified as cardiac transplant candidates are generally suffering from some form of end-stage cardiomyopathy. Cardiomyopathy is generally classified as dilated, hypertrophic, or restrictive. The etiology of cardiomyopathy is often idiopathic. Known etiologies of cardiomyopathy include the following[3,8,16]:

- Ischemic heart disease
- Viral infection
- Connective tissue disease (such as sarcosis or scleroderma)
- Neuromuscular disorders (such as muscular dystrophy)
- Cardiotoxic substances (such as alcohol, antineoplastic agents, or radiation therapy of the cardiothoracic area)
- Pregnancy
- Congenital heart disease
- Valvular heart disease
- Metabolic disorders (such as hemachromatosis)
- Genetic predisposition

In addition to end-stage cardiac disease and numerous criteria discussed under Management Trends in this chapter, donor recipient matching is a key factor related to positive transplant outcomes.

Criteria for determining a donor-recipient match for cardiac transplantation include ABO blood group compatibility, body size and weight, cytotoxicity and CMV titer. ABO typing is important because a mismatch could cause acute humoral rejection and graft loss. The donor and the recipient should also be of similar body size and weight. In most cases, the size difference should be no greater than 20% to 30%. Some centers occasionally accept hearts from smaller donors and place them heterotopically in a larger recipient. However, in recipients with elevated pulmonary vascular resistance, hearts from larger donors may be placed orthotopically. (See Figure 25-1.) Cytotoxicity is determined preoperatively through laboratory testing for panel reactive antibodies (PRA). The PRA test measures the presence of

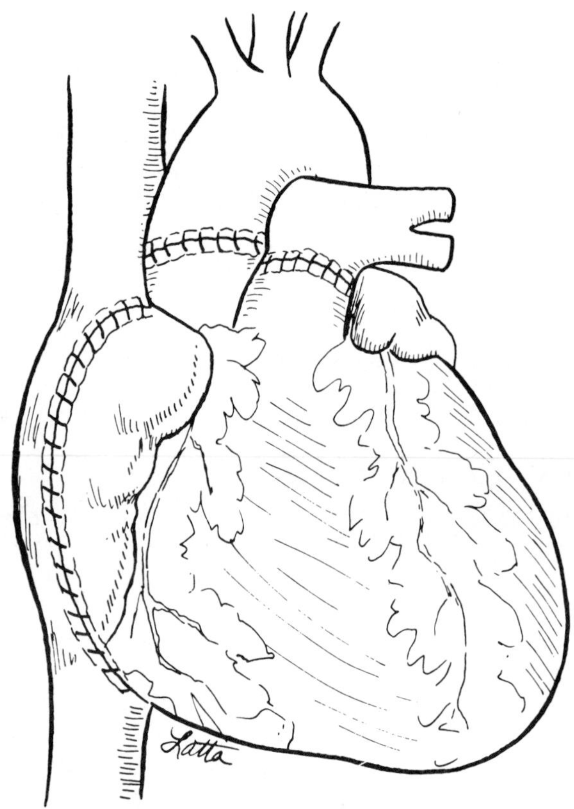

Figure 25-1 Heterotopic cardiac transplant procedure. Artwork courtesy of Carol Latta, Medical Illustrator, The Texas Heart Institute.

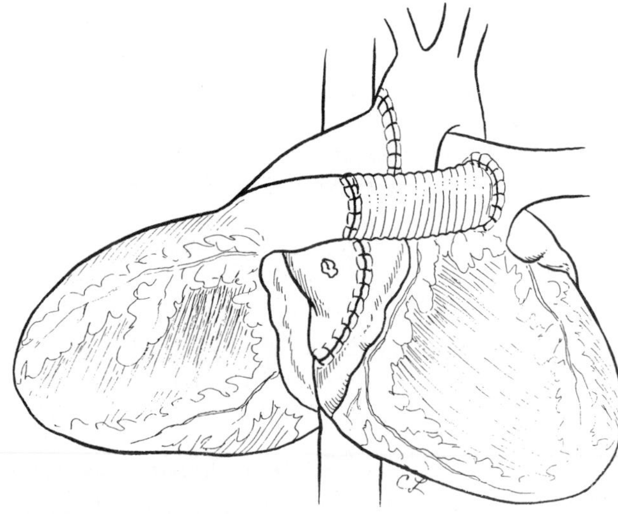

Figure 25-2 Orthotopic cardiac transplant procedure. Artwork courtesy of Carol Latta, Medical Illustrator, The Texas Heart Institute.

recipient cytotoxic antibodies against a panel of lymphocytic antigens present in a randomized population. Preformed cytotoxic antibodies develop in people who have been exposed and sensitized to tissue antigens. Thus, elevated PRA levels are found in multiparous women and in individuals who have received multiple blood transfusions. A recipient PRA greater than 5% to 10% necessitates a direct cross-matching of donor-recipient blood for antigen-antibody response. A direct cross-match between donor and recipient serum is usually performed but not always before transplant due to the length of time required for testing.

When a potential donor is identified, a well-orchestrated team goes into action. The team usually consists of procurement personnel from the donor's location and from the recipient's transplant center. Procurement personnel work closely with the donor's family, giving them information about the procedure, the timing of events, and what they may expect. During this difficult time, the donor's family is usually concerned about how the time of death is established, what paperwork needs to be completed, when they may leave the hospital, and whether they will know how the recipient fares after transplant. The procurement team must answer all these questions with patience and compassion, while managing the donor. Multiple-organ harvests are the most difficult to manage because several procurement teams may arrive at the same time.

To preserve the heart and other organs, it is important to maintain donor stability with minimal pharmacologic support. Furthermore, the donor and recipient operations must be accurately timed so that the ischemic period does not exceed 4 hours for adult hearts or 6 hours for pediatric hearts. Reducing the ischemic time helps preserve cardiac contractility. Ongoing research to develop better preservation techniques may eventually allow increased ischemic time. Such techniques might help prevent donor hearts from being wasted in that failure to find a recipient within the region could allow the heart to be given to a recipient at a more distant location.

PROCEDURE

Orthotopic heart transplantation is the most common procedure. (See Figure 25-1.) The recipient is placed on cardiopulmonary bypass, and the native heart is excised at the midatrial level, leaving the posterior right and left atrial walls and their venous connections intact. The donor heart is anastomosed at the left atrium, right atrium, and the great vessels. Epicardial pacing wires are implanted in the right atrium and exteriorized to the chest wall.

Heterotopic (piggy-back) heart transplantation is performed by placing the donor heart in the right chest cavity, then anastomosing the donor's right superior vena cava, aorta, and pulmonary artery to the corresponding vessels in the recipient.[7] (See Figure 25-2.)

In the immediate postoperative period cardiac transplant recipients require the same care given to patients undergoing other open heart surgical procedures, but there are a few additional considerations. The risk of infection is greater in these patients because they are immunosuppressed. Infection control measures vary among centers.[10] Current recommendations from the Centers for Disease Control include hospitalizing the patient in a private room, hand washing with an antiseptic soap prior to patient contact, and having anyone with an upper respiratory tract infection wear a mask when caring for or visiting the patient.[15] Additionally, all invasive lines, catheters, and chest tubes should be removed as soon as possible. The patient's nutritional status must be monitored preoperatively and postoperatively. Proper nutrients help decrease susceptibility to infection.[6]

Rejection may occur at any time after transplant. Hyperacute rejection, which occurs within minutes or hours of the operation, is believed to be caused by preformed antibodies. This form of rejection usually results in loss of the allograft. Acute rejection, which represents a cellular immune response, usually occurs within the first few weeks or months of transplantation but may still occur anytime thereafter. Clinical signs may or may not be present. Such signs include increased central venous pressure, decreased cardiac output, dysrhythmias, fever, and decreased left ventricular ejection fraction. Diagnosis is confirmed by endomyocardial biopsy. Chronic rejection, which usually manifests late in the post-transplant course, produces diffuse atherosclerotic changes in the coronary vessels. Patients frequently experience heart failure, and retransplantation may be the only option.

Immunosuppressive agents are used to prevent or to treat rejection. These agents are often combined, and doses are adjusted based on clinical findings as well as endomyocardial biopsy results. The goal of immunosuppressive therapy is to prevent rejection without compromising the patient's ability to fight infection. Cyclosporine (Sandimmune), azathioprine (Imuran), antithymocyte globulin (ATG), Orthoclone OKT3, and corticosteroids (prednisone, methylprednisolone) are the most commonly used immunosuppressive agents. New immunosuppressive medications are being investigated, several of which are undergoing clinical trials.

LENGTH OF STAY/ANTICIPATED COURSE

Length of stay after cardiac transplantation varies with each patient and is directly related to the severity of the clinical condition before transplant and to postoperative complications. On the average, cardiac transplant patients and care givers may anticipate a minimum LOS of 10 to 14 days with an average LOS of 35.8 days as noted in DRG 103: Heart Transplant.[13] Initial surgical recovery in an ICU setting typically requires a minimum of 3 days, assuming that the patient did not require intensive preoperative support. Thereafter, the patient is hospitalized in a unit that is staffed by nurses with expertise in caring for this challenging patient population.

Preparation for discharge begins before the transplant as patients and their families are informed of the process and requirements of follow-up. Patients and family members must be educated regarding the collaborative plan of care, which may include a multitude of specialists. Throughout this process, the patient and family become a vital part of the multidisciplinary team, with each member contributing to the overall plan of care and ultimate success of the transplant.

TABLE 25-1 Contraindications to Cardiac Transplant

Relative

Renal failure
Chronic obstructive pulmonary disease
Fixed pulmonary hypertension
Age
Systemic infection
Peptic ulcer disease

Absolute

Unresolved drug or alcohol dependency/addiction
AIDS
Malignancy, current
Cirrhosis

MANAGEMENT TRENDS AND CONTROVERSIES

All potential transplant recipients undergo a thorough evaluation procedure. The multidisciplinary approach includes cardiologists, transplant surgeons, transplant nurse coordinators, pulmonologists, psychiatrists, psychologists, gastroenterologists, nutritionists, social workers, physical therapists, and financial advisors. At evaluation, the goal is to determine the medical and psychosocial suitability of the potential recipient.

Cardiac transplantation is considered only when all other conventional medical and surgical therapies have failed. A thorough medical examination is required to determine which patients have the greatest potential for returning to a functional life-style and the best chance for long-term survival. A psychosocial evaluation is also performed to determine whether the family will be able to cope with the stringent postoperative medical regimen, as well as handle the financial commitment. Post-transplant management is complex and demands active participation from the potential candidate and family; therefore, everyone must understand the benefits and risks of transplantation, the alternatives to treatment, and the requirements of the transplant center so that they can make an informed decision.

Medical criteria for cardiac transplantation vary from center to center. In general, however, patients are in New York Heart Association functional class III or IV and have conditions that are refractory to conventional medical or surgical therapy. Left ventricular function, determined by left ventricular ejection fraction, is usually 20% or less. Coexisting medical conditions that might jeopardize long-term survival would preclude transplantation. (See Table 25-1.)

Whereas some centers place an age restriction on candidates, the current trend is to determine eligibility on an individual basis. Fixed pulmonary hypertension may also exclude some candidates, unless the center performs heterotopic cardiac transplantation.

Once the cardiac transplant candidate has been accepted for transplantation, the waiting period begins. The median waiting time for a donor heart is 249 days.[14] During the waiting period, all transplant candidates require careful monitoring and management at frequent intervals to assess disease progression and deterioration of other organ function. Patients who are seriously ill may require hospitalization. Recurrent admissions for heart failure, renal or hepatic dysfunction, and cardiac cachexia are common. Inotropic support may be required to maintain the candidate's transplant status. If these measures are ineffective, mechanical circulatory support may be necessary to bridge the patient to transplantation.[1,2,12] Some centers will allow candidates to wait at home if they can reach the hospital within 4 hours of being notified that a donor has been found. Others may need to move to temporary housing near the transplant center. Most centers have some form of housing available for patients and their families.

ASSESSMENT

PARAMETER	ANTICIPATED ALTERATION
History that Includes	
Onset and nature of cardiac symptoms, course of disease, previous hospitalization for increasing cardiac failure	S/S of congestive heart failure with need for hospitalization and/or inotropic support *due to progressive cardiac failure*
Diagnostic or therapeutic procedures, particularly	
• Cardiac catheterization	Confirms severe cardiac dysfunction
• Endomyocardial biopsy	Presence of myocarditis on EMC biopsy
• Cardiac surgery	May have had previous surgery or rejection for surgical intervention
Previous history of related cardiovascular problems	
• Congenital heart disease	Possible presence of previous palliative/corrective surgery or uncorrected anomalies
• Valvular disease	Rheumatic fever/heart disease/artificial valves
• Coronary artery disease; coronary artery bypass grafting	Previous surgery that increases risk of bleeding
• Peripheral vascular or cerebral vascular disease	May require corrective surgery before transplant
• Ventricular aneurysm	May or may not be present
• Septal defect	May or may not be present
• Uncontrollable risk factors for cardiovascular disease: age, sex, family history	May or may not be applicable depending on etiology and type of cardiac disease
• Controllable risk factors for cardiovascular disease: hypertension, cigarette smoking, obesity, sedentary life-style, substance abuse	May or may not be related to origin of transplant need; regardless of impact or underlying pathology, life-style modification to eliminate these factors, if present, will be required post-transplant
• Past MI	May or may not be present
• Stroke, thrombophlebitis	May or may not be present
• Angina, other signs of myocardial ischemia	Common but not in all cases
• Dysrhythmias (palpitations)	Common, may be life threatening
Other organ dysfunction that may be related to cardiac compromise	
• Pulmonary	Hypoxia with Pa_{O_2} <80 mm Hg Infiltrates on CXR Pleural effusion

• Renal	BUN elevated: >20 mg/dl Creatine elevated: >1.2 mg/dl UO decreased: <30 cc/hr
• Neurological	Somnolence Decreased mentation Confusion
• Hepatic	Abnormal liver function Ascites
Conditions that may prevent or delay cardiac transplantation	See Table 25-1
Physical Examination	
Activity tolerance	Activity restriction, presence of early fatigue
BP	Systolic BP <90 mm Hg *due to heart failure and use of afterload-reducing agents*
Pulse	Irregular rhythm, pulsus alternans, weakness pretransplant Baseline tachycardia with HR ≈100 bpm *due to denervated transplanted heart*
Peripheral perfusion	Presence of pallor, duskiness, cyanosis Cool temperature Diaphoresis Clubbing
Heart sounds	Murmurs, gallop rhythms
LOC	Decreased
Venous distention	Sacral edema, dependent edema, distention of neck veins, ascites, hepatomegaly
Presence of syndromes associated with certain types of congenital or acquired heart disease	Down or Marfan syndrome
Weight	Weight gain *due to CHF* Weight loss *due to cachexia*
Pulmonary Status	
Rate, rhythm, quality of respiration	Presence of rales, rhonchi, wheezing, shortness of breath, tachypnea, dyspnea, orthopnea
Lab and Diagnostic Tests	
Electrocardiogram	Myocardial ischemia Hypertrophy Dysrhythmia Effects of inotropic/antiarrhythmic medications Congenital heart disease, axis and ventricular hypertrophy consistent with defect
Chest x-ray	Cardiac dilatation Pulmonary vascular congestion Location and configuration of great vessels
Right-heart catheterization	Right atrial or ventricular hypertrophy, elevated intracardiac pressures, valvular disease PAP elevated: PAS >35 mm Hg, PAD >15 mm Hg PCWP elevated: >16 mm Hg PVR elevated: >97 dynes/cm/m^2 Congenital cardiac or pulmonary artery disease CO decreased: <4.0 L/min CI decreased: <2.5 L/min/m^2

Left-heart catheterization	Coronary artery disease or valvular disease Left atrial or left ventricular hypertrophy Ventricular aneurysm Septal defect Congenital cardiac or aortic disease
Echocardiogram	Valvular abnormalities Hypertrophy of specific cardiac chambers Right and left ejection fraction decreased: RVEF <40% LVEF <50% Intracardiac/great vessel shunts Possible restrictive disease Thrombus
MVo_2	Decreased: <14.5 ml/kg/min (peak Vo_2)
Radionuclide studies (if indicated)	
• Lung scan	Pulmonary infarction
• Venogram	Deep venous thrombus
• MUGA/LVPS	Decreased ejection fraction; regional wall abnormalities
• Stress thallium	Stress-induced ischemia
Electrolytes, BUN, creatinine	K^+ decreased: <3.5 meq/L Na^+ decreased: <130 meq/L BUN increased: >20 mg/dl Creatinine increased: >1.2 mg/dl
Complete blood count with differential	CBC WNL
Coagulation profile	PT, PTT increased *due to anticoagulation therapy and hepatic dysfunction due to right-heart failure*
Blood type	
Cultures (blood, urine, stool, sputum)	Negative
Serologic titers	
• Cytomegalovirus, toxoplasma, Epstein-Barr virus, legionella, herpes	May be positive or negative; beneficial in donor matching (i.e., CMV-negative recipient needs CMV-negative donor) and postop management
• HIV	Negative
• Candida antigen	Negative
Iron-binding capacity	May be decreased *due to CHF/cachexia*
Serum hepatitis antigen/antibody	Negative
Antinuclear antibody	Negative
Serum test for syphilis	Negative
Skin test for tuberculosis	Negative (<10 mm) *If positive, patient will require antituberculosis therapy for 1 year post-transplant to prevent reactivation*

Psychosocial–Emotional Assessment

Results of consultations with cardiac transplant team members, which may include • Social service worker • Physical therapist • Psychiatrist • Neurologist • Dental surgeon • Dietitian	Consensus that patient is a reasonable candidate from all consultants

Patient/family's level of anxiety regarding disease process, medical therapy used, purpose of hospitalization, need for surgery, postoperative management, and general follow-up plan of care	Increased anxiety
Patient/family's roles and activities of daily living associated with patient disease process	Role reversal/change Loss of patient independence
Patient/family's knowledge regarding search for suitable donor heart for patient	Guilt feelings regarding death of another in order for recipient to live Lack of understanding regarding how waiting list is organized and how priorities for allocating heart are set

PLAN OF CARE

INTENSIVE PHASE

The first 12 hours after cardiac transplantation are the most critical. During this period, many patient care priorities are the same as those for patients who have undergone CABG (see Guideline 20). Some factors, however, such as right-heart failure, allograft failure, hyperacute rejection, neurologic changes due to immunosuppression, and infection, are all specific to the cardiac transplant recipient.

PATIENT CARE PRIORITIES	EXPECTED PATIENT OUTCOMES
Decreased cardiac output *r/t* *Altered preload, afterload, contractility, heart rate* *Cardiac tamponade* *Rejection of transplanted organ* *Right-heart failure*	CO, CI, PAP, CVP/RAP, BP, HR, within acceptable range HR >90 bpm, SBP 100 to 150 mm Hg Peripheral perfusion adequate (distal pulses present, capillary refill <3 seconds) No alterations in mental status Absence of syncope, weakness, or dizziness UO >30 cc/hr Breath sounds clear Body weight not more than 5% of baseline Skin pink, warm, and dry Minimal edema BUN, creatinine, and total bilirubin: WNL
Alteration in cardiac rhythm *r/t* *Autonomic denervation* *Ischemia* *Electrolyte imbalance* *Altered electrical condition* *Drug toxicity* *Rejection*	NSR with minimal ectopy (PVCs <10/min, no runs >3 bpm, no atrial ectopy) Heart rate is within acceptable range (<90 bpm to improve cardiac output) No evidence of heart block Adequate oxygenation K^+ and Mg^{++}: WNL Therapeutic drug levels
High risk for infection *r/t* *Surgical interventions* *Atelectasis* *Invasive catheters and/or tubes* *Immunosuppression*	Afebrile WBC will be elevated (20,000 to 25,000/mm^3) *due to steroids* No green or yellow sputum Urine clear, without pungent odor or burning on voiding Catheter sites free of redness, tenderness, or swelling Cultures negative; or receiving appropriate antimicrobial therapy
Impaired LOC *r/t* *Anesthesia* *Cardiopulmonary bypass* *Stroke*	Neurologically intact

Plan of Care (cont'd)

Infection process
Fluid/electrolyte imbalance
Metabolic imbalance
Immunosuppression

Impaired gas exchange *r/t* *Altered O_2-carrying capacity of blood* *Alveolar-capillary membrane changes* *Altered blood flow* *Atelectasis* *Fluid overload* *Heterotopic transplant*	Clear chest x-ray, breath sounds $Sao_2 > 90\%$ $Svo_2 > 60\%$

INTERVENTIONS

Monitor hemodynamic parameters and titrate vasoactive agents according to predetermined parameters (i.e., isoproterenol, PGE_1, dopamine, and nitroprusside).

Be prepared for artificial pacing or the use of β-stimulating drugs (epinephrine, isoproterenol) in the event of bradycardia *due to ineffectiveness of atropine in the denervated transplanted heart.*

Maintain temperature within normal range.

Monitor ECG continuously for dysrhythmias.

Assess peripheral circulation (distal pulses, temperature, color, sensation) regularly.

Monitor laboratory values (CBC, cultures, serology titers, K^+, Mg^{++}, Ca^{++}) as ordered.

Monitor therapeutic serum levels (cyclosporine, digoxin, CD_3) as ordered.

Practice aseptic techniques for all dressing changes and any invasive procedure *to prevent infection.*

Observe suture lines, IV, and chest tube sites for swelling, redness, discharge, or tenderness. Report any evidence of infection to the physician immediately *to ensure optimal intervention in this immunosuppressed patient.*

Assess neurologic status routinely.

Assess breath sounds routinely.

Monitor ABGs, Sao_2, Svo_2 routinely and with any indication of compromise *to ensure prompt intervention for potential respiratory complications.*

Provide aseptic pulmonary toilet *to facilitate surgical recovery and provide immunosuppressive protection.*

Turn patient q2h when hemodynamic stability is achieved.

After extubation, perform incentive spirometry hourly, when patient is awake.

Help patient to dangle and encourage patient to progressively increase activity, as tolerated, as soon as extubated and VS stable.

INTERMEDIATE PHASE

The intermediate care phase begins when the patient reaches hemodynamic stability, which usually occurs within the first 48 hours after transplantation. Nursing goals during this phase are aimed at preventing infection, recognizing signs of early rejection, and beginning rehabilitation.

PATIENT CARE PRIORITIES	EXPECTED PATIENT OUTCOMES
High risk for infection *r/t* *Invasive catheters and/or tubes* *Immunosuppression*	Same as those in intensive phase
Alteration in cardiac rhythm *r/t* *Rejection* *Drug toxicity*	No atrial ectopy HR <90 beats/min

Plan of Care (cont'd)

Nursing Diagnosis	Expected Outcomes
Impaired skin integrity *r/t* *Surgical incisions* *Immobility/pressure* *Impaired circulation* *Invasive procedures* *Altered nutritional status* *Impaired sensation* *Immunosuppression*	Skin intact Edges of incision well approximated Nutritional status adequate
Decreased nutrition *r/t* *Immunosuppression* *Anorexia* *Nausea* *Vomiting* *Absorption disorder* *Catabolic states* *Dysphagia* *Multiorgan instability* *Stomatitis*	Body weight does not decrease >3% of baseline Serum albumin levels: WNL No nausea or vomiting
Activity intolerance *r/t* *Generalized weakness* *Fluid/electrolyte imbalance* *Prolonged bed rest* *Decreased cardiac output* *Medications* *Infection* *Pain* *CHF* *Rejection*	Not reluctant to attempt activity Full ROM Adequate muscle strength and control HR does not increase more than 20 bpm above baseline with ambulation Systolic BP does not increase more than 10 to 20 mm Hg above baseline
Body image disturbance *r/t* *Immunosuppression* *Surgical intervention*	Acceptance of body image changes
Self-care deficit *r/t* *Strict antirejection medication regime* *Follow-up assessment of transplant status* *S/S organ rejection*	Patient/family able to verbalize/demonstrate medication regime, follow-up schedule, S/S to report to physician

INTERVENTIONS

Practice aseptic techniques for all dressing changes and any invasive procedure *to provide maximum protection in light of immunosuppressed state.*

Monitor laboratory values (CBC, cultures, serology titers) *to detect any S/S of infection in a timely fashion.*

Monitor temperature.

Observe suture lines, IV, and chest tube sites for swelling, redness, discharge, or tenderness.

Remove all indwelling lines/catheters as soon as possible *to reduce risk of infection.*

Encourage patient to wear mask in public areas of hospital and to avoid crowds *to protect from exposure to infectious agents.*

Ask visitors to wash hands well.

Monitor ECG for dysrhythmias.

Use pressure-reducing mattress when patient is immobile and is hemodynamically stable *to prevent skin breakdown and reduce risk of associated infection.*

Assess skin for any signs of actual or potential breakdown. Provide early intervention *to minimize infection risk.*

Plan of Care (cont'd)

Begin physical therapy as soon as the patient is hemodynamically stable *to facilitate physical reconditioning, wound healing, pain management, and sense of recovery.*

Assess nutritional status by keeping accurate calorie count and monitoring supplements *to facilitate wound healing and general surgical recovery.*

Monitor I/O.

Weigh patient daily *to ensure adequate mobilization of presurgical fluid retention and recovery from malnourished state.*

Encourage patient to increase activity, as tolerated.

Consult with physical therapist to plan rehabilitation program through discharge phase.

Provide psychoemotional support *to facilitate patient coping with body image changes, lingering guilt or anxiety regarding receipt of a donor organ.*

Instruct patient/family regarding need for strict adherence to prescribed medication regime and follow-up care *to minimize risk of rejection.*

Instruct patient/family regarding S/S associated with organ rejection (fatigue, weight gain, dyspnea, fever) or risk associated with immunosuppression (respiratory infection, flu symptoms, need for antibiotic coverage prior to other invasive tests or procedures) *to optimize patient safety and long-term survival.*

TRANSITION TO DISCHARGE

The key to a successful outcome after cardiac transplantation involves patient education and adherence to a complex medical regimen. After extubation, cardiac transplant patients begin to learn about their medical regimen, as well as how to self-administer their drugs. Before discharge, they must also be able to identify the signs and symptoms of rejection and infection; monitor their own vital signs, weight, and diet; and understand their follow-up schedule. In most cases, phase II cardiac rehabilitation is initiated at discharge to maximize cardiac function and to reinforce behavioral changes necessary for a successful outcome.

REFERENCES

1. Abou-Awdi NL, Frazier OH: The Heartmate: a left ventricular assist device as a bridge to cardiac transplantation, *Transplant Proc* 24(5):2002-2003, 1992.
2. Abou-Awdi NL, Frazier OH: Heartmate ventricular assist system. In Quaal S, editor: *Cardiac mechanical assistance beyond balloon pumping,* St Louis, 1992, Mosby–Year Book, pp 174-190.
3. Alpert JS, Rippe JM: Cardiomyopathy, myocarditis, and rheumatic fever. In *Manual of cardiovascular diagnosis and therapy,* ed 3, Boston, 1988, Little, Brown.
4. Borel JF: The history of cyclosporine A and its significance. In White DJG, editor: *Proceedings of an international conference on cyclosporine A,* Amsterdam, 1982, Elsevier Biomedical Press, pp 5-17.
5. Chiu CJ: *Biomechanical cardiac assist,* Mount Kisco, NY, 1986, Futura.
6. Frazier OH, et al: Nutritional management of the heart transplant recipient, *J Heart Transplant* 4:450-452, 1985.
7. Gamberg P, Walton K: Heart transplant. In Sigardson-Poor KM, Haggerty LM, editors: *Nursing care of the transplant recipient,* Philadelphia, 1990, WB Saunders.
8. Hall RJ, Cooley DA, McAllister HA: Neoplastic heart disease. In Hurst JW, editor: *The heart,* ed 7, New York, 1990, McGraw-Hill.
9. Kaye MP: Personal communication, The Registry of the International Society for Heart and Lung Transplantation, Minneapolis, Minn, 1993.
10. Lange SS, et al: *Heart Lung,* 21(2):101-105, 1992.
11. Pierce GA: Organization of organ sharing in the United States and its relevance to the Middle East, *Transplant Proc* 25(3):2261-2263, 1993.
12. Shinn JA, Oyer PE: Novacor ventricular assist system. In Quaal S, editor: *Cardiac mechanical assistance beyond balloon pumping,* St Louis, 1992, Mosby–Year Book, pp 99-115.
13. St. Anthony's *DRG guidebook 1995,* Reston, Va, 1994, St. Anthony.
14. United Network for Organ Sharing (UNOS): Statistics for 1991 compiled in 1993, Richmond, Va.
15. Vaska PL: Common infections in heart transplant patients, *Am J Crit Care* 2(2):145-154, 1993.
16. Wenger NK, et al: Cardiomyopathy and specific heart muscle disease. In Hurst JW, editor: *The heart,* ed 7, New York, 1990, McGraw-Hill.

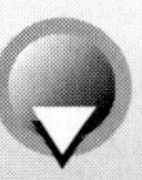

C L I N I C A L G U I D E L I N E

26

Hypertensive Crisis

Susan Flewelling Goran, MSN, RN, CCRN

DESCRIPTION

It is estimated that approximately 60 million Americans have hypertension or are borderline hypertensive.[7] Nearly one half of persons over the age of 65 have elevated systolic or diastolic blood pressure, with the consequences of increased morbidity and mortality.[3,14] Hypertension, or high blood pressure (HBP), can be defined in a variety of ways. The Joint National Committee on Detection, Evaluation, and Treatment of High Blood Pressure (JNC) defined normal blood pressure for adults age 18 years and older as a systolic reading of less than 140 mm Hg and a diastolic of less than 85 mm Hg.[7] The JNC went on to define alterations as mild, moderate, and severe. In 1992, concerned that the terms mild and moderate did not convey the seriousness of the problem, a new classification system was devised.

Stage 1: systolic 140 to 159 mm Hg
diastolic 90 to 99 mm Hg
Stage 2: systolic 160 to 179 mm Hg
diastolic 100 to 109 mm Hg
Stage 3: systolic 180 to 209 mm Hg
diastolic 110 to 119 mm Hg
Stage 4: systolic ≥210 mm Hg
diastolic ≥120 mm Hg

Hypertension may also be classified according to its etiology. *Essential* or *primary hypertension* does not have an identifiable cause and represents approximately 90% of all hypertensive patients. The remaining 10% of the hypertensive population have *secondary hypertension* in which the cause is related to renal or endocrine malfunction.

The impact of hypertension on body systems is another classification system. *Malignant hypertension* is defined by the presence of elevated systemic blood pressure with associated papilledema. *Accelerated hypertension* is characterized by fibrinoid necrosis of arterioles, clinically apparent by the presence of retinal exudates and hemorrhages. The diagnosis of either accelerated or malignant hypertension requires evidence of vascular damage.[6]

Finally, hypertension may be classified based on the urgency of treatment. *Transient hypertension* is seen in conditions such as anxiety, early dehydration, stroke, epistaxis, alcohol withdrawal, and overdoses of phencyclidine and clonidine. Treatment is focused on correcting the underlying condition rather than the hypertension per se. *Mild uncomplicated hypertension* is defined as a diastolic blood pressure (DBP) less than 115 mm Hg with the absence of end-organ damage. It does not require acute treatment but requires follow-up care. *Hypertensive urgencies* occur with elevation of diastolic blood pressure to a level that may be potentially harmful, usually defined as greater than 115 mm Hg, but without evidence of end-organ dysfunction. The treatment goal is to reduce BP gradually over a 24-hour period to a level appropriate for the patient.[6,14,15] *Hypertensive crisis or emergency* is defined without a specific level of BP elevation. The diagnosis is made on the basis of elevated BP in combination with overt signs of end-organ dysfunction, such as encephalopathy, congestive heart failure, myocardial ischemia, or renal insufficiency.[10,15] Treatment is focused on reducing BP 20% to 30% or reducing diastolic BP to 100 to 110 mm Hg within 30 minutes, and subsequently within an hour to a level that is "normal" for the patient, all within a controlled, graded manner.[8]

Hypertensive crisis is an uncommon condition, occurring in approximately 1% of all patients with hypertension, but it occurs most commonly in patients with a history of hypertension.[5] Table 26-1 summarizes the clinical syndromes that may cause hypertensive emergencies. Often the patient

TABLE 26-1 Clinical Syndromes Causing Hypertensive Crisis

Cardiovascular	Acute myocardial infarction Myocardial ischemia Unstable angina Pulmonary edema Congestive heart failure Aortic dissection
Renal	Acute renal failure
Central nervous system	Hypertensive encephalopathy Subarachnoid hemorrhage Cerebrovascular hemorrhage Cerebrovascular thrombosis or embolus
Metabolic	Pheochromocytoma Antihypertensive withdrawal Interactions between monoamine oxidase inhibitors and certain foods and/or drugs
Obstetric	Eclampsia Preeclampsia

has not been taking medication as prescribed or has been receiving inadequate therapy.[1,9] Untreated patients with malignant hypertension have a mortality rate of 80% to 90% within 1 year, usually as a result of renal failure.[8] Death rates secondary to hypertensive crisis have declined significantly during the past 25 years due to more aggressive management, widespread availability of newer antihypertensive agents, and meticulous monitoring capabilities in modern intensive care units.

The current 5-year survival rate after an episode of hypertensive crisis is 75%.[5] However, studies have shown that patients who present in hypertensive crisis with creatinine levels of greater than 3.5 mg/dl will develop progressive renal failure with its associated morbidity and mortality.[8]

PATHOPHYSIOLOGY

Arterial blood pressure is regulated by several factors, including the vasomotor tone of the arteries and arterioles, cardiac output (CO), and blood volume. Normal regulation of vasomotor tone involves neural and hormonal mechanisms. The medulla oblongata, which consists of vasopressor and depressor subdivisions, receives input from baroreceptors, atrial diastolic stretch receptors, the limbic system, midbrain, and pulmonary stretch receptors. It also is responsive to local hypoxia or hypercapnia. Stimulation of the vasopressor center results in increased sympathetic stimulation of the alpha receptors in arterial smooth muscle cells, which leads to arterial constriction, increased systemic vascular resistance (SVR), and a subsequent rise in BP since BP is the product of CO × SVR. Stimulation of the depressor area results in decreased sympathetic discharge leading to vasodilation and a decrease in BP. Hormonal regulation of arterial blood pressure is affected by adrenal medulla catecholamines and the renin-angiotensin system. Catecholamines produce an effect similar to that of the sympathetic system by causing arterial constriction and increasing pressure.

A decrease in renal perfusion stimulates the secretion of renin, which leads to the production of angiotensin I and II. This results in vasoconstriction, which increases BP, thus increasing renal perfusion. Angiotensin increases salt and water reabsorption by a direct renal mechanism as well as through stimulation of aldosterone secretion by the adrenal cortex. The result is increased blood volume. Over time, with the release of circulating vasoactive substances, there is an increase in size of the renal afferent arteriole lumen, but not the efferent arteriole. This leads to pressure diuresis, which may contribute to hypovolemia. This, in turn, further stimulates release of vasoactive substances, and a vicious cycle of hypertension continues with eventual renal impairment.

Hypertensive crisis in patients who have stopped taking their antihypertensive medications is believed to be precipitated by an abrupt increase in SVR as a result of increases in the circulating levels of vasoconstrictor substances such as norepinephrine, angiotensin II, or antidiuretic hormone.[1,4] Severely elevated BP causes vascular endothelial damage, platelet and fibrin deposition, and loss of autoregulatory function leading to end-organ ischemia. Ischemia triggers the release of vasoactive substances, which cause further vasoconstriction and tissue damage.

Blood pressure is also influenced by the level of unbound calcium. Calcium enters the cell through calcium channels which then regulate contractility. Increased contractility increases vascular tone which leads to higher BP. Decreased calcium input decreases contractility, leading to loss of vascular tone and a fall in BP.

Autoregulation of BP is a protective mechanism to prevent organ ischemia during times in which BP may drop rapidly. For example, when BP falls, cerebral vasodilatation occurs; conversely, when BP rises, cerebral vasoconstriction occurs. Normally cerebral perfusion remains a constant 60 to 70 mm Hg. When mean arterial pressure (MAP) drops below the lower limit of autoregulation, the brain extracts more oxygen from blood to compensate for the reduced cerebral blood flow. When this mechanism fails, clinical signs and symptoms such as fainting, nausea, yawning, clamminess, and syncope occur. Patients in hypertensive crisis, unlike most individuals with normal cerebral vasculature, cannot tolerate rapid reduction of BP. In chronic hypertension, normal cerebral autoregulation is impaired so that decreased cerebral blood flow occurs at a higher MAP. In both normotensive and hypertensive individuals, the lower limit of cerebral autoregulation is roughly 25% below

TABLE 26-2 Clinical Signs and Symptoms of Hypertensive Crisis

Central nervous system	Blurred vision Diplopia Hemiparesis Seizures Headache Dizziness Altered mental status Coma
Cardiac complaints	Chest pain Dyspnea Nausea/vomiting
Blood pressure	Severe elevation in BP with above clinical symptoms Diastolic BP >120-130 mm Hg

resting MAP.[4] Hyperperfusion of the brain occurs when the upper limit of cerebral autoregulation is exceeded. This results in cerebral edema, petechial hemorrhages, and microinfarcts leading to encephalopathy.

Signs and symptoms of hypertensive crisis are noted in Table 26-2.

LENGTH OF STAY/ANTICIPATED COURSE

Hypertensive crisis requires immediate reduction of BP within 1 to 3 hours, necessitating the use of potent parenteral antihypertensive agents.[6,10,15] This type of aggressive therapy is best delivered in the ICU, to provide invasive arterial monitoring, and to monitor for serious potential complications of the hypertension, such as stroke or seizures, or the vasodilator therapy, such as sudden hypotension.

Length of stay will vary related to the extent of the hypertensive crisis and any complications that may have occurred. In the absence of complications, hypertensive crisis is classified as DRG 134: Hypertension with an average LOS of 4.4 days.[13]

MANAGEMENT TRENDS AND CONTROVERSIES

The medical management of hypertensive crisis is twofold: (1) prompt reduction of blood pressure, and (2) preservation of vital organs.[9,17] In conjunction with stabilizing BP, volume status must also be addressed. Many patients with hypertension are volume-depleted as a consequence of a pressure-related diuresis.[1] Volume depletion may actually worsen hypertension. As a result, diuretics and fluid restrictions should be used only for patients who are clinically fluid-overloaded. In cases of severe volume depletion, patients should receive fluid replacement with isotonic saline solution.

Pharmacological treatment of hypertensive emergencies is the major focus of treatment. Table 26-3 summarizes common pharmacological treatment options. A reasonable goal for most hypertensive emergencies is to lower MAP by approximately 25% over a period of minutes to several hours.[9,15] Precipitous reductions in blood pressure and reductions to normotensive or hypotensive levels should be avoided as this may cause end-organ ischemia or infarction. BP should be maintained at this initial level for several days and then reduced to normotensive levels over the next few weeks.

Hypertensive emergencies complicated by other conditions require specific treatment.

Hypertensive encephalopathy. The goal of treatment in hypertensive encephalopathy is to reduce MAP gradually by no more than 20% to 25%, or to a diastolic blood pressure of 100 mm Hg during the first hour.[4] Should deterioration in neurologic function occur after reduction in BP, antihypertensive therapy should be suspected and BP allowed to increase. Treatment should be reinstituted gradually.

Cerebral infarction. Elevated BP is both a cause and effect of cerebral infarction. Due to precarious BP regulation, post-cerebral infarction, and loss of cerebral blood-flow regulation, antihypertensive therapy is not recommended except in cases of diastolic blood pressures above 130 mm Hg.[4,10] In this situation, BP should be gradually reduced by 20% to 25% during the first 24 hours.

Intracerebral hemorrhage. Rapid reduction of BP in patients with intracerebral hemorrhage may reduce the chances for further bleeding, but at the risk of precipitating cerebral hypoperfusion. Management is currently a subject of controversy, but antihypertensive therapy is generally withheld except in cases of extreme elevations of BP such as 200/130 mm Hg.[10]

Subarachnoid hemorrhage. Antihypertensive treatment in patients with subarachnoid hemorrhage is complicated by cerebral arterial spasm, which alters cerebral blood flow. No clear benefit is seen from reducing blood flow in this setting, except in extreme elevations.

Myocardial ischemia or infarction. Increased SVR in hypertension increases left ventricular wall tension, thus increasing myocardial oxygen demand and consumption. Nitrates are used to gradually reduce BP until the symptoms disappear or until DBP is about 100 mm Hg.[4,10]

Left ventricular failure. Extreme elevations in SVR seen in hypertensive emergencies cause left ventricular failure. Sodium nitroprusside with oxygen, morphine, and a loop diuretic are used in combination to simultaneously decrease both preload and afterload.

Aortic dissection. In order to decrease extension of aortic dissection, it is essential to reduce DBP quickly to 100 mm Hg or as low as can be tolerated without compromising organ perfusion.[4,10] Treatment usually includes trimethaphan

TABLE 26-3 Treatment Recommendations for Hypertensive Crises[2,16,17]

Vasodilators. Dilate arterial vessels and reduce systemic resistance.

Agent	Type of crisis	Key aspects
Sodium nitroprusside (Nipride, Nitropress)	Hypertensive encephalopathy Central nervous system events Aortic dissection Renal failure Congestive heart failure Antihypertensive withdrawal	Usual dose 0.5-10 μq/kg/min Effect is instantaneous Drug is light-sensitive and must be covered Adequate volume status is needed to prevent severe hypotension Cyanide or thiocyanate toxicity may occur with prolonged therapy.
Hydralazine (Apresoline)	Eclampsia/preeclampsia	Usual dose 10-20 mg IV Effect in 10-20 min; lasts 6 hours May produce reflex tachycardia
Diazoxide (Hyperstat)	Hypertensive encephalopathy	Usual dose 50-150 mg IV bolus repeated every 15-30 mg/min by IV infusion Effect in 1-2 minutes May aggravate angina pectoris Causes hyperglycemia, fluid retention
Nitroglycerin	Myocardial ischemia Congestive heart failure	Usual dose 5-100 μq/min as IV infusion; titrate for effect; no maximum dose limit Effect in 2-5 minutes Administer >1 μq/kg/min to decrease SVR Venous dilation effect may cause severe hypotension in hypovolemic patients

Adrenergic-inhibiting drugs. Inhibit sympathetic response at the central nervous system, peripheral nerve endings, and alpha receptors.

Agent	Type of crisis	Key aspects
Trimethaphan camsylate (Arfonad)	Aortic dissection	Usual dose 1-4 mg/min IV infusion Effect in 1-5 min May cause severe HBP rebound and circulatory collapse
Phentolamine mesylate (Regitine)	Pheochromocytoma Interactions with MAOI/food/drugs Antihypertensive withdrawal	Usual dose 5-15 mg IV Effect in 1-2 min Used locally to prevent tissue necrosis from dopamine extravasation
Labetalol (Normodyne, Transdate)	Hypertensive encephalopathy Myocardial ischemia Renal failure Antihypertensive withdrawal Interactions with MAOI/food/drugs	Usual dose 20-80 mg IV bolus every 10 min 2 mg/min IV infusion Effect in 5-10 min May cause significant postural hypotension

Angiotensin-converting enzyme inhibitors. Prevent the conversion of inactive angiotensin I to the potent vasopressor angiotensin II. The role in the treatment of hypertensive emergencies is still unclear, but is very effective in controlling hypertension. Examples are captopril and enalapril (Vasotec).

Calcium channel blockers. Verapamil, nifedipine, diltiazem, and felodopine interfere with excitation contraction coupling in smooth and cardiac muscle, reduce cardiac contractility, and promote systemic vasodilation. Role in the treatment of hypertensive emergencies is unclear, but are very effective in controlling hypertension.

Diuretic therapy. Used as an adjuvant therapy in hypertensive crisis where volume overload is clearly noted; loop diuretics such as furosemide (Lasix), ethacrynic acid (Edecrin), and bumetanide (Bumex) are used.

or sodium nitroprusside in combination with a β-adrenergic-receptor antagonist. Labetalol is also effective in such cases.

Eclampsia. BP must be reduced to prevent progression of neurologic and renal injury, although the definitive therapy is delivery of the fetus.[12] The agent of choice is hydralazine. New research has shown that labetalol may have an important role in the treatment of eclampsia, as it reduces BP without inducing fetal distress.[11]

Renal insufficiency. Therapy must reduce SVR without compromising renal blood flow or glomerular filtration. Sodium nitroprusside is effective, but it is important to be aware of the risk of thiocyanate toxicity. Labetalol is an effective alternative as well as calcium channel blockers.

Pheocromocytoma. The treatment of choice is phetolamine, given in intravenous boluses, but labetalol is also effective. Sodium nitroprusside should be reserved for refractory cases only.[1]

Other. Drugs such as cocaine, MAO/food ingestion, withdrawal syndromes, and spinal-cord syndromes may result in hypertensive emergencies which are effectively treated with labetalol, phentolamine, or sodium nitroprusside.

ASSESSMENT

PARAMETER	ANTICIPATED ALTERATION
History	Previous history of duration, severity, and level of control of preexisting hypertension. *Hypertensive crisis occurs most commonly in patients with a history of hypertension* Drug history of use of decongestants, appetite suppressants, steroids, oral contraceptives, MAOIs in combination with other drugs or food, cocaine, or amphetamines, *which may cause hypertension* Withdrawal from antihypertensives or CNS depressants *may also cause hypertension*
Physical Exam	
Cardiac	Sudden hypotension, complaints of chest pain, SOB, increased filling pressures, S_3 gallop, neck vein distention, and arrhythmias *may reflect impending cardiac compromise*
Respiratory	Shallow, ineffective respirations, abnormal breath sounds, decreased Sa_{O_2} <90%, increasing P_{CO_2} levels with decreasing pH *may reflect need for mechanical ventilation*
Gastrointestinal	Poor appetite, bloating, complaints of abdominal pain, N/V, diarrhea, and melena *may reflect mesenteric ischemia*
Renal	Oliguria, weight gain, edema *may reflect increasing renal damage*
Neurological	Severe headache, nausea, vomiting, visual disturbance, sensory and motor deficit, pupil changes, and changes in level of consciousness *may reflect hypertensive encephalopathy, subarachnoid hemorrhage, intraparenchymal hematoma, or acute ischemic stroke*
BP	BP should be measured with an appropriate size cuff, and two or more readings from both arms should be averaged before BP is accepted as elevated Devices that record automatic noninvasive blood pressure readings may be inaccurate at the extremes; thus BP should be measured with a sphygmomanometer Supine and upright BP should be obtained *as orthostasis may reflect severe dehydration, which may increase hypertension*
Funduscopic examination	May reveal papilledema, exudates, or hemorrhages
Diagnostic/Laboratory Tests	
Electrocardiography	May reveal ischemia or left ventricular hypertrophy
Chest x-ray	May show pulmonary edema and cardiomegaly *due to CHF, or mediastinal widening and blunting of the aortic arch consistent with a dissecting aneurysm*

Urinalysis and renal function tests	Urinalysis may show proteinuria, red cells, or red-cell casts in a hypertensive crisis Blood urea nitrogen (BUN) and creatinine *determine the severity of the hypertensive episode*
Urine drug screen (in selected patients)	May confirm ingestion of drugs *that induce hypertension*
CBC with differential	Histocytes and target cells indicate microangiopathic hemolytic anemia, as they pass through arterioles, *in which subendothelial collagen and fibrin protrude into the lumen secondary to necrosis of the vessel wall*
Serum electrolytes	Hypokalemia may be seen with high-renin forms of hypertension *Hypokalemia or hypomagnesemia increases the risk of arrhythmias*
Computed tomography	Should be obtained when the physical findings lead to the suspicion of focal cerebral ischemia or intracranial hemorrhage, and in evaluation of the comatose patient

PLAN OF CARE

INTENSIVE PHASE

The intensive phase of care for patients with hypertensive crisis is focused on reducing BP to safe levels as fast as possible without increasing the risk of complications. Achieving this goal typically requires the parenteral administration of potent vasodilating medication. These medications can easily reduce BP too far, contributing to an already high-risk situation. Invasive arterial monitoring is often employed to enable continuous assessment of BP so that aggressive reduction in hypertension may occur with minimal risk. As a result, hypertensive patients may be admitted to an ICU for management and stabilization of a crisis state. The advent of improved noninvasive BP monitors has resulted in some controversy regarding ICU admission for the management of hypertensive crisis. Whether admitted to an ICU or an alternate monitored unit, the need for continuous monitoring of BP, frequent assessment, and readiness to respond to potential complications of hypertensive crisis must be provided by qualified staff.

PATIENT CARE PRIORITIES	EXPECTED PATIENT OUTCOMES
Decreased tissue perfusion *r/t increased peripheral systemic vascular resistance*	Peripheral pulses: WNL CRT <3 sec Absence of peripheral edema or s/s of organ ischemia
High risk for injury *r/t* *Medication side effects* *Sensorimotor and mentation alteration*	Return to optimal arterial pressure without complications
Decreased comfort *r/t* *Invasive monitoring lines* *Chest pain from increased myocardial oxygen consumption* *Headache from increased intracranial pressure* *Possible dissecting aortic aneurysm*	Maintain optimal levels of comfort as reported by the patient
Anxiety (patient/family) *r/t* *Crisis situation* *Admission to the critical care unit* *Fear of death*	Able to rest, sleep, and communicate needs Verbalizes decreased level of anxiety
Alteration in LOC *r/t* *Altered arterial pressure* *Actual or potential increase in ICP*	Return to LOC consistent with precrisis neurologic function

Plan of Care (cont'd)

High risk for decreased cardiac output *r/t* *Dysrhythmias from electrolyte disturbances* *Hypovolemia* *Ventricular dysfunction*	CO: WNL CI: WNL
High risk for impaired gas exchange *r/t* *Decreased CNS function* *Pulmonary edema*	PaO_2 >90 mm Hg ABG: WNL Lungs clear
High risk for altered fluid balance *r/t* *Volume excess due to:* *Decreased urine output* *Left ventricular failure* *Volume deficit due to:* *Pressure-related diuresis*	Normovolemic state: CVP: WNL PCWP: WNL UO: WNL No s/s of peripheral edema Weight: WNL

INTERVENTIONS

Continuous assessment and monitoring of blood pressure *to determine efficacy of treatment.*

Record cuff pressures on both arms in sitting and lying position if possible to *determine baseline blood pressures.*

Manage invasive arterial line monitoring with alarms set within 10 mm Hg of lowest desired BP *to ensure prompt intervention for fluctuation of BP.*

Administer antihypertensive agents as prescribed, *noting any side effects, hypotension, and efficacy.*

Obtain baseline assessment of neuro, cardiac, respiratory, renal, and GI systems *for comparison if changes occur in patient status.*

Monitor for and report signs and symptoms of potential complications as described in the assessment section with emphasis on the neuro, cardiac, renal, and GI systems.

Institute seizure precautions as appropriate *to assure patient safety.*

Emphasize a calm, quiet environment with minimal stimulation and sedation as needed *to decrease patient/family anxiety and facilitate BP control.*

Carefully assess any complaints of pain, administer analgesics aggressively, and keep physician informed *to prevent increased BP and protect organ systems from ischemia and tissue damage.*

Monitor lab work for abnormalities requiring intervention *to prevent further complications and to assess efficacy of therapy.*

Administer fluids as indicated *to maintain optimal CO.*

INTERMEDIATE PHASE

The focus of the intermediate phase is the continued reduction of BP to optimal levels. The immediate threat of end-organ damage has passed, but during this phase, BP must be maintained at a level specific to each patient. Doses and types of oral agents may be tested during this period to find the combination that best maintains BP with minimum side effects. Usually, the patient has been transferred from the critical care unit to the medical-surgical floor, but this depends on the stability of BP. Patient/family education becomes a priority as the patient's BP is controlled. Patients must be allowed the opportunity to discuss their feelings related to life-style changes, dietary restrictions, and medication regimes.

PATIENT CARE PRIORITIES	EXPECTED PATIENT OUTCOMES
High risk for complications *r/t continued hypertension*	BP within patient norm
Self-care deficit *r/t hypertension and care requirements*	Patient demonstrates knowledge and self-responsibility for controlling BP

Plan of Care (cont'd)

High risk for decreased nutritional status *r/t anorexia and stress of recent crisis*	Maintain adequate nutritional status

INTERVENTIONS

Continued assessment of BP trends after crisis has been resolved *to prevent repeat hypertensive crisis.*

Administer oral antihypertensive agents as prescribed with continued assessment of side effects.

Assess patient's nutritional intake and daily weight *to assure optimal nutritional status.*

Patient/family teaching with emphasis on the following key points *to assist the patient in assuming responsibility for the maintenance of normal BP.*

- Factors contributing to HBP and the effect of HBP on end organs
- Procedure for monitoring BP with emphasis on when to notify the physician
- Importance of diet and weight control in the maintenance of normal BP
- Role of smoking in HBP—offer support for cessation
- Regular exercise as a mechanism for controlling weight, stress, and BP
- Alternatives for stress reduction with emphasis on the relationship between stress and HBP
- Antihypertensive therapy, including name, rationale, dosage, and side effects of all medications

TRANSITION TO DISCHARGE

Discharge of the patient who has entered the hospital with a hypertensive crisis may occur within several days to weeks depending upon the severity of symptoms upon admission, the difficulty in regulating BP, and complications that may have occurred either from therapy or from end-organ damage. The focus for nursing during this period is preparing the patient and family for the discharge to home. Since many patients have entered the hospital because they stopped taking their medication, one must recognize the possibility that the patient will again stop taking medication when beginning to feel well, especially if the cost of medications is an issue. The nurse must help the patient and/or family understand the importance of maintaining a therapeutic blood level of medication. Patients and families may be taught to monitor the patient's blood pressure. It should be clear to patients/families what to do if the individual is unable to take medicine, as in cases of flu or other illness that limits oral intake. Symptoms of increasing blood pressure should be reviewed with instructions to call the physician if there are concerns. If cost is an issue, efforts must be made in collaboration with social services to explore strategies to help the patient purchase medications.

Education should also be focused on a healthy living pattern with emphasis on diet, exercise, cessation of smoking, and stress reduction. Services available within the community should be shared with both patient and family.

REFERENCES

1. Calhoun D, Oparil S: Treatment of hypertensive crisis, *New Engl J Med* 323(17):1177-1183, 1990.
2. Eagan J, Stewart S, Vitello-Cicciu J: *Quick reference to cardiac critical care nursing,* Gaithersburg, Md, 1991, Aspen Publishers.
3. Elnicki M, Kotchen T: Hypertension: patient evaluation, indications for treatment, *Geriatrics* 48(4):47-61, 1993.
4. Gifford R: Management of hypertensive crisis, *JAMA* 266(6):829-835, 1991.
5. Jackson R: Hypertension in the emergency department, *Emerg Med Clin North Am* 6(2):173-196, 1988.
6. Johannsen J: Update: guidelines for treating hypertension, *Am J Nurs* 93:42-49, 1993.
7. Joint National Committee on Detection, Evaluation, and Treatment of High Blood Pressure: *1992 report, National Heart Lung, and Blood Institute,* Washington, DC, 1992, Department of Health and Human Services, NIH Publications.
8. Keller K, Lemberg L: Hypertensive crises, *Heart Lung* 20(4):421-424, 1991.
9. McKinney T, Stein J: Management of hypertensive crisis, *Hosp Pract* 27:133-151, March 1992.
10. Sanders A: Hypertension emergencies, *Am Fam Phys* 44(5):1767-1774, 1991.

11. Sibai B: Hypertension in pregnancy, *Obstet Gynecol Clin North Am* 19(4):615-630, 1992.
12. Silver H: Acute hypertensive crisis in pregnancy, *Med Clin North Am* 73(3):623-638, 1989.
13. *St Anthony's DRG guidebook 1995,* Reston, Va, 1994, St Anthony.
14. Thacker H, Jahnigen D: Managing hypertensive emergencies and urgencies in the geriatric patient, *Geriatrics* 46(10):26-37, 1991.
15. Teplitz L: Hypertensive crisis: review and update, *Crit Care Nurs* 13(6):20-36, 1993.
16. Underhill S, et al: *Cardiovascular medications for cardiac nursing,* Philadelphia, 1990, JB Lippincott.
17. Venkata C, Ram S: Management of hypertensive emergencies: changing therapeutic options, *Am Heart J* 122(1):356-363, 1991.

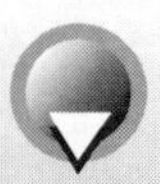

CLINICAL GUIDELINE

27

Aortic Aneurysms

Elise Dempsey, MS, RN, CCRN

DESCRIPTION

Aortic aneurysms are defined as a weakening and dilatation of a section of the aortic wall. Aneurysms are classified by their location, and treatment may vary accordingly. Thoracic aneurysms occur in the ascending and transverse portion of the thoracic aorta and may involve the aortic valve and the carotid, innominate, and subclavian arteries that branch off the aortic arch. These patients usually require prompt surgical intervention to prevent complications, especially if the aneurysm is expanding or at risk of rupture.[14] Thoracoabdominal aneurysms involve the descending branch of the thoracic aorta from above the diaphragm to some point either above or below the renal arteries. Abdominal aneurysms are usually located below the renal arteries and may involve the iliac arteries to some extent[3] (Figure 27-1). Patients with more distal aneurysms may be successfully managed with antihypertensives and β-blocker therapy before surgical intervention is required.[14] Decisions regarding surgery for abdominal or thoracoabdominal aneurysms are based on size of the distention and the development of associated signs and symptoms.

Dissection of the aorta occurs when the aortic media has been split and there is collection of blood between the intimal and medial layers of the vessel wall. Aortic dissection is classified as either acute or chronic based on the time elapsed since the occurence. Dissection is considered acute if it has occurred within the last two weeks. Most deaths occur within the first 30 days when the aorta is inflamed and friable.[2]

Aortic aneurysms are the 13th most common cause of death in the United States, affecting 6% of all women and 1.2% of all men.[8] It is possible that these numbers may underestimate the incidence of the disease because many aortic dissections are not diagnosed before death and are found at autopsy.[2] Death is usually attributed to either rupture of an infrarenal aneurysm (80% of all deaths) or a complete dissection of a thoracoabdominal aneurysm.

Two developments in health care have served to decrease the number of deaths due to aneurysmal dissection. Newer imaging techniques such as the CT scan and magnetic resonance imaging (MRI) have helped to detect dissecting aneurysms earlier and aid in prompt intervention. In addition, increased awareness and aggressive treatment of hypertension have diminished the impact of this chronic illness as a predisposing factor in aortic disease.[12] However, as the population continues to age, the incidence of infrarenal aneurysms has increased to the extent that approximately 3% of patients older than 50 years are expected to develop aneurysms.[8]

PATHOPHYSIOLOGY

Two types of pathologic processes contribute to the development of aneurysm formation. The first, and most common, is degeneration of the medical layer of the aortic vessel wall, leading to loss of elastic fibers, eventual medical necrosis, and loss of smooth muscle cells. Syndromes and disease processes considered etiologies of aneurysmal disease include Marfan syndrome, Ehlers-Danlos syndrome, and other genetically linked abnormalities. If chronic hypertension is associated with these diseases, the likelihood of aneurysm formation is increased. Hypertension alone is implicated in the development of 75% to 90% of all aneurysms.

A second pathologic process leading to aneurysmal formation can be related to various forms of aortitis. This may

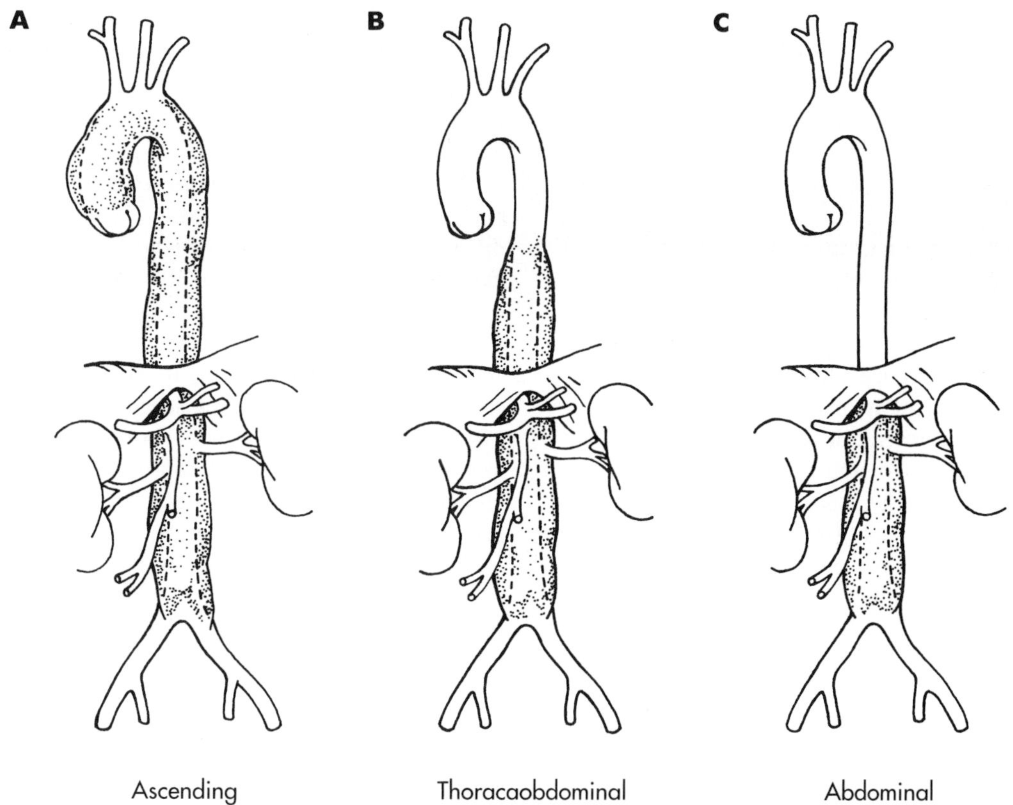

Figure 27-1 Classification of aortic aneurysms. **A,** Ascending. **B,** Thoracic abdominal. **C,** Abdominal. (Modified from Svensson LG, Crawford ED: Aortic dissection and aortic aneurysm surgery: clinical observations, experimental investigations and statistical analysis, *Curr Probl Surg* 29(12):913-1057, 1992, p 926.)

result from an inflammatory process or may be a symptom of an autoimmune disease and is characterized by interstitial fibrosis and hyperplasia. Autoimmune diseases such as systemic lupus erthythematosus, schleroderma, rheumatic arthritis, and Takayasu's disease have been known to cause aortitis and chronic inflammation.[12] Infectious organisms that may contribute to aneurysm development via inflammation of the aortic wall include *Staphylococcus epidermidis,* streptococci, and *Eshcherichia coli.*[10]

A predisposition to aneurysmal disease within families has been observed. As many as 15% of patients with aortic aneurysms have a close relative with the same disorder.[1] Because of this genetic tendency, the search for a biochemical cause of the disease has been extensive. The excessive presence of the enzyme elastase appears to be a significant etiological mechanism. This enzyme is believed to be released by activated WBCs and other sources and results in destruction of elastic fibers in the aortic wall. The resulting nonelastic and noncompliant aorta becomes dilated. Other biochemical abnormalities that have been observed include decreased levels of collagen within the aortic wall and a greater-than-normal level of collagenase activity. Cell-mediated immunity, especially in inflammatory aneurysms, may also contribute to weakening of the vessel wall.[17]

Atherosclerosis may also be found at the site of aneurysm formation, especially in the elderly. It is most often associated with lesions occurring below the renal arteries and, rather than being a contributing factor, may actually strengthen the dilated vessel and prevent further dissection.[12]

Finally, blunt trauma to the aorta may tear the vessel wall and result in the development of hematoma and dilation of the aortic arch. The proposed mechanism of injury is based on the fact that the aortic arch and diaphragm are fixed points in the thorax, and during rapid deceleration, these sites absorb the full impact of the force. Thus, tears of the aorta occur near the innominate and subclavian arteries and along the diaphragm. Therapy is focused on rapidly lowering the blood pressure, confirming the site by angiography, and stabilizing the patient for surgical repair.[12]

Most asymptomatic aneurysms are detected during routine CXR or ultrasound. Aneurysms become symptomatic when they begin to leak, rapidly enlarge, or dissect. Symptomatology is related to either direct expansile process or hypoperfusion of an organ such as cardiac ischemia or in an extremity. The pain of aortic dissection is often described as a tearing sensation but may also be described as "burning" or "cutting." The onset of pain is often associated with vigorous or rapid movement such as swinging a golf club or splitting wood. Syncope or loss of consciousness may occur with the onset of pain. The severe pain first experienced with aortic dissection may subside over a couple of hours, to be replaced by a deep ache that may lull the physician into thinking the cause of the pain has resolved. The patient will be tachycardic and may be hypertensive as a result of stimulation of the aortic arch baroreceptors and release of catecholamines. Activation of the renin-angiotensin system may also contribute to hypertension due to renal artery obstruction and resulting renal ischemia.

Ascending aortic aneurysms result in increased pressure on organs in the thoracic cavity and may disrupt blood flow through the carotid, innominate, and subclavian arteries. This may be manifested as pulse abnormalities or inconsistencies in bilateral comparisons, pain in the extremities, or the appearance of neurological insults such as transient stroke and vertebrobasilar symptoms. Dissection of the ascending aorta may also stretch the aortic valve ring, causing aortic regurgitation, and distend the pericardium, leading to cardiac tamponade and congestive heart failure. The coronary ostium may become obstructed, causing decreased coronary perfusion and possible myocardial infarction or rhythm disturbance. Pressure effects on the structures in the chest may present as hoarseness, chest and neck fullness, dysphagia, back pain, and superior vena cava syndrome.

Descending thoracoabdominal aneurysms expand and cause pressure within the thorax and abdominal cavity. This may be experienced as right or left chest pain or shoulder pain due to irritation of the diaphragm. Perfusion of the kidneys, gut, and spinal cord may be decreased, leading to renal failure, bowel ischemia, and paraplegia or paraparesis.

Abdominal aneurysms typically cause symptoms related to tenderness or backache, and a pulsatile mass may be noted in the epigastric or midabdominal area. Less frequent signs may include leg weakness and pain, nausea and vomiting, melena, and gastric retention due to decreased perfusion to the lower bowel. Flank pain due to ureteral obstruction may mimic a kidney stone.[12]

LENGTH OF STAY/ANTICIPATED COURSE

Patients with aneurysmal disease are often elderly and have associated health problems that complicate their care. The presence of chronic cardiovascular or respiratory disease can negatively influence the postoperative course and may impact whether the patient is treated medically or surgically.

Medically managed aneurysms typically fall within DRG 130: Peripheral Vascular Disorders with Cardiac Catheterization or DRG 131: Peripheral Vascular Disorders without Cardiac Catheterization.[11] The average lengths of stay for these DRGs are 7.4 days and 5.6 days, respectively. Medical treatment of distal aortic aneurysms requires aggressive management of blood pressure to diminish the forceful ejection of blood into the aorta and decrease overall aortic pressures. The patient should be monitored in intensive care until blood pressure and pain are under control. Rupture is most likely to occur within the first 3 to 5 days after dissection, making prompt surgical intervention imperative for survival. After IV vasodilators are weaned to oral medications and pain is controlled, the patient may be transferred to a medical floor. Depending on the patient, length of stay may be as high as 10 days to 2 weeks.

Patients who require surgical intervention are usually classified under DRG 110 or 111. Both refer to Major Cardiovascular Procedures, with average length of stay of 12.2 days and 7.5 days, respectively.[11] The difference between the two is whether cardiac catheterization is performed. There are dramatic differences in the course of the hospital stay between the patient who undergoes emergency surgery and the patient who has been scheduled electively. Elective surgery allows optimization of the patient's known risk factors and a more controlled approach during surgery. This allows the surgeon to plan the desired approach for repair, such as tube versus patch graft, and to consider the need for organ preservation techniques while the aorta is cross-clamped. Depending on postoperative complications, most patients undergoing elective repair of an aneurysm spend 2 to 4 days in the intensive care area and return home within 10 days to 2 weeks.

The hospital course for emergent aortic aneurysm repair is difficult to predict and depends on preoperative status of the patient and the difficulty of the surgery itself. The ultimate outcome is dependent on the degree of ischemic injury that may have ensued and the ability to prevent postoperative complications due to advanced age and associated health problems.

MANAGEMENT TRENDS AND CONTROVERSIES

A primary decision in the treatment of aortic aneurysms is whether to manage the patient medically or to proceed directly to a surgical approach. Controversy exists concerning the indications for aortic surgery in the asymptomatic patient. Guidelines have been suggested that healthy asymptomatic patients with distal aneurysms twice the size of the normal aorta or thoracic aneurysms >5 cm should undergo surgical repair.[12] Others have argued that the rate of aneurysm rupture is significant even at a size of 4 cm and that surgery should occur when aneurysms reach 4 cm or greater.[7] Medical management is aimed at preventing further expansion of the aneurysm through control of pain and blood pressure but should be replaced with surgical intervention if ineffective or signs of branch artery obstruction occur. Acute dissection of ascending aortic aneurysms should always be treated with immediate surgery because fatal rupture or cardiac tamponade may occur at any time.[14]

Management of preexisting disease in these patients can be challenging and time-consuming. However, delay of surgery in order to optimize the patient's health status invariably results in a more favorable outcome after surgery. Studies have shown that there is significant cardiac risk associated with aneurysm repair when the surgical candidate has a history of decompensated CHF, angina or myocardial infarction, abnormal resting ECG or associated diabetes, hypertension, or cerebral vascular disease.[6] If possible, the surgery should be delayed to allow optimization of cardiac status. The need for preoperative cardiac catheterization is controversial. Results have been good when coronary disease is repaired before aortic surgery.[5] In rare cases patients who have severe diffuse coronary disease, severely impaired left ventricular function, and patients whose respiratory function is so poor that survival from consecutive major procedures is unlikely may benefit from combined myocardial revascularization and aortic aneurysm repair.[16,18] Patients with chronic pulmonary disease also benefit from a delay in surgery for 2 to 4 weeks to receive aggressive bronchodilator therapy and physiotherapy and to discontinue smoking if this is necessary.[14] Preoperative renal disease should be identified before surgery if possible and measures taken during the procedure to preserve renal flow. Adequate hydration of the patient before angiography and surgery are imperative.[12] Finally, carotid artery stenosis should be evaluated before surgery to minimize the possibility of neural insult during surgery. During repair of the aortic arch, embolization of plaque can be disastrous and prolonged hypotension can greatly impair cerebral blood flow. If carotid stenosis is severe, consideration should be given to correcting this lesion before aortic repair.[4]

Major surgical considerations include selection of surgical technique to repair the vessel wall, control of hemmorhage, and preservation of the organs to prevent ischemic injury. A thoracotomy or abdominal approach is used, depending on the site of the aneurysm. Possible choices for graft repair include Dacron patches or a whole tube graft that replaces the native aorta. The latter can be bifurcated to repair the iliac arteries if involved. In some instances the surgeon may choose to place a bypass graft rather than an end-to-end anastomosis. An alternate approach is to clip the aneurysm and then support the area by encasing it in a segment of tube graft, much as a cast supports a broken bone. Repair of an ascending aorta may involve replacement of the aortic valve ring, the whole aortic valve, or a valve-graft composite, which is frequently used with Marfan syndrome. Another alternative is to use a pulmonary or aortic homograft when it is necessary to replace both the aortic valve and ascending aorta. Success rates are particularly high when this procedure is used in children or young adults who have congenital anomalies.[9]

Ascending aorta repair is challenging because of the danger of embolization and the need for preservation of brain and cardiac tissue. Most repair in this area is done with circulatory arrest compensated with the cardiopulmonary bypass pump and deep hypothermia to minimize ischemic insult. During reattachment of the aortic arch vessels or the coronary arteries, care is taken to prevent plaque from breaking loose. As a result, use of the aortic clamp is minimized when evidence of atherosclerosis is seen in the ascending aorta and arch. Even with these precautions the incidence of postoperative stroke is 15%.[14]

Distal aortic repairs may compromise perfusion to the kidney, gut, and spinal cord. Most repairs involve clamping the aorta below the renal arteries, resulting in minimal risk to vital organs. If the clamp is required above the renal arteries, a clamp time of 5 to 10 minutes can usually be tolerated well. Adequate hydration of the patient and a small dose of mannitol have been recommended to protect renal function in cases where infrarenal clamping is needed.[16]

Careful attention to the various branches from the distal aorta to the intestinal tract is important. Reattachment of the inferior mesenteric, superior mesenteric, celiac, and renal arteries is required once the graft is in place. If these branches are diseased, they may be replaced at this time to ensure optimal postoperative organ perfusion.[12]

Spinal cord ischemia is a rare but devastating complication and is usually attributed to prolonged hypotension and/or clamp time and the failure to reattach all segmental branches to the new graft.

Management of fluids and hemodynamic pressures is paramount to maintaining adequate tissue perfusion and ensuring graft patency both during and after surgery. This is accomplished through close monitoring of hemodynamic parameters, urinary output, and electrolyte levels. Stabilization of mean arterial pressure is achieved through careful titration of vasoactive medications and fluid replacement. The diagnosis of perioperative MI will require close attention to myocardial filling pressures to prevent fluid overload. All attempts are made during surgery to conserve blood. The use of cell-saving devices allows autotransfusion of lost blood and minimizes the use of donated blood.

Deep hypothermia is used to prolong the amount of time organs can be safely hypoperfused, particularly during proximal aortic surgery. A further decrease in core body temperature results from prolonged exposure of the open thorax to room air. Vasoconstriction of the peripheral blood vessels can cause pronounced hypertension and stress on the new graft site. As the surface of the body warms and cooled blood is returned to the center of the body, shivering may begin, further contributing to hemodynamic instability and an increase in myocardial oxygen demand. Careful warming of the patient and the use of paralyzing agents can minimize this complication.

Ischemic injury becomes evident later in the postoperative course. Renal failure may appear immediately, indicating atheromatous embolization during surgery. Prognosis for return to normal function in this case is poor. Renal failure that occurs 7 to 10 days after surgery is usually due to inadequate hydration or preexisting renal disease. Dialysis is often successful in reversing this type of renal dysfunction.

Bowel ischemia may present as either mild or severe. Mild ischemia involving only the muscle wall can be managed by resting the gut, ensuring adequate hydration, and administration of antibiotics. More severe ischemic damage will require surgical intervention.

Infection, although rare, is worrisome, especially if it involves the graft site. Local infection of the wound may be managed by drainage, open packing, and antibiotics. If the graft is involved, it must be replaced and the area irrigated, debrided, and drained.

Future research will be directed toward various ways to maintain organ perfusion during surgery. Increased use of cold perfusion of the kidneys and spinal cord will be attempted to increase the amount of time the aorta can be clamped. Research is also active in the development of new ways to provide retrograde perfusion via veins during circulatory arrest to ensure cerebral preservation, as well as distal perfusion techniques during thoracic surgery to prevent spinal cord injury. Some of the possible benefits may include oxygenating the brain, providing metabolic substrates, removing metabolic pathway effluent, and keeping the brain cold.[13,15]

ASSESSMENT

PARAMETER	ANTICIPATED ALTERATION
Cardiovascular Status	
HR and rhythm	Increased: >100 bpm and potential ventricular dysrhythmias or conduction defects *due to blood loss and possible involvement of coronary arteries*
MAP	Elevated: >100 mm Hg *due to catecholamines* and postop *due to aortic clamping, hypothermia, and possible shivering* Hypotensive with MAP <60 mm Hg *due to massive hemorrhage associated with aneurysm rupture*
PAP	Normal or decreased: <15 mm Hg if hypovolemic *due to hemorrhage or postoperative third spacing*
PCWP	Normal or decreased: <14 mm Hg *if hypovolemic* Increased: >16 mm Hg with CHF *due to perioperative MI or fluid overload*
SVR	Increased: >1200 dynes/sec/cm^{-5} *due to increased catecholamines and activation of aortic baroreceptors, hyperthermia, and possible shivering*
CI	WNL or decreased: <2.5 L/m/m^2 *due to myocardial depression, ischemic events, or decreased preload due to hypovolemia*
Heart sounds	May have new aortic murmur, muffled heart tone, or new S3 or S4 *due to retrograde dissection of aorta causing dilation of the aortic valve or tamponade*
Chest pain	Described as tearing or burning, sudden onset decreasing to a dull ache over time; may be felt in right or left chest and radiate to neck, arms, back, or shoulder
Peripheral pulses	Unequal pulses bilaterally, may be diminished or absent
Pulmonary Status	
RR	Dyspneic, wheezing, hoarseness, dysphagia *due to compression of bronchus, trachea, and esophagus from expanding aneurysm*
Lung sounds	Clear bilaterally or evidence of pulmonary edema *due to compromised myocardial status*
ABG	Normal or metabolic acidosis with pH <7.35 and HCO_3 <21 *due to poor tissue perfusion and shock*
Neurological Status	
LOC	Anxious, restless, transient neurological deficits, syncope *due to hemodynamic changes and cerebral perfusion deficits*
Pupils	Unequal *due to pressure on the cervicospinal nerve*

Other

Abdomen	Tender with palpable pulsatile mass *due to abdominal aneurysm*
Lower intestine	Bloody diarrhea *due to ischemic bowel*
Renal status	Hematuria, UO <30 cc/hr *due to decreased renal perfusion obstruction of the renal arteries* Flank pain and frequency *due to compression of ureters and bladder from expanding aneurysm*
Hgb/Hct	WNL or Hgb decreased <12 and Hct decreased <37 *due to blood loss*
WBC	Elevated: >10,000/mm^3 *due to stress response and/or infection*
Creatinine/BUN	WNL or creatinine increased >1.2 mg/dl and BUN increased >20 mg/dl *due to hypoperfusion from hypovolemia or obstruction*

PLAN OF CARE

INTENSIVE PHASE

Initial interventions must be geared toward achieving hemodynamic stability in the patient as evidenced by optimal cardiac output and mean arterial pressure. The nurse should also monitor the patient for signs of hemorrhage due to rupture or suture line leak. The patient with aortic aneurysm is at risk for many complications arising from hypoperfusion of organ systems. Early intervention during the intensive phase may prevent these outcomes from occurring.

PATIENT CARE PRIORITIES	EXPECTED PATIENT OUTCOMES
Decreased cardiac output *r/t* *Possible aortic valve incompetence* *Cardiac dysrhythmia* *Congestive heart failure* *Cardiac tamponade* *Hemorrhage*	MAP: WNL UO: ≤30 cc/hr CO: WNL CI: WNL Extremities pink, warm, and dry CXR: WNL Hgb and Hct: WNL
Hypertension *r/t* *Increased catecholamine levels* *Aortic cross-clamping* *Hypothermia* *Shivering*	MAP: WNL No increase in size of aneurysm No increase in postop bleeding No evidence of postop shivering
High risk for decreased perfusion of myocardium *r/t* *Hypotension* *Preexisting cardiac disease* *Stress of surgery* *Obstruction of flow through coronary arteries in ascending aortic aneurysm*	Absence or resolution of ischemia Absence of myocardial infarction
High risk for decreased perfusion of lower extremities *r/t* *Occlusion of vessel from decreased perfusion* *Dislodgement of thrombus* *Atherosclerotic plaque*	Patent vessel or graft Circulation distal to aneurysm is sufficient with good pulses and warm skin
High risk for decreased cerebral perfusion *r/t* *Arterial embolism associated with atherosclerotic plaque* *Obstruction of carotid artery flow in ascending and thoracic aortic aneurysm*	CNS function within patient norms Absence of confusion, disorientation, or restlessness No evidence of cerebral infarct

Plan of Care (cont'd)

High risk for decreased renal perfusion *r/t*
Preop renal ischemia due to obstruction of renal arteries
Intraoperative ischemia during repair

Creatinine: WNL
BUN: WNL
Electrolytes: WNL

High risk for decreased perfusion to spinal cord *r/t*
Interruption of main artery to cord
Hypotension
Embolus in descending thoracic aneurysm

Absence of paralysis
Absence of parasthesias
Autonomic, genitourinary function: WNL

High risk for ineffective breathing pattern *r/t*
Elevated diaphragm after surgery
Abdominal distention
Incisional pain
Compression of upper airway from aneurysm

ABG within patient norms
Clear lungs with full lung expansion
V_t within patient norms
NIF within patient norms

High risk for ineffective gas exchange *r/t*
Atelectasis
Pulmonary edema

ABG within patient norms
Sao_2 >90%

High risk for GI dysfunction and ileus *r/t*
Recurrence of abdominal aneurysm
Mesenteric infarction
Bowel ischemia

GI function: WNL
Bowel sounds present
Abdomen soft, nontender

High risk for decreased renal function *r/t mechanical obstruction or injury to kidney, ureters, or bladder*

UO: WNL
No presence of flank pain
No increase in urinary frequency

High risk for sexual dysfunction *r/t*
Reduced blood flow to perianal area
Interruption of internal iliac artery
Autonomic nerve damage

Sexual function: WNL
Adequate blood flow to penile, perineal tissue

INTERVENTIONS

Monitor hemodynamic parameters *to ensure adequate filling pressures and prevent hypotension and hypovolemia.*

Administer fluids and/or blood products *to maintain adequate CO and stabilize Hgb and Hct.*

Administer vasoactive agents *to maintain MAP within desired range.*

Keep BP low with vasodilators, sedatives, and maintenance of a quiet, peaceful environment *to minimize expansion of a dissection or protect a new graft.*

Warm blood and/or use a warming blanket until core temp >36.1° C *to prevent shivering.*

Administer paralyzing agents if shivering causes hypertension or SVo_2 <60%.

Observe for changes in mentation or neurological function *to discern potential cerebral perfusion deficits.*

Assess heart tones *to note any new aortic murmurs.*

Monitor 12-lead ECG and cardiac enzymes *to rule out myocardial infarction or ongoing ischemia.*

Administer antianginal medications prn in the event angina occurs.

Assess for increasing dyspnea, hoarseness, or dysphagia *to discern for signs of expanding thoracic aneurysm.*

Monitor peripheral pulses distal to the aneurysm, noting fullness, pattern, and occlusion pressure.

Monitor perfusion of extremities and onset of abrupt pain with localization to organs involved.

Monitor intake and output *to ensure adequate hydration and renal function.*

Assess for hematuria or occult blood in the stool *to discern the presence of renal or intestinal ischemia.*

Plan of Care (cont'd)

Measure abdominal girth *to note increasing distention.*

Monitor bowel sounds q4h, note return postoperatively or if bowel sounds cease *to discern recovery or insult to GI tract.*

Monitor lab results, noting abnormalities in Hgb, Hct, WBC, platelets, BUN, creatinine, and coagulation studies.

INTERMEDIATE PHASE

Once the patient has been stabilized hemodynamically and the aneurysm has either been successfully repaired or is believed to be stable, the plan of care turns to correcting complications that may have occurred and preparing the patient for self-care after discharge. Hemodynamic monitoring lines will be removed and vasoactive drugs that were required will have been weaned to an oral form. Late complications that may occur in this phase include renal failure and ischemic bowel.

PATIENT CARE PRIORITIES	EXPECTED PATIENT OUTCOMES
Self-care deficit *r/t* *Knowledge of medications* *Activity, progression* *When to notify physician*	Verbalizes knowledge of incision care and when to call the physician (as applicable) Demonstrates return to ADLs
High risk for pain *r/t surgical intervention*	Pain controlled to allow participation in self-care activities, rest, and sleep
High risk for inadequate nutrition *r/t loss of appetite or GI compromise following surgery*	No nausea or gastric distention Nutritional intake adequate for wound healing
High risk for impaired renal function *r/t ischemia or embolism of kidneys*	BUN, creatinine, UO remain WNL

INTERVENTIONS

Develop plan for gradual progression from bedrest to ambulation, monitoring patient for signs of postural hypotension or dizziness *to ensure patient safety.*

Wean patient as tolerated from IV narcotic pain medications to oral medications. Stress importance of routine use of analgesics for at least 72 hours and early notification of need for pain medication *to minimize unnecessary pain levels, maintain acceptable levels of comfort and to enhance ability to engage in recovery activities such as ambulation, respiratory therapy, and eating.*

Introduce oral intake after bowel sounds have returned. Monitor closely for abdominal distention and retention of fluids. Prevent nausea and retching *to prevent strain on suture lines or preexisting aneurysm.*

Continue to monitor for late occurrence of renal failure by daily evaluation of BUN and creatinine.

Monitor caloric intake *to ensure optimal wound healing and prevent infection.*

Instruct patient regarding medications, especially antihypertensives, *to ensure ongoing stability of aneurysm site.*

Instruct patient to notify physician for sudden occurrences of sharp pain, numbness, or syncope *to ensure patient safety if the aneurysm expands or ruptures or a new aneurysm develops.*

TRANSITION TO DISCHARGE

As the patient recovers, moving from the intensive to the intermediate phase, plans should be well underway for his or her return to the home. How quickly discharge occurs depends on the patient's age, health before hospitalization, and how traumatic the surgical experience, if any, was. Increasing strength and stamina in ambulation and self-care activities with return to prehospitalization nutritional patterns are the focal points of this phase. Patients must be followed closely to monitor existing aneurysm or for the development of new aneurysmal disease. All patients should be considered as having ongoing disease requiring long-term management and follow-up. Enlargement of an unresected but dissected aorta can be expected in 20% to 40% of patients. Five-year survival rates range between 72% and 80%.[3] Even more encouraging is that most survivors remain in either New York Heart Association functional classes I or II, indicating minimal impact on ADLs. Most aortic aneurysm patients may expect to return to their previous level of activity and quality of life.

REFERENCES

1. Cannon DJ, Read RC: Blood elastolytic activity in patients with aortic aneurysms, *Ann Thorac Surg* 34:10-15, 1984.
2. Doroghazi RM, Slater EE, DeSanctis RW: Long term survival of patients with treated aortic dissection, *J Am Coll Cardiol* 3:1026-1034, 1984.
3. Glower DD, et al: Comparison of medical and surgical therapy for uncomplicated descending aortic dissection, *Circulation* 80:39-46, 1990.
4. Hertzer NR, et al: Incidental asymptomatic carotid bruits in patients scheduled for peripheral vascular reconstruction: results of cerebral and coronary angiography, *Surg* 96:535-544, 1984.
5. Hertzer NR, Yong JR, Beven EG: Late results of coronary bypass in patients with infrarenal aortic aneurysm, *Ann Surg* 205:360-367, 1987.
6. Hinkamp T, et al: Combined myocardial revascularization and abdominal aortic aneurysm repair, *Ann Thorac Surg* 51:470-472, 1991.
7. Hollier LH, Taylor LM, Oschner J: Recommended indications for operative treatment of abdominal aortic aneurysms, *J Vasc Surg* 15:1046-1056, 1992.
8. Lilienfeld DE, et al: Epidemiology of aortic aneurysms, *Arteriosclerosis* 7:637-643, 1987.
9. McKowen RL, et al: Extended aortic root replacement with aortic allografts, *J Thorac Cardiovasc Surg* 93:366-374, 1987.
10. Reddy DJ, et al: Management of infected aortoiliac aneurysms, *Arch Surg* 126:873-878, 1991.
11. *St Anthony's DRG Guidebook 1995,* Reston, Va, 1994, St Anthony.
12. Svensson LG, Crawford ES: Aortic dissection and aortic aneurysm surgery: clinical observations, experimental investigations and statistical analysis, *Curr Probl Surg* 29(12):913-1057, 1992.
13. Svensson LG, et al: Deep hypothermia with circulatory arrest: determinants of stroke and early mortality in 656 patients, *J Thorac Cardiovasc Surg* 106:19-27, 1993.
14. Svensson LG, et al: Dissection of the aorta and dissecting aortic aneurysms: improving early and long-term surgical results, *Circulation* 82:24-48, 1990.
15. Takamoto S, et al: Distal aortic arch aneurysmectomy and coronary revascularization through a left thoracotomy, *Ann Thorac Surg* 55:151-152, 1993.
16. Taylor S, et al: Combined coronary artery bypass and abdominal aortic aneurysmectomy: appropriate management in selected cases, *South Med J* 86:974-976, 1993.
17. Webster MW, et al: Abdominal aortic aneurysm: results of a family study, *J Vasc Surg* 13:366-373, 1991.
18. Westaby S, et al: Combined cardiac and abdominal aortic aneurysm operations: the dual operation on cardiopulmonary bypass, *J Thorac Cardiovasc Surg* 104:990-995, 1992.

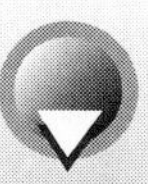

CLINICAL GUIDELINE

28

Carotid Endarterectomy

Anita Bush, PhD, RN, CCRN, CNRN

DESCRIPTION

Carotid endarterectomy (CEA) is a surgical procedure performed to prevent or reduce cerebral vascular complications due to the presence of atherosclerotic plaques in the carotid arteries.[9,32] The basic technique by which plaque is removed and a graft (synthetic or autograft) placed was introduced in 1954 by Eastcott, Pickering, and Robb.[7] CEA effectively provides treatment to prevent the recurrent transient ischemic attacks and ischemic stroke consequences of carotid artery stenosis by increasing cerebral blood flow and by removing sources of emboli.[20]

Approximately 80,000 to 100,000 carotid endarterectomies are performed each year in the United States, with an annual cost estimated at $1.2 billion, and averaging $13,000 per operation. This makes CEA the most common peripheral vascular procedure performed, and the third most common operation overall.[14,20] However, the prevalence of CEA is anticipated to decline in the future due to improved prevention and medical control of hypertension and cardiac disease, as well as economic scrutiny and the ongoing international debate about the procedure's value.[11,12,20,27,29]

PATHOPHYSIOLOGY

Carotid endarterectomy is performed to relieve symptoms, preserve neurologic function, and reduce the risk of stroke in a variety of patient conditions (see Table 28-1). Common to these conditions are reduced blood flow to cranial structures and increased risk of embolic occlusion due to the formation of plaques. This process is the leading cause of extracranial vascular disease.[15,22] Commonly, such plaques form at the carotid bifurcation, which is about the level of the jaw angle (Figure 28-1).

Blood flows through the brain at an average rate of 750 ml/min, or roughly 14% of the cardiac output. The brain receives 85% of this flow via the carotid arteries, with each carotid serving one cerebral hemisphere (Figure 28-1). Carotid supply divides further into the three major arteries of the brain, known as anterior, middle, and posterior cerebral arteries. The remaining 15% of cerebral blood supply is via the vertebrobasilar arterial system.

The clinical manifestations exhibited by the patient are directly related to those area(s) of the brain that experience reduced or obstructed supply of nutrient-rich oxygenated blood (Table 28-2).[4]

The plaques that develop are firm, platelike deposits that form within the inner wall of arteries as part of a process that begins with endothelial damage. Everyone is potentially susceptible to endothelial damage as a result of mechanical, chemical, or immunological assault on the blood vessels. Following such injury, platelets are deposited, smooth muscle proliferates, and cholesterol deposits begin to build at the site. As this matrix enlarges, it pushes the endothelium outward and begins to obstruct the vessel lumen. The plaque may rupture and pieces may break off in the high-pressure turbulent flow of an artery.[22,28] Typically this degenerative process develops over time against a backdrop of genetic predisposition and life-style factors.

LENGTH OF STAY/ANTICIPATED COURSE

As with other surgeries, LOS is dependent upon clinical indications for the procedure, general state of health, and development of complications.[6] Typically patients spend 1 to 2 days in an ICU, then 5.1 to 9.5 days in a general post-

TABLE 28-1 Patient Problems for which Carotid Endarterectomy May Be Performed
• Acute completed stroke (within first few hours) • Asymptomatic carotid stenosis • Carotid ulcerative plaques • Cerebral insufficiency • Global ischemic symptoms • Multi-infarct dementia • Progressive intellect impairment (with demonstrable arterial lesion) • Stroke in evolution (transient symptoms) • Transient ischemic attacks (hemispheric, amaurosis fugax) • Vertebrobasilar insufficiency

surgical unit, for a total LOS of 5 to 10 days in accord with DRG 478 and 479: Other vascular procedures with and without complications.[18,33,34] Those at risk for longer stays include females, the elderly, and patients undergoing CEA following a stroke.[10,20] The education, skill, and experience of the surgeon and perioperative nurses at the institution are crucial, as low surgical volume has been related to increased risk.[14]

Recent studies examining 22,500 CEA patients show an average of 1% to 2% operative mortality, 2% to 3% incidence of perioperative stroke, and a combined mortality/morbidity rate from all causes of about 6% nationwide.[20] Complication rates, however, vary widely between institutions, as well as between surgeons at the same institution, ranging from zero to 40%.[17] This contributes to widely varying lengths of stay and related health care costs.

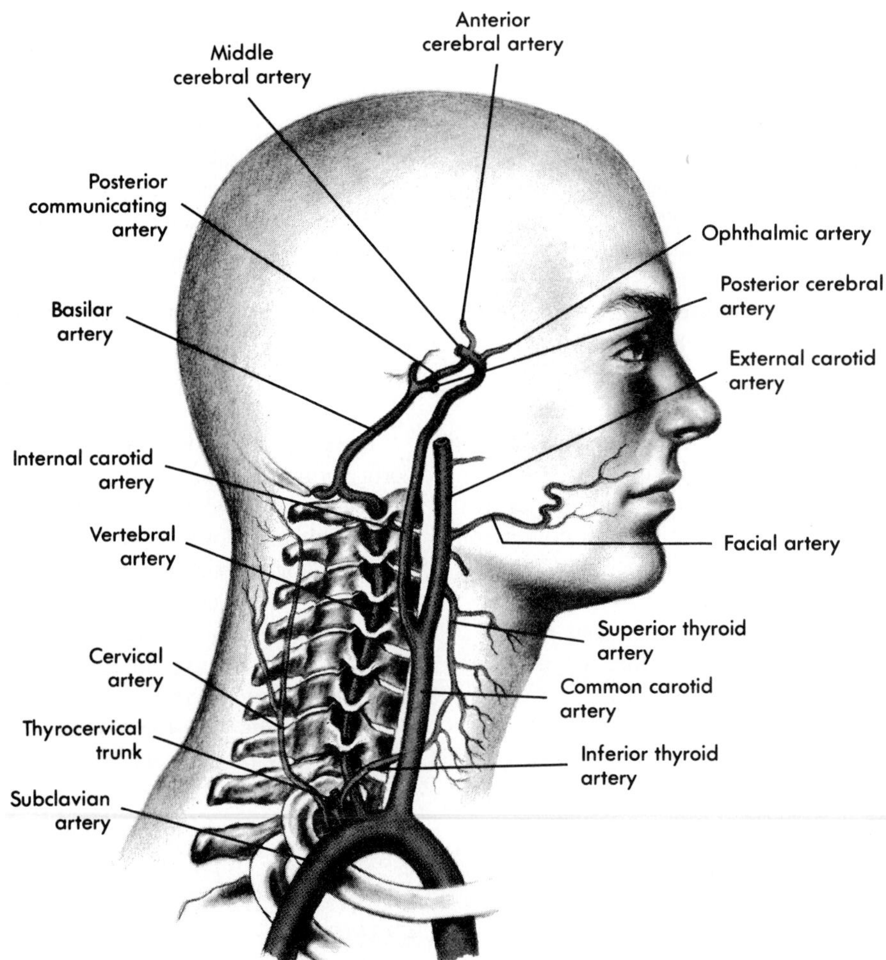

Figure 28-1 Conducting arteries of the brain. (From Phipps, et al: *Medical-surgical nursing*. In Rudy EB: *Advanced neurological and neurosurgical nursing,* ed 5, St Louis, 1995, Mosby–Year Book.)

TABLE 28-2 Correlation of Vessel Involvement with Indications of Impairment and Corresponding Definitions and Descriptions

Vessel and brain area supplied	Indications of impairment	Definitions and descriptions
Carotid arteries		
External carotid Scalp, skull, and meninges	Amaurosis fugax	Fleeting blindness in one eye
	Carotid bruit	May be secondary to radiation of a systolic murmur from the aortic region
Internal carotid Eye and eye orbit, cerebral hemispheres	Unilateral, contralateral motor and/or sensory disturbances such as:	
	• Dysphasia	*Expressive:* speech may be correctly spoken but content may not make sense *Receptive:* does not understand speech
	• Visual impairments	Highly variable, ranging from monocular blindness to subtle deficits
	• Weakness, numbness, or paralysis of arm or leg	Affects the body side opposite the intracranial lesion
	Severe, profound, global hemispheric functional deficits such as:	
	• Aphasia	Unable to speak, may not understand speech or writing
	• Unilateral, contralateral sensory loss and paralysis	Affects arm, leg, facial, and truncal half of body on side opposite the intracranial lesion
	• Visual impairment	Disturbances greater in the ipsilateral eye
Anterior cerebral artery		
Medial portion of frontal lobe to parietal sulcus, and portions of central brain structures: caudate nucleus, putamen, internal capsule	Incontinence	Loss of control over bladder elimination
	Diffuse motor and/or sensory deficits	Disturbances usually affect leg more than arm or face
	Eye-tracking disturbances	Difficulty following moving objects
	Mental status changes	Highly variable, may be subtle, but usually involve personality change, confusion, and/or impaired insight or judgement
	Return of primitive reflexes in adults, such as:	Usually affects body side opposite intracranial lesion
	• Snout	Lips pucker and protrude when lightly stroked
	• Sucking	Sucking motions of mouth and jaw when lips are lightly stroked
	• Grasping	Fingers flex when palm touched or lightly stroked
	Weakness or paralysis of the contralateral leg	May have clumsy gait or unsteady stance

TABLE 28-2 Correlation of Vessel Involvement with Indications of Impairment and Corresponding Definitions and Descriptions—cont'd

Vessel and brain area supplied	Indications of impairment	Definitions and descriptions
Middle cerebral artery		
Lateral surface of all lobes, portions of the basal ganglia and internal capsule, and macular input portion of the occipital lobe	Agnosia	Unable to recognize persons and things
	Dysphasia	See dysphasia above
	Motor deficits: weakness and/or paralysis	Disturbances affect arm and face more than leg on body side opposite the lesion
	Sensory problems such as:	Usually affecting face and arm more than leg
	• Numbness	Sensory losses
	• Hypresthesia	Increased sensation
	• Hemianopsia	Blindness in half of visual field, contributes to perceptual deficits
Posterior cerebral artery		
Inferior lateral surface of the temporal lobe, lateral & medial portions of the occipital lobe, portions of the central brain structures: pineal body, medial geniculate and lentiform nuclei	Agnosia	Unable to recognize persons and things
	Alexia	Unable to read or comprehend writing
	Mental status changes	Usually accompanied by impaired memory
	Oculomotor weakness/paralysis	
	Sensory disturbances	Contralateral to intracranial lesion
	Spatial-perceptual disturbances	Due to visual-field defects and affected eye muscles
Vertebrobasilar artery		
Basilar	Global disturbances such as:	
Pons, cerebellum, pineal body	• "Drop attacks"	Sudden weakness or paralysis of all limbs with loss of consciousness
Vertebral Spinal cord, medulla		
	• Syncope	Temporary loss of consciousness
	Motor disturbances such as:	
	• Weakness and impaired coordination	
	• Dysarthria	Difficulty forming speech sounds
	• Dysphagia	Difficulty swallowing
	• Vomiting	
	Sensory disturbances such as:	
	• Diplopia	Double vision
	• Impaired sense of touch	Mostly on face
	• Loss of pain and temperature sensation	Contralateral to the lesion
	• Vertigo	Dizziness

MANAGEMENT TRENDS AND CONTROVERSIES

Carotid endarterectomy has become an internationally controversial therapy with ongoing scientific debate about its value. At the heart of the matter are questions of efficacy, education/experience, and economics.

Efficacy

The presumed relationship between carotid atheromatous processes and cerebral infarction has led to CEA being performed to prevent strokes in both symptomatic and asymptomatic patients.[10,25] By current study methods, up to 34% of stroke patients have no warning TIA, but the rate may be much higher.[15] After a 20-year review of carotid endarterectomies, the Agency for Health Care Policy and Research published the opinion that "no properly designed prospective clinical trial has convincingly demonstrated this surgery to be superior or inferior to nonoperative management for any subsets of patients with carotid disease."[5]

Additional controversy surrounds the use of anticoagulants or antiplatelet agents pre-CEA. The questions are whether medical therapy alone might be sufficient for certain patients, and whether employing such therapies, not without their own risk, might eliminate warning TIAs.[15,27,30] Furthermore, neither anticoagulants nor antiplatelet agents affect existing plaques.

Education/Experience

There are also questions regarding who should perform CEA, at what type of institution, and using which techniques. Currently, CEA is performed by neurological surgeons, cardiovascular and peripheral vascular surgeons, and general surgeons. In a multicenter audit, there were statistical differences related to surgical complications and the surgeon's specialty.[16] Physician-specific complications within the same institution vary widely, from zero to 20% in published reports and up to 40% in internal audits.[17,19] Gibbs, et al., demonstrated that the complication rate of a single surgeon can adversely effect an institution's overall performance, raising stroke and death rate from 4% to over 14%.[17]

CEA is performed in large university hospitals as well as small community hospitals. A multicenter audit found that institutions with over 700 beds had a lower incidence of stroke and death overall, while the risks in a community hospital were much higher.[16] There are few reports from public teaching hospitals, where morbidity is often considered excessive and presumed due to the advanced disease state of the indigent and/or that they are cared for by physicians in training. However, Brien, et al., state that morbidity "is not necessarily related to the institutional volume of the procedure or the surgeon's specialty."[9] In addition, they report a significant reduction in mortality/morbidity, from 20% down to 3%, by developing, adopting, and adhering to a protocol for CEA.[9]

Widely differing techniques exist among the various surgeons and institutions. With the exception of patching to close the arteriotomy, the surgical techniques used are largely a personal matter.[29] No existing controlled studies compare the surgical variety for criteria such as where to make the skin incision, considering that vertical gives better exposure but horizontal gives better cosmetic results; whether or when to use intraoperative neurological monitoring, which some claim is excessively costly; whether to shunt routinely, selectively, or not at all, which may or may not reduce incidence of intraoperative embolization; or whether means of evaluating surgical outcome should be used, such as intraoperative or postoperative angiography, ultrasonography, or angioscopy.[15,22,29]

Economics

This controversial surgery is expensive. A major point of contention in the efficacy and education/experience debate is, of course, patient outcome and attendant costs. Resource utilization and patient selection criteria address the cost-benefit questions more directly. The need for "routine" ICU admission postoperatively has come under debate. O'Brien, et al., conclude that only about 18% of CEA patients require unique ICU services, and that the need became apparent within 2 hours of the surgery.[26] Use of intermediate care units, or longer observation in the postanesthetic care unit, is becoming the new norm.

Another question is whether CEA patients require general anesthesia (with its associated risks). Two studies using regional anesthesia for CEA have demonstrated significant cost savings without increasing mortality or morbidity.[18,33] Other investigators address the need for "routine" and costly diagnostics used for CEA patients, such as angiography, CT scanning, ultrasonography, duplex scanning, and transcranial Doppler of cerebral blood flow, to name just a few.[8,13,21,23-24,31]

ASSESSMENT

PARAMETER	ANTICIPATED ALTERATION
Respiratory Status	
Airway patency	Unable to manage secretions *due to loss of gag, swallow, or cough reflexes*
Tracheal position	Deviation or compression *due to soft tissue edema or hematoma formation*
Breathing pattern	Tachypnea or dyspnea *due to vagus nerve (CN-X) edema or manipulation* Irregular pattern *due to neurological dysfunction*
Breath sounds	Decreased quality of aeration, signs of obstruction, rales, rhonchi

Pulse oximetry and ABG	Spo_2 decreased: <95% Respiratory acidosis: • pH <7.40 • $Paco_2$ >40 mm Hg • Pao_2 <80 mm Hg *due to possible aspiration, tracheal compression, or pulmonary embolism*
Chest x-ray	Atelectasis, aspiration *due to complications of anesthesia and surgical site*

Cardiovascular Status

HR	Bradycardia *due to vagus nerve edema/manipulation* Tachycardia *due to pain, surgical stress, blood loss*
Heart rhythm	Tachybrady patterns *due to carotid sinus manipulation* Interpolated ectopy, escape beats *due to vagus nerve edema/manipulation*
BP	Impaired regulation, hypo- or hypertension *due to carotid sinus manipulation or compression by edema/hematoma and distensibility after plaque removal*
Peripheral pulses (temporal pulses for internal carotids; radial pulses for vertebral artery operations)	Diminished or hyperpulsations *due to arteriospasms, bleeding, occlusions*
Vessel patency diagnostics (completion angiography, carotid ultrasonography, Doppler flow study)	Reduced flow *due to leak* Impaired flow *due to edema, arteriospasm, thrombus, patch aneurysm*
Arterial surgical site	Edema, hematoma, excessive bleeding *due to surgical manipulation, anticoagulation therapy, loss of arteriotomy patch integrity*
Vascular autograft site	Bleeding, hematoma, distal edema, and venous distention *due to thrombus, occlusive forces*
Hct and Hgb	Decreased: Hct <37%, Hgb <12 g/dl *due to blood loss, dilutional effect*
PTT and APTT	Prolonged: PTT >70 sec, APTT >40 sec *due to intraoperative heparinization*

Neurological Status

Protective reflexes	Diminished/absent gag, swallow, cough; dysphonia *due to vagus nerve edema/manipulation or endotracheal intubation or extubation*
Glasgow coma scale	Score lower than preoperative baseline after fully recovered from general anesthesia *due to possible perioperative stroke*
EEG	New signs of localized or diffuse slowing (e.g., change in amplitude or frequency) not attributable to other causes (e.g., hypoxia, sedation) *due to perioperative ischemia, stroke, or emboli*
MRI or CT of head	Evidence of cerebral ischemia or infarction *due to possible procedure complications*
Transcerebral Doppler	Evidence of hypoperfusion *due to loss of arterial patency, occlusive forces*

PLAN OF CARE

INTENSIVE PHASE

While the need for post-carotid endarterectomy patients to receive care in an ICU setting has been challenged as no longer necessary, the nature of the procedure continues to require close or intensive monitoring for a minimum of 1 to 2 days. The following intensive plan of care reflects the care requirements associated with initial recovery regardless of patient location.

Plan of Care (cont'd)

PATIENT CARE PRIORITIES	EXPECTED PATIENT OUTCOMES
High risk for inadequate airway patency *r/t surgical site edema or hematoma*	Airway patent
High risk for ineffective breathing patterns *r/t* *Vagus nerve edema or manipulation* *Acute perioperative CNS event*	Normal respiratory rate and quality Adequate protective reflexes
High risk for impaired gas exchange *r/t* *Atelectasis* *Emboli* *Aspiration*	Adequate alveolar ventilation ABG within patient's norms
High risk for impaired circulation *r/t loss of vascular patency; occlusive forces*	Artery patent and functioning normally External pulses palpable and strong
Impaired regulation of HR and BP *r/t* *Carotid sinus manipulation/compression* *Vagus nerve edema/manipulation* *Carotid distensibility after plaque removal*	HR and BP normal or within prescribed range Hemodynamically significant cardiac rhythms are absent or controlled
High risk for altered cerebral perfusion *r/t* *Impaired circulation* *Hyperperfusion syndrome*	Neurological status is maintained or improved from preoperative level Seizures absent or controlled Headaches absent or controlled
Incisional pain and/or headache *r/t* *Surgical site trauma* *Possible impairment of cerebral perfusion*	Comfort within patient's acceptable parameters Able to rest and sleep

INTERVENTIONS

Prepare to perform or assist with emergency measures *to assure airway patency and adequate ventilation.*

Prepare to perform or assist with emergency direct arterial pressure or resuturing *to restore vascular patency and prevent hemorrhage.*

Notify physician immediately if evidence of ineffective breathing pattern or impaired gas exchange is detected.

Notify physician immediately if external pulses become absent or diminished, if hyperpulse develops, or if any sudden abnormality in the surgical site develops.

Notify physician immediately if neurological status worsens, if new deficits appear whether or not accompanied by change in vital signs, or if seizures develop.

Ongoing assessment and documentation of respiratory, cardiovascular and neurological status.

Administer prescribed supplemental humidified oxygen *to optimize gas exchange.*

Administer and titrate prescribed IV vasodilator agents, maintaining patient's BP within prescribed range, *to preserve arteriotomy patch integrity while ensuring adequate organ perfusion.*

Monitor for effects and side effects of medications and consult with physician if therapy change seems warranted.

Handle surgical site carefully during inspection, or when changing/reinforcing dressing, *to prevent inducing bradycardia due to vagal nerve or carotid sinus stimulation.*

Assist patient to change from horizontal to vertical positions slowly, *to protect from postural hypotension that may develop from impaired regulation abilities.*

Increase patient activity as patient is able to regulate HR and BP, unless medically contraindicated, *to prevent pulmonary and venous stasis.*

Elevate HOB *to relieve/prevent vascular headaches.*

Administer prescribed analgesics, monitoring effects and side effects. Consult with physician if changes in type, dosage, or frequency seem indicated.

Plan of Care (cont'd)

INTERMEDIATE PHASE

Most CEA patients survive the intensive phase. However, life-threatening complications such as intracerebral hemorrhage or embolic strokes may occur as late as 2 weeks post-CEA.[6,32] As a result, CEA patients require vigilant monitoring for potential complications even as they are prepared for discharge.

PATIENT CARE PRIORITIES	EXPECTED PATIENT OUTCOMES
High risk for orthostatic hypotension *r/t ongoing neurovascular changes and possible dehydration*	Patient able to sit, stand, and ambulate without dizziness or syncope
High risk for impaired cerebral perfusion and continued presence of neurological deficits such as:	Maximal neurological functioning
• Self-care deficits	Maximal independence in ADL, within capabilities
• Ineffective coping	Patient and family/significant others demonstrate adequate coping
Self-care deficit *r/t inadequate knowledge of health care needs*	Patient and family/significant others demonstrate adequate knowledge of health care status. Discharge plans are based on this knowledge.

INTERVENTIONS

Monitor for late onset or recurrence of procedure complications.

Maintain HOB at level that supports normal BP and prevents dizziness.

Teach patient to support head with one hand while arising from recumbent position *to reduce tension at the surgical site.*

Assist and supervise patient to change to a vertical position slowly (e.g., dangle 5 min before standing) until patient can ambulate independently and safely *to protect from injury.*

Notify physician if dizziness or postural hypotension persists beyond 48 hours.

Stay with patient with suction at bedside when initially starting po intake *to monitor swallowing ability and prevent aspiration.* Cool semisolids frequently are more easily swallowed initially than clear liquids.

Reassure patient/family that swallowing ability and voice quality are expected to normalize. Notify physician if improvement is not detected within 72 hours.

Offer cool/cold po items as diet advances *to relieve hoarseness and promote resolution of laryngeal edema.*

Determine patient/family education needs, and support services requirements, if transfer to rehabilitation facility is anticipated, *to plan for discharge.*

Plan and implement appropriate education for patient/family *to reduce knowledge deficit, improve coping, and anticipate discharge to home.*

TRANSITION TO DISCHARGE

Perioperative stroke occurs in 1% to 6% of CEA patients. The most catastrophic consequence of cerebral hyperperfusion syndrome is an intracerebral hemorrhage.[7,20] Those who survive such massive insults will require specialized rehabilitation or lifetime custodial care. The majority of CEA patients, however, recover and return to their homes and families.

While monitoring for late-occurring post-operative stroke carries through the discharge phase, nursing care is primarily that of increasing both tolerance and independence in ADL; of coordinating care with other health care team members such as PT/OT, clinical dietician, clinical pharmacist, and others; of supporting the patient/family in the face of continued or new neurological deficits; and of determining the patient's/family's educational and support services needs in anticipation of going home.

REFERENCES

1. Reference deleted in proofs.
2. Reference deleted in proofs.
3. Reference deleted in proofs.
4. AANN: *Core Curriculum for Neuroscience Nursing,* ed 3, Chicago, 1990, AANN.
5. AHCPR #91-10: *Carotid endarterectomy. Health technology assessment reports, 1990,* No. 5, Access #PB01-127118, Springfield, Va, 1991, National Technical Information Services.
6. Archie JP: Early and late geometric changes after carotid endarterectomy patch reconstruction, *J Vasc Surg* 14(3):258-266, 1991.
7. Barnett HJM, et al: Beneficial effect of carotid endarterectomy in symptomatic patients with high-grade carotid stenosis, *New Engl J Med* 325(7):445-453, 1991.
8. Bredenberg CE, et al: Operative angiography by intraarterial digital subtraction angiography: a new technique for quality control of carotid endarterectomy, *J Vasc Surg* 9(4):530-534, 1989.
9. Brien HW, et al: A review of carotid endarterectomy at a large teaching hospital, *Am Surg* 57(12):756-762, 1991.
10. Brook RH, et al: Carotid endarterectomy for elderly patients: predicting complications, *Ann Intern Med* 113(10):7747-7753, 1990.
11. Brook RH, et al: Predicting the appropriate use of carotid endarterectomy, upper gastrointestinal endoscopy, and coronary angiography, *New Engl J Med* 323(17):1173-1177, 1990.
12. Burns BJ, Willoughby JG: South Australian carotid endarterectomy study, *Med J Aust* 154(10):650-653, 1991.
13. Cook J, Thompson BW, Barnes RW: Is routine duplex examination after carotid endarterectomy justified? *J Vasc Surg* 12(3):334-340, 1990.
14. Fisher ES, et al: Risk of carotid endarterectomy in the elderly, *Am J Public Health* 79(12):1617-1620, 1989.
15. Fode NC: Carotid endarterectomy: nursing care and controversies, *J Neurosci Nurs* 22(1):25-31, 1990.
16. Fode NC, et al: Multicenter retrospective review of results and complications of carotid endarterectomy in 1981, *Stroke,* 17(3):370-376, 1986.
17. Gibbs BF, Guzzetta VJ: Carotid endarterectomy in community practice: surgeon-specific versus institutional results, *Ann Vasc Surg* 3(4):307-312, 1989.
18. Godin MS, et al: Cost effectiveness of regional anesthesia in carotid endarterectomy, *Am Surg* 55(11):656-659, 1989.
19. Gomez CR: Outcomes of carotid endarterectomy (letter), *Ann Intern Med* 114(8):703, 1991.
20. Handelsman H: *Carotid endarterectomy,* Public Health Service Publication #91-3472, Rockville, Md, 1991, Dept of Health & Human Services.
21. Jergensen LG, Schroeder TV: Transcranial Doppler for detection of cerebral ischemia during carotid endarterectomy, *Eur J Vasc Surg* 8(2):142-147, 1992.
22. Johnson SM, Anderson B: Carotid endarterectomy: a review, *Crit Care Nurs Clin North Am* 3(3):499-506, 1991.
23. Kalyanpur PB, Bell WH, Kerstein MD: Amaurosis fugax: carotid endarterectomy without an angiogram, *J La State Med Soc* 141(7):45-46, 1989.
24. Martin JD, et al: Is routine CT scanning necessary in the preoperative evaluation of patients undergoing carotid endarterectomy? *J Vasc Surg* 14(3):267-270, 1991.
25. Mayberg MR, et al: For the Veterans Affairs Cooperative Studies Program 309 Trialist Group: Carotid endarterectomy and prevention of cerebral ischemia in symptomatic carotid stenosis, *JAMA* 266(23):3289-3294, 1991.
26. O'Brien MS, Ricotta JJ: Conserving resources after carotid endarterectomy: selective use of the intensive care unit, *J Vasc Surg* 14(6):796-802, 1991.
27. Pratschner T, et al: Antiplatelet therapy following carotid bifurcation endarterectomy: evaluation of a controlled clinical trial: prognostic significance of histologic plaque examination on behalf of survival, *Eur J Vasc Surg* 4(3):285-289, 1990.
28. Ramsey JM: *Basic pathophysiology: modern stress and the disease process,* Menlo Park, Calif, 1982, Addison-Wesley.
29. Rob MT, Welten J, Eikelboon BC: Technical details in carotid endarterectomy, *Eur J Surg Suppl,* no. 555, pp 205-208, 1990.
30. Rodriguez R, et al: Antiplatelet treatment after carotid endarterectomy: a pilot study, *J Neurosurg Sci* 36(1):39-45, 1992.
31. Sawchuk AP, et al: The fate of unrepaired minor technical defects detected by intraoperative ultrasonography during carotid endarterectomy, *J Vasc Surg* 9(5):671-681, 1989.
32. Sise MJ, et al: Prospective analysis of carotid endarterectomy and silent cerebral infarction in 97 patients, *Stroke,* 20(3):329-352, 1989.
33. Slutzki S, et al: Carotid endarterectomy under local anesthesia supplemented with neuroleptic analgesia, *Surg Gynecol Obstet* 170(3):141-144, 1990.
34. *St Anthony's DRG guidebook 1995,* Reston, Va, 1994, St Anthony.

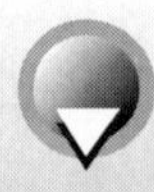

CLINICAL GUIDELINE

29

Peripheral Vascular Disease

June Howland-Gradman, MS, RN, CCRN

DESCRIPTION

The term peripheral vascular disease (PVD) is used to describe a group of diseases and syndromes that involve the arterial, venous, or lymphatic systems. PVD of the lower extremities causes chronic disability and significantly decreases quality of life. The prevalence of arterial PVD is 10% for persons over 65 years and is the most debilitating form of this disease.[21]

Arterial disease restricts blood flow through the aorta and its branches and affects an estimated 2.4 million persons in the United States. Arterial insufficiency and ischemia occur acutely in patients with arterial embolism and spasm. Chronic manifestation of the process is seen in patients with arteriosclerosis obliterans and thromboangitis obliterans. Each year approximately 200,000 people in the United States undergo surgery for arterial occlusive disease. This disease often deprives a person of doing the simplest tasks, such as walking a block or two. In the more severe stages, it may lead to chronic pain, nonhealing ulcers, gangrene, and amputation.

PATHOPHYSIOLOGY

Atherosclerosis is the predominant underlying factor contributing to PVD. This disease affects the medium and large arteries, decreasing blood flow until it becomes insufficient to meet metabolic demands. Atherosclerosis is an insidious and irreversible process. As the disease progresses, fatty streaks, fibroid plaque, calcification, and thrombus formation result in arterial wall thickening, hardening, and loss of elasticity. This process may lead to stenosis and eventual occlusion or the development of aneurysms with potential dissection.[6]

The atherosclerotic plaque may be focal or diffuse, may grow slowly, or may rapidly occlude the lumen. In the case of acute occlusion, there is insufficient time for collateral circulation to develop, resulting in sudden ischemic changes.[2,20] The extent of arterial insufficiency is relative to the location and severity of the lesion and the presence of collateral vessels.

The usual risk factors involved in development of atherosclerosis are seen in PVD patients. Patients with vascular disease often are elderly and may have one or more associated medical problems such as diabetes mellitus, chronic obstructive lung disease, coronary artery disease, or renal disease. Smoking, hyperlipidemia, and diabetes are the major risk factors associated with PVD.

Common sites for stenosis or occlusion include the aortoiliac, femoral-popliteal, and tibial arteries. The most commonly affected site is the superficial femoral artery segment. The disease process is often bilateral because of its systemic nature and tends to manifest in the later years of life.

LENGTH OF STAY/ANTICIPATED COURSE

Patients with symptoms of peripheral arterial disease can be classified into one of five stages (Table 29-1). Patients in stage III and IV are those with "critical ischemia" whose limbs may be threatened. Invasive diagnostic procedures are justified for patients in these stages.[18] The average length of stay for patients who are evaluated for peripheral vascular disorders without cardiac catheterization is 5.6 days in accord with DRG 131: Peripheral Vascular Disorders without Cardiac Catheterization.[16] Patients who need cardiac catheterization as part of their workup are hospitalized an av-

TABLE 29-1 Stages of Peripheral Arteriosclerosis[18]

Stage	Presentation	Invasive diagnostic and therapeutic intervention
0	No signs and symptoms	Never justified
I	Intermittent claudication (>1 block)	Usually justified
II	Severe claudication (<½ block) Dependent rubor Decreased temperature	Sometimes justified Not always necessary May remain stable
III	Rest pain Atrophy, cyanosis Dependent rubor	Usually indicated but may do well for long periods without revascularization
IV	Nonhealing ischemic ulcer or gangrene	Usually indicated but not always

Adapted from Veith F et al: Impact of nonoperative therapy on the clinical management of peripheral arterial disease, *Circ* 83(2):1-138, 1991.

erage of 7.4 days and classified by DRG 130: Peripheral Vascular Disorders with Cardiac Catheterization.[16] Patients who require surgical treatment are classified by DRG 110: Major Cardiovascular Procedures with Cardiac Catheterization and remain hospitalized an average of 12.2 days.[16]

MANAGEMENT TRENDS AND CONTROVERSIES

Traditional methods of therapy for PVD include peripheral vasodilators, such as nylidrin; agents that reduce blood viscosity, such as pentoxifylline (Trental); and antiplatelet agents, such as dipyridamole (Persantine), ticlopidine, and aspirin. Risk factor modification, balloon angioplasty, and arterial reconstruction may also be considered. Recently, laser angioplasty and stents have been used.

Ischemic resting foot pain, gangrenous necrosis, or other limb-threatening symptoms signal the need for surgical intervention. Extensive disease involving a long segment of occlusion may also indicate the need for surgery. Surgical intervention entails bypassing the occluded or ulcerated arterial segment by using autogenous vein or synthetic graft material such as Dacron or polytetrafluorethylene (Teflon). The procedure involves the anastomosis of the graft from an area proximal to an area distal to the disease (Table 29-2).

When a thrombus or embolus produces acute arterial occlusion, embolectomy may be performed. In this surgical procedure, a balloon-tipped catheter is inserted, usually through the femoral artery, beyond the clot. The balloon is then inflated and the catheter withdrawn, removing the clot.

Routine preoperative evaluation includes assessing the patient's risk for surgery. Cardiac, pulmonary, and renal functions are evaluated. A history of coronary and/or carotid artery disease may indicate the need for a more in-depth evaluation due to the added risk of acute MI and associated mortality.

Intraoperative angioscopy is performed routinely during peripheral vascular surgery. This technique allows the surgeon to visualize arterial plaque and thrombus within the native vessel or previous arterial bypass graft. It is also used for direct visualization of valves in the in situ vein graft and to inspect anastomotic suture lines after bypass surgery. Identifying and correcting pathological and technical errors within the lumen may prevent early graft failure and the need for additional surgery. One group has found that angioscopy proved to be more accurate for detecting technical problems than completion arteriography after bypass surgery.[4]

New nonsurgical approaches to treat arterial disease are currently being used. The role of device therapy in the management of patients with arterial occlusive disease is still being defined. Much research is now being done on mechanical devices that are used to recanalize and/or reperfuse obstructed vessels. There are more than 40 new devices currently under evaluation. However, early results indicate that the technology cannot compare with the long-term patency seen with autogenous femoro-popliteal bypass procedures.[13]

Percutaneous transluminal angioplasty (PTA) is one of the device-based approaches being used and involves insertion of a balloon catheter under local anesthesia. Mechanical inflation at the site of stenosis causes cracking of the plaque and dissecting of the intimal lining of the artery. The damage to the intimal lining necessitates the use of antiplatelet aggregating agents before and after the procedure.[12] Reendothelialization of the area smoothes the surface, however, within several days to weeks. PTA is less invasive, less expensive, and has lower morbidity than arterial bypass surgery; however, eventual restenosis rates of up to 50% have been reported.[1,11,19]

Intravascular stenting has been proposed as a means for reducing acute restenosis after PTA. Balloon expandable and self-expanding stents have proved useful in postangioplasty elastic recoil, in early cases of postangioplasty restenosis, and in angioplasty-induced dissection.[3] The bal-

TABLE 29-2 Common Vascular Operations

Surgery	Definition and rationale	Representation
Femoral-femoral bypass	Performed in high-risk patients who are initially seen with unilateral claudication or ischemia. This operation is performed only if donor artery is without marked proximal stenosis. Five-year patency rate is 65–75%.	A Femoral-femoral bypass 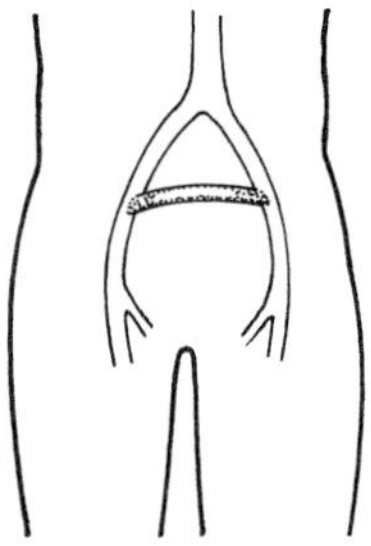
Femoropopliteal bypass	Autogenous vein grafting remains the standard operation for relieving ischemic symptoms secondary to superficial femoral artery occlusive disease. Prosthetic grafts are used only if vein is not available. Patients initially seen with this disease process may have involvement of both distal popliteal arteries and their tibial branches. Thus, bypass may extend to distal tibial vessels. Five-year patency is 80–90% with autogenous vein.	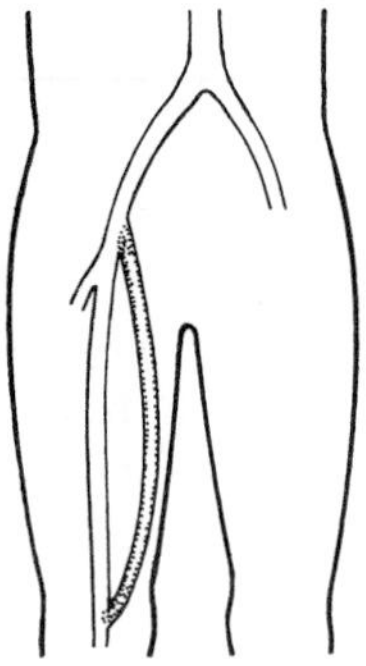 B Femoropopliteal bypass
Aortoiliac bypass	Aortoiliac occlusive disease rarely extends proximal to the renal arteries. Patient may require simultaneous reconstruction of renal or visceral arteries. Bilateral aortoiliac reconstruction using prosthetic bypass grafting offers the most desirable results. Five-year patency is 85–90%.	C Aorto-iliac bypass 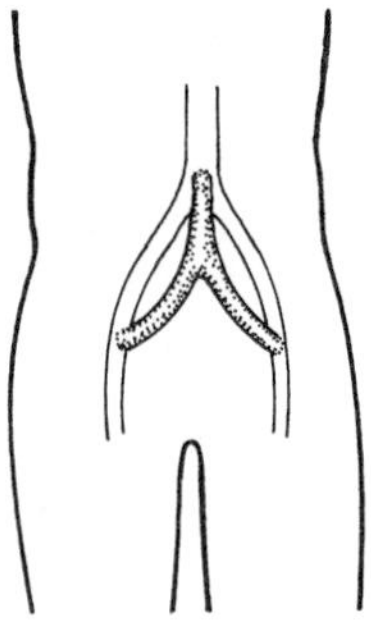
Aortobifemoral bypass	Performed more commonly than an aortoiliac bypass. Atherosclerosis usually involves iliac arteries. Graft patency is improved by initially bypassing to femoral artery level. Five-year graft patency is 85–90%.	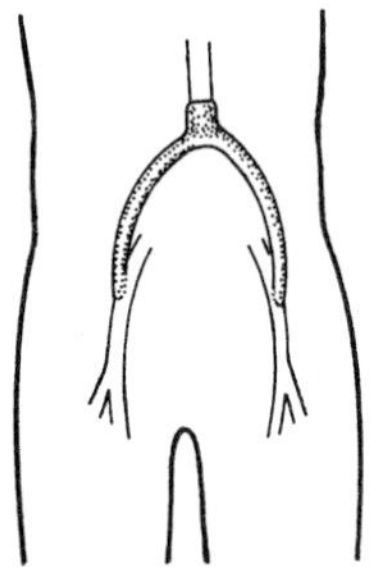 D Aorto-bifemoral bypass
Axillobifemoral bypass	Used when bilateral iliac disease requires a graft for inflow restoration. Can be performed with light general anesthesia or epidural block because subcutaneous tunneling is generally required. Lower patency rates of 50% at 5 years.	E Axillo-bifemoral bypass 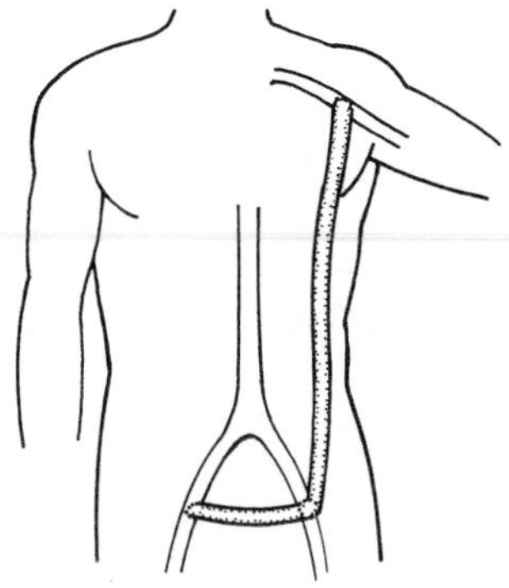

loon-expandable stent is positioned within the recently angioplastied area and expanded via an angioplasty balloon. The stent provides internal support for the artery and prevents acute elastic recoil. The role of stents in primary angioplasty procedures is still uncertain. Ongoing clinical trials are now assessing the safety, efficacy, and proper roles of self-expanding and balloon-expandable stents in the treatment of iliac and femoro-popliteal arterial disease. Stenting appears to offer some improvement in early PTA outcomes, but the long-term stenosis rates remain approximately 25% to 30%.[3] Biodegradable stents are in the very early stages of study. Such stents would provide arterial support when needed most in the early post-PTA recovery period, but would not potentially complicate intervention for late reoccurrence of stenosis.

Vascular endoscopy permits imaging of the intra-arterial disease in color and in three dimensions using fiberoptic technology. It is able to identify surface topography as it is advanced down or up the artery. The angioscope enables the physician to judge the nature of the lesion before a procedure and to follow the progress of the intervention. The angioscope cannot visualize small runoff vessels, provide information on atherosclerotic intima composition, or estimate percent stenosis. This information is best obtained with angioplasty or intravascular ultrasound.

Atherectomy is a third device-based intervention. It is unique in that it removes the plaque, leaving behind a smoother surface. This technique may decrease the risk for restenosis. Atherectomy devices drill, pulverize, or shave the plaque.[10] Adjunctive use of intra-arterial urokinase with atherectomy has made lesions complicated by thrombus easier to treat.[8]

A controversial device used to treat chronic arterial disease is the laser angioplasty catheter. This method uses a laser catheter with or without balloon angioplasty to open localized, short occlusions of the iliac artery, superficial femoral artery, and above-the-knee popliteal arteries.[15] This technique is especially useful in lesions that cannot be crossed by standard guide wire techniques.[15] The procedure may be done in the radiology department or as an adjunct to bypass surgery in the operating room. Complications of laser angioplasty are similar to those of conventional angioplasty and include embolization, vessel dissection or perforation, and thrombus or hematoma at the puncture site.[9,14,22] In addition, vasospasm, severe heatlike pain during the procedure, and thermal injury have been reported.[6] One-year patency results of 40% to 90% after hot-tipped, laser-assisted balloon angioplasty have been reported.[17] As a result, further research will be needed in this area before wide use of laser-assisted PTA can be expected.

Nonsurgical procedures require close vascular assessment. In addition, these patients are routinely placed on heparin to maintain the partial thromboplastin time (PTT) 1.5 to 2.5 times the control. Monitoring blood urea nitrogen (BUN) and creatinine levels are necessary to assess the renal effects of the contrast material used during diagnosis and intervention. Hydration is critical after laser treatment and accurate intake and output must be recorded. Hemoglobin and hematocrit levels are important to detect blood loss, especially less-obvious bleeding that may occur in the peritoneal cavity. PTA patients are placed on bed rest for about 24 hours following the procedure. The head of the bed remains flat or is elevated no higher than 30 degrees. The affected leg must be kept straight. After femoral sheath removal, the leg is kept straight for an additional 6 to 8 hours to ensure hemostasis. A pressure dressing may be applied, although some care givers challenge the effectiveness of this intervention as providing little or no help in stabilizing the wound and potentially concealing oozing or bleeding that requires further manual pressure. Range of motion exercises are to be encouraged in the feet to prevent venous stasis.[7]

ASSESSMENT

PARAMETER	ANTICIPATED ALTERATION
History	Myocardial infarction, angina, and/or cerebrovascular disease is common
Pain	Intermittent claudication: cramping, burning, aching, pain brought on by ambulation relieved by rest Rest pain: cramping, burning, stinging, aching, or sharp pain in the toes, forefoot, or heel that often appears at night Buttock or thigh pain *due to lesions in the abdominal aorta or iliac* Calf pain *due to lesions in the superficial femoral artery*
Circulation	Prolonged CRT >3 seconds, diminished pulses, cold/cool skin temperature in affected extremity, decreased toe temperature *due to arterial obstruction in the extremity*
Auscultation	Bruits over the affected vessels *due to turbulent blood flow caused by stenosis*
Color of extremities	Persistent cyanosis, elevation pallor, increased pigmentation, or dependent rubor *due to severe ischemia*

Tropic changes	Hair loss, thickened toenails, stasis dermatitis, gangrenous lesions, chronic ulcers *due to inadequate perfusion*
Nerve function	Paresthesia
Neurologic stasis	Syncope or alterations in LOC *due to cerebrovascular lesions*
Genitourinary	Impotence *due to aortic iliac occlusion*

Diagnostic Tests

Doppler ultrasound	Detects sound waves as blood moves through a vessel. Diminished sound waves *due to arterial obstruction.*
Ankle, brachial index (ABI)	Compares the BP in the limbs. Normally, ankle pressure is the same or higher than the brachial pressure. Locate posterior tibial or pedal pulse. Apply BP cuff around the ankle above the malleolus. Inflate to 20 mm Hg above current brachial SBP. Note the reappearance of Doppler signal as cuff deflates. Divide the ankle SBP by the brachial SBP to determine ratio. Normal is .08 to 1.2. Patients with arterial calcification may have an ABI >1.2
Segmental plethysmography	Measures arterial blood volume changes that occur in the lower extremities during the cardiac cycle. Blood pressure cuffs are placed on the thigh, calf, and ankle, and pulsed waveform recordings are obtained. Pulse contour and amplitude correlates with the amount of obstruction.
Exercise testing	Evaluates functional disability. Treadmill exercise for 5 minutes, until maximum limit of exertion is reached, or until symptoms develop. Ankle waveforms and ABIs are obtained before and after the test.
Arteriography	Delineates proximal site of arterial occlusion. Provides precise information of arterial inflow and outflow.

PLAN OF CARE

INTENSIVE PHASE

In the early post-procedure/postoperative period complications may occur that may affect limb perfusion or salvage. Bleeding, embolization, and hematoma formation can adversely affect blood flow to the limb. Nursing assessment focuses on maintaining adequate perfusion to prevent these complications. Admission to an ICU is not a prerequisite, but the degree of monitoring needed in this phase of care cannot be compromised.

PATIENT CARE PRIORITIES	EXPECTED PATIENT OUTCOMES
Pain *r/t decreased peripheral perfusion*	Pain free or controlled sufficiently to allow ADLs, rest, and sleep
Decreased tissue perfusion *r/t hemorrhage, distal embolization, and occlusion*	Extremity pink and warm with good pulses
High risk for hematoma or infection *r/t postop bleeding or site care*	Absence of hematoma or infection
High risk for fluid volume deficit *r/t hemorrhage*	Hgb and Hct: WNL Normal hemodynamic parameters Site clean, dry, and intact
High risk for decreased renal function *r/t decreased renal perfusion*	UO ≥30 cc/hr BUN and creatinine: WNL

INTERVENTIONS

Assess pulses q15min for a minimum of 2 to 4 hours after intervention. *Sudden loss of distal pulses, excruciating pain or decreased motor-sensory functions requires immediate attention due to graft occlusion or embolization.*

Plan of Care (cont'd)

Assess sensory and motor function of extremities. *Severe swelling accompanied by paresthesia may necessitate a fasciotomy due to compartment syndrome.*

Assess vital signs and administer medications to control blood pressure. *High systolic BP can rupture graft anastomosis and a low BP may cause loss of graft patency.*

Monitor for increase in pulse rate, decrease in BP, anxiety, restlessness, pallor, cyanosis, clammy skin, hematoma formation, swelling of extremity, bleeding from incision *due to bleeding that may require reoperation or cause acute limb ischemia secondary to graft thrombosis or distal thromboembolism as seen in 1% to 2% of patients.*

Assess incisional site for oozing, hematoma, or tenderness *due to inadequate hemostasis before or after sheath removal.*

Assess level of discomfort or pain and medicate with prescribed analgesia. Evaluate effectiveness of pain medication after each dose.

Monitor for signs and symptoms of myocardial ischemia.

Monitor UO, BUN, creatinine. Acute renal failure may occur *due to inadequate fluid volume replacement during surgery/procedure.*

Assess neurological status before, during, and after surgery/procedure.

Monitor bowel sounds, complaints of nausea, vomiting, abdominal tenderness, paralysis, or paresthesia *due to the risk of spinal cord or bowel ischemia, which may occur as complications of surgery.*

INTERMEDIATE PHASE

The goals of care during this phase focus on improving patient mobility. Early ambulation can be effective in relieving pain, improving function, and promoting optimal wellness.[5]

PATIENT CARE PRIORITIES	EXPECTED PATIENT OUTCOMES
Impaired mobility *r/t pain and recent intervention*	Ambulate without symptoms of claudication
Impaired skin integrity *r/t decreased circulation, surgical incision or procedure access site*	Skin and incisions intact Gradual healing of any peripheral ulceration
Self-care deficit *r/t lack of knowledge about disease, medications, and intervention*	Verbalizes knowledge of disease process, medications, and follow-up treatment

INTERVENTIONS

Provide information regarding disease process, risk factor reduction, drug therapy, activities, exercise program, infection control, and follow-up care.

Instruct patient regarding proper foot care, including keeping the feet protected with shoes or slippers and avoiding heating pads or hot water bottles directly on the skin *to prevent wounds that poor perfusion makes difficult to heal and that may, as a result, develop infection or gangrene.*

Use a bed cradle, sheepskin under the foot, and lamb's wool between toes; avoid tape if possible; and keep heels propped off bed surface at all times *to protect lower-extremity integrity.*

Instruct patients to report any future sexual dysfunction to their physician. Postoperative sexual dysfunction may occur in 15% to 25% of patients *due to retrograde ejaculation secondary to disturbance of pelvic autonomic nerves.*

TRANSITION TO DISCHARGE

Patient teaching before discharge should focus on atherosclerosis risk-factor reduction and incisional care. Education must stress that surgery does not "cure" peripheral arterial disease, and modification of risk factors is necessary to prevent progression. In addition, patients must be instructed regarding the importance of taking their medications regularly, including antihypertensives and oral hypoglycemics or insulin as indicated. Incisional care and signs and symptoms of infection must be reviewed before discharge. Patients must also know to inform their physician of any change in circulation to the feet, including pain, pallor, coolness, or reappearance of ulcers.

REFERENCES

1. Ahn S, et al: Reporting standards for lower extremity arterial endovascular procedures, *J Vasc Surg* 17:1103-1107, 1993.
2. Beal K, Danzig B: Lasers in vascular surgery, *Nurs Clin North Am* 25:711-718, 1990.
3. Becker G: Intravascular stents, *Circ* 83(suppl 2):I 122-136, 1991.
4. Borgini L, Almgren C: Peripheral vascular angioscopy, *AORN J* 53(3):543-550, 1990.
5. Ciaccia J: Benefits of a structured peripheral arterial vascular rehab program, *J Vasc Nurs* 11(1):1-4, 1993.
6. Emma L: Chronic arterial occlusive disease, *J Cardiovasc Nurs* 7(1):14-24, 1992.
7. Ford K: Laser assisted angioplasty in the patient with peripheral arterial disease, *J Vasc Nurs* 25(4):777-784, 1990.
8. Graor R, Whitlow R: Transluminal atherectomy for occlusive peripheral vascular disease, *J Am Coll Cardiol* 15(7):1551-1558, 1990.
9. Harrington M, et al: Expanded indications for laser assisted balloon angioplasty in peripheral arterial disease, *J Vasc Surg* 11:146-155, 1990.
10. Hinohara T, et al: Directional atherectomy: new approaches for treatment of obstructive coronary and peripheral vascular disease, *Circ* 81(suppl):79-91, 1990.
11. Hofling B, et al: Percutaneous removal of atheromatous plaques in peripheral arteries, *Lancet* 2:384-387, 1988.
12. O'Keefe S, Woods B, Beckman C: Percutaneous transluminal angioplasty of the peripheral arteries, *Cardiol Clin* 9(3):515-522, 1991.
13. Payne J: Alternatives for revascularization: peripheral atherectomy devices, *J Vasc Nurs* 10(1):2-8, 1992.
14. Perler B, et al: Percutaneous laser probe femoropopliteal angioplasty: a preliminary experience, *J Vasc Surg* 10:351-357, 1989.
15. Seeger J: Laser angioplasty, *Circ* 83(suppl 2):I 97-98, 1991.
16. *St Anthony's DRG Guidebook 1995,* Reston, Va, 1994, St Anthony.
17. Tobis J, et al: Laser-assisted versus mechanical recanalization of femoral arterial occlusions, *Am J Cardiol* 68:1079-1086, 1991.
18. Veith F, et al: Impact of nonoperative therapy on the clinical management of peripheral arterial disease, *Circ* 83(suppl 2):I 137-142, 1991.
19. Walker T, Greenfield A: Percutaneous atherectomy relieves vascular stenoses, *Diagn Imag* 10:108-112, 1988.
20. Wildus D, Osterman F: Evaluation and percutaneous management of atherosclerotic peripheral vascular disease, *JAMA* 262:3148-3154, 1990.
21. Woods B: Clinical evaluation of peripheral vasculature, *Cardiol Clin* 9(3):413-427, 1991.
22. Wright J, et al: Laser angioplasty for limb salvage: observations on early results, *J Vasc Surg* 10:29-38, 1989.

DEVICE GUIDELINE

30

Hemodynamic Monitoring

Polly E. Gardner, MN, RN, ARNP

DESCRIPTION

Hemodynamic monitoring involves placement of invasive catheters in the vascular system for the purpose of continuous or intermittent measurement of intra-arterial pressures, intracardiac pressures, pulmonary artery pressures, and oxygenation parameters. The data obtained allow prompt recognition and accurate assessment of serious circulatory changes in the critically ill patient.

Arterial catheters may be placed into the femoral, axillary, brachial, dorsalis pedis, or radial artery. The radial artery is most often the site of choice because of its easy access for catheter placement, and ease of managing site integrity and subsequent catheter manipulations. Cannulation of the femoral artery or left axillary artery is recommended for use in long-term critically ill patients because there are fewer complications associated with these sites.[45] The various arterial pressures with normal ranges and physiologic descriptions are found in Table 30-1.

Central venous catheters are inserted percutaneously or by surgical cutdown. Percutaneous placement is the preferred method. Sites of preferred insertion include the superior vena cava, subclavian vein, internal or external jugular vein, and brachial vein. Central venous catheters are placed in patients who receive multiple administrations of fluids, medications, blood products, or parenteral nutrition; frequent blood sampling; and assessment of mean right atrial pressure (RAP), also known as central venous pressure (CVP). Refer to Table 30-1 for normal values.

A pulmonary artery (PA) catheter is inserted percutaneously to measure right- and left-sided intracardiac pressures and pulmonary artery pressures. The standard four-lumen PA catheter measures RAP/CVP, pulmonary artery pressures (PAP), pulmonary capillary wedge pressure (PCWP), and cardiac output (CO). PA catheters offer various features such as continuous measurement of Svo_2, continuous measurement of CO, measurement of right-ventricular volumes and ejection fractions, and pacemaker capabilities (Figure 30-1).[4]

The multiple lumens provide a means to assess and monitor the intracardiac structures. The proximal lumen is used to monitor RAP/CVP and carries the injectate solution necessary for CO measurement. The distal lumen is used during passage of the PA catheter to measure PA and PCW pressures. For true mixed-venous oxygen saturation determination, blood samples must be collected from the distal lumen. Normal values for PA and PCW pressures are listed and explained in Table 30-1.

Cardiac output (CO) is measured with a standard PA catheter. A known volume of fluid at a known temperature is injected through the proximal lumen of the PA catheter where it enters the right atrium and mixes with blood, altering the blood temperature. As the mixture moves with the forward flow of blood through the heart, the lower temperature of blood and fluid is detected and recorded by the thermistor sensor located 4 cm from the tip of the catheter.[15] The resulting change in temperature is transmitted to the CO computer for calculation and numerical display of the CO value.

It is common practice to use 5 ml or 10 ml of iced or room-temperature injectate to obtain thermodilution CO measurements.[57] Cardiac output values are comparable using both 5 ml or 10 ml of injectate in critically ill adults

TABLE 30-1 Arterial Pressures

Pressure parameter	Normal range	Physiologic description
Systolic Arterial Pressure (BPS)	100-140 mm Hg	Highest pressure in arterial circulation associated with ventricular systole
Diastolic Arterial Pressure (BPD)	60-80 mm Hg	Lowest pressure in arterial circulation associated with ventricular diastole Reflective of arterial systemic resistance Perfusion pressure of the coronary arteries
Mean Arterial Pressure (MAP)	70-90 mm Hg	Average arterial pressure throughout the cardiac cycle Actual perfusion pressure of vital organs
Mean Right Atrial Pressure (RAP) or Central Venous Pressure (CVP)	2-8 mm Hg	Average right atrial pressure throughout the cardiac cycle Reflective of circulating volume and RV preload Does not reflect left heart status
Pulmonary Artery Systolic Pressure (PAS)	20-35 mm Hg	Pressure of blood flow from RV into PA. Approximates RV systolic pressure in the absence of pulmonic valve stenosis.
Pulmonary Artery Diastolic Pressure (PAD)	10-15 mm Hg	PA pressure during RV diastole Higher than RV diastolic pressure due to closure of the pulmonic valve PA volume is proportionately greater than RV volume during diastole resulting in higher PAD pressure. PAD approximates PCWP in the absence of mitral valve disease, with PAD 0-5 mm Hg >PCWP.
Pulmonary Artery Mean Pressure (PAM)	15-20 mm Hg	Average pulmonary artery pressure throughout the cardiac cycle.
Pulmonary Capillary Wedge Pressure (PCWP)	6-12 mm Hg	Pressure is read from the distal tip of the PA catheter when the balloon is inflated, causing the catheter to float forward into a smaller PA vessel and "wedge" occluding flow from the RV. PCWP is an indirect measure of mean left atrial pressure and LV end-diastolic pressure (LV preload) when the mitral valve is open.

with low, normal, and high CO. Controversy still exists in the clinical arena regarding the use of iced or room-temperature injectate in determining CO. However, multiple studies have reviewed the relationship of volume and temperature of injectate in critically ill patients with low, normal, and high CO; the studies have found the relationship to be highly correlated ($r > .90$) with other CO measurement techniques.* A study done with six ewes demonstrated that injectate temperature (iced and room-temperature) did not impact reproducibility of CO measurement.[37] However, the volume of injectate (5 ml) did affect accuracy and reproducibility when COs were high or low. The findings of this study are limited due to the small number of samples and repeated measures. The volume-temperature relationship also needs to be studied in a critically ill adult population.

The clinician should tailor the injectate temperature and volume to the status of the patient. An example would be to use 10 ml of iced injectate in a patient with a high or low CO to maximize the signal-to-noise ratio (described as ratio of injectate temperature to fluctuation in blood temperature) to the CO computer.

If the proximal infusion port or lumen becomes occluded, or it is difficult to inject the CO injectate within a 4-second time period, other inject ports may be used to perform CO measurement.[16,20,26-29,34,53] These injection ports may include the venous infusion port or the side port of the introducer catheter. In contrast, one study found a lower correlation ($r = .83$) when the injectate and the infusion port were compared to an independent measure using an electromagnetic flow meter.[36]

A catheter can also be placed directly into the left atrium to assess left atrial pressures. A **left atrial catheter** is placed in some cardiac surgical patients with impaired cardiac func-

*References 9, 11, 19, 23, 24, 32, 33, 42, 43, 49, 58.

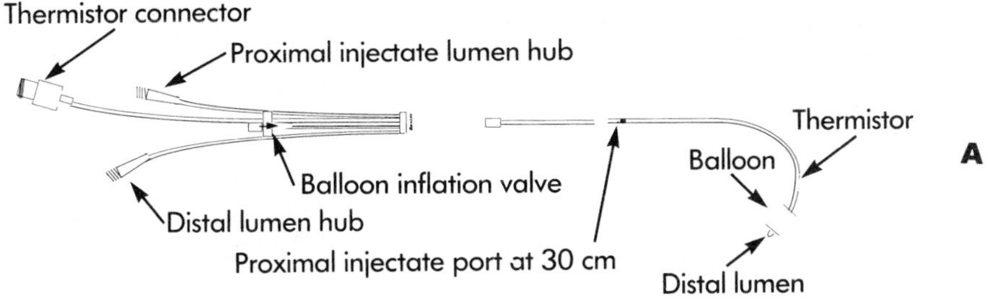

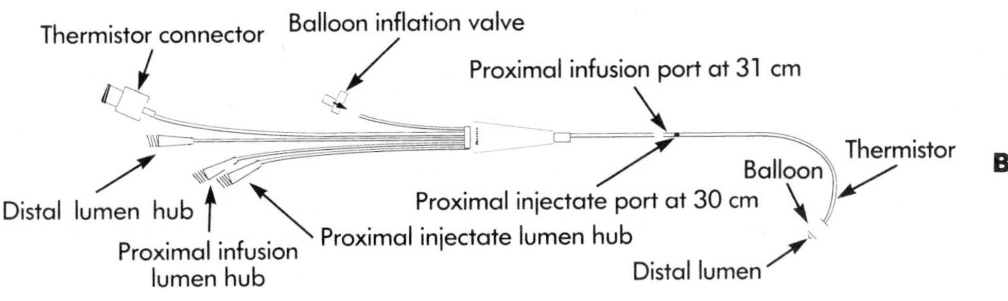

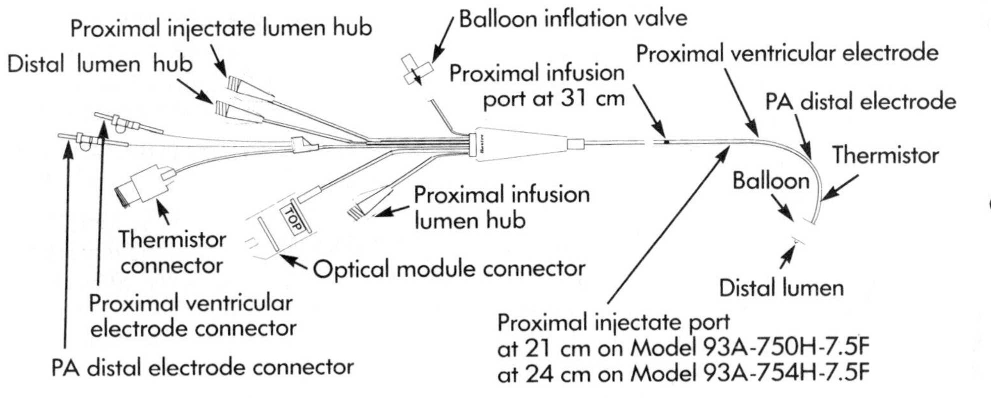

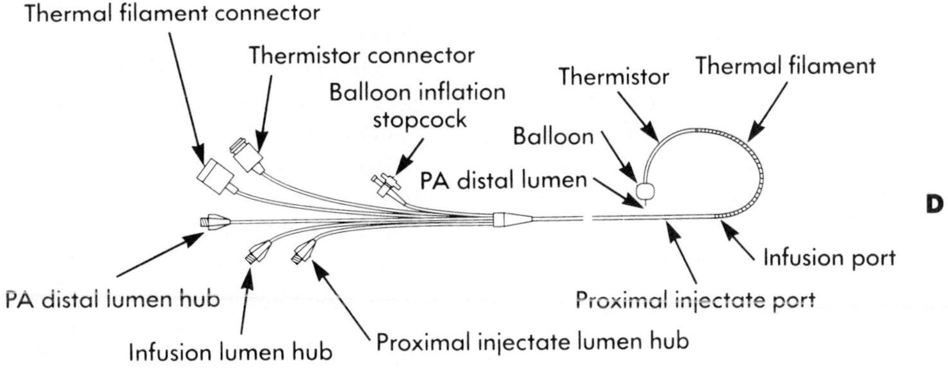

Figure 30-1 Types of pulmonary artery catheters available for clinical use. **(A),** Four-lumen catheter. **(B),** Five-lumen catheter that includes an additional infusion lumen in the right atrium. **(C),** Multifunction six-lumen catheter that combines an additional infusion lumen, right ventricular volume measurement, and continuous SvO_2 monitoring. **(D),** Six-lumen catheter with continuous cardiac output capability. (Courtesy Baxter Healthcare Corporation, Edwards Critical Care Division)

Clinical Indications For Invasive Hemodynamic Pressure Monitoring[6,21,45]

- Clinical conditions at high risk of causing sudden changes in arterial pressure
- Frequent arterial blood sampling
- Uncontrolled hypertension
- Hypovolemic and septic shock states
- Vasoactive pharmacologic support (vasopressors or vasodilators)
- Myocardial infarction complicated by left heart failure or cardiogenic shock
- Cardiogenic or noncardiogenic pulmonary edema
- Diagnosis and treatment of acute respiratory distress syndrome (ARDS)
- Perioperative fluid imbalance in selected patients
- Evaluation of circulatory syndromes (atrial or ventricular septal defects)
- Acute respiratory failure in patients with chronic obstructive pulmonary disease (COPD)
- Shock of all etiologies

tion, hemodynamic instability, low cardiac output syndrome, rapid blood loss, and volume replacement therapy. Normal left atrial pressure is similar to PCWP with an intact mitral valve and normal pulmonary function.

INDICATIONS

Placement of invasive catheters in critically ill patients is indicated when acute changes in cardiopulmonary function occur and cannot be assessed from the usual measurements of vital signs, pulse, respiration, BP, and urine output.[44,47,48] Data including RAP, PAP, PCWP, CO, oxygenation parameters, and BP can be obtained directly and the patient's response to therapy assessed rapidly. Conditions that indicate the use of invasive hemodynamic pressure monitoring are listed in the following Box.

Once these physiologic pressures are measured, derived, or calculated, data can be determined to assess more fully the hemodynamic mechanisms of preload, afterload, and contractility (see Appendix A: Hemodynamic Parameters, Formulas, and Normal Ranges). Referred to as a hemodynamic profile, the measured and calculated data provide comprehensive hemodynamic assessment to serve as a guide for intervention and evaluation in the management of critically ill patients.[1,50]

LIMITATIONS

Invasive hemodynamic monitoring is not a substitute for sound clinical assessment. Invasive assessment devices are limited by many factors including insertion location, accuracy of readings, and the clinical status of the patient. In addition, invasive hemodynamic monitoring does not provide all of the information necessary for comprehensive patient care. Clinical observation and other assessment information such as laboratory data, radiologic studies, and so forth must be considered in order to provide optimal care.

POTENTIAL COMPLICATIONS

There are three major categories of complications associated with intra-arterial cannulation. **Arterial thrombosis** is an uncommon complication of vascular cannulation since the advent of continuous heparinized flush systems.[12,21,45] A large, randomized clinical study was done to evaluate the effects of heparinized and non-heparinized flush solutions on the patency of arterial pressure lines.[2] The results of this study indicate that heparin does affect patency of arterial pressure lines over time. Other variables that affected patency of arterial pressure lines included insertion site (femoral sites have greater patency rates), anticoagulants and antithrombotics (agents increase chances of patency), catheter length (catheters greater than 2 inches showed greater patency), and gender (males have greater patency rates). The risk of arterial thrombosis remains a threat to patients in the following conditions: catheters larger than 20 gauge; tapered, polypropylene catheters; and catheters in place more than 4 days.[21,45] Emboli may occur as a result of small clots forming on the intra-arterial catheter tip. These emboli typically migrate in the direction of arterial blood flow to sites distal to the location of the catheter and may cause ischemia and necrosis. Aspiration of the clot or removal of the catheter is recommended if thrombosis is suspected.[21,45]

Infections are the most common complication of vascular cannulation. Conditions that place patients at higher risk include immunosuppression, arterial insufficiency states, catheters placed by surgical cutdown, or catheters left in place longer than 4 days. The reported infecting organisms include gram-negative rods, enterococci, or Candida.[21] Careful hand-washing and changing the equipment setup even down to the arterial catheter hub is recommended every 72 hours to minimize contamination and bacterial growth.[12,13]

Air can enter an arterial line at several locations (connections, stopcocks) within the intra-arterial catheter tubing system. The embolus rapidly follows the direction of arterial blood flow with potential insult to organs or tissues distal to the catheter site. If air is introduced while flushing the line for an extended period of time (longer than 2 to 3 seconds), the force of the 300 mm Hg of pressure on the flush solution could push the air against and overcome the normal arterial pressure gradient. Under these unique circumstances, the air embolus could reach the aorta, where it could enter the cerebral or coronary artery circulation or any other organ system between the catheter and the heart. Maintaining the integrity of the system and a continuous flush device are essential to safe arterial pressure monitoring.

Potential complications associated with the PA catheter are listed in the following Box. Laceration of the subclavian

Complications Associated With Pulmonary Artery Pressure Monitoring*

- Simple and tension pneumothoraces
- Hematoma at site of insertion
- Vessel laceration of the vein or artery, with hemorrhage and possible hemothorax
- Atrial and ventricular dysrhythmias
- Right bundle branch block (transient)
- Mechanical damage of tricuspid and pulmonic valves
- Infection
- Air embolism associated with balloon rupture
- Pulmonary artery perforation and rupture
- Pulmonary infarction
- Thrombosis
- Thrombocytopenia

*References 13, 17, 31, 39, 44-48, 51.

artery results in hemorrhage and potential hemothorax because the bleeding cannot be controlled by local pressure.[6] Although the risk of pneumothorax is low, there is a higher incidence (1% to 6%) associated when PA catheters are inserted through the subclavian vein.[6,44,45]

Atrial and ventricular dysrhythmias are the most common complication associated with insertion of a PA catheter.[45,47] These dysrhythmias may result from endocardial irritation during passage of the PA catheter. Ensuring that the balloon is fully inflated and engulfing the tip of the catheter, and limiting the time of passage from the RV to the PA, will reduce the incidence of dysrhythmias. Transient right bundle branch block can occur as the PA catheter passes through the RV.[51] The right bundle branch is located superficially in the RV endocardium and can be irritated by the passage or ongoing presence of the PA line. Prolonged PA catheterization has also been associated with mechanical damage of the tricuspid and pulmonic valves as a result of wearing of the valve cusps from repeated contact with the catheter or tearing of the valve cusps with catheter removal.[44,45]

The incidence of infection, both at the insertion site and systemically, can range from 3% to as high as 35%.[44] The number of times the integrity of catheter-tubing system is entered for blood sampling, CO measurements, and catheter repositioning influences infection risk and must be minimized. Results regarding the relationship between the infection rate and length of insertion are equivocal; increased risk or positive cultures are noted as early as 48 hours.[8]

Balloon rupture is most likely to occur if more than the manufacturer's prescribed amount of air is injected into the balloon, or if the catheter has been indwelling for a long period of time. Over time, the balloon absorbs lipoproteins from the passing blood, which soften and weaken the balloon material. As a result, even prescribed amounts of air may result in tearing of the balloon in PA catheters left in place for extended periods of time. The small amount of air introduced into the PA circulation in the event of balloon rupture is well tolerated generally. The exception is in the presence of a right-to-left intracardiac shunt where air potentially can enter the LV and produce an embolic insult systemically. As a result, it is important to guard against repeated introduction of air through the ruptured balloon. In most instances, the PA catheter is removed and, depending on patient indications, another PA catheter may be placed.

PA perforation and rupture is the most serious complication. The mortality rate is 50%, although the reported incidence is low (0.2%).[17,45] The risk of PA rupture is increased with eccentric or excessive balloon inflation, vigorous flushing with large amounts of fluid, and distal migration of the catheter. Patients at risk include older adults and those with pulmonary hypertension, mitral valve dysfunction, and receiving anticoagulant therapy.[45] Pulmonary infarction may occur if the PA catheter migrates distally and persists in a wedged position.

Thrombosis around the catheter as it sits in the vascular space is a fairly common occurrence.[44,45] Possible sequelae related to thrombus formation include pulmonary embolus, frequent contact of the PA catheter with the endocardium, and septic phlebitis.[45] The advent of the heparin-bonded catheter was heralded to prevent thromboembolic events. However, the efficacy of the heparin-bonded catheter to prevent thrombus formation is limited to 48 hours.[31]

Another associated complication reported by the literature is the incidence of thrombocytopenia induced by the heparin-bonded PA catheter and heparin flush solution.[39] It has been suggested that the catheter may cause an increase in consumption of the platelets related to the microaggregation of the catheter. The occurrence of thrombocytopenia may suggest use of a nonheparin-bonded catheter and the removal of heparin from the flush solution.

GENERAL NURSING INTERVENTIONS

Considerable knowledge and skill are needed to manage hemodynamic monitoring systems. The critical care nurse must have conceptual understanding of the cardiovascular system, the indications and limitations of pressure monitoring systems, and the clinical and technical factors that may affect the accuracy of the data measures. The activities required to establish, maintain, and monitor a pressure monitoring system are summarized in Table 30-2.

Initiating and Establishing a Pressure Monitoring System

Pressure monitoring systems are divided into two components: the electrical system and the plumbing system.[12,14] The electrical system consists of the amplifier, the oscilloscope or screen, the processor or display, and the analog or graphic recorder. The mechanical signal received from the transducer is increased or amplified by the amplifier. The signal is displayed on the oscilloscope as a pressure waveform and numerically on the digital display. The pres-

TABLE 30-2 General Nursing Interventions Associated with Pressure Monitoring Systems*

General considerations	Related nursing interventions
Initiation and establishment of equipment components of pressure monitoring system	Understand the two components: electrical system and plumbing system Assemble and set up pressure monitoring system Calibrate using the five-step process Set alarms
Maintenance and prevention of complications	Identify technical factors that may affect pressure measurements Monitor/care for insertion site Monitor system for malfunction Rezero system every shift following patient transfers, changes in fluid dynamics of system (i.e., blood sampling), system manipulation, or during system malfunction Use distal port of PA catheter only for continuous assessment of the PA waveform to detect any changes in catheter position (i.e., wedged position)
Analysis and interpretation of hemodynamic data	Obtain and calculate data that evaluate preload, afterload, and contractility Identify clinical factors that may affect pressure measurements Monitor trends and response to treatment measures Collaborate with the physician regarding any abnormalities of hemodynamic data
Differentiation of waveform or pressure abnormalities and associated clinical indications	Assess dynamic response of system every shift Document baseline atrial pressure waveforms Analyze pressure waveforms to determine and compare pressure values and changes in patient condition
Evaluation of the effects of mechanical ventilation and body positioning	Read pressure measurements at end-expiration; height of pressure wave during spontaneous breathing, and trough of pressure wave during mechanical ventilation Compare intracardiac measurements in flat, supine position with those measurements in desired back-rest elevations up to 60°. Assure reference point is releveled to phlebostatic axis with position changes.

*References 5, 7, 10, 13, 22, 25, 30, 35, 38, 52, 54-56.

sure waveform is recorded on graph paper by the analog recorder. The purpose of the electrical system is to process and display pressure waveforms and numerical data, and for obtaining derived hemodynamic indices including PVRI and SVRI.

The purpose of the plumbing system is to carry the mechanical signal to the transducer. The plumbing system consists of a variety of parts including the vascular catheter, noncompliant pressure tubing, a continuous flush device, two or three stopcocks, a pressure transducer, an infusion pressure bag, and flush solution.[12] Depending on the institution, the flush solution may contain heparin to maintain catheter patency. The infusion pressure bag must be maintained at 300 mm Hg to enable the continuous flush device to deliver solution at a rate at 1 to 3 ml/hr.[4,13,14] This plumbing system is in direct contact with the patient's vascular system; thus strict adherence to aseptic technique in handling the system is essential. Current recommendations are to change the flush solution every 24 hours and the system parts every 72 hours.[12]

Assembly of pressure monitoring systems will vary with the type of equipment used and institutional resources. Nurses must follow their institutional protocols for set-up and insertion of pressure monitoring systems. Calibration of pressure monitoring systems involves a five-step process as follows:

- Step 1 Zeroing the catheter-tubing-transducer system to atmospheric pressure
- Step 2 Defining and establishing the reference position-phlebostatic axis

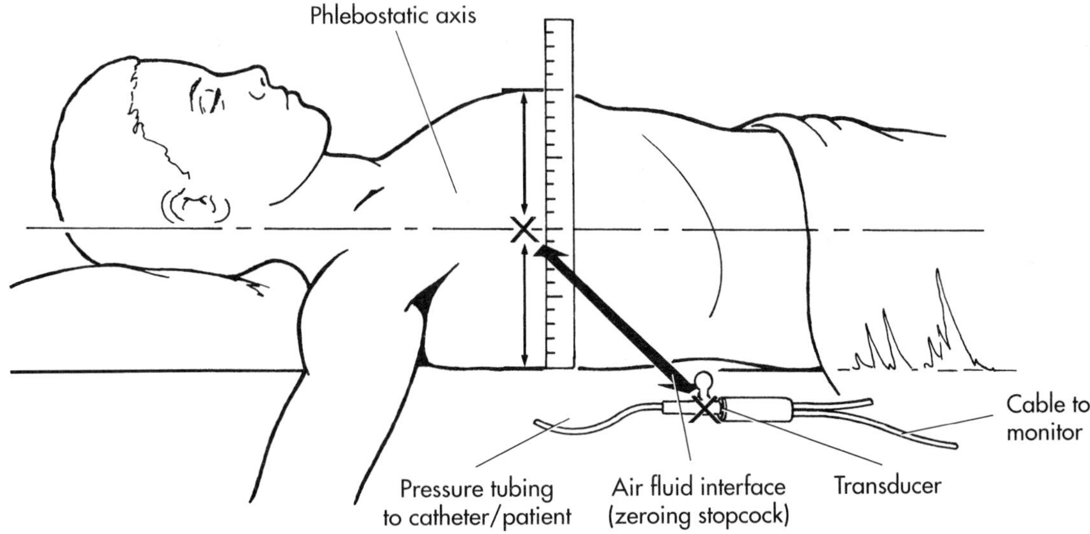

Figure 30-2 Measurement of the patient's chest to determine the phlebostatic axis/midchest position *(X)* so that the air-fluid interface of the transducer *(zeroing stopcock x)* may be properly positioned at this point or level with this point. In this way, the two "open ends" (hemodynamic catheter tip and zeroing stopcock) are at the same level, allowing proper adjustment to atmospheric pressure.

- Step 3 Leveling to phlebostatic axis
- Step 4 Assessing sensitivity of the transducer
- Step 5 Optimizing dynamic response characteristics

The process of zeroing is achieved by turning the stopcock open to atmospheric air and off to the patient. Zeroing the catheter-tubing system provides a zero baseline relative to atmospheric pressure and compensates for the hydrostatic weight effect of fluid in the catheter-tubing system.[12,13,50] The purpose of zeroing ensures that only the pressures within the vessels or heart chambers are measured. Zeroing is recommended every shift, or after patient transfer, system manipulations, or apparent malfunction of the pressure monitoring system.

Opening the stopcock in the catheter-tubing system defines the air-fluid interface. The air-fluid interface is the part of the catheter-tubing-transducer system that is maintained at the reference position.[13,14] The standard reference position in the supine position is the phlebostatic axis. The phlebostatic axis is the junction of the frontal and transverse planes located at the fourth intercostal space adjacent to the sternum midway point between the anterior and posterior chest. The mid-axillary point should not be used as a landmark. The midchest reference point and mid-axillary point are different in patients with large and asymmetrical chests.[3] The phlebostatic axis should be marked to ensure consistency in measuring to the same reference level.

The air-fluid interface of the zeroing stopcock is leveled or positioned to the phlebostatic axis (Figure 30-2). If the air-fluid interface is placed higher than the phlebostatic axis, the resultant pressure measurements will be underestimated due to the decrease in hydrostatic pressure. If the air-fluid interface is placed lower than the phlebostatic axis, the resultant pressure measurements will be overestimated due to an increase in hydrostatic pressure.[12] Every inch of discrepancy between the air-fluid interface and the pressure source results in error of 2 mm Hg.[13,14] Leveling with a carpenter's level/ruler is recommended prior to obtaining all pressure measurements.

Calibration of the pressure monitoring system ensures the sensitivity of the transducer and verifies that the monitoring system is reproducing the mechanical signal and measuring the pressure accurately.[12] Contemporary monitoring systems are calibrated internally to the pressure scale selected.

Assessment of the dynamic response of the catheter-tubing-transducer system is performed by activation of the "fast-flush" device (interflow), producing a square wave on the oscilloscope. An optimal dynamic response is characterized by the presence of two or three rapid oscillations from the top to the bottom of the pressure tracing at the end of the squared-off waveform, followed by return to the baseline waveform pattern.[12,13] An underdamped response is characterized by more than three oscillations, resulting in overestimation of systolic pressure. An overdamped response is characterized by "blunting" of the square wave pattern, resulting in underestimation of systolic pressure and overestimation of diastolic pressure. The dynamic response characteristics of the catheter-tubing-transducer system will be compromised with the presence of air bubbles, more than four feet of pressure tubing, and use of compliant, distensible tubing.[12]

Finally, high and low alarm limits must be set and activated. Alarms will indicate disconnection of the system or changes in patient condition that necessitate evaluation of the patient.

Maintenance and Prevention of Complications

The critical care nurse is the primary operator of the pressure monitoring system and therefore must be aware of the *technical factors* that influence date accuracy as follows:

- Zero baseline not established or maintained
- Inconsistent reference level position
- Overdamped or underdamped dynamic response

In addition, the nurse is responsible for routine *maintenance* activities that ensure patient safety, catheter integrity, and data accuracy as follows:

- Maintain catheter patency by protecting the site and using continuous heparinized flush systems.
- Ensure proper placement of central line catheters by assessment of chest radiograph film and characteristic waveforms and pressures.
- Ensure transducer accuracy by proper zeroing and testing of dynamic system response.
- Protect the system from leaks, disconnection, or introduction of air.
- Assess proper function of amplifier/monitor and recorder.
- Reduce the risk of infection by aseptic site care, use of occlusive dressings, application of anti-microbial ointment to the insertion site, and changing the flush solution every 24 hours and the plumbing system every three days.
- Notify physician if complications arise.

The use of transparent polyurethane dressing versus gauze dressing has been debated. Recent studies suggest that the risk of bacterial colonization of peripheral and central catheters is less with gauze dressing that is changed every 24 hours than with a transparent dressing.[8,18] As a result, many institutions have changed their protocols to apply sterile dry gauze dressings to central catheter sites.

If long-term catheterization is anticipated, a compressed-collagen-silver-impregnated cuff can be placed around a central line catheter or introducer and positioned just under the skin.[6] This cuff provides a physical barrier to the ingrowth of bacteria from the skin. To date, these cuffed catheters have shown less colonization than standard catheters.

Analysis and Interpretation of Hemodynamic Data

Clinical decisions about preload, afterload, and contractility are based on data obtained from arterial and PA catheters. Parameters directly measured include BP, MAP, RAP, PAP, PCWP, CO, and SvO_2. Derived parameters are calculated from specific formulas and include PVR or PVRI, SVR or SVRI, CI, SV or SVI, RVSWI, and LVSWI (Appendix A). Indexing of hemodynamic parameters is recommended because treatment decisions should be based on the individual's body surface area.

Interpretation of data also involves analysis of the pressure waveforms. The **arterial pressure waveform** is divided into three components: systolic peak, diastolic low, and nicrotic notch (closure of the aortic valve) (Figure 30-3). Changes occur in the contour of the arterial pressure waveform as it moves from the proximal aorta toward the periphery. As the arterial pressure wave moves distally, the systolic pressure can increase as much as 15 to 20 mm Hg, and the diastolic pressure decreases. However, the mean arterial pressure remains relatively constant, providing a more accurate index of central aortic pressure.

Comparison of direct arterial pressures and auscultated pressures is often made in the clinical setting. The two techniques, however, do not measure the same function. An intra-arterial catheter directly measures pressure, while the auscultatory method using a cuff measures flow.[14,15] Therefore, an indwelling arterial line will measure pressure more accurately. If comparison of the pressures between the indwelling line and cuff is done, more often the indwelling pressures will be higher. It is acceptable to have a line pressure difference up to 20 mm Hg greater than the cuff pressure.

Atrial pressure reflects the filling pressure or preload of the heart. Both the RAP and PCWP waveforms are atrial waveforms, as they measure mean pressure in the right and left atria, respectively.

The contours of the atrial waveform may provide useful information in determining accuracy of readings and potential pathology.[40] There are five mechanical components of an atrial waveform (Figure 30-4).[41] The *a* wave reflects the increase in atrial pressure during atrial contraction and correlates with electrical depolarization of the atrial chambers seen as the P wave on the ECG. The *c* wave represents closure of the atrio-ventricular valves (tricuspid and mitral) and follows the QRS complex on the ECG. The measured distance between the *a* and *c* waves is the same as the PR interval on the ECG. The *x* descent is the downstroke of the *a* and *c* waves and represents the decrease in atrial pressure following atrial contraction. The *v* wave, the second upstroke, represents filling of the atria during ventricular systole and corresponds to the T wave on the ECG. The downstroke of the *v* wave is the *y* descent and represents rapid, passive emptying of the atria immediately after the tricuspid or mitral valve opens.[41]

The mean atrial pressure is determined by bisecting the *a* and *v* waves so that there is equal area above and below the bisection. A dual-channel strip chart recorder can be used to identify the atrial pressure waves (*a*, *c*, and *v* waves) by correlating them to the electrical events on the ECG.

Abnormalities and Clinical Indications

Changes in the configuration of waveforms occur with mechanical and clinical factors. An **underdamped arterial pressure waveform** (Figure 30-3) may be due to systemic or pulmonary hypertension, arteriosclerosis, aortic regurgitation, pressure tubing exceeding four feet, and poor dynamic response in the system.[12] Causes of elevated pulmonary artery pressure include atrial and ventricular septal defects, hypoxemia, and obstructive lung disease.[50] High

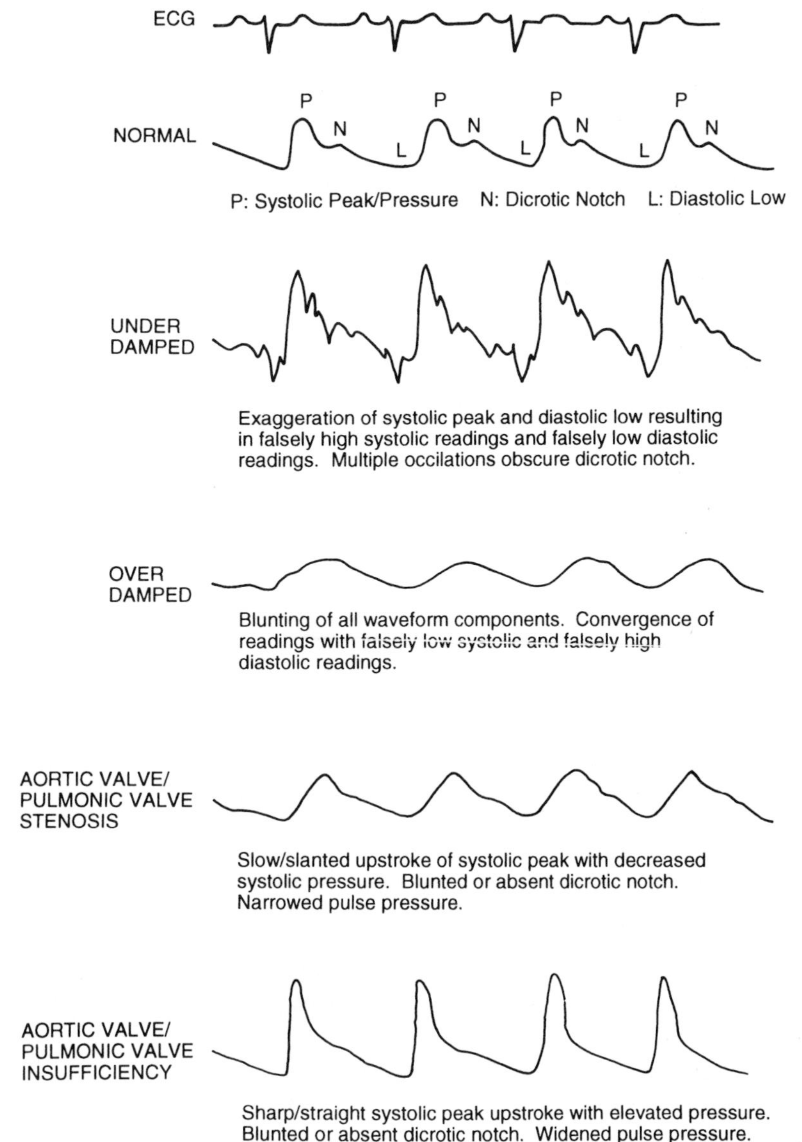

ECG
P
N
L
NORMAL
P: Systolic Peak/Pressure N: Dicrotic Notch L: Diastolic Low
UNDER DAMPED
Exaggeration of systolic peak and diastolic low resulting in falsely high systolic readings and falsely low diastolic readings. Multiple occilations obscure dicrotic notch.
OVER DAMPED
Blunting of all waveform components. Convergence of readings with falsely low systolic and falsely high diastolic readings.
AORTIC VALVE/ PULMONIC VALVE STENOSIS
Slow/slanted upstroke of systolic peak with decreased systolic pressure. Blunted or absent dicrotic notch. Narrowed pulse pressure.
AORTIC VALVE/ PULMONIC VALVE INSUFFICIENCY
Sharp/straight systolic peak upstroke with elevated pressure. Blunted or absent dicrotic notch. Widened pulse pressure.

Figure 30-3 Normal and abnormal arterial pressure waveforms. (Courtesy of Nancie Urban)

diastolic PA pressures are seen with tachycardia and pulmonary embolus. A decrease in PA pressures may be associated with hypovolemia.

Insufficiency of the aortic or pulmonic valves may produce arterial waveforms with characteristics similar to the underdamped pressure waveform. The regurgitation of blood into the ventricle during diastole increases the volume load in the ventricle while decreasing aortic volume and pressure. The waveform depicts a rapid, sharp upstroke with elevated systolic pressures, and a rapid downstroke with low diastolic pressures. A widened pulse pressure is produced. The dicrotic notch may be blunted or absent, caused by the lack of proper closure of the valve. The appearance of the pressure waveform associated with valve insufficiency differs from the mechanically underdamped pressure waveform in that it lacks the multiple oscillations seen in the latter.

An **overdamped arterial pressure waveform** (Figure 30-3) is more common and is caused by air bubbles within the catheter-tubing-transducer system. Clinical causes of an overdamped waveform include hypotension, vasodilatation, hypovolemia, and dysrhythmias. Aortic or pulmonic valve stenosis also may produce an arterial pressure waveform that appears overdamped. A stenotic valve may produce a pressure waveform with a slowed or slanted systolic peak. The lowered systolic pressure is due to difficulty in ejecting blood through the stenotic valve and the resulting decrease in CO. The dicrotic notch may be blunted since stenotic valves do not snap shut briskly, which is the phenomenon that produces the dicrotic notch normally. The decreased systolic pressure produces a narrowed pulse pressure. Despite the overdamped appearance, the arterial pressure waveform of aortic or pul-

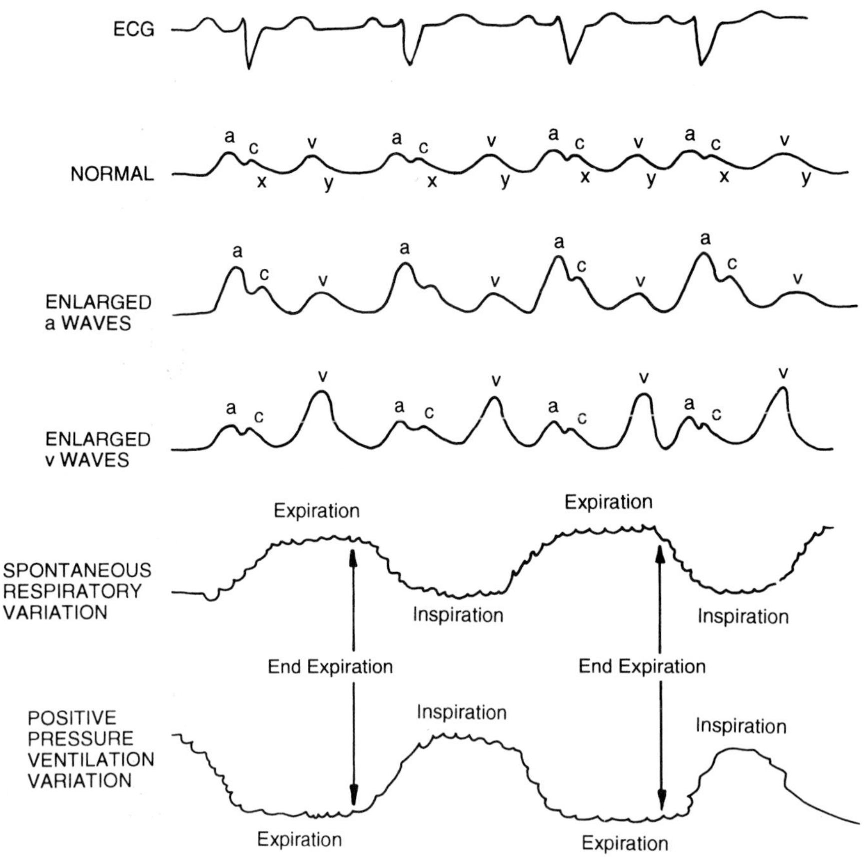

Figure 30-4 Normal and abnormal atrial pressure waveforms. (Courtesy of Nancie Urban)

monic stenosis still depicts a distinct systolic peak and diastolic low.

Analysis of the atrial waveform may be helpful to diagnose certain pathologies.[40,41] An elevated *a* wave results from conditions that increase resistance to ventricular filling and is associated with ventricular failure or tricuspid or mitral stenosis (Figure 30-4). An elevated *v* wave occurs in conditions that cause a reflux of blood in the atria during ventricular systole, such as tricuspid or mitral regurgitation.

Elevated *a* and *v* waves occur with conditions caused by a combination of resistance and reflux, such as cardiac tamponade, constrictive pericarditis, hypervolemia, and chronic ventricular failure. Along with changes in the pressure waveforms, changes in atrial pressure signal physiologic changes, as summarized in Table 30-3.

The PCWP is lower than the PAD by 1 to 5 mm Hg when pulmonary function is normal and the mitral valve is competent. When the PAD exceeds the PCWP by more than 5 mm Hg, the cause may be tachycardia, pulmonary hypertension, cor pulmonale, or pulmonary embolus.[13] The PCWP never exceeds the PAD pressure except in the following conditions: left atrial myxoma, pulmonary embolus, mitral regurgitation, or stenosis.[48] It is recommended that comparison of the gradient between the PAD pressure and

TABLE 30-3 Pathology Associated with Changes in Atrial Pressure

Atrial pressure change	Associated pathology
Decreased atrial pressure RAP <2 mm Hg PCWP <6 mm Hg	Hypovolemia Vasodilation Increased CO
Increased atrial pressure RAP >10 mm Hg PCWP >14 mm Hg	Hypervolemia Vasoconstriction Decreased CO Ventricular failure Positive pressure ventilation Cardiac tamponade
Increased RAP specific	Tricuspid stenosis or insufficiency Pulmonic stenosis or insufficiency Pulmonary embolus COPD
Increased PCWP specific	Mitral stenosis or insufficiency Aortic stenosis or insufficiency LV aneurysm

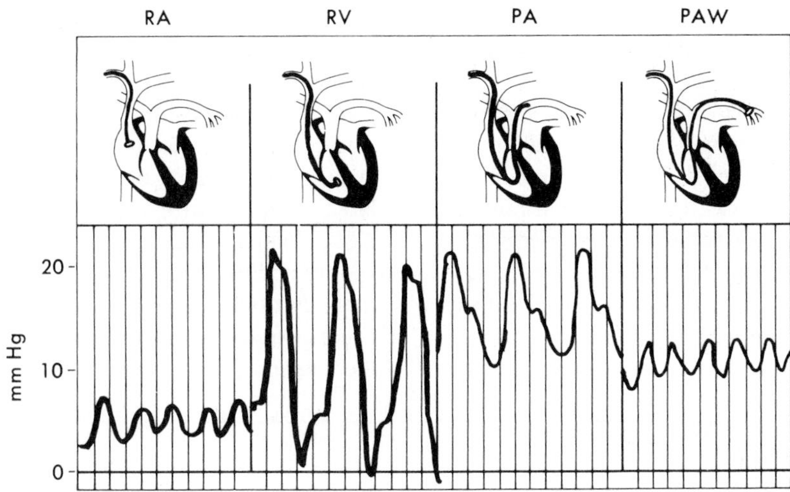

Figure 30-5 Corresponding pressure waveforms as PA catheter passes through the different chambers of the heart. (From Daily: *Techniques in bedside hemodynamic monitoring,* ed 5, St Louis, 1994, Mosby–Year Book.)

the PCW pressure be done to assess and evaluate ongoing changes in the patient's condition.[13,14]

To determine the PCWP, the clinician must inflate the balloon at the distal tip of the catheter, which allows the catheter to float forward to wedge in a small vessel segment in the PA vasculature.[47] To ensure that the balloon is fully inflated and in proper position, it is recommended that 1.25 to 1.5 ml of air be used to inflate the balloon and produce a "wedge" or atrial waveform.[4] If less air is required to achieve wedge, the catheter has migrated forward and needs to be withdrawn. It is also recommended that the balloon not be inflated for more than four respiratory cycles to prevent pulmonary ischemia or vessel trauma.[14] An inflated balloon with 1.5 ml of air generates 500 mm Hg or more of pressure against the vessel wall.[14] Deflation of the balloon is achieved by removal of the syringe from the balloon inflation valve. The elastic recoil of the balloon will expel the air. Manual withdrawal of air from the balloon may apply negative pressure and damage or tear the balloon. The syringe must *never* be left secured on the balloon inflation valve.[4] Removal of the syringe allows full, passive deflation of the balloon and prevents accidental inflation with patient movement. Proper placement of the PA catheter is confirmed by the return of the PA waveform on the oscilloscope.

The pressure waveforms produced during passage of the PA catheter throughout the right atrium (RA), through the right ventricle (RV), in the pulmonary artery (PA), and into the wedge position are depicted in Figure 30-5. The left atrial waveform is similar to the RAP waveform except that it is slightly damped and phase-delayed due to pulmonary vascular and catheter-tubing transmission.

Effects of Ventilation and Body Positioning

Because pressure measurements are read and recorded at end-expiration of the respiratory cycle, the clinician must be aware of the influence of spontaneous breathing and mechanical ventilation on the pressure waveform. Proper placement of the PA catheter in physiologic zone 3 (at or below level of the LA) minimizes the effect of spontaneous or mechanical ventilation on pulmonary artery pressures. During normal inspiration, respiratory variation is due to a fall of intrathoracic pressure. PA and PCW pressures follow pressure in the lung. During the inspiratory phase, PA pressures fall. Conversely, during expiration, intrathoracic pressure rises and PAP and PCWP rise. To be consistent, the pressures are read at *end-expiration*. Therefore, the pressure waveform is read just before it begins to fall (Figure 30-4).

Mechanical ventilation delivers positive pressure during the inspiratory cycle. Therefore, PAP and PCWP will rise with inspiration. During expiration (passive exhalation) PAP and PCWP decrease. The pressure waveform is read at *end-expiration* just before it begins to rise (Figure 30-4).

Pressure measurements are read at end-expiration of the respiratory cycle because end-expiration is determined to have the least variation in intrathoracic pressure and is easy to estimate clinically. Removing a patient from the ventilator to record pressure measurements is *not* recommended as it may pose a physiologic threat of decreasing oxygenation.

It is common practice to position the patient supine and flat while measuring intracardiac pressures. Some patients with respiratory dysfunction or increased intracranial pressure may not tolerate this practice. Research has shown in a wide variety of critically ill patients that accurate PAP and PCWP can be measured in the supine position with the legs extended and backrest elevations up to 45°, provided that the phlebostatic axis was the reference level.[25] Left atrial pressures can be measured in backrest elevations up to 30°.[38] Individuals vary in their response to position change.

Therefore, measurements obtained with backrest elevation should be compared with those obtained in the flat, supine position.[54,55,56]

Measurements obtained in patients in lateral recumbent positions have yielded variable results because of an inconsistent and undefined reference level. The 90-degree lateral position with the backrest flat was the only lateral position in which reliable PA pressures could be measured.[22] Recently, a study conducted in 16 adult patients found a consistent zero reference level in 30-degree left lateral positions.[52] The left atrial location was determined by comparison of echocardiography and estimating one half the distance between the left sternal border and bed surface. Further study is needed in larger and more variable critically ill patient populations to establish and confirm a reference level in lateral positions.

The challenge of monitoring critically ill patients is the evaluation of trends of hemodynamic data rather than isolated values. As treatment measures are implemented, the nurse compares the patient's response to the expected response and evaluates for continued or different therapy options. Physician consultation and intervention is sought with acute changes in the patient's condition or when changes in the course of therapy are needed.

TROUBLESHOOTING

The majority of troubleshooting situations are common to both arterial and atrial pressure monitoring systems. Problems associated with hemodynamic monitoring, with their most common causes and corrective actions, are as follows:

Problem: Overdamped Pressure Tracing (Figure 30-3)

CAUSE	CORRECTIVE ACTION
Air bubbles in pressure tubing or transducer	Eliminate air bubbles by flushing system *or* aspirate air bubbles to clear.
Collection of blood in and around transducer	Engage interflow device to flush the transducer and gently tap against palm of hand. *Do not* use hemostats, pens, or other hard devices that may damage transducer resistance wires. If blood remains, replace the transducer.
More than three stopcocks between catheter and transducer	Remove additional stopcock(s).
Catheter is wedged against vessel wall	Catheter must be repositioned by physician (or RN if protocol allows) to withdraw and manipulate PA catheter, and to reassess waveform and the required ml to inflate balloon to a wedge position.
Kinked catheter internally or at insertion site	Manipulation of PA catheter using fluoroscopy is managed by the physician to straighten the catheter. Kinks at insertion site can be managed by the RN by placing gauze under the catheter to straighten. Often a kinked catheter will need to be replaced.
Excessive tubing length (>4 ft) and loose connections	Use nondistensible tubing (not to exceed 60 in) from vascular catheter to transducer. Secure all connections.
Clot of fibrin deposition on catheter tip	If fibrin is suspected on the tip of the catheter, attempts to aspirate can be made. However, more often the vascular catheter needs to be replaced.

Problem: Underdamped Pressure Tracing (Figure 30-3)

CAUSE	CORRECTIVE ACTION
Excessive tubing length (>4 ft)	Use nondistensible tubing less than 4 ft in length. Assess dynamic response. Place in-line filtering device if necessary.
Excess number of stopcocks or connectors	Remove extra, unnecessary stopcocks and connectors (~3 per line).

Problem: Absence of PCWP Tracing

CAUSE	CORRECTIVE ACTION
Balloon rupture	If rupture is suspected, place patient in Trendelenburg's position, notify physician, and assess for respiratory distress. Label balloon port DO NOT WEDGE. Obtain chest radiograph film and ABG if necessary. PA catheter will need to be replaced.
Improper positioning of PA catheter	Use 1.25 to 1.5 ml of air to inflate the balloon. If balloon is inflated without change in waveform, the catheter needs to be advanced.

Problem: Catheter Whip (Fling) Artifact

CAUSE	CORRECTIVE ACTION
Location of distal tip of PA catheter near pulmonic valve is subject to valvular turbulence	Inform physician to reposition the catheter into PA. Review placement on x-ray film.
Looping of PA catheter in right ventricle, or excessive external noise	Inform physician to withdraw excessive catheter. Review placement on x-ray film.
Hyperdynamic heart	Record pressures using the mean.

Problem: Migration of the PA Catheter Into the Right Ventricle

CAUSE	CORRECTIVE ACTION
Accidental or spontaneous withdrawal of catheter into RV	Inflate balloon fully to engulf tip of catheter. Reposition PA catheter by advancing if protocol allows or notify physician. Withdraw catheter into right atrium with balloon deflated if dysrhythmias are compromising the patient's condition.

Problem: Inappropriate Pressure With Proper Pressure Waveform

CAUSE	CORRECTIVE ACTION
Inaccurate reference points—zeroing stopcock not properly leveled to phlebostatic axis	Measure phlebostatic axis and mark the identified area with black ink. Level zeroing stopcock to phlebostatic axis with carpenter's level. Measure hemodynamic values.
Inaccurate calibration	Rezero the system. Calibrate monitor scale or recorder. Assess dynamic response.
Change in patient condition	Consider possible causes.

Problem: Overwedging or Spontaneous Wedge

CAUSE	CORRECTIVE ACTION
Catheter migration	Instruct patient to cough. Turn onto side or straighten arm to dislodge the catheter. Withdraw the catheter in 1 to 2 cm increments until PA waveform is restored or until excess coiling of catheter is withdrawn as assessed in chest x-ray film.

Small pulmonary veins	Notify physician to reposition the catheter. Maintain balloon wedge volume at 1.25 to 1.5 ml of air as evidence of optimal catheter placement.

SUMMARY

Hemodynamic monitoring provides quantitative information about the patient's response to hemodynamic instability and treatment measures. The information obtained from arterial and pulmonary artery catheters must be precise and timely. The critical care nurse must understand the complexities and limitations of the monitoring equipment so that the information is not under- or overinterpreted. The challenge for the nurse is the integration of the data base with clinical data to provide the foundation for therapeutic decisions.

REFERENCES

1. Alspach JG: *Core curriculum for critical care nursing,* Philadelphia, 1991, WB Saunders.
2. American Association of Critical-Care Nurses: Evaluation of the effects of heparinized and nonheparinized flush solutions on the patency of arterial pressure monitoring lines: the AACN Thunder Project, *Am J Crit Care* 2(1):3-15, 1993.
3. Bartz B, Maroun C, Underhill SL: Differences in midanterioposterior level and midaxillary level in patients with a range of chest configurations, *Heart Lung* 12:308, 1988.
4. Baxter Healthcare Corporation, Edwards Critical-Care Division: The Swan-Ganz heparin flow-directed thermodilution catheter, 1985.
5. Chulay M, Miller T: The effect of backrest elevation on pulmonary artery and pulmonary capillary wedge pressures in patients after cardiac surgery, *Heart Lung* 13(2):138-140, 1984.
6. Clark CA, Harmon EM: Hemodynamic monitoring: pulmonary artery catheters. In Taylor RW, Civetta JM, Kirby RR, editors: *Techniques and Procedures in Critical Care,* Philadelphia, 1990, JB Lippincott.
7. Clochesy JM, Hinshaw AS, Otto CW: Effects on change in position on pulmonary artery and pulmonary capillary wedge pressures in mechanically ventilated patients, *National Intravenous Therapy Association* 7:223-225, 1984.
8. Corona ML, et al: Infections related to central venous catheters, *Mayo Clin Proc* 65:979-986, 1990.
9. Davidson LJ, et al: Effect of volume and temperature of injectate on thermodilution cardiac output measurement using an open system of injection, *Prog Cardiovasc Nurs* 2:86-91, 1987.
10. Dobbin K, et al: Pulmonary artery pressure measurements with elevated pressures: effect of backrest elevation and method of measurement, *Am J Crit Care* 1(2):61-69, 1992.
11. Elkayam U, et al: Cardiac output by thermodilution technique: effect of injectate volume and temperature on accuracy and reproducibility in the critically ill patient, *Chest* 84:418-422, 1983.
12. Gardner RM: Hemodynamic monitoring: from catheter to display, *Acute Care* 12:3-33, 1986.
13. Gardner PE, Woods SL: Hemodynamic monitoring. In Underhill SL, et al, editors: Cardiac nursing, ed 2, Philadelphia, 1989, JB Lippincott.
14. Gardner PE: Pulmonary artery pressure monitoring, *AACN Clin Iss Crit Care Nurs* 4(1):98-119, 1993.
15. Gardner PE: Cardiac output—theory, technique, and troubleshooting, *Crit Care Clin N Am* 1(3):577-588, 1989.
16. Gibney R, Ryan H: Thermodilution cardiac output measurements, *Crit Care Med* 12:614-615, 1984 (letter).
17. Hannan AT, Brown M, Bigman O: Pulmonary artery catheter-induced hemorrhage, *Chest* 85:128-131, 1984.
18. Hoffman KK, et al: Transparent polyurethane film as an intravenous catheter dressing: a meta-analysis of the infection risks, *JAMA* 267(15):2072-2076, 1992.
19. Hruby IM, Woods SL: Effect of injectate temperature on measurement of thermodilution cardiac output in cardiac surgery patients, *Circulation* 68:III-223, 1983 (abstract).
20. Hunn D, et al: Thermodilution cardiac output values obtained by a centrally placed introducer sheath and right atrial port of a pulmonary artery catheter, *Crit Care Med* 18:438-439, 1990.
21. Kaye WE, Dubin HG: Vascular cannulation. In Taylor RW, Civetta JM, Kirby RR, editors: *Techniques and procedures in critical care,* Philadelphia, 1990, JB Lippincott.
22. Kennedy GT, Bryant A, Crawford MH: The effect of lateral body positioning on measurements of pulmonary artery and pulmonary artery wedge pressures, *Heart Lung* 13:155-158, 1984.
23. Killpack AK, et al: Effect of injectate volume and temperature on measurement of thermodilution cardiac output in acutely ill patients, *Circulation* 64:IV-165, 1981 (abstract).
24. Larson C, Woods SL: Effect of injectate volume and temperature on thermodilution cardiac output measurement in critically ill patients, *Circulation* 66:II-98, 1982 (abstract).
25. Laulive JL: Pulmonary artery pressure and position changes in the critically ill adult, *Dimens Crit Care Nurs* 1(1):28-34, 1982.
26. Lee DW, Stevens GH: Comparison of thermodilution cardiac output measurements by injection of the proximal lumen vs. side port of the Swan-Ganz catheter, *Heart Lung* 14:126-127, 1985.
27. Martin C, et al: Thermodilution cardiac output measurements in pulmonary artery vs CVP catheter, *Crit Care Med* 11:460-461, 1983.
28. Mault JR, et al: Central venous catheter vs. proximal port injection site for thermodilution cardiac outputs, *Crit Care Med* 11:224, 1983 (abstract).
29. Medley RS, DeLapp TD, Fisher DG: Comparability of the thermodilution cardiac output method: proximal injectate vs. proximal infusion lumens, *Heart Lung* 21:12-17, 1992.
30. Miller R, Chulay M: Effect of change in body position on pulmonary artery pressures in critically ill patients. In *Proceedings of the AACN International Intensive Care Nursing Conference*, London, 1982, American Association of Critical Care Nurses, p 32.
31. Mollenholt P, Eriksson I, Anderston T: Thrombogenicity of pulmonary artery catheters, *Intensive Care Med* 13:57-59, 1987.
32. Nelson LD, Anderson HB: Patient selection for iced versus room-temperature injectate for thermodilution cardiac output determinations, *Crit Care Med* 13:182-184, 1985.
33. Pelletier C: Cardiac output measurement by thermodilution, *Can J Surg* 22:347-350, 1979.
34. Pesola GR, Ayala B, Plante L: Room-temperature thermodilution cardiac output: proximal injectate lumen vs. proximal infusion lumen, *Am J Crit Care* 2:132-133, 1993.
35. Prakash R, et al: Hemodynamic effects of postural changes in patients with acute myocardial infarction, *Chest* 64(1):7-9, 1973.
36. Renner LE, Meyer LT: Injectate port selection affects accuracy and reproducibility of cardiac output measurements with multiport ther-

modilution pulmonary artery catheters, *Am J Crit Care* 3(1):55-61, 1994.

37. Renner LE, Morton MJ, Sakuma GY: Indicator amount, temperature, and intrinsic cardiac output affect thermodilution cardiac output accuracy and reproducibility, *Crit Care Med* 21(4):586-597, 1993.
38. Retailliau MA, McGregor-Leding M, Woods SL: The effect of backrest position on the measurement of left atrial pressure after cardiac surgery, *Heart Lung* 14(5):477-483, 1985.
39. Rull JRV, et al: Thrombocytopenia induced by pulmonary flotation catheters, *Intensive Care Med* 10:29-31, 1984.
40. Schriner DK: Using hemodynamic waveforms to assess cardiopulmonary pathologies, *Crit Care Clin N Am* 1(3):563-575, 1989.
41. Sharkey SW: Beyond the wedge: clinical physiology and the Swan-Ganz catheter, *Am J Med* 83:111-122, 1987.
42. Shellock FG, Riedinger MS: Reproducibility and accuracy of using room-temperature versus ice-temperature injectate for thermodilution cardiac output determination, *Heart Lung* 12:175-176, 1983.
43. Shellock FG, et al: Thermodilution cardiac output determination in hypothermic postcardiac surgery patients: room-versus ice-temperature injection, *Crit Care Med* 11:668-670, 1983.
44. Sise MJ, et al: Complications of flow-directed pulmonary artery catheters: a prospective analysis in 219 patients, *Crit Care Med* 9:315-318, 1981.
45. Sladen A: Complications of invasive hemodynamic monitoring in the intensive care unit. In Ravitch MM, Steichen FM, editors: *Current problems in surgery,* Chicago, 1988, Yearbook Medical Publishers.
46. Sprung CL, et al: Risk of right bundle-branch and complete heart block during pulmonary artery catheterization, *Crit Care Med* 17:1-3, 1989.
47. Swan JJC, Ganz W: Complications of flow-directed balloon-tipped catheters, *Ann Intern Med* 91:494, 1979 (editorial).
48. Swan JJC: Monitoring the seriously ill patient with heart disease (including use of Swan-Ganz catheter). In Hurst JW, et al, editors: *The heart, arteries and veins,* ed 7, New York, 1990, McGraw-Hill.
49. Swinney RS, et al: Iced versus room-temperature injectate for thermodilution cardiac output, *Crit Care Med* 8:265, 1980.
50. Thelan LA, Davie JK, Urden LD: *Textbook of critical care nursing. Diagnosis and management,* St Louis, 1990, Mosby–Year Book.
51. Thompson IR, et al: Right bundle branch block and complete heart block caused by the Swan-Ganz catheter, *Anesthesiology* 51:359-362, 1979.
52. VanEtta DJ, Gibbons E, Woods SL: Estimation of left atrial location in supine and 30° lateral positions, *Am J Crit Care* 2:264, 1993.
53. Vicari M, Ogle V: Comparison of measurements of cardiac output from the side port vs. the proximal lumen of the Swan-Ganz catheter: follow-up study, *Heart Lung* 16:379-380, 1987.
54. Woods SL, Grose BL, Laurent-Bopp D: Effect of backrest position on pulmonary artery pressures in acutely ill patients, *Cardiovasc Nurs* 18:19-24, 1982.
55. Woods SL, Grose BL, Laurent-Bopp D: Effect of backrest position on pulmonary artery pressures in acutely ill patients, *Circulation* 62:III-184, 1980.
56. Woods SL, Mansfield LW: Effect of body position upon pulmonary artery and pulmonary capillary wedge pressures in noncritically ill patients, *Heart Lung* 5(1):83-90, 1976.
57. Woods SL, Osguthorpe S: Cardiac output determination, *AACN Clin Iss Crit Care Nurs* 4(1):81-97, 1993.
58. Woog RH, McWilliam DB: A comparison of methods of cardiac output measurement, *Anesthesiology Intensive Care* 11:141-146, 1983.

DEVICE GUIDELINE

31

Pacemakers: Temporary and Permanent

Lisa Cerino-Toth, BSN, RN
Nancie Urban, MSN, RN, CCRN

DESCRIPTION

A pacemaker is an electronic device that delivers stimuli to the cardiac muscle to maintain heart rate and cardiac output when the native pacemaker of the heart is unable to do so. A pacing system consists of a power source, known as the pulse generator, that contains electronic circuitry responsible for delivering appropriately timed stimuli and for sensing intrinsic cardiac activity. The system also contains a unipolar or bipolar electrode/lead catheter that is placed in contact with the endocardium of the right atrium or right ventricle. Alternatively, the electrode/lead may be sutured directly to the epicardium of either atria or ventricle. The tip of the lead, the electrode, is the conductive portion of the lead system that makes direct contact with the cardiac muscle and transfers electrical stimuli and intrinsic information between the pulse generator and the heart. (See Figure 31-1.) The primary difference between temporary and permanent pacing is the location of the pulse generator. (See Figures 31-2 and 31-3.) New developments in temporary pacemakers have significantly narrowed the gap between pacing options and functions between this and the permanent or implantable approach to cardiac pacing.[18] With the exception of rate-modulation capabilities, temporary pacemakers now offer most pacing capabilities, including DDD and some overdrive pacing functions.

In addition to permanent/implantable and traditional temporary pacing, noninvasive transcutaneous pacing has gained acceptance as a safe and effective approach to providing pacing support in emergency situations. First introduced in the early 1950s, noninvasive transcutaneous pacing was poorly received due to significant patient discomfort.[34] The recent increased interest in noninvasive approaches to all manner of high-tech assessment and intervention techniques makes the recent advances in noninvasive transcutaneous pacing an important innovation. This technology has been demonstrated to be highly effective in the emergent management of bradydysrhythmias, resulting in increased use of this technology in emergency situations, including inclusion in the latest Advanced Cardiac Life Support (ACLS) protocols.[36] Combined with defibrillation capability, noninvasive transcutaneous pacemakers have been shown to be effective using the same electrode patches used for defibrillation, with resulting increase in speed of response.[12] On the horizon is increased use of this technology to overdrive supraventricular tachydysrhythmias. Early reports of modifying current noninvasive transcutaneous pacing technology for this application in emergency situations have demonstrated encouraging results.[17]

Pacemaker Function

Capture occurs when the stimulus delivered by the pulse generator is adequate to depolarize the cardiac muscle. A single-chamber pacemaker will depolarize either the atrium or the ventricle, resulting in a large p wave or large QRS following the respective pacing artifact. A dual-chamber pacemaker will depolarize both the atrium (usually the right atrium) and the ventricle (usually the right ventricle) as needed.

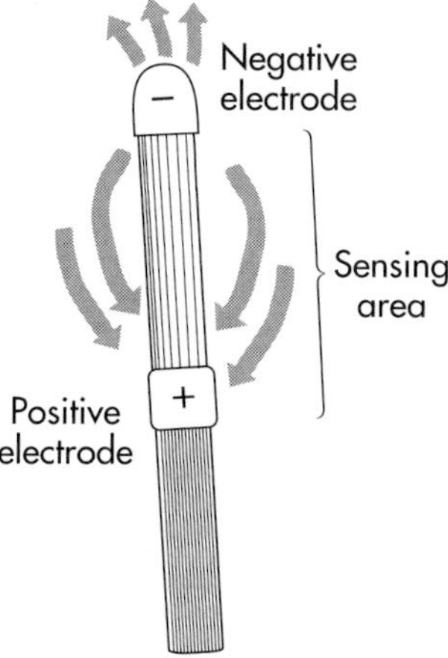

Figure 31-1 Pacing and sensing segments of a bipolar pacing catheter. The negative/distal electrode delivers the pacing stimulus. The positive/proximal electrode completes the electrical circuit. The sensing area is located between the electrodes. (From Thelan, et al: *Critical Care Nursing,* ed 3, St Louis, 1992, Mosby–Year Book.)

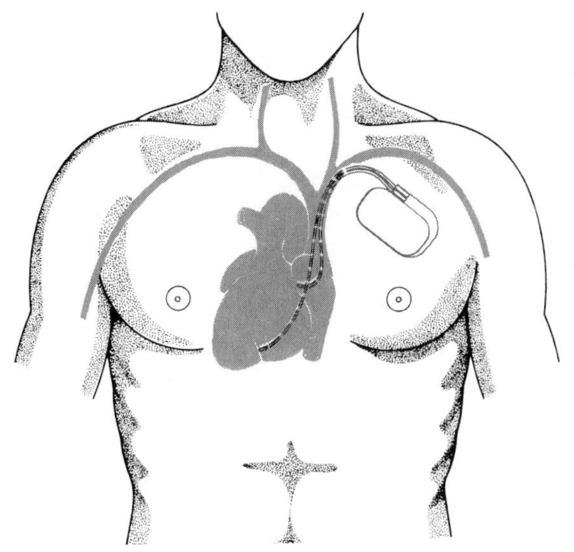

Figure 31-2 Placement of a permanent pacemaker generator. (From Lewis, et al: *Medical–surgical nursing,* ed 3, St Louis, 1992, Mosby–Year Book.)

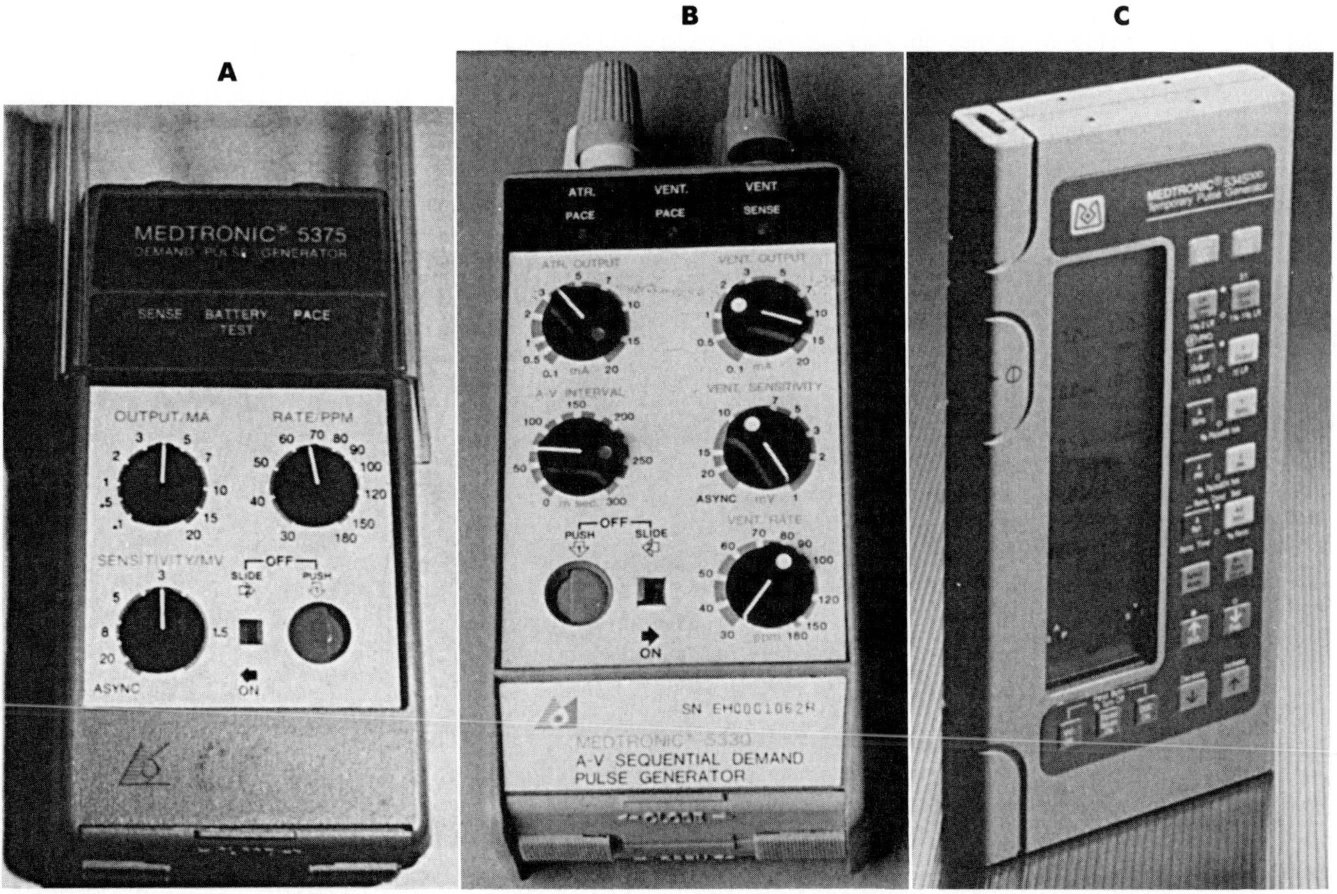

Figure 31-3 Temporary pacemaker models. **A,** VVI. **B,** AV sequential. **C,** DDD. (Courtesy of Medtronic, Inc, Minneapolis.)

TABLE 31-1 The NASPE/BPEG Generic (NBG) Pacemaker Code

Position	**I***	**II***	**III***	**IV**	**V**
Category	Chamber(s) paced	Chamber(s) sensed	Response to sensing	Programmability, rate modulation	Antitachyarrhythmia function(s)
	0 = None A = Atrium V = Ventricle D = Dual (A + V)	0 = None A = Atrium V = Ventricle D = Dual (A + V)	0 = None T = Triggered I = Inhibited D = Dual (T + I)	0 = None P = Simple programmable M = Multiprogrammable C = Communicating R = Rate modulation	0 = None P = Pacing (antitachyarrhythmia) S = Shock D = Dual (P + S)
Manufacturers' designation only	S = single (A or V)	S = single (A or V)			

*Used exclusively for antibradyarrhythmia function.
Used with permission: Bernstein AD, et al: The NASPE/BPEG generic pacemaker code for antiarrhythmia and adaptive rate pacing and antitachyarrhythmia devices, *PACE Pacing Clin Electrophysiol* 10:794-799, 1987.

Sensing occurs when the circuitry of the pacemaker recognizes specific intrinsic electrical activity, which resets the timing mechanisms of the pacemaker, resulting in inhibition of the pacing stimulus. This is a critical principle in understanding how artificial pacemakers function. Sensing must be understood in context with sensing or "seeing" intrinsic rhythm, as opposed to the common misconception that pacemakers "sense when they are supposed to fire." Artificial pacemakers *automatically* fire at their programmed rate unless an intrinsic heartbeat occurs faster than the preset rate or interval of the artificial pacemaker. The purpose of sensing is to allow intrinsic conduction and to prevent potentially life-threatening competition between the artificial pacemaker and the native pacemaker of the heart. As a result, it is imperative that an artificial pacemaker recognize intrinsic electrical activity that occurs faster than the underlying, escape rate of the pacemaker. Most pacemakers, both temporary and permanent, are designed to sense intrinsic cardiac activity and lose this ability only when a magnet is placed over the device.

A magnet may be used in follow-up of permanent pacemaker function in those patients who rarely use their pacemaker. The magnet blocks the ability of the pacemaker to sense intrinsic cardiac activity, resulting in fixed, automatic firing of the pacemaker. Removal of the magnet returns sensing function. Although a routine and generally safe assessment technique, use of a magnet on a pacemaker is not without risk. For example, there have been case reports of pacemaker malfunctions such as prolonged inhibition of the pacemaker in a pacemaker-dependent patient.[6] Complications such as this are very rare and do not imply that magnets should not be used to assess pacemaker integrity. However, the rare potential for complications does suggest that such assessment techniques are best performed under carefully monitored conditions by personnel who fully understand the function of pacemaker devices.

The North American Society for Pacing and Electrophysiology (NASPE) has collaborated with the British Pacing and Electrophysiology Group (BPEG) over the years to develop a coding system for pacemakers that uniformly describes the numerous functions of these devices. In 1987, this group published the latest version of the NASPE/BPEG generic (NBG) code, which includes five letters describing pacing, sensing, response to sensing, programmability, and antitachyarrhythmia functions.[5] Table 31-1 summarizes the components of the NBG code. The most recent update from the NASPE/BPEG collaboration expands on the pacemaker-focused NBG code to describe the capabilities of various implanted cardiovertor/defibrillators. Known as the NASPE/BPEG Defibrillator Code (NBD), it includes details regarding shock location, antitachycardia pacing, means of tachycardia detection, and antibradycardia pacing location.[4] This code indicates the latest technological advances in both pacing and implantable defibrillator technology by combining the features of both devices. Table 31-2 summarizes the NBD code.

Single-Chamber Pacemakers

The most common single-chamber pacemakers include the following:

- AAI: atrial pacing, atrial sensing, inhibited by intrinsic atrial activity (p waves).
- VVI: ventricular pacing, ventricular sensing, inhibited by intrinsic ventricular activity (QRS complexes).
- VVIR: identical to the VVI pacemaker with the addition of some form of rate-responsive technology.

Although not as "physiologic" as dual-chamber pacemakers, single-chamber pacemakers have been used effectively in a variety of settings. For example, single-chamber atrial and ventricular pacing has been used successfully to overdrive and convert supraventricular tachycardias and ventricular tachycardia, respectively.[16,31] VVI and VVIR pacing have also been suggested as equally therapeutic to dual-chamber pacing in patients with sick sinus syndrome.[32] On the other

TABLE 31-2 The NASPE/BPEG Defibrillator (NBD) Code

I	II	III	IV
Shock chamber	Antitachycardia pacing chamber	Tachycardia detection	Antibradycardia pacing chamber
0 = None A = Atrium V = Ventricle D = Dual (A + V)	0 = None A = Atrium V = Ventricle D = Dual (A + V)	E = Electrogram H = Hemodynamic	0 = None A = Atrium V = Ventricle D = Dual (A + V)

Used with permission: Bernstein AD, et al: North American Society of Pacing and Electrophysiology policy statement: the NASPE/BPEG defibrillator code, *PACE Pacing Clin Electrophysiol* 16:1776-1780, 1993.

hand, AAI pacing has been suggested as optimal for patients with sick sinus syndrome who do not demonstrate heart block at the junctional level.[20] Single-chamber endocardial pacing has been associated with fewer complications and acceptable support of CO in children.[11]

Dual-Chamber/AV-Sequential Pacemakers

Although effective in maintaining heart rate, single-chamber ventricular pacemakers do not maintain atrioventricular (AV) synchrony. The resulting compromise in CO may produce symptoms of heart failure, fatigue, dizziness, and chest discomfort in select patients, a phenomenon known as *pacemaker syndrome*.[22] As a result, dual-chamber or AV-sequential pacing becomes an important option. Dual-chamber pacemakers ensure AV synchrony and optimal CO by pacing both an atrium and a ventricle or by responding to intrinsic atrial and ventricular activity in ways that ensure an appropriate response in the alternate chamber or by inhibiting pacing stimuli when necessary. Coded as DDD, this type of pacemaker will pace both the atrium and the ventricle, sense in both chambers, and either be triggered to fire or be inhibited as appropriate.

Rate Responsiveness

Rate responsiveness, or rate modulation, is an important feature of contemporary pacemaker technology. This capability is available in single- and dual-chamber pacemakers and ensures appropriate chronotropic response to changes in physical or physiologic status. Specialized sensor systems (biosensors) have been incorporated into these pacemaker devices, enabling them to increase or decrease the rate of pacemaker firing as needed. Sensors include mechanical, chemical, thermal, and electrical devices.[27] Examples of sensors include the accelerometer, which is sensitive to a wide range of physical movement, the minute volume sensor, and the QT-interval sensor.[1,21] Unfortunately, single-sensor devices have not demonstrated optimal results. As a result, considerable effort is being made to develop devices that combine the information from multiple sensors in more complex algorithms to more optimally match chronotropic response of the pacemaker to patient need.[21] In one example, the Topaz group has demonstrated considerable success in combining activity and QT-interval sensors in a VVI pacemaker.[9] See Figure 31-4 for illustrations of all pacing modes reviewed.

Programmability

Programmability is a function of temporary and permanent pacemakers. In both situations, this feature refers to the ability to noninvasively change the pacing parameters or settings based on the specific needs of the patient. Pacing rate, energy output (milliamps, or mA), and sensitivity are common programmable parameters in all pacemakers. Dual-chamber pacemakers may also have their AV delay and refractory periods reprogrammed. Reprogramming pacing mode, pulse width, tachycardia response, and rate responsiveness are currently specific to permanent pacemakers. In addition, information regarding electrode/lead integrity and pacemaker use is available via telemetried devices. These functions allow optimal pacing, troubleshooting pacemaker problems, and treatment of pacemaker-induced complications. Reprogramming a pacemaker is painless and poses little risk to the patient. Transtelephonic monitoring is also routine for pacemaker patients to ensure close, ongoing monitoring of pacemaker function.

INDICATIONS

The use of pacemaker technology for either temporary or permanent pacing falls into one of three categories: therapeutic, diagnostic, or prophylactic. The therapeutic indications for artificial pacing include the following:

- Bradydysrhythmias[7]
- Tachy-brady syndrome (sick sinus syndrome)
- Heart block
- Overdrive for ventricular tachydysrhythmias
- Conversion of atrial flutter or other reentry atrial tachycardias

The diagnostic indications for using a pacemaker are focused primarily in the sophisticated assessment of dysrhythmia risks in select patients and include the following:

- Electrophysiology studies
- Evaluation of dysrhythmias
- Evaluation of antidysrhythmic drug therapy

The prophylactic indications for temporary or permanent

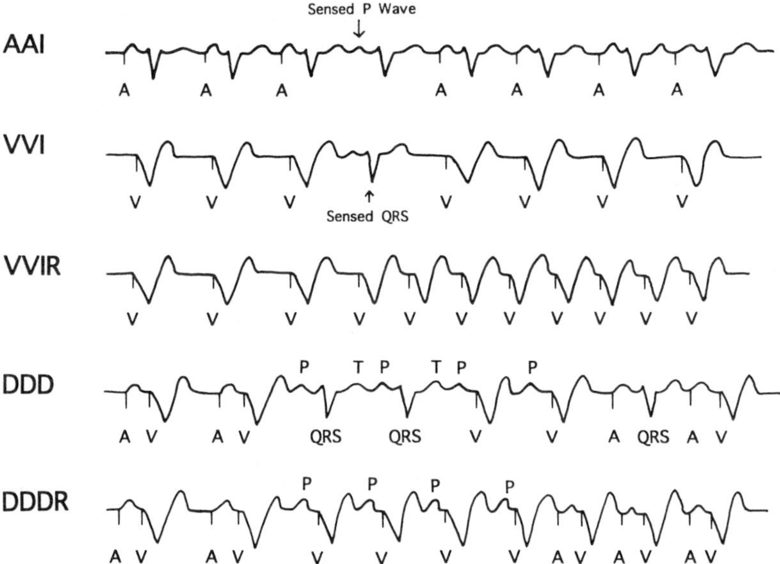

Figure 31-4 Summary of various pacing modes. **AAI,** Atrial pacing that senses intrinsic atrial activity (p waves). **VVI,** Ventricular pacing that senses intrinsic ventricular activity (QRS complexes). **VVIR,** Ventricular pacing that senses intrinsic QRS complexes and increased rate of ventricular pacing in response to physical activity. **DDD,** AV sequential pacing that senses intrinsic atrial and ventricular activity (p waves, QRS complexes, or both). **DDDR,** AV sequential pacing that will exceed response to increased intrinsic atrial rate to increase AV pacing rate per increased activity.

pacing are specific and selective. The two primary prophylactic uses for pacemakers are as follows:

- The immediate postoperative period following cardiac surgery (especially valve repair or replacement procedures, but also coronary artery bypass grafting procedures and cardiac transplantation[23,29])
- Cardiac drug toxicities

In addition to the indications for temporary or permanent pacing, there are specific indications for the type of pacemaker and the type of approach for pacemaker insertion. The approach to pacemaker insertion depends primarily on the acuity of the situation. Approaches infjclude external/transcutaneous pacing, epicardial pacing, and transvenous endocardial pacing. The techniques and indication for each type of pacemaker are summarized in Table 31-3.

Once a temporary or permanent pacemaker is positioned, the minimal amount of energy needed to stimulate the heart muscle consistently is determined. The energy setting of the pacemaker generator will usually be set at double or triple the minimum threshold stimulus to ensure an adequate safety margin for maintaining pacemaker capture. The mode of pacing will be selected based on the needs of the individual patient. The sensitivity of the pacemaker will also be adjusted to ensure that the pacemaker adequately senses appropriate intrinsic electrical activity to prevent competition. Finally, the rate is set to maintain an adequate CO for the patient.

LIMITATIONS AND POTENTIAL COMPLICATIONS

Artificial pacemakers are capable of maintaining adequate heart rate (single-chamber pacemakers) and atrial kick that optimizes CO (dual-chamber AV-sequential pacemakers). However, anything less than a DDDR pacemaker will not fully replace the physiologic action of intrinsic cardiac rhythm.

Potential complications for temporary and permanent pacemakers are similar in many respects. However, each type of pacemaker does carry unique risks. Potential complications of temporary pacemakers include the following:

- Higher risk for lead displacement
- Higher risk for disconnection
- Microshock potential
- Accidental setting changes

Permanent pacemakers carry slightly different risks, most of which are associated with differences in the type of pacemaker catheters used and the fact that permanent pacemaker patients are more likely to be exposed to external, competing signals that may affect their pacemaker function. The potential complications of permanent pacemakers are as follows:

- Higher risk for ventricular perforation (including malposition within the left ventricle, free wall perforation, and diaphragmatic pacing[15])
- Higher risk for lead fracture or twisting, known as twiddler's syndrome[37]

TABLE 31-3 Techniques and Indications for Pacemakers

Pacemaker type	Technique	Indication
External/ transcutaneous pacemaker (produces ventricular pacing)	• Anterior and posterior electrodes placed on thorax • Rate, sensing, and energy output set as ordered • Sedation administered for painful chest wall stimulation with pacing	• Emergency situations • High-risk situations such as asystole or extreme bradycardia • Temporary only
Transthoracic pacemaker (produces ventricular pacing)	• Subxyphoid insertion of a long needle into the ventricle • Pacing wire threaded via needle to achieve direct endocardial contact • Attached to a standard temporary generator	• Last resort in emergency situations • Asystole that is unresponsive to drugs or external pacing • Temporary only • Used only until a more stable pacing system can be established
Transvenous pacing (produces atrial, ventricular, or AV sequential pacing)	• Pacing lead inserted via subclavian or jugular vein into right ventricle • Single-lead wire or multilumen balloon-tipped lead may be used • Direct contact with endocardium • Fluoroscopy is needed with hardwire, non–balloon-tipped leads to reduce risk of ectopy and ventricular perforation • Permanent pulse generator implanted under the skin in the chest or abdomen • Temporary pulse generator allows external control of multiple parameters (rate, energy output, sensitivity, AV delay, refractory periods, etc.)	• Most common type of pacemaker • Temporary or permanent
Epicardial pacing (usually for ventricular pacing, but atrial pacing is possible)	• Pacing leads are sewn or screwed into the epicardium for permanent pacing • Pacing leads are loosely looped through the epicardium for temporary pacing • Requires surgical opening/entering of chest for placement (sternotomy or thoracotomy)	• Technique of choice in cardiac surgery • Temporary or permanent

- Pacemaker erosion
- Pacemaker generator displacement
- Reset (failure to fire) due to electrical interference

Concerns about external suppression of pacing function have long been associated with permanent pacemakers. Although historical sources of such interference have been successfully compensated for, new forms of potential electrical interference have been noted. External electrical interference is more likely with unipolar-lead systems.[3] Reports of contemporary sources of electrical interference note the use of transcutaneous electrical nerve stimulation (TENS) in somewhat rare and select cases.[8,28] Another study examined the effect of a growing technology in our society on pacemaker function: electronic article surveillance (EAS), otherwise known as antitheft devices.[10] EAS devices that used radiofrequency and pulsed electromagnetic technology were not found to significantly influence pacemaker performance, but devices that used continuous magnetic fields were noted to produce prolonged inhibition in 7 out of 10 dual-chamber pacemakers.[10] On another note, presence of a pacemaker has long been considered a contraindication for magnetic resonance imaging (MRI). However, a recent study demonstrated that MRI of the head could be safely performed in a pacemaker patient as long as the pacemaker was programmed to a fixed-rate mode and the device had been implanted long enough for adequate scar tissue to have formed to prevent lead movement.[19]

Both types of pacemakers share a number of potential complications. Most of these complications are associated with the invasive nature of pacemaker insertion and are temporary risks. The more common complications seen in temporary and permanent pacemakers include the following:

- Infection at the insertion site or the leads
- Generator malfunction

TABLE 31-4 Description of the Programmed Intervals of Pacemakers

Interval	Description
Automatic interval (A-A or V-V)	The rate at which a pacemaker will automatically fire without intrinsic activity. Measured as the distance between two atrial or two ventricular pacing artifacts. Usually equal to the minimum rate of the pacemaker. 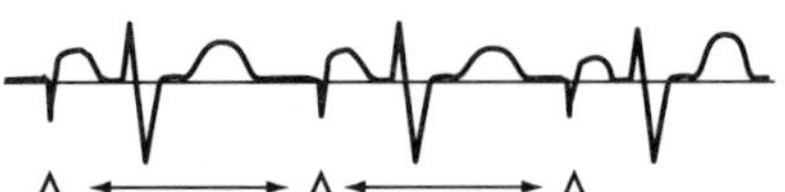 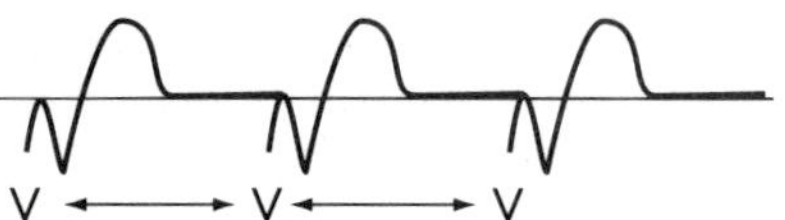
Escape interval	The rate at which a pacemaker first fires following an intrinsic beat. This rate is often equal to the automatic rate of the pacemaker. The escape interval may be set at a slower rate (hysteresis) to allow intrinsic activity to occur whenever possible. Once activated, the automatic interval of the pacemaker is maintained. 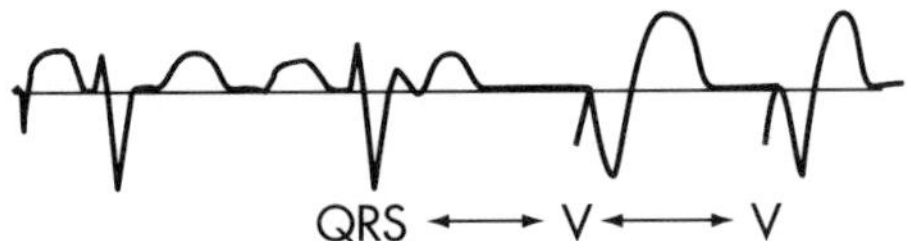
A-V interval (A-V delay)	Time delay between an atrial and ventricular pacing stimulus. Applies to AV pacemakers. The ventricular pacemaker is triggered by the firing of the atrial pacemaker, but it does not fire until after the programmed delay expires. An intrinsic QRS occurring before the A-V delay is completed will inhibit the ventricular pacemaker. 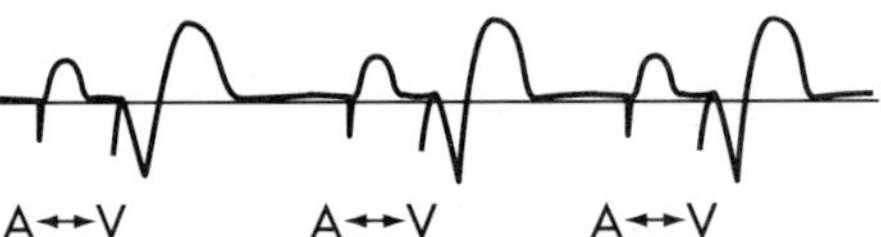
V-A interval	Time interval between a ventricular pacing artifact or an intrinsic QRS and the subsequent firing of the atrial pacemaker. Applies to AV pacemakers. The V-A interval added to the A-V delay will equal the automatic ventricular interval or rate of the pacemaker (V-V interval). 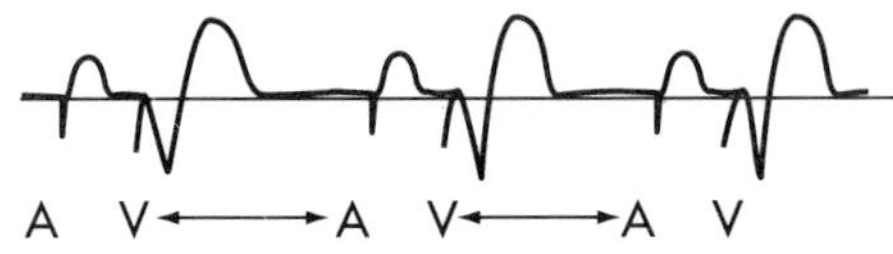

- Lead fracture or insulation break
- Ventricular ectopy for 24 to 48 hours after insertion
- Atrial and ventricular ectopy during insertion
- Increased myocardial resistance that results in gradually increasing minimum thresholds
- Pneumothorax or hemothorax during insertion

Significantly more rare, superior vena cava occlusion secondary to thrombosis has been reported but appears to have minimal impact on patient safety.[25] In addition, increased platelet aggregability has been noted in patients with VVI pacemakers, which may be related to the thromboembolic events noted on occasion in these patients.[13] However, more research will be needed to determine the clinical significance of these findings and whether or not platelet-inhibiting drugs should be administered to pacemaker patients.

GENERAL NURSING INTERVENTIONS

Accurate analysis of pacemaker function on the ECG is a major nursing intervention.[14,26] This includes the ability to accurately evaluate the function of noninvasive transcutaneous pacing function as well as more traditional modes of pacing.[2] In order to accurately analyze the ECG of a pacemaker, one must understand the intervals by which pacemakers are programmed. Pacemakers *automatically* fire at their programmed intervals unless they sense intrinsic elec-

TABLE 31-5 General Nursing Interventions Associated with Cardiac Pacing

General considerations	Nursing interventions—temporary pacing	Nursing interventions—permanent pacing
Initiation of pacing	Ensure battery function Tighten terminal connections Threshold and sensing testing per physician order	Reinforce information about the device with patient and family
Maintenance and prevention of complications	Monitor/care for insertion site Minimize motion of extremity or torso at site of insertion Check pulse distal to insertion site to ensure perfusion Keep box and wires dry Keep plastic cover over dials Check battery status and replace when low Check thresholds q24h or as ordered Check consistency between settings of pacemaker and those recorded in the chart Check ECG for appropriate pacing and sensing	Monitor/care for insertion site Minimize motion of extremity at site of insertion Observe for catheter displacement • Changes in QRS complex in v leads • Loss of capture • Failure to sense Discharge planning to include function and type of pacemaker
Evaluation of effectiveness	Ensure pacemaker unit is functioning properly • Fires at preset rate • Each pacemaker stimulus produces myocardial response • Senses intrinsic beats • Absence of competition • Observe for dysrhythmias • Notify physician if malfunction is noted Evidence of adequate CO, VS WNL, lungs clear, tolerates activity within patient norms[24]	Same as temporary pacemaker

trical activity prior to their automatic firing rate. The specific intervals of pacemakers are described in Table 31-4. The general nursing interventions associated with temporary and permanent cardiac pacing are described in Table 31-5.

Patient education is another essential nursing intervention for pacemaker patients. Patient responses to permanent pacemaker implantation may run the gamut from fearfulness, which places them at risk of becoming "cardiac cripples," to feeling as though they are invincible.[30] At either extreme, pacemaker patients may place themselves at unnecessary risk for complications. Ensuring that pacemaker patients enjoy an active life following the implantation is a function of careful education and follow-up. Provision of education and educational materials in both the inpatient and outpatient settings has been suggested as useful in ensuring optimal adjustment to pacemaker implantation.[33] Structured teaching programs have also been shown to be effective in increasing knowledge of safe and active lifestyle following pacemaker implantation in both adults and children.[35]

TROUBLESHOOTING

Pacemaker malfunctions generally fall into one of three categories: loss of capture, oversensing, or undersensing. The following discussion offers suggestions for determining the cause of a malfunction, as well as actions to correct the problem. Independent action to correct pacemaker malfunctions is important, especially when the malfunction places the patient at

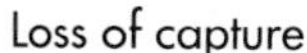

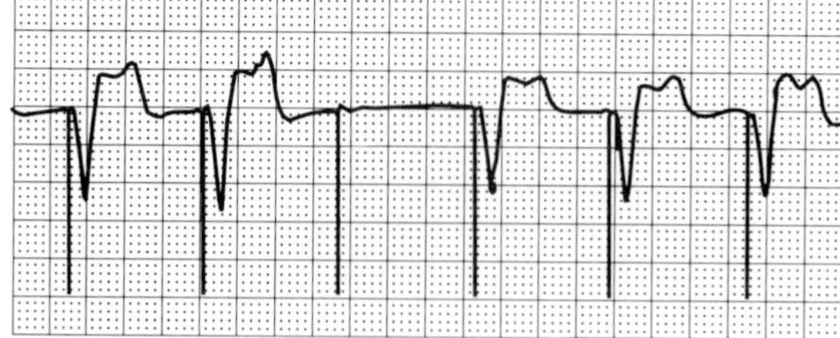

Oversensing

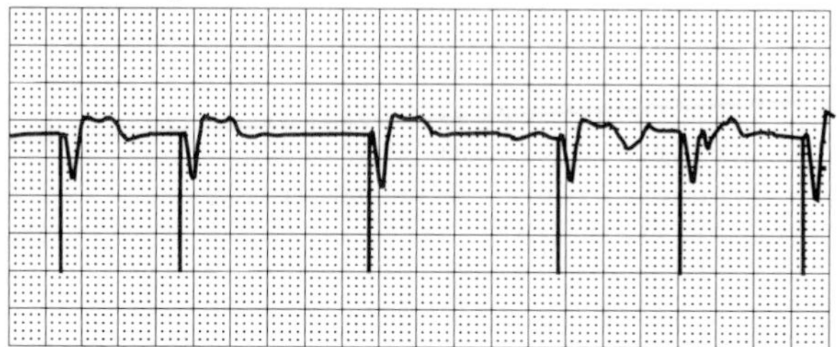

Undersensing

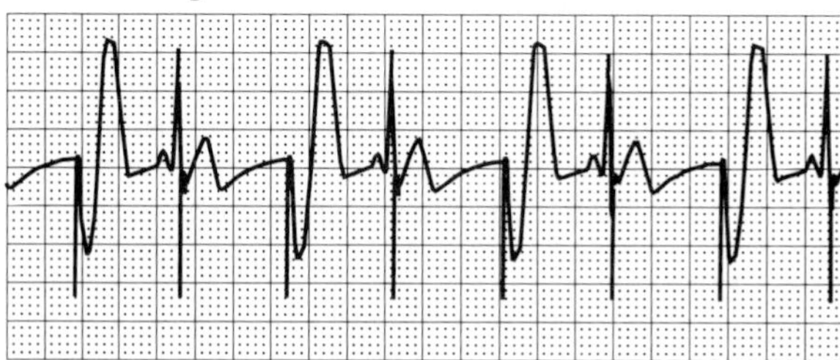

Figure 31-5 Pacemaker malfunctions.

risk. However, communication with the physician is essential, especially when the problem cannot be corrected promptly and may require invasive intervention.

Problem: Loss of Pacemaker Capture

Loss of pacemaker capture is visible as a pacemaker artifact without the appropriate complex. Loss of atrial capture would be seen as an atrial pacemaker artifact without a p wave following it. A ventricular pacemaker artifact without a QRS would be an example of loss of ventricular capture. (See Figure 31-5.) Loss of pacemaker capture may have serious consequences for pacemaker-dependent patients, necessitating supportive interventions pending pacemaker correction.

CAUSE	CORRECTIVE ACTION
Lead dislodgement Lead perforation Lead fracture	Assess chest x-ray for possible lead displacement Reprogram pacemaker amplitude and/or pulse width Reposition patient to left side
Inadequate energy output (MA)	Increase MA to maximum
Low battery	Change battery (temporary pacer) Change generator (permanent pacer)

Increased myocardial resistance	Reposition patient to left side
Decreased myocardial responsiveness	Reassess minimum threshold and increase MA as needed Assess drug levels and electrolytes Reprogram pacemaker amplitude and/or pulse width

Problem: Pacemaker Oversensing

Seen as the absence of a pacing artifact when firing of the pacemaker should have occurred based on the automatic interval of the pacemaker and the absence of an inhibiting intrinsic beat. As a result, the ECG will demonstrate pauses, some of which may be prolonged. This phenomenon may also occur as failure of the pacemaker to fire at its automatic interval due to internal device failure. Clinically, the absence of pacemaker firing may produce significant bradycardic symptoms in the patient. (See Figure 31-5.)

CAUSE	CORRECTIVE ACTION
Lead displacement Lead fracture	Assess chest x-ray for possible lead displacement Reposition the patient to left side
Electromagnetic interference (EMI)	Isolate EMI and distance patient from source Caution patient to avoid direct contact with MRI scans and other pulsatile high-energy sources (radio towers, running car alternator, etc.)
Pacemaker cross talk (proximity of leads producing a self-inhibiting signal loop)	Switch from bipolar to unipolar mode (may need an indifferent external lead with temporary pacemaker) Switch from dual- to single-chamber pacing mode Decrease pacemaker sensitivity
Myopotential inhibition (extreme skeletal muscle activity, such as shivering, seizures, hypokalemia with tall T waves)—more common with unipolar pacemakers	Decrease pacemaker sensitivity Correct causative muscle activity Switch to bipolar pacing, if possible Increase pacemaker refractory periods
Generator failure Generator power loss	Change generator (permanent pacer) Change battery (temporary pacer)

Problem: Pacemaker Undersensing

Results in the appearance of pacing artifacts in competition with intrinsic cardiac rhythm. (See Figure 31-5.) The pacemaker fails to sense or "see" the intrinsic activity and may fire in a fixed pattern at its automatic interval. The greatest risk to the patient with an undersensing pacemaker is the potential for a pacemaker artifact to occur at a vulnerable time during the cardiac cycle (such as R-on-T phenomenon) and produce life-threatening dysrhythmias (such as ventricular tachycardia or ventricular fibrillation).

CAUSE	CORRECTIVE ACTION
Lead displacement	Assess chest x-ray for possible lead displacement Turn patient to left side
Presence of magnet over permanent generator	Use magnet for minimal time to check pacemaker function
Increased myocardial resistance Generator failure Generator setting error	Increase pacemaker sensitivity Change generator (permanent pacer) Change battery (temporary pacer) Turn pacemaker off if underlying rhythm produces adequate CO to protect patient from competition

SUMMARY

Managing pacemaker technology and supporting patients who require these interventions are increasingly common challenges for critical care nurses. As the generators become progressively more sophisticated, patients' physiologic needs may be more optimally met with either permanent or temporary devices. Critical care nurses can best respond to certain continued improvement in pacemaker technology by maintaining a firm foundation of knowledge regarding the key functions and principles associated with this technological support device. Ability to interpret the NASPE/BPEG pacemaker code and measure the primary pacing intervals (A-A, V-V, V-A, A-V) are the cornerstones to safe and accurate interpretation of pacemaker function and malfunction. In addition, standard attention to patient response, both physical and psychoemotional, will ensure that pacemakers are optimally programmed and patients are maximally able to enjoy full and active lives.

REFERENCES

1. Abrahamsen AM, et al: Rate responsive cardiac pacing using a minute ventilation sensor, *PACE Pacing Clin Electrophysiol* 16:1650-1655, 1993.
2. Appel-Hardin S: The role of the critical care nurse in noninvasive temporary pacing, *Crit Care Nurs* 12(3):10-19, 1992.
3. Astridge PS, et al: The response of implanted dual chamber pacemakers to 50 Hz extraneous electrical interference, *PACE Pacing Clin Electrophysiol* 16:1966-1974, 1993.
4. Bernstein AD, et al: North American Society of Pacing and Electrophysiology policy statement: the NASPE/BPEG defibrillator code, *PACE Pacing Clin Electrophysiol* 16:1776-1780, 1993.
5. Bernstein AD, Camm AJ, Fletcher RD: The NASPE/BPEG generic pacemaker code for antiarrhythmia and adaptive rate pacing and antitachyarrhythmia devices, *PACE Pacing Clin Electrophysiol* 10:794-799, 1987.
6. Bierman PQ, Roche DA, Carlson LG: Abnormal permanent pacemaker inhibition by a magnet: a case study, *Heart Lung* 22:148-150, 1993.
7. Buysman JR: Pacemaker therapies for bradycardias. In Conover M, editor: *Understanding electrocardiography,* ed 6, St Louis, 1992, Mosby, pp 424-447.
8. Chen D, et al: Cardiac pacemaker inhibition by transcutaneous electrical nerve stimulation, *Arch Phys Med Rehabil* 71:27-30, 1990.
9. Connelly DT: Initial experience with a new single chamber, dual sensor rate responsive pacemaker: the Topaz study group, *PACE Pacing Clin Electrophysiol* 16:1833-1841, 1993.
10. Dodinot B, Godenir JP, Costa AB: Electronic article surveillance: a possible danger for pacemaker patients, *PACE Pacing Clin Electrophysiol* 16:46-53, 1993.
11. Esperer HD, et al: Permanent epicardial and transvenous single and dual chamber cardiac pacing in children, *Thorac Cardiovasc Surg* 41:21-27, 1993.
12. Falk RH, Battinelli NJ: External cardiac pacing using low impedance electrodes suitable for defibrillation: a comparative blinded study, *J Am Coll Cardiol* 22:1354-1358, 1993.
13. Fazio S, et al: Platelet aggregability in patients with a VVI pacemaker, *PACE Pacing Clin Electrophysiol* 16:254-256, 1993.
14. Feeney MK: Electrocardiographic interpretation of pacemaker rhythms, *AACN Clin Iss Crit Care Nurs* 2:159-169, 1991.
15. Ghani M, et al: Malposition of transvenous pacing lead in the left ventricle, *PACE Pacing Clin Electrophysiol* 16:1800-1807, 1993.
16. Gillis AM, et al: A prospective randomized comparison of autodecremental pacing to burst pacing in device therapy for chronic ventricular tachycardia secondary to coronary artery disease, *Am J Cardiol* 72:1146-1151, 1993.
17. Grubb BP, et al: The use of external, noninvasive pacing for the termination of supraventricular tachycardia in the emergency department setting, *Ann Emerg Med* 22:714-717, 1993.
18. Hickey CS, Baas LS: Temporary cardiac pacing, *AACN Clin Iss Crit Care Nurs* 2:107-117, 1991.
19. Inbar S, et al: Case report: nuclear magnetic resonance imaging in a patient with a pacemaker, *Am J Med Sci* 305:174-175, 1993.
20. Katritsis D, Camm AJ: AAI pacing mode: when is it indicated and how should it be achieved? *Clin Cardiol* 16:339-343, 1993.
21. Katritsis D, Shakespeare CF, Camm AJ: New and combined sensors for adaptive rate pacing, *Clin Cardiol* 16:240-248, 1993.
22. Kleinschmidt KM, Stafford MJ: Dual chamber cardiac pacemakers, *J Cardiovasc Nurs* 5(3):9-20, 1991.
23. Markewitz A, et al: Longterm results of pacemaker therapy after orthotopic heart transplantation, *J Cardiac Surg* 8:411-416, 1993.
24. Martin M, Aragon D: Temporary DDD pacing: evaluating hemodynamic performance, *Dimensions Crit Care Nurs* 11(4):191-199, 1992.
25. Mazzetti H, et al: Superior vena cava occlusion and/or syndrome related to pacemaker leads, *Am Heart J* 125:831-837, 1993.
26. McErlean ES: Dual chamber pacing, *AACN Clin Iss Crit Care Nurs* 2:126-131, 1991.
27. Morton PG: Rate responsive cardiac pacemakers, *AACN Clin Iss Crit Care Nurs* 2:140-149, 1991.
28. O'Flaherty D, Wardill M, Adams AP: Inadvertent suppression of a fixed rate ventricular pacemaker using a peripheral nerve stimulator, *Anaesthesia* 46:687-689, 1993.
29. Otaki M: Permanent cardiac pacing after cardiac operations, *Artif Organs* 17:346-349, 1993.
30. Paluso KA: Cardiac pacemaker interactions in medical and nonmedical environments, *Phys Assist* 17:57-58, 67-69, 73-74, 1993.
31. Roman-Smith P: Pacing for tachydysrhythmias, *AACN Clin Iss Crit Care Nurs* 2:132-139, 1991.
32. Sgarbossa EB, Pinski SL, Maloney JD: The role of pacing modality in determining long term survival in sick sinus syndrome, *Ann Intern Med* 119:359-365, 1993.
33. Stewert JV, Sheehan AM: Permanent pacemakers: the nurse's role in patient education and follow up care, *J Cardiovasc Nurs* 5(3):32-43, 1991.
34. Teplitz L: Transcutaneous pacemakers, *J Cardiovasc Nurs* 5(3):44-57, 1991.
35. Verderber A, Fitzsimmons L, Shively M: Research connections: physiologic and psychologic responses to cardiac pacemakers, *J Cardiovasc Nurs* 5(3):77-79, 1991.
36. Waggoner PC: Transcutaneous cardiac pacing, *AACN Clin Iss Crit Care Nurs* 2:118-125, 1991.
37. Wong JK, House RJ: Pacemaker twist: twiddler's syndrome. *Australas Radiol* 37:286-287, 1993.

DEVICE GUIDELINE

32

Intra-aortic Balloon Pump

Susan Flewelling Goran, MSN, RN, CCRN

DESCRIPTION

The intra-aortic balloon (IAB) is a volume-displacement device positioned in the descending aorta 2 to 3 cm distal to the left subclavian artery. With timed inflation and deflation, the IAB increases oxygen supply to the myocardium and decreases ventricular work load, which decreases oxygen (O_2) demand.[12] The IAB is "timed" in synchrony with the cardiac cycle. During cardiac diastole, when the aortic valve is closed and the coronary arteries are being perfused, the balloon inflates, displacing arterial blood volume to the coronary arteries and increasing their perfusion pressure.[11] The balloon is timed to deflate just prior to systole, during the isovolumetric contraction of wall tension phase of ventricular systole. Deflation at this precise moment causes a potential space in the ascending aorta as previously trapped blood moves forward down the aorta. As a result, afterload is decreased, which allows systole to occur at a lower pressure. This action also decreases myocardial O_2 demand and consumption (MVO_2). When the ventricles are in systole, the balloon is at rest or deflated. When the ventricles are in diastole, the balloon is at work or inflated (Figure 32-1). This is known as the principle of *counterpulsation*.[15]

The IAB was first introduced in the clinical arena for the treatment of cardiogenic shock by Dr. Adrian Kantrowitz in 1967.[10] Initially, insertion and removal of the balloon required a surgical team to graft the IAB into the femoral artery and repair the artery post-removal. Percutaneous insertion of the IAB was introduced in the late 1970s, along with other improvements in balloon technology, which resulted in increased use of this treatment modality.[5,10]

Intra-aortic balloon pump (IABP) therapy consists of two components—the balloon catheter, and the drive unit or pump.[9] The polyurethane catheter is a 30- to 40-cc balloon mounted on a vascular catheter that may be inserted surgically or percutaneously. The balloon is typically inflated with helium.[9] Helium has been chosen most often because it moves swiftly when shuttled in and out of the balloon catheter. In addition, helium dissipates quickly, which reduces the risk of a gas embolus in the event that the balloon ruptures. Double-lumen balloon catheters are fitted with a central lumen located inside the helium channel. The central lumen, which leads to the catheter tip, allows for the use of a J-tip guide wire to assist insertion. The central lumen also allows monitoring of central arterial pressure. Typically, percutaneous IABs are inserted via a sheath placed in the femoral artery. However, sheathless balloons are the latest advance in catheter technology. These balloons are easier to insert with less obstruction of the femoral artery. In cases where direct visualization of the femoral artery is required, a surgical cutdown must be done. Femoral cutdown employs the anastomosis of a tubular graft to the artery through which the balloon is passed. Upon discontinuation of the IAB, the graft is removed and the artery closed. For patients undergoing cardiac surgery with the chest already opened, the balloon may be inserted in the aorta through a direct aortic incision. Transthoracic placement may be more comfortable for the patient awaiting transplantation but obviously requires a return trip to the OR for removal.

The balloon pump console is the drive unit that shuttles gas, usually helium, in and out of the balloon catheter causing balloon inflation and deflation. Although pump features differ depending on the vendor, all contain the common ingredients of an ECG and arterial monitor, timing and triggering controls, a gas source, and a pneumatic pump or drive system.[15]

The IABP system requires a signal to activate balloon

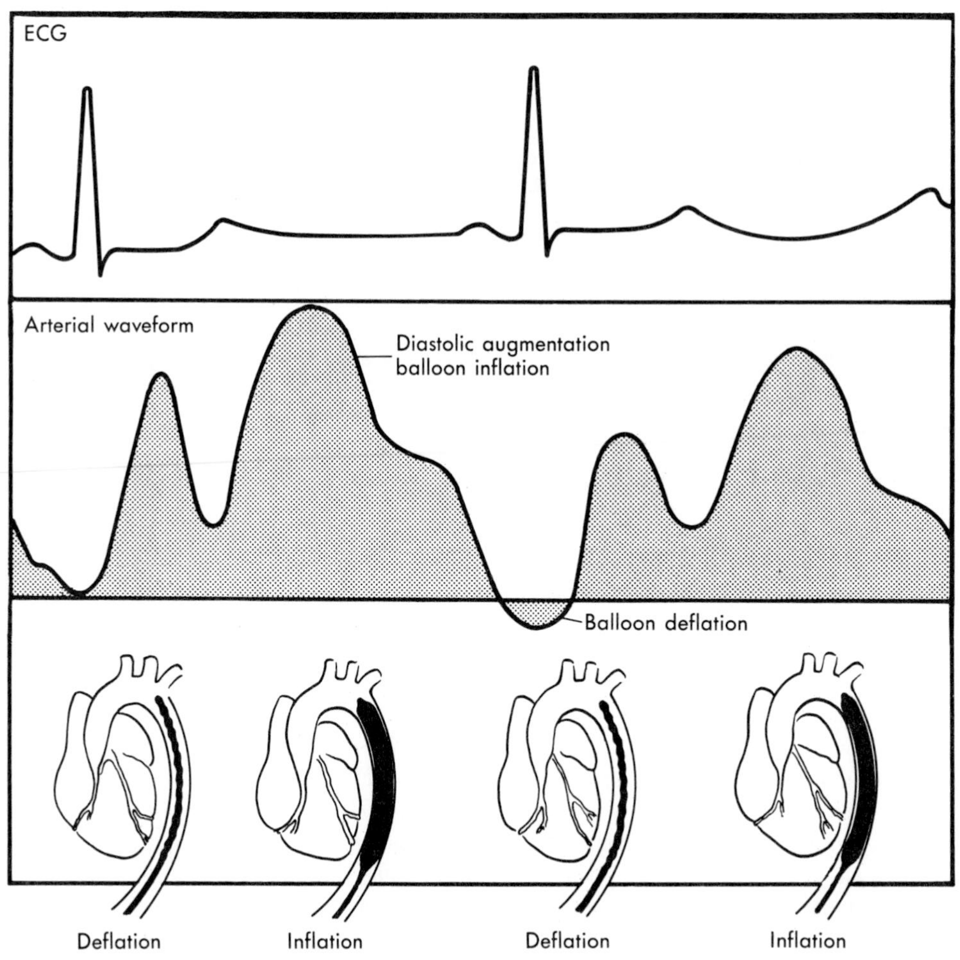

Figure 32-1 Two counterpulsation cycles. The balloon is inflated during diastole, thus "augmenting" diastolic pressure. Deflation occurs during isovolumetric contraction. Because balloon inflation displaces intra-aortic balloon volume, aortic end-diastolic pressure is "lowered" during IAB deflation. (From Quaal SJ: *Comprehensive intra-aortic balloon pumping,* ed 2, St Louis, 1993, Mosby–Year Book.)

inflation and deflation. Traditionally, this trigger signal is the R wave of the ECG, but trigger signals are also available from the arterial waveform, ventricular pacing spikes, or an internal triggering signal. If the trigger signal is lost, the pump is unable to operate. Triggering should not be confused with timing. Timing occurs when the operator determines the exact point on the arterial waveform where inflation and deflation should occur. Triggering is automatic based on the signal chosen by the operator. Timing is selective based on the skill of the operator.

INDICATIONS

The IABP is used primarily to provide hemodynamic support for patients with imminent or frank cardiac failure refractory to medical interventions. The major indications for use of the IABP include:

- Acute myocardial infarction
- Weaning from cardiopulmonary bypass
- Ventricular aneurysm
- Cardiogenic shock
- Unstable angina
- Post-infarction angina
- Ventricular dysrhythmias post-MI
- Mitral regurgitation
- Ventricular-septal defect
- Papillary muscle rupture
- Left ventricular failure
- Cardiac support for noncardiac surgery[5]
- Bridge to cardiac transplantation
- Prevention of acute restenosis in PTCA

Contraindications are usually classified as either relative or absolute, depending on their severity and the level of patient crisis. The most significant relevant contraindications include:

- Bleeding disorders
- History of severe peripheral vascular disease

The absolute contraindications for use of the IABP are the following:

Potential Complications Associated with IABP
Vascular complications
Limb ischemia
Loss of pulses
Peripheral emboli
Pseudoaneurysm
Compartment syndrome
Aortic dissection
Aortic rupture
Intimal hematoma
Hematological complications
Bleeding
Thrombocytopenia
Central nervous system complications
Delirium
Spinal cord necrosis
Paralysis
Other complications
Infection
Mesenteric ischemia
Renal emboli
Improper timing
Inability to wean
Balloon leak and entrapment

- Abdominal aortic aneurysm
- Aortic valve incompetence
- Metastatic cancer
- Aortic dissection

LIMITATIONS

Limitations of IABP therapy relate to the degree of cardiac compromise in the patient. The effectiveness of the IABP is dependent on the baseline arterial pressure and cardiac rhythm of the patient. The IABP augments the existing arterial pressure. As a result, augmentation improves as arterial pressure improves. In addition, the more stable the rhythm, the better the IABP will perform. While contemporary IABP devices trigger from irregular rhythms quite well, the IABP cannot fully compensate for the hemodynamic consequences of rapid, irregular dysrhythmias. A final limitation of the IABP relates to its use as a "bridge to transplant." While the IABP may enable stabilization in a pre–cardiac-transplant patient, the mobility limitations associated with most applications of this device make this form of ventricular assist a poor choice. In the event that the patient is severely compromised hemodynamically or will require prolonged support waiting for a transplant, more-advanced ventricular assist devices are indicated.

TABLE 32-1 Clinical Benefits of IABP Counterpulsation

Physiological effects	Clinical indications
Inflation	
Increased coronary perfusion pressure	Decreased chest pain
Increased systemic perfusion pressure	Improvement in mentation
Increased myocardial O_2 supply	Increased urine output Improved skin color Decreased dysrhythmias
Deflation	
Decreased afterload Systolic unloading	Improved ABG Decreased pulmonary congestion
Decreased myocardial O_2 demand	Decreased filling pressures (CVP, PCWP)
Decreased myocardial O_2 consumption	Decreased SVR, PVR
Improved ejection fraction	Improved CO, CI

POTENTIAL COMPLICATIONS

Complication rates with the use of the IAB have been the subject of extensive research.[13,16,17,18] Current complication rates range from 14% to 45%, although the mortality rate of IABP therapy is less than 1%.[10] Complications may occur during balloon insertion, counterpulsation, balloon removal, post-balloon removal, and post-discharge, including IAB rupture and entrapment.[3] The potential complications most often associated with IABP therapy are listed in the following Box.

Research has also identified predisposing factors that increase the risk for complications as follows: female sex, insulin-dependent diabetes, IABP support for more than 60 hours, previous history of peripheral vascular disease, percutaneous IAB insertion, and an ankle-arm index of less than 1.0.[6,10,14] Although the majority of research focuses on vascular complications, recent research has also identified height as a predisposing factor for balloon leak.[4] Statistical analysis of patient height versus incidence of IAB leak showed a significant difference between patients greater than 170 cm tall and those less than 170 cm tall. The data support the recommendation to insert 34-cc balloons instead of 40-cc balloons in patients under 5′4″ tall.[4]

GENERAL NURSING INTERVENTIONS

The role of the nurse in the care of patients requiring IAB therapy varies with the institution. In many locations, the responsibility for console management and timing lies with

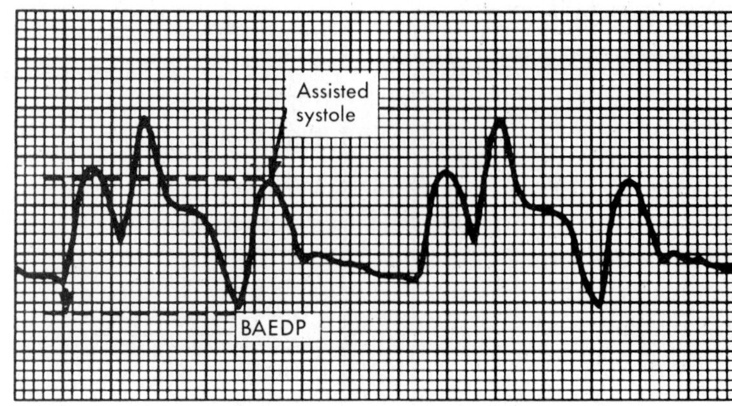

Figure 32-2 Landmarks of proper IAB deflation. BAEDP should be lower than UAEDP. Point 2 assisted systole should ideally be lower than, but definitely not higher than, patient systole. (From Quaal SJ: *Comprehensive intra-aortic balloon pumping,* ed 2, St Louis, 1993, Mosby–Year Book.)

the nurse; but specially trained technicians, respiratory therapists, perfusionists, or other assistive personnel may hold this responsibility in other institutions. In any setting, it is vitally important that collaboration occur between all members of the health care team to ensure the best possible patient outcome.

Nurses caring for the IABP patients have three major areas of responsibility: (1) monitoring for effectiveness, (2) prevention and recognition of complications, and (3) family/patient education and support.

Monitoring Effectiveness

Monitoring effectiveness of IAB therapy involves recognition of the clinical indicators of optimal counterpulsation (Table 32-1). Timing the IAB to ensure optimal increase in myocardial oxygen supply while reducing myocardial oxygen demand is another aspect of monitoring IABP effectiveness. Evaluation and adjustment of timing is based on assessment of the arterial waveform. The IABP is set in a 1:2 or 1:3 ratio to assist the operator in the identification of arterial waveform landmarks. Optimal IAB inflation occurs immediately upon the close of the aortic valve when ventricular diastole begins.[8] This action displaces blood back toward the aortic valve and forward down the aorta, increasing aortic pressure during ventricular diastole. As a result, the arterial waveform demonstrates an upstroke at the dicrotic notch, peaking at 10 to 15 mm Hg greater than the systolic pressure (Figure 32-2). Optimum deflation occurs just prior to the next ventricular systole.[8] Rapid deflation causes a "potential space" in the ascending aorta, which reduces aortic volume and associated afterload. As a result, ventricular systole effectively occurs at a lower pressure. This is observed on the arterial waveform as an IABP end diastolic pressure 5 to 15 mm Hg lower than the patient's diastolic pressure, and a lowered assisted peak systolic pressure[8] (Figure 32-2).

The third area of monitoring effectiveness involves weaning the patient from IABP support. Weaning is considered when the patient becomes hemodynamically stable with minimal pharmacological support.[2] Stability is evidenced by a CI of greater than 2.0 L/min/m^2; PCWP less than 20 mm Hg; systolic BP greater than 100 mm Hg with minimal or no vasopressor support; adequate peripheral perfusion; and absence of angina, dysrhythmias, or other indicators of myocardial ischemia. Weaning may be accomplished by decreasing the assist ratio or by reducing IAB volume. The ratio method begins by decreasing to a 1:2 ratio of one balloon cycle for two cardiac cycles. If the patient remains stable, the ratio is further decreased to 1:3, 1:4, or 1:8 as tolerated by the patient and in accord with the capability of the console. Weaning may also occur by gradually decreasing IAB volume until the balloon is only "fluttering" with each counterpulsation. When weaning by this method, it is important to inflate the balloon to full volume for 5 minutes every hour to prevent clot formation. During weaning the nurse must closely assess the patient's tolerance of each step in the process before proceeding further. If weaning is successful, the patient is prepared for balloon removal.

Prevention and Recognition of Complications

Although not always possible, a thorough baseline patient assessment prior to IAB insertion is helpful in timely recognition of vascular and other complications of IABP therapy. Ongoing nursing assessment and interventions associated with prevention and recognition of the most common potential complications are listed in Table 32-2.

Another complication easily corrected by nursing is suboptimal timing. Timing should be assessed at least at the beginning of each shift, at times of change in patient condition, and with activation of IABP console alarms. Timing errors, physiologic effects, and clinical signs and symptoms are described in Table 32-3.

Education for nurses, physicians, and others who may be involved in operating the IABP is vital to optimal IABP

TABLE 32-2 General Nursing Interventions for Potential Intraaortic Balloon Pump (IABP) Complications

Complication	Nursing assessment/intervention
Limb ischemia *r/t disruption in perfusion associated with presence of IAB in femoral artery*	Assess pulse, color, temperature of limb preinsertion of balloon Upon insertion, check peripheral pulses q15min × 2 hrs, then q30min × 2 hrs Assess pulses, color, and limb temperature q1h to q2h until IAB removal Prevent flexion of the affected hip and knee
Peripheral embolism or thrombosis *r/t clot formation on the balloon, prolonged bedrest, dislodgment of plaque or clots during insertion*	Frequent limb assessment as above Administer anticoagulation as ordered Do not allow the balloon to remain dormant longer than 30 min Passive ROM; frequent repositioning Assess for deterioration in mental status, renal function, and neurological or gastro-intestinal functioning
Bleeding at the insertion site	Observe insertion site for bleeding When catheter is removed, hold direct pressure for 30 to 45 min or until hemostasis is achieved
Thrombocytopenia *r/t destruction of platelets from IAB turbulence*	Daily PT, PTT, platelets, and HCT Observe for bleeding of gums and mucous membranes Test stool, gastric drainage, and urine for blood
Infection *r/t disruption in skin integrity*	Routine assessment of temperature Dressing changes with strict sterile technique Monitor WBC, differential Assess the site for signs of inflammation/infection Culture drainage from insertion site prn
Aortic dissection *r/t IAB insertion, effects of IAB action within aorta*	Monitor complaints of back pain Assess changes in VS, especially in combination with c/o back pain Provide sedation for agitated patients Prepare for circulatory collapse and removal of IAB as indicated
Immobilization *r/t catheter positioned in femoral artery*	Turn and provide back care q2h Administer analgesics or muscle relaxants prn Provide distraction Encourage relaxation techniques Assess the need for pressure-relieving bed or mattress
Cardiac status deterioration	Assess for optimum balloon timing Establish treatment plan for anginal pain Assess for c/o back pain Report deterioration trends to physician
Anxiety *r/t sounds of balloon console, interrupted sleep patterns, and fear of death*	Review the causes of the sound variations with patient/family Respond to alarms STAT Provide uninterrupted rest periods Encourage patient/family to express their fears Provide frequent information Administer sedation prn

TABLE 32-3 Effects and Indications of Improper Timing

Timing error	Physiologic effects	Clinical signs and symptoms
Early inflation 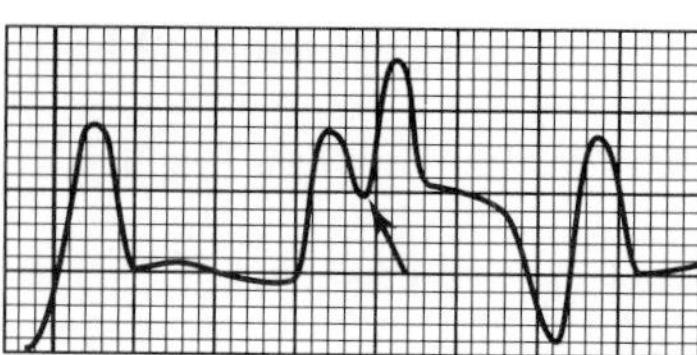 IAB inflation occurs without ventricular systole complete. Inflation point precedes the dicrotic notch occurring too high on the systolic peak.	Increased preload Decreased SV, SVI Increased myocardial O_2 demand Increased MVo_2 Possible damage to aortic valve Possible aortic regurgitation	Increased filling pressure (PCWP) Increased HR Decreased BP Deterioration of ABG Decreased CO, CI Increased pulmonary congestion
Late inflation 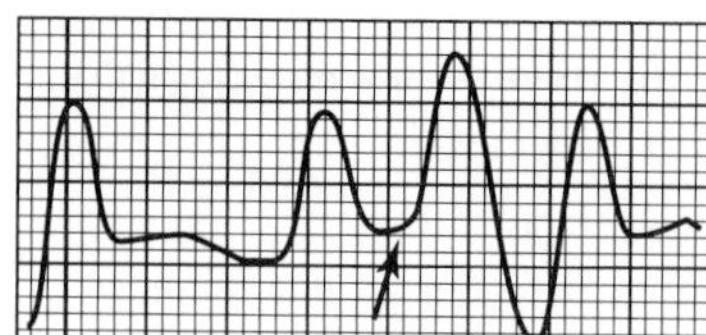 IAB inflation occurs after ventricular diastole has started. Inflation point occurs after the dicrotic notch revealing the notch or producing a U-shaped inflation point.	Lack of improvement in coronary artery perfusion Lack of improvement in systemic perfusion	Continued evidence of myocardial ischemia Inability to achieve hemodynamic stability Continued need for maximum pharmacological support
Early deflation 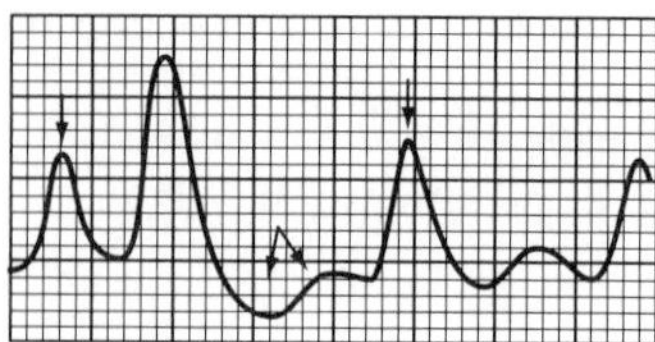 IAB deflated before ventricles ready for systole. Diastolic baseline raises to level of unassisted cardiac cycle. Assisted systolic peak equal to unassisted peak.	Decreased coronary artery filling pressure Aortic blood volume and associated diastolic pressure rises to levels associated without IABP support Loss of afterload reduction Loss of systolic unloading Myocardial O_2 demand not decreased	Evidence of myocardial ischemia may return—chest pain, dysrhythmias, ST-, and T-wave changes May continue to need maximum vasodilator support to reduce afterload
Late deflation 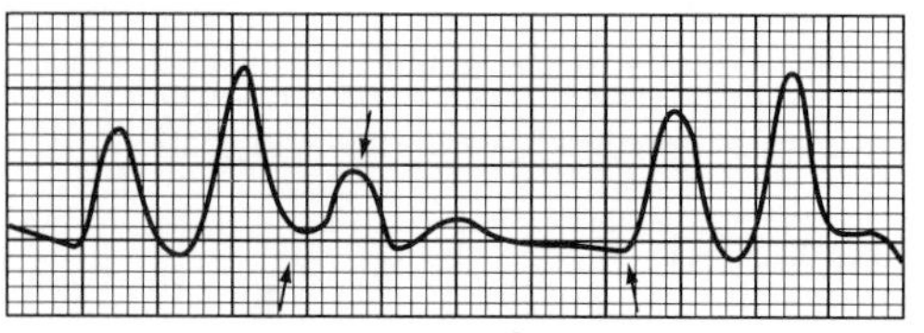 IAB still inflated as ventricular systole begins. Diastolic point of IAB higher than unassisted diastolic point. Systolic peak following IAB may be compromised.	Increased afterload Increased myocardial workload Increased myocardial O_2 demand Increased MVo_2 Impaired ventricular outflow	Decreased BP Increased HR Increased filling pressure (PCWP) Decreased CO, CI Increased SVR Chest pain Changes in LOC

support and the prevention and treatment of IAB complications. Critical care nurses must be well educated prior to caring for IAB patients. Instruction should include theory regarding counterpulsation and assessment of hemodynamic outcomes as well as hands-on practice. Many institutions provide integrated courses for physicians, nurses, and technicians to assure an adequate level of knowledge. Information regarding assessment of potential long-term vascular complications associated with the IAB must also be shared with nurses who will provide care to the IABP patient post-discharge from the ICU. Similar information may also be necessary as part of the discharge instructions to the patient and family.

Patient/Family Education and Support

Patient and family support remain another area of importance for the nurse. As with most patients in the critical care unit, the family of a patient requiring IABP support fear for the survival of their loved one. Patients, also afraid of dying, need the support of their significant others. It is vital for the nurse to ensure time for the patient and family to be together. Increased flexibility of visiting hours may be needed to enhance overall patient outcome since family members are often able to reassure and calm the patient. Family members also can be encouraged to help remind the patient not to bend the affected leg at the hip, or other key aspects of patient care. Families of IABP patients also have been shown to benefit from education that helps them understand what the IABP is and how it helps the patient.[7] The patient and family should be kept aware of changes in condition and therapy expectations. They also should have input into care goals. Providing an opportunity to consult with clergy, social workers, or other professionals may assist the family in obtaining needed support. In turn, they may be better able to support the patient and cooperate with the health care team.

TROUBLESHOOTING

Problems that interfere with the optimum benefits of IABP therapy arise from the IAB catheter, the console, or patient conditions. To provide for optimal patient outcome, basic troubleshooting techniques are an important aspect of care. The most common problems requiring troubleshooting intervention include the following:

Problem: Decreased Augmentation

CAUSE	CORRECTIVE ACTION
Decreased volume displacement as noted by decreased diastolic augmentation pressure on arterial waveform	Assure accurate waveform: check for air bubble in intransducer, flush dampened waveform, and assess hemodynamic status of patient Assure adequate helium in system: refill balloon if necessary and assess for an IAB leak Assure proper balloon placement: check x-ray for position of IAB tip 2 to 3 cm below aortic arch and reposition by MD

Problem: Console Alarms

CAUSE	CORRECTIVE ACTION
Loss of trigger	Validate proper trigger mode Replace detached electrodes Correct electrical interference Check pacer timing as indicated Institute internal trigger for cardiac arrest
Low helium	Assure helium tank opened Replace helium tank prn
Gas loss/low pressure	Assure helium line connections secure Assess for leak in IAB catheter as evidenced by blood in catheter or connecting tubing (blood may be seen as black flecks) Notify physician and prepare for balloon removal if blood present Dispel excess moisture from helium line
High pressure/catheter	Assess for internal/external catheter kink Assure IAB unwrapped completely at time of insertion Dispel excess moisture from helium line

System failure	Switch to another console Notify biomedical department and/or manufacturer

Problem: Patient Dysrhythmias

CAUSE	CORRECTIVE ACTION
Atrial fibrillation	Optimize timing per manufacturer's guidelines Decrease assist frequency to 1:2 if rapid ventricular rate Assess for hemodynamic changes
Paced rhythms	Assure appropriate trigger mode Filter pacer spikes for R-wave trigger Trigger on spike prn
Ventricular fibrillation	Defibrillate; pump is electrically isolated
Cardiac arrest	Initiate internal trigger or turn IABP off Do not allow balloon to lay dormant for more than 30 minutes Hand-inflate balloon every 5 minutes if internal trigger not used

Problem: Catheter Entrapment

CAUSE	CORRECTIVE ACTION
Undiagnosed catheter leak or intraluminal clot formation	Observe for signs of balloon rupture: blood in IAB or connecting tubing, decreased augmentation, or gas leak alarms If unable to remove balloon percutaneously, prepare patient for surgical removal

SUMMARY

Patients requiring the cardiac support provided by an IAB are severely compromised and present a complex nursing challenge. Maximum patient benefits can be afforded with skilled and knowledgeable care. Continuous assessment for the prevention of complications must be balanced with the assessment of IAB effects. Optimal timing can increase myocardial O_2 supply while decreasing O_2 demand, providing significant clinical improvements. Nursing interventions also must be directed toward relieving patient pain—emotional, physical, and spiritual—while encouraging family members to work as partners with the health care team to ensure positive patient outcomes.

REFERENCES

1. Reference deleted in proofs.
2. Bavin T, Self M: Weaning from intra-aortic balloon pump support, *Am J Nurs*, pp 54-59, October 1991.
3. Brodell G, et al: Intra-aortic balloon pump rupture and entrapment, *Cleve Clin J Med* 56(7):740-742, 1989.
4. Cox P, et al: *Plaque abrasion and intra-aortic balloon leak,* Presented at 58th Annual Scientific Assembly of the American College of Chest Physicians, Chicago, Oct 29, 1992. Publication pending.
5. Georgeson S, Coombs A, Eckman M: Prophylactic use of the intra-aortic balloon pump in high-risk cardiac patients undergoing noncardiac surgery: a decision analytic view, *Am J Med* 92:665-678, 1992.
6. Goran S: Vascular complications of the patient undergoing intra-aortic balloon pumping, *Crit Care Nurs Clin North Am* 1(1):459-468, 1989.
7. Goran S: Family perceptions of the intra-aortic balloon pumping experience, *Crit Care Nurs Clin North Am* 1(1):475-479, 1989.
8. Gould K: Perspectives on intra-aortic balloon pump timing, *Crit Care Nurs Clin North Am* 1(1):469-474, 1989.
9. Joseph D, Bates S: Intra-aortic balloon pumping: how to stay on course, *Am J Nurs* 90:42-47, 1990.
10. Kantrowitz A, Cardona R, Freed P: Percutaneous intra-aortic balloon counterpulsation, *Crit Care Clin* 8(4):819-837, 1992.
11. Kern M, et al: Enhanced coronary blood flow velocity during intra-aortic balloon counterpulsation in critically ill patients, *J Am Coll Cardiol* 2(2):359-368, 1993.
12. Kern M, et al: Augmentation of coronary blood flow by intra-aortic balloon pumping in patients after coronary angioplasty, *Circulation* 87(2):500-510, 1993.
13. Lazar J, et al: Outcome and complications of prolonged intra-aortic balloon counterpulsation in cardiac patients, *Am J Cardiol* 69:955-958, 1992.
14. Miller JS, et al: Vascular complications following intra-aortic balloon pump insertion, *Am Surg* 58:232-238, 1992.
15. Quaal S: *Comprehensive intraaortic balloon counterpulsation,* ed 2, St Louis, 1993, Mosby–Year Book.
16. Opie J: Hemorrhage control after removal of surgically implanted intra-aortic balloon pump, *Society of Thoracic Surgeons* 49:326-327, 1990.
17. Orr E, et al: Paraplegia following intra-aortic balloon support, *J Cardiovasc Surg* 30:1013-1014, 1989.
18. Riggle K, Oddi M: Spinal cord necrosis and paraplegia as complications of the intra-aortic balloon, *Crit Care Med* 17(5):475-476, 1989.

DEVICE GUIDELINE

33

Mechanical Circulatory Support Devices

S. Jill Ley, MS, RN, CCRN

DESCRIPTION

Mechanical circulatory support devices assume cardiac pumping functions, ensuring delivery of cardiac output (CO) to vital organs in cases of severe myocardial dysfunction. Temporary cardiac assist devices help maintain end-organ function while reducing myocardial oxygen demands, allowing time for either recovery of native heart function or cardiac transplantation. Depending on patient need and the particular device used, right, left, or biventricular cardiac support may be provided.

For most mechanical support systems, blood is diverted from a failing ventricle via inflow cannulae to the assist device, which then pumps blood back to the great vessels (aorta or pulmonary artery) via outflow cannulae, thus ensuring systemic or pulmonary perfusion. When ventricular recovery is anticipated, inflow cannulae are placed in the atria. Direct cannulation of the left ventricular (LV) apex is also possible and may improve inflow to the device. However, this approach is reserved for patients awaiting cardiac transplantation when the ventriculotomy is not a concern for ventricular recovery. Cannulae may be entirely implanted, as with the Novacor left-ventricular assist system (LVAS), or exit the chest or abdomen for connection to external devices (centrifugal or pneumatic pumps). Figure 33-1 illustrates several cannulation approaches that may be used during mechanical circulatory support.

More than a dozen different mechanical support systems are currently being evaluated. Although most systems are available only under research protocol as an investigational device, centrifugal ventricular assist devices (VADs) and the Abiomed system have been approved for general use by the Food and Drug Administration (FDA). Some information presented here may be generalized to other than the four devices mentioned. However, the reader is referred elsewhere for additional information regarding other circulatory support systems.[9]

Three types of centrifugal pumps (Medtronic-Biomedicus, Sarns-3M, and St. Jude Medical) have been approved by the FDA for cardiopulmonary bypass, with demonstrated safety and wide availability for temporary ventricular support. These devices operate by way of centrifugal force whereby a rapidly rotating impeller contained within a pump head creates kinetic energy, similar to a cyclone, propelling nonpulsatile blood flow through the system (Figure 33-2). The pump head is electromagnetically coupled to the device console, where pump flow is regulated by adjusting pump speed, which is measured in revolutions per minute (rpm).[5]

The Thoratec pneumatic VAD alternately compresses and evacuates air behind a blood-pumping sac, thus delivering pulsatile blood flow to the patient. A small air hose connects these external prosthetic ventricles to their drive console, which supplies power and air to the system (Figure 33-3). Console adjustments allow for support in one of several operation modes. The volume, or full-to-empty, mode is most commonly used. This mode automatically adjusts the device rate and flow to patient requirements while delivering a constant stroke volume of 65 cc.[2]

The Novacor LVAS is an electrically driven pump that is totally implanted within the abdomen and connected to its external console via an extension cable (Figure 33-4).

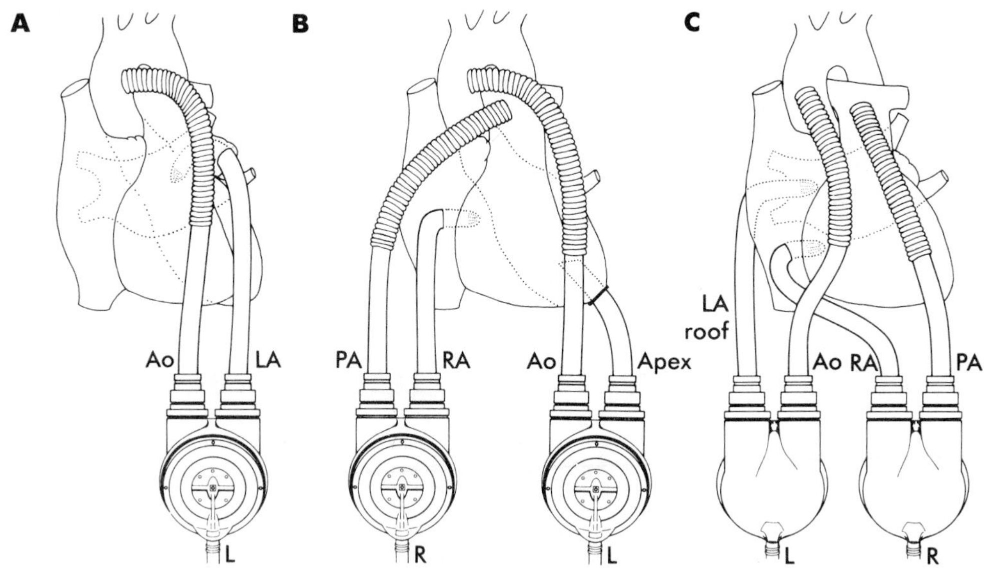

Figure 33-1 Cannulation approaches for univentricular or biventricular support. Inflow cannulation from the left heart is via the left atrial appendage **(A),** left ventricular apex **(B),** or LA roof via the interatrial groove **(C),** with return blood flow to the aorta. Right-heart cannulation is from the right atrium to the pulmonary artery (**B** and **C**). (Reprinted by permission of the *New England Journal of Medicine*. From Farrar DJ, et al: *N Engl J Med* 318:333, 1988.)

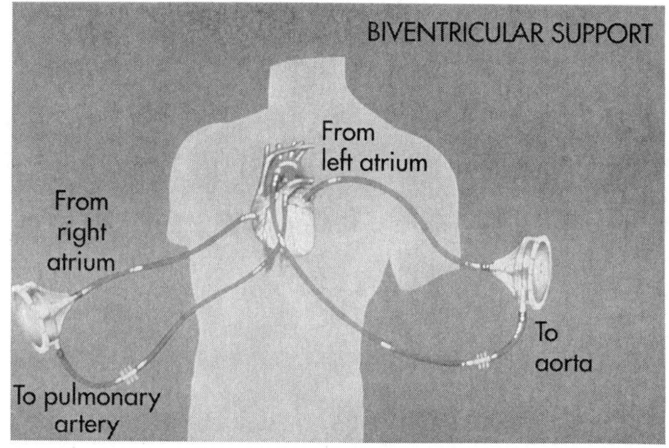

Figure 33-2 Cannulation and pump-head configuration for biventricular support with centrifugal VAD system. (Courtesy, Medtronic-Biomedicus, Eden Prairie, Minn.)

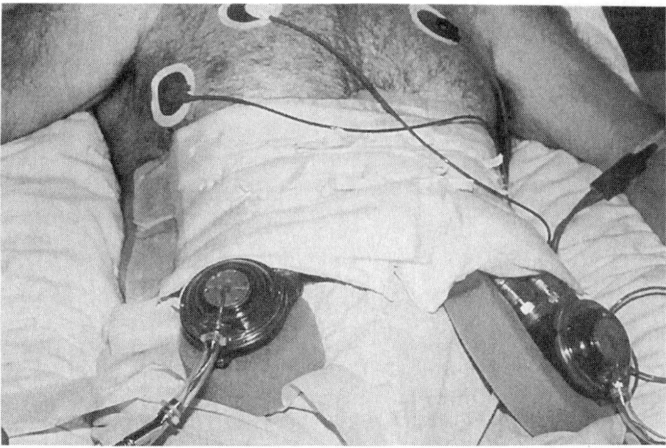

Figure 33-3 Patient with biventricular Thoratec VADs in place. (Courtesy, Thoratec Laboratories, Berkeley, Calif.)

The device uses dual pusher plates that symmetrically compress a blood sac in synchrony with LV events, delivering pulsatile blood flow from the LV apex to the aorta. Although primarily used as a bridge to transplant, this system may eventually be capable of long-term, permanent support for patients with end-stage heart failure.[8]

The Johnson & Johnson Hemopump is a unique, nonpulsatile device that incorporates a small pump and a fluid-purging system inside a soft silicone cannula placed within the LV apex. Rapid pump rotation at 25,000 rpm uses axial flow principles, similar to a jet turbine, pulling blood from the left ventricle and propelling it into the aorta.[6] A cable connects the device to its console, allowing for seven pump-speed adjustments and regulation of the fluid purging-system that ensures lubrication of the device (Figure 33-5).

INDICATIONS

Three groups of patients have been identified as potential candidates for mechanical circulatory support:

- Patients who cannot be weaned from cardiopulmonary bypass following cardiac surgery
- Patients in cardiogenic shock believed reversible with myocardial rest or treatment, such as acute myocardial

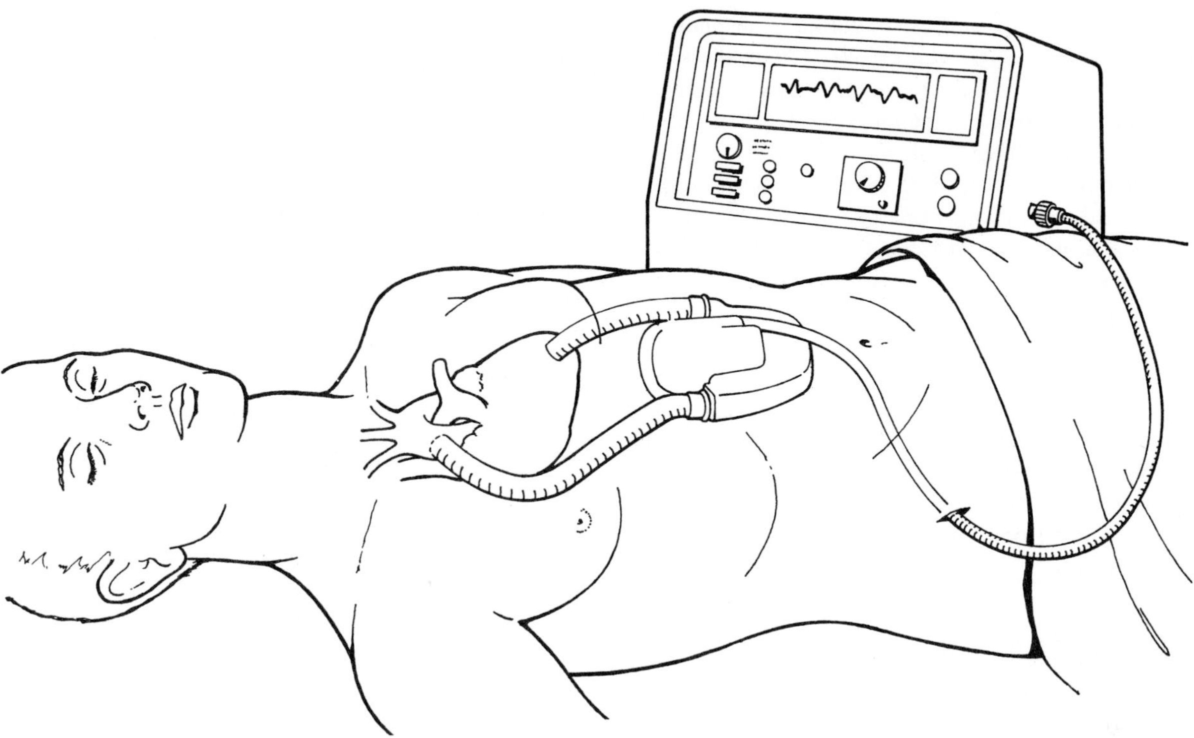

Figure 33-4 Anatomic placement of Novacor LVAS with console connection. (Redrawn from Reedy JE, et al: Progress in cardiovascular nursing, 4:1-9, 1989.)

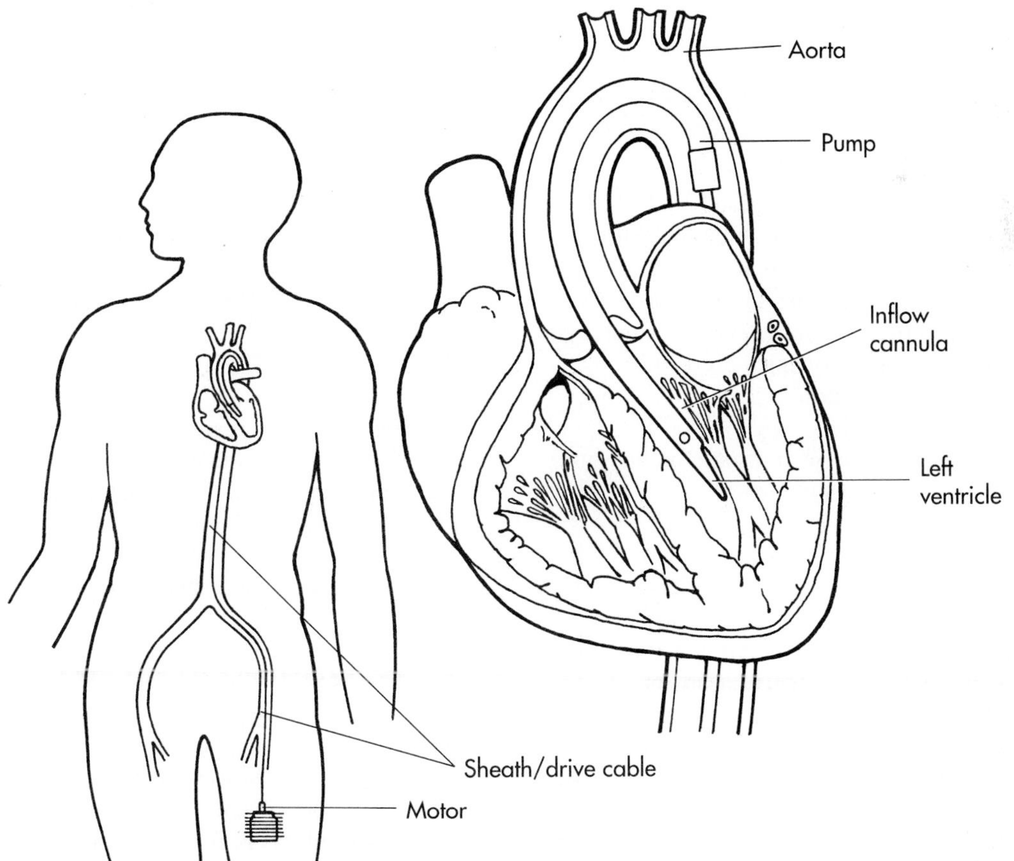

Figure 33-5 Anatomic placement of Johnson & Johnson Hemopump system via femoral artery cannulation. (Redrawn from Rutan PM, et al: *Crit Care Nurs Clin N Am* 1:529, 1989.)

infarction (MI), myocarditis, or cardiac transplant rejection
- Patients awaiting cardiac transplantation who deteriorate prior to location of a suitable donor.

Hemodynamic criteria have also been established for device insertion. Listed as follows, these criteria are seen despite optimum preload and maximal pharmacologic support[4]:
- CI <2 L/min/m^2
- MAP <60 mm Hg
- SBP <90 mm Hg
- RAP >20 mm Hg
- SVR >2100 dynes/sec/cm^{-5}
- UO <20 cc/hr

Additional selection criteria for postcardiotomy patients include an appropriate surgical repair and control of excess bleeding prior to VAD insertion. Bridge-to-transplant candidates must be free from standard contraindications to cardiac transplantation.

CONTRAINDICATIONS

The relative contraindications for the use of any type of ventricular support device include the following[4]:
- Renal failure
- Advanced age
- Infection

The absolute contraindications have been identified as follows[4]:
- Active malignancy
- Severe neurologic deficit
- Sepsis
- Hepatic failure
- Multiorgan failure

There are additional contraindications based on the specific device that may be used. For example, contraindications for use of the Novacor LVAS include fixed pulmonary hypertension and a body surface area (BSA) less than 1.5 m^2.[7] The Johnson & Johnson Hemopump device is contraindicated in the presence of the following[6]:
- Cardiac transplant candidates
- Significant blood dyscrasia
- Known or suspected aortic wall disease or aneurysm
- Aortic valve stenosis or insufficiency
- Prosthetic aortic valve

LIMITATIONS

Ventricular support devices, although able to provide temporary replacement function for a native heart, present significant limitations. Patients are essentially "tethered" to the hospital, in most cases in a literal sense, via attachment to a drive unit. Even if a totally implanted device can be used, the need for close monitoring for potential complications results in the need for hospitalization. In addition, these devices are primarily used as a bridge to cardiac transplantation. As a result, use of these devices is limited to those patients who are also reasonable transplant candidates. Current technology, with its external drive units and high risk for complications over time, significantly limits the application of this form of ventricular support. Ventricular support devices are clearly temporary interventions and not for long-term or permanent support at this time.

TABLE 33-1 Potential Complications of Mechanical Circulatory Support

Device	Characteristics	Potential complications
Centrifugal	Heparinization required Short-term support only (days) No size limitations	Hemolysis Unstable sternum
Pneumatic	Low-dose oral anticoagulation possible Long-term support possible (months) Size restriction (≥30 kg)	Risk of infection increases with long-term support
Novacor LVAS	Low-dose oral anticoagulation possible Long-term support possible (months) Left-sided support only Size restriction (BSA >1.5 m^2)	Risk of infection increases with long-term support Potential abdominal pocket infection Right ventricular failure
Hemopump	Heparinization required Femoral cannulation Intracardiac placement Left-sided support only Short-term support only (≤7 days)	Hemolysis Vascular injury Aortic valve or endocardial injury Right ventricular failure Cannula displacement

POTENTIAL COMPLICATIONS

According to registry data compiled for all support systems, the most frequent complications precluding device weaning include bleeding, disseminated intravascular coagulation (DIC), renal and biventricular failure, cyanosis secondary to unrecognized patent foramen ovale, inadequate CO, and inflow cannula obstruction.[3] Device-specific differences reveal that bleeding is more common with centrifugal devices,

TABLE 33-2 General Nursing Interventions During Mechanical Circulatory Support: Monitoring Guidelines

General considerations	Related nursing interventions
Nonpulsatile support system	Monitor MAP rather than SBP/DBP Anticipate ↓ peripheral pulses; assess skin color, temperature, capillary refill Pulse oximeter and Doppler invalid
Right-sided support system	Thermodilution CO inaccurate Calculate CO using Fick formula Monitor for s/s left-sided failure: ↓ perfusion, ↓ MAP, ↑ LAP/PCWP, ↓ / – CVP
Left-sided support system	Assess patient contribution to CO: thermodilution CO – VAD flow = patient CO Monitor for right-sided failure: ↓ perfusion, ↓ MAP, ↓ / – LAP/PCWP, ↑ CVP
Return of cardiac function	Improved pulsations from native heart on arterial pressure tracing ↑ patient CO/MAP, ↓ filling pressures Tolerance of ↓ device support Tolerance of ↓ pharmacologic support Minimal/absent dysrhythmias ABGs within normal limits
Worsening cardiac function	Decreased/absent pulsations from native heart on arterial pressure tracing ↓ patient CO/MAP, ↑ filling pressures Require ↑ device/pharmacologic support to maintain hemodynamic parameters ↑ cardiac dysrhythmias Worsening metabolic acidosis/hypoxemia

and infection occurs more frequently with pneumatic systems. Factors associated with in-hospital death for the recovery group (postcardiotomy and cardiogenic shock patients combined) included renal failure, perioperative MI, and infection. Factors precluding transplantation in the bridge-to-transplant group were bleeding; biventricular, renal, respiratory, or multiorgan failure; and infection. Additional device-specific characteristics and potential complications are listed in Table 33-1.

GENERAL NURSING INTERVENTIONS

Nursing care of the patient receiving mechanical circulatory support requires an understanding of the unique pathway for blood flow created by a device insertion and its impact on assessment parameters. Placement of a right-sided device creates an alternative pathway for thermodilution CO injectate, making this an invalid assessment parameter for RVAD patients.

Patients receiving unilateral circulatory support are at risk for failure of the contralateral ventricle, which occurs in up to 36% of patients.[1] Continuous monitoring of both right- and left-sided filling pressures in the immediate postoperative period allows for rapid assessment of this risk. Treatment may include traditional cardiac support measures, such as volume loading, inotropic support, and afterload reduction, or may require return to the operating room for placement of a second device yielding biventricular support.

A dampened arterial pressure waveform may be evident in patients with severe myocardial dysfunction. The decreased systolic and diastolic events associated with nonpulsatile support may yield a flat arterial waveform tracing. The mean arterial pressure (MAP) should be followed for hemodynamic assessments and titration of vasoactive medications in this situation. Additional monitoring guidelines that are unique to these patients are listed in Table 33-2.

Nursing care measures to promote optimal patient outcomes focus on four major areas: pulmonary hygiene, activity progression, nutritional support, and psychosocial support. Because device stability is enhanced with long-term support systems such as the Novacor LVAS and the Thoratec VAD, protocols for progression in these areas are generally more aggressive than with short-term systems.[7] Pulmonary hygiene measures are instituted to promote adequate oxygenation and decrease infection. This includes ventilatory adjustments to optimize arterial blood gases (ABGs), followed by prompt extubation and incentive spirometry as tolerated.

Activity progression varies considerably with the type of device used, but should be progressed as tolerated for recovery. Patients with short-term devices may tolerate active and passive range-of-motion exercises, with attention paid to proper patient positioning to ensure device stability. Long-term support devices permit more aggressive activities, including progressive ambulation, stationary bicycling, and use of light weights, while maintaining poststernotomy precautions.

TABLE 33-3 General Nursing Interventions During Mechanical Circulatory Support: Preventing Complications

Complication	Related nursing interventions
Bleeding	Monitor for excess bleeding: assess CT output q30min to q60min until stable Monitor lab values (PT, PTT, platelets, fibrinogen, Hgb, Hct) as ordered Note signs of excessive bleeding from lines/incisions Administer blood products as ordered Replace volume promptly to avoid hemodynamic instability Prepare for surgical reexploration if CT output remains excessive after coagulation tests normalized
Thromboemboli	Initiate anticoagulation promptly when initial postoperative bleeding is controlled Adjust anticoagulation as ordered to maintain desired coagulation parameters Monitor for s/s of embolic event: assess neurologic status/peripheral perfusion q2h to q4h
Infection	Monitor for s/s infection: assess temperature q2h to q4h, monitor WBC as ordered, assess line sites/incisions for evidence of infection, remove invasive lines and tubes ASAP, note quality of sputum/urine Administer antibiotic therapy as ordered Follow universal precautions, frequent hand washing, strict aseptic technique Sterile dressing changes to device exit site(s) daily Initiate enteral or parenteral nutrition promptly with progression to oral diet as tolerated
Multiorgan failure	Monitor for s/s of impaired renal function: ↑ BUN/creatinine, ↓ UO Monitor for s/s of impaired hepatic function: jaundice, dark urine, ↑ PT/PTT, ↑ bilirubin/liver enzymes Monitor for s/s of impaired gas exchange: refractory hypoxemia, abnormal breath sounds, abnormal CXR findings Assess and optimize cardiac support to increase end-organ perfusion Initiate supportive measures/treatment for sepsis as indicated

Benefits of nutritional support include reversed protein catabolism, improved wound healing, and promotion of immunocompetence. Initiation of either enteral or parenteral nutrition occurs within 48 hours after device placement, with progression to oral dietary intake as tolerated. Careful assessment of patient tolerance to increased fluid intake is warranted with any method of nutritional support, and may require the addition of diuretic therapy to prevent fluid overload.

Given the emergent nature of acute myocardial failure, patients and families are often unprepared psychologically for the institution of mechanical support. Important nursing interventions focus initially on relief of fear and anxiety through open, honest communication. Factual information about the device and regular progress reports are essential in the early stages of mechanical support. Available support systems within the institution, such as social services, clergy, or meeting former VAD patients, should be explored with patients and families, as well as calling on previously effective coping strategies.

For patients facing long-term hospitalization while waiting for transplantation, feelings of powerlessness may be overwhelming. Additionally, feelings of guilt and uncertainty occur during the wait for an organ donor, and should be discussed and acknowledged as expected occurrences in this situation. Providing opportunities for patients to exert control over their environment (dietary choices, visiting hours, daily schedules, etc.) may limit these feelings. In addition, becoming knowledgeable about their device and participating in maintenance activities is an additional strategy that has been advocated by some centers.[7]

Monitoring for and preventing complications of mechanical circulatory support are critical to achieving optimal patient outcomes. Although some complications may be transient with proper intervention, such as immediate postoperative bleeding, infectious complications or multiorgan failure are associated with high mortality and often prevent ventricular recovery or transplantation. Current practices vary regarding isolation procedures for these patients. Although some centers advocate reverse isolation, there is no evidence that its use decreases infectious complications or improves patient outcomes.[7] Assessment parameters and nursing interventions that focus on prevention of common complications are addressed in Table 33-3.

TROUBLESHOOTING

Troubleshooting device- or patient-related complications during mechanical support is a final important aspect of nursing care. Two major areas of concern include correction of inadequate CO and emergency support measures. Low CO in patients receiving biventricular support is usually due to factors other than impaired contractility, because the devices can assume 100% of cardiac pumping function. However, physiologic principles apply in that the pumps cannot deliver an adequate stroke volume if inadequately filled or ejecting against high afterload. Although the CO may be inadequate or even absent, cardiac compressions are contraindicated for these patients because dislocation of the device and possible ventricular damage may result. Troubleshooting during mechanical circulatory support focuses on the problem of decreased CO with probable causes and corrective actions as follows:

Problem: Decreased Cardiac Output

CAUSE	CORRECTIVE ACTION
Device malfunction	Assess for sights and sounds of proper device function and console controls Note decreased/absent device sounds, blank or inappropriate console signals Initiate emergency corrective measures or switch to another console as indicated in collaboration with biomedical department
Hypovolemia	Assess for signs of decreased preload: low filling pressures, decreased UO, I < O, weight loss, flat neck veins, thirst Assess centrifugal devices for excess "chatter" (increased movement and vibration of device tubings) Administer blood products or colloids as ordered
Increased afterload	Assess for signs of high afterload: increased SVR/PVR, decreased pulses, cool and clammy skin, cyanotic nail beds, increased BP (decreased if pump output severely impaired) Administer vasodilator therapy as ordered
Decreased afterload	Assess for signs of excessive vasodilation: low SVR, hot and flushed skin, bounding pulses, low BP Evaluate possible etiology, including allergic reaction or sepsis Administer vasopressor therapy as ordered
Cardiac arrest	Do not initiate chest compressions Assess and treat underlying problem Initiate console adjustments/device troubleshooting to optimize blood flow through the device
Ventricular tachycardia or fibrillation	Assess patient response to rhythm change: may be well tolerated with maintenance of CO via device For nonemergent cardioversion or defibrillation, administer sedation prior to countershock Place paddles on chest to avoid contact with metal surfaces of device Cardiovert/defibrillate according to standard procedure

SUMMARY

Current results with use of mechanical circulatory support devices are encouraging: approximately 45% of patients in the recovery group tolerated device weaning, with 25% eventually being discharged from the hospital.[3] More than 85% of these patients were in NYHA Class I-II, indicating excellent recovery and potential for return to normal activities. For patients in the bridge-to-transplant group, 69% were able to receive a transplant and 66% were discharged from the hospital.[3] Outcomes for these patients following transplantation are equivalent to the cardiac transplant population as a whole, indicating appropriate allocation of organ donors for this group of patients. Nursing care for patients requiring mechanical circulatory support is critical to achieving optimal patient outcomes. Only through an in-depth understanding of both the patient and the device technology can the nurse provide safe, appropriate, and effective care to these challenging patients.

REFERENCES

1. Farrar DJ, et al: Thoratec VAD system as a bridge to heart transplantation, *J Heart Transplant* 9:415-423, 1990.
2. Ley SJ, Hill JD: Thoratec ventricular assist device. In Quaal SJ, editor: *Cardiac mechanical assistance beyond balloon pumping,* St Louis, 1993, Mosby–Year Book.
3. Pae WE: Ventricular assist devices and total artificial hearts: a combined registry experience, *Ann Thorac Surg* 55:295-298, 1993.
4. Pennington DG, et al: Panel 1: patient selection, *Ann Thorac Surg* 47:77-81, 1989.
5. Quaal SJ: Centrifugal ventricular assist devices, *AACN Clin Iss Crit Care Nurs* 2:515-526, 1991.
6. Rountree WD: The hemopump temporary cardiac assist system, *AACN Clin Iss Crit Care Nurs* 2:562-574, 1991.
7. Shinn JA, et al: Nursing care of the patient on mechanical circulatory support, *Ann Thorac Surg* 55:288-294, 1993.
8. Shinn JA, Oyer PE: Novacor ventricular assist system. In Quaal SJ, editor: *Cardiac mechanical assistance beyond balloon pumping,* St Louis, 1993, Mosby–Year Book.
9. Smith RG, Cleavinger M: Current perspectives on the use of circulatory assist devices, *AACN Clin Iss Crit Care Nurs* 2:488-499, 1991.

UNIT

III

Respiratory System

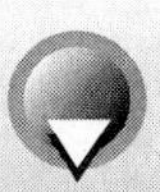

CLINICAL GUIDELINE

34

Acute Respiratory Failure

Pamela Becker Weilitz, MSN(R), RN

DESCRIPTION

Acute respiratory failure (ARF) results from major abnormalities in ventilation, gas exchange, perfusion, or pulmonary compliance resulting in hypoxemia, hypercapnia, or both.[9] The respiratory system is unable to supply oxygen adequately to maintain metabolism and/or cannot sufficiently eliminate carbon dioxide, resulting in respiratory acidosis. Clinically, there is a sudden deterioration in the patient's arterial blood gas (ABG) values indicating acute pulmonary insufficiency: a respiratory rate of >20 breaths per minute, a $Pa{O_2}$ <60 mm Hg with an $Fi{O_2}$ >.50 and a $Pa{CO_2}$ >45 mm Hg.[9]

PATHOPHYSIOLOGY

ARF can develop from a primary respiratory failure related to an acute lung injury or resulting from exacerbation of underlying lung disease. The disease processes leading to ARF, categorized by etiology, are identified in Table 34-1.

Patients with COPD are at particular risk of developing acute respiratory failure. Risk factors include airway obstruction, decreased expiratory flow, excessive secretions, bronchospasm, and mucosal edema. Prolonged, severe COPD may lead to cor pulmonale, right heart failure, and increased pulmonary vascular resistance due to degenerative, fibrotic perivascular changes in the lungs. This results in a permanent increase in pulmonary vascular resistance and a severe increase in right ventricular afterload. The right heart fails while attempting to pump against extremely high pulmonary pressures.

Acute respiratory distress syndrome (ARDS) is an extreme form of respiratory failure. ARDS is ARF refractory to oxygen therapy, with increased pulmonary capillary pressure, or increased pulmonary capillary permeability, and diffuse pulmonary edema.[22] See Guideline 35 regarding ARDS.

ARF may present as hypoxic respiratory failure, ventilatory respiratory failure, or a combination. **Hypoxic respiratory failure** is characterized by profound hypoxemia that responds poorly to oxygen therapy as a result of overwhelming lung disease such as pneumonia or pulmonary edema. Hypoxia, the greatest threat to the patient, is caused by alveolar hypoventilation, right-to-left shunting, impaired diffusion, decreased inspired oxygen, increased oxygen consumption ($V{O_2}$), and ventilation-perfusion (V/Q) mismatching.[59] Hypercapnia is the hallmark of **ventilatory respiratory failure,** stemming from failure of the ventilatory pump, abnormal gas exchange, and alterations in breathing patterns.[17] Ventilatory respiratory failure often occurs over time with an insidious rise in the arterial carbon dioxide level. Although hypoxia may be present, it usually responds well to oxygen therapy.

Alveolar hypoventilation may result in hypoxia. Alveolar ventilation (V_A) is the volume of inspired air available for gas exchange each minute. Factors influencing V_A include minute ventilation (respiratory rate × tidal volume) and dead-space ventilation (that portion of ventilation that does not participate in gas exchange), and carbon dioxide production ($V{CO_2}$). $V{CO_2}$ is dependent on factors influencing oxygen consumption: temperature, oxygen delivery, and tissue utilization of oxygen.[9] Alveolar ventilation is altered by changes in respiratory rate, tidal volume, dead-space ventilation, acid-base status, and carbon dioxide production, and is reflected in the $Pa{CO_2}$.

Hypoventilation is an arterial partial pressure of carbon dioxide ($Pa{CO_2}$) above 45 mm Hg resulting from a decreased minute ventilation (V_E) and alveolar gas exchange. The imbalance between carbon dioxide production and elimination results in an increasing $Pa{CO_2}$ and a decreasing $Pa{O_2}$.

Ventilation-perfusion (V/Q) mismatching is a common cause of hypoxemia.[5] Areas of the lung that receive similar amounts of ventilation and blood flow have matched ven-

TABLE 34-1 Disease Processes Leading to Acute Respiratory Failure

Impaired alveolar ventilation

COPD: emphysema, bronchitis, asthma, cystic fibrosis
Restrictive lung disease: interstitial pulmonary fibrosis, pleural effusion, pneumothorax, obesity, diaphragmatic paralysis, kyphoscoliosis
Neuromuscular defects: Guillain-Barré syndrome, myasthenia gravis, multiple sclerosis, muscular dystrophy
Respiratory center depression: drug-induced cerebral infarction, endocrine and metabolic disorders, e.g. encephalitis

Diffusion disturbances

Pulmonary/interstitial fibrosis
Pulmonary edema
ARDS
Anatomic loss of functioning lung tissue

Ventilation or perfusion disturbances

Pulmonary emboli
Atelectasis
Pneumonia
Emphysema
Chronic bronchitis
Bronchiolitis
ARDS

Right-to-left shunting

Atelectasis
Pneumonia
Pulmonary edema
Pulmonary emboli
Oxygen toxicity

Adapted from Swearingen PL, Sommers MS, Miller K: *Manual of critical care,* St Louis, 1988, Mosby–Year Book.

TABLE 34-2 DRGs Related to ARF

DRG #	Name of DRG	Average LOS (days)
79	Respiratory infections and inflammations, age >17 years with CC	10.7
80	Respiratory infections and inflammations, age >17 years without CC	7.4
87	Pulmonary edema and respiratory failure	7.5
88	Chronic obstructive pulmonary disease	6.9
89	Simple pneumonia and pleurisy, age >17 years with CC	8.0
92	Interstitial lung disease with CC	8.1
96	Bronchitis and asthma, age >17 years with CC	6.2
97	Bronchitis and asthma, age >17 years without CC	4.9
99	Respiratory signs and symptoms with CC	4.1
100	Respiratory signs and symptoms without CC	2.8
475	Respiratory system diagnosis with ventilator support	13.7

CC: Complication or comorbid condition
(Source: *St Anthony's DRG guidebook 1995*, Reston, Va, 1994, St Anthony.

tilation/perfusion. V/Q mismatching may result from vascular occlusion such as pulmonary emboli, low cardiac output, or hypoxic vasoconstriction or gravity resulting in a decrease or absence of blood flow to ventilated alveoli.[1] This wasted ventilation or ventilation in excess of perfusion is referred to as dead-space ventilation. When the ratio of ventilation to perfusion is extremely high, physiological dead space is the result.[1] The other extreme of V/Q mismatching is intrapulmonary shunt.

Intrapulmonary shunting is that portion of the pulmonary blood flow not exposed to functioning alveoli. It provides an index of the lungs' efficiency at gas exchange.[24] When blood perfuses an area with essentially no ventilation, the blood is "shunted" past the lung. Hypercarbic and hypoxemic blood is returned to the left side of the heart for distribution to the systemic arterial circulation.[1] Clinical examples of intrapulmonary shunt include mucous plugging, bronchial obstruction, and fluid-filled alveoli. Measures of intrapulmonary shunt include the alveolar-arterial (A-a) oxygen gradient, the arterial/alveolar ratio (a/A), and the $Pa{O_2}/Fi{O_2}$ ratio. The alveolar-arterial oxygen tension difference is a measure of the efficiency of oxygen transfer from the lung to the arterial blood. The A-a gradient is determined by calculating the alveolar air using the alveolar air equation (see the Box on p. 341).

A more accurate measure of intrapulmonary shunt is determined by calculating the arterial/alveolar (a/A) ratio. The a/A ratio is determined by dividing the partial arterial pressure of oxygen ($Pa{O_2}$) by the alveolar oxygen ($PA{O_2}$), derived from the alveolar air equation (see Box). A normal a/A ratio is greater than .75; less than .75 indicates an increased intrapulmonary shunt.[24]

Calculating the a/A Gradient

Alveolar-arterial oxygen gradient

$$P(A - a)O_2 = PAO_2 - PaO_2$$

where
$$PAO_2 = [(P_B - PH_2O) \times FiO_2] - PaCO_2/RQ,$$
P_B = barometric pressure (760 mm Hg),
PH_2O = water vapor pressure (47 mm Hg),
FiO_2 = fraction of inspired oxygen (.21 room air),
$PaCO_2$ = measured partial pressure of arterial carbon dioxide,
RQ = respiratory quotient (0.8).

After calculating the alveolar air, subtract the measured partial pressure of the arterial oxygen from the alveolar air. On room air the normal A-a gradient is about 10 mm Hg. As shunting increases, the gradient widens, indicating a problem with getting oxygen into the blood.

Arterial-alveolar ratio

$$a/A \text{ ratio} = \frac{PaO_2}{PAO_2}$$

where
PaO_2 = measured partial pressure of arterial oxygen,
PAO_2 = alveolar air.

The a/A ratio should be .75 or greater. An a/A ratio of less than .75 indicates increased shunting.

Diffusion impairment occurs when the alveolar capillary membrane becomes thickened, impairing gas diffusion across the alveolar-capillary membrane. This can result from interstitial fibrosis, interstitial pneumonia, or collagen-vascular diseases such as scleroderma or hyaline membrane disease.

LENGTH OF STAY/ANTICIPATED COURSE

ARF is a common and frequent terminal complication of severe COPD.[16] Length of stay is variable, from days to weeks. DRG 87: Pulmonary edema and respiratory failure, averages a length of stay of 7.8 days.[20] Respiratory failure may represent the primary diagnosis or a complication or comorbidity of another DRG. A listing of possible DRGs related to ARF may be found in Table 34-2.

If respiratory failure is treated early, the patient may require only the recommended 7.5 days of hospitalization, with 3 to 5 days in the intensive care unit and 3 to 4 days on mechanical ventilation. If the respiratory failure is severe (e.g., severe COPD with bacterial pneumonia, or respiratory failure as a result of congestive heart failure) the patient may require prolonged mechanical ventilation and possibly weeks or months of hospitalization. The goal of therapy is reversal of the hypoxemia and hypercapnia and correction of the underlying problem.

MANAGEMENT TRENDS AND CONTROVERSIES

Management of the patient with ARF should include respiratory muscle rest, correction of hypoxia and acidosis, controlling shock, treatment of infection, and nutritional repletion.[17] The decision to institute mechanical ventilation should take into consideration the cause of ARF, the potential responsiveness to therapy, the degree of airflow limitation, functional and nutritional status, and patient/family advance directives for health care.[11,16]

The first priority is to correct hypoxemia. This may be done with administration of oxygen therapy or, in many instances, the use of mechanical ventilation. Since effective oxygenation is the first and highest priority, 100% oxygen should always be used after successful intubation, until adequate oxygenation has been documented.[19] Mechanical ventilation will provide a controlled oxygen delivery and support respiratory muscle fatigue. The modes of mechanical ventilation most often used for patients in respiratory failure include assisted mandatory ventilation (AMV), synchronized intermittent mandatory mechanical ventilation (SIMV), and pressure support ventilation (PSV). (See Guideline 41 on mechanical ventilation.) After ventilatory support has been initiated and the patient stabilized, the goal is to maintain adequate gas exchange without complications, while the primary cause of the respiratory failure is treated or allowed to resolve.[19]

The goal for reversing respiratory acidosis is to improve carbon dioxide removal and increase the efficiency of the respiratory muscles. Providing mechanical ventilatory support will help reverse respiratory acidosis. Monitoring arterial carbon dioxide level ($Paco_2$) and pH will determine if ventilation is adequate.

Bronchodilator therapy is initiated to treat bronchospasm. Intravenous aminophylline is given to achieve a serum level of 10 to 20 μg/ml with daily serum levels to monitor the patient. Nebulized beta agonists are used to open peripheral airways and maximize bronchodilatation. Steroid therapy may be used to reduce airway edema and swelling. Therapy may be systemic, as in prednisone, or by metered dose inhaler (MDI) such as beclomethasone dipropionate.

Chest physiotherapy includes chest percussion, postural drainage, and vibration and is indicated for patients who have difficulty clearing secretions, with expectorated sputum production greater than 25 to 30 cc every 24 hours or infiltrates on chest radiograph.[2] In addition, coughing and deep-breathing exercises are used to help promote lung expansion and mobilize secretions. If the patient is unable to mobilize secretions, suctioning may be necessary. Adequate fluid intake is also helpful in keeping secretions from becoming thick and increasing the risk of airway plugging.

Antibiotics are initiated in patients with a known infection or who are suspected of an underlying infection as evidenced by sputum changes, increased temperature, or positive sputum cultures.

Intravenous (IV) fluids are used to maintain fluid balance, prevent dehydration, and prevent secretions from becoming thick and tenacious. Fluid intake ranges from 4 to 6 liters per day, if not contraindicated by cardiac or renal impairment.

Patients with COPD are generally malnourished,[18] most likely due to an increase in resting energy expenditure.[10] Malnutrition and ARF in the patient with COPD have been shown to have deleterious effects, especially in successful weaning from mechanical ventilation.[10] Malnutrition has been associated with decreased inspiratory muscle strength, diaphragmatic mass, and ventilatory drive, and increased risk of nosocomial pneumonia. Laaban et al. report that ventilatory support was required more frequently in patients with COPD and ARF who presented with malnutrition on admission (66%) than those with normal nutritional status (35%).[10] The goal of nutritional support is to restore lean body mass. Nutritional assessment should be done early in the acute illness and aggressive nutritional support initiated.[10]

ASSESSMENT

PARAMETER	ANTICIPATED ALTERATION
Arterial blood gases (ABG)	
• pH	Decreased: <7.35
• Pao_2	Decreased: <60 mm Hg
• $Paco_2$	Increased: >45 mm Hg
• Sao_2	Decreased: <90%
	Initially the patient may show respiratory alkalosis. With increasing work of breathing and respiratory muscle fatigue, respiratory acidosis will develop rapidly. Note: hypoxemia, not hypercapnia, is the greatest threat to the patient.
Minute ventilation	5 to 10 L/min normally but increased >10 L/min as work of breathing increases
A-a gradient	Widened
a/A ratio	Decreased: <.75
Pao_2/Fio_2 ratio	Decreased: <286

Respiratory Status

Rate	Tachypnea
Lung sounds	Crackles, wheezes *due to bronchospasm and increased secretions* Hyperresonate chest on percussion in patients with emphysema or advanced COPD *due to air trapping.*
Breathing pattern	Labored Use of accessory muscles of respiration Dyspnea on exertion or at rest *due to increased work of breathing*
Secretions	Purulent sputum *in patients with chronic bronchitis or an acute infectious process*
Cough	Productive
Pulmonary artery pressure	Normal to elevated PAD >15 *due to underlying lung disease*
Chest radiograph	Infiltrates

Pulmonary function	Decreased FEV_1 *in patients with asthma or chronic bronchitis* Increased FRC, TLC; decreased VC, FEV_1 *in patients with emphysema*
Cardiovascular Status	
HR	Tachycardia
Rhythm	Cardiac dysrhythmias, especially atrial *due to cardiac strain associated with increased pulmonary vascular resistance*
BP	Decreased *due to vasodilatation*
Extremities	Digital clubbing *due to chronic hypoxemia* Pedal edema *in patients with chronic bronchitis and cor pulmonale* Cyanosis *due to peripheral vasoconstriction*
Cardiac output	Normal to decreased: <4 L/min *as heart rate increases*
Hemoglobin	Elevated: >18 g/dl *due to underlying COPD and increased production of red blood cells to increase arterial oxygen levels*
Hematocrit	Elevated: >52% *due to underlying COPD*
Neurological Status	
LOC	Restlessness Anxiety Confusion Lethargy Coma *Due to decreased oxygen levels*
Other	
Subjective s/s	Fatigue Headache
Weight	Weight gain/loss *If the patient is malnourished there will usually be a history of weight loss. If the patient has cardiovascular compromise, as in congestive heart failure or pulmonary edema, there may be a weight gain.*
Malnourishment	Poor skin turgor Decreased body weight Decreased albumin levels Decreased lymphocyte count Altered mental status Brittle and split nails Flaky, dry skin with spots or bruises Spongy, tender gums that bleed easily Hypothermia

PLAN OF CARE

INTENSIVE PHASE

Patients with acute respiratory failure require intensive nursing care due to the life-threatening nature of the illness. The focus of care is monitoring and promoting effective gas exchange, breathing pattern, and airway clearance.

PATIENT CARE PRIORITIES	EXPECTED PATIENT OUTCOMES
Impaired gas exchange *r/t alveolar hypoventilation, right-to-left shunting, or ventilation/perfusion mismatch*	Adequate oxygenation • PaO_2 60 to 100 mm Hg • SaO_2 >92%

Plan of Care (cont'd)

	Adequate ventilation • pH 7.35 to 7.45 • $Paco_2$ 35 to 45 mm Hg or corrected to patient baseline Absence of signs and symptoms of hypoxia such as restlessness, light-headedness, dizziness, and cyanosis
Ineffective breathing pattern *r/t increased work of breathing and use of accessory muscles of respiration*	Maintain effective breathing pattern through use of diphragmatic breathing and pursed-lip breathing
Ineffective airway clearance *r/t* *Retained secretions* *Bronchospasm* *Bronchial edema*	Patent airway Clear breath sounds on auscultation Baseline respiratory rate pattern, and depth Clear chest radiograph
Inability to sustain spontaneous ventilation *r/t increased work of breathing and respiratory muscle fatigue*	Able to sustain spontaneous ventilation
Anxiety *r/t* *Dyspnea* *Disease process and prognosis* *Limited understanding of diagnostic procedures*	Patient demonstrates decreased level of anxiety Patient uses breathing techniques to reduce dyspnea Patient/family verbalize understanding of disease process and its relationship to therapy used Patient/family participate in planning and implementation of care
High risk for infection *r/t* *Retained secretions* *Use of respiratory equipment* *Impaired pulmonary defense mechanisms secondary to COPD*	Absence or resolution of pulmonary infection No clinical manifestation of pulmonary infection Chest radiograph, sputum and culture, and sensitivity show no evidence of infection
Nutrition: less than body requirements *r/t prolonged debilitating lung disease*	Patient maintains a positive nitrogen balance Weight maintained/gained Absence or resolution of any signs of malnutrition Regular elimination

INTERVENTIONS

Provide supplemental oxygen therapy to maintain $Sao_2 > 92\%$.

Encourage pursed-lip breathing to *improve oxygenation and control breathing pattern.*

Provide humidification *to help keep secretions thin and reduce risk of airway plugging.*

Administer bronchodilators per order *to treat bronchospasm.*

Monitor lung sounds q1h to q2h for any increase/decrease of abnormal/adventitious breath sound such as crackles, wheezes, or gurgles.

Monitor breathing pattern q1h to q2h for rate, rhythm, sternal retraction, use of accessory muscles of respiration, *which indicate increased WOB.*

Position to promote V/Q stabilization, with good lung down *to promote increased perfusion and improved oxygenation.*

Promote airway clearance using measures to remove secretions:

- Chest physiotherapy and postural drainage if >30 cc's of secretions per 24 hrs, or infiltrate by chest radiograph
- Turn and position q2h
- Cough and deep breathe q2h to q4h
- Incentive spirometry q2h to q4h

Provide adequate hydration (4 to 6 quarts per day unless contraindicated by heart failure) *to facilitate removal of secretions.*

Monitor fluid balance and daily weights *to determine fluid volume overload.*

Provide mechanical ventilation as ordered *to maintain adequate gas exchange and provide respiratory muscle rest.*

Assist patient to quantify dyspnea/breathlessness by using shortness of breath scale 0 to 10 *to show progress and help reduce anxiety.*

Plan of Care (cont'd)

Prevent physiological factors that promote restlessness and anxiety.
Encourage verbalization of anxiety or fear related to dyspnea, course of therapy, diagnostic procedures, and plan of care.
Perform treatments in unhurried manner, allowing rest periods between treatments *to reduce breathlessness.*
Involve patient/family in planning for care *to help reduce anxiety.*
Use strict aseptic technique in airway care and other procedures *to decrease risk of infection.*
Monitor visitors for signs of infections; e.g., colds.
Establish optimal caloric and fluid intake with physician and dietitian.
Schedule treatments to mobilize secretions at least 1 hour before meals.
Provide conditions conducive to eating:

- Oral hygiene before and after meals and prn
- Position patient for comfort and within easy reach of food
- Assist with feeding as needed
- Encourage family to participate in feeding
- Remove evidence of sputum or anything that may hinder the patient's appetite

If the patient is receiving enteral nutrition:

- Ensure patency and proper location of feeding tube *to prevent aspiration*
- Place patient in semi-Fowler's position before feeding *to reduce risk of aspiration*
- Administer bolus or continuous feedings as indicated

Monitor for abdominal cramps, diarrhea, constipation, nausea, and glucosuria *to assess patient tolerance.*

INTERMEDIATE PHASE

Once the patient no longer requires intensive care, the individual will be transferred to a medical-surgical or pulmonary care area. If prolonged mechanical ventilation and weaning are required, the patient may be transferred to a ventilation rehabilitation unit or hospital.[11,13] Retrospective studies comparing the length of stay, cost, and outcomes of patients cared for on a specialized unit or hospital versus the intensive care unit (ICU) have shown decreased cost,[4,7,8,12,15] improved patient/family satisfaction, increased multidisciplinary planning, and increased success in weaning the patient from mechanical ventilation.* Patients like the relaxed, homelike setting and increased visiting options.[4,15] What is still needed are prospective, randomized studies to determine which care setting (ICU, ventilator rehabilitation unit, or general medical-surgical care unit) results in the best outcomes for the patient.[6]

The care priorities for the patient in the intermediate phase are a continuation of those in the ICU with the addition of extensive patient education and discharge planning for home care.

PATIENT CARE PRIORITIES	EXPECTED PATIENT OUTCOMES
High risk for dysfunctional ventilator weaning *r/t disease process and slow recovery*	Patient able to maintain spontaneous ventilation Patient/family understand the weaning plan
High risk for impaired health maintenance *r/t knowledge deficit*	Patient/family verbalize understanding of medication, dietary, activity, and therapeutic procedures for home

INTERVENTIONS

Assess patient/family level of understanding and ability to provide home care regimens.
Instruct the patient/family on measures *to prevent respiratory infection:*

- Promoting adequate nutrition
- Use of good handwashing
- Recognizing signs and symptom of respiratory infection such as sputum changes, febrile state, increase in shortness of breath, cough or fatigue

Teach patient/family breathing exercises *to promote control of breathing:*

- Pursed-lip breathing

*References 4, 7, 8, 12, 14, 15, 21.

Plan of Care (cont'd)

- Diaphragmatic breathing
- Orthopneic positioning

Teach patient/family medication regimen, including medications, action, frequency, schedule, and side effects.

Describe plan for follow-up visits, including purpose, when and where to come, whom to see, what specimens to bring, and what laboratory and radiograph tests are planned.

Provide opportunity for and encourage patient/family questions and verbalization of anxiety regarding discharge regimen.

Provide information regarding community health agencies such as the American Lung Association, Better Breathing clubs, Meals on Wheels, transportation and social services.

TRANSITION TO DISCHARGE

The patient and family need to learn about the care that will be needed for discharge from the hospital. Nursing care priorities will focus on reducing the patient's and family's anxiety, and teaching the care measures necessary for discharge. It is important that the patient and family have a good understanding of the care measures necessary to prevent recurrent episodes of ARF. Key points to be taught before discharge include breathing techniques such as pursed-lip and diaphragmatic breathing; signs and symptoms of infection such as sputum color change, temperature, and shortness of breath; how to prevent an infection; when to call the physician; medication regimen; an exercise plan; a nutritional plan; energy conservation techniques; and available community resources. Getting the patient with COPD involved in a pulmonary rehabilitation program will help teach the importance of exercise, techniques for self-care, and how to plan the activities of daily living to decrease the work of breathing and incidents of breathlessness.[5]

REFERENCES

1. Ahrens TS, Nelson G: Pulmonary anatomy and physiology. In Kinney MR, Packa DR, Dunbar SB, editors: *AACN clinical reference for critical-care nursing,* ed 3, St Louis, 1993, Mosby–Year Book.
2. American Association of Respiratory Care: AARC guidelines: postural drainage therapy, *Respir Care* 36(12):1418-1426, 1993.
3. Reference deleted in proofs.
4. Daly BJ, et al: Development of a special care unit for chronically critically ill patients, *Heart Lung* 20:45-51, 1991.
5. Dettenmeier PA: *Pulmonary nursing care,* St Louis, 1992, Mosby–Year Book.
6. Elpern EH, et al: The non-invasive respiratory care unit: patterns of use and financial implications, *Chest* 99:205-208, 1991.
7. Gracey DR, et al: Outcomes of patients admitted to a chronic ventilator-dependent unit in an acute-care hospital, *Mayo Clin Proc* 67:131-136, 1992.
8. Indihar FJ: A 10-year report of patients in a prolonged respiratory care unit, *Minn Med* 74:23-27, 1991.
9. Kandra TG, Rosenthal M: The pathophysiology of respiratory failure, *Int Anesthesiol Clin* 31(2):119-147, 1993.
10. Laaban JP, et al: Nutritional status of patients with chronic obstructive pulmonary disease and acute respiratory failure, *Chest* 103(5):1362-1368, 1993.
11. Lanken PN; ATS Bioethics Task Force: Withholding and withdrawing life-sustaining therapy, *Am Rev Respir Dis* 144:726-731, 1991.
12. Leister DZ, Batterden RA: The evolution of a long-term ventilator unit, *J Nurs Adm* 22:46-50, 1992.
13. Lundberg JA, Noll ML: The long-term acute care hospital: a new option for ventilator-dependent individuals, *AACN Clin Iss Crit Care Nurs* 1:280-288, 1990.
14. O'Donohue WJ: Chronic ventilator-dependent units in hospitals: attacking the front end of a long-term problem, *Mayo Clin Proc* 67:198-199, 1992.
15. Patterson PA, Elpern EH, Silver MR: Advances in patient care management: the NRCU, *Crit Care Nurse* 11:42-45, 1992.
16. Rieves RD, et al: Severe COPD and acute respiratory failure, *Chest* 104(3):854-860, 1994.
17. Rochester DF: Respiratory muscles and ventilatory failure: 1993 perspective, *Am J Med Sci* 305(6):394-402, 1993.
18. Rose W: Total parenteral nutrition and the patient with chronic obstructive pulmonary disease, *Journal of Intravenous Nursing* 15(1):18-23, 1992.
19. Schuster DP: Physiologic basis for mechanical ventilation. In Scharf SM, editor: *Cardiopulmonary physiology in critical care,* New York, 1993, Marcel Dekker.
20. *St Anthony's DRG guidebook 1995,* Reston, Va, 1994, St Anthony.
21. Stoller JK: Caring for the hospitalized ventilator-dependent patient outside the ICU: united and stand, or divided and fall? *Cleve Clin J Med* 58:537-539, 1991.
22. Thompson JM, et al: *Mosby's clinical nursing* ed 3, St Louis, 1993, Mosby–Year Book.
23. Reference deleted in proofs.
24. Weilitz PB: Weaning a patient from mechanical ventilation, *Critical Care Nurse* 13(4):33-41, 1993.

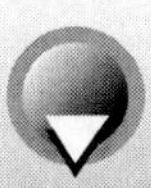

CLINICAL GUIDELINE

35

Acute Respiratory Distress Syndrome

Kay Knox Greenlee, MSN, RN, CCRN

DESCRIPTION

The term *adult respiratory distress syndrome* (ARDS) was introduced by Ashbaugh and Petty in 1967 to describe a syndrome of acute respiratory failure that had been referred to by a variety of terms, including shock lung, trauma lung, and Da Nang lung.[2] At the American-European consensus conference on ARDS, it was decided to use the term *acute* rather than *adult*.[4] In ARDS, direct or indirect injury to the alveolar capillary membrane results in pulmonary edema with normal cardiac function. Therefore, ARDS is frequently referred to as noncardiogenic pulmonary edema. ARDS is characterized by $PaO_2/FiO_2 \leq 200$ mm Hg, regardless of PEEP; radiographic evidence of bilateral pulmonary infiltrates seen on frontal chest radiograph; and PAWP ≤ 18 mm Hg when measured or no clinical evidence of left atrial hypertension.[4]

ARDS affects approximately 150,000 to 200,000 patients per year.[6,30] The mortality of this syndrome is extremely high, 30% to 100% depending on the number of other organs involved.[33] Despite improved clinical management and research efforts, the mortality rate has not changed over the past 25 years. The major contributor to increased mortality is the lack of clear understanding of the mechanisms involved and hence the lack of specific therapy.[7] The critically ill patients in the 1990s survive long enough to develop ARDS. The cause of death in patients with ARDS is not usually a result of refractory hypoxemia or respiratory acidosis but rather is related to the associated conditions.[20]

PATHOPHYSIOLOGY

The hallmark of ARDS is diffuse alveolar damage. Hypotension, trauma, and septic shock, among others, have been suggested as precipitating factors of ARDS. Although the mechanisms and mediators of diffuse alveolar damage may vary depending on the precipitating events, once the pulmonary capillary membrane is injured the pathogenesis follows a similar pattern, as described in Figure 35-1. Some of the mechanisms and mediators identified include neutrophil activation, complement activation, alveolar macrophage stimulation, platelet activation, and release of humoral vasoactive substances.

Neutrophil activation results in an inflammatory response in the pulmonary vasculature. Many of the other mechanisms and mediators lead to further neutrophil aggregation within the pulmonary vasculature, which in turn increases the inflammatory response. Free oxygen radicals, proteases, arachidonic acid metabolites (prostaglandins and leukotrienes), and platelet-activating factors are released from the neutrophils. These substances result in further injury to the vascular endothelium. The complement system, which is part of the immune system, when activated, supports and amplifies the inflammatory/immune response by releasing vasoactive and bioactive substances that can attack the host.[30]

Alveolar macrophage stimulation can result in injury to the alveoli through release of oxygen radicals, proteolytic enzymes, interleukin, and tumor necrosis factor. Platelet activation causes the release of substances such as arachi-

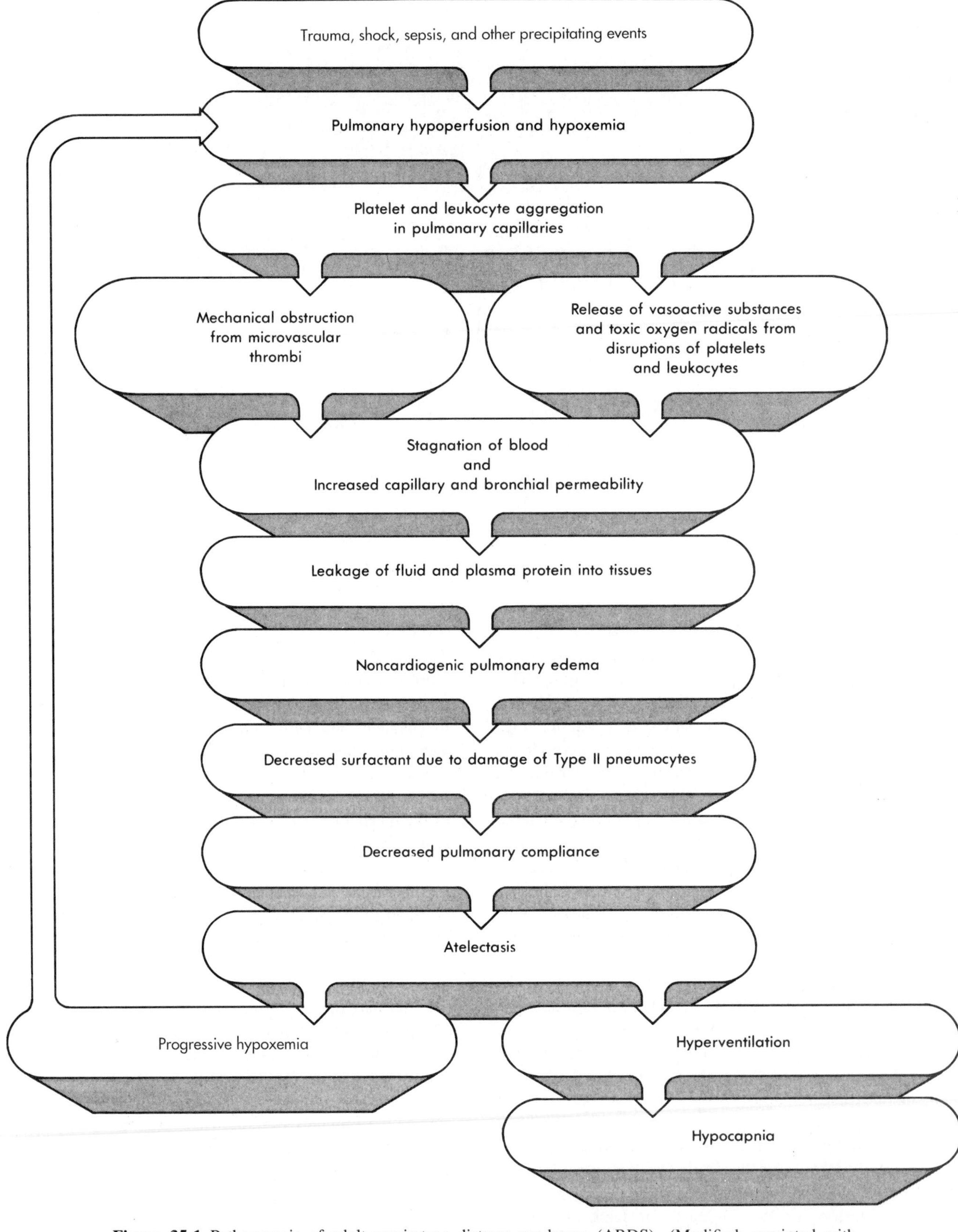

Figure 35-1 Pathogenesis of adult respiratory distress syndrome (ARDS). (Modified; reprinted with permission from the February issue of Nursing 82; copyright © 1982, Springhouse Corporation, 1111 Bethlehem Pike, Springhouse, PA 19477; all rights reserved.)

Precipitating Events for ARDS

Direct injury

Aspiration
Diffuse pulmonary infection
Infection
Near drowning
Toxic inhalation
Lung contusion

Indirect injury

Sepsis syndrome
Severe nonthoracic trauma
Hypertransfusion for emergency resuscitation
Cardiopulmonary bypass

donic acid metabolites, serotonin, platelet-activating factor, and platelet-derived growth factor. These vasoactive substances may result in early pulmonary hypertension and embolization within the pulmonary vasculature. Finally, humoral substances such as histamine and bradykinin increase capillary permeability and promote interstitial edema and fluid exudation into the alveoli.

The stages of ARDS have been labeled differently by authors to describe the physiologic changes that occur. Coalson describes the phases as exudative and reparative.[9] Modig and Putterman describe the stages as latent, acute interstitial edema, acute intraalveolar edema, and subacute chronic phase.[21,23] Most cases of ARDS occur within 24 hours of the precipitating events (62%) identified in the preceding Box. However, 20% occur 24 to 48 hours after the event and 7% occur 48 to 72 hours after the event.[11]

After the precipitating event occurs, lymphatic flow increases, but no obvious clinical changes occur. As damage to the pulmonary capillaries begins, the endothelial pores widen, allowing protein-rich fluids to leak into the interstitium. Type I alveolar epithelial cells and Type II surfactant-producing cells are damaged or impaired, affecting the ability to maintain adequate surface tension and leading to alveolar collapse. Substances that have flooded into the alveoli begin to adhere to the alveolar surface, resulting in a thickening of the alveolar septum. This thickening, and the fibrosis of the alveolar structure that can occur, results in impaired diffusion of oxygen, increased vascular resistance, and decreased lung compliance.

The clinical manifestations vary with each phase.[11] Initially, there may be no clinical signs and the chest x-ray will appear normal. As the injury progresses, the patient will begin to hyperventilate and cough. The chest x-ray will show fine lung reticular infiltrates and the Pa_{O_2} will begin to fall. Within 12 to 24 hours, lung compliance decreases and the x-ray shows diffuse alveolar and interstitial infiltrates. Crackles are heard during auscultation and the patient will become tachypneic. The terminal phase of ARDS results in severe hypoxemia, hypercapnia, and decreased compliance.

Many of the patients seen in the critical care setting are at risk for developing ARDS, as the list of precipitating events in the accompanying box demonstrates. The most lethal and common cause of ARDS is sepsis with or without positive blood cultures. Aspiration is also a common cause of ARDS. With patients experiencing major trauma resulting in direct injuries, or those who experience severe hypotension, emergency surgery, and multiple transfusions, ARDS usually develops within the first 24 hours. Fat embolism is also identified as one of the causes of ARDS, although the prognosis is much better, with survival as high as 90%. It is unclear whether direct lung damage occurs with drug overdoses or whether the complications of hypotension and aspiration result in the development of ARDS. Although cardiopulmonary bypass remains on the list of risk groups, the number of cases has decreased, possibly because of decreased pump times and/or changes in the oxygenation process while the patient is on the pump.

LENGTH OF STAY/ANTICIPATED COURSE

The length of stay for patients with ARDS depends heavily on the precipitating event and the timing of the diagnosis and subsequent treatment. The ultimate outcome depends on the degree of lung injury, effectiveness of respiratory support, and prevention of further injury.[22]

ARDS is a form of respiratory failure and would most likely be classified as DRG 475: Respiratory System Diagnosis with Ventilator Support, with an average length of stay of 13.7 days.[26]

MANAGEMENT TRENDS AND CONTROVERSIES

The care of patients with ARDS is primarily supportive. The focus is to provide oxygen at the lowest level possible, to obtain a Pa_{O_2} of at least 60 to 70 mm Hg. Patients with ARDS will require mechanical ventilation to administer consistent oxygen concentrations, to accomplish hyperinflation of the lung, to assist in opening collapsed alveoli, and to prevent small-airway closure at the end of expiration. Positive end expiratory pressure (PEEP) is usually added when the Fi_{O_2} is greater than 50% and without achieving a Pa_{O_2} of 70 mm Hg. These interventions assist in keeping alveoli open to improve effectiveness of gas exchange.

The best level of PEEP needs to be determined in relation to cardiac output. Even though the Pa_{O_2} may improve with increasing levels of PEEP, PEEP may cause a decrease in cardiac output, resulting in decreased delivery of oxygen to the tissues. Currently, PEEP is used as a support measure to improve gas exchange. Use of PEEP prophylactically does not prevent the development of ARDS. However, new modes of ventilatory therapy are being explored as ways to further improve gas exchange. The alternatives include inverse ratio ventilation[19] and airway pressure release ventilation[28] used to decrease inspiratory pressure but increase mean airway pressure with longer inspiratory time. Continuous-flow ventilation and intermittent-flow expiratory ventilation are used to decrease dead-space ventilation.[15] Adequate oxygenation may also be improved by focusing on the factors that affect delivery and consumption of oxygen. Efforts should be made to decrease oxygen consumption, such as lower fever, decrease anxiety, and limit muscle activity. Positioning of the patient to facilitate lung expansion and ventilation perfusion matching can also positively affect oxygenation.[25] Preventing hypothermia, increasing 2,3-diphosphoglycerate (2,3-DPG), avoiding alkalosis, and maintaining normal hemoglobin are nursing activities to improve oxygenation by maintaining a favorable oxyhemoglobin dissociation curve. 2,3-DPG is a highly charged anion formed in the erythrocyte. It binds to deoxygenated hemoglobin, causing release of oxygen to the tissues.[29] 2,3-DPG is decreased in stored blood. If multiple transfusions become necessary, the potential impact of 2,3-DPG depletion on gas transport must be considered.

Fluid management is important to ensure adequate cardiac output and blood flow to major organs. Although controversy exists as to the most appropriate fluids to use in the patient with ARDS, maintaining the lowest possible pulmonary artery wedge pressure with adequate cardiac output is necessary to improve outcomes for the patient with ARDS. Colloids have been used to increase colloidal osmotic pressure to draw fluid from the interstitium into the capillaries.[14] Crystalloids are recommended, by others, to avoid the increased edema resulting from albumin crossing the impaired alveolar membrane.[5] Use of packed RBCs is appropriate with low cardiac output and low hematocrit. This measure will improve not only cardiac output but also oxygen-carrying capacity. Use of diuretics to decrease pulmonary capillary wedge pressure is indicated, even though the edema is in the airspaces. Beta-adrenergic agonist therapy may be used to accelerate the removal of excess liquid in airspaces to interstitium, where the lymphatic and circulatory systems can disperse excess fluid.

Additional treatment may be focused on attempting to decrease the pulmonary hypertension that results and/or limiting the inflammatory response. These therapies are less definitive in terms of the effect on patient outcomes, but may include prophylactic aerosolized antibiotics, immunotherapy to strengthen the immune system by injecting serum from immunized patients, and surfactant therapy. Endotracheal administration of surfactant therapy has been successful in hyaline membrane disease (HMD), where the amounts of surfactant are inadequate. Surfactant therapy has been studied in a small number of patients with ARDS. There is a reported trend toward decreased mortality without statistical significance.[31,32] However, larger sample sizes are needed to determine if surfactant really works in ARDS.[27]

The focus on current and future research on ARDS primarily relates to early diagnosis and appropriate therapy. Developing scoring mechanisms and identification of markers for the diffuse lung injury that occurs with ARDS has been attempted in hopes that treating the lung injury early would decrease the resulting respiratory failure of ARDS. However, the research on measurement of blood-borne mediators of lung injury has not been useful in predicting which patients will develop ARDS.[17]

Therapies to stop the specific mechanisms of diffuse alveolar damage are being investigated, including antioxidants (*N*-acetylcysteine, L-2 oxothiazolidine-4-carboxylate), inhibitors of arachidonic acid metabolites (5-lipoxygenases), anticytokines, antiendotoxins, monoclonal antibodies, cell adhesion molecules, and cycloxygenase inhibition.[18] Therapies to improve gas exchange are also being investigated. Extracorporeal carbon dioxide removal ($ECCO_2R$) is a form of extracorporeal membrane oxygenation (ECMO) therapy that is also being investigated as a means of maintaining tissue oxygenation.[12] The intravascular oxygenator (IVOX) delivers oxygen via several hundred gas-permeable hollow fibers placed in the vena cava. As gas flows through the fibers, oxygen is added and carbon dioxide is removed.[13] This therapy does not require an extracorporeal circuit or pump, which is the greatest advantage over $ECCO_2R$.[10]

Additional drugs are being evaluated to determine if patient outcomes can be improved. Ketoconazole, an antifungal agent, has demonstrated decreased frequency of ARDS in patients with systemic sepsis.[33] Nitric oxide is being evaluated for improvement on ventilation/perfusion matching by decreasing pulmonary artery pressures and intrapulmonary shunting.[24] Corticosteroids had been used in patients at high risk for ARDS and with ARDS. However, studies conducted in the mid-1980s indicate that corticosteroids have no significant role in prevention or early treatment.[18] More recent studies have reported clinical improvement and survival when corticosteroids are used in later stages.[8,16] NSAIDs are being studied as a result of a small study that demonstrated decreased incidence, high rate of reversal, and improved survival for patients with ARDS.[32]

Research will continue in the area of pathogenesis of ARDS in an effort to identify the most appropriate therapy. Early identification and treatment are key to successful patient outcomes. Assessment of the patient's condition is critical for early recognition and to determine patient response to therapeutic interventions.

ASSESSMENT

PARAMETER	ANTICIPATED ALTERATION
ABG	Initial respiratory alkalosis *due to increased respiratory effort to meet oxygen demands* • pH >7.40 • $PaCO_2$ ≤35 to 40 mm Hg • PaO_2 <60 mm Hg • HCO_2 22 to 26 mEq/L • SaO_2 <95% • SpO_2 <90% Subsequent respiratory acidosis *due to patient fatigue and respiratory failure* • pH <7.40 • $PaCO_2$ >45 mm Hg • PaO_2 <60 mm Hg • HCO_2 22 to 26 mEq/L • SaO_2 <95% • SpO_2 <90%
Pulmonary Status	
Rate	Tachypnea Dyspnea
PAP	Increased: >35/15/20 mm Hg (PA S/D/M) *due to pulmonary edema*
PCWP	WNL: <18 mm Hg but *pulmonary artery diastolic to wedge pressure gradient greater than 5 mm Hg*
Chest x-ray	Infiltrates in dependent lung
FiO_2	Increase percent needed to maintain adequate oxygenation
Shunted perfusion/total perfusion (Qs/Qt)	Increased shunt: >10% Increase dead-space ventilation
Static compliance	Decreased: <50 mg/cm H_2O
Oxygen delivery	Decreased: <900 ml/min
Oxygen consumption	Increased: >250 ml/min
Cardiovascular Status	
Heart rate	Tachycardia
Rhythm	Regular
Mean arterial pressure	Hypotension MAP <70 mm Hg
Cardiac index	*Normal to increased unless myocardium is depressed due to pathogenesis of ARDS*
Systemic vascular resistance	Decreased: <800 dynes/sec/cm^{-5} in septic shock Increased: >1200 dynes/sec/cm^{-5} in hypervolemic vasoconstriction
Pulmonary vascular resistance	Increased: >97 dynes/sec/cm^{-5}
Neurological Status	
LOC	Anxious Restless Confused

Other

Hgb	WNL
Hct	WNL

PLAN OF CARE

INTENSIVE PHASE

The patient with acute respiratory distress syndrome requires intensive care for close observation and support of the respiratory system. Care is directed to effectively clear the airway, improve gas exchange, and promote an effective breathing pattern.

PATIENT CARE PRIORITIES	EXPECTED PATIENT OUTCOMES
Ineffective airway clearance *r/t* *Intubation* *Mechanical ventilation* *Retained secretions*	Clear lungs Secretions managed/removed Improved ABG Patent airway
Impaired gas exchange *r/t* *Ventilation perfusion mismatch* *Shunting* *Interstitial edema* *Alveolar collapse*	Improved ABG Improve ventilation/perfusion relationship
Ineffective breathing pattern *r/t* *Increased work of breathing* *Anxiety* *Hypoxemia* *Pain*	Normal/improved pattern Pain relief
Inadequate nutrition *r/t* *Intubation* *Increased metabolic need*	Maintain weight Adequate intake Maintain anabolic state
Anxiety *r/t dyspnea, fear of dying*	Decreased anxiety evidenced by relaxed facial expression, stable vital signs Reduced respiratory effort
Impaired communication *r/t intubation*	Able to communicate needs effectively
High risk for infection *r/t compromised defense mechanisms*	Free of infection: afebrile, WBC: WNL, clear sputum
Pain/discomfort *r/t intubation, increased work of breathing*	Indicate feeling of comfort
Impaired physical mobility *r/t deconditioning, prolonged bed rest*	Mobility maintained/increased No skin breakdown
Dyspnea *r/t disease process*	Absent or reduced levels of dyspnea
High risk for pulmonary complications, such as tracheal/laryngeal injuries, super infections, atelectasis, pneumothorax, subcutaneous emphysema, air embolization *r/t disease process and clinical deterioration*	Free of complications or complications promptly noted and treated

INTERVENTIONS

Provide mechanical ventilation with oxygen therapy *to optimize gas exchange.*

Monitor ventilator settings, including rate, mode, volumes, oxygen, and pressures, *to ensure accurate settings in collaboration with respiratory therapists.*

Monitor patient's response to mechanical ventilation.

Plan of Care (cont'd)

Monitor ABGs with ventilatory changes and with changes in patient status. *ABG must be used to monitor acid–base balance in addition to oxygenation status.*
Monitor Spo_2 per pulse oximetry.
Decrease oxygen consumption and reduce oxygen demand.
Administer paralytic drugs as needed *to decrease oxygen demand/consumption and/or facilitate ventilatory support.*
Prevent shivering, tachycardia, tachypnea, pain, and increased muscle activity, *which increase oxygen demand/consumption.*
Maintain temperature within normal range.
Maintain patent airway.
Suction airway based on assessment. Preoxygenate before each suction pass. If Spo_2 not maintained >90% with suctioning, consider hyperinflation.
Note type and amount of secretions suctioned.
Position patient with good lung down *to facilitate oxygenation.*
Turn patient side to side *to help mobilize secretions and prevent complications.*
Humidify inspired air *to decrease irritation and facilitate secretion removal.*
Provide chest physiotherapy as needed *to facilitate secretion removal.*
Administer fluids *to maintain adequate cardiac output.*
Monitor hemodynamic parameters, specifically cardiac output and index in context with mechanical ventilation and PEEP.
Monitor weights.
Monitor I/O.
Collaborate with dietitian daily to determine caloric needs *to maintain anabolic state.* Consider enteral nutrition with decreased carbon dioxide byproduct with metabolism, such as Pulmocare.
Consider therapeutic mattress *to prevent skin breakdown secondary to prolonged bed rest and impaired tissue perfusion.*
Control and manage environment *to ensure safety and comfort.*
Interact with patient *to maintain orientation and instill hope.*
Enhance communication through alternate mechanism, such as write board, letter board, signal, or gesture messages.
Prevent infection by ensuring ventilator circuits are changed every q24h to q48h, changing suction equipment daily, monitoring invasive lines sites, and using aseptic technique with respiratory and wound care.
Provide analgesia and sedation as needed *to maintain comfort and decrease oxygen demand/consumption.*
Provide reassurance.

INTERMEDIATE PHASE

If the patient survives the intensive phase of care, recovery will depend on the precipitating event and the patient's length of time in the acute phase. Specific to the respiratory system, nursing care will focus on weaning from the ventilator and assisting the patient to adapt to changes resulting from the acute illness.

PATIENT CARE PRIORITIES	EXPECTED PATIENT OUTCOMES
Ineffective breathing pattern *r/t* *Increased work of breathing* *Return to spontaneous breathing* *Activity progression*	Normal/improved pattern Maintain spontaneous ventilation
Impaired physical mobility *r/t deconditioning and resulting weakness*	Activity with minimal SOB
Dyspnea *r/t activity progression and disease process*	SOB to level agreed upon

Plan of Care (cont'd)

INTERVENTIONS

Collaborate with physical therapy to increase strength of respiratory muscles and gradually return to activities of daily living with increased range of motion exercises, chair activity, and short ambulation.

Ensure adequate sleep/rest periods by scheduling activity and cares *to promote physical healing and strength.*

Teach shortness of breath scale; rate shortness of breath from 0 to 10, similar to pain scale: 0 = no SOB, 10 = severe SOB. Use scale to monitor patient's tolerance during weaning exercises and activity progression.

TRANSITION TO DISCHARGE

As the patient moves from the intermediate phase and usually out of the critical care setting, the focus of nursing care is to prepare the patient for discharge. This involves assisting the patient to establish self-care regimens, using adaptive techniques to compensate for any residual effect of the ARDS experience. Approximately one third of adult survivors show abnormalities, such as restrictive defects, impaired gas exchange, desaturation with exercise, and evidence of obstructive lung disease. These changes may not persist over time and are usually mild. The prognosis for patients who survive the intensive phase of ARDS is favorable: 83% are clinically normal, 73% have normal lung volumes, 74% have normal ABGs, 48% have decreased $Pa{O_2}$ with exercise.[1] Given these statistics, nursing care during the transition phase is focused on increasing activity tolerance and assisting the patient to return to prehospital routines.

REFERENCES

1. Alberts W, et al: The outlook for survivors of ARDS, *Chest* 84:272-274, 1983.
2. Ashbaugh DB, et al: Acute respiratory distress in adults, *Lancet* 2:319-323, 1967.
3. Bernard GR, et al: Effects of a short course of ibuprofen in patients with severe sepsis, *Am Rev Respir Dis* 137:A138, 1988.
4. Bernard GR, et al: The American-European consensus conference on ARDS, *Am J Respir Crit Care Med* 149:818-824, 1994.
5. Brigham K, et al: Correlation of oxygenation with vascular permeability surface area but not with lung water in humans with acute respiratory failure and pulmonary edema, *J Clin Invest* 72:339-349, 1983.
6. Case SC, Sabo CE: Adult respiratory distress syndrome: a deadly complication of trauma, *Focus* 19(2):116-121, 1992.
7. Casey LC: Role of cytokines in the pathogenesis of cardiopulmonary-induced multisystem organ failure, *Ann Thorac Surg* 56:S92-96, 1993.
8. Chinn A, et al: High dose corticosteroids for rescue treatment of fibroproliferation in late ARDS, *Am Rev Respir Dis* 147:A349, 1993.
9. Coalson JJ: Pathophysiologic features of infant and adult respiratory distress syndromes. In Shoemaker WC, et al, editors: *Textbook of critical care medicine,* Philadelphia, 1989, WB Saunders.
10. East TD: The magic bullets in the war on ARDS: aggressive therapy for oxygenation failure, *Respir Care* 38(6):690-702, 1993.
11. Farrell MM: The challenge of adult respiratory distress syndrome during interleukin-2 immunotherapy, *Oncol Nurs Forum* 19(3):475-480, 1992.
12. Gattinoni L, et al: Low frequency positive pressure ventilation with extracorporeal CO_2 removal in severe adult respiratory failure: clinical results, *JAMA* 256:881-886, 1986.
13. Gentilello LM, et al: The intravascular oxygenator (IVOX): preliminary results of a new means of performing extrapulmonary gas exchange, *J Trauma* 35(3):399-404, 1993.
14. Hausser CJ, Shoemaker WC, Turpin E: Oxygen transport responses to colloid and crystalloid in critically ill surgical patients, *Surg Gynecol Obstet* 150:811-816, 1980.
15. Hazelzet JA, et al: New modes of mechanical ventilation for severe respiratory failure, *Crit Care Med* 21:S366-367, 1993.
16. Hooper RG, Kearl RA: Established ARDS treated with a sustained course of adrenocortical steroids, *Chest* 97:138-143, 1990.
17. Hudson LD: The prediction and prevention of ARDS, *Respir Care* 35(2):161-173, 1990.
18. Hudson LD: Pharmacologic approaches to respiratory failure, *Respir Care* 38(7):754-764, 1993.
19. Marcy TW, Marini JJ: Inverse ratio ventilation in ARDS: rationale and implementation, *Chest* 100:494-504, 1991.
20. Matthay MA: The adult respiratory distress syndrome, *West J Med* 150:187-194, 1989.
21. Modig J: AARDS: pathogenesis and treatment, *Acta Chir Scan* 152:241-249, 1986.
22. Petty TL, Ashbaugh DG: The adult respiratory distress syndrome, *Chest* 60(3):233-239, 1971.
23. Putterman C: Adult respiratory distress syndrome: current concepts, *Resuscitation* 16(2):91-105, 1988.
24. Rossaint R, et al: Inhaled nitric oxide for the adult respiratory distress syndrome, *N Engl J Med* 328(6):399-404, 1993.
25. Schmitz TM: The semi-prone position in ARDS: five case studies, *Crit Care Nurs* 11(5):22-33, 1991.
26. *St Anthony's DRG Guidebook 1995,* Reston, Va, 1994, St Anthony.
27. Steinberg KP: Surfactant therapy in the adult respiratory distress syndrome, *Respir Care* 38(4):365-372, 1993.
28. Stock MC, Downs JB, Frolichter DA: Airway pressure release ventilation, *Crit Care Med* 15:462-466, 1987.

29. Stone K: Respiratory physiology. In Clochesty J, et al, editors: *Critical care nursing*, Philadelphia, 1993, WB Saunders.
30. Vaughan P, Brooks C: Adult respiratory distress syndrome: a complication of shock, *Crit Care Clin North Am* 2(2):235-253, 1990.
31. Weg J, et al: Safety and efficacy of aerosolized surfactant in human sepsis-induced ARDS, *Chest* 100:137S, 1991.
32. Wiedemann H, et al: A multi-center trial in human sepsis-induced ARDS of an aerosolized synthetic surfactant, *Am Rev Respir Dis* 145:A184, 1992.
33. Yu M, Tomasa G: A double blind, prospective, randomized trial of ketoconazole, a thromboxane synthetase inhibitor, in the prophylaxis of the adult respiratory distress syndrome, *Crit Care Med* 21(11):1635-1642, 1993.

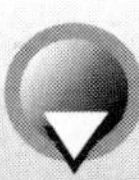

C L I N I C A L G U I D E L I N E

36

Pulmonary Embolism

Jacqueline Morgan, MSN, RN

DESCRIPTION

A pulmonary embolus is a thrombus that originates elsewhere in the body and travels via the venous system through the right side of the heart and lodges in the pulmonary arterial system. The occlusion to blood flow in the pulmonary circulation results in clinical manifestations dependent upon the degree of occlusion. The larger the embolus, the larger the occlusion, causing increasing hemodynamic compromise. Many small emboli may go unrecognized, whereas large emboli can cause pulmonary infarction and death. Pulmonary embolism is, in actuality, a sequel or side effect of other patient problems and can vary in severity.

Pulmonary embolism (PE) occurs in over 650,000 patients annually and is fatal in approximately 38% of symptomatic patients.[3] Reports may vary as to its actual occurrence, and often the diagnosis of pulmonary embolism is made postmortem.

The key to survival is early recognition of risk factors and preventative treatment. However, even when all risk factors are considered, pulmonary emboli still have the potential to develop. In such instances early recognition of signs and symptoms hopefully will lead to early diagnosis and treatment. Signs and symptoms may mimic those of other conditions; thus the risk factors for pulmonary embolus should always be considered.

PATHOPHYSIOLOGY

Over 90% of pulmonary emboli originate from clots or thrombi that form in the veins of the lower extremities, the calf muscle being the most frequent site.[6,19] These thrombi can be made up of platelets, thrombin, and red and white blood cells. Other emboli may be composed of air, fat, amniotic fluid, tumors, or particles from sites of infection (see the following Box).

A large percentage of pulmonary emboli originate from a deep-vein thrombosis (DVT). These thrombi are the result of one of three identified venous states, which were identified in 1858 and are known as Virchow's triad: venous stasis, abnormalities or injury to vessel walls, and alterations in the blood coagulation process. Despite the many medical advances that have been made since 1858, patients still develop DVTs and resultant pulmonary emboli.

The most common predisposition to the development of DVT is venous stasis. Prolonged bed rest and immobility frequently present in the critical care setting cause venous dilatation in the deep calf muscles, leading to pooling of blood in this area and thereby increasing the risk of developing pulmonary embolism.[17] Venous return to the heart from the lower extremities also may be impeded by conditions such as a pelvic mass. Impeded flow, combined with the body's natural clotting mechanism, results in thrombi formation.

The second factor, vein wall injury, results from direct trauma. To heal the site of injury, a thrombus forms naturally to prevent blood loss from the site. Platelets and fibrin collect at the site of injury to form the clot or thrombus. In cases of vascular abnormalities, leukocytes also may accumulate at the site. "White thrombi" are composed mainly of platelets and leukocytes, while "red thrombi" are composed mainly of fibrin. In either case, it is the tails of these thrombi that dislodge to become pulmonary emboli.[4]

The third origin of thrombi is directly related to defects in coagulopathic properties. Certain disease states such as sickle cell anemia, polycythemia, and malignancy result in abnormal hypercoagulability.

The Origins of Pulmonary Emboli

- Deep vein thrombosis
  - Venous stasis from prolonged bedrest
  - Hypercoagulopathic states
- Air embolism
  - Trauma
  - Improper care/insertion of IV catheters
- Fat embolism
  - From fractures of large bones (e.g., pelvis)
- Amniotic fluid embolism
  - Fragments of fluid clots
  - Fragments of placenta
- Septic embolism
  - From infectious sites (e.g., endocarditis)
- Tumor embolism
  - From origins of malignancy
- Right atrium ventricle
  - Clots within the chambers
  - Clots upon the valves
  - Clots among the arteries

Pulmonary emboli can also be composed of fat, air, calcium, amniotic fluid, tumor fragments, and foreign materials. Fat emboli usually originate from bone marrow at the site of a large fracture such as of the hip or pelvis. These fat emboli travel to the capillaries of the lung causing inflammation and interstitial edema. Air can be introduced through trauma or improperly inserted or handled central venous catheters. Emboli also can be the result of a site of infection. Bacterial debris from a septic area can loosen and become emboli. Pregnancy and the postpartum period also bring with them the threat of pulmonary emboli, as parts of the amniotic sac can become emboli.[1,14]

Regardless of its origin, an embolus travels via systemic circulation through the right side of the heart and lodges in the pulmonary circulation. The site of occlusion causes disruption in circulation distal to the embolus. The lack of circulation to the area affects proper gas exchange, and with a large enough embolus, this will become evident with arterial blood gas analysis. The lack of gas exchange causes dead space.

The size and location of emboli play a part in both the clinical picture of the condition as well as its treatment. If an entire branch of an artery is affected, pulmonary infarction can occur. Pulmonary infarction occurs in only about 10% of emboli due to collateral circulation that can develop. However, patients with underlying pulmonary disease are at greater risk due to their decreased ability to form the circulation patterns. There are several signs and symptoms that are particularly indicative of infarction. They include the sudden onset of pleuritic chest pain, hemoptysis, fever, and an increased sedimentation rate, the latter two of which are associated with an inflammatory process.[17] The person afflicted with an embolism causing obstruction but no infarct may not necessarily manifest hemoptysis, fever, or an increased ESR.

Pulmonary embolism can be categorized according to the following manifestations: an embolism at the bifurcation of the bronchi, multiple emboli, and those that cause occlusion but not infarction.[15] The most deadly is the pulmonary embolism that occurs near the area of bifurcation because it can affect blood flow to more than one of the lobar arteries. There also can be patients who suffer from multiple emboli. These emboli usually are very small and can go unnoticed until a large embolus occurs. Such patients generally have a long history of venous thrombosis and its risk factors. Emboli that cause occlusion but not infarction are the most common of the four types of emboli. This type of emboli is the most difficult to diagnose because it presents a clinical picture similar to other conditions. Despite the difficulty in diagnosis, they are the most easily treated when detected.

LENGTH OF STAY/ANTICIPATED COURSE

The length of stay and anticipated course depend upon the type of treatment that is necessary as well as the amount of time it takes to stabilize the patient hemodynamically. The length of stay is longer for patients with large pulmonary emboli that require radical treatment such as surgery, as opposed to successful treatment with anticoagulants. Infection of the involved lobes may also further complicate matters and increase length of stay. DRG 78: Pulmonary embolism has an average length of stay of 9.2 days.[15]

MANAGEMENT TRENDS AND CONTROVERSIES

Recognition and Diagnostics

Early recognition of signs and symptoms of a pulmonary embolus is the key to early treatment. First, it is important that a patient's medical and surgical history is screened for risk factors (see following Box). Together with these risk factors, a thorough assessment of both subjective and objective data is necessary to uncover the condition. Finally, diagnostic tests and procedures will be ordered to verify and classify the diagnosis.

A ventilation perfusion (VQ) scan is a key diagnostic study in the evaluation of a pulmonary embolus. VQ scanning usually is performed with little or no risk.[16] Both ventilation and perfusion are scanned separately and compared with the ratios of each that normally are found in the various lung fields. Since pulmonary emboli cause dead space, which is ventilation without perfusion, a higher VQ ratio is obtained. This difference in the ratio is known as a mismatch. During the ventilation phase of the scan, a patient inhales a radio-labeled gas that is followed under x-ray. The perfusion scan requires the injection of a radioactive isotope. Despite the reliability of a VQ scan, there is a possibility that the results can be falsely interpreted or the scan itself

Risk Factors of Pulmonary Embolism

- History of DVTs
- Increased age
- Burns
- Trauma
- Pregnancy
- Recent surgery (especially orthopedic or gynecologic)
- Obesity
- Prior history of PE
- Malignancy
- Stasis states:
  - Immobility
  - Bedrest
- Hypercoagulopathic states:
  - Sickle cell anemia
  - Polycythemia vera
- Disease states:
  - CHF
  - MI
  - COPD
  - Atrial fibrillation

can be indeterminant. In the event that the VQ scan is indeterminant, further diagnostic study is required if the signs and symptoms of pulmonary embolus persist.

The test that provides the most definitive diagnosis of pulmonary embolus is a pulmonary angiogram. Unlike a VQ scan, an angiogram is an invasive procedure and carries with it some risks, which include allergic reaction to the injected dye, cardiac perforation from the inserted catheter, and dysrhythmias. However, in some instances an angiogram is necessary to diagnose the embolus, usually because the severity of the signs and symptoms necessitate quick results. An angiogram is also performed in cases when preventative anticoagulation at the time of suspected embolus is contraindicated. Finally, as mentioned earlier, an angiogram will be used to verify indeterminant VQ scans.

During an angiogram a catheter is inserted and threaded to the right and left main pulmonary arteries. Contrast is injected and followed under fluoroscopy as it travels through the pulmonary circulation. An angiogram is considered positive when it shows a filling deficit or sharp cut-offs in flow. Despite the risks mentioned, the actual rate of negative effects of an angiogram is as low as 4%.[1]

Once a diagnosis of pulmonary embolus is made, whether it is definitive or suggestive, treatment is necessary to prevent further complications. Treatment usually is dependent on the severity of the embolus and its subsequent hemodynamic effects. The patient's past medical and surgical history, including medications and allergies, must be taken into consideration. Of course, the more unstable the patient, the more aggressive the therapy will be.

Medical Management

The first line of treatment in the majority of pulmonary emboli is anticoagulation. The drug of choice is heparin. Heparin often is started even before the embolus is confirmed. Thus the heparin can prevent the coagulation of other emboli or multiple emboli from developing. Heparin enhances the action of one of the body's natural inhibitors of the clotting cascade and also prevents the formation of fibrin. It has been shown that white thrombi are best controlled by drugs that affect platelets and their formation as compared to red thrombi, which respond to anticoagulants because of their high fibrin content.[17] The patient is medicated with an initial bolus dose and then placed on a continuous heparin infusion. During heparin therapy the patient's PTT is closely followed to track the anticoagulatory effects. The goal of therapy is to keep the PTT ½ to 2½ times the normal, although this range may vary.

Coumadin is an oral anticoagulant that has an effect on the Vitamin K clotting factors. The clotting factors with the shortest half-lives are eliminated by Coumadin first, and a subsequent period of hypercoagulopathy is possible shortly after initiating this medication, thus making it necessary to continue heparin until the desired effects of Coumadin are obtained, usually within 2 to 3 days.[11] When a patient is on Coumadin it is necessary to monitor PT. As is true with heparin, the goal is to prolong bleeding, which is proof of anticoagulation. Patients often are discharged home on Coumadin. This fact needs to be considered when planning education for discharge. Heparin and Coumadin have a long history of use in the presence of pulmonary embolism. However, both drugs take time to achieve their desired effects. In patients who are significantly compromised, these medications may not work fast enough.

Since 1989, thrombolytic agents that are used to treat myocardial infarction have been used to treat pulmonary emboli. Both streptokinase and urokinase have been approved and used in treatment. The risk of severe hemorrhage and continued bleeding may not allow some patients to be candidates for this therapy, which is the primary reason these drugs have not been more widely accepted. Other factors exist for avoidance of use and most often are based on patient history (see following Box). Both drugs act to increase the amount of plasmin generated, leading to lysis and anticoagulation. TPA, used to treat patients with acute MI, is a third thrombolytic under investigation regarding its efficacy for treatment of pulmonary embolus. Its actions are similar to both streptokinase and urokinase, and it has the same risk factors. Recent studies have investigated the benefits of directly injecting these medications onto the emboli themselves during angiography. This direct injection reduces many of the bleeding problems associated with systemic infusion.[2] A study done by researchers at Brigham and Women's Hospital was aimed at determining the proper dosage of thrombolytics for treating emboli. Research is necessary to make the practitioner more comfortable with

Contraindications to Thrombolytics

- Active/recent history of bleeding
- CVA with and/or without hemorrhage
- Spinal disease
- Recent head trauma or surgery
- Surgery or burn within 10 days
- Biopsy or other internal procedure
- Uncontrolled hypertension
- Coagulation defects

the use of thrombolytics. It is hoped that as practitioners gain more knowledge, these agents will become more widely used.[7,8]

Surgical Treatment

If thrombolytic therapy and any type of anticoagulation are contraindicated, the only treatment for a massive pulmonary embolism is surgery. Embolectomies carry with them many risks; however, they may be the only treatment for those patients with greater than 50% of pulmonary circulation impaired, or for those who have not responded to treatment aimed at reversing hypotension. The procedure has improved greatly since its introduction in 1908 by Trendelenburg, especially since the introduction of cardiopulmonary bypass. This type of embolectomy requires a sternotomy. A second approach is performed much like an angiogram in that a catheter is introduced into a vein and threaded to the lungs. This catheter is equipped with a suction tip used to break apart the embolus. Despite these advances, there is still not an impressive survival rate from the surgery. A mortality rate of 27% has been reported for the latter surgical procedure, and a 33% mortality rate for the open embolectomy.[4]

Another invasive intervention that is used depends upon the patient's potential for developing further emboli. When the potential is high and the patient is not a candidate for anticoagulants, vena cava interruption may be considered as a means to block thrombi from systemic circulation. The earliest procedure to interrupt flow from the vena cava was to totally sever the vena cava or place clips to narrow its lumen.[13,17] However, the possibility of development of collateral circulation around the occluded area remains; thus the potential for emboli remains. Recently there has been a move to interrupt vena cava flow by inserting filters. The primary goal is not to cease blood flow but to trap clots that eventually will dissolve. Several types of filters have been developed; the type used generally is decided upon by the physician or institution. The patient is placed under fluoroscopy in a procedure much like an angiogram. Various filters such as bird's nest, umbrella, and the popular Greenfield filter are used.[4,6,18] With any interruption in venous flow, there is the possibility of chronic venous stasis in the lower extremities, causing edema.

Prevention

In addition to the actual treatment choices for the diagnosis of pulmonary embolism, much research has been done in the area of primary prevention of emboli and the prevention of recurring emboli. The primary preventative strategies and equipment all aim at the various risk factors that lead to the development of a pulmonary embolus. These strategies, for the most part, have been aimed at preventing venous stasis and hypercoagulopathy.

Nurses play a major role in the prevention of venous stasis, and many nursing interventions are aimed at the effects of immobility and prolonged bed rest. Early ambulation after surgery, simple elevation of the legs, and various exercises aid in venous return. Exercise and movement squeeze the veins in the leg by muscle contraction, increasing venous return.

Many patients who have undergone orthopedic surgery or who have been on prolonged bed rest will routinely receive low-dose subcutaneous heparin (2500 to 5000 units). The premise is that even in low doses, heparin can still have enough of an effect on the coagulation cascade to prevent thrombi. One minor risk or side effect of this drug is hematoma formation at the injection site.[11] A more detrimental side effect is a resultant thrombocytopenia that is thought to be caused by a heparin-induced platelet antibody.[1,11]

A very common means of prevention with little if any risk is the use of mechanical devices that help reduce venous stasis. These devices include elastic stockings and gradient-pressure stockings. These gradient stockings are attached to a pump that systematically applies gentle pressure to the calf muscles, alternating with the thighs. Besides preventing venous stasis by increasing emptying and providing a pulse flow, the stockings increase local fibrinolytic activity, the mechanism of which is unknown.[11] These devices may be used in conjunction with subcutaneous heparin injections.

To prevent hypercoagulopathy, it is important for the nurse to encourage po fluids if the patient is able, or to maintain IV fluids as ordered. Fluids also are used during the acute stages of pulmonary embolism to increase right ventricle and diastolic pressures. Dextran also has been used as a prophylaxis because it interferes with platelet function and is a plasma volume expander. Its major drawback is that it must be watched closely to ensure that the patient does not become fluid overloaded. It may also cause an allergic reaction.[1,2,13]

Nursing research also has been directed toward the prevention of pulmonary emboli. One area of interest is the ways in which a thrombus is dislodged and released into circulation. Sudden movement and trauma are two such ways. Also being researched is the role of the Valsalva maneuver during defecation as a possible trigger of dislodgement. Squatting has been shown to cause vasodilation of the extremities; when the individual stands up, a pressure gradient develops that may lead to dislodgement.[12]

ASSESSMENT

PARAMETER	ANTICIPATED ALTERATION
Pulmonary Status	
Rate and rhythm	Sudden onset of dyspnea Tachypnea (RR >25) Abnormality dependent on size of embolus and degree of occlusion
ABG	Mild/small PE • CO_2 decreased: <35 mm Hg • pH increased: >7.45 • *Due to hyperventilation secondary to tachypnea* Massive PE • Pao_2 decreased: <80 mm Hg • Respiratory acidosis *due to increased dead space* • Increased a-A gradient
Chest x-ray	Possible pleural effusion Possible atelectasis *due to decreased surfactant production* Possible infiltration Westermark's sign (decreased vascular markings on side of embolus) Elevated diaphragm on PE side
Lung sounds	Crackles on affected side
Cough	Hemoptysis in case of infarction
Cardiovascular Status	
HR	Sinus tachycardia
Hemodynamic parameters	
• MAP	Hypotension: <70 mm Hg
• PVR	Increased: >97 dynes/sec/cm^{-5}
• CO	Decreased: <4 L/min
• CVP	Increased: >30 mm Hg
Neck veins	JVD
Heart sounds	Fixed split of S_2
Color	Peripheral cyanosis
ECG	Nonspecific ST changes Right bundle branch block Peaked T waves *due to increased pressure in right atrium*
Pain	C/O pleuritic pain
Other Parameters	
Neurological status	Decreased LOC in presence of hypoxemia
GI/GU	Oliguria
Other	Fever Increased ESR

PLAN OF CARE

INTENSIVE PHASE

The intensity of care required by the patient with pulmonary embolus is determined by the impact of the insult on the respiratory and cardiovascular systems. The goals of the intensive

Plan of Care (cont'd)

phase of care are focused on preserving hemodynamic stability and adequate oxygenation. This care may not require admission to an intensive care unit unless the patient presents with life-threatening compromise to ventilatory or hemodynamic capability.

PATIENT CARE PRIORITIES	EXPECTED PATIENT OUTCOMES
Impaired gas exchange *r/t* *VQ scan mismatch* *Interstitial edema* *Atelectasis*	Improved ABG Improved perfusion Reduction/absence of crackles Improved chest x-ray
Ineffective breathing pattern *r/t* *Anxiety* *Hypoxemia* *Pain*	Improved pattern Calm demeanor Improved ABG Pain-free
Decreased CO *r/t* *Dehydration* *RV failure* *Stasis*	Improved CO Good skin turgor Stable VS Improved circulation: PaO_2 >60 mm Hg
Decreased peripheral tissue perfusion *r/t* *Thrombus development* *Venous stasis*	Absence of DVT Improved circulation: CRT <3 sec
Activity intolerance *r/t hypoxemia*	Manages ADL with minimal assistance Improvement in exercise and active ROM
Potential for bleeding *r/t anticoagulants*	PT/PTT within prescribed levels No evidence of active bleeding

INTERVENTIONS

Assess medication and health history for predisposition for hypercoagulability.

Monitor respiratory rate and rhythm *to evaluate status and progress.*

Administer oxygen as ordered.

Administer fluids as ordered *to maintain CO.*

Administer cardiotonic and/or vasoactive drugs as ordered *to maintain adequate blood pressure and organ perfusion.*

Monitor ABG maintaining PaO_2 >60 mm Hg *to ensure adequate oxygen delivery to vital organs.*

Monitor hemodynamic parameters *to ensure appropriate response to fluids and cardiovascular medication.*

Administer anticoagulants as ordered *to decrease the risk of re-embolization.* Assess potential medical or surgical contraindications for anticoagulant therapy prior to initiation.

Monitor APTT *to ensure therapeutic heparin administration.*

Begin warfarin administration prior to discontinuation of heparin *to prevent reembolization.*

Monitor PT *to ensure therapeutic warfarin administration.*

Prevent venous stasis by the following actions:

- ROM *to enhance circulation*
- Reposition immobilized patients q2h *to enhance circulation and mobilize secretions*
- Ambulate postoperative patients as early as possible *to increase venous return, mobilize secretions, and aid in pain management*
- Ensure patient does not cross legs/ankles, *to prevent venous stasis*
- Monitor skin under mechanical devices and over bony prominences *to prevent breakdown*

Monitor I/O *to ensure adequate hydration.*

Monitor chest x-rays and ECG.

Monitor clinical S/S, sedimentation rate, and WBC *to identify potential infection early and ensure prompt intervention.*

Plan of Care (cont'd)

INTERMEDIATE PHASE

If the patient survives the initial crisis following pulmonary embolization, the focus turns to preventing recurrence, weaning form supplemental oxygen, and maintaining therapeutic anticoagulation. Follow-up VQ scans, chest x-rays, and ECGs will be used to aid in evaluating progress and to ensure that multiple PE have not occurred. Patient anxiety related to the PE and follow-up care also must be addressed as the patient is prepared to move toward discharge.

PATIENT CARE PRIORITIES	EXPECTED PATIENT OUTCOMES
High risk for impaired gas exchange *r/t potential reembolization*	ABG within patient norms Weaned from ventilator and supplemental oxygen
High risk for ineffective breathing pattern *r/t pulmonary trauma and possible mechanical ventilation*	Free from dyspnea Weaned from ventilator and supplemental oxygen Improved activity tolerance
Self-care deficit *r/t lack of knowledge about medications, especially anticoagulants; disease process; ongoing recovery regime*	Verbalizes action, dose, schedule and side effects of all medications Verbalizes S/S of new PE, adverse effects of anticoagulants, and importance of follow-up lab work
Anxiety *r/t fear of reembolization*	Verbalizes realistic expectations of recurrence Demonstrates calm state Able to rest/sleep
High risk for bleeding *r/t anticoagulation therapy*	Free of overt bleeding PT within therapeutic range No evidence of bruising, petechiae, tarry stools

INTERVENTIONS

Monitor pulse oximetry or ABG with changes in oxygen delivery dose or mode *to ensure tolerance of weaning process.*

Monitor VS and level of consciousness ongoing.

Monitor APTT while on heparin and PT while on warfarin *to ensure therapeutic dose and minimize hemorrhagic risks.*

Guaiac stools and urine *to detect presence of occult blood.*

Pattern ADL according to tolerance level *to optimize reconditioning and return to maximum independence.*

Initiate teaching regarding anticoagulant medication and importance of follow-up lab work *to ensure safety and compliance with dose, schedule, and follow-up monitoring of bleeding times.*

Teach patient S/S of bleeding associated with anticoagulant use, including black, tarry stools, bleeding from gums, excessive bruising, petechiae *to protect patient from possible complications.*

TRANSITION TO DISCHARGE

The focus of discharge planning is twofold. Patients need instruction on the medications they will be taking at home, as well as preventative measures to avoid DVT and subsequent emboli. Patients discharged home on Coumadin must be made aware of the risk of active bleeding and should be advised to report excessive bruising, discolored areas of the skin, and any changes in color and consistency of stools and urine. They also should be advised to use safe measures when performing ADL; for example, using a soft-bristled toothbrush to avoid bleeding, and taking extreme caution when shaving. Patients on Coumadin should be provided with a medical-alert bracelet to inform other health care providers, especially in the case of an emergency, that they are taking this medication. Advise these patients to make their dentist aware that they are on the medication before having dental work done.

The other aspect of education focuses on the signs and symptoms of a DVT such as redness, swelling, and pain in the deep calf muscle. They should be taught to avoid tight-fitting clothing, and to take part in some sort of regular exercise as tolerated to enhance circulation and promote venous return. Instruct them to avoid crossing their legs, and advise them to elevate their legs when sitting in a chair to prevent venous stasis and promote venous return.

Prevention may be the key to avoiding pulmonary emboli, since even with great medical advances in the detection and treatment of PE there are still many times when they prove to be fatal. The nurse is often the first person alerted to the signs and symptoms of DVT and subsequent pulmonary embolus, and thus can have a great impact on its prevention. Nursing research should focus further on preventative nursing measures and patient education to lead to early detection and treatment.

REFERENCES

1. Currie D: Pulmonary embolism: diagnosis and management, *Critical Care Nursing Quarterly* 13(2):41-49, 1990.
2. Dickinson S, Bury G: Pulmonary embolism: anatomy of a crisis, *Nursing* 19(4):34-42, 1989.
3. Doyle J, Johantgen M, Vitello-Cicciu J: Vascular disease. In Kinney MR, Packa DR, Dunbar SB, editors: *AACN clinical reference for critical care nursing,* St Louis, 1993, Mosby–Year Book.
4. Fahey V: Life-threatening pulmonary embolism, *Critical Care Quarterly* 8(2):81-88, September 1985.
5. Fishman A: *Pulmonary diseases and disorders,* New York, 1980, McGraw-Hill.
6. Fuller E: Treating and preventing blood clots, *Patient Care* 16(20):87-97, 1982.
7. Golhaber SZ: What role for thrombolysis is there in patients with pulmonary embolism? *Journal of Critical Illness* 7(2):192-199, 1992.
8. Goldhaber SZ: Thrombolysis in venous thromboembolism, *Chest* 97(4)(suppl):176-180, 1990.
9. Reference deleted in proofs.
10. Reference deleted in proofs.
11. Hoyt D, Swegle J: Deep-vein thrombosis in the surgical intensive care unit, *Surg Clin North Am* 71(4):811-830, 1991.
12. Kollef M, Neelon-Kollef R: Pulmonary embolism associated with the act of defecation, *Heart Lung* 20(5):451-454, 1991.
13. Meloche A: PE: pulmonary embolism, *Canadian Nurse* 8(7):23-26, 1986.
14. Sisson MC: Amniotic fluid embolism, *Crit Care Nursing Clin North Am* 4(4):667-673, 1992.
15. *St Anthony's DRG guidebook 1995,* Reston, Va, 1994, St Anthony.
16. Stratton M: Ventilation perfusion scintigraphy in diagnosis of pulmonary embolism, *Focus on Critical Care* 17(4):287-293, 1990.
17. Thomas M: Acute pulmonary embolism, *Focus on Critical Care* 10(4):21-28, 1983.
18. Trulock E: Approaches to deep venous thrombosis and pulmonary embolism in aging, *Geriatrics* 43(2):101-106, 1988.
19. Vermilya S: Future indications for thrombolytic therapy with tissue plasminogen activator, *Journal of Emergency Nursing* 15(2):207-210, 1989.

CLINICAL GUIDELINE

37

Pleural Compromise

Bev Ryan, MSN, RN, CCRN
Anne Aloi, MSN, RN

DESCRIPTION

The term *pleural compromise* describes a collection of conditions that interfere with the mechanics of respiration either through direct interruption of the pleura or through a space-occupying lesion. Pleural effusions, pneumothorax, chylothorax, and hemothorax are the more commonly seen conditions causing pleural compromise

A **pleural effusion** is an accumulation of fluid within the pleural space. The etiology of pleural effusions is varied and summarized in Table 37-1. It occurs in 25% to 50% of individuals with congestive heart failure, pneumonia, malignancy, and pulmonary emboli. Conditions that lower serum protein, thereby decreasing oncotic pressure, may lead to pleural effusions. Malignant pleural effusions are seen in patients with primary lung and breast tumors.[4] Pleural effusions occur in up to 27% of hospitalized AIDS patients, due to infection and/or hypoalbuminemia.[7]

A **pneumothorax** is a collection of gas or air within the pleural space resulting in partial or total collapse of the lung. Pneumothorax may be spontaneous, iatrogenic, or traumatic in origin. Primary spontaneous pneumothorax occurs most frequently in tall, thin young males. Its incidence is 9 per 100,000 individuals each year, and it carries a high recurrence rate.[1] Secondary spontaneous pneumothorax is associated with underlying pulmonary diseases. Causes of iatrogenic pneumothorax include central line placement, bronchoscopy, nasogastric tube insertion, and thoracentesis. Mechanical ventilation, especially with high levels of positive end expiratory pressure (PEEP), has a 3% to 5% incidence of pneumothorax.[1]

Hemothorax is a collection of blood in the pleural space, usually the result of blunt or penetrating chest trauma. It is seen in patients with malignancies or tuberculosis, which cause pleural inflammation and rupture of blood vessels. Hemothorax may also be due to iatrogenic causes such as central venous line insertion. Traumatic hemothorax is often associated with pneumothorax. In the setting of chest trauma with multiple costal fractures, the incidence of hemothorax is 32.8%, pneumothorax is 25.5%, and hemopneumothorax is 41.7%. Five percent of chest trauma cases will require thoracotomy for ongoing evacuation of blood.[10]

Chylothorax is the accumulation of chyle within the intrapleural space. 30% to 50% occur as a result of thoracic surgery or trauma; the remaining cases are due to malignancies or idiopathic reasons. Post-traumatic development occurs within 2 to 10 days. Accumulation is usually large and the fluid has a characteristic milky appearance. The mortality rate from chylothorax is up to 50%.[9]

The impact of pleural compromise relates to the size of the disturbance, the rate of accumulation, and the cardiopulmonary status of the patient. A small pleural effusion or pneumothorax in a normal individual would be asymptomatic, but either would cause fulminant respiratory failure in a patient with severe chronic obstructive pulmonary disease (COPD).

A major complication from a hemothorax is the development of an empyema. A persistent organized clot following a hemothorax forms a "peel" on the pleural surfaces, causing fibrosis, lung damage, and impaired gas exchange. When this occurs, decortication is necessary in an effort to restore normal lung function.[8] Despite these complications, 85% of patients with hemothorax and retained blood are free of pleural abnormalities.[14]

TABLE 37-1 Common Etiologies of Pleural Effusions

Disease process	Incidence
Bacterial pneumonia	30%-40%
Pulmonary embolism	30%-50%
Pancreatitis	20%
Esophageal perforation	60%
Abdominal surgery	50%
Subphrenic abscess	80%
Other etiologies with unknown incidence	
Congestive heart failure	
Asbestos/radiation exposure	
Cirrhosis	
Nephrotic syndrome	
Peritoneal dialysis	
Tuberculosis	
Connective tissue disease	
Uremia	
Neoplastic disease	
Drug-induced	
Ascites	

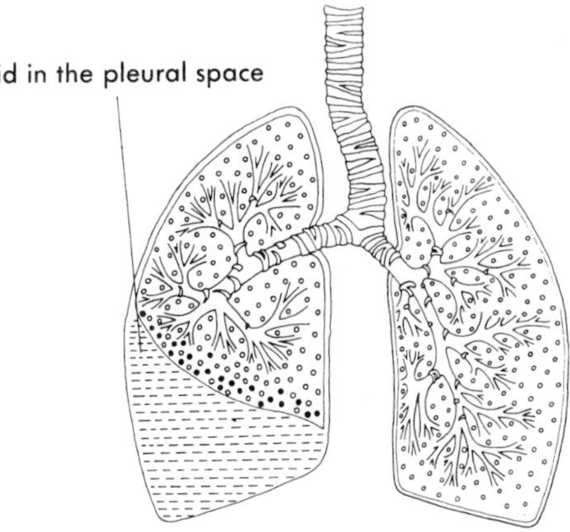

Figure 37-1 Illustration of pleural effusion. (From Thelan, et al: *Critical care nursing,* ed 2, St. Louis, 1993, Mosby–Year Book.)

PATHOPHYSIOLOGY

The pleura is a two-layered serous membrane. The visceral layer surrounds the lungs and the parietal layer lines the entire thoracic cavity. Between the two layers is a potential space containing 5 to 15 cubic centimeters of serous fluid. During respiration the elastic recoil of the chest wall opposes the natural tendency of the lungs to collapse. This opposition of forces creates a negative pressure within the pleural space and helps maintain the full expansion of the lungs. The pressure in the pleural space varies, remaining negative during a normal respiratory cycle. Pleural pressure becomes positive during forceful expiration, Valsalva maneuver, and positive pressure ventilation. Disruption of pleural integrity will cause a loss of negative pressure in the pleural space. During inspiration, the pleural pressure decreases from the resting level of -6 cm H_2O to -12 cm H_2O. This pressure gradient favors the flow of gas into the lungs. During expiration, pleural pressure increases up to -8 cm H_2O and gas flows out of the respiratory tract.

The fluid normally present in the intrapleural space provides lubrication, eliminating friction between the opposing layers of pleura. The blood supply to the parietal pleura is systemic in origin; the supply to the visceral layer is pulmonary. Systemic circulation pressure is higher than pulmonary circulation pressure. The resultant hydrostatic pressure gradient promotes fluid movement of pleural fluid. Fluid moves from the high-pressure system (systemic) into the low-pressure system (pulmonary). The visceral pleura is very vascular, enhancing this resorption of fluid.

Another source of fluid within the pleural space is the lymphatic drainage. Two liters of chyle drain into the venous system daily via numerous anatomical variations of the thoracic duct. Chyle is composed of electrolytes, proteins, glucose, urea, white blood cells, and fats. Blockage of the thoracic duct diverts lymphatic flow into the mediastinum, eventually disrupting the pleura. Accumulation may restrict lung expansion and precipitate cardiovascular collapse.

Any condition disrupting the pleural space impairs its ability to maintain full lung expansion. Fluid or air within the pleural space displaces lung volume and causes a partial or total collapse of the lung.

Pleural effusions are caused by an increase in production of fluid, an increase in capillary permeability, a decrease in absorption, or a change in the normal hydrostatic or colloidal pressure gradient. Effusions are differentiated by the chemistry and cellular characteristics of the pleural fluid. Exudative effusions are due to an increased capillary permeability and are commonly seen with neoplastic diseases and infectious processes. Transudates are serous and due to changes in the hydrostatic pressure gradient. (See Fig. 37-1.)

As long as the pleura is intact, the alveolar pressure remains higher than intrapleural pressure. Any rupture in the alveolar wall allows for gas movement from the alveoli into the intrapleural space. The resultant lung collapse is accompanied by a decrease in vital capacity, total lung capacity, and functional residual volume. (See Fig. 37-2.) The severity of hypoxemia is related to the degree of intrapulmonary shunting and perfusion of the nonventilated portion of the lung.

A pneumothorax from any cause may convert to a tension pneumothorax, a life-threatening emergency. Tension occurs via a ball-valve mechanism that allows air to enter the pleural space during inspiration but prevents its escape during expiration. Pleural pressure steadily increases, causing progressive collapse of the underlying lung, decreased venous return, decreased cardiac output, mediastinal shift,

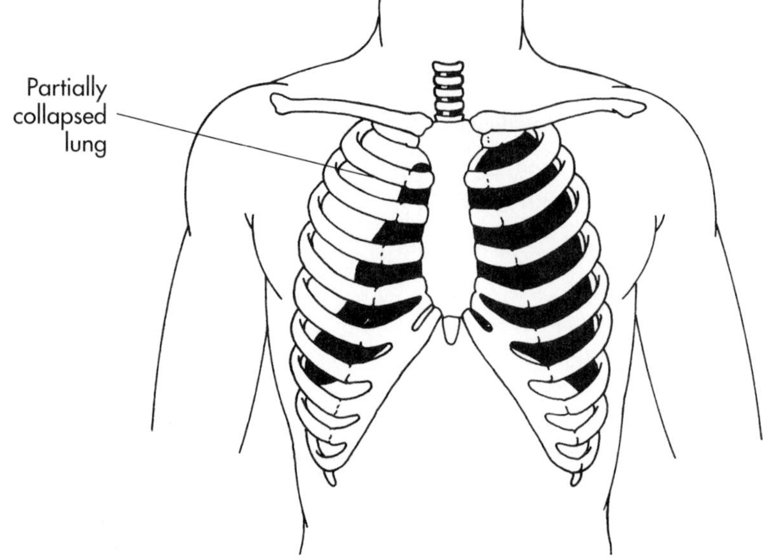

Figure 37-2 Simple pneumothorax. One lung is partially collapsed; the other structures are unaffected.

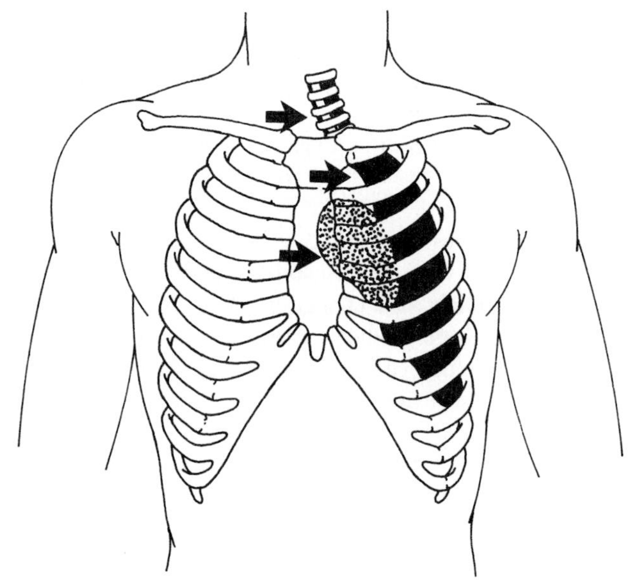

Figure 37-3 Right tension pneumothorax. One lung is completely collapsed, and the resulting pressure compromises structures in the left chest.

and, if allowed to continue, cardiovascular collapse. (See Fig. 37-3.)

LENGTH OF STAY/ANTICIPATED COURSE

The most important factor in anticipating the patient's course is the presence of underlying pulmonary disease in association with the severity and etiology of the insult. Interruption of pleural integrity is potentially life threatening. Length of stay ranges from outpatient therapy to prolonged hospitalization. Complications from pleural injury can prolong hospitalization and convalescence. Continued separation of the pleural layers impedes healing, resulting in a chronic air leak. The resulting communication between lung and pleura is a bronchopleural fistula. Bronchopleural fistulas are seen as a complication of mechanical ventilation and its associated barotrauma. DRG length of stay data are found in Table 37-2.[11]

MANAGEMENT TRENDS AND CONTROVERSIES

The chest x-ray remains the mainstay of diagnosis of pleural compromise. There is an increasing utilization of ultrasonography and CAT scans, particularly in the critically ill. Ultrasound is helpful in localizing pleural fluid for diagnostic thoracentesis and can be easily accomplished at the bedside. It is useful in diagnosis of the anterior pneumothorax, which may be missed on a portable chest film.

Treatment of pleural compromise depends on the presenting symptoms. Chest tube thoracostomy is standard for the symptomatic patient. The size of the tube depends on the type of fluid to be drained and physician preference. Recently, small-caliber tubes known as *pigtail catheters* have been used successfully in management of pleural effusions.[2] They offer the advantage of less-traumatic insertion and decreased discomfort for the patient. Because the small-caliber tubes are more likely to become obstructed, these catheters cannot be used to drain viscous fluid. A small-caliber tube known as the *Heimlich flutter valve* is a one-way valve that allows exit of air while prohibiting air reentry. It is used for patients with a symptomatic but self-

TABLE 37-2 Diagnosis Related Group Length of Stay

DRG #	Label	Age >17 without complications or comorbidity	Age >17 with complications or comorbidity
86/85	Pleural Effusion	4.9	8.2
95/94	Pneumothorax	4.9	8.5
80/79	Respiratory infections and inflammations	7.4	10.7
82	Respiratory neoplasms	8.9	8.9
84/83	Major chest trauma	4.3	7.2

Source: *St Anthony's DRG Guidebook 1995,* Reston, Va, 1994, St Anthony.

limiting pneumothorax.[3] This type of apparatus would not be used in a tension pneumothorax.

Within the past decade the routine practice of stripping and sealing chest tubes has been questioned. Research demonstrating levels of suction approaching -400 cm H_2O during chest tube stripping suggests that this practice is hazardous and should not be routinely employed. Complications associated with the increased suction include lung damage by invagination into the eyelets, excessive suture line tension, and dislodgement of suture line clips.[13]

Chest tube clamping, once commonly practiced, is contraindicated in most situations. Clamping of a chest tube may precipitate a tension pneumothorax. Chest tubes may be clamped to determine readiness for removal, to change the collection system, or to determine the origin of an air leak.[6]

The ideal dressing used around chest tube sites is controversial. The most common type is an occlusive dressing with petroleum gauze wrapped firmly around the tube to prevent air leakage. This type of dressing has been found to cause skin breakdown and may increase the incidence of infection. Other options include a dry, sterile gauze and leaving the site open to air.[6]

Another trend in the management of the patient with pleural compromise is the use of autotransfusion in patients with a hemothorax, either traumatic or surgical. This involves the collection, filtration, and reinfusion of the patient's blood. One advantage of this procedure is an increased oxygen-carrying capacity as compared with banked blood. Fewer acid–base and electrolyte imbalances are other advantages to autologous blood transfusions. Disadvantages include the presence of particulate matter and debris in the collected blood. The use of a blood filter reduces the risk of microemboli.[6,12]

ASSESSMENT

PARAMETER	ANTICIPATED ALTERATION
Pulmonary Status	
Rate	Tachypnea Dyspnea Use of accessory muscles
Chest expansion	Asymmetric Bulging of interspaces *due to mass effect of large effusions or pneumothorax*
Breath sounds	Diminished/absent over affected area *due to lack of air movement*
Percussion	Pleural effusion: dullness Pneumothorax: hyperresonance
Tracheal position	Pneumothorax (without tension): deviation toward the contralateral side—*increased pressure within the thorax pushes the intrathoracic structures away* Pleural effusion, hemothorax: deviation to the contralateral side—*space-occupying fluid pushes the structures toward the contralateral side*
Subcutaneous emphysema	Crepitus over chest, neck, face may be the first sign of a pneumothorax—*air takes the path of least resistance, dissecting through the fascial planes*

Vocal fremitus "99"	Decreased in tension pneumothorax, pleural effusions, hemothorax—*air or fluid causes a decreased conduction of sound*
Peak airway pressure	Increased Increased resistance to manual ventilation *due to a decrease in lung volume and loss of elastic recoil*
Chest x-ray	Pleural effusion: obliteration of costophrenic angle Pneumothorax: lack of vascular markings, mediastinal shift, subcutaneous air
ABG	Variable related to the size of compromise, baseline status of the patient Initially: • Pao_2 Decreased: <60 mm Hg • $Paco_2$ Decreased: <35 mm Hg • Respiratory alkalosis Subsequent: • Pao_2 Decreased: <60 mm Hg • $Paco_2$ Increased: >45 mm Hg • Respiratory acidosis pH <7.35 • Metabolic acidosis *r/t hypoperfusion, shock state*
Chest tubes	Occlusive dressing dry and intact Tube secure with connectors taped Water seal chamber filled according to manufacturer's instructions Suction chamber filled according to order and bubbling gently Pneumothorax: Air bubbles in water seal chamber, diminishing in intensity over several days and stopping *Initial correction of a pneumothorax results in a rapid release of air through the chest tube; over several days, the defect should heal and the air leak stop* Pleural effusion: no evidence of air bubbles Chylothorax: milky white drainage

Cardiovascular Status

Neck veins	JVD
Color	Cyanosis
Peripheral perfusion	Cold, clammy skin *due to hypoperfusion/shock*
Heart sounds	Distant Displaced PMI *due to mediastinal shift*
HR	Tachycardia Bradycardia *indicating severe cardiovascular compromise/hypoxemia*
BP	Pneumothorax: hypertension *due to pain/anxiety* Tension pneumothorax: • Hypotension *due to the mediastinal shift compressing the great vessels, decreasing cardiac output* • Pulsus paradoxus Hemothorax: hypotension *due to a decrease in circulating blood volume*
ECG	Decreased R wave, QRS amplitude Precordial T wave inversion Phasic voltage alternans *due to shift in position of heart within the chest cavity*
Cardiac output	Decreased *in shock states, tension pneumothorax*

Neurologic

LOC	Signs and symptoms *due to hypoxemia:* • Restlessness • Agitation

- Confusion
- Disorientation
- Obtundation
- Coma

Other

Hgb	Decreased with hemothorax
Hct	Decreased with hemothorax

PLAN OF CARE

INTENSIVE PHASE

The etiology of pleural compromise will result in the need for intensive care more than the pleural compromise itself. The patient's cardiopulmonary status before the pleural compromise determines the intensity of care required. Monitoring the respiratory and cardiovascular status of the patient is the focus of care. Management of pain is also very important during the intensive phase.

PATIENT CARE PRIORITIES	EXPECTED PATIENT OUTCOMES
Impaired gas exchange *r/t ventilation perfusion mismatch*	Improved ABGs, $Pa{O_2}$ within patient norms Reexpansion of lung Alert and oriented
Ineffective breathing pattern *r/t* *Pain* *Anxiety* *Disruption of normal mechanics of respiration*	Improvement/relief of pain Normal/improved pattern of breathing Restoration of normal intrapleural pressures
Pain/discomfort *r/t* *Pneumothorax* *Thoracentesis* *Chest tubes* *Trauma*	Indicate improvement/relief of discomfort Able to rest/sleep Able to participate in care
Anxiety *r/t* *Dyspnea* *Fear* *ICU environment*	Decreased anxiety as evidenced by relaxed facial expression, stable vital signs, reduced respiratory effort
Decreased tissue perfusion *r/t* *Decreased CO* *Decreased circulating blood* *Volume* *Compression of great vessels*	Normal CO: • Stable vital signs • Adequate peripheral pulses • Urine output >30 cc/hr • Normal mentation • Skin warm and dry
High risk for infection *r/t invasive therapy*	Free of nosocomial infection as evidenced by wound site without drainage or inflammation; normal WBC, temperature, heart rate

INTERVENTIONS

Monitor respiratory status for rate, rhythm, depth, use of accessory muscles, oxygen saturation, breath sounds q4h.

Monitor ventilator setting, including rate, mode, volumes, $Fi{O_2}$ q4h.

Monitor peak inspiratory pressures (mechanically ventilated patients) q1h to q4h. *An increase in airway pressure may indicate the development of a new or expanding pneumothorax. Increased airway pressures cause barotrauma and may precipitate a pneumothorax.*

Plan of Care (cont'd)

Monitor ECG for dysrhythmias.
Provide oxygen as ordered.
Manually ventilate intubated patient in preparation for emergency thoracotomy.
Provide reassurance and explain all procedures.
Monitor cardiac output q12h & prn. *Decreased cardiac output may be indicative of blood loss or tension pneumothorax.*
Monitor pulmonary artery pressures hourly. *A dampened PA waveform may indicate the development of a pneumothorax.*
Monitor chest tubes for air leak, fluctuation, water level q8h. *Bubbling during forceful exhalation or during delivered ventilator breaths indicates a continuing air leak. Water evaporates from the suction chamber, decreasing the effective suction.*
Monitor chest tube for amount and type of drainage q8h.
Maintain integrity of chest-drainage system by taping all connections and ensuring all points between the patient and the water seal are airtight.
Maintain drainage system below the level of the chest tube insertion site *to facilitate drainage and prevent retrograde flow of air/fluid into the pleural space.*
Adjust suction on chest tube to maintain continuous gentle bubbling if suction ordered.
Administer analgesia and sedation as needed *to maintain comfort, minimize work of breathing, and prevent splinting.*
Assist patient in turning side-to-side q2h *to prevent atelectasis, promote reexpansion of lung, and prevent complication.*
Elevate head of bed if patient condition allows *to promote drainage, aid reexpansion of lung, and relieve dyspnea.*
Administer fluid, blood as needed *to maintain normal blood pressure, hematocrit >30%.*
Maintain occlusive dressing with petroleum gauze and sterile gauze *to reduce the risk of infection and air leak.*

INTERMEDIATE PHASE

Recovery from pleural compromise depends on the etiology and extent of the insult. The nurse focuses on assessment of the respiratory system, observing for signs and symptoms of reaccumulation of fluid or recurrence of a pneumothorax. During this time, chest tubes are discontinued and the patient is weaned from mechanical ventilation.

PATIENT CARE PRIORITIES

High risk for ineffective breathing pattern *r/t*
Disease process
Potential complications
Exacerbation

EXPECTED PATIENT OUTCOMES

Normal/improved pattern of breathing
Resolution of pleural compromise

INTERVENTIONS

Clamp chest tube as ordered before removal *to assess patient tolerance and possible recurrence of pneumothorax.*
Administer analgesics before removal of chest tube.
Place petroleum gauze, occlusive dressing over chest tube site *to prevent air entry into the pleural space.*
Monitor dressing for bleeding and reinforce as necessary.
Maintain dressing until chest tube site is closed *to prevent air entry into the pleural space.*
Explain to patient the importance of notifying nurse of onset of dyspnea, sudden pain.

TRANSITION TO DISCHARGE

During the convalescent phase of hospitalization, the focus is on education and preparation for discharge. Residual deficits are identified and a plan to optimize activity tolerance is established. Patient and family are provided with information regarding etiology and pathophysiology. Precipitating factors of pleural compromise are reviewed and life-style changes, such as smoking cessation, are emphasized. Patients discharged with significant pulmonary deficits should be assisted in identifying any necessary environmental changes.

Proper education and support permits some patients to be discharged with small-caliber chest tubes. Candidates for home care include patients with recurrent pneumothoraces or malignant pleural effusions unresponsive to pleurodesis. Instruction includes chest tube management and identification of complications and emergencies.[5]

REFERENCES

1. Anthonisen NR, Filuk RB: Pneumothorax. In Fishman AP, editor: *Pulmonary diseases and disorders,* ed 2, New York, 1988, McGraw-Hill, pp 2171-2179.
2. Burns J: Caring for the patient with a pigtail drainage catheter, *Nurs* 92 22(6):52-53, 1992.
3. Connor PA: When and how do you use a Heimlich flutter valve? *Am J Nurs* 87(3):288-290, 1987.
4. Feinsilver SH, Houston MC, Sahn SA: Fast-track effusion care, *Patient Care* 26(1):92-108, 1992.
5. Garvey CM: Home management of chest tubes, *Caring* 11(9):78-82, 1992.
6. Gross SB: Current challenges, concepts, and controversies in chest tube management, *AACN Clin Iss Crit Care Nurs* 4(2):260-275, 1993.
7. Joseph J, Strange C, Sahn S: Pleural effusions in hospitalized patients with AIDS, *Ann Intern Med* 118(1):856-860, 1993.
8. Kinasewitz GT, Fishman AP: Pleural dynamics and effusions. In Fishman AP, editor: *Pulmonary diseases and disorders,* ed 2, New York, 1988, McGraw-Hill, pp 2117-2136.
9. Morey LB, Dungan JM: Chylothorax: a complication of thoracic trauma or surgery, *Dim Crit Care Nurs* 11(3):184-190, 1992.
10. Safarov IS: The treatment of pneumothorax and hemothorax in multiple rib fractures and associated trauma, *Klin Khir* (4):43-46, 1992.
11. *St Anthony's DRG Guidebook 1995,* Reston, Va, 1994, St Anthony.
12. Sympson GM: CATR: a new generation of autologous blood transfusion, *Crit Care Nurse* 11(4):60-64, 1991.
13. Teplitz L: Update: are milking and stripping chest tubes necessary? *Focus Crit Care* 18(6):506-511, 1991.
14. Winterbauer RH: Nonneoplastic pleural effusions. In Fishman AP, editor: *Pulmonary diseases and disorders,* ed 2, New York, 1988, McGraw-Hill, pp 2150-2154.

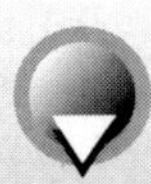

CLINICAL GUIDELINE

38

Thoracic Trauma

Cindy Goodrich, MS, RN, CCRN

DESCRIPTION

The leading cause of death for individuals less than 40 years of age is trauma.[12] Thoracic trauma is commonly seen in the multiple-injured patient and is frequently associated with life-threatening conditions. Twenty-five percent of all civilian trauma-related deaths in North America are due to thoracic trauma.[11,23] It has been identified as a contributing factor in an additional 25% to 50% of deaths.[24] Many of these deaths occur after the individual is admitted to the hospital. Thoracic trauma involves injuries to the chest wall, lungs, pleura, heart, great vessels, tracheobronchial tree, and esophagus. Mechanisms of injury include both blunt and penetrating trauma. Motor vehicle accidents account for 70% to 80% of all blunt thoracic injuries.[32] Other common causes include accidents involving motorcycles, falls, and bicycles. Penetrating chest injuries frequently result from blast injuries, gunshot wounds, stab wounds, and impalement of foreign bodies. Survival from thoracic trauma is dependent on early recognition and prompt intervention. The majority of thoracic injuries do not require extensive surgical intervention, being treated by observation, tube thoracostomy, pain control, and support of respiratory function. Only 10% to 15% of thoracic injuries will require an open thoracotomy.[11,17,18,30]

Long-term disability has been associated with severe thoracic injuries, having significant economic and social impact.[30] Employment time may be lost depending on the patient's preexisting health history and severity of the thoracic injury.

PATHOPHYSIOLOGY

Thoracic trauma results in disruption of chest wall integrity and/or alteration in the functioning of underlying structures such as the lungs or heart. Life-threatening thoracic injuries include flail chest, tension pneumothorax, massive hemothorax, aortic disruption, and cardiac tamponade. Potentially life-threatening injuries include myocardial and pulmonary contusions, tracheobronchial disruption, rib fractures, and traumatic diaphragmatic rupture.

Blunt trauma involves injuries in which there is no communication between the internal structures and the outside environment as a result of the primary impact. Direct and indirect damage to the chest wall and underlying structures occurs. Mechanisms of blunt trauma include direct impact, rapid deceleration, and compression forces.[10,16] Direct impact occurs when the chest wall comes in contact with a blunt object such as a steering wheel. Localized damage to the rib cage or underlying structures may occur, resulting in rib fractures, myocardial or pulmonary contusions, or pneumothorax. The force most commonly involved in falls and high-speed motor vehicle accidents is deceleration. In this situation, the body stops suddenly, but the internal structures continue in a forward motion. Severe compression of the chest may result in rib fractures, flail chest, or rupture of the heart or diaphragm.[10] When dealing with blunt thoracic injuries, it is important to remember that the severity of injury may not be reflected by the outward appearance of the patient's chest. Significant internal injuries may be present in individuals with only minor chest wall abrasions.

Penetrating injuries disrupt the integrity of the chest wall and underlying structures, resulting in direct and indirect injury. Structures in the path of the penetrating object will be directly affected. Indirect damage to adjacent structures occurs as energy is given off to the tissues. The velocity and mass of the penetrating object as well as its path will be the true predictors of the amount of resultant damage.

The final outcome of both blunt and penetrating trauma is an alteration in the normal physiology of respiration and circulation. The specific pathophysiology of each type of thoracic injury is unique. This chapter will focus on injuries involving the chest wall and pulmonary system that commonly result after blunt thoracic trauma. The specific injuries to be covered include rib fractures, flail chest, pulmonary contusion, and tracheobronchial disruption. Pneumothorax and hemothorax are covered in Guideline 37 on pleural compromise. Cardiac contusion and cardiac tamponade are discussed in Guideline 21 on cardiac trauma.

Rib fractures are the most common injury resulting from blunt thoracic trauma.[6,11] These injuries are often significant, resulting in impairment of ventilation, retainment of secretions, atelectasis, and pneumonia.[11] Rib fractures vary greatly in their severity. Intrathoracic and intra-abdominal organ injury are frequently associated with multiple rib fractures. Significant force is required to fracture the upper ribs because they are protected by the scapula, clavicle, humerus, and muscles of the back and shoulders.[6,11] Fractures of the first and second ribs often are associated with significant injury to the head, spinal cord, neck, lungs, tracheobronchial tree, and great vessels.[11] A mortality rate of 50% is associated with fractures of these ribs due to the high incidence of severe concurrent injuries.[11]

The most frequent sites of fractures are the middle ribs, 4 through 9. Fractures may result from a direct blow to the chest wall. Compression of the chest by anteroposterior forces may result in mid-shaft rib fractures. Serious intrathoracic injuries may be seen with rib fractures, including pneumothorax, hemothorax, pulmonary or myocardial contusion, lung laceration, and tracheobronchial or great vessel disruption.[10] Fractures of the lower ribs, 9 through 12, often are associated with injuries to the spleen, liver, and kidney.

Flail chest is a common life-threatening injury, occurring in 10% to 20% of trauma admissions.[28] This injury involves a disruption of the chest wall resulting from direct impact or severe compression. Damage may result as the chest wall directly impacts an immobile object such as a steering wheel during a motor vehicle accident. Compression injury with crushing is seen frequently in industrial and farm accidents. Chest compressions during CPR also may produce a flail chest. Other associated injuries must be suspected due to the great amount of force needed to produce a flail chest.[6] This injury is commonly associated with pulmonary contusions.

A flail chest occurs when two or more sites on two or more adjacent ribs are fractured, or when a free-floating sternum is produced. The integrity of the chest wall is disrupted and the chest wall no longer moves as a single unit. The flail segment does not respond to the actions of the respiratory muscles, but instead moves according to changes in intrapleural pressure.[15] During inspiration, intrapleural pressure becomes more negative than atmospheric pressure, and the flail segment moves inward. Intrapleural pressure becomes more positive during expiration, exceeding atmospheric, and the flail segment moves outward.[6] The flail segment moves in opposition to the rest of the rib cage during respiration. This is referred to as paradoxical chest wall movement. The bellows function of the chest wall is altered and damage to underlying structures such as the lungs frequently occurs.[36] This paradoxical chest wall movement along with pain will interfere with alveolar ventilation, resulting in atelectasis.[6] Three types of disturbances in ventilation occur after flail chest. They include (1) increased work of breathing and ineffective chest expansion due to paradoxical chest wall movement, (2) damage to underlying lung tissue which may result in pulmonary contusion, and (3) pain from fractures that reduces ventilation.[17] The most significant physical abnormality and a predictor of mortality is the amount of underlying pulmonary injury that is present.[9,17] Initially this injury may be overlooked if multiple injuries are present or the patient is able to compensate effectively. Unfortunately, in many cases the flail may not be noticeable until respiratory muscle splinting is lost 8 to 24 hours postinjury.[8]

Pulmonary contusion is the most common potential life-threatening thoracic injury seen in North America.[11] It generally results from blunt trauma and frequently is associated with flail chest. A high index of suspicion and careful assessments are needed to identify this potentially lethal thoracic injury. Pulmonary contusion results when a portion of the lung forcefully impacts the chest wall. This is commonly seen when the anterior chest hits an immobile object such as a steering wheel during a motor vehicle accident. It is also caused by situations that increase pressure within the pulmonary vascular system. Examples of this mechanism include compression of the chest wall or blast injuries.[5] In both situations, forces are transmitted to the lung(s), resulting in damage to lung tissue, alveoli, and airways. This disruption of lung architecture leads to interstitial and alveolar hemorrhage. Blood and fluid accumulate within the interstitial spaces and alveoli. Varying degrees of edema and atelectasis occur, leading to airway obstruction and increased pulmonary vascular resistance (PVR). Pulmonary blood flow and compliance decrease, intrapulmonary shunting increases, and hypoxemia occurs during the first 24 to 48 hours.[3,13,38] Pulmonary contusions may range from small localized areas of hemorrhage to massive areas of damage involving one or both lungs. Careful monitoring and close observation will allow for early detection of the respiratory compromise that is seen in these individuals. It is important to remember that the full extent of lung damage may not be seen until 48 hours postinjury. Uncomplicated lung contusions may resolve within 10 days to 2 weeks.[35]

Tracheobronchial disruption is a less common life-threatening injury resulting from both blunt and penetrating trauma to the neck and chest.[34] Blunt trauma is caused by direct impact or when shearing forces are applied to the trachea or mainstem bronchus. Penetrating injuries occur when the wall of the tracheobronchial tree is punctured by a penetrating object such as a knife or rib.[14] The incidence of this injury has risen dramatically as motor vehicle accidents have become more prevalent.[29] Tracheobronchial injuries may vary in severity from minor tears to complete transections.[2]

Injury to the tracheobronchial tree may take place at any level. Tracheal tears generally occur vertically in the membranous portion near the carina. Commonly, the mainstem bronchus is injured within 1 inch of the carina. This injury frequently is missed on clinical exam, and many of these patients die before ever reaching the hospital due to their associated injuries. Those admitted to the hospital have a 30% mortality rate.[11] The clinician must have a high index of suspicion to identify this injury. In many cases these patients present with few symptoms, or attention is diverted to associated injuries. Concurrent injuries to the esophagus, larynx, and aorta and its major branches are seen frequently. This often-fatal injury is identified within the first 24 hours in less than 30% of cases.[15] Unrecognized injuries may present later as a tracheal stenosis.[2] Emphasis must be placed on early diagnosis so that prompt, definitive life-saving treatment is instituted.

LENGTH OF STAY / ANTICIPATED COURSE

The length of stay and anticipated course for patients with thoracic trauma will depend on the severity of the injury, associated injuries, and the pre-trauma pulmonary status of the individual. Elderly individuals and those with a history of pulmonary disease may require more aggressive interventions and longer hospitalizations.[14] DRG 83: Major chest trauma with CC is assigned an average LOS of 7.2 days, and DRG 84: Major chest trauma without CC is assigned an average LOS of 4.3 days.[33]

The impact of blunt thoracic trauma on long-term disability is still under investigation. Research studies report contradictory results regarding the long-term outcomes of these individuals.[4,19,20,22] Early identification of all injuries and prompt interventions will provide these patients with the greatest chance for optimal recovery.

MANAGEMENT TRENDS AND CONTROVERSIES

The initial management of all patients with thoracic trauma centers around management of airway, breathing, and circulation. The number-one priority is to establish and maintain a patent airway while providing cervical spine control. This is followed by support of breathing and ventilation. Lastly, circulation is maintained and shock states are treated. Successful management of these individuals involves rapid assessment and prompt intervention as problems are identified. The clinician must maintain a high index of suspicion to identify all life-threatening injuries and complications. The specific management of rib fractures, flail chest, pulmonary contusion, and tracheobronchial disruption is discussed below.

Rib Fractures

The major concern with rib fractures is the presence of life-threatening associated injuries. Fractures of the first and second ribs are often accompanied by injuries to the lungs, great vessels, spinal cord, and tracheobronchial tree. Once life-threatening injuries have been treated, management of rib fractures is initiated. The goal of treatment should be to provide adequate pain control so that effective ventilation is achieved. Proper analgesia will reduce the occurrence of splinting, retained secretion, and hypoventilation that frequently accompany rib fractures. This will decrease the risk of serious complications such as atelectasis and pneumonia. Oral or parenteral narcotics usually are effective for treatment of simple rib fractures. In patients with more severe injuries, intercostal nerve blocks and continuous epidural analgesia will help to enhance ventilatory function.[25] It is no longer accepted practice to use binders or to tape the chest wall.[11] These procedures have been found to restrict chest wall motion, leading to increased splinting, retention of secretions, and hypoventilation.[6,10] Some individuals will need to be hospitalized so that aggressive treatment can be initiated to prevent ventilatory impairment. Criteria for hospitalization include (1) age, (2) preexisting cardiopulmonary disease, (3) jagged rib fractures, (4) severity of associated injuries, and (5) extent of respiratory compromise.[6] Surgical intervention for simple rib fractures is usually unnecessary and most will heal within 6 weeks.[10]

Flail Chest

The management of flail chest has been extremely controversial over the past decades. Historically, external stabilization of the flail segment was the emphasis of treatment. Elaborate traction devices, wrapping, and placement of sandbags over the flail segment were tried to eliminate the paradoxical movement that occurs during respiration.[28] Internal splinting with positive pressure ventilation and intubation became the accepted treatment for flail chest in the late 1950s. This was an effective method for treating the respiratory dysfunction associated with flail chest, but in many cases the complications outweighed the benefits. In 1975, Trinkle and associates published a study demonstrating that mortality could be decreased by using selective intubation and mechanical ventilation.[36] They theorized that the most important aspect of flail chest was the resultant pulmonary injury. These authors strongly advocated early treatment aimed at minimizing pulmonary injury so that the need for ventilator treatment would be decreased. Currently, management centers around treatment of the underlying pulmonary injury. Only those who cannot adequately ventilate should be intubated. Treatment goals for flail chest include (1) respiratory support with selective intubation and mechanical ventilation, (2) aggressive pulmonary hygiene, and (3) adequate pain management.

The choice of respiratory support depends upon many factors. All individuals with flail chest should receive humidified supplemental oxygen therapy. Indications for intubation and mechanical ventilation include respiratory failure, shock, severe head injury, severe associated injuries requiring a surgical procedure, preexisting pulmonary disease, age of 65 years or greater, and inability to maintain a patent airway.[10,17,31] Weaning the patient off the ventilator will depend on resolution of gas exchange abnormalities associated with the pulmonary injury, not the disappearance of paradoxical chest wall movement.

Aggressive pulmonary hygiene should involve suctioning, postural drainage, early mobilization, incentive spirometry, and turning, coughing, and deep breathing.[13] These will help support existing respiratory function and prevent complications such as pneumonia and atelectasis.

Pain associated with flail chest frequently results in shallow breathing, atelectasis, splinting, and hypoventilation. Adequate pain management will help improve ventilation and gas exchange.[25] Conventional pain management for thoracic trauma has involved the use of parenteral narcotics and intercostal nerve blocks.[26] More recently, the use of continuous epidural fentanyl analgesia has gained popularity for the treatment of multiple rib fractures and blunt thoracic trauma.[25,26] Mackersie demonstrated relief of pain and improved ventilatory function using this method of pain management in patients with multiple rib fractures.[26]

Fluid management is of great importance in these individuals. The amount and type of intravenous fluids will be dependent on the patient's condition. If shock is present, adequate amounts of crystalloid intravenous fluids should be given to restore hemodynamic stability. In a nonshock state, it is important to control the administration of fluids so that overhydration is prevented in these individuals who already have a compromised pulmonary status. Fluid restriction and the use of diuretics are no longer acceptable practices for reducing or preventing pulmonary contusion or ARDS because of the limited research data available.[10,11] The use of hemodynamic monitoring is helpful in optimizing the fluid status of these individuals.

There has been renewed interest in surgical stabilization of the flail segment when severe flail chest is present. However, it remains controversial as to whether the risks outweigh the benefits. The majority of patients do not require surgical stabilization. However, if a thoracotomy is performed for the treatment of associated injuries, surgical stabilization should be considered.[27] Chest wall deformity often results in patients treated nonsurgically. The significance of this in terms of producing long-term restrictive defects is still under investigation.[1]

Lung Contusion

Treatment goals for lung contusion are aimed at (1) maintenance of acceptable alveolar ventilation and arterial oxygenation, and (2) prevention of complications. Management involves maintaining a patent airway, providing adequate ventilatory support, administration of supplemental oxygen, aggressive pulmonary hygiene, fluid management, and control of pain.

Management begins with establishment and maintenance of a patent airway. Airway obstruction may result secondary to retainment of bloody secretions, clots, and dead tissue. Frequent suctioning and irrigation with saline as needed for thick secretions are essential to avoid obstruction of endotracheal and tracheostomy tubes. Emergency equipment including airway adjuncts should always be kept readily available at the bedside.

The usefulness of early intubation and mechanical ventilation for patients with lung contusion still remains controversial. In the mid-1970s Trinkle and associates introduced the concept of selective intubation for patients with flail chest and pulmonary contusion.[36] Patients without respiratory impairment can be managed successfully with supplemental oxygen as long as oxygenation and ventilation are maintained. Those who develop progressive ventilatory failure and hypoxemia will require intubation and mechanical ventilation. Signs of ventilatory failure and hypoxemia such as $Pa{O_2}$ <60 mm Hg on 50% oxygen, respiratory rate >24/min, and/or tidal volume of <5 ml/kg are some indications that early intubation and mechanical ventilation are warranted.[7] The addition of PEEP may be useful in those individuals who continue to demonstrate respiratory compromise. Simultaneous independent mechanical ventilation (SIMV) may be considered when there is unilateral lung damage. This will allow for the delivery of a different volume of gas to each lung, resulting in improved oxygenation of the affected lung.[37] High-frequency jet ventilation has been used when bilateral pulmonary contusions are present. Small tidal volumes and high respiratory rates are used to keep alveoli well-ventilated with this type of ventilatory therapy.[37]

Aggressive pulmonary hygiene is instituted early to mobilize and clear bloody secretions. Mobilization of secretions is accomplished through humidification of inspired gases and proper hydration. Pain medication is administered so that the patient can cough and effectively clear airway secretions. Incentive spirometry and chest physiotherapy will assist in the prevention or treatment of atelectasis and pneumonia.

It is important to monitor fluid status closely in these patients so that overhydration is prevented. Fluid overload may lead to increased pulmonary edema and further lung damage. Fluid status may be monitored closely by evaluating central venous pressure or by using pulmonary artery pressure monitoring.

Tracheobronchial Disruption

The clinician's number one priority in tracheobronchial disruption is to secure and maintain a patent airway. In the unstable patient who presents with airway obstruction or massive hemoptysis, this will involve placement of an endotracheal or tracheostomy tube. Fiberoptic bronchoscopy-guided intubation can be helpful when more difficult cases are encountered. Administration of 100% oxygen should be carried out before and after these procedures. Caution should be exercised in those individuals who have a suspected partial or complete tracheal transection. Blind intubation of the distal portion of the trachea is often difficult, and a partial transection may be converted to a full transection during this procedure. In this situation, fiberoptic intubation or the placement of a tracheostomy tube are the preferred methods of airway management.[21]

ASSESSMENT

PARAMETER	ANTICIPATED ALTERATION
Pulmonary Status	
Airway patency	Partial or complete obstruction Stridor
Rate	Dyspnea Tachypnea Increasing hyperpnea Bradypnea
Chest wall	Ecchymosis, abrasions, lacerations: *suspect damage to underlying stuctures*
Integrity and appearance	Deformity
Breathing pattern	Accessory muscle usage Labored
Tracheal position	Deviated *due to tension pneumothorax or hemothorax*
Symmetry of chest expansion	Paradoxical movements *due to flail segment moving in opposition to chest wall during breathing* Splinting Asymmetrical
Secretions	Hemoptysis *due to damage to tracheobronchial tree or to lung tissue* Change in color *due to presence of infection* Ineffective cough resulting in retention of secretions
Palpation	Point tenderness Crepitus/subcutaneous emphysema *due to air leaking into subcutaneous tissue from injury to lung, airway, or esophagus* Rib or sternal deformity *due to displacement of bone fracture*
Breath sounds	Absent Decreased Localized wheezing *due to possible obstruction* Click on inspiration *due to rib or sternal fracture*
Bowel sounds	Middle to lower lung fields *due to diaphragmatic tear with herniation of abdominal contents into the thoracic cavity*
Cardiovascular Status	
HR	Tachycardia
BP	Hypotensive: MAP <70 mm Hg
Neck veins	Distended *due to increased right-sided heart pressures; e.g., pericardial tamponade, tension pneumothorax* Flat *due to decreased fluid volume; e.g., hemorrhage*
Skin color	Pale, ashen Cyanotic
Heart sounds	Shifted to right or left *due to deviation of cardiac structures with severe pneumothorax*

Neurological Status	
LOC	Anxiety Confusion Restlessness

Laboratory Studies	
ABG	Hypoxemia with PaO_2 decreased: <60 mm Hg Hypocapnia with $PaCO_2$ decreased: <35 mm Hg *due to initial compensatory hyperventilation* Hypercapnia with $PaCO_2$ increased: >45 mm Hg *due to severe chest wall injury and extensive lung injuries*
Intrapulmonary shunt Common estimates of intrapulmonary shunt include:	Increased: >10% *due to reduced alveolar function with decreased oxygen exchange*
• PaO_2/FiO_2 ratio	Decreased: <300
• Arterial/alveolar ratio	Decreased: <60%
• Alveolar-arterial gradient	Increased: >10 mm Hg
Pulmonary compliance	Decreased *due to stiff lung tissue, which may result from damaged alveoli and/or fluid accumulation*

Diagnostic Studies	
Chest x-ray	Fractured ribs or sternum Subcutaneous air Mediastinal air Widened mediastinum Progressive development of radiologic densities that do not conform to anatomical segments Atelectasis Recurrent or isolated pneumothorax Hemothorax Pneumomediastinum
SpO_2	Progressive desaturation
End-tidal CO_2	Increases as patient fatigues
Pain	Chest pain that increases upon inspiration/palpation *due to rib fractures, flail chest*
Chest tube	Persistent air leak

PLAN OF CARE

INTENSIVE PHASE

Patients experiencing thoracic trauma require intensive nursing care due to the high risk of respiratory compromise. Therefore, the priorities of care focus on airway clearance, breathing pattern, and gas exchange. Additional priorities of care include cardiac function, pain, and anxiety, which must be addressed to prevent further compromise to the respiratory system.

PATIENT CARE PRIORITIES	**EXPECTED PATIENT OUTCOMES**
Ineffective airway clearance *r/t* *Airway obstruction* *Trauma* *Tracheobronchial disruption* *Impaired cough* *Retained secretion, clots, tissue*	Secured and patent airway

Plan of Care (cont'd)

Ineffective breathing pattern *r/t* *Unstable chest wall segments* *Loss of bellows function of thoracic cage* *Lung tissue injury* *Pain*	Symmetrical chest expansion Respiratory rhythm and rate: WNL Absence of accessory muscle usage Tidal volume ≥10 ml/kg Pao_2 >80 mm Hg on room air Improved ABG Deep breaths without pain Pain relieved
Impaired gas exchange *r/t* *Impaired lung tissue* *Pulmonary contusion* *Decreased lung tissue perfusion* *Persistent air leak from tracheobronchial disruption*	Pao_2 >80 mm Hg on room air Improved oxygen saturations Respiratory rate 12 to 20/min A-a gradient <10 mm Hg Svo_2 60-80%
Decreased cardiac output *r/t* *Alteration in intrathoracic pressure*	CO: WNL Heart rate 60 to 100 bpm Normal sinus rhythm Svo_2 60 to 90% Palpable peripheral pulses Capillary refill time <3 seconds Urine output >0.5 to 1.0 ml/kg/hr
Pain *r/t* *Intubation* *Rib fractures* *Alteration in chest wall integrity* *Improper positioning*	Rates pain on 0 to 10 scale as decreased or absent Absence of nonverbal signs of pain: guarding, moaning, vital sign changes, diaphoresis, grimacing
High risk for infection *r/t* *Retained secretion* *Splinting/pain on breathing* *Vascular line placement*	Absence of infection Normothermic Normal WBC Body fluid cultures negative
Inadequate nutrition *r/t* *Increased metabolic demand* *Insufficient intake*	Positive nitrogen balance Minimal weight loss Fluid and electrolyte balance Increased albumin
Anxiety *r/t* *Traumatic event* *Threat of death* *Pain* *Dyspnea* *ICU environment* *Compromised ability to communicate if intubated*	Verbalizes decreased anxiety Physiologic signs of anxiety will be decreased: heart rate, blood pressure, respiratory rate Able to communicate needs/concerns

INTERVENTIONS

Protect cervical spine in all patients with uncleared spines or in which spinal cord injury has been identified.

Monitor airway patency, respiratory effort, breathing pattern, tidal volume, and other pulmonary function tests *for adequacy of ventilation.*

Suction based on assessment *to maintain patent airway and remove retained secretions.*

Protect airway from inadvertent removal or malpositioning, *which may dislodge the tube, thus increasing the risk of hypoxemia or extending an existing tracheal tear.*

Administer high-flow, humidified supplemental oxygen *to maximize respiratory function.*

Anticipate the need for aggressive ventilatory support with intubation and mechanical ventilation *to correct hypoxemia and support ventilatory efforts.*

Plan of Care (cont'd)

Monitor the patient for need for sedation and neuromuscular blocking agents *to decrease oxygen consumption and allow for adequate ventilation and effective breathing pattern.*

Assess for subcutaneous emphysema, crepitus, hemoptysis, dyspnea, and accessory muscle usage *indicating the presence of associated injuries or the worsening of identified injuries.*

Monitor for signs and symptoms of a tension pneumothorax (tracheal deviation, chest pain, dyspnea, hypotension, decreased breath sounds on affected side).

Monitor amount of air evacuated from chest drainage *to determine the presence of persistent air leaks indicating tracheobronchial disruption.*

Assess and document trends in arterial blood gases, pulse oximetry, intrapulmonary shunting, and A-a gradients *indicating adequacy of gas exchange.*

Observe and document respiratory rate and rhythm, chest excursion, breathing effort, and use of accessory muscles *to determine if respiratory distress is present.*

Position properly *to optimize lung expansion and ventilation/perfusion matching of uninjured lung tissue.*

Use aggressive pulmonary hygiene including suctioning, chest physiotherapy, incentive spirometry, postural drainage, early mobilization, turning, coughing, and deep breathing *to prevent atelectasis, retained secretion, and pneumonia.*

Instruct patient how to splint chest wall while coughing, deep breathing, and turning *to facilitate removal of secretions.*

Provide adequate hydration *to decrease viscosity of secretions.*

Monitor and trend hemodynamic measurements such as cardiac output, right atrial pressure, pulmonary artery pressure, and pulmonary artery wedge pressure *to indicate the effectiveness of fluid and drug therapy.*

Administer warmed intravenous crystalloid fluids and blood through large-bore IVs for volume replacement in shock states *to maintain adequate cardiac output and delivery of oxygen to the tissues.*

Closely monitor IV fluid infusions *to prevent fluid overload, which may lead to pulmonary complications such as ARDS.*

Measure intake and output and daily weights, *monitoring for serial trends.*

Administer pain medications *to provide patient comfort, improve ventilation, and assist with pulmonary hygiene* as ordered. Consider use of continuous analgesia, patient-controlled analgesia, and epidural narcotic infusions.

Assess for verbal and nonverbal manifestation of pain and evaluate patient's response to pain medications using a scale of 0 to 10 (0 = no pain, 10 = worst pain) *so that level of pain relief can be trended.*

Collaborate with dietitian *to develop strategies aimed at early nutrition.*

Monitor for signs and symptoms of infection *that may indicate the presence of pneumonia or vascular line infection.*

Monitor body cultures and CXR results as available *to assess for the presence of infection.*

Encourage verbalization of questions and concerns *to decrease anxiety.* Use alternative means of communication if necessary.

Explain all procedures and treatments in simple and easy-to-understand language *to decrease anxiety.*

INTERMEDIATE PHASE

The focus of care during the intermediate phase is to maintain adequate respiratory function. Management of pain and increasing mobility are key priorities of care to maintain effective airway clearance and breathing pattern.

PATIENT CARE PRIORITIES

Ineffective breathing pattern *r/t*
Chest wall deformity
Decreased energy/fatigue
Pain

EXPECTED PATIENT OUTCOMES

Effective breathing pattern
Spontaneous ventilation
Weaned off supplemental oxygen
Reports decreased pain on breathing

Plan of Care (cont'd)

Pain *r/t* *Alteration in chest wall integrity* *Rib fractures*	Rates pain on 0 to 10 scale as decreased or absent Absence of nonverbal signs of pain: guarding, moaning, vital sign changes, diaphoresis, grimacing
High risk for activity intolerance *r/t* *Pain* *Weakness/fatigue*	Verbalizes increased comfort while performing activities Verbalizes activities that increase fatigue Participates in required physical activities
Impaired physical mobility *r/t* *Pain* *Decreased strength/endurance* *Chest wall injury*	Improved physical mobility

INTERVENTIONS

Monitor and document any continued shortness of breath, dyspnea, and feelings of chest tightness *to determine emerging complications or disability.*

Continue aggressive pulmonary hygiene *to help resolve problem areas of lung tissue and improve thoracic muscle strength.*

Provide adequate nutritional support *to improve respiratory muscle strength.*

Monitor and document patient's level of tolerance for activities.

Monitor respiratory rate, pulse, amount of dyspnea, pain, diaphoresis *to indicate activity tolerance.*

Encourage patient to report activities that increase pain and fatigue.

Teach patient and family the use of relaxation techniques.

Plan activities collaboratively with patient and family *to promote independence and minimize fatigue.*

Set realistic, attainable goals for activity progression.

Monitor and document patient's current sleep pattern and provide rest periods between activities.

Provide comfort measures prior to sleep that the patient has found helpful in the past.

Coordinate nursing activities *to allow for rest periods and minimal interruptions during sleep.*

Encourage and assist with active and passive range-of-motion exercises *to develop muscle strength and endurance.*

Provide encouragement and positive reinforcement during activity progression.

Develop a plan with patient and family to increase mobility in collaboration with physical therapy.

TRANSITION TO DISCHARGE

Once the patient is no longer critical, preparation for discharge should begin. Deformities of the chest wall may begin to become apparent in those patients with multiple rib fractures and flail chest. Some respiratory compromise may be present manifested by dyspnea, activity intolerance, and abnormal spirometry. Chronic pain associated with chest wall injury may also be a persistent problem for some individuals. Nursing care during this phase of trauma recovery is focused on identification of effective pain-management strategies, continued pulmonary hygiene, strengthening of pulmonary function, and progression of activity. Preparation for discharge should focus on developing realistic self-care routines and activity progression in those with some residual respiratory disability.

REFERENCES

1. Ali J: Torso trauma. In Hall JB, Schmidt GA, Wood LD, editors: *Principles of critical care,* New York, 1992, McGraw-Hill.
2. Baldino WA, Cernaianu AC: Tracheal and bronchial disruptions, *Trauma Q* 6(3):19-26, 1990.
3. Baldino WA, Cilley JH: Flail chest and pulmonary contusion, *Trauma Q* 6(3):13-18, 1990.
4. Beal SL, Oreskovich MR: Long-term disability associated with flail chest injury, *Am J Surg* 150:324-326, 1985.
5. Bongard FS, Lewis FR: Crystalloid resuscitation of patients with pulmonary contusion, *Am J Surg* 148:145-151, 1984.
6. Boyd AD: Chest wall trauma. In Hood RM, Boyd AD, Culliford AT, editors: *Thoracic trauma,* Philadelphia, 1989, WB Saunders.
7. Brunko MW, Rosen D: Blunt and penetrating chest trauma. In Callaham ML, editor: *Current practice of emergency medicine,* ed 2, Philadelphia, 1991, BC Decker.
8. Cernaianu AC, Field CK: Complications and errors in thoracic trauma, *Trauma Q* 8(1):34-48, 1991.
9. Cilley JH, Mure AJ: Chest wall injuries, *Trauma Q* 6(3):1-11, 1990.
10. Cogbill TH, Landercasper J: Injury to the chest wall. In Moore EE, Mattox KL, Feliciano DV, editors: *Trauma,* ed 2, Norwalk, Conn, 1991, Appleton & Lange.
11. Committee on Trauma, American College of Surgeons: *Advanced trauma life support instructor manual,* Chicago, 1993, American College of Surgeons.
12. Committee on Trauma Research: *Injury in America: a continuing public health problem,* ed 3, Washington DC, 1986, National Academy Press.
13. Eddy AC, Carrico CJ, Rusch VW: Injury to the lung and pleura. In Moore EE, Mattox KL, Feliciano DV, editors: *Trauma,* ed 2, Norwalk, Conn, 1991, Appleton & Lange.
14. Hammond SG: Chest injuries in the trauma patient, *Nurs Clin North Am* 25(1):35-43, 1990.
15. Hood RM: Trauma to the chest. In Sabiston DC, Spener FC, editors: *Gibbons surgery of the chest,* ed 4, Philadelphia, 1983, WB Saunders.
16. Hurn PD, Hartsock RL: Blunt thoracic injuries, *Crit Care Clin North Am* 5(4):673-686, 1993.
17. Jackimczyk K: Blunt chest trauma, *Emerg Med Clin North Am* 11(1):81-96, 1993.
18. Kish C, et al: Indications for early thoracotomy in the management of chest trauma, *Ann Thorac Surg* 22:23, 1976.
19. Kishikawa M, et al: Pulmonary contusion causes long-term respiratory dysfunction with decreased functional residual capacity, *J Trauma* 31(9):1203-1210, 1991.
20. Landercasper J, Cogbill TH, Lindesmith LA: Long-term disability after flail chest injury, *J Trauma* 24:410, 1984.
21. Lipper BL, Klapholz A, Iberti TJ: Recognizing tracheobronchial injuries, *Hospital Physician* 25(3):53-56, 1990.
22. Livingston DH, Richardson JD: Pulmonary disability after severe blunt chest trauma, *J Trauma* 30(5):562-567, 1990.
23. Lo Cicero J, Mattox KL: Epidemiology of chest trauma, *Surg Clin North Am* 69(1):15-19, 1989.
24. Lickhard CG: Thoracic trauma, *Crit Care Q* 9:32, 1986.
25. Mackersie RC, et al: Continuous epidural fentanyl analgesia: ventilatory function improvement with routine use in treatment of blunt chest injury, *J Trauma,* 27(11):1207-1212, 1987.
26. Mackersie RC, et al: Prospective evaluation of epidural and intravenous administration of fentanyl for pain control and restoration of ventilatory function following multiple rib fractures, *J Trauma* 31(4):443-451, 1991.
27. Manzano JL, et al: Internal costal fixation of fractured ribs in a six-year-old patient, *Crit Care Med* 10:67, 1982.
28. Pate JW: Chest wall injuries, *Surg Clin North Am* 69(1):59-70, 1989.
29. Pate JW: Tracheobronchial and esophageal injuries, *Surg Clin North Am* 69(1):111-123, 1989.
30. Pickard LR, Mattox KL: Thoracic trauma: general consideration and indications for thoracotomy. In Moore EE, Mattox KL, Feliciano DV, editors: *Trauma,* ed 2, Norwalk, Conn, 1991, Appleton & Lange.
31. Sankarans S, Wilson RF: Factors affecting prognosis in patients with flail chest, *J Thorac Cardiovasc Surg* 60:402, 1970.
32. Shorr RM, et al: Blunt thoracic trauma: analysis of 515 patients, *Ann Surg* 206(2):200-205, 1987.
33. *St Anthony's DRG guidebook 1995,* Reston, Va, 1994, St Anthony.
34. Symbas PN, et al: Rupture of the airways from blunt trauma: treatment of complex injuries, *Ann Thorac Surg* 54:117-183, 1992.
35. Symbas PN, Gott JP: Delayed sequelae of thoracic trauma, *Surg Clin North Am* 69(1):135-142, 1989.
36. Trinkle JK, et al: Management of flail chest without mechanical ventilation, *Ann Thorac Surg* 19:355-363, 1975.
37. Van Way CW: Advanced techniques in thoracic trauma, *Surg Clin North Am* 69(1):143-155, 1989.
38. Wilson RF: Accidental and surgical trauma. In Shoemaker WC, et al, editors: *Textbook of critical care,* ed 2, Philadelphia, 1989, WB Saunders.

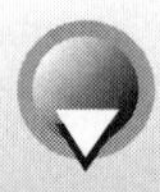

CLINICAL GUIDELINE

39

Pulmonary Surgery

David Strider, MSN, RN, MSB, CCRN
Christine Morrison, MSN, RN, CCRN
Kathleen Quinn, BSN, RN, MBA, CCRN
Arlene Yuan, MSN, RN, CCRN

DESCRIPTION

Pulmonary surgery involves the resection of lung airways, parenchyma, or pleura in patients with certain types of lung cancer, infection, or recurrent pneumothoraces. Such surgery is performed on more than 70,000 patients per year in the United States.[35] Pulmonary surgery is indicated if the identified lung lesion cannot be adequately suppressed with chemotherapy, antibiotics, or radiation treatments and if there is a low probability of postoperative recurrence if the lesion is surgically resected. The potential to stabilize or improve the patient's pulmonary function must be weighed against the inherent physiologic risks and discomfort associated with any thoracic surgery. It is essential for the nurse to have knowledge of the anatomy and physiology of the pulmonary system in providing care for surgical thoracic patients.

PATHOPHYSIOLOGY

Indications

The most common indication for pulmonary surgery is **lung cancer,** which now ranks as the major cause of malignancy-related death in men and women, and accounts for more than 145,000 deaths annually.[32,39] If untreated, lung neoplasms invade surrounding lung parenchyma, airways, pleura, and adjacent thoracic organs, leading to inadequate gas exchange and localized organ dysfunction, with subsequent multisystem organ failure followed by death. Therefore, surgical interventions are required to prevent or reverse these compromising conditions.

Despite multifaceted research efforts and characterization of modifiable risk factors, the 5-year survival for lung cancer has risen only from 8.5% to 15% in the last 25 years.[3] Current smokers are 9 to 12 times more likely to die from lung cancer than nonsmokers.[27] Increased lung cancer risks are also associated with exposure to asbestos, radon, arsenic, nickel, chloromethyl ether, cadmium, and beryllium.[33]

Most lung tumors can be characterized as small cell, non–small cell (NSC), or bronchial adenoma. (See Table 39-1.) Staging of lung cancer provides the clinician with better diagnostic and prognostic indicators and helps delineate treatment options. Such staging describes the neoplasm in terms of tumor size and location, spread to regional lymph nodes, and metastasis to distant organs.[26,31,37] Seventy percent of patients initially diagnosed with lung cancer have lesions that are not completely resectable.[33] For the remaining 30% who *are* candidates for lung tumor resection, average postoperative 5-year survival rate ranges from 25% to 35%.[36]

Pulmonary conditions other than cancer may require surgical intervention. These conditions include bronchiectasis, empyema, and spontaneous pneumothorax. **Bronchiectasis** refers to dilatation of the bronchi, with infection distal to a bronchial obstruction. Pooled mucopurulent secretions in the obstructed bronchus lead to bronchial wall infection and subsequent damage to its muscle and elastic tissue. Patients who are refractory to aggressive antibiotic therapy may require localized resection of the bronchiectatic region.[30]

An **empyema** is an infected pleural space that may be

TABLE 39-1 Major Lung Cancer Types in the United States[6,7,8]

Parameter	Small cell	Non–small cell	Bronchial adenomas
Prevalence as percentage of all patients with lung cancer	20%-25%	70%-75%	3%-5%
Specific cancer subtypes	Also referred to as *oat cell*	Adenocarcinoma Squamous cell cancer Large cell cancer	Adenoid cystic Carcinoid Mucoepidermoid
Usual treatment	Chemotherapy, radiation treatments	Surgical resection in early stages, chemo/radiation therapy in advanced stages	Surgical resection
Five-year survival rate	<1%	25%-35%	70%-90%

caused by a bronchopleural fistula, severe bronchopulmonary infection, or infradiaphragmatic sepsis. Initial treatment for empyema includes aggressive antibiotic therapy and thoracostomy tube drainage of the infected pleural space. Surgical treatment is reserved for patients refractory to therapy.

Spontaneous pneumothoraces may occur after rupture of subpleural cysts, emphysematous blebs or bullae, or after a torn pleural–vascular adhesion. Conventional treatment involves thoracostomy tube placement; however, surgical stapling through a limited axillary thoracotomy incision or thoracoscopy may also resolve spontaneous pneumothoraces.[16]

In addition to a thorough history and physical exam, the need for pulmonary surgery is determined by a diagnostic workup that may include chest radiographs, flexible bronchoscopy, percutaneous aspiration needle biopsy, and computerized axial tomography.[12] Not every patient with resectable lung lesions is a surgical candidate, due to preexisting respiratory, cardiac, or hepatorenal insufficiency. Tests frequently performed to assess preoperative lung function include forced expiratory volume in 1 second (FEV_1), forced vital capacity, and exercise studies.[24] Relative contraindications to pulmonary resection include unstable angina, congestive heart failure, and myocardial infarction within 6 months. Patients with metastases to nodes of the contralateral lung or to distant organs are usually not surgical candidates.[8]

Surgical Procedures

Pulmonary surgical procedures include lobectomy, segmentectomy, wedge resection, bronchial sleeve resection, pneumonectomy, and decortication. The indications, procedure descriptions, and potential complications vary for each procedure.

Lobectomy is indicated for primary lung tumors confined to a single lobe of the lung, allowing for conservation of as much functional lung tissue as possible while still removing the cancer and its nearest lymph nodes. Other less frequent indications include pulmonary tuberculosis, bronchiectasis, lung infections, fungal diseases, and large solitary metastatic tumors.[37]

The surgical procedure involves identification of the diseased lobe, dissection of the lobe from the rest of the lung, ligation of arteries and veins supplying the lobe, and bronchial stump closure. (See Figures 39-1*A* and 39-1*B*.) The space once occupied by the resected lobe is filled by a combination of diaphragm elevation, mediastinal shift, closer rib approximation, and some expansion of the remaining lung. One or two chest tubes are placed to create suction in the space where the lung was and allow the above events to happen.[20]

Operative mortality rates range from 3% to 5%, with the major causes of death being sepsis, cardiopulmonary insufficiency, pulmonary embolism, and pulmonary edema. Nonfatal complications include atelectasis and pneumonia, dysrhythmias, empyema, pleural effusions, bronchopleural fistula, and persistent pneumothorax.[37].

Segmentectomy is the removal of an individual bronchovascular segment of a lobe, and is indicated for small and peripherally located lung tumors when the patient has pulmonary insufficiency and removal of the entire lobe cannot be tolerated. This procedure differs from a wedge resection in that a segmentectomy removes the lung mass and the segmental lymph nodes draining the tumor. A segmentectomy can also be used to resect solitary metastatic tumors of the lung.[37]

Separation of the diseased segment from the remaining lobe requires the stapling of lung tissue after segmental arteries, veins, and bronchioles have been identified, ligated, and divided. A segmentectomy is technically more difficult than a lobectomy and significant air leaks are common in the immediate postoperative period. Two chest tubes are placed and remain in the pleural space until drainage has ceased and any air leak is resolved.[20]

The most common major complication is a prolonged air

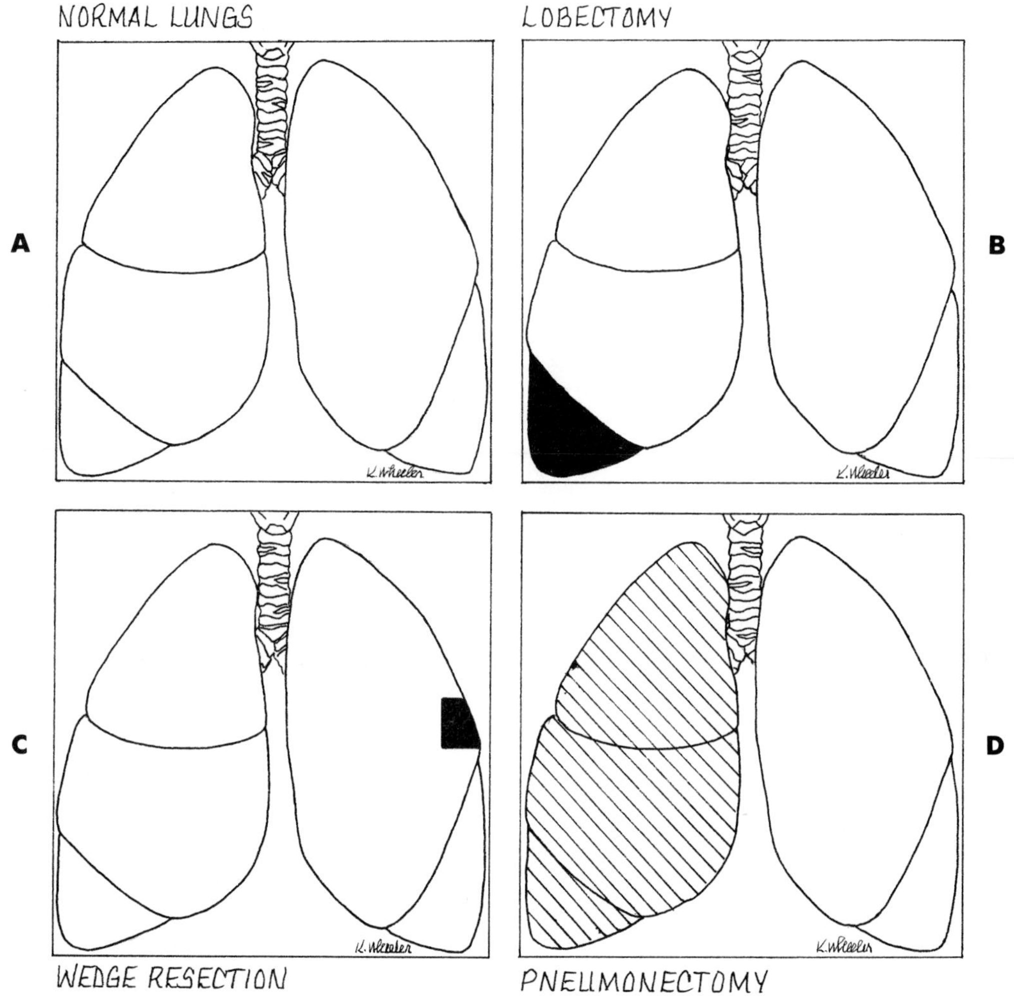

Figure 39-1 Select pulmonary procedures as compared to normal lungs (**A**); Lobectomy (**B**); Wedge resection (**C**); and Pneumonectomy (**D**). Shaded areas represent sections of lung tissue removed.

leak caused by bronchopleural fistula and empyema. The mortality rate is 1% to 5% and is usually related to the patient's underlying pulmonary function.[37] The expected LOS is 5 to 8 postoperative days.

Wedge resection is indicated for resection of small, peripherally located lesions when removal of adjacent lymph nodes is not desired. Peripheral granulomas, pulmonary blebs, benign tumors, and, rarely, primary or metastatic malignancies can be removed by wedge resection. This procedure may also be used for biopsy in diffuse lung disease and for patients with early malignancies who cannot tolerate a lobectomy.[37]

The operative procedure involves identifying the diseased section of the lobe, removing the area and a margin of normal lung tissue, and closing the remaining lung tissue. (See Figure 39-1*C*.) Mechanical stapling devices are commonly used for wedge resections, and a chest tube is inserted into the pleural space.[30]

The mortality rate for wedge resection is less than 1%. The most common complication is atelectasis caused by retention of pleural secretions. The expected LOS is 4 to 6 days. The chest tube drainage and air leak frequently resolve earlier than for lobectomy and segmentectomy, and the chest tube can usually be removed by the second or third postoperative day.

Bronchial sleeve resection is used to remove a lobe when the origin of the bronchus is involved with tumor. A "sleeve" or segment of main bronchus is removed, and the distal bronchus with its attached lobe is salvaged and sewn back to the proximal bronchus. A sleeve resection is frequently used to circumvent the necessity of a pneumonectomy in patients with severe pulmonary insufficiency who have bronchial carcinoma involving the origin of the right upper lobe, and less frequently in patients with left upper lobe neoplasms.[37]

The procedure involves removing the section of the main bronchus with its attached lobe that contains tumor and anastomosing the remaining distal bronchus to the proximal bronchus, being careful to minimize the interruptions of the bronchial arterial supply. Bronchoscopy is often used during and after the procedure to assess the adequacy of the bronchial lumen and remove excessive secretions.[37]

Perioperative mortality rates are 2% to 3%, and the expected LOS is 7 to 10 days. Several complications that are unique to bronchial sleeve resection include kinking of bronchial anastomosis; circumferential stenosis or granuloma formation; bronchial suture line dehiscence, which results in bronchopleural fistula with empyema or bronchovascular fistula with bleeding; and kinking of pulmonary artery.

Pneumonectomy is indicated for lung tumors that involve the mainstem bronchus or the beginning of a lobar bronchus that cannot be removed by a simpler procedure, such as lobectomy or wedge resection.[30] The assessment and staging of the patient's cancer must verify that the tumor and involved nodes are surgically resectable and potentially curable. Pneumonectomy is also indicated for massive hemoptysis, empyema, bronchopleural fistula, or tuberculosis that has not responded to medical therapy and results in a continuous source of infection.[37]

The mortality rate from pneumonectomy varies from 5% (a simple pneumonectomy) to 15% (pneumonectomy with extended chest wall resection).[41] The mortality rate is consistently higher in right pneumonectomies than left pneumonectomies, because the patient loses greater respiratory capacity in a right pneumonectomy than in a similar procedure to the left lung (the right lung has a greater alveolar surface area than the left lung).[7]

The surgical approach is usually through a posterolateral thoracotomy incision, in the area of the fifth rib.[20] The pleura is opened, and the pulmonary artery and veins are exposed, ligated or stapled, and divided. The bronchus is then exposed and dissected free from surrounding structures. (See Figure 39-1*D*.) The bronchus is closed with staples or simple interrupted sutures, and the bronchial suture line is checked for air leaks by covering it with saline. The surgeon observes for air bubbles while the anesthesiologist ventilates the remaining lung. Selected mediastinal lymph nodes are then dissected and removed for tumor staging.[30] After the surgeon has closed the incision, the patient is turned from the decubitus to the supine position. Pressure in the resected thoracic cavity is adjusted to atmospheric pressure by venting the operative space with a needle. This prevents severe displacement of the mediastinum to the contralateral side. Over time, the resected pneumonectomy space fills with fluid and congeals as a fibrin mesh. This fluid–gelatinous matrix helps stabilize the mediastinum during the first two postoperative weeks. There are usually no chest tubes in pneumonectomy patients. Positioning of the postoperative pneumonectomy is important in maintaining mediastinal stability. The average LOS is 7 to 10 days.[41]

Postoperative complications of pneumonectomy include supraventricular dysrhythmias, bleeding, atelectasis, chylothorax, and empyema. Postoperative bleeding is difficult to evaluate because of the absence of chest tubes in the pneumonectomy patient. Pulmonary edema may be a fatal complication of pneumonectomy and may result from hyperpermeability and increased filtration gradients across the pulmonary microcirculation. The severity of pulmonary edema during the postpneumonectomy period may also be influenced by the amount of perioperative intravenous fluids infused.[34]

Additional complications specific to the postpneumonectomy patient are tension pneumothorax, cardiac herniation, bronchopleural fistula, and left recurrent laryngeal nerve damage. Following pneumonectomy, "significant mediastinal shift may occur either toward the operated or the unoperated side."[11] Shift toward the unoperated side is due to excess positive pressure in the pneumonectomy space, whereas shift toward the operative side is related to excess negative pressure in the pneumonectomy space. Mediastinal position should be followed closely by chest x-ray because mediastinal shifts can lead to hemodynamic compromise.[11]

Cardiac herniation is an uncommon but potentially fatal complication of pneumonectomy, and may occur when a portion of the pericardium has been removed along with the pulmonary resection. The heart becomes displaced through the opening in the pericardium, resulting in sudden cardiovascular collapse. Although early diagnosis and treatment may achieve correction of this defect, mortality rates still range from 40% to 50%.[42]

Bronchopleural (BP) fistula, due to an abnormal communication between the bronchial stump and the pleural cavity, may follow a pneumonectomy (6% incidence). Patients with this complication often have serosanguineous sputum caused by the postoperative chest drainage through the stump leak. An empyema often follows because bacteria has a direct abnormal entry into the pleural cavity. The mortality of postpneumonectomy BP fistula approximates 50%.[42]

The left recurrent laryngeal nerve travels beneath the aortic arch and back up the mediastinum to the left vocal cord in the neck. If the pneumonectomy includes dissection of nodes in this area, the recurrent laryngeal nerve could be damaged during the surgery. Once this nerve has been damaged, the patient is hoarse, less able to cough, less able to clear secretions, and at higher risk for aspiration.[14]

Decortication consists of the removal of a restrictive, fibrous membrane or tissue layer from the pleural surface of the lung. This procedure is used in the treatment of a fibrothorax resulting from either an organized hemothorax or empyema. Decortication facilitates the release of the trapped, encased lung, permitting lung reexpansion and subsequent improvement in pulmonary function.[37] Decortication may be indicated if lung expansion does not occur after thoracentesis and chest tube drainage of the pleural collection.

The surgical procedure involves a posterolateral thoracotomy incision with blunt dissection of infected parietal and visceral pleura and removal of "restrictive" fibrous or tissue membrane from the pleural surface of the lung. This is followed by insertion of chest tubes and surgical closure of the space.[37]

Because the entire operation involves extensive peeling of inflamed and fibrotic tissue off the undersurface of the ribs and the outside of lung tissue, it can result in significant intraoperative and early postoperative bleeding and air leaks. LOS approximates 7 days; incidence of nonfatal complications approximates 10%, and includes postoperative bleeding secondary to the vascularity of the visceral pleural surface, sepsis (wound infection and recurrence of empyema), and persistent air leak.

The mortality rate has been reported at 8%, and is usually related to sepsis or hemorrhage from injury to the lung or chest wall vessels. Successful outcomes of greater than 90% should be expected after decortication for a chronic empyema, and greater than 95% for a clotted hemothorax.[37]

Operative procedures that facilitate a more definitive diagnosis and staging of a pulmonary lesion include mediastinoscopy, mediastinotomy, and exploratory thoracotomy. **Mediastinoscopy** involves a suprasternal incision with insertion of fiberoptic instruments to visualize and perform a biopsy on the paratracheal, tracheobronchial, and subcarinal lymph nodes. If the aortopulmonary nodes must be evaluated, the surgeon may perform an **anterior mediastinotomy.** This procedure involves a short transverse, or "hockey stick," incision over the second costal cartilage and adjacent rib on the affected side. In most cases, a pleural chest tube is not needed for mediastinoscopy or mediastinotomy. An **exploratory thoracotomy** permits the evaluation and biopsy of lung tumors and nodes in the hilar area. The usual approach is by a posterolateral parascapular incision; pleural chest tubes are inserted at the end of the procedure.[12]

LENGTH OF STAY/ANTICIPATED COURSE

Table 39-2 shows how pulmonary surgery is classified by Diagnostic Related Group (DRG), with the respective national average length of stay for those patients to which the DRG applies.[17]

Advances in thoracoscopy, more sophisticated anesthetic techniques, better postoperative analgesics, aggressive physical therapy, proactive postoperative nursing management, and careful screening and selection of pulmonary surgical candidates can only support the continued decrease in LOS for these patients. Health care trends suggest that, despite the continued shortening LOS for each pulmonary surgical procedure, there will be a steady increase in average age and the number of preoperative comorbidity factors for each operative candidate. Discharge criteria for these patients will still include the removal of all pleural chest tubes, radiographic evidence of reexpansion of the remaining lung, absence of infection, and return to the preoperative cardiopulmonary baseline.[35,37]

TABLE 39-2 Diagnostic Related Groups for Pulmonary Surgery

DRG #	Name of DRG	Average LOS (days)
75	Major Chest Procedures (noncardiac)	12.4
76	Other Respiratory System with Operation, and with postoperative complications or comorbidities	13.9
77	Other Respiratory System with Operation, and without postoperative complications or comorbidities	6.0

Source: *St Anthony's DRG Guidebook 1995*, Reston, Va, 1994 St Anthony.

MANAGEMENT TRENDS AND CONTROVERSIES

Postoperative pulmonary hygiene is an important intervention for the management of patients requiring pulmonary surgery. However, controversy exists about the most appropriate method of pulmonary hygiene. Clinicians continue to question the efficacy of routine incentive spirometry and chest physiotherapy for every postoperative pulmonary surgical patient. Although incentive spirometry (IS) may improve respiratory muscle strength, endurance, and functional residual capacity, no studies demonstrate a significant reduction in atelectasis or improvement in oxygenation after IS in extubated, post-thoracotomy patients. "Stacked," one-way valve inspiratory spirometry maneuvers (STIS) have been shown to increase the volume and duration of an inspiratory effort in small groups of intubated and extubated adult patients, although no significant improvements in oxygenation have been noted following this maneuver.[2,40] In the STIS maneuver, the patient continues to breathe in through the spirometer, but is unable to exhale (one-way valve) until the end of the maneuver. More research is needed to determine the efficacy of alternative IS maneuvers in post-thoracotomy patients.

Chest physiotherapy (CPT) in the form of postural drainage with chest percussion, may cause dysrhythmias, exacerbate incisional pain, and cause mucus plugs to lodge in the larger airways of post-thoracotomy patients.[15] The combination of CPT with bronchodilators may improve O_2–CO_2 exchange in post-thoracotomy patients who are unable to clear copious amounts of respiratory secretions (such as patients with bronchitis, bronchiectasis, or cystic fibrosis), and obviate the need for bronchoscopy.

Frequent turning helps mobilize pulmonary secretions and decrease postoperative atelectasis. Most clinicians still turn recovering partial lung resection patients such that the "good lung" (unaffected lung) is down, to maximize dependent pulmonary blood flow to the unaffected lung and permit the operative lung to fully expand. Pneumonectomy patients are turned with the remaining lung up, to maintain expansion of this lung and facilitate fluid accumulation in the resected hemithorax. Preoperative ventilation/perfusion mismatches may cancel out any position-related improvements in oxygenation in post-thoracotomy patients.[4]

Management of chest tube drainage and hydration are also important to consider in the management of patients requiring pulmonary surgery. Consistent postoperative stripping of the pleural chest tube may be detrimental to the pulmonary surgical patient because the extremely high negative pressure (up to -400 cm H_2O) associated with such stripping can actually entrap and injure lung tissue adjacent to the chest tube eyelets. Periodic pleural chest tube stripping may also dislodge small fibrin clots over pleural air leaks, thus resulting in a persistent leak.[23,35] Milking the pleural chest tubes ("milking" involves the manual squeezing and releasing of chest tubes) will help maintain patency and break up any clots or fibrin in the chest tube itself, while avoiding the high negative intrapleural pressure associated with stripping.[25]

Conservative fluid repletion is usually achieved during the post-thoracotomy period with isotonic crystalloid, and diuretics may be given to mobilize fluid administered during the perioperative period. Some patients may be prophylactically digitalized to decrease the likelihood of atrial fibrillation.[35,37]

For the past 80 years, thoracoscopic surgery has been performed for the diagnosis of diseases of the pleura and "minor" therapeutic interventions, such as lysis of pleural adhesions and small pleural and lung biopsies.[43] Recent technological developments in optical techniques and video imaging have broadened the clinical applications of thoracoscopy.[21,22]

Current indications of thoracoscopic surgery include use for pleural biopsy, diagnosis of effusions or pleurodesis for recurrent effusions, drainage of hemothoraces or early empyemas after chest drainage has failed, lung biopsy, resection of primary lung lesions or peripheral nodules, excision of pulmonary blebs, mediastinal biopsy, excision of selected mediastinal masses or cysts, pericardial biopsy, and partial pericardiectomy. Other indications include thoracic sympathectomy for autonomic nerve disorders of the upper extremities, splanchnicectomy for chronic visceral pain (such as pancreatitis), and esophagectomy for achalasia. The indications for thoracoscopy will grow and change as thoracic surgeons increase their expertise and as technology continues to improve.

Thoracoscopy is still major thoracic surgery and is technically difficult to perform, yet it is conducted through minimal invasive access.[43] The technique requires general anesthesia and a double-lumen endotracheal tube to allow single-lung ventilation while the appropriate surgical procedure is performed in the space provided from deflation of the other lung.[9,21,43] Two to five incisions (1 to 2 cm each) are made in the thorax to introduce the diagnostic telescope and its attached camera and other endoscopic instruments. When completed, a small-bore chest tube is placed in one incision for drainage, and the remaining incisions are closed. Frequently, if no bleeding or air leaks are present, no chest tube is used.[6,28]

The technologic advances of video thoracoscopy have significant implications for the postoperative recovery of these selected patients. The several small incisions used, rather than one large thoracotomy incision, decreases the severity and duration of postoperative pain. Analgesia requirements are less. Opiates are needed for the first 24 hours, and may be delivered through a patient-controlled analgesia (PCA) pump. After 24 hours, analgesia may be administered alone or in combination with a nonsteroidal antiinflammatory medication.

Extubation is performed in the operating room or recovery room. Consistent pulmonary hygiene (coughing and deep breathing, use of IS) is easier to maintain postoperatively due to decreased pain, and such pulmonary hygiene reduces postoperative atelectasis and supports early ambulation.

There is minimal need for an ICU bed for recovery, unless the patient has predisposing medical problems requiring monitoring after general anesthesia or has postoperative cardiopulmonary complications. Patients will normally require a stay of 4 to 8 hours in a post-anesthesia care unit to recover from anesthesia. LOS approximates 2 to 3 days for thoracoscopy, with discharge 12 to 24 hours after chest tube removal. Chest tubes are usually removed 24 hours after the surgical procedure. Return to preoperative ADLs occurs within 10 to 14 days, much earlier than for thoracotomy.[28]

ASSESSMENT

PARAMETER	ANTICIPATED ALTERATIONS
General appearance	Cachexia *due to catabolism associated with rapid tumor growth* Chest rise may be asymmetric *due to impaired air exchange in affected* lung
Tracheal position	Trachea may be shifted away from midline *due to pneumothorax, mediastinal shift,* or *extensive unilateral atelectasis*

Subcutaneous emphysema	The presence of subcutaneous emphysema is abnormal *due to bronchial or pleural air leak*
Chest x-ray	Post-thoracotomy patients may have basilar atelectasis *due to perioperative nitrogen washout, bronchiolar obstruction, surfactant loss, or compression by the adjacent abdominal viscera* Hilar engorgement and cardiomegaly may be *due to fluid overload* Pneumothorax may be seen, *which could be secondary to absence of a complete pleural seal or due to bleb rupture postoperatively* Pleural effusions may be evident
Chest tubes	The presence of an air leak *due to lack of a complete pleural seal* Sanguineous drainage of more than 100 cc/hour for more than 3 hours *due to coagulopathy and/or a leaking thoracic vessel* Sudden cessation of early postoperative chest tube drainage or multiple clots in the chest tube signify the need to "milk" the drainage tube (not strip) more frequently[25] Continuous drainage of white, milky fluid in the chest tube *due to chylothorax, which involves a thoracic duct leak with loss of large amounts of protein-rich lymphatic fluid*
Respiratory rate	Tachypnea *due to hypoxemia, blood loss, pain, or agitation* Bradypnea *due to residual anesthesia, narcotic analgesia, or severe carbon dioxide retention.*
Auscultation of lung sounds	Adventitious lung sounds postoperatively may include rhonchi (static secretions in larger airways), crackles (pulmonary edema, infiltrates), and wheezes (endobronchiolar obstruction) Absence of air movement *due to atelectasis or pneumothorax*
ABG	Acidosis: pH <7.32 *due to hypercapnia, rapid rewarming, renal insufficiency, or severe hyperglycemia* Hypercapnia: $Pa_{CO_2} >45$ mm Hg *due to postoperative hypoventilation* Hypoxemia: $Pa_{O_2} <65$ mm Hg or $Sa_{O_2} <92\%$ *due to fluid overload, atelectasis, hypoventilation, or depressed cardiac output*
Sputum	Copious amounts of sputum *due to bronchiectasis or chronic bronchitis* The first few tracheal suctioning passes on any postoperative thoracotomy patient will usually yield large amounts of sputum *due to intraoperative stasis of secretions* Yellow-green secretions *due to concomitant pneumonia* Pink secretions *due to pulmonary edema or a traumatic intubation*
Heart rate and rhythm	Atrial fibrillation may occur after pulmonary resection *due to decreased stroke volume, increased left atrial irritability, increased left atrial pressure, hypoxemia, hypokalemia, or mediastinal instability*
Pain	Varying degrees of incisional and chest tube–related pain Other possible causes of thoracic pain include angina, pleuritis, pericarditis, gastritis or esophagitis, and pulmonary embolus Assess patient's response to analgesic therapy
Paresthesias	Numbness, hyperesthesia, and "pins and needles" sensation anterior to the incision *due to intercostal nerve injury, which is very common with any thoracotomy, thoracoscopy, or chest tube and which affects the distribution (dermatome) of the nerve anteriorly*

PLAN OF CARE

INTENSIVE PHASE

The patient requiring pulmonary surgery requires close monitoring during the immediate postoperative period. The focus of care relates to airway, gas exchange, and breathing pattern. Monitoring for complications during the intensive phase of the illness is key to successful recovery.

PATIENT CARE PRIORITIES	EXPECTED PATIENT OUTCOMES
Impaired gas exchange and ineffective airway clearance *r/t* *Intubation* *Anesthesia* *Atelectasis* *Mechanical ventilation* *Surgical site bleeding* *Pain* *Retained secretions* *Fluid volume overload or pulmonary edema* *Bronchospasm* *Pulmonary embolus* *Bronchopleural fistula* *Recurrent left laryngeal nerve damage**	Adequate oxygenation and ventilation Effective breathing patterns Patent airway, ability to clear secretions Improved breath sounds, with air movement present in all remaining lung fields Chest tube drains will maintain "space" drainage (no chest tube with pneumonectomy) Chest tube drainage will remain less than 25 cc/hr after first 8 hours
Impaired or ineffective breathing patterns *r/t* *Infection* *COPD* *Pleural effusion* *Incisional pain* *Anxiety* *Hypoxia* *Persistent air leak* *Abrupt absence of chest tube drainage (happens infrequently with pleural chest tube secondary to fibrinolysis in pleural space)* *Kinking/dehiscence at bronchial anastomosis (specific for bronchial sleeve resection)*	Normal/improved respiratory rate and pattern, with respiratory rate of 14 to 24/min and spontaneous tidal volume of 7 cc/kg Satisfactory pain relief Arterial blood gases and SaO_2 will remain within normal limits: • SaO_2 >91% • $PaCO_2$ <49 mm Hg (pt. may be CO_2 retainer) • PaO_2 >65 mm Hg Diminishing/absent air leak Improving chest x-ray Absence of ventilation/perfusion defects Patent chest tube drains
High risk for decreased CO *r/t* *Postoperative bleeding with subsequent hypovolemia* *Dysrhythmias* *Tension pneumothorax* *Fluid volume overload* *Myocardial ischemia* *Bronchopleural fistula** *Mediastinal shift** *Cardiac herniation** *Sepsis* *Pulmonary embolus*	Achieve hemostasis within 24 hours after operation Achieve and maintain hemodynamic stability Maintain adequate tissue perfusion Maintain adequate intravascular fluid volume
Decreased comfort *r/t* *Incisional pain*	Pain-free Demonstrate ability to maintain clear airway

*Specific for pneumonectomy.

Plan of Care (cont'd)

Pulmonary hygiene *Repositioning* *Increased work of breathing*	Maintain normal respiratory rate (14 to 24 breaths/minute) Maintain normal respiratory volume and symmetry of chest muscles
Decreased gastric motility *r/t* *Anesthesia* *Narcotics* *Ileus* *Immobility*	Maintain gastric motility and normal peristalsis Protected from aspiration
High risk for decreased nutrition *r/t* *Dyspnea* *NPO status* *Infection/sepsis* *Pain*	Maintain and attain positive nitrogen balance and aerobic metabolism
Anxiety *r/t* *Communication problems* *Sleep pattern disturbances* *Diagnosis/uncertainty regarding prognosis* *Dyspnea* *Pain* *Intubation*	Obtain relief from pain Clearly communicates needs Regains orientation to environment within 24 hours Maintains vital signs within normal limits: • SBP 90 to 150 mm Hg • HR 60 to 100 bpm • Temp: <38.0° C Maintains at least 2-hour-periods of rest/comfort during night Indicate feelings of comfort

INTERVENTIONS

Provide mechanical ventilation to facilitate adequate O_2–CO_2 exchange.

Adjust Fio_2 to maintain ABG within normal limits ($Paco_2$ <4 mm Hg, Pao_2 >65 mm Hg) *to decrease atelectasis associated with oxygen-induced nitrogen washout.*

For pneumonectomies, set tidal volume to 6 cc/kg body weight because of presence of single lung. (For other pulmonary surgical procedures, set initial ventilator tidal volume at 12 cc/kg.)

Monitor patient's response to ventilator settings and changes in settings *to maintain adequate ventilation and detect complications.*

Maintain oxygen saturation of 91% or greater *to ensure adequate tissue oxygenation.*

Suction airway only as needed *to maintain patent airway and clear secretions.*

For postpneumonectomy patients, insert suction catheter only to designated cm markings *to prevent trauma to tracheal or bronchial suture line.*

Administer IV fluids *to maintain adequate stroke volume and CO and decrease viscosity of respiratory secretions.*

Monitor cardiac rhythm *to assess for onset of dysrhythmias.*

For pneumonectomies, turn patient only on the affected side (affected side down) q2h *to promote adequate expansion of the remaining lung and mobilize secretions.*

For patients with partial lung resections, turn patient with the affected side up, q2h *to promote adequate reexpansion of the affected lung.*

Humidify air *to facilitate loosening of secretions.*

Assess breath sounds q2h for first 8 hours and then q4h *to evaluate patency of airway and presence of adventitious sounds.*

Assist patient with incentive spirometry, coughing, and deep breathing q1h to q2h for first 8 hours after extubation and then q4h *to facilitate expansion of remaining lobes and mobilization of secretions.*[19]

If patient is unable to clear copious secretions and is hemodynamically stable, consider CPT and bronchodilator/mucolytic nebulizer treatments *to facilitate mobilization of secretions.*

Plan of Care (cont'd)

Elevate head of bed 30° after extubation *to promote adequate breathing pattern and facilitate diaphragmatic excursion*. Reverse Trendelenberg position may also facilitate the work of spontaneous breathing by decreasing the pressure of the abdomen on the diaphragm.

Note amount and color of secretions *to identify infection or bleeding*.

Perform neurological checks on admission and every hour until awake *to assess recovery of neurological integrity as patient reacts from general anesthesia*.

Orient patient to time and place, and explain all interventions *to relieve anxiety and promote safe and secure environment*.

Administer analgesics and anxiolytics as needed *to control postoperative incisional pain, pain associated with chest tubes, anxiety and to facilitate pulmonary hygiene and mobility*.

If patient-controlled analgesia is used, ensure that patient understands how to administer analgesic.

If epidural analgesia is used, assess sensorimotor status of lower and upper extremities every hour for first 12 hours and then q2h.

Other analgesic therapy may include nonsteroidal antiinflammatory drugs (Ketorolac), parenteral narcotics such as morphine or demerol, intrapleural Bupivicaine, and regional or paravertebral blocks.[13]

Assess respiratory rate and rhythm q1h while patient is on ventilator and 2 hours immediately after extubation, and q2h for 8 hours *to assess for adequate O_2–CO_2 exchange*.

Assess chest tube drainage for color, consistency, and air leaks *to maintain evacuation of pleural drainage and encourage lung reexpansion*.

"Milk" (do not "strip") chest tubes only when excessive drainage is present *to prevent blood from collecting within the pleural space.[25] Bleeding and air leaks that normally follow decortication will gradually subside if the lung surface is allowed to reexpand fully to the underside of the ribs*.

Facilitate frequent postoperative chest x-rays *to confirm adequate drainage of the pleural space by the chest tubes*.

INTERMEDIATE PHASE

Successful recovery from the intensive phase following pulmonary surgery changes the focus of care during the intermediate phase. The priorities of care are to help the patient obtain adequate nutrition and increased mobility. The high risk of infection requires aggressive treatment aimed at prevention and monitoring to make an early determination of the presence of infection.

PATIENT CARE PRIORITIES	EXPECTED PATIENT OUTCOMES
High risk for infection *r/t* *Thoracotomy incision* *Atelectasis* *Invasive lines* *Debilitated state* *Compromised immune status* *Recurrent empyema*	Free of infection Temperature: WNL WBC: WNL 4000 to 12,000 Negative sputum culture Intact skin integrity with approximation of incision
High risk for inadequate nutrition *r/t* *Debilitated state* *Intubation* *Increased metabolic need* *Dyspnea and increased work of breathing* *Pain and associated anorexia* *Nausea*	Maintain adequate nutrient intake Maintain weight at admission weight (or "target weight," if patient in CHF upon admission) Maintain anabolic state Administer antiemetics as needed

Plan of Care (cont'd)

High risk for impaired gas exchange *r/t* *Atelectasis* *Persistent air leak* *Pulmonary embolus* *Bronchopleural fistula* *Retained secretions* *Hypoventilation* *Interstitial edema*	Sa_{O_2} >91% RR of 14 to 24 Absence of subcutaneous emphysema and resolution of chest tube air leak Absence of ventilation/perfusion deficits Ability to mobilize and clear secretions Clear lung sounds Reexpansion of remaining lung(s), as documented by chest radiograph Adequate hydration
Impaired physical mobility *r/t* *Decreased strength and endurance* *Incisional pain*	Intact skin integrity Regain preoperative level of mobility
High risk for ineffective coping *r/t* *Prognosis* *Acceptance of illness* *Separation from support systems*	Verbalize acceptance of illness and understanding of prognosis
Knowledge deficit *r/t* *Outcome of surgery* *Prognosis* *Disease process* *Postoperative management*	Verbalize understanding of disease process and postoperative routines

INTERVENTIONS

Clean surgical incision twice a day *to decrease risk of infection.*

Assess wound for signs of redness, infection, swelling, or drainage *to detect possible infection early.*

Monitor WBC and temperature *to assess for infection.*

Advance diet as tolerated, to promote wound healing and endurance. *Delay po nutritional advancement if patient is receiving epidural analgesic infusion; such therapy may limit gastric motility and peristalsis.*

Assess response to diet daily *to determine if more aggressive means of nutrition is needed.*

Provide dietary and/or pharmacologic aids *to promote normal bowel function.*

Provide physical therapy *to promote regaining of physical strength and endurance.*

Reposition patient frequently *to prevent skin breakdown over bony prominences.*

Begin discharge teaching *to facilitate home self-care management.*

Assess chest tube drainage every four hours *to determine if there is a change in the amount or color of drainage and if there is an air leak.*

Evaluate chest tube drainage for signs of pleural infection, renewed bleeding, or chylothorax.

Monitor for indications for pleural chest tube removal, including absence of an air leak and chest tube drainage <50 cc in a 24-hour period.

Maintain occlusive dressings around pleural chest tube sites *to preserve the integrity of the system and decrease the risk of infection.*

Assess nature, location, and relief of pain after analgesics have been administered. Utilize PO analgesics such as acetaminophen/oxycodone or meperidine tablets *to maintain adequate levels of comfort so patient can effectively cough, move, and sleep.*

Instruct patient on use of incentive spirometer, coughing, and deep breathing *to facilitate the removal of secretions and promote lung expansion.* Consider CPT with bronchodilator/mucolytic therapy for patients unable to mobilize secretions.

Provide ongoing emotional support to patient and family.

Monitor patient for dysrhythmias, such as atrial fibrillation or atrial flutter.[29]

TRANSITION TO DISCHARGE

Discharge teaching should begin before admission with patient instruction regarding self-care activities and expectations upon discharge. The patient will continue many of the interventions initiated in the hospital (such as coughing, deep breathing, use of incentive spirometry) and attempt to regain the level of independence that existed before surgery.

The priorities for discharge teaching are activities, medications, wound care, diet, and follow-up call. Discharge activities may include the progressive use of the arm and shoulder on the ipsilateral surgical side. Set restrictions on strenuous activities such as heavy lifting. Most patients are restricted to weights of 10 pounds or less for 4 weeks after thoracotomy. Patients are also asked to refrain from driving for 4 weeks.

Patients are encouraged to resume their normal activities of daily living as soon as possible within these limitations. The time frame for returning to work depends on the nature of the work and the condition of the patient. A general rule of thumb is 4 weeks. The medication regimen consists of pain medication and medications the patient took before admission.

Wound care should be kept as simple as possible. The incision should be assessed and cleaned by the patient or significant other twice a day. The patient may get the incision wet in the shower as long as there are no surgical staples.

The discharge diet instructions should include high-protein foods to promote wound healing. The surgeon will usually see the patient for a postoperative checkup at 4 to 6 weeks. The patient should be encouraged to see his or her primary care physician within 2 weeks after discharge. The nurse should instruct the patient and significant others on the signs and symptoms of infection and on individuals to call if problems should arise at home.

REFERENCES

1. Reference deleted in proofs.
2. Baker WL, Lamb VJ, Marini JJ: Breath-stacking increases depth and duration of chest expansion by incentive spirometry, *Am Rev Resp Dis* 141:343-346, 1990.
3. Boring CC, Squires TS, Tong T: Cancer statistics, 1992, *Cancer* 42(1):19-39, 1992.
4. Chang SC, et al: Effect of body positioning on gas exchange in patients with unilateral central airway lesions, *Chest* 103(3):787-791, 1993.
5. Reference deleted in proofs.
6. Coltharp W, et al: Videothoracoscopy—improved techniques and expanded implications, *Ann Thorac Surg* 53:776-779, 1992.
7. Cottrell JJ, Ferson PF: Pre-operative assessment of the thoracic surgical patient, *Clinics in Chest Medicine* 13(1):47-53, 1992.
8. Dales RE, et al: Preoperative prediction of pulmonary complications following thoracic surgery, *Chest* 104(1):155-159, 1993.
9. Daniel T: Benign diseases of the lung. In Levine BA, et al., editors: *Current practice of surgery,* New York, 1993, Churchill Livingstone.
10. Reference deleted in proofs.
11. Elefteriades JA, Geha AS: Problems following noncardiac thoracic surgery. In *House officer guide to ICU care: the cardiothoracic surgical patient,* Rockville, Md, 1985, Aspen, 159-167.
12. Epps ME: Diagnostic testing for patients with lung cancer, *Nurs Clin North Am* 27(3):615-625, 1992.
13. Eng J, Sabanthan S: Post-thoracotomy analgesia, *J R Coll Surg Edinb,* 38:62-66, 1993.
14. Greenfield LJ, editor: *Complications in surgery and trauma,* Philadelphia, 1984, JB Lippincott.
15. Hammon WE, Connors AE, McCaffree DR: Cardiac arrhythmias during post-operative drainage and chest percussion of critically ill patients, *Chest* 102(6):1836-1841, 1992.
16. Hazelrigg SR, et al: Thoracoscopic stapled resection for spontaneous pneumothorax, *J Thorac Cardiovasc Surg* 105(3):389-393, 1993.
17. Health Systems International: *Diagnostic Related Groups manual,* 1993.
18. Reference deleted in proofs.
19. Johnson NT, Pierson DJ: The spectrum of pulmonary atelectasis: pathophysiology, diagnosis, and therapy, *Respir Care* 31(11):1107-1120, 1986.
20. Langston WG: Surgical resection of lung cancer, *Nurs Clin North Am* 27(3):665-679, 1992.
21. Lewis R, et al: One hundred consecutive patients undergoing video-assisted thoracic operations, *Ann Thorac Surg* 54:421-426, 1992.
22. Lewis R, Caccavale R, Sisler G: Imaged thoracoscopic lung biopsy, *Chest* 102:60-62, 1992.
23. Long BC, Phipps WJ, Cassmeyer VL: *A nursing process approach,* St Louis, 1993, Mosby–Year Book, pp 560-575.
24. Marshall M, Olsen GN: The physiological evaluation of the lung resection candidate, *Clin Chest Med* 14(2):305-318, 1993.
25. Morrison CC, Tribble C: *Mediastinal and pleural chest tubes: TCV-PO clinical protocol,* Charlottesville, Va, 1994, UVA Health Sciences Center, pp 1-3.
26. Mountain CF: A new international staging system for lung cancer, *Chest* 89(4)(suppl):225S-233S, 1986.
27. Mulshine JL, et al: Initiators and promoters of lung cancer, *Chest* 103(1)(suppl):4S-8S, 1993.
28. Nicholson C, Coleman C, Mack M: Are you ready for video thoracoscopy? *Am J Nurs* 93(3):54-57, 1993.
29. Nishimura H, et al: Cardiopulmonary function after pulmonary lobectomy in patients with lung cancer, *Ann Thorac Surg* 55:1477-1484, 1993.
30. Pichlmaier H, Schildberg FW, editors: *Thoracic surgery,* New York, 1989, Springer Verlag.
31. Roth JA, Ruckdeschel JC, Weisenburger TH: *Thoracic oncology,* Philadelphia, 1989, WB Saunders.

32. Samet JM: The epidemiology of lung cancer, *Chest* 103(1)(suppl):20S-29S, 1993.
33. Seale DD, Beaver BM: Pathophysiology of lung cancer, *Nurs Clin North Am* 27(3):603-613, 1992.
34. Shapira OM, Shahian DM: Postpneumonectomy pulmonary edema, *Ann Thorac Surg* 56:190-195, 1993.
35. Shekleton M, Litwak K: *Critical care nursing of the surgical patient,* Philadelphia, 1991, WB Saunders.
36. Shields TW: Lung cancer and the solitary pulmonary nodule. In MG Khan, editor: *Cardiac and pulmonary management,* Philadelphia, 1993, Lea and Febiger, pp 902-935.
37. Shields TW: *General thoracic surgery,* ed 3, Philadelphia, 1989, Lea and Febiger.
38. *St Anthony's DRG Guidebook 1995* Reston, Va, 1994, St Anthony.
39. Strauss GM, Gleason RE, Sugarbaker DJ: Screening for lung cancer re-examined, *Chest,* 103(4):337S-341S, 1993.
40. Strider D, et al: Stacked inspiratory spirometry reduces pulmonary shunt in patients post coronary artery bypass *Chest* 106(2):391-395, 1994.
41. Wahi R, et al: Determinants of perioperative morbidity and mortality after pneumonectomy, *Ann Thorac Surg* 48(1):33-37, 1989.
42. Wolfe WG, editor: *Complications in thoracic surgery,* St Louis, 1992, Mosby–Year Book.
43. Wood D: Thoracoscopic surgery, *Respir Care* 38(4):388-397, 1993.

ACKNOWLEDGMENTS

The authors of this chapter acknowledge significant assistance from the following individuals: Thomas M. Daniel, M.D., Professor of Thoracic and Vascular Surgery, University of Virginia Health Sciences Center; Donna Johansen, Program Support Technician, Model Hospital Project, University of Virginia Health Sciences Center; and Karen Wheeler, Health Unit Coordinator, TCV Acute Care Unit, University of Virginia Health Sciences Center.

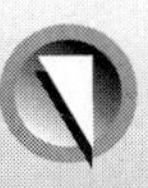

TRANSPLANT GUIDELINE

40

Lung Transplantation

Jeanette T. Thompson, BSN, RN, CCTC

DESCRIPTION

In 1963, Dr. James Hardy of the University of Mississippi performed the first human lung transplant, in a patient with bronchogenic carcinoma. This patient lived for 18 days before succumbing to renal failure and malnutrition.[17] Over the next 20 years, nearly 40 lung transplant procedures were performed, without long-term success. Those patients surviving longer than 2 weeks had poor outcomes related to impaired bronchial healing.[3,29] Factors contributing to bronchial healing, such as high-dose prednisone and vascular supply, were studied. The studies resulted in modification of postoperative treatment and surgical techniques. These findings led to the first successful single and double lung transplants, performed by Dr. Joel Cooper in 1983[36] and 1986,[35] respectively.

With improvement of the surgical technique and introduction of the major immunosuppressive agent cyclosporine in the late 1980s, isolated lung transplantation has become a proven, viable therapy for selected patients with end-stage lung disease.[10] According to The Registry of the International Society for Heart and Lung Transplantation, more than 1600 single and double lung transplants have been performed since 1981.[30] The Registry reports current 1-year and 2-year actuarial survival rates of 73% and 69%, respectively, for single lung transplants, and 70% and 63%, respectively, for bilateral lung transplants (Figure 40-1).

PATIENT SELECTION

The recipient selection process is the core of a successful transplant program. Although selection criteria, listed in Table 40-1, may vary from one institution to another, the essentials are similar in most transplant centers.[9] The timing of the transplant is critical. Basically, transplantation is reserved for those individuals whose life expectancy is 2 years or less, who have not suffered from any secondary organ failure, and who are well enough to withstand such a major operation. Single and bilateral lung transplantation is being offered to patients with restrictive, obstructive, and pulmonary hypertensive diseases. Patients with septic lung diseases, such as cystic fibrosis and bronchiectasis, require bilateral lung transplantation because the remaining native lung would infect the newly transplanted graft. Likewise, the presence of an infectious component in a patient with emphysema and pulmonary fibrosis would be an indication to perform a bilateral rather than a single lung transplant. Patients with pulmonary hypertensive diseases may benefit from either a single or a bilateral lung transplant, depending on organ availability.

Predicting those individuals who are approaching the "transplant window"[23] is based upon clinical manifestations selective to the disease process. Important factors to consider in the patient with obstructive lung disease include deterioration of pulmonary function tests, increased hospital admissions for exacerbations, weight loss, decline in exercise tolerance, hypercarbia, and oxygen desaturation with exercise. In patients with chronic obstructive pulmonary disease (COPD), the rate of progression is less predictable. For example, the patient with COPD might have a forced expiratory volume in 1 second (FEV_1) of less than 30% for many years. Investigators at the Hospital for Sick Children in Toronto studied factors predicting mortality in patients with cystic fibrosis.[20] This study, following 673 patients over a 12-month period, concluded that patients with an FEV_1 less than 30% predicted, and Po_2 less than 55 mm Hg or a Pco_2 greater than 50 mm Hg, had a 50% chance of dying

A

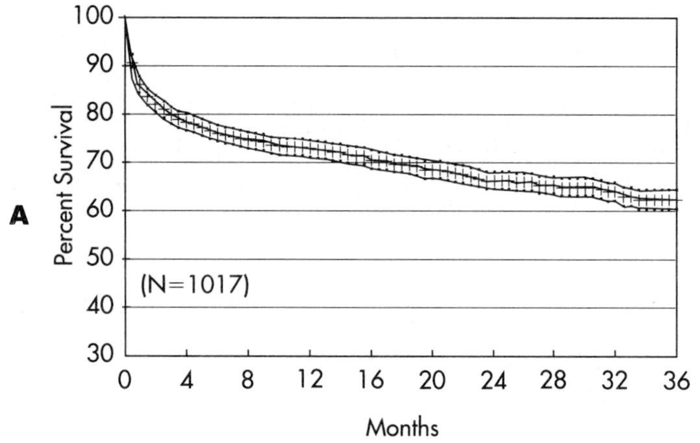

B

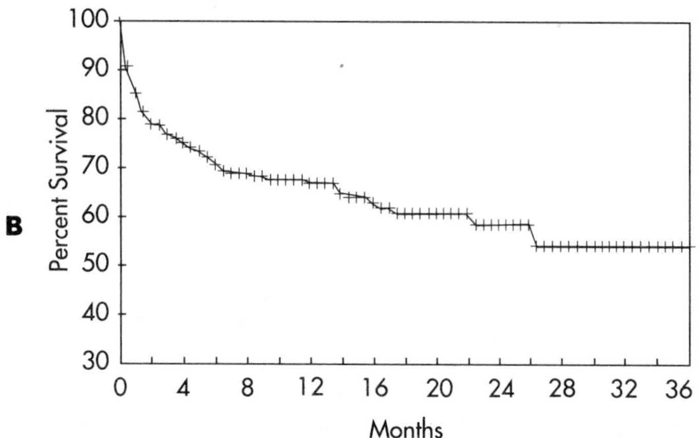

Figure 40-1 Actuarial survival following **(A)** single and **(B)** bilateral lung transplantation reported to the Registry of the International Society for Heart and Lung Transplantation (**A,** reprinted with permission; **B,** adapted with permission.[32])

TABLE 40-1 Selection Criteria for Lung Transplantation Candidates
• Life expectancy less than 18-24 months • No other systemic illness • Ambulatory and motivated • Minimal usage of daily steroids • No history of major psychosocial problems • Adequate financial and emotional support • No major coronary artery disease • Nonsmoker for at least 1 year

within 2 years. Weight-to-height ratio of less than 70% was also a predictor of death. This study helps predict life expectancy and therefore assists with the selection of appropriate candidates for transplantation.

D'Alonzo's study helped define optimal timing of transplantation for candidates with pulmonary hypertension.[5] This national prospective study found that factors associated with poor survival were New York Heart Association functional class of III or IV, presence of Raynaud's phenomenon, elevated mean right arterial pressure, elevated mean pulmonary artery pressure, decreased cardiac index, and decreased diffusing capacity for carbon monoxide (DLCO).

Patients with pulmonary fibrosis present differently from patients with obstructive lung disease. They have a restrictive pathophysiology in which a decreased total lung capacity, usually less than 60%, and a decline in forced vital capacity are seen. Because pulmonary fibrosis can progress extremely rapidly, referral for transplantation is recommended at an earlier stage for these patients.

PROCEDURE

The last 10 years have brought new developments in the field of pulmonary transplantation. The old surgical procedure—en bloc double lung transplant that entailed a tracheal anastomosis—has been replaced by a newer technique called the bilateral sequential single lung transplant. This operation is performed through an anterior bilateral thoracotomy ("clam shell") approach, and both lungs are replaced separately, with the "worse" lung being removed first. The advantages of this new technique include fewer airway complications due to the separate bronchial anastomosis, reduction of the need for total cardiopulmonary bypass, and improved access to lungs that reduces intraoperative and postoperative hemorrhage.[8,28]

LENGTH OF STAY/ANTICIPATED COURSE

Postoperative nursing management of the lung transplant patient can be very challenging. Following transplantation, the patient is admitted to the intensive care unit for multisystem monitoring and mechanical ventilation. Ideally, extubation should be accomplished within the first 24 hours.

In uncomplicated cases, patients are transferred out of the ICU on postoperative day 2 or 3 and remain on the ward until postoperative day 14 or 15, when they are discharged to their local accommodations. Lung transplantation is an operating-room procedure identified for DRG 75: Major chest procedures. The average LOS is 12.4 days.[33]

For the next 8 to 12 weeks, the patient participates in pulmonary rehabilitation 4 to 5 days a week. The program consists of aerobics, strengthening, and flexibility. The goals are to work the cardiovascular system 30 to 40 minutes to reach the patient's target heart rate, as predicted by age. The major complaint initially is musculoskeletal weakness, rather than pulmonary limitations. Blood pressure, heart rate, oxygen saturation, perceived exertion, speed, grade, and distance are documented daily. When patients are medically stable and have reached their individual pulmonary rehabilitation goals, they are released to their home towns.

MANAGEMENT TRENDS AND CONTROVERSIES

The transplant team screens referrals on the basis of the selection criteria listed in Table 40-1. After the team has determined a patient to be an acceptable candidate for transplantation, the evaluation process begins. A 3-day hospital admission for formal evaluation is recommended because of the candidate's severe end-stage lung disease and consequent disability. The evaluation includes a series of laboratory tests and various procedures used to determine whether the patient has any medical or psychological contraindications to transplantation. Routine laboratory studies include hematologic and biochemical studies to rule out dysfunction of other organs, and immunologic studies to identify cytomegalovirus, human immunodeficiency virus (HIV), *herpes simplex* virus, *Epstein-Barr* virus, *varicella zoster* virus, and hepatitis profile. HLA typing and ABO/Rh studies are conducted.

Cardiac evaluation consists of a resting radionuclide ventriculogram and a two-dimensional echocardiogram with Doppler studies. Candidates over the age of 40 undergo coronary angiography to rule out coronary artery disease. A computed tomography scan of the chest is done in patients with COPD to exclude severe bullous disease and bronchiectasis, because the presence of either condition mandates consideration of bilateral lung transplantation. A ventilation and perfusion lung scan is performed to determine which is the "better" lung. In the bilateral lung transplant procedure, the "worse" lung can be removed first; in the single lung transplant procedure, the worse lung is replaced by the newly transplanted graft, leaving the better lung behind. The ventilation and perfusion scan is omitted for patients with pulmonary hypertension. In most cases when single lung transplant is being considered for patients with pulmonary hypertension, the right lung is preferred because it has a larger vascular surface area, and it is easier to institute cardiopulmonary bypass through the right chest.

The pulmonary evaluation includes a 6-minute walk to determine the patient's endurance and oxygen needs. Most lung transplant candidates are malnourished before transplantation; therefore, a dietary consult is included to assess their nutritional needs. A social worker and psychologist perform a psychosocial evaluation to assess emotional stability and compliance. The patient's financial status is also reviewed. Prospective candidates are also evaluated by the nurse coordinators, and preoperative and postoperative education is presented. It is important for the nurse and the transplant team to assess the capacity of the patient to comprehend and process the information given and the patient's ability to comply with the rigorous postoperative medical regimen. The multidisciplinary team—social workers, psychologists, lung transplant coordinators, pulmonologists, surgeons, dietitians, anesthesiologists, and therapists—holds conferences to discuss the potential candidates and any contraindications they may have. Often, a final decision on a particular candidate is deferred until issues such as relocation, insurance, financial capability, and support can be addressed.

Absolute contraindications to lung transplantation are malignancy (remission less than 5 years), high-dose corticosteroid therapy, significant coronary artery disease, active cigarette smoking, irreversible organ dysfunction (excluding the lungs), psychosocial issues such as noncompliance or lack of support of a significant other, and a history of drug or alcohol abuse. Ventilator dependency is a relative contraindication; some institutions will transplant patients who require ventilator support if the candidates are currently listed and are being followed at the transplant center.[11]

Many major transplant centers require patients to relocate after they are accepted into the program. The purpose for relocation is to allow participation in pulmonary rehabilitation. The advantages of pulmonary rehabilitation for patients with end-stage lung disease have been documented.[6] Patients who have end-stage parenchymal lung disease attend rehabilitation 3 to 5 days a week and are monitored using a bicycle ergometer and treadmill. Six-minute walks are performed routinely to assess changes in exercise capacity. For patients with pulmonary hypertension, preoperative rehabilitation is deferred because of the risk of sudden death from extreme elevation of pulmonary artery pressures. The ultimate goal of pretransplant rehabilitation is to try to optimize the patient's endurance and muscular strength, thereby making the patient better able to withstand surgery and allowing earlier extubation. In this way, postoperative recovery time can be minimized. At the University of North Carolina Hospitals, cystic fibrosis patients awaiting transplantation have demonstrated a consistent improvement in their 6-minute walks and lower extremity ergometry,[2] despite their severe respiratory compromise. In addition to the goals stated above, patients are continuously assessed during exercise, thereby allowing for early identification and treatment of exacerbations.

The waiting period for donor lungs continues to increase. The prospect of dying before transplantation can be extremely stressful for the candidates and their families. Support groups for patients and their families can assist in coping with the stresses that accompany transplantation and relocation. The nurse can take an active role in organizing speakers for the support group to help facilitate the education process. Another helpful adjunct to reduce anxiety is to prepare the patient for realistic postoperative expectations. One way of accomplishing this is for the nurse to provide ICU tours and an explanation of the equipment used in the postoperative period.

The United Network of Organ Sharing (UNOS) reports that 1161 patients are listed for isolated lung transplantation.[38] As the waiting list continues to grow, organ availability continues to be compromised. The supply does not meet the demand. One factor influencing organ donation is lack of education of health care professionals. Critical care nurses play an especially important role in the process of organ donation. Often, the nurse working in the critical care

TABLE 40-2 Criteria for Donor Lungs
• Age less than 55 • Normal chest roentgenogram • Adequate gas exchange (Pa_{O_2} >300 mm Hg on Fi_{O_2} 1.0 and 5 cm PEEP H_2O) • Normal bronchoscopy (no evidence of pus or aspiration) • Normal appearance • Viral studies negative for HIV and hepatitis B surface antigen

HIV = human immunodeficiency virus

setting is the first to identify a potential donor.[24] Therefore, it is imperative that the nurse have a clear understanding of brain death and organ retrieval. (See Appendix E.)

The selection of donor lungs is critical to the outcome of the transplant. Donor lungs are not always suitable for transplantation. Unsuitability can be related to contusions from motor vehicle accidents, or infection related to aspiration or prolonged ventilation.[39] Bronchoscopy is performed on all donors, and a sputum specimen is obtained for Gram stain and culture. Criteria for donor lungs are listed in Table 40-2.

ABO blood group compatibility and height are the two most important factors when considering donor lungs for a potential recipient. Thoracic dimensions acquired from a chest X-ray may be helpful for recipient-donor matching. The measurements are right and left vertical (apex of the lungs to the level of the diaphragm) and horizontal (costophrenic angle to costophrenic angle). The outer chest circumferences of the donor and the recipient are compared, and measurement is taken at the nipple line. While these measurements are helpful, height, age, sex, and race are determinants of lung volumes and, hence, lung size. Large lungs often can be reduced by performing a right middle lobectomy or lingulectomy to fit the recipient,[18] but small lungs cannot be expanded.

Postoperatively, bedside nurses are frequently the first to identify the various pulmonary complications recipients sustain following lung transplantation. Increase in extracellular fluid related to reperfusion injury, infection, and disruption of the pulmonary lymphatics can be challenging problems even for the experienced ICU nurse. Reperfusion injury usually occurs in the early postoperative phase, with fluid accumulation in the allograft (Figure 40-2). This phenomenon can be related to graft ischemia, preservation techniques, or lymphatic disruption. With increased lymphatic drainage, the graft is more vulnerable to fluid overload, which can result in pulmonary edema. Noncardiogenic pulmonary edema can cause hypoxemia. Increased ventilator support, diuretics, and fluid restriction may be required. Intake and output need to be documented accurately every hour. The nurse needs to be astute in reporting changes in breathing patterns, renal function, hemodynamics, and laboratory values.

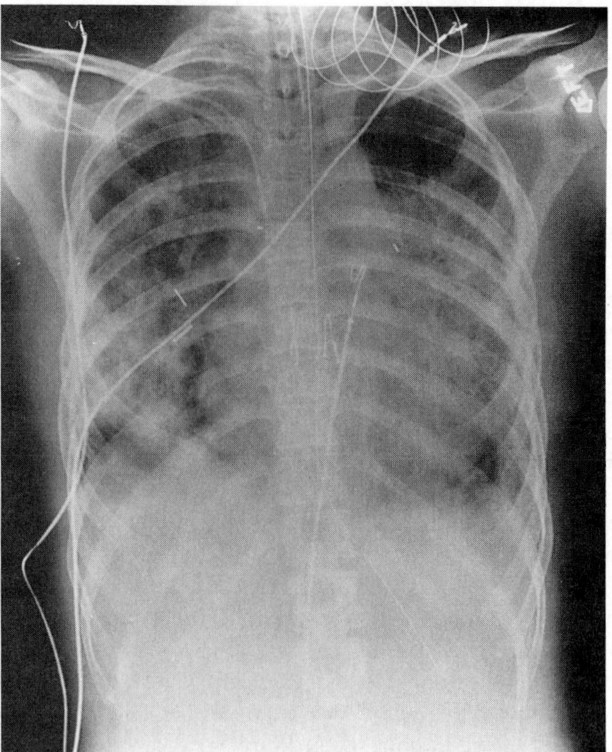

Figure 40-2 Chest X-ray demonstrating severe reperfusion injury after bilateral lung transplantation. This patient went on to complete recovery.

It is not unusual for transplant patients to experience two or three rejection episodes during the first postoperative month. In the single lung transplant patient, lung perfusion scans are often helpful in determining rejection by identifying a reduced perfusion or blood flow to the transplanted lung.[9] Making the distinction between rejection and infection is critical because the treatment for each is different. Transbronchial biopsy is the most helpful tool for diagnosing rejection but is not absolutely reliable.[37] Clinical signs and symptoms the nurse can recognize include fever, increase in alveolar-arterial oxygen gradient, decrease in spirometry, decrease in exercise tolerance, arterial oxygen desaturation or requirement of increased oxygen needs during exercise, dyspnea, fatigue, and radiographic changes. If the transbronchial biopsy is negative and infection is ruled out by the lavage specimens, rejection is suspected in the presence of clinical symptoms and treatment is instituted. Treatment for an acute rejection episode consists of a bolus of methylprednisolone intravenously over 3 consecutive days, for a total of 1 to 2 g, depending on weight. If the patient has a positive response to the first dose of steroids, the diagnosis of a rejection episode is strengthened even in the presence of a negative histologic report, and steroid therapy is continued.

Transplant recipients have an increased susceptibility to opportunistic lung infections. Manifestations of rejection

TABLE 40-3 Prophylactic Antibiotics

Medication	Dose	Organism
Acylovir	200 mg bid	HSV
Nystatin oral suspension	500,000 units qid	*Candida*
Trim-Sulfa	1 tablet bid M-W-F	PCP

HSV = *herpes simplex* virus; PCP = pneumocystis carinii; Trim-Sulfa = trimethoprim-sulfamethoxazole

can often be confused with infection in lung transplant patients. Therefore, diagnosis is confirmed by transbronchial biopsy, bronchoalveolar lavage, and microbiology. To prevent opportunistic infections, a standard protocol of prophylactic antibiotics is utilized (Table 40-3).

Viral infections such as cytomegalovirus (CMV) are a significant cause of morbidity and mortality in lung transplant recipients.[41] Immunosuppressive therapy reaches its peak 6 to 12 weeks after transplantation, and this is when CMV usually presents. CMV is a herpes virus infection to which 50% to 80% of the population acquire antibodies, usually during childhood or adolescence. In persons with a normal host defense, CMV rarely causes sickness.[15] The lung is the primary site of infection in lung transplant recipients, although the virus can affect the liver or GI tract. The virus is transmitted by donor organs and body fluids such as urine, semen, breast milk, saliva, blood, and vaginal secretions. To try to prevent the occurrence of this complication, CMV seronegative blood products are given to all recipients. When possible, CMV seronegative recipients receive organs from CMV seronegative donors. This can reduce the incidence of CMV infection. The current treatment is ganciclovir (DHPG), an antiviral agent, at a dose of 2.5 to 5 mg/kg twice a day for 14 to 21 days.

Bacterial infections are usually primary pulmonary but can also be catheter related. Foley catheters and central lines are discontinued as soon as possible. Donor bronchial washings are assessed immediately following surgery. If organisms are identified on Gram stain or culture, empiric antibiotic coverage is started in the recipient. Cystic fibrosis recipients receive antibiotics 7 to 10 days postoperatively. Their antibiotics are directed toward their most recent respiratory tract culture sensitivities. All other transplant patients are treated with antibiotics to cover skin flora for 3 days postoperatively.

Posttransplant lymphoproliferative disease (PTLD) can be a complication of immunosuppressive medication (Table 40-4). The tumor is often related to the Epstein-Barr virus.[34] Diagnosis usually is made by open lung biopsy. Treatment modalities include reduction of the immunosuppressive agents, surgical intervention, chemotherapy, and radiation. Children have a three times greater risk of developing PTLD than their adult counterparts.[1] In pediatric patients, Epstein-Barr virus titers are monitored on a monthly basis to detect any changes.

TABLE 40-4 Immunosuppressive Protocol

Triple drug therapy	
Cyclosporine	Implemented during the implantation of the donor graft
Azathioprine	On call to the operating room
Methylprednisolone	Controversial regarding when it should be started, due to risk of infection and interference with airway healing
Cytolytic induction	Anti-thymocyte globulin is used to replace prednisone in the initial postoperative phase

Obliterative bronchiolitis (OB) is a form of chronic rejection that may be significant to the lung transplant population.[21,25] OB is progressive scarring of the small airways involving the terminal and respiratory bronchioles. Its etiology is unknown, but some investigators have hypothesized that OB is related to repeated acute rejection episodes[32] or CMV pneumonia.[16,19] The occurrence of OB has been reported to be as high as 50% in the heart-lung transplant population,[14] with a higher incidence in the pediatric-isolated lung population than in the adult population.[26] Pulmonary function tests reveal a restrictive and obstructive process. OB is diagnosed histologically by open lung biopsy or by transbronchial biopsy. Patients often experience a nonproductive cough, dyspnea, and a recurrence of pulmonary bacterial infections.[12,16] Early diagnosis is important in the clinical outcome of OB. Frequent monitoring of pulmonary function tests is imperative to assist in establishing the diagnosis. The extent of pulmonary damage from OB depends on treatment and early detection. Progression of OB may be arrested with augmented immunosuppression. If pulmonary function continues to deteriorate because of OB, the only treatment may be retransplantation.

ASSESSMENT

Immunosuppressive therapy increases the patient's susceptibility to infection. Rejection is possible due to the foreign allograft. Two to three rejection episodes are common during the first month. The following parameters and diagnostic procedures are necessary to determine the presence of infection or rejection.

PARAMETER	ANTICIPATED ALTERATION
Pulmonary function	Decrease in spirometry (FVC, FEV_1). *Patients are instructed to notify the nurse coordinator if spirometry falls by 10% in a 24-hour period.* Dyspnea Cough/sputum production
Laboratory data	Leukopenia. *Viral infections such as cytomegalovirus can cause leukopenia.*[15] Leukocytosis. *Often, elevation in WBC is correlated with rejection.*[27] CMV-specific IgM titer positive. *Antibody can be detected in the patient's blood when there is an active infection.*[40]
Temperature	Increase of 1° from patient's normal temperature
Chest x-ray	Changes from baseline. *Infiltrates and consolidation are noted in an infectious process. Perihilar flare often suggestive of rejection.*[31]
Chest auscultation	Decreased airflow to the transplanted graft Adventitious sounds
Wound and line insertion sites	Redness, swelling, and purulent drainage around IV and incision sites
Bronchoscopy with bronchial alveolar lavage (BAL) and transbronchial biopsy (TBB)	Positive BAL cultures and positive TBB. *Infection organisms isolated in BAL fluid and TBB identify opportunistic infections such as herpes, PCP, and CMV. TBB may assist in diagnosing rejection.*
Lung perfusion scan for single lung recipients	Decrease perfusion to the transplanted graft
Exercise tolerance	Decreased
Fatigue	Increased

PLAN OF CARE

INTENSIVE PHASE

The patient is admitted to an intensive care unit following lung transplantation. The focus of care is supportive to the respiratory system and monitoring other systems for complications associated with the postoperative period.

PATIENT CARE PRIORITIES	EXPECTED PATIENT OUTCOMES
High risk for decreased CO *r/t transplantation*	Stable hemodynamic status, including: • MAP 60 to 80 • CVP 6 to 12 • Chest tube drainage <100 cc/hr • Cardiac index >2.2 • Urine output >30 cc/hr • Heart rate <100 bpm
Ineffective airway clearance *r/t denervated graft*	Adequate cough reflex to mobilize secretions Respiratory rate and pattern: WNL Clear bilateral breath sounds
Impaired gas exchange *r/t disruption of pulmonary lymphatics and reperfusion injury*	No signs of pulmonary edema such as decreased oxygen saturations, increased work of breathing, copious secretions, chest x-ray changes, elevated CVP/PA, edema, rales
High risk for pulmonary infection, line and incision infection *r/t immunocompromised host*	No signs or symptoms of infection No fever No dyspnea Nonproductive cough

Plan of Care (cont'd)

	Negative sputum cultures WBC: WNL Clear lungs on auscultation No changes in chest x-ray ABG: WNL Sao_2 >92%
High risk for bronchial complications (i.e., dehiscence or ischemia) *r/t hypotension and/or steroids*	Peak airway pressures <45 No bronchial stricture. *Avoid inotropes and vasoconstrictors because of increased risk of airway necrosis and dehiscence.*[22]
High risk for rejection *r/t foreign graft*	Demonstrates no signs and symptoms of rejection Sao_2 >92% Minimal chest tube drainage Clear chest x-ray Temperature ≤98.6° F Successful weaning from the ventilator. *Increased ventilatory support and oxygenation is often required during rejection.*
Discomfort *r/t postoperative pain and sleep deprivation*	Participate in activity progression and chest physiotherapy without being limited by pain. *Generally, an epidural is used to administer analgesics without reducing respiratory function.* Sleep throughout the night without complaints

INTERVENTIONS

Monitor vital signs, I/O every hour. *Renal status is often compromised postoperatively by cardiopulmonary bypass or the use of aminoglycosides and intravenous cyclosporine.*

Chest physiotherapy q2h to q4h *to prevent atelectasis and pneumonia. The transplanted lung is more vulnerable to infection because of impaired mucociliary clearance,*[7] *airway denervation,*[13] *and postoperative pain.*

Post-extubation, coach patient to cough and deep breathe *to prevent mucus plugging.*

Position single lung transplant patients operative side up *to allow for gravitational drainage, to mobilize secretions, and to reduce postsurgical edema.*

Turn double lung transplant patients side to side and prone *to facilitate mobilization of secretions.*

Monitor respiratory function: rate, breath sounds, blood gases, airway pressures, and tidal volumes.

Assess for signs and symptoms of increased extracellular fluid and pulmonary edema.

Monitor temperature and WBC daily.

Obtain sputum cultures daily and note color, consistency, and amount.

Compare chest x-rays daily *to detect changes such as atelectasis or pneumonia.*

Monitor oxygen saturations continuously and report any change from baseline.

Auscultate lungs to assess breath sounds q2h and prn *to detect any changes.*

Document peak airway pressures hourly. *Elevated airway pressure increases the risk of barotrauma and impairment of the airway anastomosis.*[28]

Fiberoptic bronchoscopy should be performed at 1 week and 3 weeks after transplantation *to assess airway viability and monitor for rejection.*

Adhere to isolation procedures. *Modified isolation is a requirement for all patients.*

Discontinue IV lines and Foley catheter as soon as possible.

Monitor pain control and administer analgesics prn. *Pain medication must be sufficient to allow the patient to endure physiotherapy without compromising respiratory function.*

Ensure uninterrupted sleep from 11 PM to 6 AM if patient is hemodynamically stable.

Plan of Care (cont'd)

INTERMEDIATE PHASE

The lung transplant patient is transferred out of the ICU on postoperative day 2 or 3 and remains hospitalized until postoperative day 14 or 15. Most patient care priorities are similar to those in the intensive phase. Nursing care is directed toward self-care, increasing activity, and preparing for discharge.

PATIENT CARE PRIORITIES	EXPECTED PATIENT OUTCOMES
High risk for infection or rejection *r/t foreign graft and immunocompromised host*	Free of infection or rejection, such as decline in SaO_2, decline in exercise tolerance, decrease in FVC or FEV_1, chest x-ray changes, fever, increase in oxygen needs during exercise, or positive sputum cultures
High risk for inadequate nutrition *r/t paralytic gastric ileus from mobilization of the omentum*	Bowel function restored to pre-admission status Progression to oral intake (usually 5 to 7 days postop)
Self-care deficit *r/t lack of knowledge regarding transplant medications and ongoing care*	Demonstrate knowledge and self-care capability with medications, activity, monitoring blood pressure, pulse, weight, and spirometry function
High risk for anxiety *r/t the total transplant experience: infection, rejection, and separation from support systems*	Verbalizes feelings of fear and anxiety; identifies and utilizes effective coping mechanisms

INTERVENTIONS

Monitor temperature q4h.

Monitor activity and report desaturation or increased fatigue. *Decreased exercise tolerance with desaturation can be a manifestation of rejection and/or infection.*

Teach patient to monitor and document daily spirometry readings and note a decrease by 10% in a 24-hour period. *Lung function (FVC and FEV_1) is the most important measurement to detect rejection or infection.*

Monitor lab values and cultures daily.

Monitor cyclosporine levels daily.

Limit visitation to immediate family members.

Adhere to protective isolation requirements. *Private rooms with positive-negative airflow systems are used by most centers to prevent infection by opportunistic organisms.*

Encourage small, frequent meals and advance diet as tolerated.

Consult dietitian.

Monitor bowel function by auscultation; offer laxatives prn as ordered.

Discontinue total parenteral nutrition when diet is tolerated.

Discontinue nasogastric tube when oral intake is initiated.

Monitor patient's ability to self-medicate and educate patient to adverse reactions of all medications.

Provide patient with medication chart with doses and times.

Have patient demonstrate measurement and daily documentation of blood pressure, pulse, weight, and spirometry function.

Reinforce parameters to call the nurse coordinator after discharge regarding signs and symptoms of rejection and infection, blood pressure parameters, and weight gain or loss of two to three pounds in 24 hours.

Encourage verbalization of fear and anxiety.

Normalize environment as much as possible and encourage family visits. *The presence of a significant other whom the patient trusts decreases the anxiety level.*

Reinforce patient's assessment of family strengths, positive self-concept, and progress.

Explain typical course and possible complications.

TRANSITION TO DISCHARGE

Lung transplant patients should be well informed and educated about self-care, including medications, prior to discharge. Clinic appointments are scheduled with the transplant team every 6 weeks (in between 3-month bronchoscopies) for the first year. Transbronchial biopsies and bronchoscopies are performed every 3 months for the first year. Most lung transplant centers do not continue to perform routine surveillance bronchoscopies or transbronchial biopsies after the first year posttransplant. Formal pulmonary function tests are scheduled monthly for the first year and every 3 months for the remainder of the patient's life. More frequent transbronchial biopsies and bronchoscopy and pulmonary function tests can be indicated if the patient has symptoms of infection or rejection.

Patients are required to keep a diary with daily measurements of FVC and FEV_1, temperature, blood pressure, heart rate, and weight.

Limitations for the first 6 to 10 weeks include:

- No lifting of objects greater than 10 pounds
- Avoidance of strenuous activities such as tennis, bowling, pushing a vacuum cleaner or a lawn mower
- No driving for 6 weeks *to give the sternum time to heal*
- Faithful use of a sunscreen in appropriate weather. *Patients on immunosuppressants are photosensitive and are at a higher risk of developing skin cancers.*

Lung transplantation is not a cure, but it may offer an improved quality and quantity of life for selected end-stage lung disease patients. Many advancements have been made in the area of lung transplantation in the last decade, but several unknowns still remain. A Toronto Lung Transplant Group survey[4] of 20 consecutive recipients from their institution who were at least 6 months posttransplant found that 50% were working, and an additional 30% were active as homemakers or students. Out of this group, 70% reported their overall life satisfaction to be good to excellent. This survey represents the majority of lung transplant recipients, in that most patients return to a productive and normal life-style independent of oxygen after transplant.

Long-term actuarial survival will continue to improve as more research is conducted in obliterative bronchiolitis, infection, and lymphoproliferative disease, which contribute to increased postoperative morbidity and mortality in transplanted patients. Nurses can contribute to the success of lung transplantation by assisting in recipient selection, donor management, education, research, and pre- and postoperative care. The ultimate challenge is the enhancement of patient care, with the goal of a smooth recovery and a return to a healthy life-style.

REFERENCES

1. Armitage JM, et al: Posttransplant lymphoproliferative disease in thoracic organ transplant patients: ten years of cyclosporine-based immunosuppression, *J Heart Lung Transplant* 10:877-887, 1991.
2. Arnold CD, et al: Benefits of an aerobic exercise program in CF patients waiting for double lung transplantation, *Pediatr Pulmonol* 6(suppl):287, 1991.
3. Cooper JD: The evolution of techniques and indications for lung transplantation, *Ann Surg* 212:249-256, 1990.
4. Craven J, the Toronto Lung Transplant Group: Psychiatric aspects of lung transplant, *Can J Psychiatry* 35:759-764, 1990.
5. D'Alonzo GE: Survival in patients with primary pulmonary hypertension, *Ann Intern Med* 115:343-349, 1991.
6. Dear CL, Grossman RF, Maurer JR: Preoperative rehabilitation of patients awaiting lung transplantation, *Ann Thorac Surg* 42:394-398, 1986.
7. Dolovich M, et al: Mucociliary function in patients following single lung or lung-heart transplantation, *Am Rev Respir Dis* 35:A363, 1987 (abstract).
8. Egan TM, Detterbeck FC: Technique and results of double lung transplantation, *Chest Surg Clin N Am* 3:89-111, 1992.
9. Egan TM, Kaiser LR, Cooper JD: Lung transplantation, *Curr Probl Surg* 26:675-751, 1989.
10. Egan TM, et al: Isolated lung transplantation for end-stage lung disease: a viable therapy, *Ann Thorac Surg* 53:590-596, 1992.
11. Flume PA, et al: Lung transplantation for mechanically ventilated patients, *J Heart Lung Transplant* 13(1 Part 1):15-21, 1994.
12. Flume PA, et al: Infectious complications in lung transplantation: cystic fibrosis (CF) versus non-CF, *Am Rev Respir Dis* 147:A601, 1993 (abstract).
13. Glanville A, et al: Bronchial hyperresponsiveness after human cardiopulmonary transplantation, *Clin Sci* 73:299-303, 1987.
14. Glanville A, Baldwin J, Burke C: Obliterative bronchiolitis after heart-

lung transplantation: apparent arrest by augmented immunosuppression, *Ann Intern Med* 107:300-304, 1987.
15. Green A, Claibourne C: A nursing challenge: cytomegalovirus in the transplant recipient, *Focus Crit Care* 16:349-354, 1989.
16. Griffith BP, et al: Immunologically mediated disease of the airways after pulmonary transplantation, *Ann Surg* 208:371-378, 1988.
17. Hardy JD, et al: Lung homotransplantation in man, *JAMA* 186:1065-1074, 1963.
18. Haydock DA: Lung transplantation: analysis of thirty-six consecutive procedures performed over a twelve-month period, *J Thorac Cardiovasc Surg* 103:329-340, 1992.
19. Keenan RJ, et al: Similarity of pulmonary rejection patterns among heart-lung and double-lung transplant recipients, *Transplantation* 51:176-180, 1991.
20. Kerem E, et al: Prediction of mortality in patients with cystic fibrosis, *New Engl J Med* 326:1187-1191, 1992.
21. Kramer MR, et al: The diagnosis of obliterative bronchiolitis after heart-lung and lung transplantation: low yield of transbronchial lung biopsy, *J Heart Lung Transplant* 12:675-681, 1993.
22. Malen J, et al: Tissue and organ transplantation, *Crit Care Nurs Clin N Am* 4:111-130, 1992.
23. Marshall SE, et al: Selection and evaluation of recipients for heart-lung and lung transplantation, *Chest* 98:1488-1494, 1990.
24. Martin S: Pediatric critical care: nurses' perceptions and understanding of cadaver organ procurement, *Crit Care Nurse,* pp 74-81, February 1993.
25. Maurer JR, et al: Late pulmonary complications of isolated lung transplantation, *Transplant Proc* 23:1224-1225, 1991.
26. Métras D, et al: Lung transplantation in children, *J Heart Lung Transplant* 11:S282-S285, 1992.
27. Muirhead J: Heart and heart-lung transplantation, *Crit Care Nurs Clin N Am* 14:97-108, 1992.
28. Pasque MK, et al: Improved technique for bilateral lung transplantation: rationale and initial clinical experience, *Ann Thorac Surg* 49:785-791, 1990.
29. Pearson G: Lung transplantation, *Arch Surg* 24:535-538, 1989.
30. Registry of the Internal Society for Heart and Lung Transplantation: tenth official report—1993, *J Heart Lung Transplant* 12:541-548, 1993.
31. Shennib H, Nguyen D: Bronchoalveolar lavage in lung transplantation, *Ann Thorac Surg* 51:335-340, 1991.
32. Shumway SJ: Immunosuppression in lung transplantation, *Chest Surg Clin N Am* 3:145-155, 1993.
33. *St Anthony's DRG guidebook 1995,* Reston, Va, 1994, St Anthony.
34. Starnes VA, et al: Heart, heart-lung, and lung transplantation in the first year of life, *Ann Thorac Surg* 53:306-310, 1992.
35. The Toronto Lung Transplant Group: Experience with single lung transplantation for pulmonary fibrosis, *JAMA* 259:2258-2262, 1988.
36. The Toronto Lung Transplant Group: Unilateral lung transplantation for pulmonary fibrosis, *New Engl J Med* 314:1140-1145, 1986.
37. Trulock EP, et al: The role of transbronchial lung biopsy in the treatment of lung transplant recipients: an analysis of 200 consecutive procedures, *Chest* 102:1049-1054, 1992.
38. UNOS: Patients waiting for transplants: number of patient registrations on the national waiting list 9/30/93, *UNOS Update* 9, September-October 1993.
39. Winton TL: Lung transplantation: donor selection, *Semin Thorac Cardiovasc Surg* 4:79-82, 1992.
40. Wreghitt TG, et al: Cytomegalovirus infections in heart and heart-and-lung transplant recipients, *J Clin Pathol* 41:660-667, 1988.
41. Zeevi A, Uknis ME, Spichty KJ: Proliferation of cytomegalovirus-primed lymphocytes in bronchoalveolar lavages from lung transplant patients, *Transplantation* 54:635-639, 1992.

DEVICE GUIDELINE

41

Mechanical Ventilation

Kay Knox Greenlee, MSN, RN, CCRN

DESCRIPTION

Mechanical ventilation supports the pulmonary system in providing gas exchange to supply tissues with oxygen. A positive or negative force is generated to inflate the lungs, thus initiating inhalation, the active phase of respiration. When the force is discontinued, the passive phase of respiration, exhalation, follows. Mechanical ventilation is a support device frequently used in the critical care setting. The nursing staff in collaboration with other members of the health care team, is responsible for monitoring the patient's response to mechanical ventilation and, therefore, must have a good working knowledge of the indications, potential complications, and general nursing interventions related to mechanical ventilation.

INDICATIONS

Mechanical ventilation is necessary when conservative means cannot rectify the clinical picture of acute respiratory failure. Specifically, mechanical ventilation is indicated when the patient has inadequate ventilation, inadequate oxygenation, or both. Mechanical ventilation is used in conditions that result in the following:

- Inadequate lung expansion
- Respiratory muscle fatigue
- Excessive work of breathing
- Unstable ventilatory drive

Mechanical ventilation is also used postoperatively to prevent respiratory acidosis, poor lung expansion, or respiratory muscle fatigue in the high-risk patient.[8] The patient with a closed head injury may require mechanical ventilation to maintain low P_{CO_2}, which results in lower intracranial pressure.

The goals of mechanical ventilation are to maintain cardiopulmonary homeostasis within acceptable physiologic limits for a period of time, decrease the myocardial workload, and improve efficiency of ventilation and/or oxygenation by manipulating the ventilatory pattern and parameters.[1] Mechanical ventilation is accomplished with the use of three types of ventilators that generate a force to inflate the lungs: positive-pressure, negative-pressure, and high-frequency ventilators. The type of ventilator used is determined by the physical condition or indication for the need for mechanical ventilation.

Positive-pressure ventilators deliver positive pressure to inflate the lungs and expand the chest and cycle by preset volume, pressure, or time. Negative-pressure ventilators apply a negative pressure to the trunk to create pressure changes that result in chest and lung expansion. High-frequency ventilators use less positive pressure but significantly higher rates than traditional types of positive-pressure ventilators.

The most frequently used ventilator in the critically ill adult is the volume-cycled positive-pressure ventilator. This guideline will focus on this type of mechanical ventilator. Volume-cycled ventilators are preferred by most clinicians because they reliably deliver the preset tidal volume as well as the desired F_{IO_2}% concentration. A volume-cycled ventilator delivers a constant tidal volume in the presence of changes in airway resistance or in compliance (distensibility) of the lungs or thorax. It terminates inspiration after a preset volume is delivered. This preset volume is delivered regardless of the pressure needed to do so. However, when excessive pressures are generated in the airway, a pressure alarm limit is activated, and inspiration ends prematurely.

Several modes of ventilation are available using the volume-cycled ventilators, including controlled ventilation, assist-control ventilation, and intermittent mandatory ventilation. Adjuncts to mechanical ventilation include positive end expiratory pressure, continuous positive airway pressure, pressure support ventilation, and inverse ratio ventilation. The mode and/or adjunct chosen depends on specific patient needs.

With **controlled ventilation,** the patient is not permitted to (or cannot) initiate inspiratory effort. The ventilator delivers a preset tidal volume at a preset rate, with the patient unable to generate a breath from the machine. This method is used for patients who have tachypnea and marked respiratory distress, in which the patient's breathing pattern is not in synchrony with the machine. To block out patient effort, pharmacological agents such as opioid (morphine sulfate), neuroblocker (pancuronium), and benzodiazepines (Midazolam) are required.

With **assist-control ventilation,** the patient can initiate each breath by creating negative pressure in the lungs through muscle contraction. The ventilator responds to this pressure by delivering a positive pressure breath at the preset tidal volume. In addition, the ventilator automatically delivers positive pressure breaths if the patient does not initiate a breath within a preset time. Assist control ventilation can result in hypocapnia due to hyperventilation because the patient can initiate an unlimited number of breaths at the preset tidal volume.

With **intermittent mandatory ventilation (IMV),** the patient is allowed to spontaneously breathe humidified, oxygenated air from the ventilatory system at whatever rate and volume the patient chooses. Intermittent positive-pressure breaths are delivered from the ventilator at preset intervals and volume to ensure adequate alveolar ventilation. IMV is particularly useful for patients who have been intubated for a prolonged period of time and in whom the respiratory muscles are weak. IMV allows the patient to actively contract his or her own respiratory muscles and gradually build muscle strength. This mode of ventilation is generally used for gradually weaning a patient from artificial ventilation. Most ventilators deliver the IMV breaths in synchrony with the patient's own effect. This is referred to as **synchronized intermittent mandatory ventilation (SIMV)** and decreases the chance of stacking breaths, which creates larger-than-desired tidal volumes.

With **positive end expiratory pressure (PEEP),** positive pressure is maintained above atmospheric pressure throughout the ventilatory cycle. PEEP is used to improve oxygenation by increasing the function residual capacity (FRC). By increasing FRC, PEEP expands collapsed alveoli and further expands under ventilated alveoli, thus increasing surface area and exposure time for the diffusion of oxygen.

Continuous positive airway pressure (CPAP) refers to PEEP applied in conjunction with spontaneous ventilation. With CPAP all patient breaths are spontaneous, with no interposed mechanical ventilator breaths. The patient breathes humidified, oxygenated air from the ventilatory system at whatever rate the patient chooses. During the expiratory phase, the patient exhales to the preset positive end-expiratory pressure level. CPAP is useful for patients who do not require assistance in maintaining an adequate tidal volume but who benefit from an increased end-expiratory pressure used to improve oxygenation, such as those with sleep apnea or neuromuscular disorders. CPAP can be delivered using a mask to improve oxygenation, without the invasive procedure of intubation. The CPAP mask may be uncomfortable because of the pressure required to create a seal.

Pressure support is available on the microprocessor ventilators. Positive pressure is added to each inspiration the patient takes while the patient is on an IMV mode or on CPAP. The patient's tidal volumes are thus augmented, and the mandatory IMV rate of the ventilator can be decreased so that the patient does more of the work of breathing with less effort.

Inverse ratio ventilation occurs when the time for inspiration is longer than that for expiration, which is the reverse of the normal I/E ratio. Normal I/E ratios on mechanical ventilation range from 1:2 to 1:4. During IRV the I/E ratio is brought closer together and possibly reversed (1:1 to 2:1) to improve hypoxemia that has not responded to increased FiO_2 and PEEP therapy.[1] The patient requires sedation and possibly paralysis during this adjunctive therapy to reduce anxiety and provide comfort.[16]

LIMITATIONS

Mechanical ventilation is limited in that it is supportive therapy, not curative. The initiation of mechanical ventilation is usually with the intent that it will be temporary. However, in some cases the patient cannot be weaned. When weaning is no longer possible, decisions must be made to determine if the patient wishes to continue on mechanical ventilation long term or chooses to discontinue the treatment.

Long-term mechanical ventilation may occur in the hospital, home, or long-term care facility. The location is determined by the patient's overall condition, availability of support systems, and the facility resources available. The success of any long-term program depends on a multidisciplinary approach and a committed support team.

Discontinuation of mechanical ventilation may occur when death is imminent and continuation would only prolong the process. Discontinuation may also occur for patients whose death is neither imminent nor inevitable, but the futility of continued mechanical ventilation is recognized or the patient requests the treatment be discontinued. The process of discontinuing mechanical ventilation is collaborative between the health care team and the patient or family. The treatment plan should address the process of decision making, explanation and reassurance, delay between decision and action, support, and timing for withdrawal of mechanical ventilation.[6]

Complications

Complications r/t artificial ventilation

Hypoventilation
Hyperventilation
Infection
GI abnormalities

Complications r/t positive pressure ventilation

Decreased venous return
Barotrauma
Auto PEEP
Fluid retention

POTENTIAL COMPLICATIONS

Complications of mechanical ventilation can be categorized into two major groups: complications related to artificial ventilation and complications related to positive pressure ventilation (see the preceding Box). The nursing interventions directed toward prevention of complications are listed in Table 41-1.

The primary complications associated with artificial ventilation include hypoventilation, hyperventilation, and infection. Hypoventilation may result in atelectasis and respiratory acidosis. Hyperventilation may increase the risk of barotrauma and result in respiratory alkalosis. The patient requiring artificial ventilation is at risk for infection because of the artificial airway. The airway bypasses the natural defense mechanisms of the respiratory system, including the mucociliary blanket and the ability to warm and humidify the inhaled air. Risk of respiratory infection increases with age, obesity, ineffective airway clearance, altered breathing pattern, inadequate nutritional intake, and impaired physical mobility.

The primary complications related to positive pressure ventilation include decreased venous return, barotrauma, and auto-PEEP. The positive pressure created within the intrathoracic cavity results in decreased venous return. This can lead to decreased cardiac output and/or hypotension. The risk for hemodynamic compromise is especially high for the hypovolemic patient.

Barotrauma is injury to the tracheobronchial tree. Patients at risk for barotrauma include those with COPD, emphysematous blebs, and chest trauma, especially when high-volume and/or high-pressure settings are needed to meet ventilatory demands. Barotrauma can result in the development of a tension pneumothorax. The signs of barotrauma include acute increase in airway pressure, respiratory distress, unequal breath sounds, decreased or distant breath sounds, crepitant rales during inspiration or expiration, unilateral chest expansion, asymmetrical chest movements, tracheal deviation, decreased cardiac output and BP, tachycardia with weak pulse, increased CVP, distended neck veins, and cyanosis.

Auto-PEEP refers to air and pressure trapped in the lung as a result of inadequate expiration time. Auto-PEEP can increase the risk of barotrauma and further decrease venous return.

In addition to the complications of mechanical ventilation, long-term outcomes for the patient have been studied. The factors of disease, severity of illness, age, duration of therapy, and previous health have been evaluated to determine influence on patient outcomes following mechanical ventilation. Nonoperative patients admitted to ICU on a ventilator had a 52% chance of dying, usually within the first week.[9] Mortality following mechanical ventilation of greater than 3 days ranged from 40% to 79%.[5] Several studies have been done to determine the influence of age; the results have been controversial. Using an index of age plus days of mechanical ventilation, mortality rates were compared. Patients with an index ≥ 100 had a mortality rate of 93%, whereas patients with an index <100 had a mortality rate of 75%.[5] However, in another study patients 70 years of age and younger and 70 years of age and older experienced mortality rates of 57% and 59%, respectively.[12] Others have concluded that the only factor influencing the patient outcome was the reason for mechanical ventilation. Patients with ventilatory insufficiency had better survival rates at 57% than those with oxygen impairment, who had survival rates of 24%.[13] Mechanical ventilation carries with it some degree of risk; however, the factors influencing outcomes are not definitive.

GENERAL NURSING INTERVENTIONS

Several nursing interventions are key to the effective use of mechanical ventilators. These interventions, listed in Table 41-1, include those necessary to monitor for effectiveness of the therapy and to prevent complications of mechanical ventilation.

Whenever possible, the initiation of mechanical ventilation should include preparing the patient for the procedure. Anxiety will be reduced if the patient has an understanding of the sensations experienced, such as relief of dyspnea, big lung inflations, noise of the ventilator, and the sound of alarms.[2] The patient and family must understand that the patient will be unable to speak while intubated and another method of communication needs to be established.

When the airway has been established, use the manual resuscitation bag to support the patient's respiratory efforts. After the patient has been prepared for the sensation and demonstrates a comfortable breathing pattern, convert to the mechanical ventilator for ongoing ventilatory support.

The patency of the airway is key to accomplishing effective mechanical ventilation. The intervention most often used to maintain patency is suctioning. Endotracheal suctioning has been the focus of nursing research over the past several years. A variety of studies have investigated the

TABLE 41-1 General Nursing Interventions Associated with Mechanical Ventilation

General considerations	Related nursing interventions
Monitor effectiveness	
Assess airway patency	Suction, as described in the following Box, Guidelines for Suctioning, based on assessment.
Assessment of air movement	Auscultate breath sounds q4h
Assess gas exchange	Monitor arterial blood gases (ABG) Monitor oxygenation with Spo_2 Monitor $ETCO_2$
Provide method of communication	Provide paper and pencil Use word/letter board
Assessment of respiratory effort	Use scale of 0 to 10 to quantify shortness of breath 0 = No SOB and 10 = Worst imaginable SOB[4]
Prevention of complications	
Improper positioning of endotracheal tube	Secure tube with tape or holder Note landmarks of proper positioning Chest x-ray verification
Accidental extubation	Evaluate need for restraint—chemical and/or physical Allow enough slack by adjusting tubing on support arms of ventilator to accommodate patient's movements Keep resuscitator bag connected to oxygen and syringe to remove cuff air at bedside If extubation occurs, hand ventilate patient with oxygen mask, and resuscitator bag Teach the patient about the interventions used to prevent extubation and the consequences of an unplanned extubation
Fistulas	Use of minimal air leak or minimal occlusive pressure to decrease amount of pressure exerted on tracheal tissue Deflate cuff when repositioning tube (suction pharynx before deflation)
Pressure sores	Inspect mouth, nose, tracheostomy site, and beneath tape for pressure sores, redness, or skin breakdown Avoid pressure areas around mouth and nose from ET tube Retape as needed to keep tape and skin below dry
Potential infection	Oral hygiene q2h to q4h to decrease risk of nosocomial infection Change water used to lubricate and clear suction catheter q8h to q24h Place end of suction tubing from canister in clean container when not in use and change q24h Maintain asepsis of ventilator connector when disconnected Change suction canister q24h Change ventilator circuit q24h to q72h Monitor for signs of infection—elevated temperature, change in vital signs, change in secretions (amount, color, odor) If oral airway present, remove and clean q8h to q12h
Barotrauma	Monitor for signs and symptoms of tension pneumothorax
Fluid retention	Monitor daily weights for weight gain Impaired breathing pattern Decreased cardiac output Monitor I/O, skin color, temperature, moisture Monitor HR, BP, and Sao_2
Gastrointestinal bleeding and malfunction	Monitor for abdominal pain, nausea and signs of bleeding Insert NG tube if gastric distention is present Consider use of H_2 blocker to decrease risk of stress ulcers
Pyschological concerns	Provide method for patient to communicate Work with patient to address anxiety and fear Explain safety procedures and alarms systems to reassure patient Encourage patient participation in care to promote sense of hope and independence

Guidelines for Suctioning

- Use suction no greater than 150 mm Hg
- Use catheter not greater than one half the diameter of the artificial airway
- Hyperoxygenate before, during, and after endotracheal suctioning[14]
- Provide three hyperoxygenation/hyperventilation breaths with 100% oxygen and 150% tidal volume before, during, and after endotracheal suctioning[14]
- Use of the ventilator is preferable for hyperoxygenation/hyperventilation (there are instances where it is necessary to use a manual resuscitator bag)[14]
- Limit the number of suction passes to only those necessary to limit changes in MAP, CO, HR, and ICP[14]
- Limit the time of each suctioning pass to less than 15 seconds

Data collected from Stone K: Ventilator versus manual resuscitation bag for delivering hyperoxygenation before endotracheal suctioning, *Annu Rev Nurs Res* 7:27-29, 1990.

techniques implemented to minimize the most common complication of suctioning—hypoxemia. Hyperoxygenation, hyperinflation, and the use of adapters are the most common variables studied. The results are as varied as the methods and populations used in the studies. The procedure supported by research conducted thus far is outlined in the preceding Box.

Further research is needed to determine the amount of preoxygenation necessary and the most appropriate method of hyperventilation to minimize hypoxemia without compromising other patient responses, such as intracranial and hemodynamic pressures and the effects of using endotracheal tube adapters beyond decreasing hypoxemia.[15]

Assessment of respiratory effort, using a scale, provides a subjective quantitative measure that can be correlated with physiologic parameters used to evaluate patient response. The scale is very effective in evaluating the patient's response to ventilator setting changes during the weaning process.

Nursing interventions are also key during the discontinuation of mechanical ventilation and are listed in Table 41-2. When the indication for mechanical ventilation has been resolved, the process of discontinuing mechanical ventilation begins. This is referred to as *weaning*. Weaning is viewed as a process beginning with the evaluation of readiness to wean, assessing the tolerance to weaning, removal of the mechanical ventilator, and, finally, evaluation of airway status with consideration given to removal of the artificial airway.

Weaning from mechanical ventilation involves psychological, physiological, and environmental adjustments. The majority of patients wean from a mechanical ventilator with relative ease. Others require more interventions and time to be successful. Consideration should be given to the amount of time the person has been mechanically ventilated; the longer mechanical ventilation is used, the more difficult it may be to wean.

A variety of studies has been conducted to determine readiness for weaning and predictability of successful weaning. Although the results of these studies have provided us with information about the factors that prevent weaning and methods of weaning used in the clinical setting, a predictor of successful weaning has not been determined. Young and Tobin[18] evaluated the ratio of respiratory frequency to tidal volume and the CROP index (thoracic compliance, respiratory rate, oxygenation, and inspiratory pressure) as predictors of the outcome of weaning. The frequency/tidal volume ratio was the best predictor of successful weaning. Several tools have been developed to assist the nurse to determine the patient's ability to wean. The Morganroth[11] tool calculates an adverse factor score and a ventilator score. In combination, these were more predictive of successful weaning than either score separately. The wean score instrument developed by Dettenmeier[7] has been found to be useful, but reliability across populations has not been determined. The Burns wean assessment program is a tool designed to assist the critical care nurse in the weaning process.[3] General, respiratory, and mechanical factors that impede weaning are assessed, and, with computer support, the nurse is given information to develop an appropriate plan of care for the patient.

The method of weaning is one of the environmental factors to be considered during the weaning process. The methods of weaning include T-piece, CPAP, IMV, and PS.

The T-piece method is often used for patients who require short-term ventilation. The patient is removed from the mechanical ventilator and placed on a T-piece for a specified period of time. As the time of spontaneous breathing increases respiratory muscle strength and endurance are increased, enabling the patient to maintain spontaneous ventilation. The spontaneous breathing period is exercise for the respiratory muscles and the patient must be allowed periods of rest between exercise sessions.

Continuous positive airway pressure (CPAP) can be added to the T-piece method to increase the FRC and to decrease the complication of atelectasis. It does increase work of breathing. This increased WOB could be minimized with the use of pressure support.

Intermittent mandatory ventilation (IMV) is the most common method of weaning. The number of breaths delivered by the ventilator is gradually decreased. The patient increases the number of spontaneous breaths. This method is good for patients who can't tolerate large drops or abrupt changes in the ventilator settings. IMV has been favored because of better maintenance of respiratory muscle tone, more similar to normal ventilation requiring less sedation, improved distribution, and less cardiovascular disturbance.[15]

Pressure support ventilation (PSV) decreases the work of breathing by augmenting the patient's inspiratory effort. The patient is more comfortable and has been shown to spend less time weaning.

TABLE 41-2 General Nursing Interventions Associated with Determining Readiness and Discontinuing Mechanical Ventilation

General considerations	Related nursing interventions
Physiologic readiness	Measured ventilation mechanics • Rate less than 30/min • ABG within patient norms • Vital capacity 10 to 15 ml/kg or greater than 1 liter • Tidal volume greater than 6 ml/kg • Maximal inspiratory flow greater than −25 to −30 cm H_2O • Static compliance >40 ml/cm H_2O • Dead space to tidal volume ratio (V_D/V_T) <0.6 • Maximum voluntary ventilation (MVV) >2 times resting minute ventilation • Negative inspiratory force >−20 mm H_2O • Minute ventilation <10 L/min Measured oxygenation parameters • A-a Do_2 <350 on 100% • Shunt factor (Q_s/Q_t) <20% • Pao_2 >80% on 60% • PEEP <5 cm H_2O • a/A ratio >.75 Assessed • Secretions • Breathing pattern • Cough and gag reflex intact • Position required • Position for comfort, consider HOB elevated for better lung expansion • Pain • Sleep/rest • Nutrition • CNS: no seizures, adequate drive as measured by minute ventilation, able to protect airway • Metabolic: adequate caloric intake for resting energy, plus disease requirements • Renal: equal intake output, stable electrolytes, no edema or controlled, stable weight • CV: stable, transport is dependent on cardiac output with adequate hemoglobin and hematocrit • Muscle strength
Psychologic readiness	Anxiety • Explain when changes are made • Explain monitoring/assessments to be done Fear • Explain safety features/alarms • Pulse oximetry • Provide mechanism for communication Knowledge • Explain weaning process • Power resources/control • Reinforce progress • Use support systems
Environmental readiness	Select appropriate method of weaning Create a comfortable environment Provide access to personnel

TABLE 41-2 General Nursing Interventions Associated with Determining Readiness and Discontinuing Mechanical Ventilation—cont'd

General considerations	Related nursing interventions
Patient response during weaning	Compare patient parameters to baseline • Respiratory rate • Vital signs • ABG • Oxygenation (Spo_2) • Shortness of breath • Diaphoresis • Use of accessory muscles • Coordination of effort Return patient to prewean settings or mode if significant changes occur indicating weaning failure[10,17] • Altered breathing pattern • Increased dyspnea • Use of accessory muscles • Prolonged expiration • Asynchronous movements of chest/abdomen • Retractions • Shortened inspiratory time • Increased rate, >30/min or > 10/min over baseline • Restlessness/irritability • CV deterioration: diastolic BP >100 mm Hg, fall in systolic BP, HR >110 bpm or >20 bpm over baseline, excessive changes in HR or BP, arrhythmias, angina, change in ST segment • Decreased LOC • Tidal volume <250 to 300 ml • $Paco_2$ increased by 8 mm Hg
If SOB occurs during weaning[4]	Decrease effort and improve function • Use previous method to decrease SOB: position pursed lip breathing, slow deep breathing, relaxation, distraction • Inspiratory muscle training • Bronchodilators Decrease drive and perception of SOB • Sedation, opiods • Oxygen • Coaching • Large tidal volumes Relaxation and biofeedback
Discontinue mechanical ventilation	Monitor patient's ability to maintain spontaneous ventilation
Removal of artificial airway	Procedure • Position patient in high Fowler's • Set up oxygen • Suction patient via ET tube and orally • Deflate cuff and resuction if needed • Remove tape/holder • Have patient breathe deeply and cough, remove tube at peak of inhalation • Apply oxygen Monitor for stridor Evaluate swallowing ability to decrease risk of aspiration

Failure to wean from the mechanical ventilator is often related to one or more of the parameters used to determine readiness to wean. Nutrition, muscle weakness, method of weaning and cardiac failure are some of the more common reasons for failing to wean. When the patient fails to wean, it is important that the factors identified in Table 41-2 be reassessed. Nursing care must be directed toward optimizing readiness to wean successfully.

TROUBLESHOOTING

The final consideration in the care of the patient being mechanically ventilated is troubleshooting. In general, there are two areas to problem solve: high-pressure alarm and low-volume alarm. A high-pressure alarm indicates that the set volume of air cannot be delivered with an acceptable amount of pressure; a low-volume alarm indicates that the amount of air exhaled through the ventilator is lower than the volume delivered. The causes and corrective actions for these claims are as follows.

When a patient experiences respiratory distress while being mechanically ventilated, the patient's ability to maintain adequate ventilation must be the first consideration during troubleshooting. If the problem cannot be corrected immediately, the patient should be removed from the mechanical ventilator and artificially ventilated using a resuscitator bag until the problem is corrected.

Problem: High-Pressure Alarm

CAUSE	CORRECTIVE ACTION
Kinked endotracheal tube	Check endotracheal tube for kinks Tape endotracheal tube to maintain alignment
Kinked ventilator tubing	Check ventilator circuit for kinks Use circuit holder or other mechanism to protect tubing from tension of kinks
Retained secretions	Suction prn based on assessment
Pneumothorax	Assess for presence of breath sounds Assess symmetry of respiratory effort Notify physician prn

Problem: Low-Pressure Alarm

CAUSE	CORRECTIVE ACTION
Ventilator tubing disconnected from endotracheal tube	Check tubing and reconnect prn Secure connections Support ventilator circuit to prevent tension on tubing
Ventilator tubing disconnected from ventilator	Check connections to ventilator Maintain proximity between ventilator and patient/bed
Cuff leak	Assess for presence of cuff leak Protect patient from potential aspiration Contact physician if patient is unable to maintain minute volume, is at risk of aspiration, or requires reintubation

SUMMARY

Mechanical ventilation is used in the treatment of many of the respiratory diseases addressed in other guidelines in this text. Mechanical ventilation has been identified as one of the top research topics within the critical care setting. The use of mechanical ventilation within critical care is commonplace, yet the research related to specific outcomes is limited. The purpose of guidelines specific to mechanical ventilation is to support the patient and extend the decision-making capabilities of the bedside nurse using a technology commonly seen in the critical care environment.

REFERENCES

1. Ahrens TS: Mechanical support of ventilation. In Kinney MR, Packa DR, Dunbar SB, editors: *AACN's clinical reference for critical-care nursing,* St Louis, 1993, Mosby–Year Book.
2. Boggs RL, Wooldridge-King M: *AACN Procedure manual for critical care,* ed 3, Philadelphia, 1993, WB Saunders.
3. Burns SM, et al: Weaning from mechanical ventilation: a method for assessment and planning, *AACN Clin Iss Crit Care Nurs* 2(3):372-387, 1991.
4. Carrieri-Kohlman V: Dyspnea in the weaning patient: assessment and intervention, *AACN Clin Iss Crit Care Nurs* 2:462-473, 1991.
5. Cohen IL, Lambrinos J, Fein A: Mechanical ventilation for the elderly patient in intensive care, *JAMA* 269:1025-1029, 1993.
6. Daly BJ, et al: Withdrawal of mechanical ventilation: ethical principles and guidelines for terminal weaning, *Am J Crit Care* 2(3):217-223, 1993.
7. Dettenmeier PA, et al: Reliability testing of an instrument to predict an optimal weaning period for patients on mechanical ventilation, *Am Rev Respir Dis* 139:A99, 1989.
8. Kersten LD: *Comprehensive respiratory nursing: a decision making approach,* Philadelphia, 1989, WB Saunders.
9. Knaus WA: Prognosis with mechanical ventilation: the influence of disease, severity of disease, age and chronic health status on survival from acute illness, *Am Rev Respir Dis* 140, S8-S13, 1989.
10. Knebel AR: When weaning from mechanical ventilation fails, *Am J Crit Care* 1(3) 19-29, 1992.
11. Morganroth ML, et al: Criteria for weaning from prolonged mechanical ventilation, *Arch Intern Med* 144:1012-1016, 1984.
12. O'Donnell A, Bohner B: The outcome in patients requiring prolonged mechanical ventilation, *Chest* 100:29S, 1991.
13. Pesau B, et al: Influence of age on outcome of mechanically ventilated patients in an intensive care unit, *Crit Care Med* 20:489-492, 1992.
14. Stone K: Ventilator versus manual resuscitation bag for delivering hyperoxygenation before endotracheal suctioning, *AACN Clin Iss Crit Care Nurs* 1(2):289-299, 1990.
15. Stone KS, Turner B: Endotracheal suctioning, *Ann Rev Nurs Res* 7:27-49, 1989.
16. Weilitz PB: New modes of mechanical ventilation, *Crit Care Nurs Clin North Am* 1(4):689-695, 1989.
17. Weilitz PB: Weaning a patient from mechanical ventilation, *Crit Care Nurs* 13(4):33-41, 1993.
18. Yang KL, Tobin MJ: A prospective study of indexes predicting the outcome of trials of weaning from mechanical ventilation, *N Engl J Med* 324(21):1445-1450, 1991.

UNIT

IV

Gastrointestinal System

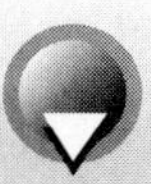

CLINICAL GUIDELINE

42

Peritonitis

Peg Snyder, MN, RN, CCRN

DESCRIPTION

Peritonitis is inflammation of the peritoneum from microbial invasion or contact with an irritant. Peritonitis may be classified as primary, secondary, or tertiary.

Primary peritonitis is peritoneal infection that occurs without an identifiable intra-abdominal lesion as the source. The infecting organism is transmitted by the lymph and blood from an area of colonization or infection such as the genitourinary or respiratory tract. Primary peritonitis occurs most frequently in persons with ascites due to cirrhosis, nephrotic syndrome, congestive heart failure, or impaired host immunity due to age, disease, radiation therapy, or pharmacotherapy. Patients with indwelling peritoneal catheters for peritoneal dialysis also are at risk. Primary peritonitis previously was more common in children, but while the pediatric case incidence appears to be declining, the disease is occurring more frequently in adults.[7] Spontaneous bacterial peritonitis occurs in approximately 10% to 25% of cirrhotic patients with ascites.[4]

Secondary peritonitis results from contamination of the peritoneal cavity by infectious substances from a ruptured, inflamed, or infected abdominal or pelvic organ.[2] Etiologies of secondary peritonitis are outlined in the following Box.

Tertiary peritonitis is a progression of secondary peritonitis and refers to persistent, diffuse peritonitis despite treatment with appropriate antibiotics and surgery. Tertiary peritonitis is more likely to occur in patients with marked impairment of host defense mechanisms who are unable to eradicate or localize an intra-abdominal infection. Tertiary peritonitis is associated with the development of multiple organ dysfunction syndrome (MODS).

PATHOPHYSIOLOGY

The peritoneum is a serous membrane lining the inner abdominal wall (parietal peritoneum) and reflecting back onto the abdominal organs (visceral peritoneum). The peritoneum has a surface area roughly equivalent to that of the skin (1.7 m^2) and defines a large potential space, the peritoneal cavity. Normally this space contains <50 ml of free fluid. The fluid is sterile, clear, yellow, and contains <3000 cells/mm^3, primarily macrophages and lymphocytes.

The introduction of irritants, bacteria, or other microorganisms into the peritoneal cavity stimulates local defense mechanisms that mechanically clear bacteria and other particulates from the peritoneal cavity, phagocytize and destroy invading microorganisms, and sequester and isolate bacteria for later clearance by phagocytic cells. Mechanical clearance of bacteria and particulates begins within minutes after inoculation into the peritoneal cavity. Cephalad flow of intraperitoneal fluid carries matter to the diaphragmatic surface for absorption into the lymphatics. Contraction of the diaphragm and decreased intrathoracic pressure during respiratory inspiration promote fluid flow into the thoracic lymph where caudally directed flow is prevented by one-way valves. Lymphatic drainage of bacteria and their products (particularly endotoxins) into the bloodstream activates the inflammatory and immune responses resulting in the systemic manifestations of peritonitis. In addition to mechanical clearance, the peritoneal inoculum is further reduced by resident macrophages that adhere to and ingest bacteria.

Microbial invasion of the peritoneum generates a local inflammatory response, which includes hyperemia of the peritoneal vasculature, increased capillary permeability, and

Etiologies of Secondary Peritonitis

Inflammation
Intestine
Diverticulitis
Inflammatory bowel disease
Appendicitis

Other organs
Cholecystitis
Pancreatitis
Salpingitis
Puerperal sepsis

Perforations
Neoplasms
Foreign body
Peptic ulcer
Tears
Strangulation
Adhesions
Hernia
Volvulus
Intussusception
Closed-loop obstruction of colon

Trauma
Blunt rupture of viscus
Penetrating injury
Iatrogenic
Biopsy
Endoscopy
Leaking anastomosis
Catheter perforation

Vascular
Embolus
Mesenteric ischemia
Portal or mesenteric venous thrombosis

Modified from Wilson SE: Secondary bacterial peritonitis. In Wilson SE, Finegold SM, Williams RA, editors: *Intra-abdominal infection,* New York, 1982, McGraw-Hill; and Ellis H: Acute secondary peritonitis. In Schwartz SI, Ellis H, editors: *Maingot's Abdominal Operations,* Norwalk, Conn, 1989, Appleton & Lange, pp 2, 9.

exudation of fluid from the intravascular to the peritoneal space. The details of the peritoneal inflammatory response are not well understood at this time, but are believed to be similar to induced inflammation in experimental animals.[8] The fluid exudate includes activated complement components that opsonize bacteria and attract neutrophils. Within 2 to 4 hours neutrophils replace macrophages as the predominant phagocytic cell line. Activated macrophages also release cytokines, including tumor necrosis factor (TNF), interleukins, and macrophage-colony stimulating factor (M-CSF). These cytokines further mediate the inflammatory response. The exudative fluid is rich in fibrinogen, which becomes converted to fibrin by tissue thromboplastins and procoagulant cytokines. Fibrin deposition sequesters bacteria and adheres to bowel loops and omentum, effectively walling off the offending organism.

Paradoxically, the local defensive responses to peritoneal bacterial invasion may adversely affect the host. Systemic absorption of bacteria from the lymphatics results in bacteremia and may cause sepsis. Massive fluid shifts from the intravascular space to the peritoneal cavity cause intravascular volume depletion which, if severe enough, may lead to hypovolemic shock. Intraperitoneal fluid dilutes opsonins and phagocytic cells. Fibrinous adhesions limit access of host defense mechanisms and exogenously administered antibiotics to bacteria, and form bases for abscesses and permanent fibrous adhesions.

The systemic response to peritonitis can be divided into two phases: the neuroendocrine phase typical in any traumatic insult, with release of catecholamines, adrenocortical hormones, aldosterone, and antidiuretic hormone; and the septic phase.

The fluid shifts in peritonitis may be massive—up to 4 liters in 24 hours. Severe intravascular volume depletion or inadequate compensatory responses may result in hypovolemic shock. The depletion of circulating volume triggers release of catecholamines, stimulates the renin-angiotensin-aldosterone system, and promotes the release of antidiuretic hormone. Vasosconstriction preserves mean arterial pressure and shunts blood from the renal and mesenteric beds to sustain perfusion of more vital organ systems. Aldosterone and antidiuretic hormone promote retention of sodium and water by the kidneys. During this phase, the hemodynamic manifestations of hypovolemia prevail, with a reduced cardiac output and increased systemic vascular resistance.

If the bacterial inoculum is large, and fluid resuscitation restores circulating volume, the septic phase emerges. The hemodynamic pattern of early sepsis includes an increased cardiac output and decreased systemic vascular resistance. Systemic activation of the immune and inflammatory responses results in circulating mediators that influence vascular tone, capillary permeability, and cellular metabolism. An ongoing septic pattern in patients who have been appropriately treated with surgery and antibiotics may indicate progression to tertiary peritonitis.

Systemic responses to peritonitis place certain organ systems at particular risk for dysfunction. Hypovolemia results in decreased renal perfusion and the potential for prerenal failure. Sepsis may precipitate acute lung injury and acute respiratory distress syndrome (ARDS) and further renal damage. Sepsis, with ongoing stimulation of the inflammatory and immune responses, is the most common cause of MODS.

Patients are also at risk for a later complication of peritonitis, the development of intra-abdominal abscesses, which are collections of pus walled off by fibrinous adhesions, omentum, loops of bowel and mesentery, or other abdominal organs. Untreated abscesses may act as sources for ongoing sepsis.

The microbiology of peritonitis varies with the type. Spontaneous bacterial peritonitis in cirrhotic patients frequently is caused by a single enteric organism, usually *Escherichia* or *Streptococcus* species.[4] Secondary peritonitis and abscesses are polymicrobial with aerobic and anaerobic bacteria acting synergistically. Cultures generally yield facultative Gram-negative bacilli, particularly *E. coli* and obligate anaerobes, especially *Bacteroides fragilis*.[1] Bacterial virulence is also enhanced by the presence of adjuvants such as hemoglobin, fecal matter, gastric secretions, and necrotic tissue. Bacterial cultures from patients developing tertiary peritonitis often yield *Staphylococcus epidermidis, Pseudomonas* species, and *Candida* species, microbes historically considered to be innocuous. These bacteria may colonize the GI tract and translocate due to altered barrier function or impaired host immunity.[7]

Pain is the hallmark symptom of secondary peritonitis and is characterized by visceral and somatic components. Visceral pain is mediated through the autonomic nervous system; arises from inflamed, distended, or injured abdominal organs; and is crampy, poorly localized, and associated with nausea and vomiting. The somatic component of abdominal pain is due to irritation of the parietal peritoneum and is mediated through somatic nerve fibers. Somatic pain is sharper and localizes to the area of inflammation. The somatic pain of peritonitis is associated with the signs of rebound tenderness and abdominal rigidity from reflex abdominal muscle spasm. The onset of pain in peritonitis may be acute or gradual and generally is described as severe and constant. Because movement aggravates the pain, the patient will often lie still with the knees and hips flexed to reduce tension on the abdominal wall.

Because of the reliance on clinical signs and symptoms, diagnosis of secondary peritonitis may be difficult in patients with diminished levels of responsiveness or masking of pain by analgesics. Delayed diagnosis often occurs in postoperative abdominal surgical patients who normally may be expected to have many of the signs and symptoms of peritonitis.

LENGTH OF STAY / ANTICIPATED COURSE

The length of stay and patient outcome vary markedly depending on the etiology of peritonitis, patient immune status and general health at onset, and timeliness of diagnosis and intervention. At the present time, it is difficult to compare outcomes from different treatment strategies because there are no widely accepted definitions of peritonitis or methods for patient stratification based on severity of illness.[5] Peritonitis falls within DRG 188: Other digestive diseases with complications; or DRG 189: Other digestive diseases without complications. The average length of stay is 6.8 days and 3.7 days, respectively.[9]

With appropriate therapy, full recovery without residual dysfunction may be expected. One complication may be the formation of permanent fibrous adhesions that later result in intestinal obstruction. Delayed therapy or peritonitis in an already compromised host may result in prolonged hospitalization, and organ failure with associated high mortality.

MANAGEMENT TRENDS AND CONTROVERSIES

The medical management of secondary peritonitis is directed at rapid restoration of circulating volume with crystalloid solution, antimicrobial therapy, and early surgical intervention. Initial antimicrobial therapy for community-acquired intra-abdominal infection consists of single-agent or combination therapy directed against facultative Gram-negative bacilli and obligate anaerobes. Intraoperative culture and Gram stain of peritoneal fluid are used to guide subsequent adjustments in antimicrobial therapy. Antifungal therapy generally is not required unless the host is immunocompromised or the peritonitis persists or recurs.[1]

The guiding principles of surgical intervention for peritonitis are: (1) identify and eliminate the infectious focus, (2) reduce bacterial and adjuvant contamination of the peritoneal cavity, and (3) prevent recurrent or ongoing sepsis.

In diffuse peritonitis the surgical approach is usually a vertical midline incision. For localized peritonitis of known etiology (e.g., appendicitis) the surgical approach may be directly over the site of inflammation. Elimination of the infectious focus is achieved by closing, excluding, or resecting the diseased viscus. Gentle debridement of loculations in the cavitary margins, aspiration of grossly purulent exudate, and saline lavage of the peritoneal cavity reduce the bacterial inoculum and remove adjuvants such as blood, feces, and necrotic tissue. Drains are placed if a well-defined abscess cavity is identified intraoperatively. Delayed closure of the skin and subcutaneous tissues may be done to avoid wound infection in heavily contaminated cases. Proposed methods to prevent recurrent or persistent infection include continuous postoperative lavage, planned relaparatomy, and laparostomy (abdomen left open). None of these methods is of proven benefit in rigorously conducted studies.[3]

Intra-abdominal abscesses are managed by ultrasound- or CT-guided percutaneous drainage, or surgical drainage. Antibiotic therapy is adjusted based on culture results, and other supportive measures are provided as indicated by patient condition.

Tertiary peritonitis responds poorly to the classical therapies of surgery and antibiotics, and at this time the best treatment is prevention by aggressive intervention for secondary peritonitis. Based on the postulated role of the gut as a source of ongoing bacteria and toxins, suggested therapies for tertiary peritonitis include nutritional measures to promote gut mucosal barrier function, or selective decontamination of the gut.[6,8]

ASSESSMENT

PARAMETER	ANTICIPATED ALTERATION
Abdomen	
Inspection	Abdominal distension *due to ileus and increased peritoneal fluid*
Auscultation	Diminished or absent bowel sounds
Percussion	Hyperresonance *due to gas-filled bowel loops*
Palpation	Abdominal tenderness, diffuse or localized Rebound tenderness Voluntary guarding initially progressing to rigidity *due to reflex muscle spasm*
X-ray	Gas-filled bowel loops, air-fluid levels *due to ileus* Free air under the diaphragm on upright film *due to duodenal perforation* (less frequent with other types of perforation)
Ultrasound/CT	Increased volume of peritoneal fluid Abscess(es) Other lesion-specific changes depending on cause of peritonitis
Pulmonary Status	
Respirations	Rapid and shallow *due to pain and abdominal distension*
ABG	Hypoxemia and metabolic acidosis *if stimulation of immune and inflammatory responses have resulted in acute lung injury and anaerobic metabolism with lactic acid production*
Chest x-ray	Elevated hemidiaphragm Effusion *if subphrenic abscess develops* Other findings consistent with ARDS *if acute lung injury occurs*
Cardiovascular Status	
HR	Tachycardia >100 bpm *due to pain and hypovolemia*
MAP	Decreased: <70 mm Hg *due to hypovolemia*
CO/CI	Initially normal: 4.0 to 7.0 L/min; 2.5 to 4.0 L/min or decreased: 4.0 L/min; 2.5 L/min *due to hypovolemia* Increased in early phase of sepsis Decreased in later phases of sepsis *due to myocardial depression by circulating cytokines*
SVR	Initially increased: >1200 dynes/sec/cm^{-5} *due to catecholamine response to hypovolemia* Subsequently may be decreased: <800 dynes/sec/cm^{-5} *due to sepsis*
Neurologic Status	
LOC	Initially alert, restless *due to pain* Subsequently may become confused with a diminished LOC *due to hypoxemia, hypovolemia, or metabolic changes associated with sepsis*
Hct	WNL or may be increased: >47% to 52% *due to dehydration*
WBC with differential	Increased: >10,000/mm^3 with shift to the left in an immunocompetent host
Peritoneal fluid	Cloudy Fecal matter, bile, blood *if peritonitis due to perforation of the GI tract* >500 cells/mm^3 following a 1-liter saline peritoneal lavage[7] Positive Gram stain and cultures

PLAN OF CARE

INTENSIVE PHASE

Care of the patient in the intensive phase is focused on reestablishing intravascular fluid volume, treating pain, and managing complications related to the local and systemic effects of peritoneal inflammation. Rapid assessment and diagnosis of peritonitis is important to ensure early surgical intervention as appropriate.

PATIENT CARE PRIORITIES	EXPECTED PATIENT OUTCOMES
Decreased intravascular fluid volume *r/t* *Fluid shift in peritoneal space* *Vomiting* *Decreased oral intake* *NG suction*	Intravascular volume deficit sufficient to maintain tissue perfusion Hemodynamic parameters: WNL
Ineffective breathing pattern *r/t* *Abdominal pain and splinting* *Abdominal distension*	ABG within patient norms Lungs clear to auscultation Ventilation pattern normal Spo_2 >92%
Pain *r/t* *Inflammation and abdominal distension* *Laparotomy incision*	Pain relief
Inadequate nutrition *r/t* *Increased caloric requirements* *Ileus* *Prolonged NPO status*	Maintain lean body weight Intake of adequate kilocalories, minerals, vitamins to meet metabolic and tissue repair needs Positive nitrogen balance
Altered bowel elimination *r/t ileus*	Restoration of peristalsis and appropriate elimination pattern
High risk for metabolic acidosis *r/t anaerobic metabolism with lactic acid production*	pH: WNL
High risk for ongoing systemic infection *r/t* *Impaired immune response* *Abscess formation*	Infection prevented Body temperature: WNL Negative cultures
High risk for wound infection *r/t* *Contaminated surgical procedure* *Impaired immune response* *Decreased nutrition*	Wound healing without purulent drainage, dehiscence
High risk for multiple organ dysfunction syndrome (MODS) *r/t* *Hypovolemia* *Systemic inflammatory and immune response stimulation*	Organ function: WNL Prompt recognition of and intervention for organ dysfunction

INTERVENTIONS

Replace intravascular volume *to maintain perfusion to tissues.*

Monitor response to fluid resuscitation: hemodynamic parameters, body weight, intake and output.

Position with head of bed elevated *to promote lung expansion, relieve pressure from distended abdomen, and reduce abdominal pain.*

Coach frequent deep breathing *to promote lung expansion and mobilization of secretions.*

Assist patient to chair sitting when hemodynamically stable *to prevent pulmonary and other complications of immobility and deconditioning.*

Plan of Care (cont'd)

Administer analgesics and sedatives and evaluate patient response.

Collaborate in planning alternative routes, agents, or therapies *for pain management as needed.*

Provide nutrition as prescribed. Parenteral nutrition may be the best means for patients with surgery to the GI tract, but early enteral nutrition *promotes return of peristalsis, may assist in maintaining gut mucosal barrier function, and is less expensive.*

Insert NG tube and apply and maintain suction *to drain and decompress the upper GI tract.*

Avoid excessive use of neuromuscular blocking agents, *to promote return of peristalsis.*

Administer antimicrobial agents at prescribed intervals *to maintain serum, intraperitoneal, and tissue levels.*

Maintain asepsis in wound and drain management.

Monitor and report signs and symptoms of ongoing infection—elevated body temperature, leukocytosis, purulent drainage, ongoing abdominal pain, reddened or poorly healing surgical wound.

INTERMEDIATE PHASE

The intermediate phase of care of patients surviving the acute, critically ill phase of peritonitis will focus on recovery of normal GI function, nutritional support, and reversal of deconditioning. Patients with surgical incisions will require appropriate wound management, which will be more complex for patients with wounds that are to heal by granulation or with multiple abscess drains. Patients suffering additional organ failure as a result of peritonitis also will require care specific to recovery of function of the involved organs.

PATIENT CARE PRIORITIES	EXPECTED PATIENT OUTCOMES
GI dysfunction *r/t* *Abdominal surgery* *Narcotics and sedatives* *Prolonged period without enteral nutrition* *Immobility*	Normal bowel motility and elimination
Inadequate nutrition *r/t catabolic state*	Maintain lean body weight Positive nitrogen balance
Activity intolerance *r/t deconditioning*	Able to perform self-care and ambulation (level of independence varies with premorbid functional status)
High risk for wound infection *r/t* *Decreased nutrition* *Dirty surgical procedure* *Wound electively left open to heal by granulation*	Wound heals without signs and symptoms of infection

INTERVENTIONS

Promote enteral nutrition as soon as possible *to reduce gut atrophy.*

Avoid excessive use of narcotics or sedatives *to promote/maintain normal gut motility.*

Collaborate with physical therapy *to develop a schedule of progressive increase in activity and self-care.*

Maintain asepsis in all wound and drain management.

Monitor for signs and symptoms of wound infection: fever, purulent drainage, redness, swelling, tenderness of incision.

TRANSITION TO DISCHARGE

The focus of care in this phase will be to provide nutrition and promote increased activity and self-care. Patients with incompletely healed surgical wounds will require teaching for management of the dressing changes and signs of infection to report. Oral analgesics should be adequate to meet comfort needs. Patients who do not develop organ dysfunction from severe intra-abdominal sepsis should recover without complications. Patients who develop organ failure secondary to peritonitis may have some residual effects depending on the system involved and the severity of the insult.

REFERENCES

1. Bohnen JMA, et al: Guidelines for clinical care: anti-infective agents for intra-abdominal infection, *Arch Surg* 127:83-89, 1992.
2. Ellis H: Acute secondary peritonitis. In Schwartz SI, Ellis H, editors: *Maingot's abdominal operations,* Norwalk, Conn, 1989, Appleton & Lange, pp 341-351.
3. Farthmann EH, Schoffel U: Principles and limitations of operative management of intra-abdominal infections, *World J Surg* 14:210-217, 1990.
4. Hallak A: Spontaneous bacterial peritonitis, *Am J Gastroenterol* 84:345-350, 1989.
5. Nystrom PO, et al: Proposed definitions for diagnosis, severity scoring, stratification, and outcome for trials on intra-abdominal infection, *World J Surg* 14:148-158, 1990.
6. Poole GV, Muakkassa FF, Griswold JA: Pneumonia, selective decontamination, and multiple organ failure, *Surgery* 111:1-3, 1992.
7. Rotstein OD, Meakins JL: Diagnostic and therapeutic challenges of intra-abdominal infections, *World J Surg* 14:159-166, 1990.
8. Rotstein OD, Simmons RL: Intra-abdominal infection. In Abrams JH, Cerra FB, editors: *Essentials of surgical critical care,* St. Louis, 1993, Quality Medical Publishing, pp 419-426.
9. *St Anthony's DRG guidebook 1995,* Reston, Va, 1994, St Anthony.

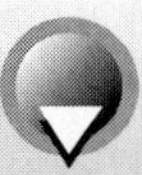

CLINICAL GUIDELINE

43

Acute Pancreatitis

Joanne M. Krumberger, MSN, RN, CCRN

DESCRIPTION

Acute pancreatitis is characterized by a process in which there is premature activation of pancreatic enzymes normally produced by the pancreas. This disease can be mild in presentation or can develop into a fulminant form. In the mild form, or edematous pancreatitis, edema of glandular and interstitial tissue predominates. The fulminant form is characterized by generalized pancreatic necrosis with disruption of vessels in and around the pancreas. Necrotic pancreatic tissue may also initiate an inflammatory response process that extends beyond the pancreas. This can lead to the release of substrates into the circulation, which can trigger systemic complications.

The incidence of acute pancreatitis in the United States ranges from 54 to 238 instances per million population per year.[11] In 5% to 15% of patients, the disease takes on a fulminant course, and 20% to 60% of these patients die or face potentially lethal complications.[3] Overall mortality rates are reported between 10% and 20%.[26] They are most commonly a result of multisystem complications.

PATHOPHYSIOLOGY

Acute pancreatitis is characterized by premature activation of pancreatic enzymes. The pancreatic enzymes trypsin, chymotrypsin, elastase, and carboxypeptidase are secreted into the duodenum as part of the endocrine function of this gland. These enzymes are essential to the digestion of proteins, fats, and carbohydrates. The pancreas normally has protective mechanisms to prevent these enzymes from autodigesting pancreatic cells. The same cells that secrete proteolytic enzymes into the acini of the pancreas also secrete a substance known as trypsin inhibitor. Normally, trypsin inhibitor prevents activation of trypsin as well as other digesting enzymes within the pancreas itself. Once in the duodenum, the pancreatic enzymes are activated by the enzyme enterokinase, which causes a cycle of local inflammation and, potentially, necrosis.

Although the exact mechanism of acute pancreatitis is unknown, etiologic factors have been identified and theories developed to explain how activation of pancreatic enzymes occurs. Etiologies of acute pancreatitis are reviewed in Table 43-1. Mechanical factors cause obstruction or damage to the pancreatic duct system, leading to pancreatic injury. Metabolic factors affect the secretory functions of the pancreatic cell. Miscellaneous factors include ischemic injury to the pancreas and infections.[4,14,15,25] Pancreatitis is also associated with certain drugs and with abdominal trauma, and may follow endoscopic retrograde angiography (ERCP).

Gallstone disease and alcoholism account for 70% to 80% of instances of acute pancreatitis.[5] Gallstone pancreatitis is thought to be caused by a transient obstruction of the ampulla of Vater by a migrating stone. Alcohol is known to increase stimulation of pancreatic enzymes and may also cause obstruction of acinar ductules and trap pancreatic enzymes within the pancreas.

Clinical manifestations of acute pancreatitis are listed in Table 43-2. The only universal sign for acute pancreatitis is severe abdominal pain. This pain is believed to be due to edema and distention of the pancreatic capsule, to obstruction of the biliary tree, or to a chemical burn of the peritoneum by pancreatic enzymes.[10] Vomiting is frequently present and usually does not relieve the pain. Other gastrointestinal findings are variable and mimic other diseases. In severe pancreatitis, the patient may exhibit signs of hypovolemic shock due to sequestration of fluids within the peri-

TABLE 43-1 Precipitating Events for Acute Pancreatitis

Mechanical

Biliary tract disease
Cholelithiasis
Pancreatic cancer
Duodenal disease
Pancreatic duct obstruction
Following trauma (abdominal)
Pregnancy
Radiation
Retrograde pancreatography

Metabolic

Alcoholism
Hypercalcemia
Hyperlipoproteinemia
Diabetic ketoacidosis
Hyperparathyroidism
Drugs (acetaminophen, furosemide, opiates, salicylates, steroids)

Miscellaneous

Hepatitis B
Mumps
Campylobacter
Atheroembolism
Low-flow states (shock)
Following transplantation

toneum.[3,15] Hemorrhagic pancreatitis may cause bleeding into the peritoneum and associated clinical signs. A bluish discoloration of the flanks (Grey Turner's sign) or around the umbilical area (Cullen's sign) indicates this condition.[6,18] Because the signs and symptoms of acute pancreatitis are nonspecific, accurate diagnosis requires laboratory and radiographic confirmation.

Complications of acute pancreatitis include almost every organ system and impact significantly on the morbidity and mortality of this disease.[13,17,26] These complications are thought to result from the inflammation of the pancreas, leading to generalized pancreatic necrosis. The substrates released from this process, as well as the activated pancreatic enzymes, can trigger systemic complications.

Sixty percent of deaths are associated with pulmonary complications, including hypoxemia, atelectasis, and acute respiratory distress syndrome.[3,7] Cardiovascular effects are also common and can include hypotension, decreased cardiac output, and increased systemic vascular resistance. Pancreatic ischemia causes the release of a substance called *myocardial depressant factor,* which is thought to be responsible for impairment of cardiovascular function.[9]

Hypocalcemia is a common metabolic complication and is associated with the fulminant form of acute pancreatitis.[8]

TABLE 43-2 Clinical Manifestations of Acute Pancreatitis

- Pain
- Vomiting
- Nausea
- Fever
- Abdominal distention
- Abdominal guarding
- Abdominal tympany
- Hypoactive/absent bowel sounds
- Severe disease
  - Signs of hypovolemic shock
  - Rebound tenderness
  - Ascites
  - Jaundice
  - Palpable abdominal mass
  - Grey Turner's sign
  - Cullen's sign

Septic complications include a wide range of conditions, such as pancreatic abscess, infected pancreatic necrosis, and infected pseudocyst. Bacterial translocation of host gastrointestinal bacteria with episodes of hypotension and bowel hypoperfusion have been implicated as the etiology of sepsis syndrome in this patient population.[24] Coagulation problems have also been documented.[19] Elevated levels of fibrinogen and factor VIII contribute to the development of a hypercoagulable state.

LENGTH OF STAY/ANTICIPATED COURSE

The length of stay for patients with acute pancreatitis depends on the type of pancreatitis the patient develops (edematous interstitial pancreatitis or necrotizing fulminant acute pancreatitis) and the development of systemic complications as a result of enzyme activation. Determining the severity of acute pancreatitis is important to differentiate between mild and severe disease.[1]

Ranson's prognostic signs are the most widely used indicators in the United States to predict the severity of disease and associated mortality. These signs are listed in the following Box. Patients with less than three signs within 48 hours of admission had a 1% mortality rate, patients with three to four signs had a 16% mortality rate, patients with five to six signs had a 40% mortality rate, and patients with more than six signs had a 100% mortality rate.[22] The acute physiologic and chronic health evaluation (APACHE II) and the multiple organ system failure (MOSF) scores have also been used in evaluating the severity of acute pancreatitis.[28] Serum markers to distinguish necrotizing pancreatitis from interstitial acute pancreatitis have not been reliable.[1]

Acute pancreatitis falls within DRG 204: Disorders of

Ranson's Prognostic Signs[22]

At diagnosis

Age >55 years
WBC count >16,000/mm^3
Blood glucose >200 mg/dl
LDH >350 IU/L
SGOT >250 IU/L

During initial 48 hours

Hct decrease >10%
Serum Ca^{++} level <8 mg/dl
BUN rise >5 g/dl
Base deficit >4 mEq
Estimated fluid sequestration >6000 ml

Compiled from Ranson JH: Risk factors in acute pancreatitis, *Hosp Pract* 20:69-73, 1985.

pancreas except malignancy. The average length of stay is 7.3 days.[27]

MANAGEMENT TRENDS AND CONTROVERSIES

There are no known therapies or medications that are curative for acute pancreatitis. Initial treatment is directed at hemodynamic stabilization, supportive interventions, and therapies to decrease pancreatic secretion.

Fluid stabilization is an initial priority in all forms of acute pancreatitis. Hypovolemia and shock are major causes of death early in the disease. Colloids and Ringer's lactate are the most commonly ordered fluids. Higher doses of fresh-frozen plasma have theoretical support because they replenish plasma fibronectin, which, when diminished, is associated with the severe form of acute pancreatitis.[19] Intravenous albumin may be administered to restore fluid balance in the intravascular compartment.

Electrolyte replacement is also important. Hypocalcemia is the most common imbalance seen in acute pancreatitis and is associated with severe disease. The pathogenesis is unclear. The formation of calcium soaps in areas of pancreatic and parapancreatic fat necrosis may cause a sequestration of calcium, leading to hypocalcemia.[8] Because one half of calcium is bound to albumin, total calcium may be falsely lowered. Values of ionized calcium rather than total calcium should be measured, or the total calcium should be corrected for hypoalbuminemia.

Patients who remain hypotensive after fluid and electrolyte replacement may require cardiac support drugs to reverse the effects of myocardial depressant factor released from ischemic pancreatic cells. Dopamine in low to moderate dose ranges (2 to 19 μg/kg/min) is thought to be the drug of choice because it supports myocardial contractility and may decrease pancreatic inflammation by decreasing pancreatic microvascular permeability through stimulation of β-adrenergic receptors.[12]

Supplemental oxygen is almost always necessary to maintain an adequate PaO_2 in these patients. The exact mechanism to explain this phenomenon of impaired gas exchange is unclear, but is thought to be related to the activation of trypsin and its action on pulmonary vasculature. Other associated complications may include pleural effusion or atelectasis. Ventilatory support may be required with severe disease.

Pain control is a high priority in the management of this patient population. Non–opiate-containing analgesics have been recommended because they do not cause spasm of the sphincter of Oddi, which is thought to be a cause of pain. Recent clinical trials, however, have found morphine to be a very effective pain reliever with minimal effects on the sphincter.[11] Assisting the patient into a position where the knees and hips are flexed also may promote comfort.

Aggressive nutritional support is essential to support anabolic processes and to promote restoration of damaged pancreatic tissue. Total parenteral nutrition has been recommended as the therapy of choice.[14] The use of lipid emulsions is controversial because it is thought to increase pancreatic exocrine secretion. Enteral feedings are generally not recommended because they stimulate enzyme secretion as well. In severe cases of acute pancreatitis, patients are generally kept NPO and an NG tube may be placed if there is an associated ileus or vomiting.

Peritoneal lavage has been used for the treatment of systemic complications, although the benefits of this therapy are controversial. The goal is to remove the vasoactive substances (trypsinogen, kinins, phospholipase A, and prostaglandins) released by the damaged pancreas into the peritoneal fluid before they can trigger systemic complications. Peritoneal lavage for greater than 7 days has been found to decrease the incidence of complications and mortality.[23]

The type and timing of surgical intervention in acute pancreatitis is controversial.[2,21,29] Surgical therapy may be performed to modify the early course of the disease or to treat specific complications such as pancreatic abscess or pseudocyst. Surgical therapies include pancreatic drainage, pancreatic resection, and biliary procedures.

ASSESSMENT

PARAMETER	ANTICIPATED ALTERATION
Pain	Severe, unrelenting upper abdominal pain *due to edema and distension of the pancreatic capsule, a chemical burn of the peritoneum by enzymes, or obstruction of the duodenum or biliary tree*

	LUQ pain *due to a lesion in the tail of the pancreas* RUQ pain *due to a lesion in the head or body of the pancreas*
GI Status	
Grey Turner's sign	Bluish discoloration of the flanks *due to blood in the retroperitoneum*
Cullen's sign	Bluish discoloration around umbilicus *due to blood dissecting beneath the anterior abdominal muscles*
Vomiting	Usually protracted
Bowel sounds	Hypoactive *due to the effects of enzyme-induced inflammation on the bowel*
Abdomen	Rigidity and rebound tenderness *due to peritoneal inflammation by activated enzymes*
Cardiovascular Status	
HR	Tachycardia: >100 bpm
MAP	Decreased: <70 mm Hg
PCWP	Decreased: <8 mm Hg Tachycardia, hypotension, and decreased preload *due to loss of intraperitoneal fluid and diminished ventricular filling*
CI	Decreased: <2.5 L/min/m^2 *due to release of myocardial depressant factor from ischemic pancreatic cells*
SVR	Increased: >1200 dynes/sec/cm^{-5} *due to vasoconstriction associated with hypovolemia*
Serum Pancreatic Enzymes	
Amylase	Increased: >250 Somogyi units *due to activation of pancreatic proteoloytic enzymes and inflammation (with inflammation, amylase enters the bloodstream at an increased level)* Serum amylase begins to rise in 3 to 6 hr Rises to >250 SU within 8 hours in 75% of patients Peaks in 20 to 30 hr *The height of the increase and rate of fall do not correlate with the severity of the disease, prognosis, or rate of resolution; an increase >7 to 10 days is associated with intrapancreatic complications such as pseudocyst or ascites*[16,20]
Lipase	Increased: >110 units/L *due to activation of pancreatic proteoloytic enzymes*
Serum Tests	
Ca^{++}	Decreased: <2 mg/dl *due to sequestration of calcium in areas of parapancreatic fat necrosis associated with severe disease*[8]
Total bilirubin	Increased: >1.0 mg/dl *due to biliary tract obstruction*
WBC count	Elevated: >10,000/mm^3 *due to the body's natural stress response or early sign of infection*
Glucose	Elevated: >200 mg/dl *due to the stress response or β cell damage in the pancreas*
Albumin	Decreased: <3.2 g/dl *due to extravasation of protein-rich fluids into the extracellular space*
AST/ALT	Elevated *when pancreatitis is due to alcohol or with obstructions of the biliary tree*
Hgb/Hct	May be decreased with hemorrhagic acute pancreatitis *due to bleeding in and around the pancreas*
K^+	Decreased: <3.6 mEq/L *due to loss of electrolytes with vomiting*

ABG	Arterial Pao_2 decreased: <60 mm Hg *due to injury of the lung vasculature by circulating pancreatic enzymes*
Radiographic Studies	
CT	Pancreatic enlargement, cystic lesions in the pancreas, pancreatic abscess, fluid collection *due to intrapancreatic complications associated with inflammation*
Ultrasonography	Pancreatic enlargement, distention of the common bile duct, pancreatic mass, or pancreatic pseudocyst *due to intrapancreatic complications associated with inflammation*
Other	
Endoscopic retrograde cholangiography	Abnormalities of the pancreatic duct or biliary tract or presence of biliary stones *due to gallstone pancreatitis (usually not performed in the acute inflammation stage; may exacerbate inflammation)*

PLAN OF CARE

INTENSIVE PHASE

Nursing care of the patient in the intensive phase is directed at restoring fluid volume and halting the stimulation of pancreatic enzymes. Because fulminant acute pancreatitis can potentially affect all body systems, patients are at risk for multisystem organ dysfunction. Therefore, support of all body systems is a priority until the cycle of enzyme stimulation and pancreatic inflammation is reversed.

PATIENT CARE PRIORITIES	EXPECTED PATIENT OUTCOMES
Fluid volume deficit *r/t* *Fluid sequestrations in abdominal cavity* *Vomiting* *Pancreatic vascular disruption by inflammatory process*	MAP: WNL PCWP: WNL CVP: WNL Urine output: WNL Stable Hct/Hgb
Pain *r/t* *Interruption of blood supply to pancreas* *Pancreatic edema or distension* *Peritoneal irritation by activated pancreatic enzymes*	Verbalize pain relief after analgesia (using pain rating scale)
Impaired nutrition *r/t* *Prolonged NPO status and hypomotility of intestine* *Nausea and vomiting* *Impaired nutrient metabolism* *Altered production of digestive exocrine enzymes* *Alcoholism*	Positive nitrogen balance Serum albumin: WNL Total protein: WNL
Impaired gas exchange *r/t* *Pulmonary complications of pancreatic inflammation and mediated responses* *Fluid overload during intravascular rehydration* *Atelectasis from diaphragmatic splinting due to pain*	Pao_2: WNL Sao_2: >90% RR within patient norms Absence of effusions, areas of consolidation, ARDS on chest x-ray
Ineffective breathing pattern *r/t* *Hypoxemia* *Pain* *Ascites* *ARDS* *Pleural effusion* *Microemboli*	RR within patient norms $Paco_2$: WNL No use of accessory muscles

Plan of Care (cont'd)

Electrolyte imbalance *r/t* *Vomiting* *Parapancreatic inflammation* *Fluid sequestration* *Fatty acids combined with calcium* *NG suction*	Ca^{++}: WNL K^{+}: WNL
Decreased CO *r/t* *Release of pancreatic myocardial depressant factor* *Decreased preload*	CI: WNL
High risk for infection *r/t* *Compromised defense mechanisms* *Peritonitis, inflammation, pancreatic pseudocyst, and infection caused by leakage of pancreatic enzymes into peritoneum*	WBC: WNL Absence of fever Resolving abdominal pain, rigidity, abdominal mass

INTERVENTIONS

Collaborate with physicians to restore fluid volume with colloids, crystalloids, or blood products as appropriate. *There is theoretical support for the use of fresh-frozen plasma because it contains components of the plasma antiprotease system and replenished plasma fibronectin, which is depleted in acute pancreatitis. PRBCs may be required with vascular interruption of the pancreas.*[20]

Monitor for signs and symptoms of fluid volume deficit and outcomes of fluid replacement therapy, including BP, pulse, intake and output, preload indicators, skin turgor, capillary refill, mucous membranes, and urine output. *BP and pulse are the most sensitive noninvasive clinical signs of volume status. PCWP is the most sensitive measure of the adequacy of volume status and left ventricular filling pressure.*

Monitor Hct, Hgb, Cullen's sign, and Grey Turner's sign *because decreasing blood counts and these signs indicate internal bleeding and hemorrhagic pancreatitis.*

Measure for increasing abdominal girth q4h.

Administer blood products as ordered.

Perform respiratory assessment and correlate with ABG analysis, pulse oximetry, and chest x-ray results *for early detection of impaired gas exchange associated with acute pancreatic inflammation.*

Monitor Spo_2 and assist the patient in coughing, deep breathing, and secretion removal *to maximize ventilation and perfusion matching.*

Position patient with good lung down *to facilitate oxygenation.*

Administer oxygen therapy. If hypoxemia persists, consult physician for possible mechanical assistance or ventilation.

If microemboli are suspected, monitor results of coagulation studies.

Perform peritoneal lavage *to clear activated mediators and enzymes from the peritoneal cavity.*

Monitor serum amylase and lipase levels.

Monitor serial blood glucose levels.

Perform a comprehensive assessment of pain using a pain rating scale *to evaluate level of pain and effects of analgesics.*

Administer pain medications *to provide optimal pain relief.*

Maintain NPO as long as patient reports abdominal pain *to decrease pancreatic exocrine secretion.*

Maintain bed rest *to decrease pancreatic exocrine secretion.*

Assist patient to most comfortable position. *Knee-to-chest position often decreases intensity of the pain.*

Evaluate use of physical measures to augment narcotic-induced pain relief such as progressive muscle relaxation, massage, and other measures *to increase patient comfort.*

Plan of Care (cont'd)

Assess patient anxiety *because it may heighten pain perception.*
Administer sedatives with analgesics.
Assess nutritional status through laboratory analysis of nitrogen balance, albumin, and total protein.
Monitor weight daily.
Administer total parenteral nutrition *because it allows for complete rest of the pancreas and, therefore, inhibits pancreatic exocrine secretion.*
Avoid lipid therapy *because hyperlipidemia is associated with severe pancreatitis.*
If enteral feedings are ordered, elemental tube feedings (such as Vivonex, Vital) should be administered into the jejunum (distal to the duodenum) *to prevent pancreatic exocrine secretion.*
Administer somatostatin as ordered *to decrease metabolism of pancreatic cells and production of enzymes.*
Administer supplemental insulin and/or enzymes preparations as ordered.
Monitor serum Ca^{++} and K^{+} and replace as necessary.
Monitor CO *because myocardial depressant factor released from ischemic pancreatic cells may cause decreased contractility.*
Promote optimum preload *to improve contractility while minimizing heart failure.*
Administer positive inotropic medications *to support myocardial contractility.*
Prevent infection by monitoring invasive line sites, and use aseptic techniques with all procedures.
Monitor for signs and symptoms of GI complications, including increasing abdominal pain, abdominal distention/rigidity, or abdominal mass.
Administer antibiotics as ordered *to prevent or combat secondary infection and secondary abscess formation.*
Prepare patient for surgical procedure as necessary.

INTERMEDIATE PHASE

Most patients with acute pancreatitis develop the mild self-limiting form and recover without formidable complications. Functional recovery of the pancreas after acute pancreatitis is not well studied. Some studies indicate that up to two thirds of patients show endocrine and exocrine functional loss after necrotizing pancreatitis.[2]

PATIENT CARE PRIORITIES	EXPECTED PATIENT OUTCOMES
Impaired nutrition *r/t prolonged stress state*	Weight return to baseline or ideal weight Positive nitrogen balance Albumin: WNL
Glucose imbalance *r/t effects of pancreatic inflammation on islet cells of pancreas.*	Glucose: WNL
Impaired gas exchange *r/t the effects of pancreatic enzymes on pulmonary vessels, prolonged immobility*	Pa_{O_2} returned to baseline

INTERVENTIONS

Continue maneuvers to promote optimal ventilation/perfusion matching.
Monitor serum amylase, lipase, and pain *to evaluate effect of NPO status.*
Monitor serial blood glucose levels.
Monitor for signs of hyperglycemia: polydipsia, polyuria, polyphagia, weakness.
Provide adequate nutritional intake.
Monitor weight daily.
Administer supplemental pancreatic enzyme preparations (pancreatin [Viokase], pancrealipsase [Cotasym]) and/or insulin as needed.
Monitor patterns of pain episodes to initiate pain management measures before pain becomes severe.

TRANSITION TO DISCHARGE

The focus of this phase is to prepare the patient for discharge. Some patients may be left with permanent damage to the pancreas. These patients will require medications to support glucose metabolism or pancreatic enzymes to maintain nutrient metabolism. The patient/family need sufficient information to comply with the discharge regimen as well as post-discharge medication and dietary regimens.

If diabetes is present, the patient/family will require teaching on how to control this disease. As appropriate, teaching about the hazards of continued alcohol intake may be required. A referral to Alcoholics Anonymous or community resources that can assist in making life-style changes necessary to prevent recurrence of acute pancreatitis may be recommended. Patients with biliary disease may need teaching regarding dietary modifications, including avoidance of spicy foods, heavy meals (eat smaller, more frequent meals), alcohol, tea, and coffee.

Rarely, patients develop chronic pancreatitis as a result of acute pancreatitis. Pain and malnutrition are major areas of concern. Teaching related to the analgesic medication regimen and comfort measures for management of pain episodes are nursing priorities.

REFERENCES

1. Banks PA: Predictors of severity in acute pancreatitis, *Pancreas* 6(1):S7-S12, 1991.
2. Beger HG: Surgical management of necrotizing pancreatitis, *Surg Clin North Am* 69:529-547, 1989.
3. Brown A: Acute pancreatitis, *Focus Crit Care* 18:121-130, 1991.
4. Carr-Locke DL: Acute gallstone pancreatitis and endoscopic therapy, *Endoscopy* 22:180-183, 1990.
5. Carter DC: Pancreatitis and the biliary tree: the continuing problem, *Am J Surg* 155:10-17, 1988.
6. Chung MA, Oung C, Szilagyi, A: Cullen's sign: it doesn't always mean hemorrhagic pancreatitis, *Am J Gastroenterol* 87(8):1026-1028, 1992.
7. Guice K, et al: Pancreatitis-induced acute lung injury, *Ann Surg* 7:71-77, 1988.
8. Hauser CJ: Calcium homeostasis in patients with acute pancreatitis, *Surgery* 94:830-835, 1983.
9. Horton JW, Burnweit CA: Hemodynamic function in acute pancreatitis, *Surgery* 103:538-546, 1988.
10. Jeffres C: Complications of acute pancreatitis, *Crit Care Nurse* 9:38-50, 1989.
11. Jones ML, Neoptolemos JP: Recent advances in the treatment of acute pancreatitis, *Surg Ann* 22:235-255, 1990.
12. Karanjia JD, et al: The anti-inflammatory effect of dopamine in alcoholic hemorrhagic pancreatitis in cats, *Gastroenterology* 101:1635-1641, 1991.
13. Krumberger JM: Acute pancreatitis, *Crit Care Clin North Am* 5(1):185-201, 1993.
14. Latifi R, McIntosh K, Dudrick S: Nutritional management of acute and chronic pancreatitis, *Surg Clin North Am* 71:579-595, 1991.
15. Loos F: Acute pancreatitis, *Can Crit Care Nurse J* 6:5-11, 1989.
16. Lott JA: The value of clinical laboratory studies in acute pancreatitis, *Arch Pathol Lab Med* 115:325-326, 1991.
17. McFadden DW: Organ failure and multiple organ system failure in pancreatitis, *Pancreas* 6(1):S37-S43, 1991.
18. Meyers MA, Feldberg M, Oliphant M: Grey Turner's signs and Cullen's signs in acute pancreatitis, *Gastrointest Radiol* 14:31-37, 1989.
19. Nhumoni CS, Agarwal J, Jain JK: Systemic complications of acute pancreatitis, *Am J Gastroenterol* 83:597-603, 1988.
20. Panteghini M, Pagani F: Clinical evaluation of an algorithm for the interpretation of hyperamylasemia, *Arch Pathol Lab Med* 115:355-358, 1991.
21. Poston G, Williamson R: Surgical management of acute pancreatitis, *J Surg* 77:5-11, 1990.
22. Ranson JH: Risk factors in acute pancreatitis, *Hosp Pract* 20:69-73, 1985.
23. Ranson JH: Long peritoneal lavage decreases pancreatic sepsis in acute pancreatitis, *Ann Surg* 211:708-715, 1990.
24. Runkel NS, et al: The role of the gut in the development of sepsis in acute pancreatitis, *J Surg Res* 51:18-23, 1991.
25. Singh M, Simsek H: Ethanol and the pancreas, *Gastroenterology* 98:1051-1062, 1990.
26. Sleisenger M, Fordtran J: *Gastrointestinal diseases,* ed 4, Philadelphia, 1989, WB Saunders.
27. *St Anthony's DRG Guidebook 1995,* Reston, Va, 1994, St Anthony.
28. Tran DD, Cuesta MA: Evaluation of severity in patients with acute pancreatitis, *Am J Gastroenterol* 87(5):604-608, 1992.
29. Widdison AL, Alvarez C, Reber HA: Surgical intervention in acute pancreatitis, *Pancreas* 6(1):S44-S51, 1991.

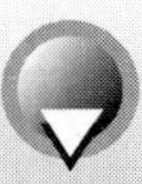

C L I N I C A L G U I D E L I N E

44

Pancreatic Surgery

Patricia J. Forg, BS, RN, CNN
Jacqueline Pearson, BA

DESCRIPTION

Pancreatic surgery carries a considerable risk of morbidity and mortality. Surgical complications are associated primarily with exocrine pancreatic secretions leaking from the remaining pancreatic remnant to the peripancreatic region and possibly into the abdominal cavity. Diabetes mellitus is another complication, which results from removal of the islet cells and loss of endocrine function. Surgery is performed for the treatment of adenocarcinomas, benign tumors of the pancreas, complications of pancreatitis (which include hemorrhagic pancreatitis unresponsive to pharmacologic suppression of enzyme excretions) abscess, pseudocyst, and pancreatic ascites, recurrent relapsing chronic pancreatitis, and trauma caused by motor vehicle accidents.

The major types of surgical procedures of the pancreas are (1) pancreatoduodenectomy, also known as the *Whipple procedure,* which is the standard operative procedure for treatment of resectable malignant tumors in the head of the pancreas,[1,13,15] tumors invading contiguous organs including adenocarcinomas, beta or alpha cell tumors, and cystadenocarcinomas; (2) the pylorus and duodenal bulb-preserving pancreatoduodenectomy (a modification of the Whipple procedure) as an alternative procedure for patients with localized noninvasive lesions;[15,21] (3) a simple resection of the involved pancreatic tissue for noninvasive islet cell tumors; and (4) debridement of devitalized pancreatic or peripancreatic tissue as a result of infection.[12]

Tumors of the head of the pancreas, pyloric antrum, duodenum, upper jejunum, distal portion of the common bile duct, and regional lymph nodes are removed with the pancreatoduodenectomy (Whipple) procedure. The remaining portion of the common bile duct is sutured to the end of the jejunal segment, and the remaining pancreas is anastomosed to the side of the jejunal loop (pancreaticojejunostomy).

Palliation of symptoms may be the only realistic goal of surgery.[18] If a Whipple operation is not possible, as the majority of pancreatic cancers are unresectable, then a palliative operative procedure is performed. The three areas of palliation include relief of biliary obstruction, relief of duodenal obstruction, and chemical splanchnicectomy. The standard palliative operation includes cholecystojejunostomy or choledochojejunostomy to divert bile from the gallbladder into the jejunum, gastroenterostomy, and a chemical splanchnicectomy for pain relief.[11]

The pylorus and duodenal bulb-preserving pancreatoduodenectomy is a modification of the Whipple procedure, with preservation of the stomach, pylorus, and proximal 1 to 2 cm of duodenum.[13,15] This procedure can mean less postgastrectomy complications such as delayed gastric emptying, dumping syndrome, diarrhea, and suboptimum nutrition, as well as gastrointestinal hemorrhage due to marginal ulcer that can result with the Whipple procedure. This procedure should be used with caution[15] as it is unproven as a curative procedure for cancer but remains an excellent therapeutic option for benign disease.

PATHOPHYSIOLOGY

The pancreas has two main functions. The exocrine function secretes pancreatic enzymes for the purpose of digestion and the endocrine function produces insulin and glucagon. Surgical removal of the pancreas results in the loss of exocrine function leading to severe impairment of digestion and absorption of nutrients. The loss of the endocrine function, and the loss of glucagon and islet cells that secrete insulin, results in uncontrolled blood sugars (diabetes) and therefore the possible need for exogenous insulin replacement.

Early detection of pancreatic carcinoma is practically impossible and is usually asymptomatic until advanced stages of the disease.[18] Pain, weight loss, and jaundice are characteristic symptoms. The absence of jaundice may indicate the tumor is occluding the common bile duct, or the presence of a primary tumor of the bile duct at the ampulla of Vater. The etiology is unknown but risk factors include age (usually over 50), male gender, cigarette smoking, history of chronic pancreatitis, diabetes mellitus, and exposure to some industrial carcinogens. A high-fat, high-protein diet also is noted to be an associated risk factor. It can affect either the head or tail of the pancreas or both. The carcinoma may spread and invade the surrounding structures—liver, biliary tract, and duodenum. Metastases are carried by lymphatic and blood circulation. Adenocarcinoma occurs in the head of the pancreas about 70% of the time.[2]

Acute pancreatitis is a diffuse inflammation of the pancreas most commonly caused by alcohol ingestion and biliary calculi causing ductal obstruction (see Guideline 43). Hemorrhagic pancreatitis, one complication of acute pancreatitis, causes tissue necrosis extending into the vasculature. Repeated attacks of acute inflammation can progress to a chronic stage called chronic pancreatitis which is most often caused by persistent alcohol ingestion.[5]

Pancreatic pseudocyst is a common complication of severe pancreatitis where extravasation of pancreatic juice, glandular necrotic debris, tissue, and blood encapsulates and forms a localized pocket of fluid. As the lesion enlarges to 5 cm or more, the pseudocyst may block pancreatic juice, thus interfering with digestion or compressing surrounding structures such as the portal vein or bile ducts. If these pockets remain infection-free, they usually resolve on their own. The accumulation of enzyme-rich drainage in the peritoneal cavity can become infected and lead to pancreatic abscess, the most serious complication. The pseudocysts can occasionally rupture and cause a generalized peritonitis.[7] These large pseudocysts require treatment, usually consisting of external drainage, internal drainage, and/or resection of that portion of the pancreas where the pseudocyst is located.[12]

LENGTH OF STAY/ANTICIPATED COURSE

About 25,000 cases of pancreatic cancer occur each year. It is the third leading cause of death due to cancer in middle-aged men. For example, 90% of patients with pancreatic ductal adenocarcinoma will die of their disease within 1 year,[20] and nonfunctioning islet cell carcinoma has a 5-year survival rate of 50%.[6]

One in 10,000 people in the U.S. are diagnosed each year with acute pancreatitis and, for alcoholics, this incidence increases to 1 in 100. Mortality rate is about 12% to 15% for acute pancreatitis, 20% to 50% for hemorrhagic pancreatitis,[3] and 30% for pancreatic pseudocyst. Complications of acute pancreatitis range from mild pancreatic edema to pancreatic and peripancreatic necrosis,[5] and death occurs from respiratory failure, bronchopulmonary infections, and sepsis.[14] The operative mortality rate for pancreatoduodenectomy is 4% or less. The leading causes of death from this procedure are postoperative sepsis, hemorrhage and cardiovascular events.[22] Common postoperative surgical complications of pancreatoduodenectomy are shock, hemorrhage, renal failure, and pancreatic or biliary fistula. Fistulas are treated with wound suction and usually close spontaneously with adequate nutrition and electrolyte balance. Morbidity is 50%, with problems such as delayed gastric emptying (DGE) which occurs in one third of the patients who require a nasogastric (NG) tube for 10 or more days. This, in turn, prolongs the hospital stay. Insulin-dependent diabetes mellitus (IDDM) is the greatest drawback to pancreatic resection.[8] The incidence of IDDM after subtotal pancreatectomy where 80% to 95% of the pancreas is removed is 74% to 90%. In procedures where more than 95% of the pancreas is removed, the incidence of IDDM is even higher.

In a study of 45 patients undergoing pancreatoduodenectomy for cancer, the mean postoperative length of stay in the hospital was 27 days, with a range of 8 to 83 days. Of the 45 cancer patients studied, 19 had no postoperative complications whereas 26 did, such as DGE, abscess, or fistula.[20]

Postoperatively, a NG tube is in place until the first bowel movement. Nutrition is supported by total parenteral nutrition and hypocaloric glucose until oral intake can be resumed. Pain during the first week is mostly from the surgical wound. Pain during the second and third weeks is reduced, but analgesics are still needed due to remaining diseased tissue. Pain may intensify when oral intake and bowel movements begin. A Foley catheter and abdominal percutaneous drains are commonly in place. Sleep is often significantly disturbed.[20]

Pancreatic surgery falls within DRG 191: Pancreas, liver, and shunt procedures with complications; and DRG 192: Pancreas, liver, and shunt procedures without complications; with average lengths of stay of 18.2 days and 8.9 days, respectively.[19]

MANAGEMENT TRENDS AND CONTROVERSIES

Irradiation and chemotherapy may be used to shrink pancreatic tumors and achieve pain relief following pancreatic resection. Low cure rates and a low overall survival rate of 5% associated with pancreatoduodenectomy have resulted in increasing use of total pancreatectomy as a definitive treatment for cancer.[20] This surgery results in less frequent anastomotic disruption but often produces a brittle type of diabetes requiring exogenous insulin replacement. There is controversy surrounding the selection of patients for pylorus and duodenal bulb-preserving pancreatoduodenectomy as well as total pancreatectomy in combination with the Whipple procedure. Total pancreatectomy eliminates the potential morbidity of a pancreatic leak occurring at the site of the pancreaticojejunostomy. Octreotide may be given perioperatively to inhibit exocrine pancreas excretion of enzymes from the pancreatic remnant, which may help prevent complications such as abscesses and fistulas following resection.[4]

Surgery can ameliorate pain, but the resulting diabetes is difficult to manage. Autotransplantation affords insulin production by reimplanting intraportal or renal subcapsular injection of dispersed islet cell tissue[8] as prophylaxis of the secondary surgical complication of diabetes mellitus. Patients may remain insulin-independent for years. However, prevention of diabetes cannot be guaranteed after autotransplantation.

Surgical management of patients with pancreatitis is controversial because morbidity is so high. Accurate diagnosis of pancreatitis is essential so the value of early therapeutic surgery can be considered. Clinical, radiographic, and laboratory findings can reasonably establish the difficult diagnosis of pancreatitis. Diagnostic laparotomy is recommended to exclude extrapancreatic disease.[12] Sixty percent of nonalcoholic patients diagnosed with acute pancreatitis have gallstones. The gallstones mechanically interfere with the function of the pancreas, causing acute pancreatitis. For example, a stone may be impacting at the ampulla of Vater. Early surgical removal or cholecystectomy is done and the patient usually recovers without complications.[12] Surgical intervention may be indicated for complications of acute pancreatitis, including hemorrhage, abscess formation requiring mandatory surgical drainage of pus, and pseudocyst formation with an operation required to prevent complications and eliminate symptoms. A pseudocyst may be drained percutaneously as well. Surgical intervention for hemorrhagic pancreatitis may include debridement of necrotic pancreatic tissue, a choledochotomy, insertion of a T-tube for common bile duct obstruction, and placement of large drains near the pancreas. (See Guideline 43.)

Surgery for chronic pancreatitis usually is performed to relieve pain and/or a biliary obstruction, duodenal obstruction, or pancreatic duct hemorrhage. Identification of lesions can be performed through endoscopic retrograde cholangiopancreatography (ERCP), a method combining endoscopic and radiographic examination of the biliary and pancreatic ductal systems. It is also useful to diagnose cancer of the pancreas. Surgical procedures for pain relief include lateral pancreaticojejunostomy and resection.[10]

Trauma may cause formation of a persistent pancreatic fistula or delayed formation of a pseudocyst. Fistulas can be treated surgically by implantation of the pancreatic duct or tract into the duodenum or jejunum. A pseudocyst simply can be drained externally or internally with a cystogastrostomy or cystojejunostomy.

Whenever pancreatic surgery is performed, a NG tube attached to suction is commonly used to remove gastric contents and reduce stimulation of pancreatic secretion. A jejunostomy may be placed for feedings to prevent duodenal stimulation of pancreatic function and/or bypass duodenal obstruction. DGE after pancreatoduodenectomy is seen in one third of all patients.[22] Erythromycin, a motilin agonist, improves gastric emptying and thereby reduces the incidence of DGE. Bethanecol, metoclopramide, and cisapride may also help with DGE. A nutritionally balanced diet, insulin therapy, pancreatic enzyme replacement, rest, analgesia, and emotional support are needed for continued long-term management.

ASSESSMENT

PARAMETER	ANTICIPATED ALTERATION
Pain	Epigastrium, midback, or hypochondrium pain (may be severe) *due to cancer (late symptom)* Steady pain or pain that peaks after a meal or alcohol intake, radiating to the back *due to pancreatitis*
Skin	Jaundice *due to bile duct occlusion* Decreased turgor *due to malnutrition* Pruritus *due to bile duct occlusion*
GI	Weight loss, anorexia, early satiety, nausea, vomiting, and diarrhea *due to malabsorption and decreased food intake* Clay-colored stools *due to bile duct occlusion* Abdominal mass on palpation in the epigastrium, liver, and spleen, with possible ascites *due to tumor associated with pancreatic cancer*
Temperature	Elevated *due to pancreatitis and/or abscess formation*

Serum Tests

Albumin	Decreased: <4.5 g/dl *due to impaired GI ability to absorb nutrients*
Transferrin	Decreased: <30% *due to impaired GI ability to absorb nutrients*
Glucose	Elevated: >200 mg/dl (sudden) *due to cancer*
Alkaline phosphatase	Elevated: >85 ImU/ml *due to common bile duct obstruction*
Bilirubin (total)	Elevated: >1.0 mg/dl *due to common bile duct obstruction or hepatic metastasis*
Amylase	Elevated: >400 IU/L *due to pancreatitis*
Lipase	Elevated: >110 U/L *due to acute pancreatitis*
K^+	Elevated: >5 mEq/L *due to excess tissue destruction*
Ca^{++}	Decreased: <9 mg/dl *due to acute pancreatitis*
WBC	Elevated: >10,000 mm^3 *due to pancreatitis and/or abscess formation*

Radiographic Exams

Ultrasound, CT, ERCP with biopsy from ampullary region[9,17]	Presence of tumors, bile duct obstruction, chronic inflammation, exocrine insufficiency, and pseudocysts With contrast, identifies areas of necrosis Biopsy reveals malignant or benign cells
Upper GI series	Invasion (filling defect) *due to tumor*
Angiography of pancreas[9]	Distortion of pancreatic vessels by tumor, and increased vascularization within tumor (may be normal in acute pancreatitis 14% to 21% of the time)[3]
Transhepatic cholangiogram	Common bile duct obstruction
Chest and abdominal films	Subdiaphragmatic mass or left pleural effusion *due to pseudocyst*

PLAN OF CARE

INTENSIVE PHASE

Care of the patient after pancreatic surgery focuses on replacing fluids lost during surgery, and preventing postoperative complications. If there is a history of peritonitis prior to surgery, the patient is also at risk for ARDS, MI, CHF, and DIC. (See Guidelines 16, 17, 35, and 59.)

PATIENT CARE PRIORITIES	**EXPECTED PATIENT OUTCOMES**
Fluid volume deficit *r/t* *Dehydration* *Hemorrhage secondary to leakage of pancreatic enzymes* *Digestive acids during and after surgery* *NG fluid loss* *Third spacing* *Risk of hemorrhage increases if there is preoperative presence of fat malabsorption*	BP within patient norms HR: WNL Normal skin turgor Moist mucous membranes Absence of GI hemorrhage Abdomen soft, pain free Hct: WNL Hgb: WNL
Pancreatic insufficiency and altered serum glucose *r/t* *Excessive production/release of enzymes* *Insulin* *Glucagon (initially)* *Decreased production of insulin and glucagon (later)*	Glucose: WNL
Pain *r/t* *Incision* *Wound infection* *Anxiety*	Reports tolerable pain Body relaxed Absence of signs of infection

Plan of Care (cont'd)

High risk for decreased CO *r/t hypovolemia*	CVP: WNL CO: WNL Urine output: WNL HR: WNL Absence of MI, CHF, DIC
High risk for peritonitis *r/t* *Leakage of irritating enzymes and exudate in peritoneum during surgery* *Severe wound infection*	Afebrile Absence of abdominal pain Absence of abdominal distension Anastomosis intact
High risk for liver dysfunction *r/t* *Obstruction of splenic vein by tumor causing splenomegaly and segmental portal hypertension with bleeding esophageal varices* *Obstruction of hepatic veins causing Budd-Chiari Syndrome (thrombosis of hepatic veins)*	Bilirubin: WNL ALT: WNL AST: WNL PT: WNL APTT: WNL Absence of hepatomegaly Absence of icteric sclera
High risk for GI complications *r/t* *Gastric retention* *Ileus* *Bowel obstruction* *Marginal ulcers at anastomotic site* *Mesenteric thrombosis*	Bowel sounds: WNL within 24 to 48 hrs Absence of abdominal distension Absence of abdominal pain
High risk for impaired skin integrity *r/t* *Wound and skin irritation* *Breakdown that may result from contact with irritating pancreatic drainage*	Wound intact, without erythema, pain, and drainage Skin intact, without signs of irritation, swelling Adequate intake of nutrients

INTERVENTIONS

Assess vital signs q1h to q2h until stable.

Monitor preload indicators (CVP, PCWP) *to assess state of hydration and prevent dehydration.*

Monitor appearance of mucous membranes, poor skin turgor, dull sunken eyes, and level of consciousness q2h to q3h for the first 24 to 48 hours *to assess state of hydration.*

Monitor daily weights.

Measure I/O q1h *to assess state of hydration.*

Monitor Hct and Hgb q4h to q6h and more frequently if signs of bleeding occur.

Administer IV fluid and, if hemorrhage occurs, administer blood and blood products *to replace volume.*

Monitor serum amylase qd.

Monitor serial blood glucose levels q4h to q6h.

Monitor urine glucose and acetone q1h.

Monitor LOC.

Monitor respirations for Kussmaul pattern *to determine evidence of diabetes.*

Administer glucose/insulin prn.

Administer prophylactic antibiotics *to decrease potential infection related to peritonitis.*

Monitor for fever, general abdominal discomfort, and nausea and vomiting *to detect early signs of peritonitis.*

With signs of peritonitis, assist with careful insertion of drains into the operative area, *which may reveal exudate indicative of anastomotic rupture and/or formation of fistulas.*

Assist in dye studies *to document further anastomotic defect.*

Monitor incision for discomfort, drainage, redness, induration, swelling, and separation *to detect early signs of wound infection.*

Plan of Care (cont'd)

Keep skin around wound dry. Apply a protective agent on skin that repels drainage *to protect skin.*

Apply peristomal (stomahesive) pad around wound *to form an occlusive protective covering.*

Monitor for reddened and excoriated skin.

Monitor skin around any sump drains.

Assess nature of pain (intensity, location, character, and quality).

Administer analgesics to control pain.

Monitor liver functions tests (total protein, serum albumin, fibrinogen, PT, coagulation studies, and transaminase levels) q6h to q12h.

Monitor for hepatomegaly, jaundice, icteric sclera *to detect liver dysfunction.*

Assess bowel sounds and abdominal distension, and maintain NG tube patency, *as intestinal obstruction can cause increased pressure and disrupt anastomosis.*

Administer enteral feedings or hyperalimentation *to provide nutritional support.*[16]

INTERMEDIATE PHASE

As the patient moves into the third postoperative day, it is important to maintain and provide optimum nutrition to promote wound healing, prevent infections, and prevent weight loss. The nurse is still watchful for GI complications and continued regulation of pain and serum glucose. Liver function continues to be monitored, as well as skin integrity.

PATIENT CARE PRIORITIES	EXPECTED PATIENT OUTCOMES
Impaired nutrition *r/t prolonged absence of nutritional intake and abnormal metabolism of nutrients caused by pancreatic dysfunction*	Albumin: WNL Positive nitrogen balance Weight within patient norms
High risk for infection *r/t development of intra-abdominal or wound abscess due to inadequate drainage and collection of fluid*	Absence or resolution of intra-abdominal abscess, wound infection, and/or abscess Afebrile WBC: WNL
High risk for impaired tissue integrity *r/t* *Pancreatic and duodenal fistula (including biliary fistula) resulting from partial anastomotic disruption* *Distal obstruction* *Total disruption of anastomosis caused by inadequate blood supply to the jejunal limb* *Pancreatic fistula* *Abscess* *Pseudocyst*	Pancreatic and duodenal membrane intact (without leaks, hemorrhage or thrombus) Absence or resolution of fistula formation

INTERVENTIONS

Determine presence of preoperative weight loss or gain, patient's dietary and beverage intake history.

Assess present nutritional status, including daily weight, appearance and character of skin, mucous membranes, and muscle mass. *Inability to meet protein-calorie requirements is due to surgical reduction of mucosal surface, delayed gastric emptying, or insufficient nutrient exposure. Gut malabsorption is due to lack of the pancreatic enzyme lipase. Stress of major surgery or sepsis can increase energy expenditure by 20 to 50%.*[16]

Monitor intake of nutrients.

Administer pancreatic enzymes before meals as ordered.

Monitor for digestive disturbances q12h to q24h such as indigestion, steatorrhea, and weight loss.

Administer insulin as ordered.

Plan of Care (cont'd)

Maintain continuous, patent NG suction system *to decrease potential for infection related to intra-abdominal abscess.*

Monitor for potential intra-abdominal abscess as evidenced by spiking fevers, increasing abdominal pain and tenderness, presence of pleural effusion (elevated diaphragm, collection of fluid in abdomen, and distended bowel).

Administer antibiotics as ordered *to prevent or treat intra-abdominal abscess if present.*

Monitor for continued larger volume of NG drainage (400 to 600 cc) for more than 5 to 8 days.

Monitor for skin breakdown *due to activation of bile and pancreatic enzymes present.*

Administer skin care around any fistula, including application of protein powder or agents *to protect the skin.*

Monitor for presence of obstruction via abdominal radiography and upper GI series with contrast media.

Monitor for signs of subhepatic abscess and/or obstructive jaundice *indicating anastomotic disruption.*

TRANSITION TO DISCHARGE

Before discharge, the patient and/or family must be able to demonstrate understanding of the medication regimen, dietary management modifications, and activity progression. If part of the stomach has been removed, dumping syndrome can impair nutrition. The patient also may have chronic nausea, vomiting, anorexia, and early satiety. Methods to optimize nutrition must be explained. Reduction or absence of pancreatic enzymes will predispose patients to malabsorption and diarrhea. Enzyme replacements and antidiarrheal medications are prescribed. Instruct patient in proper timing and dosage of pancreatic enzyme supplements. The nurse should include a discussion with the patient regarding the importance of dietary modifications, including avoidance of fatty foods, alcohol, tea, and coffee. If appropriate, explain the hazards of continued alcohol intake and its effect on pancreatic pathology.

If the patient now requires exogenous insulin therapy, he/she will need to be taught to check glucose levels via a glucometer. Instruction regarding self-administered insulin injections is also a priority. Return demonstrations by the patient or family on glucometer blood testing and injections help reinforce what has been learned.

Instruction regarding methods for pain management and self-care for wounds and drains is given. Assessment of pain is individualized to each patient, and more pain analgesia may be required than preoperatively. The patient should be able to recognize signs and symptoms necessitating medical attention, such as infection, increasing weight loss, and poor glycemic control. Provide the patient with instruction on whom to call if a problem arises and the plan for follow-up visits. The nurse needs to perform an assessment of the patient's and/or family's potential compliance with the discharge regimen as a whole. The patient will need to adjust psychologically to serious illness, and referrals for counseling should be offered. If carcinoma is present, the patient may benefit from a referral from home to hospice care.

REFERENCES

1. Bagg A: Whipple's procedure: nursing guidelines, *Crit Care Nurse* 8(5):34-45, 1988.
2. Brantley L: Cancer head of the pancreas, *Surgical-Technologist* 16(5):24-27, 1984.
3. Brown A: Acute pancreatitis: pathophysiology, nursing diagnoses, and collaborative problems, *Focus Crit Care* 18(2):121-130, 1991.
4. Buchler M: Inhibition of pancreatic secretion to prevent postoperative complications following pancreatic resection, *Acta Gastroenterol Belg* 56:271-278, 1993.
5. Calleja G, Barkin J: Acute pancreatitis, *Med Clin North Am* 77(5):1037-1056, 1993.
6. Evans D, et al: Nonfunctioning islet cell carcinoma of pancreas, *Surgery* 114(6):1175-1181, 1993.
7. Fain J, Amoto-Vealey E: Acute pancreatitis: a gastrointestinal emergency, *Crit Care Nurse* 8(5):47-63, 1988.
8. Farney A, et al: Autotransplantation of dispersed pancreatic tissue combined with total or near total pancreatectomy for treatment of chronic pancreatitis, *Surgery* 110(2):427-437, 1991.
9. Freeney P: Incremental dynamic bolus computed tomography of acute pancreatitis, *Int J Pancreatol* 13(3):147-158, 1993.
10. Kalvaria I, Toskes P: Chronic pancreatitis: treatment guidelines, *Physician Assistant* 14(5):62-74, 1990.
11. Laytock R, et al: *Pancreas essentials of surgery,* Baltimore, 1988, Williams & Wilkins.

12. Ranson J: The role of surgery in the management of acute pancreatitis, *Ann Surg* 211(4):382-393, 1990.
13. Robertson AJ: Whipple's procedure; Is It Justified? *Aust N Z J Surg* 63(7):535-540, 1993.
14. Ruiz F, et al: Respiratory complications in severe acute pancreatitis, *Rev Med Chil* 120(8):893-898, 1992.
15. Sharp K, et al: Pancreatoduodenectomy with pyloric preservation for carcinoma of the pancreas: a cautionary note, *Surgery* 105(5):645-653, 1989.
16. Shikora S, Blackburn G: Nutritional consequences of major gastrointestinal surgery, *Surg Clin North Am* 71(3):509-521, 1991.
17. Smith J, Davies B: An inside view. . .endoscopic retrograde cholangiopancreatography, *Nursing Mirror* 157(22):30-33, 1983.
18. Spross J, Manolatos A, Thorpe M: Pancreatic cancer: nursing challenges, *Semin Oncol Nurs* 4(4):274-284, 1988.
19. *St Anthony's DRG Guidebook 1995,* Reston, Va, 1994, St Anthony.
20. Ulander K, et al: Needs and care of patients undergoing subtotal pancreatectomy for cancer, *Cancer Nurs* 14(1):27-33, 1991.
21. Yamauchi H, Nitta A, Namiki T: Carcinoma of the papilla of Vater accompanied by noninvasive adenomatous component (NAC), *Tohoku J Exp Med* 170(3):147-156, 1993.
22. Yeo C, et al: Erythromycin accelerates gastric emptying after pancreaticoduodenectomy, *Ann Surg* 218(3):229-238, 1993.

TRANSPLANT GUIDELINE

45

Pancreas Transplantation

Patricia J. Forg, BS, RN, CNN

DESCRIPTION

Insulin-dependent diabetes mellitus (IDDM) is well recognized as a major disease and can result in devastating secondary health problems and a life span one-third shorter than that of the general population.[37] Fifty percent of insulin-dependent diabetics will have one or more secondary complications occurring approximately 15 to 20 years after onset of their diabetes.[16] These secondary complications include coronary artery disease (CAD), peripheral vascular disease (PVD), peripheral and autonomic neuropathy, retinopathy, infections, and nephropathy.

IDDM accounts for 25% of all people with end-stage renal disease (ESRD) who require dialysis or renal transplantation. ESRD is a major cause of morbidity and mortality in patients with IDDM of longer than 15 years duration.[30] The course of nephropathy is more stressful in patients with IDDM because of the impact of disease on other organ systems. Death in patients with diabetic ESRD is most often caused by cardiovascular catastrophe, cerebrovascular catastrophe, and infection, in that order.

IDDM also affects one's psychosocial well-being and can lead to personality disorders due to dependency on others and difficulty obtaining employment. People with IDDM report that they receive 2.5 times more job refusals in their lifetime than do nondiabetic siblings.[11] Further, they risk loss of employment and health insurance secondary to illness or have difficulty obtaining health insurance.

The goal of pancreas allograft transplantation is to normalize glucose metabolism and prevent the secondary complications of IDDM. Pancreatic transplantation offers long-term metabolic control that is superior to what can be achieved by any other method of control.[14] The first pancreas transplantation surgical procedure was performed in 1966 at the University of Minnesota.[17] When successful, transplantation results in normal or near-normal glucose metabolism without the need for exogenous insulin.[27] Pancreas allograft transplantation is accomplished, most commonly in the United States, by the surgical implantation of a whole cadaver pancreas allograft into a specially selected diabetic recipient. The pancreas can be transplanted alone, in combination with a kidney allograft (simultaneous transplantation), or after a kidney allograft. As of December 1992, 126 people are on the waiting list for pancreas-alone cadaver organs and 781 are waiting for the simultaneous cadaver kidney and pancreas organs.[38] From October 1987 to November 1992, 109 pancreas transplantation procedures and 1604 simultaneous kidney and pancreas transplantation procedures were done in the United States, according to the Pancreas Transplant Registry in Minnesota.

PATHOPHYSIOLOGY

IDDM is characterized by the absence of endogenous insulin and the presence of chronic hyperglycemia. The primary defect in IDDM is inadequate insulin secretion by pancreatic beta cells. It is characterized as an autoimmune process because of the presence of islet cell antibodies, although this process is not well understood.[4,16] The defect is thought to be caused by a progressive autoimmune destruction of pancreatic islet cells by islet cell antibodies and DR3, DR4 histocompatibility antigens on chromosome 6. This defect is found in 95% of people with IDDM.[30]

Hyperglycemia is managed by the administration of exogenous insulin by intermittent injection or infusion pump. If glycemic control is poor, microvascular complications may occur. Disturbance in the microcirculation is a major cause of both disability and mortality in individuals who have diabetes. The microvasculature transports and exchanges nutrients as well as waste products within the body and depends on adequate blood flow rate. IDDM is thought to cause changes in these normal hemodynamic functions. Blood flow elevation, combined with capillary hypertension, directly affects increased organ perfusion, with potential for the eventual complications of retinopathy, neuropathy, and nephropathy.[16]

Researchers speculate that retinal vasculature debility is strongly affected by past glycemic control. This indicates that the overall metabolic dysfunction of diabetes, including persistent hyperglycemia and its effects, may account for retinal changes and blindness even in the absence of other secondary complications.[16]

The histological findings of neuropathy include loss of both large and small myelinated nerve fibers, accompanied by varying degrees of demyelination; connective tissue proliferation; and thickening and reduplication of capillary basement membranes with capillary closure.[30] The patient experiences decreased sensation and decreased motor control of muscles.

The pathology of diabetic nephropathy begins with glomerular basement membrane thickening, which progresses to sclerosis of the glomeruli and interstitial fibrosis. The peak incidence of development of overt proteinuria occurs 15 to 20 years after the onset of diabetes, followed by uremia in another 6 years.[23]

Diabetes is an independent risk factor for arteriosclerotic cardiovascular disease (ASCVD). Lipid abnormalities occur in 25% to 75% of adults. High-density lipoprotein, cholesterol, and triglycerides are often elevated in IDDM[30] and there is abnormal fat metabolism and lipid deposition in vessel walls.[36]

Ideally, pancreas transplantation should be performed in diabetic patients before histologic evidence of complications is manifested.[5] Prevention of the progression of secondary complications is not achieved if severe stages of complications exist.[14] The secondary complications of IDDM, clinical signs, and benefits of pancreas transplantation are summarized in Table 45-1.

PATIENT SELECTION

A pancreas transplant may be appropriate only if the complications of diabetes are more serious than the side effects of antirejection treatment.[34] Because pancreas transplantation is not a life-saving procedure, appropriate patient selection is critical to ensure a low mortality risk and improvement in quality of life.[40] Three groups of patients outlined in the following Box have been identified who would qualify and benefit from pancreas transplantation.

Contraindications to transplantation include the presence of uncorrectable malignancy, psychosis, ongoing peripheral gangrene, severe coronary insufficiency with angina or inoperable CAD, severely incapacitating peripheral neuropathy, and an upper age limit of 50 to 60 years.[37] Some transplant centers also exclude candidates who have suffered amputation as a result of severe PVD or who have documented severe disease by Doppler examination, candidates who actively engage in cigarette smoking, and candidates in whom diabetic retinopathy is the only diagnosed secondary complication.

PROCEDURE

The pancreas for implant is obtained from cadaver donors. The donor and recipient must be ABO compatible. Contraindications to donation include alcoholism, chemical dependency, metabolic or endocrine-related coma, pancreatic trauma, abnormal pancreatic function, diabetes, or chronic pancreatitis. Massive obesity and recurrent acute pancreatitis may also be contraindications. The condition of the pancreas is the single most important factor at the time of procurement if the donor history is negative.[9,26] It is essential to maintain donor hemodynamics, normothermia, and euglycemia with insulin drip during procurement.

The procurement of the pancreas includes the removal of the pancreas; the spleen, which serves as a handle for the surgeon; and a segment of duodenum, including the ampulla of Vater. Procurement is safely and routinely done with liver procurement.[22] Excess handling of the pancreas is avoided to protect against edema, which may hinder graft function. The pancreas is stored in University of Wisconsin solution (UW solution) and can be preserved for up to 24 hours awaiting transplantation.

The donor pancreas for pancreas allograft transplantation can either be the whole pancreas allograft or a segment of it from a cadaver donor or a segment of a pancreas from a living related donor (LRD). LRD pancreas transplants are more difficult than cadaver donor transplants; however, there may be a lower incidence of rejection with the LRD.[33] Living donors need to be highly motivated, medically able to tolerate surgery, and not at risk for developing diabetes. Most centers do not perform LRD transplants due to the adverse risks to the living donor. Whole organ technique is preferred for the following reasons:

- Greater mass of islet cells
- Less risk of vascular thromboses
- Anastomosis of whole grafts to the bladder is technically easier than anastomosis of segmental grafts[21]
- Less bleeding
- Less risk of pancreatitis
- Easier and safer management of the exocrine secretions
- No risk to a living donor

For the recipient, the surgical procedure for pancreas allograft transplantation is through a midline intra-abdominal or extraperitoneal Gibson incision, and the pancreas is placed mid-abdominal or in the right or left iliac fossa (the patient's own native pancreas is left in place and untouched). The head of the pancreas is placed inferior toward the urinary bladder of the recipient. The donor blood vessels are

TABLE 45-1 Clinical Manifestations of Diabetic Complications

Complication	Clinical signs and symptoms	Effect of pancreas transplant
Poor glycemic control	Elevated glycosated hemoglobin, hyperglycemia, insulin reactions	Glycosated hemoglobin levels return to normal within 1-3 months Majority have normal oral glucose tolerance tests
Microvascular disease		
Retinopathy	Lesions seen on retina Microaneurysm, hemorrhages seen	No consistent beneficial effect has been reported Transplantation before complication recommended[2]
Neuropathy: peripheral	Impaired sensation or excruciating pain Bilateral loss of motor and sensory nerve function increases in proportion to duration of diabetes Unilateral neuropathy occurs unrelated to the duration of disease Sexual dysfunction	Progression may be halted, possibly improved although still present Impact may be greater if transplantation performed at an early stage of disease[18,39]
Neuropathy: autonomic	Diabetic diarrhea, postural hypotension, gustatory diaphoresis, gastroparetic vomiting, cystopathy, slowed cardiorespiratory response	Indices stabilize GI function may stabilize or improve[1]
Nephropathy	Proteinuria, uremia, end-stage renal disease	Protects native or transplanted kidney from diabetic lesions
Macrovascular		
Atherosclerosis Cerebrovascular disease	Lesions on coronary arteriogram, silent myocardial infarction Early death	Unknown
Microvascular		
Peripheral vascular disease	Buttock, calf or thigh pain Decreased skin temperature and discoloration, nonhealing ulcer, and amputation Evidenced by vascular Doppler exam	Increased skin temperature Increased Po_2 to skin Unknown regarding amputation
Psychosocial	Dependency Depression	Increased quality of life, pleased to be free of insulin and dietary restrictions, increased sense of well-being

anastomosed to the recipient iliac vein and iliac arteries to establish blood supply to the pancreas. To manage pancreatic exocrine secretions, the preferred and most widely used procedure is to anastomose the pancreas to the dome of the bladder by using a bridge fashioned from the donor duodenum segment. (See Figure 45-1.) The urinary drainage of the excocrine secretions into the bladder and mixed with urine allows early detection of rejection by monitoring amylase concentrations in the urine. The recipient collects urine over time (2 to 12 hours) and amylase is reported in U/hr. If concentrations are low compared to the trend or established baseline, rejection is suspected. Another way to detect rejection is by allograft biopsy via cystoscopy-directed biopsy technique or by a percutaneous approach using CT guidance.[25] The ability to identify rejection early enables early diagnosis and treatment of rejections and greatly contributes to higher graft survival rates. Disadvantages of the bladder drainage approach include acute or chronic mild to severe hematuria, duodenal ulcers and ischemia, leaks, dysuria, urinary tract infections, space loss of bicarbonate, and cystitis. Reflux pancreatitis may also occur due to reflux of urine back into the pancreas, causing irritation.

A second method that has been used to manage exocrine drainage is to inject the exocrine drainage ducts with a synthetic polymer. This prevents the exocrine secretion from draining or even being formed.

Candidates for Pancreas Transplantation

I. Insulin-dependent diabetics who have minimal secondary complications of diabetes and no renal impairment. Criteria for selection:
- Evidence of albuminuria (proteinuria of 1 g/24 hr), an indicator that early nephropathy will otherwise progress
- A creatinine clearance of 60 ml/min so the nephrotoxic effects of cyclosporine can be tolerated[33]
- Evidence of glucose control; signs and symptoms of hypoglycemic reactions are recognized by the patient

II. Insulin-dependent diabetics with renal failure who have undergone a previous successful kidney transplant but who have minimal other secondary complications of diabetes

III. Insulin-dependent diabetics who have minimal secondary complications of diabetes and renal failure (candidates for simultaneous pancreas and kidney transplantation)

Another method is to allow exocrine secretions to be drained into the intestine (enteric drainage). The Roux-en-Y procedure placement involves anastomosis of the distal divided end of the small bowel to the head of the pancreas. The proximal end is anastomosed to the small bowel below the anastomosis. In whole-pancreas allografts, the donor duodenum is anastomosed into the side of the Roux-en-Y limb of the recipient's jejunum.[8] The draining enzymes are harmless to the bowel and this procedure offers the most physiological way of handling them. However, the Roux-en-Y procedure has a greater risk of bacterial contamination and infection in the early postoperative period.[41] The recipient also can convert to this method if the bladder drainage fails or if any of the bladder complications become unmanageable.

LENGTH OF STAY/ANTICIPATED COURSE

Upon admission, the patient is prepared in the usual manner for abdominal surgery. Blood samples are drawn for final cross-match for antibodies with the donor. Type and cross-match are ordered for four units of blood, but generally transfusion is not needed unless preoperative hemoglobin and hematocrit are low. Prophylactic antibiotics such as cefotaxime and vancomycin are given. An intravenous (IV) insulin drip sometimes is required to keep serum glucose at normal levels. The patient should be assessed for recent illness, including vomiting, fatigue, dehydration, recent retinal bleeding, marked glycosuria, or ketonuria.

The surgical transplantation of the donor pancreas takes approximately 3 to 4 hours. Following surgery, the recipient is usually recovered in a critical care unit because of the need for the close monitoring of this high-risk patient. Once hemodynamically stable, the patient is moved to the specialized transplant unit.

The length of stay in the acute care hospital is approximately 10 to 17 days, with an average length of stay of 12 to 14 days. In one study, 25% of patients studied had no postoperative complications and were released after 12 to 14 days. Others stayed longer because of a variety of problems, including rejections, infections, drug toxicities, and surgical complications.[12] HCFA classifies pancreas transplant under DRG 191 and 192: Pancreas, Liver and Shunt Procedures with or without complications, with an average LOS noted as 18.2 or 8.9 days, respectively.[31]

The need for rehospitalization occurs in a majority of the post-transplant population, usually within the first 6 months. The primary reason for rehospitalization is for the treatment of acute rejection.[12] It is common to see a rejection episode 3 to 4 weeks after transplantation. Other admissions are due to occurrence of infections secondary to immunosuppression, wound complications, pancreatitis, pancreatic reflux, significant hematuria leading to acute anemia, bladder leak, or leakages of the duodenal segment possibly requiring surgical revisions.

Allograft survival rates following simultaneous kidney and pancreas transplantation are now approaching those achieved by renal allografts alone.[6] The success of pancreas transplantation is measured by how many allografts are functioning 1 year after transplantation. Statistics published over the last few years reflect a 70% graft survival rate.[38] One of the major factors influencing allograft survival is patient compliance with the medical regimen. Rejection is the major cause of graft loss.

MANAGEMENT TRENDS AND CONTROVERSIES

Today, pancreas transplantation is successful because there are improved methods for diagnosis of rejection with bladder-drained exocrine secretions and cystoscopically directed biopsy, improved immunosuppression to prevent and treat rejection, and improved patient care management.

Most centers use OKT-3, ATGAM, and/or methylprednisolone for induction of immunosuppression and to treat acute rejection. A combination of cyclosporine, azathioprine, and prednisone is used to maintain immunosuppression. Corticosteroids can be irritating to the stomach and can cause ulcers. Antacids such as sucralfate, aluminum hydroxide, Maalox, or Ranitidine are administered to control or neutralize stomach acids. Cisapride or Reglan may help gastroparesis. Also, the immunosuppressed patient is at particular risk for viral and bacterial infections. Various antiviral preparations such as cytomegalovirus immune globulin, ganciclovir, and acyclovir are given to help reduce the severity of secondary viral infections, particularly cy-

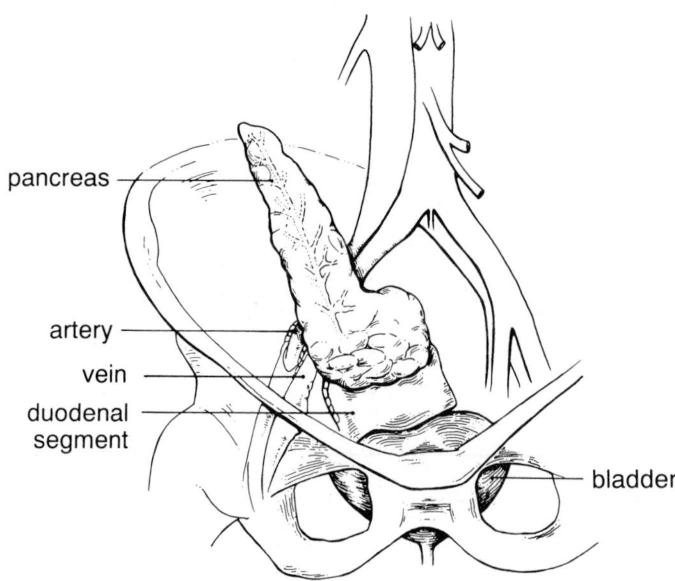

Figure 45-1 Completed pancreas transplant into the pelvis.

tomegalovirus. Trimethoprim/sulfamethoxazole is given to treat or prevent urinary tract infections and lung infection caused by pneumocystis. Fluconozole is usually prescribed to treat fungal infections of operative sites or urine. Clotrimazole trouches or Nystatin suspension prevent thrush of the mouth during the first months following transplantation surgery. Cephalexin, Ciprofloxacin, and Vancomycin are commonly prescribed for bacterial infections. Preventive nursing measures include proper administration of medications, meticulous hand washing, IV site care, wound and Foley catheter care, and strict adherence to pulmonary hygiene regime.[9] Fevers of 37.8° C or more should be noted and blood, throat, and urine cultures obtained.

Maintaining adequate fluid balance is essential. A newly transplanted kidney may enter a diuresis phase, especially with the simultaneous kidney/pancreas transplant because of short preservation time. The diabetic patient is prone to osmotic diuresis and is at risk for excess fluid loss by urination, as well as loss through nasogastric suctions. In contrast, there may be a period of acute tubular necrosis during which urine output is low, and hence there is danger of fluid overload. Hypovolemia must be avoided because blood flow through the newly grafted pancreas and kidney must be adequate to ensure adequate pressure and perfusion.

It is well documented that a person with IDDM complicated by ESRD will greatly benefit from combined renal and pancreatic transplantation primarily because with renal failure, the need for a renal transplant exists. Because the recipient will need to take immunosuppressive therapy for prevention of rejection of the kidney allograft, the pancreas should be transplanted to gain the benefits it has to offer. For a transplantation candidate who is preuremic and whose creatinine clearances are normal, there may be controversy in regard to the benefits of pancreas transplantation. Many endocrinologists argue that if the patient can maintain blood sugar control with intensive insulin management, the benefits of transplantation surgery, with the associated risks and required immunosuppression, are questionable. Cyclosporine induces a decrease in creatinine clearance, but the decline is seen in the early post-transplantation period and usually does not progress. The major drawback to pancreas transplantation in nonuremic, non-kidney transplant recipients is the need, at this time, for long-term immunosuppression.[32] When the severity of the side effects of the immunosuppressive medications are reduced, transplantation may be a more viable alternative for these patients.

Controversy also revolves around the influence of pancreas transplantation on diabetic retinopathy. There are insufficient studies to substantiate improvement of retinopathy. Longer follow-up is needed and assessment needs to be done up to 3 to 4 years after transplantation. There is no clear advantage at this time of having a pancreas transplantation procedure done to avoid the progression of retinopathy.

There is a growing body of evidence that the quality of life can significantly improve following transplantation. In a study by Gross and Zehrer,[13] it was found that almost all patients (92%) with a functioning pancreas and kidney transplant reported improved health since transplant. In contrast, 78% of the kidney-only transplant group reported they were more healthy. Although the majority of kidney transplant patients feel more healthy after transplant, the addition of a pancreas transplant appears to elevate patients' perceptions of their overall health and health-related quality-of-life outcomes.[13] Patients are also more inclined to have renal and pancreas transplantation because the advantages of a combined operation include the most efficient use of funds to cover the medical costs.[34]

More of the combined pancreas–renal transplant recipients reported working full-time, good health, a better sex life, and a slightly better quality of life.[24] Quality of life is better after simultaneous pancreas and renal transplantation than renal transplantation alone, mainly because patients are freed from the day-to-day management of diabetes: injections, dietary restrictions, blood glucose self-monitoring, hypoglycemia, and a rigid, socially incapacitated lifestyle.[34,35] More studies are needed to fully evaluate the quality of life in pancreas-only recipients.

Alternative methods of pancreatic tissue transplantation are being explored. Research is underway to find ways to successfully transplant the islet cells instead of a whole or segmental pancreas. Islet cells are isolated and injected into the liver, spleen, or renal capsule of the recipient. This potentially can avert the surgical problems associated with the revascularization of the pancreas and the management of its exocrine secretions. In animal models, islet cell transplants have been successful in reversing the diabetic state and in preventing the development of diabetic complications. An adequate number of purified intact cells are required. Currently, several donor pancreases are needed to collect enough cells. A potential source of cells includes cryopreserving the cells to be used at a later time.[28]

Rejection that occurs approximately 2 to 4 weeks after transplantation is also possible. Few, if any, recipients of islet cell allografting have been rendered permanently insulin independent for more than a few months. There are no early markers for rejection. It may be feasible to encapsulate the transplanted cells, creating a barrier from the recipient's immune system.[28] As technology and techniques advance, islet cell transplantation may become a viable option for the diabetic in the future.

In 1989, Lafferty[20] reported a study in which diabetic kidney transplant recipients were implanted with human fetal pancreas (HFP) tissue, an alternate source of islet cells. These cells were implanted under the transplanted kidney capsule at the same time as the kidney transplant in order to reverse the diabetic condition. Cultured HFP has been transplanted to the liver of the diabetic patient through the umbilical vein and the development of a serum C-peptide response (a measurement of graft insulin production) in patients has been reported.[20] HFP tissue can grow and function in humans, although clinical improvement, when seen, occurs only slowly and usually is not seen before 3 to 6 months after grafting.[20] To benefit from a sustained reduction in insulin requirements, a more than 1:4 donor equivalent of fetal tissue is needed. Further studies are needed regarding this type of transplantation. Due to cadaver donor shortages, it is important to explore other avenues of donor sources.

ASSESSMENT

PARAMETER	ANTICIPATED ALTERATION
Preoperative	
Patient knowledge	Knowledge may range from limited to well educated Education affords the patient more knowledge and promotes feeling of being more comfortable and confident managing self-care at home[29]
Laboratory values	
• Glucose	Increased: >105 mg/dl *r/t diabetes*
• Creatinine	Increased: >1.2 mg/dl
• K^+	Increased: >5.0 mEq/L *r/t renal dysfunction*
• Albumin	Decreased: <3.8 g/dl *due to possible proteinuria secondary to renal dysfunction; may be at surgical risk due to poor nutrition*
Secondary diabetic complications	Each patient has an individual degree of severity or progression of one or more secondary complications: • Retinopathy • Peripheral neuropathy • Gastroparesis • PVD • Nephropathy
Postoperative	
Laboratory values	
• Serum amylase	Increased: >90 mg/dl *seen early (pancreas preservation injury, self-limiting) or later (may indicate rejection or reflux pancreatitis)*

• Urine amylase	Will be slow to rise during the first week *r/t pancreatic allograft function* Each patient will establish a unique baseline average of 2000 to 6000 U/hr; can be as high as 15,000 U/hr
• Serum glucose	Elevated: >120 mg/dl *due to corticosteroids initially, then normal levels after a few days, when steroid dose reduced* *May elevate if TPN is being given*
• Serum creatinine	WNL: 0.3 to 1.2 mg/dl or declining daily *if kidney transplanted* May elevate slightly *because of cyclosporine toxicity or impending graft rejection.*
• CO_2	WNL: 24 to 31 mEq/l or decreased *due to bicarbonate losses in urine from duodenal segment* and hyperkalemia *r/t renal dysfunction and cyclosporine*
• WBC	Increased: >12,000 mm^3 *due to corticosteroids or infection* Decreased: <4000 mm^3 *due to immunosuppression or viral syndrome*
• Hct	Decreased: <35% *due to anemia secondary to uremia or severe hematuria*
Acid–base balance	Metabolic acidosis *due to excretions of pancreatic secretions rich in bicarbonate*
Chest x-ray	Lungs clear. Acute pulmonary edema *due to renal dysfunction, OKT-3 administration* Infection *r/t immunosuppression.*
Ultrasound	Abnormal *due to surgical complication, allograft, or bladder dysfunction*
Nuclear medicine flow scan	Abnormal *due to surgical complication, allograft, or bladder dysfunction*
Cystogram	Abnormal *due to surgical complication, allograft, or bladder dysfunction*
Pancreatic biopsy	Abnormal *due to surgical complication, allograft, or bladder dysfunction*
Renal function	Adequate urine output for level of function Normal or near-normal levels of BUN and creatinine
Cardiovascular	Unchanged ECG Hypertension *due to side effects of cyclosporine, prednisone, or cardiovascular disease* Orthostatic hypotension *due to established diabetic cardiovascular disease or fluid deficits due to dehydration, loss of bicarbonate from pancreatic graft* Difficulty assessing peripheral veins
LOC	Anxious *due to possible rejection and complications of surgery* Mentally alert Corticosteroid-induced psychosis, mood swings
Secondary diabetic complication	Usually little acute change from preoperative status of retinopathy, neuropathies Nephropathy Gastroparesis *due to prolonged ileus and extended postoperative nausea and vomiting*

PLAN OF CARE

INTENSIVE PHASE

The intensive care phase consists of the immediate postoperative transplantation period and usually is of approximately two days duration. The recipient is recovered and care is managed in the critical care setting. Nursing staff is assigned on a 1:1 basis due to the high level of monitoring required for possible postoperative complications and fluid and electrolyte imbalance.

PATIENT CARE PRIORITIES	EXPECTED PATIENT OUTCOMES
High risk for allograft vascular thromboses *r/t surgical complications*	Adequate blood flow as seen on ultrasound or nuclear flow scans

Plan of Care (cont'd)

	Thromboses prevented or surgical repair of vessel patency is attempted Repair can only be accomplished if diagnosed within 1 to 2 hours after operation
High risk for silent MI, arrythmias, HTN, and potential sudden death *r/t cardiovascular and metabolic stress of procedure*	MI prevented or diagnosed early ECG stable, hypertension controlled, stable vital signs
High risk for postoperative hemorrhage *r/t surgical technique or excessive hematuria*	Improved and stable Hgb and Hct
High risk for electrolyte imbalance *r/t control of glucose and possible renal impairment and pancreatic function*	Glucose controlled with IV insulin as needed Hyperkalemia prevented
High risk for bladder obstruction *r/t clogged Foley, surgical complications*	Urine flow through foley is unobstructed Some hematuria present No bladder pressure or pain reported by patient Problems identified and repaired early
Pain *r/t surgical incision*	Pain relieved
High risk for fluid volume deficit *r/t acute diuresis*	Adequate hydration and fluid balance noted by adequate intake and output, normal CVP
High risk for fluid excess *r/t initial dysfunction of the transplanted kidney*	Lungs clear, weight stable
Impaired renal function *r/t delayed graft function if patient received a kidney transplant in addition to pancreas transplant*	Renal function maintained or improved indicated by serum creatinine Hyperkalemia prevented
Anxiety *r/t success of procedure and fear of rejection*	Decreased anxiety evidenced by relaxed nonverbal expressions, calm respirations, and vital signs
High risk for deep vein thrombosis (DVT) *r/t bed rest, surgical site of allograft implantation*	DVT prevented No calf pain or swelling
High risk for bladder anastomotic leak *r/t surgical complications*	Bladder integrity maintained
High risk for infection *r/t immunosuppression and surgical intervention*	Afebrile or postoperative fever quickly reduced Fluid cultures negative Infection prevented or adequately treated and resolved
High risk for inadequate nutrition *r/t nausea, vomiting, or ileus*	Nausea and vomiting controlled Adequate nutrition maintained Bowels functioning
High risk for decubitus *r/t possible decreased peripheral vascular blood flow in the diabetic tissue and bed rest*	Decubiti prevented Skin integrity maintained with normal appearance

INTERVENTIONS

Monitor for allograft vascular thrombosis as evidenced by gross hematuria of a currant jelly color, severe pain in the iliac fossa, absence of blood flow on nuclear imaging flow scan, a rapid rise in serum amylase, and a decrease in urinary amylase levels.

Administer 325 mg aspirin qd or heparin *to prevent thrombosis.*

Monitor ECG closely *for evidence of myocardial infarction.*

Assess vital signs q15min for 3 to 4 hours, then q1h for 8 hours.

Observe for signs and symptoms of internal hemorrhage, including acute abdomen, change in vital signs and mental status, decreasing Hct and Hgb, and increased abdominal girth. *Hemorrhage usually occurs from blood vessel anastomotic site.*

Assess electrolytes related to graft function, including serum electrolytes, q12h, timed collections for urine amylase (q9h or q12h) around the clock.

Plan of Care (cont'd)

Monitor serum bicarbonate levels and administer replacement bicarbonate.

Monitor serum glucose q1h and administer IV insulin if needed by algorithm *to maintain serum glucose at normal levels.*

Maintain patency of Foley catheter and irrigate as needed *to prevent obstruction by clogging, which can cause urinary retention and undue pressure on bladder anastomoses. Also helps to prevent reflux pancreatitis.*

Administer pain medication. Instruct patient on the use of patient-controlled analgesic (PCA) device.

Replace fluid deficit by 1cc of fluid per cc of urine output as recommended initially.

Observe CVP readings and urine output q1h.

Hemodialysis or diuretics *for fluid excess.*

Assess for signs of anxiety: sweaty palms, increased HR. Providing reassurance and information to patient and family about the function of the allograft *will help relieve anxiety.*[7]

Apply antiembolic stockings and pneumatic compression device until out of bed and ambulating *to prevent DVT.*

Check for peripheral pulses *to ensure vessel patency.*

Administer IV immunosuppression (for example, methylprednisolone, azathioprine, ATGAM, or OKT-3). Observe for side effects of each medication and report. *OKT-3 produces a first-dose syndrome caused by cytokines and evidenced by influenza-like symptoms, high fever, chills, headache, diarrhea, and vomiting.*[19]

Closely monitor urine output. *A decrease in output may be indicative of a bladder leak.*

Monitor for change of vital signs, fever, suprapubic pain, tenderness, abdominal distention, or urine drainage from wound.

Maintain bladder decompression with a Foley catheter for approximately 7 days after transplantation.

A cystogram may be performed before the catheter is removed *to rule out extravasation. A Foley catheter may be left in for an extended period of time, allowing a leak to seal itself. Surgical correction of the leak may be required.*

Assess surgical wound and IV sites for any signs or symptoms of infection; monitor chest x-ray reports, urine, sputum, and wound cultures; viral titers (cytomegalovirus); WBC; and sudden rise in glucose or amylase.

Educate patient regarding infection control practices *because infection is a major cause of morbidity and mortality in the immunosuppressed patient.*

Administer prophylactic antibiotics or therapeutic dosages as prescribed: Bactrim *for pneumocystosis carinii (PCP),* Vancomycin *for urinary tract infections commonly caused by staphylococcus.*

Ambulate frequently. Check feet and bony areas for redness and skin breakdown *to prevent decubiti.*

INTERMEDIATE PHASE

The intermediate care phase for the pancreas transplantation recipient usually starts on the third day after transplant and can continue for up to 7 to 21 days depending on the stability of the recipient. If no complications occur, the recipient can be ready for discharge in another 4 to 7 days. During this phase, the recipient is often transferred to a specialized transplant unit.

PATIENT CARE PRIORITIES	EXPECTED PATIENT OUTCOMES
High risk for muscle wasting *r/t bed rest and corticosteroids*	Keep active and maintain muscle tone
Dehydration/postural hypotension *r/t fluid management, bicarbonate loss, and diabetic vessel disease*	Maintain good hydration Optimum serum bicarbonate levels maintained Patient aware of safety measures for self-ambulation

Plan of Care (cont'd)

High risk for loss of allograft function *r/t rejection*	Rejection episodes identified and treated early Markers for rejection normalized
High risk for inadequate nutrition *r/t NPO status*	Nutrition optimum TPN if needed Serum albumin: WNL
High risk for altered bowel patterns or bowel perforation *r/t steroids*	Regular bowel movements Active bowel sounds
High risk for ileus *r/t gastroparesis, pain medications*	Absence of nausea and vomiting
High risk for inadequate immunosuppression, rejection, or toxicity *r/t drug dosing or GI dysfunction*	Adequate immunosuppression per serum drug and CD3 levels *to prevent rejection and minimize side effects*
High risk for infection *r/t immunosuppression*	Infection prevented or minimized with help from prophylactic antibiotics
High risk for wound complications *r/t fluid accumulation, pancreatic weeping*	Usually abates 1 to 2 days after operation May continue for several weeks
High risk for duodenal graft complications or leak *r/t anastomotic site, bleeding, necrosis*	Resolution by conservative management and Foley catheter or surgical intervention Absence of abdominal pain and wound drainage
Hematuria *r/t biopsy procedures, exocrine drainage, bladder ulcers, or bleeding at site of anastomoses*	Hematuria self-limiting but if persistent, cystoscopy
High risk for urinary obstruction and reflux pancreatitis *r/t obstruction, hematuria, clogged Foley*	Obstruction avoided Foley drainage unobstructed

INTERVENTIONS

Encourage ambulation. *Muscle wasting can occur from corticosteroid administration in addition to bed rest. Ambulation will help maintain muscle strength.* Activity is advanced with physical therapy prn.

Measure daily postural blood pressure and pulse. *May indicate dehydration, diabetic vascular disease, or autonomic neuropathy.*

Assess skin turgor and mucous membranes.

Administer po or IV fluids up to 4 liters per day.

Monitor daily Hct, BUN, creatinine, HCO_3^-.

Continue intake and output.

Assess graft function by checking blood sugars, serum amylase, electrolytes, CBC and platelets regularly.

Collect timed urine for amylase BID and monitor results. *A decrease of 25% × 2 may indicate rejection.*

Monitor urine pH collections. *Amylase is alkaline and increases pH readings. With diminished pancreatic function may see decreased amylase, consequently a decrease in pH.*

Observe and report any signs and symptoms of rejection, including fever, allograft swelling and tenderness, decreased urinary amylase, decreased urine pH, increased glucose, decreased c-peptide and blood flow per nuclear scan, and increased creatinine (if kidney/pancreas).

Administer antirejection medications. *An increase in serum glucose can be caused by steroid-induced insulin resistance or an indication of late rejection; most likely, rejection cannot be reversed.*

NPO for 5 days to clear diet and advanced as tolerated by day 7. *TPN can cause hyperglycemia; therefore, limit dextrose content.*

Monitor serum albumin, prealbumin.

Assess food tolerance with start of regular diet and perform calorie counts. *Diet is liberalized from a diabetic and renal failure diet to a regular diet. Patients frequently have many questions.*

Plan of Care (cont'd)

Once bowel sounds are present, DC NG. *NG tube avoided if no history of gastroparesis.*

Provide adequate fluid and stool softeners *to prevent constipation which may cause intestinal perforation.*

Administer immunosuppressive therapy as ordered. *(Each transplant center is unique and protocols to manage immunosuppression may differ. One example to establish adequate immunosuppression and prevent rejection: antilymphocyte antibody such as ATGAM or OKT-3 beginning the day of surgery and qd, adjusted for leukopenia, methylprednisolone, azathioprine, cyclosporine started when creatinine is less than 2.5 mg/dl (if kidney/pancreas). Daily CsA trough levels at 200 to 300 whole blood HPLC. Discontinue antilymphocyte antibody therapy at 10 to 14 days when adequate CsA trough level.)*

Administer prophylactic antibiotics such as acyclovir, co-trimoxazole, and bactrim *to prevent secondary infections from immunosuppression.*

Infection control interventions same as intensive phase.

Wound drains if placed are removed over several days. Measure and record amount of wound drainage. Dressing reapplied if drainage present. Assess for signs of healing and infection.[3]

Observe for hematuria after cystoscopically directed biopsy procedure. Some hematuria is normal and should clear in 1 to 2 days. Some soreness of urethra may occur.

Foley catheter 7 to 10 days. Complete bladder emptying q2h *to keep decompressed.* Watch for urinary retention. Replace catheter if necessary.

Observe for symptoms of a duodenal leak: abdominal pain, distension, decreased urine output. Pain subsides with Foley catheter placement. *CT cystogram true positive indicates that the urine leaks from the bladder through a pinhole usually in the duodenal segment along the anastomosis into the abdomen. This complication can occur in about 10% of recipients but is significant and can account for a high rate of graft loss.*[15]

Monitor for hematuria *due to bleeding from duodenocystostomy.*

Monitor Hct, cystoscopy, and fulgaration of any bleeding sites, surgical repair of duodenal segment, conversion to Roux-en-y, or removal of graft.

Monitor for increased serum amylase and lower abdominal pain that abates with placement of a Foley catheter *due to reflux pancreatitis.*

TRANSITION TO DISCHARGE

The goal for discharge is to prepare the patient to be able to go home safely, be physically and psychologically ready, and be provided with support for long-term follow-up care. The patient needs to be well educated in self-care. This involves learning of medications, signs and symptoms of rejection and infection, infection control, diet, performing blood pressure and glucometer checks, keeping patient records, long-term follow-up clinic visits, activity, wound care, and what to do and whom to call if an emergency or problem arises.

The majority of the discharge teaching is done during the intermediate care phase of the hospitalization, with last-minute review a day or two before discharge. The largest cause of long-term graft failure in the renal transplant population is noncompliance. Usually, the recipient does not take his or her immunosuppressive medications or does not call when there may be a complication. Education is continued and reinforced in the outpatient clinic. It is helpful for the patient to also have written materials that he or she can refer to for information. Stress important information. Simply stating "I want you to listen carefully to this" will highlight for the patient what is most important.[10]

Involve family and significant others and evaluate learning. Stipulation must be given for the blind, deaf, or learning-impaired patient. Creative approaches to patient teaching may include Braille lettering on pill bottles, pill organizers, and digital or speaking thermometers or blood pressure machines.[36] Also, written materials need to be easy to read and the print should be larger because many diabetics have retinopathy and may have difficulty reading small print.

Family members can be extremely helpful in reinforcement of instruction, recognizing potential complications, and for psychosocial support. They should be encouraged to be involved as much as is appropriate. The transplant team social worker is also available to provide counseling and support. Support groups of transplant recipients to meet and exchange personal interactions, experiences, suggestions, and ideas can also be helpful to both patients and families.

The transplant recipient is generally observed in the outpatient setting 2 to 3 times per week for 2 to 3 months after transplant. Frequency of visits then declines to quarterly and then annually as long as the recipient is stable. The function of the graft is evaluated at each visit, and frequent laboratory testing is done to measure urinary and serum amylase, CBC, platelets, CsA trough levels and electrolytes. Glycosated Hgbs are tested every 3 months.

Nutrition is also assessed in the outpatient setting. Recipients follow a regular diet. Emphasis is placed on weight control and maintenance. Lipids are monitored and a low-cholesterol, low-fat diet is prescribed if necessary; otherwise there are no restrictions.

As an outpatient in long-term follow-up care, secondary complications of IDDM are monitored to see if each condition improves, worsens, or remains stable. Immunosuppression dosages are tapered over approximately 1 year to maintenance doses.

REFERENCES

1. Abell T, et al: Improvement in autonomic and GI function and gastric emptying in pancreas-kidney transplantation vs. kidney transplantation alone, *Jean Hamburger Memorial Congress* A 210, Paris, 1992.
2. Abendroth D, et al: Evidence for reversibility of diabetic microangiopathy following pancreas transplantation, *Transplant Proc* 21(1):2850-2851.
3. Bartucci MR, Loughman KA, Moir EJ: Kidney-pancreas transplantation: a treatment option of ESRD and type I diabetes, *ANNA Journal* 19(5):467-474, 1992.
4. Benjamini E, Leskowitz S: *Immunology, a short course,* ed 2, New York, 1991, John Wiley & Sons.
5. Bentley FR, Jung S, Garrison RN: Neuropathy and psychosocial adjustment after pancreas transplant in diabetics, *Transplant Proc* 22(2):691-695, 1990.
6. Cosimi AB, Conti DJ: Pancreas transplantation, *Compr Ther* 15(5):56-61, 1989.
7. Cunningham N, Boteler S, Windham S: Renal transplantation, *Crit Care Nurs Clin North Am* 4(1):79-88, 1992.
8. DeMayo E, et al: Pancreas transplantation. In *Nursing care of the transplant recipient,* Philadelphia, 1990, WB Saunders.
9. Donlan K, et al: Pancreas transplantation: a nursing overview, *Urol Nurs* 11(4):9-15, 1991.
10. Drumm DA, Schade DS: How communication disorders destabilize diabetes, *Clin Diabetes* 16-22, 1986.
11. Fisher J: Diabetics need not apply, *Diabetes Care* 12(2):659-660, 1989.
12. Frohnert PP, et al: Morbidity during the first year after pancreas transplantation, *Transplant Proc* 22(2):577, 1990.
13. Gross CR, Zehrer CL: Impact of the addition of a pancreas to quality of life in uremic diabetic recipients of kidney transplants, Jean Hamburger Memoral Congress A 140, Paris, 1992.
14. Groth C: Is there an indication for pancreatic transplantation? *Transplant Proc* 21(1):2757-2758, 1989.
15. Gruessner RWG, et al: Complication occurring after whole organ duodenopancreatic transplantation: relation to the allograft duodenal segment, *Transplant Proc* 22(2):578-579, 1990.
16. Hernandez C: The pathophysiology of diabetes mellitus: an update, *Diabetes Educator* 15(2):162-169, 1989.
17. Kelly WD, et al: Allotransplantation of the pancreas and duodenum along with the kidney in diabetic nephropathy, *Surgery* 61:827-837, 1967.
18. Kennedy W, et al: Effects of pancreatic transplantation on diabetic neuropathy, *N Engl J Med* 322(15):1031-1036, 1990.
19. Kreis H, Legendre C, Chatenoud L: OKT3 in organ transplantation, *Transplant Rev* 5(4):181-199, 1991.
20. Lafferty K, et al: Is there a future for fetal pancreas transplantation? *Transplant Proc* 21(1):2611-2613, 1989.
21. Marsh C, et al: Combined hepatic and pancreaticoduodenal procurement for transplantation, *Surg Gynecol Obstet* 168:254-258, 1989.
22. Marsh CL, et al: Pancreaticduodenal allograft procurement in combination with liver allograft procurement, *Transplant Proc* 21(1):2767-2768, 1989.
23. Mauer SM, et al: Pathology of diabetic nephropathy, *Complications Diabetes Mellitus* 95-102, 1989.
24. Molzahn A: Quality of life after organ transplantation, *J Adv Nurs* 16(9):1042-1047, 1991.
25. Perkins JD, et al: The value of cystoscopically directed biopsy in human pancreatic duodenal transplantation, *Clin Transplant* (3):306-315, 1989.
26. Perkins JD, et al: Pancreas transplantation at Mayo: II. Operative and perioperative management, *Mayo Clin Proc* 65:483-495, 1990.
27. Pozza G, et al: Endocrine responses of type 1 (insulin-dependent) diabetic patients following successful pancreas transplantation, *Diabetologia* 24:244-248, 1983.
28. Ricordi C, Starzl TE: Cellular transplants, *Transplant Proc* 23(1):73-76, 1991.
29. Sigardson-Poor K, Bartell L: *Nursing care of the transplant recipient,* Philadelphia, 1990, WB Saunders.
30. Sperling M, et al: *Physician's guide to insulin dependent (type 1) diabetes, diagnosis, and treatment,* Alexandria, Va, 1988, American Diabetes Association.
31. *St Anthony's DRG Guidebook,* 1995, Reston, Va, 1994, St Anthony.
32. Sutherland DER, Kendall DM, Moudry Munns KC: Pancreas transplantation in nonuremic type I diabetic recipients, *Surgery* 104:453-464, 1988.
33. Sutherland D: Coming of age for pancreas transplantation, *West J Med* 150(3):314-318, 1989.

34. Sutherland D: Who should get a pancreas transplant? *Diabetes Care* 11(8):681-685, 1988.
35. Tattersall R: Is pancreas transplantation for insulin-dependent diabetics worthwhile? *N Engl J Med* 321(2):112-114, 1989.
36. Trusler L: Management of the patient receiving simultaneous kidney-pancreas transplantation, *Crit Care Nurs Clin North Am* 4(1):89-95, 1992.
37. Tyden G, Groth C: Pancreas Transplantation. In Makowka, L, editor: *The handbook of transplantation management,* Austin, 1991, RG Landes, 300-321.
38. UNOS Research Department: Number of waiting list registrations and median waiting time (in days) to transplant, by organ 1988, 1989, 1990 and 1991, *UNOS Updates,* 9(1):29-30, 1993.
39. Van Der Vleit J, et al: The effect of pancreas transplantation on diabetic polyneuropathy, *Transplantation* 45(2):368-370, 1988.
40. Velosa J, et al: Pancreas transplantation at Mayo: I. Patient selection, *Mayo Clin Proc* 65:475-482, 1990.
41. Zehrer J, et al: When your diabetic patient has a pancreas transplant, *Nursing 88,* 18(3):108-109, 1988.

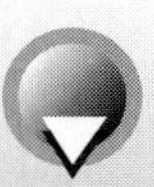

CLINICAL GUIDELINE

46

Liver Failure

Sandra A. Kucharski, MS, RN, CCRN

DESCRIPTION

Liver failure or hepatic failure are somewhat nonspecific terms used to describe a syndrome that manifests itself when the liver fails to carry out its broad range of metabolic responsibilities. It can result from an acute or chronic process.

Acute or fulminant hepatic failure is the term used to describe severe, acute liver failure associated with the development of hepatic encephalopathy within 2 to 8 weeks from the onset of jaundice in a patient without previous liver disease.

Chronic liver failure is characterized by continuous, progressive hepatocellular destruction that eventually leads to cirrhosis. Cirrhosis is a process in which the normal microcirculation, gross vascular anatomy, and hepatic architecture have been destroyed to varying degrees. It is characterized by structurally abnormal nodules in the liver, and an increase in fibrosis throughout the liver.

Liver failure is an important cause of prolonged morbidity and mortality with a significant socioeconomic impact. Liver disease is the fourth leading cause of death in persons aged 25 to 49 years in the United States, and it is estimated that the annual cost of delivering health care to patients with cirrhosis exceeds four billion dollars annually.[5]

PATHOPHYSIOLOGY

To facilitate an understanding of the principal manifestations of liver failure, major functions of the liver are presented in Table 46-1.[2]

The liver responds to injury in one of two ways. Either there is a process of vigorous, orderly, hepatic regeneration and normal structure and function are restored; or there is a process of disorderly regeneration resulting in disorganized structure and loss of function.[5] The type and severity of injury are important determinants of the type of regeneration, if any, that will occur.

The difference between acute and chronic liver failure is in the extent and rate of hepatocellular injury, and the degree of portal hypertension. Portal hypertension is a syndrome characterized by an increase in portal pressure above the normal range of 3 to 6 mm Hg.[10]

In fulminant hepatic failure, the injury is sudden and severe. Liver failure is due to massive hepatocellular necrosis and altered function of the hepatocyte. Fulminant hepatic failure can be caused by infections, such as viral hepatitis; drug reactions and toxins; vascular or ischemic injury, including shock; and other rare disorders.[9] Acute viral hepatitis is responsible for three fourths of all reported cases of fulminant hepatic failure each year, with an associated mortality rate of 70% to 90%.[3]

The pathophysiology of fulminant hepatic failure is not completely understood. The mechanisms responsible for the massive hepatocellular necrosis may vary with the etiology. Potential mechanisms include an immune-mediated mechanism for viral and infectious causes, a cytotoxic mechanism for drug- and toxin-related etiologies, and an ischemic mechanism for those conditions related to decreased hepatic perfusion.

In chronic liver disease, the manifestations of hepatic failure are due not only to altered hepatocyte function, but to the disorganized hepatic architecture as well. Cirrhosis is the terminal stage of chronic liver disease resulting from a variety of causes. These include persistent viral or parasitic infections, prolonged use of alcohol, exposure to drugs and toxins over time, primary disease of the intrahepatic ducts,

TABLE 46-1 Basic Functions of the Liver

Functions	Mechanism
• Metabolism of food substrates	
Carbohydrate metabolism	Stores glucose as glycogen (glycogenesis) Breaks down glycogen to form glucose (glucogenolysis) Forms glucose from some amino acids (gluconeogenesis) Secretes glucose into the blood
Lipid metabolism	Synthesizes cholesterol and triglycerides Excretes cholesterol in the bile Oxidizes fatty acids to produce energy
Protein metabolism	Forms new nonessential amino acids by transamination
• Synthesis of plasma proteins	Produces albumin and globulin Produces plasma transport proteins that transport steroid and thyroid hormones, vitamins, and cholesterol in the blood Produces clotting factors I (fibrinogen), II (prothrombin), V, VII, IX, X, XI, XIII
• Storage and metabolism of vitamins and minerals	Stores vitamin A, D, E, K, folic acid, selenium, copper, iron, vitamin B_{12} Activates vitamin D in conjuction with the kidney
• Detoxification of endogenous and exogenous materials	Phagocytosis by the Kupffer cells Detoxifies ethanol, bilirubin, ammonia Excretes cholesterol and other molecules in bile Produces urea, uric acid, and other molecules less toxic than parent substance Chemically alters hormones and drugs
• Secretion of bile	Secretes bile into the hepatic ducts

and certain inborn errors of metabolism such as hemochromatosis and Wilson's disease.

In cirrhosis, there are progressive changes in the cell populations and in the composition and distribution of connective tissue, or extracellular matrix.[8] The extracellular matrix is composed of collagens, noncollagenous proteins, and glycoaminoglycans. Normally, there are repetitive cycles of synthesis and degradation in the extracellular matrix.

During hepatic injury, there is an increase in the production and release of cytokines or growth factors causing a transformation and proliferation of lipocytes (fat-storing or Ito cells). The result is that collagen synthesis is increased and collagen degradation is decreased. In addition, there is a change in the type of collagen produced and the location where it is deposited.[8] The extracellular matrix is replaced by a pathological matrix characterized by a distorted lobular and vascular architecture, changes in portal hemodynamics, and disturbances in hepatic microcirculation resulting in impaired liver function.

The clinical manifestations of hepatic failure include those resulting from liver dysfunction (encephalopathy, coagulopathy, portal hypertension, ascites, jaundice, infection, malnutrition) as well as complications occurring in other organ systems. Major complications of fulminant hepatic failure and chronic liver failure are listed in the following Box.

Hepatic encephalopathy is a complex neuropsychiatric syndrome characterized by changes in personality, intellect, neuromuscular function, and level of consciousness. The pathogenesis of hepatic encephalopathy is obscure. Hypotheses have been proposed suggesting that plasma and cerebral accumulation of ammonia, synergistic actions of multiple neurotoxins, alteration in the concentration of neurotransmitter substances, or the gama-aminobutyric acid/benzodiazepine receptor complex (GABA/BZ) may be involved.[1]

In the early stages of hepatic encephalopathy, the patient may demonstrate subtle personality changes, fluctuating moods, and a decreased attention span. If the encephalopathy progresses, there is impairment of motor and intellectual functions, confusion, and disorientation. With further progression, stupor and coma are seen.

In fulminant hepatic failure, hepatic encephalopathy is related more to hepatic insufficiency than to portal systemic shunting of blood. Also, the encephalopathy associated with fulminant hepatic failure can be complicated by increased intracranial pressure and cerebral edema, a picture rarely seen in chronic liver disease.

Major Complications of Liver Failure

- Hepatic encephalopathy
- Coagulopathy
- Portal hypertension
- Gastrointestinal (GI) bleeding
- Functional renal failure
- Infection
- Impaired nutrient metabolism

The liver has a primary role in maintaining hemostasis. It synthesizes factors I (fibrinogen), II (prothrombin), V, VII, IX, X, XI, and XIII; fibrinolytic factors, which are inhibitors of coagulation; and vitamin K.[3] With severe hepatocellular necrosis there is impaired synthesis of these coagulation factors. In fulminant hepatic failure, levels of plasminogen activator and plasminogen are reduced, and levels of fibrin and fibrin degradation products are increased. Platelet counts less than 80,000 per mm^3 are often seen. Circulating platelets are smaller than normal, in both size and number, suggesting an impaired release of new platelets from the bone marrow and delayed clearance of old platelets by the reticuloendothelial system. There are abnormalities in both platelet aggregation and adhesion.[9]

Portal hypertension is a syndrome characterized by an increase in portal pressure above the normal range of 3 to 6 mm Hg,[7] and the formation of collateral vessels which shunt portal blood into the systemic circulation. Portal hypertension is associated with splanchnic and peripheral vasodilatation, with decreased arterial pressure and decreased peripheral resistance.

In cirrhosis, the distorted hepatic vascular bed leads to increased intrahepatic resistance, causing an increased resistance to portal blood flow that results in an increase in portal pressure. Clinically significant portal hypertension develops when the difference between the portal pressure and the inferior vena cava pressure (the portal pressure gradient) is raised above 12 mm Hg. This leads to the formation of collateral vessels in areas where veins draining the portal system are juxtaposed to veins draining the inferior vena cava. These areas include the submucosa of the esophagus, the stomach, the rectum, and the abdominal wall. This collateral circulation shunts up to 80% of the blood into systemic veins, thereby reducing resistance to portal flow. Although portal pressure is decreased through shunting, portal hypertension is maintained by an increase in portal blood flow, the result of a marked arteriolar vasodilatation in splanchnic organs draining the portal vein.

The development of portal hypertension is significant for two reasons. First, because blood is shunted away from the liver, the detoxifying and filtering functions of the liver are bypassed. As a result, gut-derived antigens, bacteria, drugs, and gut hormones may enter systemic circulation. Second, bleeding from esophageal and/or gastric varices may result. The precise mechanism that triggers varices to bleed is not well understood, but is thought to be related to portal pressures greater than 12 mm Hg.[7] Bleeding from esophageal or gastric varices is a major complication of portal hypertension.

Gastrointestinal (GI) bleeding is another complication of both fulminant hepatic failure and chronic liver disease, although the etiology of each differs. In fulminant hepatic failure, bleeding is related to a coagulopathy; in chronic liver disease, bleeding is due primarily to portal hypertension, and complicated by coagulopathy.

Ascites is the accumulation of excess fluid in the peritoneal space and is associated with pronounced renal sodium retention. It is seen most often in patients with advanced cirrhosis and portal hypertension and implies a poor prognosis.

Complex pathophysiologic mechanisms are involved in ascites formation. These include a distorted hepatic vasculature, resulting in sinusoidal portal hypertension; decreased oncotic pressure from inadequate hepatic synthesis of albumin; increased hepatic lymph production; leakage of hepatic and intestinal lymphatics; and splanchnic venous pooling and peripheral vasodilation.[4]

Ascites formation progressively depletes intravascular volume, which in turn activates intrathoracic and arterial mechanoreceptors, signalling the kidneys to retain salt and water. Salt and water replenish the vascular space and permit continuous ascites formation, creating a vicious cycle.

A progessive oliguric renal failure, better known as hepatorenal syndrome, often complicates severe liver failure. This functional renal failure is characterized by reduced glomerular filtration rate, concentrated urine, and low urinary sodium.

The pathogenesis of the hepatorenal syndrome is not known. Morphological changes in the kidneys that usually account for typical functional disturbances seen with acute renal failure are minimal or inconsistent. Frequently, hepatorenal syndrome is precipitated by treatment measures or other complications that reduce effective blood volume; e.g., aggressive diuretic therapy, lactulose administration, paracentesis, GI tract bleeding, sepsis, or surgery. It can, however, occur without a clearly defined precipitating event.

Spontaneous bacteremia often complicates severe liver disease and can prove fatal in and of itself, or as a precipitant of hepatic encephalopathy, GI tract hemorrhage, or functional renal failure.

The liver plays a major role in host defense. Almost 90% of the reticuloendothelial system is located within the liver. It includes Kupffer cells, which clear the blood of potentially harmful substances such as bacteria and gut-derived endotoxins from the portal system.

A significant consequence of fulminant hepatic failure and chronic liver disease is depression of the hepatic reticuloendothelial system. Susceptibility to infection may also be related to impaired synthesis of complement, altered polymorphonuclear leukocyte function, and decreased neutrophil adherence.

Jaundice is clinically manifested by a yellowish discoloration of the skin, mucous membranes, and plasma. The pathogenesis of jaundice in both fulminant hepatic failure and chronic liver disease is related to inability of the liver cells to conjugate bilirubin.

Jaundice is a hallmark manifestation of fulminant hepatic failure; however, in chronic liver disease, it usually is accompanied by other signs of hepatic failure (ascites, coagulopathy, and encephalopathy). When jaundice is associated with other signs of hepatic failure, the severity of the jaundice generally is directly proportional to the severity of liver disease.

Since the liver plays such a central role in the initial handling of many nutrients, alterations in carbohydrate, lipid, protein, and vitamin metabolism are seen frequently.

In fulminant hepatic failure and advanced chronic liver disease, hypoglycemia is observed. It is related to either a failure of gluconeogenesis or decreased glycogenolysis.

In chronic liver disease, hepatic fibrosis impairs glycogenesis, and hyperglycemia is seen. Portosystemic shunting, impaired hepatic degradation, and increased concentrations of ammonia and amino acids stimulate glucagon secretion, causing an increase in plasma glucagon levels. Insulin levels are increased, resulting in part from hepatic degradation. Although plasma insulin levels are elevated, they are not increased in proportion to glucagon, so there is a decrease in the effective insulin-glucagon ratio. This results in catabolism of skeletal muscle and hepatic gluconeogenesis.

Ketone production is decreased in chronic liver disease. A significant reduction in ketone production deprives the tissues of an important source of energy and can worsen malnutrition.

In addition, there are increased levels of aromatic amino acids because of reduced hepatic clearance and the catabolism of skeletal muscle. There is also a decrease in plasma levels of branched-chain amino acids. It is hypothesized that changes in amino acid concentrations cause disturbances in neurotransmission and contribute to the pathogenesis of hepatic encephalopathy.

Patients with chronic liver disease often have low levels of folate, thiamine, and vitamin B_{12}, as well as deficiencies of the fat-soluble vitamins A, D, E, and K. These vitamin and mineral deficiencies are related to poor diet, alterations in the metabolism of precursors, and malabsorption. Clinically, the consequences of these vitamin and mineral deficiencies are manifested as bleeding tendencies (vitamin K), bone disorders (vitamin D), peripheral neuropathy (thiamine), and megaloblastic anemia (folate and vitamin B_{12}).

LENGTH OF STAY/ANTICIPATED COURSE

There are no statistically reliable criteria to help predict anticipated courses or responses to treatment. There are, however, several classification systems that quantify the severity of liver disease.

Child's classification (grades A, B, C), introduced to assess operative risk in patients with liver disease, is based on five variables—serum bilirubin levels, serum albumin levels, the absence or extent of ascites, encephalopathy, and nutrition. Each parameter in grade A is given one point, in grade B two points, in grade C three points, and a score is totaled. There are two problems with this grading system: (1) patient findings may be a mix of variables from grades A, B, and C; and (2) observers may disagree about the subjective criteria of ascites, encephalopathy, and nutritional status.

The Pugh system is a modification of the Child grading system. Nutritional status was deleted from the Child criteria, and prolongation of prothrombin time (PT) was added. Each criterion is allotted either one, two, or three points depending on the results, and again the points are totaled to give a score. The Pugh score has some short-term prognostic value in patients with cirrhosis.

Length of stay for patients with hepatic failure is directly related to the underlying etiology, the patient's age, the presence of other preexisting medical conditions, and the occurrence of complications. Hepatic failure requiring intensive care often is associated with multisystem organ failure and high mortality.

Liver failure falls within DRG 202: Cirrhosis and alcoholic hepatitis; DRG 205: Disorders of the liver except malignancy/cirrhosis and alcoholic with complications; and DRG 206: Disorders of the liver except malignancy/cirrhosis and alcoholic without complications. The average lengths of stay are 8.7 days, 8.4 days, and 4.6 days, respectively.[11]

MANAGEMENT TRENDS AND CONTROVERSIES

The cornerstone of treatment in liver failure is supportive care. Management of hepatic encephalopathy is directed toward normalizing the patient's mental status. Precipitating factors such as electrolyte and acid-base disturbances, hypoglycemia, hypoxia, anemia, hypotension, hemorrhage, infection, and renal failure must be identified and corrected. Measures then are taken to decrease the body's nitrogenous load by minimizing absorption from the GI tract.

Lactulose, which promotes fecal nitrogen excretion, is given three to four times daily to produce two to four stools per day. During lactulose therapy, it is important to monitor electrolyte and volume status to avoid hyponatremia and dehydration. Neomycin is often administered in combination with lactulose to treat hepatic encephalopathy. By suppressing bacterial flora in the intestine, biotransformation of nitrogenous substances in the intestine is reduced. Neomycin is given orally, enterally, or by retention enema two to three times daily. However, since neomycin can cause ototoxicity and nephrotoxicity, lactulose is the preferred drug.

Cerebral edema is treated with osmotic diuretics in an effort to decrease intracranial pressure. Nursing measures to minimize increases in intracranial pressure should also be instituted. (See Guideline 1.)

Symptomatic coagulopathy associated with liver failure may be treated with vitamin K, fresh frozen plasma, and platelets. Nursing interventions directed at preventing injury related to coagulopathy are also a priority.

Acute variceal bleeding is managed with IV infusions of vasopressin. Vasopressin is used to constrict splanchnic arterioles, increase resistance to blood flow to the gut, and reduce portal pressure. Nitroglycerin often is used concomitantly with vasopressin because it enhances portal pressure reduction through vasodilation of collateral vessels, ameliorates the vasoconstrictor-related side effects of vasopressin, and causes a systemic vasodilatation with reflex splanchnic vasoconstriction resulting in decreased portal blood flow.

Sclerosing agents such as sodium tetradecyl, sodium morrhuate, ethanolamine, and ethanol can be injected directly into the varices via endoscopy to control variceal bleeding. Blood products are transfused as needed.

Propranolol is the most commonly used agent for chronic management of portal hypertension. It reduces portal venous pressure and the risk of the first and recurrent episodes of variceal hemorrhage in patients with cirrhosis.

Surgically created portosystemic shunts are no longer frequently used as the leader in the management of portal hypertension due to the increasing use of sclerotherapy, pharmacotherapy, and hepatic transplantation. Shunts, which divert all or part of the portal blood flow away from the liver, lower portal pressure and are effective in prevention of recurrent variceal hemorrhage. However, they are adversely associated with post-shunt hepatic failure and encephalopathy.

The mainstays of therapy for patients with ascites are sodium and water retention and diuretics. Therapeutic paracentesis may be performed. Hepatorenal syndrome usually does not reverse itself unless liver injury improves. In fulminant hepatic failure, ultrafiltration and hemodialysis may be used until hepatocellular regeneration occurs. In chronic liver disease, treatment is directed toward early correction of intravascular volume deficits to improve renal function.

There is no specific device or technique to provide temporary support to the failing liver. Liver transplantation has evolved as the major therapeutic intervention for patients with fulminant hepatic failure and chronic advanced liver disease. Despite its success as a life-saving procedure, liver transplantation remains controversial when considered for patients with alcoholic liver disease, viral hepatitis, or neoplastic disease of the liver.[6,12] Although rare, primate-to-human xenotransplantation of the liver has also sparked controversy, since it involves sacrifice of the primate to obtain the donor organ.

ASSESSMENT

PARAMETER	ANTICIPATED ALTERATION
Patient History	
Exposure	Environmental or occupational exposure to toxins or synthetic chemicals Recent use of prescription, nonprescription, or illicit drugs. Evidence of an allergic drug reaction. Contact with persons with viral hepatitis
Travel	Recent travel to underdeveloped countries
Transfusions/injections	Recent blood transfusions, injections, needle use, tatoos, dental work
Alcohol	Past or present history of prolonged and excessive alcohol consumption
Anesthetic agents	Halothane or methoxyflurane
Physical Exam	
Neurologic	Hepatic encephalopathy *due to diminished hepatic function, increased ammonia levels* Asterixis: an irregular, flaplike tremor of the hands *due to metabolic abnormalities*
Cardiac	Tachycardia: HR >100 bpm *due to vasodilatation, sepsis, ARDS, hypotension* Systolic hypotension *due to vasodilatation* Increased CI, CO, decreased SVR *thought to be due to circulating vasodilators*
Pulmonary	Hypoxia *due to formation of arteriovenous shunts; pulmonary vasodilatation; ventilation perfusion mismatch*

	Tachypnea: RR >20/min *due to ascites* Hypocapnia *due to increased central nervous system sensitivity to ammonia; hypoxia; increased levels of lactate and pyruvate; hypokalemia* Pleural effusions *due to protein malnutrition; leak from the abdominal cavity to the pleural cavity*
Metabolic	Fever: T >38° C *due to infection; sometimes of unknown etiology*
GI	Abdominal distension *due to ascites*
Skin	Jaundice *due to impaired bilirubin metabolism* Edema, ascites *due to decreased oncotic pressure* Spider angiomas on face, neck, forearms, and dorsum of the hands. "Paper money skin" (numerous small vessels randomly scattered through skin). Palmar and plantar erythema. *The cause of these vascular abnormalities is unknown.* Excessive bruising *due to coagulopathy* Pruritis *due to metabolic abnormalities*

Laboratory Studies

Serum total bilirubin	Increased: >1.0 mg/dl *due to inability of liver to conjugate bilirubin*
Aspartate aminotransferase (AST: formerly SGOT)	Increased: >40 IU/L *due to increased permeability of cell membrane, or hepatocellular necrosis*
Alanine aminotransferase (ALT: formerly SGPT)	Increased: >35 IU/L *due to hepatocellular necrosis*
Albumin	Decreased: <3.2 g/dl *due to decreased synthesis of albumin*
Globulin	Decreased: <2.3 g/dl *due to decreased protein synthesis*
Total protein	Decreased: <6 g/dl *due to decreased protein synthesis*
PT	Prolonged: >12.5 sec *due to deficiency of factors II, V, VII, and X*
Blood ammonia	Normal or increased: >110 μg/dl *due to increased amino acids*
Alkaline phosphatase	Increased: >85 ImU/ml *due to reduced excretion in bile*
BUN	Decreased: <10 mg/dl *due to inability of the liver to produce urea from nitrogen* Increased: >20 mg/dl *due to functional renal failure*
Creatinine	Increased: >1.2 mg/dl *due to decreased excretion by kidney in hepatorenal syndrome*
K^+	Decreased: <3.5 mEq/L *due to diuretic therapy, lactulose therapy, NG suction, or vomiting*
Na^+	Decreased: <136 mEq/L *due to hemodilution*
Ca^{++}	Decreased: <9.0 mg/dl *due to hemodilution or large-volume blood transfusions*
Urine Na^+	Decreased: <40 mEq/L/day *due to inability of kidneys to concentrate urine*

Imaging

Ultrasound	Obstruction or dilatation of portal vein, altered intrahepatic anatomy, ascites, neoplastic or inflammatory masses
CT scan	Changes in liver size, shape, and parenchymal density
Liver biopsy	Macroscopic and microscopic changes in hepatic architecture, fibrosis, fatty infiltration, inflammation

PLAN OF CARE

INTENSIVE PHASE

The primary goal of the intensive phase is to manage the patient's fluid balance, prevent complications related to liver dysfunction, and support the failing liver.

Plan of Care (cont'd)

PATIENT CARE PRIORITIES	EXPECTED PATIENT OUTCOMES
High risk for fluid volume deficit *r/t active fluid loss (overly aggressive diuresis, variceal bleeding, diarrhea)*	Moist mucous membranes Normal skin turgor Balanced I/O Absence or resolution of bleeding Normal or improved Hgb and Hct
Excess fluid volume *r/t hypoproteinemia*	Improved albumin levels Normal or improved serum and urine electrolytes and osmolarity Decreased edema, ascites Improved cardiac filling pressures Abdominal girth remains stable or decreases in size
High risk for impaired breathing pattern *r/t ascites, encephalopathy, GI bleeding*	Normal or improved breathing pattern Pa_{O_2} and Pa_{CO_2} levels: WNL
High risk for coagulation abnormalities *r/t decreased hepatic synthesis of clotting factors*	No undetected bleeding PT: WNL APTT: WNL
High risk for infection *r/t depression of the reticuloendothelial system, invasive treatments and procedures*	No signs/symptoms of infection WBC: WNL Cultures demonstrate no growth, or normal flora

INTERVENTIONS

Monitor Hct, emesis, stools, NG aspirate, BP, HR *to detect loss of blood.*
Administer IV fluids, blood, and blood products *to restore intravascular volume.*
Monitor intake and output q1h *to prevent hypovolemia.*
Assist with insertion of gastroesophageal balloon tube and monitor for potential complications, i.e.:

- Aspiration of gastric contents *due to collection of secretions, above the esophageal balloon*
- Ischemic necrosis of the esophagus *due to prolonged inflation of the esophageal balloon*
- Laryngeal obstruction *due to upward migration of the esophageal balloon*

Administer IV vasopressin and monitor for ischemia, MI, and small-bowel necrosis *due to the vasoconstrictor effects of the drug.*
Administer antacids and H_2 blockers *to reduce risk of GI bleeding.*
Prepare the patient for endoscopic variceal sclerosis if planned.
Restrict sodium and fluid intake *to prevent dilutional hyponatremia.*
Administer diuretics judiciously *as overly aggressive diuresis can lead to dehydration, acute tubular necrosis, and hepatorenal syndrome.*
Administer salt-poor albumin *to enhance osmotic pull and movement of ascitic fluid into the intravascular space.*
Assist with paracentesis and monitor for hypovolemia and shock post-procedure *as removal of a large volume of fluid from the peritoneal space can cause fluid to shift from the intravascular space into the peritoneal cavity.*
Measure abdominal girth *to monitor progression of ascites.*
Administer positive inotropic agents *to improve CO and renal perfusion.*
Limit drugs metabolized by the liver *to decrease the demands on the liver.*
Monitor CVP, PCWP, CO, CI, SVR *to determine hemodynamic status and response to treatment.*
Maintain bed rest *to decrease the metabolic demands of the liver.*
Elevate the head of the bed *to relieve pressure on the diaphragm due to ascites.*
Encourage the patient to cough and deep breathe, and reposition the patient q1h to q2h *to facilitate full diaphragmatic excursion and lung expansion.*
Administer supplemental O_2 as ordered *to maintain Pa_{O_2} WNL.*

Plan of Care (cont'd)

Administer analgesics that do not cause respiratory depression *to prevent further impairment of breathing pattern.*

Assess for dyspnea, tachypnea, and shallow breathing, *which would indicate hypoxemia or hypercapnia.*

Monitor T and WBC *to assess for signs of infection.*

Obtain culture specimens as indicated and monitor the results *to determine the presence of an infection.*

Avoid injections *to prevent bleeding into the tissues.*

Administer vitamin K *to aid in the synthesis of prothrombin.*

Provide a safe environment *to prevent trauma and hematoma formation.*

Monitor PT, APTT, Hgb, Hct, and platelet levels *to determine extent of coaguloapathy.*

INTERMEDIATE PHASE

The primary goal of the intermediate phase is to manage the precipients of liver failure and prevent further hepatic decompensation.

PATIENT CARE PRIORITIES	EXPECTED PATIENT OUTCOMES
High risk for altered thought processes *r/t hepatic encephalopathy*	Improved mentation, LOC, behavior, neuromuscular functioning Ammonia levels: WNL
High risk for progressive liver failure *r/t viral hepatitis or infection; drug reaction or exposure to toxins*	Increased albumin Decreased AST/ALT Decreased bilirubin Absence of clotting abnormalities, encephalopathy
High risk for inadequate nutrition *r/t impaired nutrient metabolism*	Sufficient protein intake for hepatic regeneration Stable or improved blood ammonia levels Absence of hepatic encephalopathy

INTERVENTIONS

Avoid dietary indiscretion, infection, dehydration, sedatives, tranquilizers, narcotics, acid-base and electrolyte disturbances, and aggressive diuresis *which can increase ammonia production.*

Administer lactulose as ordered *to promote the excretion of nitrogen.*

Administer neomycin as ordered *to decrease nitrogen-forming intestinal bacteria.*

Administer a low-protein diet (40 g/day or less) *to maintain nitrogen balance.*

Monitor plasma ammonia levels to titrate protein intake *so as not to increase ammonia to unacceptable levels.*

Maintain a safe environment using physical restraint as needed *to protect the patient from harm.*

Reorient the patient frequently to time, place, and person, and explain procedures simply and clearly *to elicit cooperation.*

Avoid administering drugs that are metabolized primarily in the liver *to minimize demands placed on the liver.*

Assess for progressive jaundice and encephalopathy as it *indicates worsening liver function.*

Monitor changes in serum bilirubin, albumin, transaminase levels, and PT, which may *indicate deterioration in the metabolic and synthetic functions of the liver.*

Assist with liver biopsy.

Titrate dietary protein intake to toleration for nitrogen load and administer one half of the total calories as carbohydrates *to spare protein.*

Consider the patient's food preferences. Offer foods in four to six small meals daily *to encourage food intake.*

Administer vitamin and mineral supplements as ordered *to correct vitamin and mineral deficiencies.*

TRANSITION TO DISCHARGE

During the transition to discharge, nursing care is directed toward patient and family education. Generally, the patient and family will need information about dietary and fluid restrictions, drug therapy, and signs and symptoms to report to the physician. These include hematemesis, melena, weight gain, edema, increased abdominal girth, infection or fever, changes in mentation or behavior, and jaundice, all of which may herald hepatic decompensation. Patients whose liver dysfunction is related to alcohol use should be instructed to avoid alcohol; referral to a detoxification program may be indicated. The patient also should be instructed to avoid any drugs not prescribed by the physician, including over-the-counter drugs such as analgesics. The discharge setting should be evaluated and home care services arranged as needed.

REFERENCES

1. Basile AS, Jones EA, Skolnick P: The pathogenesis and treatment of hepatic encephalopathy: evidence for the involvement of benzodiazepine receptor ligands, *Pharamacol Rev* 43:27-71, 1991.
2. Basman N, Baker A: Basic functions of the liver. In Gitnick G, editor: *Diseases of the liver and biliary tract,* St Louis, 1992, Mosby–Year Book, p 39.
3. Douglas D, Rakela J: Fulminant hepatitis. In Kaplowitz N, editor: *Liver and biliary diseases,* Baltimore, 1992, Williams & Wilkins, p 279.
4. Dudley FJ: Pathophysiology of ascites formation, *Gastroenterol Clin North Am* 21:215-235, 1992.
5. Gressner AM: Liver fibrosis: perspectives in pathobiochemical research and clinical outlook, *Eur J Clin Chem Clin Biochem* 29:293-311, 1991.
6. Lucey MR, Beresford TP: Alcoholic liver disease: to transplant or not to transplant? *Alcohol Alcohol* 27:103-108, 1992.
7. MacArthur P: The pathogenesis of variceal rupture, *Gastrointest Endosc Clin North Am* 2:1-15, 1992.
8. Rajkind M, Greenwel P: Pathophysiology of liver fibrosis. In Gitnick G, editor: *Diseases of the Liver and Biliary Tract,* Boston, 1992, Mosby–Year Book, p 707-716.
9. Shanna CB, Gollan JL: Fulminant hepatic failure. In Taylor MB, editor: *Gastrointestinal emergencies,* Baltimore, 1992, Williams & Wilkins, pp 227, 235.
10. Scholnerich J: Portal hypertension in chronic liver disease, *Hepatogastroenterology* 38:346-348, 1991.
11. *St Anthony's DRG working guidebook 1995,* Reston, Va, 1994, St Anthony.
12. Van Thiel DH, et al: Liver transplantation for alcoholic liver disease, viral hepatitis, and hepatic neoplasms, *Transplant Proc* 23:1917-1921, 1991.

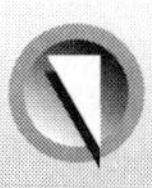

TRANSPLANT GUIDELINE

47

Liver Transplantation

Mary A. Doucet, MS, RN, CCRN

DESCRIPTION

Death from end-stage liver disease affects more than 26,000 people annually and is one of the leading causes of death in the United States.[6] Liver transplantation is generally considered the treatment of choice for patients with end-stage liver disease who are unresponsive to medical management and without contraindications to the procedure.[9,16]

In 1963, Starzl performed the first human liver transplant.[21] Initial survival rates were poor and did not improve until the advent of cyclosporine in the 1980s. The availability of effective immunosuppressive agents, along with advances in surgical techniques and organ preservation, have contributed to improved survival. One-year survival rates have been reported to be as high as 91%[12] and as low as 45%.[5] Factors that may affect patient survival are age, physical condition, and diagnosis at the time of transplantation. Two-, three-, and five-year survival rates are reported to be between 75% and 85%.[9,20]

In 1990, 2656 liver transplants were performed in the United States.[9] Estimations of the number of people who could benefit from liver transplantation are over 15,000 people a year. However, as organ donation rates stabilize, waiting lists continue to grow.

PATIENT SELECTION

Potential donors must meet certain criteria at the time of death to be considered for organ donation. Urine, blood, and sputum cultures are performed to rule out infection. The donor's liver is assessed for traumatic injury, and liver function is measured by blood chemistries, enzymes, bilirubin, and clotting factors. The major considerations for matching donor and recipient are body size and blood type. The donor's weight should be within 20 pounds of the recipient's weight in order to accommodate the transplanted donor liver. Donor and recipient ABO blood groups are the only histocompatibility requirements. The ideal match for liver graft survival is an identical ABO. However, in emergency situations, livers have been transplanted across ABO groups.[11] A major problem associated with crossing ABO groups is graft-versus-host disease (GVHD). GVHD is due to passive transfer of donor lymphocytes in the allograft that produce antibodies against the recipient's ABO antigens.[4] This hemolytic process is usually self-limiting, does not injure the allograft, and can be medically treated.[16]

Patient selection and evaluation for transplantation is based on a multidisciplinary assessment. The assessment includes the patient's level of liver dysfunction, degree of hepatic deterioration, and psychological and psychosocial suitability.[16] The most frequent indications for transplant are listed in the following Box.

PROCEDURE

Two surgical approaches have been used. In the first approach, heterotopic liver transplant, an additional liver is grafted into a human without removing the diseased liver. In orthotopic transplantation, the most common and technically difficult surgery, the diseased liver is removed and replaced with a donor liver (allograft).

Before the surgery, large-bore IV catheters are inserted for rapid fluid replacement, along with arterial and pulmonary artery lines for pressure and fluid management. The incision is made in two parts: bilateral subcostal abdominal and a midline incision extending up to the xiphoid.

The diseased liver is dissected until the vena cava, hepatic

Indications for Liver Transplantation

- Chronic active hepatitis
- Primary and secondary biliary cirrhosis
- Biliary atresia
- Sclerosing cholangitis
- Chronic viral, drug, autoimmune, or alcoholic-induced liver disease
- Portal vein thrombosis (Budd-Chiari syndrome)
- Primary hepatic malignancies
- Fulminant hepatic failure (viral, drug, or metabolic disease)
- Metabolic liver disease

artery, portal vein, and biliary system are clearly identified. Then the portal vein is clamped and the inferior vena cava is clamped above and below the liver, interrupting venous return to the heart.[12] A veno–venous bypass system is used to prevent hemodynamic instability and portal hypertension during this phase. The system consists of a centrifugal blood pump and large-bore cannulation of femoral and axillary veins to shunt blood away from the operative area and back to the heart.[11] Once the veno–venous system is activated, it is maintained throughout the hepatectomy and graft procedure.

The diseased liver is removed, the allograft is inserted, and an arterial anastomosis, three venous anastomoses, and biliary duct reconstruction are completed. The biliary duct can be anastomosed in one of two ways: common bile duct to common bile duct with a T-tube stent (Figure 47-1*A*) (choledochocholedochostomy) and common bile duct to jejunum (Roux-en-Y choledochojejunostomy) (Fig. 47-1*B*). Common bile duct to common bile duct anastomoses is the preferred method and is used when no anatomical or ductal disease exists. Before the abdomen is closed, two or three Jackson–Pratt drains are inserted under the diaphragm and near the biliary anastomosis and placed outside the wound. These drains remain in place for 3 to 4 days following surgery. The T-tube stent, inserted in the common bile duct, is brought out through a stab wound and allowed to drain for 4 to 6 weeks after surgery.

The surgery takes approximately 8 to 15 hours to complete. Complications that can occur during and after surgery are related to hematologic, metabolic, anastomotic, and circulatory problems. Two major threats to postoperative recovery are rejection and infection. Mild to moderate acute rejection is usually seen 7 to 15 days after transplant in 30% to 70% of patients.[1] Acute rejection, diagnosed by laboratory and liver biopsy studies, indicates allograft dysfunction and is initially treated with steroids.[11]

Long-term immunosuppression to prevent rejection puts these patients at risk for developing bacterial, fungal, or viral infections after liver transplant. Common types of bacterial infections seen in this patient population are pneumonia, abdominal abscess, and bacterial cholangitis. In general, prophylactic broad-spectrum antibiotic therapy is given in the immediate postoperative period and specific antibiotic therapy is initiated once the organism has been identified through culture results.

Oral fungal infections are usually associated with patients receiving immunosuppressants and antibacterial drugs and are treated with Mycostatin oral suspension. Fungal sepsis is usually related to a long operative time with bowel manipulation and is treated with Amphotericin B.[11] Opportunistic viruses such as herpes virus and cytomegalovirus (CMV) cause significant infections in liver transplant patients.[10] Herpes virus is treated with acyclovir. At present, there is no specific drug treatment for CMV. Prophylaxis of CMV with acyclovir and treatment of CMV with ganciclovir are currently being investigated.[10]

LENGTH OF STAY/ANTICIPATED COURSE

The patient should be assessed for signs of infections and rejection. A low-grade temperature, pulmonary congestion, inflamed incision or positive culture reports from blood, invasive lines, bile, or urine drainage may indicate the presence of infection. A sudden change in the color or consistency of bile, urine, stool, or the presence of jaundice, general malaise, low-grade temperature, a rise in serum bilirubin after a downward trend, and a rise in alkaline phosphatase may suggest allograft dysfunction.[11] A liver biopsy is necessary to confirm rejection.

The length of stay after liver transplantation is usually 3 to 4 weeks. If the allograft is functioning normally, signs and symptoms of end-stage liver disease should gradually be reversed.

Liver transplantation falls within DRG 480: Liver Transplant, with an approximate LOS of 34.7 days.[17]

MANAGEMENT TRENDS AND CONTROVERSIES

Current management trends in liver transplantation are directed toward developing transplant protocols for specific liver disease based on indices that would predict the best time for transplantation and improve outcomes,[5,9,15] producing safe and effective immunosuppressive therapy, and developing new surgical procedures to help alleviate the shortage of organs.

The current immunosuppressive therapy regimen used in many centers for liver transplant patients consists of cyclosporine, prednisone, and azathioprine. In spite of this therapy, the incidence of acute rejection ranges from 30% to 70%,[1] and is conventionally treated with steroid boluses. Steroid-resistant rejection that is diagnosed by a liver biopsy is usually treated with the T-cell specific antigen, monoclonal antibody, OKT3.[11] Two new drugs that are being used for "rescue" therapy in persistent rejection are FK 506,

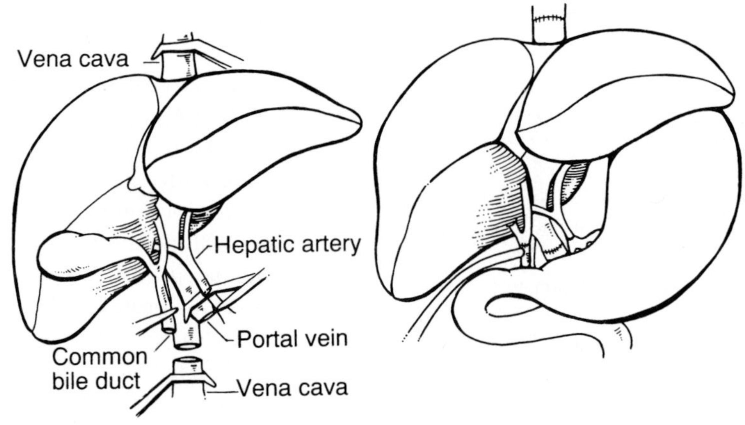

Figure 47-1 Sites of vascular and biliary anastomosis of recipient graft during liver transplantation.

a relatively new drug that reduces the immunoregulatory cytokine IL-2 that may correlate with rejection, and RS 61443, an antimetabolite that affects lymphocytes.[1,2]

New operative procedures have been developed to help with the shortage of organs. Examples include reduced-size liver allograft to facilitate placement of a larger liver into a smaller recipient, and the split-grafting technique (using a single donor organ for two recipients).[2,5,8] Other controversial techniques are being investigated, such as living-related-donor liver grafts[3] (resecting 35% or less of a related adult donor liver and grafting it into a child with end-stage liver disease)[18]; and xenografting (using organ or tissue from a different species), such as baboon donor livers, as an alternative to the ever-increasing human donation organ shortage.[2,14,19]

ASSESSMENT

PARAMETER	ANTICIPATED ALTERATION
Cardiovascular Status	
HR	Tachycardia: >100 bpm *due to sympathetic stimulation related to stress of surgery*
Rhythm	Potential for ventricular ectopy *due to K^+ shifts during the initial postoperative phase and hypothermia*
MAP	Decreased: <70 mm Hg *due to third-space fluid loss, hemorrhage, myocardial ischemia, fulminant graft failure, or sepsis* Increased: >100 mm Hg *due to inability of the liver to detoxify norepinephrine, hypervolemia, chronic hypertension, or side effects of cyclosporine therapy*
CI	Decreased: <2.5 L/min/m^2 *due to third-space fluid loss, hemorrhage, reduced myocardial contractility, or sepsis* Increased: >4.5 L/min/m^2 *due to hyperdynamic phase of septic shock or normal postoperative course*
SVR	Increased: >1200 dynes/sec/cm^{-5} *due to inability of the liver to detoxify norepinephrine, hypothermia, hypervolemia, or as a side effect of cyclosporine therapy* Decreased: <800 dynes/sec/cm^{-5} *due to vasodilation during rewarming phase; hypovolemia related to third-space fluid loss or bleeding; hyperdynamic phase of septic shock*
RAP	Increased: >12 mm Hg *due to hypervolemia, ascites*
PAP	Increased: >25/13/10 mm Hg *due to hypovolemia* Decreased: <25/13/10 mm Hg *due to hypovolemia, third-space loss, or hemorrhage*

PCWP	Increased: >18 mm Hg *due to hypervolemia*
PVR	Increased: >97 dynes/sec/cm^{-5} *due to hypervolemia*
LVSWI	Decreased: <50 g/m^2/beat *due to decreased myocardial contractility*

Coagulation

PT	Increased: >1½ times control
APTT	Increased: >1½ times control
Platelets	Decreased: <50,000 mm^3 *due to initial inability of liver to synthesize these factors*
Hgb	Decreased: <12 g/dl *due to hemorrhage*
Core body temperature	Decreased: <36.1° C *due to cold surgical suite, cold IV solutions, and open abdominal cavity during lengthy surgical procedure*

Respiratory Status

ABG	Metabolic alkalosis
pH	Increased: >7.45
$Paco_2$	WNL
Pao_2	Decreased: <80 mm Hg
HCO_3^-	Increased: >28 mEq/L
Sao_2	Decreased: <95% *due to massive administration of blood products, diuretics, corticosteroids, or hypokalemia*
Chest x-ray	Bilateral infiltrates and pleural effusions *due to effects of anesthesia/surgery, large donor liver, or ascites* Elevated right diaphragm *due to inadvertent clamping of right phrenic nerve*

Liver Graft Status

ALT/AST	Increased: >1000 U/L *due to ischemia resulting from organ retrieval damage, inadequate preservation, or implantation problems within the first 24 hours after transplant*
Serum bilirubin	Increased: >0.3 mg/dl (direct) Increased: >1.0 mg/dl (total) *due to liver dysfunction allograft rejection*
Alkaline phosphatase	Increased: >85 ImU/ml *due to allograft rejection*
Blood glucose	Increased: >105 mg/dl *due to the transplanted liver's attempt to regulate metabolism, physiologic stress, steroid therapy, or sepsis* Decreased: <70 mg/dl *due to nonfunctioning allograft, shock, or sepsis*
Hct	Decreased: <37%
Hgb	Decreased: <12 g/dl *due to bleeding*
WBC	Decreased: <5000/mm^3 *due to azathioprine therapy* Increased: >10,000/mm^3 *due to infection*
Lymphocytes	Increased: >40% *due to allograft rejection*
Platelet count	Decreased: <50,000/mm^3 *due to hypersplenism, anemia, or drug therapy*
PT	Increased: >12.5 seconds *due to depletion of coagulation factors, allograft rejection*
APTT	Increased: >40 seconds *due to bleeding*
K^+	Decreased: <3.5 mEq/L *due to diuretics, steroid therapy, metabolic alkalosis* Increased: >5.0 mEq/L *due to massive transfusions of blood products*
Ca^{++}	Decreased: <9.0 mg/dl *due to massive transfusions of blood products*

Mg^{++}	Decreased: <1.5 mEq/L *due to massive transfusions of blood products and cyclosporine therapy*[13]
T-tube drainage	Change in bile color or consistency, or decreased drainage *due to allograft dysfunction*
Liver biopsy	Lymphatic infiltrates in portal tracts, central veins *due to allograft rejection*

Neurological Status

LOC	Anxious, restless, confused, comatose *due to hypoglycemia, hepatic-metabolic encephalopathy, CVA, cerebral air embolism, drug toxicity*

Renal Status

BUN	Increased: >20 mg/dl *due to cyclosporine causing renal artery spasms, nephrotoxic antibiotics, hypotension, hypovolemia, or hepatorenal syndrome*
Creatinine	Increased: >1.2 mg/dl *due to cyclosporine causing renal artery spasms, nephrotoxic antibiotics, hypotension, or hepatorenal syndrome*
Na^+	Decreased: <136 mEq/L *due to excessive water intake* Increased: >145 mEq/L *due to water loss from diuretic therapy*

PLAN OF CARE

INTENSIVE PHASE

The first 24 to 48 hours after surgery are usually spent in the intensive care unit. During this time the focus of care is directed toward identifying and correcting signs of altered cardiovascular tissue perfusion, electrolyte/acid–base imbalances, and impaired gas exchange.

PATIENT CARE PRIORITIES	EXPECTED PATIENT OUTCOMES
Decreased cardiovascular tissue perfusion *r/t* *Hypovolemia* *Hypothermia* *Bleeding* *Hypertension* *Loss of clotting factors*	Normal/improved CI and SVR Clotting profile: WNL
Alterations in electrolyte and acid–base imbalance *r/t* *Hyper/hypokalemia* *Hyper/hypocalcemia* *Hyper/hypomagnesemia* *Metabolic alkalosis*	Serum K^+: WNL Ca^{++}: WNL Mg^{++}: WNL Normal acid–base balance
Impaired gas exchange *r/t* *Atelectasis* *Ascites* *Hypervolemia* *Large donor liver* *Right phrenic nerve injury* *Pleural effusion* *Pneumonia*	Improved ABG Decreased work of breathing
High risk for liver transplant complications *r/t* *Ischemia* *Hepatic artery/vein thrombosis* *Biliary anastomotic problems* *Rejection* *Infection*	Normal allograft function Control rejection No infection

Plan of Care (cont'd)

High risk for impaired skin integrity *r/t* *Length of surgery* *Preoperative nutritional status*	Skin remains intact

INTERVENTIONS

Monitor BP, P, RR, CVP, PAP, CI, SVR for signs and symptoms of hypovolemia *related to loss of fluid and/or rewarming of body temperature; hypotension related to bleeding and/or rewarming of body temperature; hypertension related to cyclosporine therapy.*

Administer volume expanders *to maintain CO.*

Administer vasoactive drugs *to maintain contractility and CO.*

Monitor coagulation profile to assess degree of coagulation and administer blood products as ordered *to improve clotting factors, support CO.*[11]

Institute rewarming measures *to prevent increased oxygen demand and consumption.*

Monitor K^+, Ca^{++}, and Mg^{++} levels *to assess for hyper/hypokalemia, hyper/hypocalcemia, hyper/hypomagnesemia.*

Monitor ABG results *to assess acid–base balance and oxygenation status.*

Inspect chest for bilateral expansion. *Right diaphragm paralysis will prevent full expansion of right lung.*

Administer chest physiotherapy, incentive spirometer, and exercises involving coughing and deep breathing if indicated *to facilitate secretion removal.*

Monitor for changes in sensorium and changes in skin and mucous membrane color. *Graft failure produces mental status changes as well as jaundice.*

Provide pain medication as needed *to maintain comfort level.*

Monitor Jackson–Pratt drains for amount (approximately 500 ml/day, initially) and type of drainage. *Drainage should change from sanguineous to serous and decrease in amount.*

Monitor T-tube drainage for color, consistency, and amount (approximately 500 ml/day, initially). Bile should be thick and dark green. *Decreased bile production indicates graft dysfunction.*

Inspect incision sites, puncture sites, and all drains *for bleeding.*

Administer immunosuppressive drugs *to decrease acuity of acute rejection episodes.*

Monitor daily weight, skin turgor, and peripheral edema *to assess hydration.*

Monitor urine output for amount and color *to assess hydration and the results of diuretic therapy. Dark amber urine may indicate graft dysfunction.*

Monitor cyclosporine levels for toxicity.

Assess for changes in LOC and for responsiveness, tremors, or seizures. *Changes in mental status may indicate cyclosporine toxicity, metabolic imbalance, and graft failure.*

Inspect oral mucosa for breakdown. *May be a sign of fungal infection or herpes simplex virus.*

Monitor T for low-grade elevation *because this may be sign of infection.*

Assess skin integrity at least daily and use pressure relief measures as necessary. *Patients are at risk for skin breakdown caused by lengthy surgery and poor preoperative nutritional state.*

INTERMEDIATE PHASE

In the intermediate phase of care, the patient is extubated, monitoring lines are removed, and the patient progresses to a general surgical or transplant unit. This move usually takes place within 2 days after transplantation. The patient care priorities during this phase include monitoring for allograft rejection, infection, impaired physical mobility, and fear of rejection.

PATIENT CARE PRIORITIES	EXPECTED PATIENT OUTCOMES
High risk for allograft rejection *r/t recipient's immune response to allograft*	Effective control of immune response to allograft

Plan of Care (cont'd)

High risk for infection r/t *Immunosuppression therapy* *Decreased nutrition* *Opportunistic organisms*	Absence of infection
High risk for impaired physical mobility r/t *Degree of illness* *Prolonged immobility* *Steroid therapy*	Ambulates in hallway without assistance Performs basic ADLs independently
Fear *r/t organ rejection*	Verbalizes concerns regarding rejection and actions to optimize self-care

INTERVENTIONS

Decrease or change in color, amount, and consistency of bile drainage; jaundice; increased PT; low-grade fever; and increased ALT/AST, bilirubin, and alkaline phosphatase *may indicate allograft rejection.*

Inspect incision site *because edematous, hard, tender incision may indicate infection.*

Consult dietitian for evaluation of calorie and protein needs. *Catabolic effects of steroids as well as baseline malnutrition may necessitate increased dietary protein to maintain positive nitrogen balance.*

Inspect oral mucosa for breakdown *because this may be a sign of fungal infection or herpes simplex virus.*

Consult physical therapist for strengthening exercises. *Muscle weakness caused by length of time immobilized, chronic disease, and steroid therapy can delay recovery.*

Provide time for support, and allow verbalization of fears and feelings. *The only alternative to certain death from graft failure at this time is retransplantation.*

Consult psychiatric clinical nurse specialist, clergy, social service, volunteer transplant recipients. *Altered mood, depression, and body image changes are not unusual after transplantation.*

Teach signs and symptoms of organ rejection and importance of taking immunosuppressive medication. Survival depends, in part, on understanding of the illness, compliance with the plan of care, and reporting potential problems as soon as possible.

TRANSITION TO DISCHARGE

The ultimate goal in liver transplantation is to assist the patient and family to achieve independence and comfort with the health care regimens before going home. Liver transplant patients face many challenges. Their survival depends on an understanding of their illness and compliance with treatment. Helping the patient and family to achieve this goal by fostering self-care during this transition period is an extremely important priority for the nurse. The recovery phase of liver transplantation might involve life-threatening complications and patients do not usually recover without some degree of liver impairment. In spite of this, studies show substantial improvement in the quality of life after transplant, with ability to return to a normal life (including childbirth) and work.[3,7,21]

REFERENCES

1. Asher NL: Immunosuppression and rejection in liver transplantation. *Transplant Proc* 25(2):1744-1745, 1993.
2. Bismuth H, Azoulay D, Dennison A: Recent developments in liver transplantation, *Transplant Proc* 25(3):2191-2194, 1993.
3. Boone P, Kelly S, Smith CD: Liver transplantation: living-related donations, *Crit Care Nurs Clin North Am* 4(2):243-248, 1992.
4. Burdick JF: An anatomy of rejection, *Transplant Rev* 5(2):81-90, 1991.
5. Delmonico FL, et al: The high-risk liver allograft recipient. *Arch Surg* 127:579-584, 1992.
6. Hahn RA, et al: Excess deaths from nine chronic diseases in the United States, 1986, *JAMA* 20:2654, 1990.
7. Hicks FD, Larson JL, Ferrans CE: Quality of life after liver transplant, *Res Nurs Health* 15:111-119, 1992.

8. Hockerstedt K: Liver transplantation: present results and problems, *Ann Med* 24(5):325-328, 1992.
9. Keeffe EB: Liver transplantation—challenges for the future, *West J Med* 155:541-543, 1991.
10. Kizilisik TA, Preiksaitis JK, Kneteman NM: Cytomegalovirus disease in liver transplant recipients: impact of acyclovir prophylaxis, *Transplant Proc* 25(3):2282-2283, 1993.
11. Kramer DJ, Selby RR, Murray GC: Perioperative intensive care of liver transplant patients. In Rippe JM, et al, editors: *Intensive care,* ed 6, Boston, 1991, Little, Brown.
12. Mora NP, et al: Survival after liver transplantation in 300 consecutive patients: the influence of age, clinical status and pretransplant disease. *Transplant Proc* 24(5):156-157, 1992.
13. Pillon LR: Cyclosporine: a nursing focus on immunosuppressive therapy, *Dimensions Crit Care Nurs* 10(2):68-73, 1991.
14. Post SG: Baboon livers and the human good, *Arch Surg* 128(2):131-133, 1993.
15. Sheil AGR: Quandaries and controversies in liver transplantation, *Transplant Proc* 24(6):2375-2378, 1992.
16. Smith SL, Ciferni ML: Liver transplantation, *Crit Care Nurs Clin North Am* 4(1):131-148, 1992.
17. *St Anthony's DRG Guidebook 1995,* Reston, Va, 1994, St Anthony.
18. Starzl TE, et al: Homotransplantation of the liver in humans, *Surg Gynecol Obstet* 117:659, 1963.
19. Starzl TE, et al: Baboon-to-human liver transplantation, *Lancet* 341(8837):65-71, 1993.
20. Szpakowski JL, et al: Liver transplantation experience with 100 cases, *West J Med* 155:494-499, 1991.
21. Tater RE, Switatla J, Arria A: Quality of life before and after orthotopic hepatic transplantation, *Intern Med* 151:1521-1526, 1991.

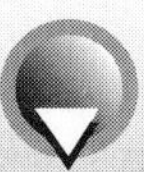

C L I N I C A L   G U I D E L I N E

48

Acute Upper Gastrointestinal Bleeding

Andrea D'Amato Quinn, MS, RN, CCRN, CS

DESCRIPTION

Acute upper gastrointestinal bleeding (UGIB) is a potentially life-threatening event. It is defined as bleeding that originates from an area above the ligament of Treitz, which is located about the level of the proximal duodenum. UGIB is not a disease entity itself; rather, it is a clinical presentation associated with a pathological process. Approximately 50 to 100 episodes of UGIB requiring hospitalization occur per 100,000 population each year; about 10% of those who bleed die.[12] Despite major advances in diagnostic and therapeutic modalities, the mortality rate has remained essentially unchanged over the last 30 years. Risk for mortality increases with age (>60 years), recurrent bleeding during hospitalization, and concurrent cardiac, respiratory, hepatic, or renal impairment.[16]

PATHOPHYSIOLOGY

The most common causes of acute UGIB necessitating critical care management are Mallory-Weiss tear, esophageal varices, gastric and duodenal ulceration, and erosive gastritis (Table 48-1). Mallory-Weiss tear is a linear mucosal laceration located at the junction of the distal esophagus and stomach. It is associated with excessive alcohol use and usually is caused by severe retching.

Esophageal varices are a collection of thin-walled, friable collateral veins. From 90% to 95% of varices develop secondary to portal hypertension associated with alcoholic liver disease. Varices develop as a compensating mechanism to return splanchnic blood to the inferior vena cava in the presence of portal hypertension or obstructed blood flow through the portal-hepatic system. Acute, massive bleeding from varices may develop as a result of an increase in the pressure within the varices, or from irritation (mechanical or chemical) of the friable vessel wall.

Gastric and duodenal ulcers (peptic ulcers) invade the submucosal and muscular layers of the GI tract, eroding vessels and causing subsequent bleeding. Duodenal ulcers occur more frequently than gastric ulcers. They are caused by high levels of gastric acid or inadequate production of acid-neutralizing bicarbonate, leading to acid penetration through the mucosal surface and erosion of underlying tissue, including GI muscular layers and blood vessels.[14]

Gastric ulceration is associated with changes in the permeability of the gastric mucosa to hydrogen ions (acid) causing acid infiltration into underlying tissue and subsequent tissue erosion. Drugs known to irritate gastric mucosa, such as aspirin and anti-inflammatory agents, also promote acid invasion through the mucosal surface. The reflux of bile salts from the duodenum into the stomach also can irritate and injure gastric mucosa and promote ulceration.[14] Although specific mechanisms for the formation of gastric and duodenal ulcers are different, ulcers are formed when there is a disruption in the delicate balance between erosive agents (acid and bile) and protective factors (mucous, bicarbonate, mucosal permeability). When this disruption exists, mucosal tissue is injured and erosion into underlying tissue layers, including blood vessels, occurs.

Emerging evidence suggests a relationship between the presence of *Helicobacter pylori,* a gram-negative bacteria,

TABLE 48-1 Major Causes of Acute Upper GI Bleeding with Treatment Options

Cause	Description	Treatment
Mallory-Weiss tear	Linear mucosal tear at junction of distal esophagus and stomach. Associated with alcohol use. Caused by severe retching.	Bleeding may stop spontaneously without treatment Vasoconstriction with vasopressin Endoscopic thermal coagulation Surgical oversewing of laceration
Esophageal varices	Thin-walled, friable collateral veins. 90-95% develop secondary to portal hypertension associated with alcoholic liver disease.	Vasoconstriction with vasopressin Tamponade therapy Injection sclerotherapy Decompressive shunt • Selective: Portocaval Mesocaval • Nonselective: Splenorenal • TIPS (transjugular intrahepatic portosystemic shunt) Surgical devascularization
Gastric and duodenal ulcers (peptic ulcer)	Erosions of submucosal and muscular layers of GI tract. Occur most commonly in the duodenum. Caused by imbalance between erosive agents (acid and bile) and protective factors (mucous, HCO_3^-, mucosal permeability).	Conservative medical therapy: • Histamine blockers (cimetidine, ranitidine, famotodine) • Cytoprotective agents (sucralfate) • Antacids Other pharmacologic therapy (omeprazole, prostaglandin analogues, antibiotics) Injection with vasoconstrictive agents such as epinephrine Endoscopic thermal coagulation Intravascular embolization Surgical repair: • Oversew or resection of ulcer • Partial gastrectomy • Partial or total vagotomy
Erosive gastritis	Superficial erosions of stomach, often in the antrum. Does not penetrate into muscularis. Generalized versus localized area of tissue affected.	Prophylactic (histamine blockers, antacids, cytoprotective agents, prostaglandin analogues) Surgical (oversewing, gastrectomy)

and the development of gastric ulcers. It is suggested that the organism initiates inflammatory changes in the mucosal surface of the stomach, altering mucosal resistance to acid. Current clinical trials using antibiotic therapy to eliminate the bacteria demonstrate promising results.[15]

Erosive gastritis, also referred to as acute mucosal erosion, involves only the superficial layers (epithelial, vascular, and minor muscular layers of the mucosal surface) of the GI tract. Curling's ulcers and Cushing's ulcers, associated with burns and head injury, respectively, are representative of erosive gastritis. Interruption of the protective gastric mucosal barrier caused by drugs, alcohol, and ischemia exposes mucosal tissue to gastric acid causing injury to surface tissues and bleeding.

Rapid loss of a large volume of blood from the GI tract causes massive loss of intravascular volume and red blood cells (RBCs). This loss of volume and RBCs (Hgb) reduces cardiac output (CO) and oxygen transport, which threatens end-organ perfusion.

Oxygen delivery (Do_2) to organs and tissues is dependent upon CO and arterial oxygen content (Cao_2) ($Do_2 = CO \times Cao_2$). CO is determined by preload, afterload, contractility, and heart rate. Any alteration in preload, afterload, or contractility, singly or in combination, affects CO and thereby Do_2. Additionally, Do_2 to organs depends upon the amount of O_2 available in the arterial circulation. Arterial oxygen saturation (Sao_2), partial pressure of arterial oxygen (Pao_2), and hemoglobin (Hgb) contribute to total CaO_2. SaO_2 and Hgb make the most significant contribution to CaO_2, so alteration in either of these values will significantly alter O_2 delivery to the tissue.

As blood is lost from the intravascular space, as with acute UGIB, O_2 delivery is reduced. This reduction is caused by changes in CO and CaO_2. CO is reduced primarily through reduction of preload (filling pressures); CaO_2 is reduced primarily through the loss of Hgb from RBC loss, resulting in a reduced O_2 carrying capability. The end result to the patient is life-threatening changes in tissue perfusion from the massive loss of intravascular volume.

The transfusion of multiple units of blood can result in a significant coagulation disorder, further complicating patient management. Severe depletion of coagulation factors occurs as a consequence both of bleeding itself as well as repletion of blood volume with banked blood, which is devoid of active clotting factors and platelets. The patient has diffuse oozing from mucous membranes, wounds, and puncture sites. PT, APTT, and TT are elevated; fibrinogen and platelets are decreased. Platelets are transfused to maintain platelet count at 100,000/mm^3 and adequate hemostasis. Fresh frozen plasma (FFP) is transfused to replace coagulation proteins. FFP is preferred over cryoprecipitate therapy because it contains more clotting factors (II, V, VII, IX, XI) than cryoprecipitate (VIII and fibrinogen). For the patient at high risk for transfusion-related coagulopathy, it is recommended to administer 4 U platelets and 1 U FFP for every 5 U blood transfused.[7] An additional cause of coagulopathy in patients with UGIB is disseminated intravascular coagulation (DIC). DIC may develop as a consequence of hypotension associated with massive bleeding and shock, or secondary to a transfusion reaction.

Hypocalcemia can exacerbate coagulopathy associated with massive blood transfusion. Calcium (Ca^{++}) is a requisite factor in the coagulation cascade and is inactivated in banked blood. Ca^{++} is replaced to maintain ionized Ca^{++} within normal parameters in the presence of massive transfusions.

Signs and symptoms associated with UGIB result from either blood loss or the body's compensatory reaction to volume loss mediated via the sympathetic nervous system (SNS). Hematemesis, a bloody vomitus or NG aspirate, may appear as fresh blood or as "coffee ground" material. Rapid and massive UGIB usually appears as bright, red blood. When blood is exposed to digestive enzymes from the stomach and/or duodenum, the hematemesis appears dark red or black; this is often referred to as "coffee ground" material. Melena, appearing as black, tarry, or maroon stool, is the passage of digested blood and waste products from the large intestine. The presence of digested blood is an irritant to the GI tract and causes the frequent diarrhea episodes associated with GI bleeding. Hematocrit (Hct) and Hgb values are slow to reflect acute blood loss and may appear deceptively normal in the face of total body fluid deficit, or conversely, deceptively abnormal in the face of massive resuscitation with fluids other than RBCs. Other laboratory values that are affected by UGIB include coagulation parameters (PT, APTT, platelets, ionized Ca^{++}). PT and APTT abnormalities usually are associated with massive blood replacement and/or accompanying liver disease. Platelets are lost to the body during bleeding and are not contained in banked blood. Ca^{++} depletion is associated with transfusion of multiple units of blood without adequate supplemental replacement.

TABLE 48-2 Clinical Classification of Hemorrhage

Class	Total blood volume loss	Clinical signs and symptoms
1	<15%	HR normal or <100 bpm supine Capillary refill <3 sec Urine output normal: >30 ml/hr Orthostasis Apprehension
2	15-30%	HR increased: >100 bpm Capillary refill increased: >3 sec BP normal supine Decreased pulse pressure RR increased Urine output decreased: 25-30 ml/hr
3	30-40%	HR increased: >120 bpm BP decreased Cool, pale skin RR increased Urine output decreased: 5-15 ml/hr
4	>40%	HR increased: >140 bpm BP profoundly decreased: MAP <55 Confused, lethargic Urine output minimal

Adapted from Klein D: Physiologic response to traumatic shock, *AACN Clin Iss Crit Care Nurs* 1:508, 1990.

Sympathetic nervous system response to decreased circulating volume produces physiologic changes aimed at supporting perfusion to central organs (head, heart) at the expense of peripheral organs (skin, skeletal muscle, splanchnic, and renal). (See Table 48-2.)

Increased heart rate (HR) is the first noticeable response to decreased volume. As preload decreases, the body attempts to increase CO by increasing HR. As volume deficit persists or worsens, orthostasis occurs. Orthostasis is defined as an increase in HR >20 bpm and/or a decrease of 10 mm Hg or greater in systolic BP with upright position changes. These changes result from the inability of the body to make compensatory vascular and hemodynamic changes with changes in postural position. Orthostasis occurs with intravascular volume deficits of 10% to 20% (500 to 1000 ml).[16]

Decreased perfusion to the skin, muscle, splanchnic system, and kidneys recruits additional volume into the vascular space to improve perfusion to the head and heart. This decreased perfusion peripherally produces the cool skin, decreased capillary refill, and decreased urine output associated with hypovolemia. It is important to emphasize that decrease in systolic BP is a late response, and represents the failure of the body's compensatory mechanisms to support perfusion.

LENGTH OF STAY/ANTICIPATED COURSE

Morbidity and mortality of UGIB depend on volume and rate of blood loss, comorbidity, age, and effectiveness of treatment measures. Length of hospitalization will vary depending on how rapidly baseline hemodynamics are reestablished, the presence of concomitant and/or complicating disease processes, and care needs subsequent to additional therapeutic interventions, such as endoscopic or surgical procedures. Bleeding should be stopped or controlled within 24 hours of admission to the ICU. Usually at day 1 or day 2 after bleeding is controlled, the patient is transferred to intermediate care.[5]

Acute UGIB falls within DRG 174: GI hemorrhage with complications; or DRG 175: GI hemorrhage without complications. The average lengths of stay are 6.2 and 3.9 days, respectively.[18] Additional interventions, such as surgery, will affect in-hospital care needs, discharge teaching, and, potentially, length of stay.

MANAGEMENT TRENDS AND CONTROVERSIES

Volume resuscitation is the mainstay of treatment for acute UGIB. Crystalloids (normal saline and Ringer's lactate) are most commonly used to replace intravascular volume when blood loss is less than 25%. For blood loss greater than 30%, it is necessary to replace both intravascular volume and oxygen-carrying capability.[9,11] Therefore, both crystalloids and RBCs are indicated. The use of colloid solutions such as 5% albumin and hetastarch for volume replacement remains controversial. Colloid solutions increase intravascular oncotic pressure, which promotes pulling of interstitial fluid into the vascular space.[10] Theoretically, this increased oncotic pull decreases the amount of fluid needed to replace intravascular volume losses. Colloid solutions are expensive and not as readily available as crystalloids. Although, potentially, complications such as leakage of fluid into the extravascular space and peripheral edema are increased with the use of crystalloids, there is a paucity of research that consistently demonstrates the benefit of one solution over the other.[3,6] However, some preliminary results demonstrate improved oxygen delivery in surgical patients resuscitated with colloids.[17]

End points of successful volume resuscitation have traditionally included filling pressures (CVP, PCWP), HR, urine output, BP, skin temperature, and capillary refill. In cases of mild to moderate blood loss, these parameters probably are adequate. However, in the face of severe blood volume loss, in addition to the traditional measures of intravascular volume, O_2 delivery should be determined to evaluate the adequacy of both volume and RBC replacement.[8] Elevated serum lactate levels and/or unexplained metabolic acidosis may be indicative of inadequate volume resuscitation and inadequate O_2 delivery.

Vasopressors and inotropic agents should not be used to support BP until volume replacement is well underway. Use of these agents in the presence of intravascular volume depletion will actually decrease tissue perfusion by causing vasoconstriction and thus further reducing blood flow.

Intravenous vasopressin (Pitressin) is used in conjunction with volume replacement in the presence of active bleeding. Vasopressin is a smooth-muscle vasoconstrictor, and this vasoconstriction decreases blood flow through the splanchnic bed. Vasoconstriction assists with hemostasis by decreasing blood flow to the area while natural formation of a thrombus at the site of bleeding occurs. Vasopressin is administered intravenously (IV) with an initial bolus of 20 U over a period of 20 to 30 minutes, followed with a continuous infusion of 0.2 to 0.8 U per minute.[4] Vasopressin produces notable untoward systemic side effects, such as bradydysrhythmias, coronary ischemia, and decreased renal perfusion; thus critical care monitoring is required throughout its use. An increased incidence of side effects is noted when vasopressin is administered at a dose greater than 0.6 U per minute.[4] Concurrent administration of nitroglycerin (IV or topical) can decrease or minimize the side effects associated with vasopressin administration.

Once volume replacement and hemostatic maneuvers are underway, treatment is aimed at identifying the source of bleeding and prevention of recurrent bleeding episodes. Precise identification of the source of acute UGIB is requisite for appropriate interventions to stop the bleeding and to prevent recurrence. Endoscopy, arteriography, and radioisotopic scanning are diagnostic procedures commonly used to identify the source of UGIB. Gastric lavage with a large-bore orogastric tube such as an Ewald or Edlich tube is used to help stop bleeding and clean the stomach of blood and clots in preparation for endoscopy. Room-temperature lavage fluid (normal saline or tap water) has been shown to be more effective than iced fluids to stop bleeding.[2]

Endoscopy provides direct visualization of the esophagus, stomach, and proximal duodenum for both diagnostic and interventional purposes. A major advantage of endoscopy is that it can be performed easily at the bedside using a flexible endoscope, and the patient requires only light sedation to conduct the procedure. If endoscopy confirms esophageal or gastric varices as the source of active bleeding, a tamponade tube (Sengstaken Blakemore or Minnesota tube) may be placed to help stop the bleeding by means of direct pressure at the bleeding site. Endoscopic interventions include injection with sclerosing or vasoconstrictive agents; thermal techniques such as laser photocoagulation, electrocoagulation, and heat probe coagulation; and application of topical agents at the site of the bleeding vessel(s).

Arteriography and radioisotopic scanning are useful to identify the bleeding source only when the patient is actively bleeding. Intravascular injection with vasoconstricting (e.g., epinephrine) or embolizing agents or devices (e.g., Gelfoam or a stainless steel coil) are alternative interventions used when the exact site of bleeding has been located via arteriography or isotopic scanning.

Lactulose often is used as a cathartic to prevent or minimize digestion and absorption of blood from the GI tract. Absorbed by-products of digested blood increase serum ammonia levels, which can lead to the development or worsening of encephalopathy. Lactulose usually is administered at 30 to 60 ml/hr until diarrhea occurs, then 30 ml every 4 to 6 hours.

Other interventions used to treat active UGIB and prevent recurrent bleeding episodes are more specifically related to the diagnosis, or to the cause of bleeding. Bleeding from Mallory-Weiss tear may stop spontaneously without treatment. Interventions used to treat persistent bleeding include IV vasopressin, endoscopic thermal coagulation, and surgical oversewing of the laceration.

Acutely bleeding esophageal varices are treated initially with IV vasopressin and tamponade therapy to stop or control the bleeding. The esophagogastric tamponade tube has two balloons (gastric and esophageal) which can be inflated to apply direct pressure on the bleeding varices. The inflated gastric balloon also decreases blood flow to the esophageal varices by compressing vessels that feed the vessels in the esophagus. This maneuver is often sufficient to stop esophageal bleeding. In the event that the esophageal varices continue to bleed, the esophageal balloon is inflated to a pressure of 35 to 40 mm Hg.

Injection sclerotherapy may be used to treat bleeding varices or to prevent initial or recurrent bleeding. The sclerosing agent causes the varix to contract; it also causes an inflammatory reaction, subsequent thrombus formation, fibrosis, and scar tissue at the varix site.

Selective (splenorenal) and nonselective (portocaval, mesocaval) shunts are surgical procedures aimed at treating or preventing bleeding from esophageal varices by decreasing portal venous pressure. These procedures provide an alternate route for splanchnic blood flow to return to the vena cava to decrease portal pressure. The splenorenal shunt connects the splenic vein to the left renal vein, which drains directly into the inferior vena cava. With this procedure, a portion of the splanchnic circulation bypasses the portal vein, thus reducing portal venous pressure. The remainder of splanchnic blood flow drains through the portal system and the liver. Total shunt procedures divert blood flow from the portal vein directly into the vena cava. Although both selective and nonselective shunts serve to decrease portal venous pressure, there is a higher incidence of subsequent encephalopathy.

A new procedure—transjugular intrahepatic portosystemic shunt (TIPS)—is an interventional radiologic technique used to accomplish the same goal as surgical shunts. In this procedure, a catheter is threaded retrograde from the jugular vein to the portal vein. A stent is threaded through the liver parenchyma and connected to the portal vein. The stent provides a conduit for blood flow through an otherwise obstructed route from the portal vein to the hepatic vein and into the inferior vena cava.[1]

Other surgical procedures may be used to control bleeding from esophageal varices. These procedures do not affect portal venous pressure, but serve to control bleeding by devascularizing the esophagus. This devascularization may be accomplished by surgical ligation (tie-off) of the varices, or transection of the esophagus to interrupt blood flow to the varices.

Histamine blockers (cimetidine, ranitidine, famotodine), cytoprotective agents (sucralfate), and antacids are the mainstays of conservative medical therapy for peptic ulcers. Each of these agents alters the exposure of gastric/duodenal tissue to luminal acid, allowing the ulceration to heal. Histamine blockers provide protection and treatment for peptic ulceration by inhibiting acid secretion. Sucralfate protects the mucosal surface from erosive agents by binding to proteins in ulcerated tissue and forming a protective barrier between the luminal contents and the mucosal surface. Additionally, sucralfate exhibits trophic effects on the gastric mucosa, effecting re-epithelialization of ulcerated areas. Antacids protect tissue and promote ulcer healing by neutralizing luminal acids.[15]

Emerging pharmacologic therapies for the treatment of peptic ulcer disease include omeprazole, an agent that inhibits the secretion of H^+/K^+-ATPase and thereby suppresses acid secretion from the parietal cells; prostaglandin analogues (misoprostol) which are believed to stimulate the secretion of mucus and bicarbonate, inhibit the secretion of acid, and enhance mucosal blood flow; and agents to treat *H. pylori,* such as colloidal bismuth and antibiotics (amoxicillin, ampicillin, erythromycin, ciprofloxacin metronidazole, and tetracycline).[15]

Acutely bleeding ulcers may be treated by injection with vasoconstricting agents, endoscopic thermal therapy, or intravascular embolization as described previously. Surgery may be performed to control or prevent ulcer bleeding or to treat perforation. The ulcer defect may be closed by a simple oversewing procedure or resected. Partial gastrectomy (removal of the distal portion of the stomach) removes the major mass of parietal cells that are responsible for the secretion of acid. With a partial gastrectomy, the remaining portion of the stomach is anastomosed to either the duodenum (Billroth I) or the jejunum (Billroth II). Acid secretion also may be reduced by means of a partial or total vagotomy procedure. Stimulation of the vagus nerve increases acid secretion; thus total or partial interruption of vagal stimulation to the stomach serves to decrease acid production.

Treatment measures for erosive gastritis are similar, in part, to those used to treat peptic ulcers. Treatment is primarily prophylactic (histamine blockers, cytoprotective agents, antacids, and prostaglandin E) and supportive care. Surgical interventions such as oversewing of erosions and total gastrectomy have been used.[12]

ASSESSMENT

PARAMETER	ANTICIPATED ALTERATION
Cardiovascular Status	
HR	Cardiovascular changes reflect intravascular volume changes and the body's attempt to maintain CO Tachycardia: >100 bpm *due to compensatory SNS response to decreased intravascular volume. Rate depends on the severity of the volume deficit and the ability of the body to compensate.*
BP	*Initial:* SBP elevated: >120 mm Hg (initially DBP slightly elevated: >80 mm Hg) (decreased pulse pressure) *due to compensatory mechanisms* *Subsequent:* Decreased systolic, diastolic, and MAP
MAP	Decreased: <70 mm Hg *due to hypovolemic shock*
Filling Pressures	
CVP	Decreased: <5 mm Hg *due to decreased intravascular volume*
PAM	Decreased: <15 mm Hg *due to decreased intravascular volume*
PCWP	Decreased: <8 mm Hg *due to decreased intravascular volume*
CO/CI	Decreased <5 L/min; <2 L/min/m^2 *due to decreased intravascular volume*
SVR	Increased: >1200 dynes/sec/cm^{-5} *due to peripheral vasoconstriction (SNS compensation)*
Hct/Hgb	
	Initially normal: Hct 35% to 45%; Hgb 12 to 15 g/dl *due to loss of equal amounts of RBCs and plasma. As the body compensates for volume loss by shifting interstitial fluid into the vascular space, volume resuscitation begins to take effect. Hct and Hgb values decrease in 12 to 48 hr, reflecting the loss of RBCs.*
Respiratory Status	
RR	Increased: >20 breaths/min *due to SNS compensation*
$PaCO_2$	Decreased: <35 mm Hg *due to tachypnea*
PaO_2	Decreased: <60 mm Hg *due to fluid overload or aspiration*
SaO_2	Decreased: <90% *due to fluid overload or aspiration*
Secretions	Increased *due to fluid overload and increased alveolar fluid accumulation*
Neurologic Status	
Mental status	Anxiety, restlessness, confusion *due to decreased cerebral perfusion and/or encephalopathy*
Neuromuscular activity	Tremors, seizures, coma *due to encephalopathy*

Renal

UO	Decreased: <30 ml/hr *due to decreased intravascular volume and decreased renal perfusion*
BUN	Increased: >40 mg/dl *due to decreased intravascular volume and the absorption of protein by-products (blood) through the digestive tract*
Urine: plasma osmolarity ratio	Increased: >2:1 *due to decreased intravascular volume resulting in reabsorption of water into the vascular space, leading to high solute-to-water composition of urine*
Specific gravity	Increased: >1.020 *due to decreased intravascular volume resulting in reabsorption of water into the vascular space, leading to high solute-to-water composition of urine*

PLAN OF CARE

INTENSIVE PHASE

Care of the patient with UGIB during the intensive phase is focused on reestablishing fluid volume status to stabilize hemodynamic parameters, and control of local and/or diffuse bleeding. Acute bleeding should be controlled within 24 hours. Once the source and etiology of the UGIB have been identified, definitive treatment can be implemented.

PATIENT CARE PRIORITIES	EXPECTED PATIENT OUTCOMES
Fluid volume deficit *r/t blood volume loss*	Hemodynamic parameters: WNL or within patient norms Cessation/control of blood volume loss Normal/improved urine output, urine:plasma osmolarity ratio, and specific gravity Hct: WNL Hgb: WNL
Decreased tissue perfusion *r/t hypovolemia*	MAP within patient norms Mental status within patient norms Urine output: WNL Peripheral pulses ≥+2 Skin temperature warm Capillary refill <3 sec
Coagulation defect *r/t multiple transfusions and/or underlying liver disease*	Control of local and/or diffuse bleeding PT: WNL APTT: WNL Platelets: WNL Bleeding time: WNL Ionized Ca^{++}: WNL
Altered thought process and neuromuscular function *r/t encephalopathy*	Serum ammonia: WNL Normal mental status Absence of confusion, disorientation Absence of tremors, seizures Absence of self-imposed injury
High risk for fluid volume excess *r/t rapid fluid replacement*	Pulmonary: • Absence of rales, shortness of breath, tachypnea • Sao_2 >94%; Pao_2: WNL or within patient norms Cardiovascular: • Absence of peripheral edema • Absence of increased MAP, CVP, PAM, PCWP, HR • Cardiac rhythm: WNL

Plan of Care (cont'd)

	Renal: Normal plasma-to-urine osmolarity ratio, specific gravity, BUN
Pain *r/t ulcers, and diagnostic and interventional procedures*	Reports comfort
Patient anxiety *r/t hypovolemia, discomfort, and fear*	Anxiety level decreased/controlled
Family anxiety *r/t fear about patient prognosis and lack of knowledge*	Anxiety level decreased/controlled Understanding of patient status and treatments
High risk for impaired gas exchange *r/t aspiration*	Pao_2: WNL or within patient norms Sao_2 >94% or within patient norms $Paco_2$: WNL or within patient norms
High risk for hypothermia *r/t rapid volume replacement*	Normothermic

INTERVENTIONS

Monitor HR, MAP, CVP, PAM, PCWP, CO/CI orthostasis, Hct, Hgb, BUN, urine-to-plasma osmolarity ratio, Na^+, K^+, Cl^-, HCO_3^-, peripheral pulses, skin color, and T *to assess patient response to fluid and blood product replacement.*

Monitor PT, APTT, platelets, bleeding time, and ionized Ca^{++} *to assess coagulation status.*

Measure I/O from all sources *to assess fluid balance.*

Measure or estimate blood volume loss from NG aspirate and vomitus.

Monitor amount and frequency of melanotic stool.

Administer RBCs, platelets, fresh frozen plasma, cryoprecipitate *to restore blood and coagulation factor losses.* Monitor for transfusion reaction.

Administer Ca^{++} and vitamin K *to promote normal coagulation.*

Elevate lower extremities *to increase venous return and filling pressures.*

Avoid the Trendelenburg position *to decrease risk of aspiration and to avoid blunting of normal baroreceptor response to hypovolemia.*

Lavage NG tube with tap water or normal saline until clear returns are achieved *to promote cessation of bleeding and to evacuate clots.*

Assess RR, breath sounds, Pao_2, $Paco_2$, Sao_2, and secretions *to monitor for fluid excess and/or aspiration.*

Assess mental status and neuromuscular function *to monitor for signs and symptoms of encephalopathy.*

Keep head of bed elevated 30 degrees and/or maintain patient in side-lying position if tolerated *to reduce the risk of aspiration.*

Warm IV fluids and blood products when administering at rate >150 ml/hr or if patient temperature is <35° C *to prevent hypothermia.*

Assist with diagnostic and interventional procedures as indicated (endoscopy, angiography, sclerotherapy, insertion of esophagogastric balloon tamponade tube).

Avoid IM injections *to prevent intramuscular bleeding with coagulation abnormality.*

Administer lactulose *to treat elevated serum ammonia or encephalopathy.*

Administer pain medication and/or sedatives *to reduce discomfort and anxiety.*

Provide information to patient/family regarding patient status, diagnostic procedures, and interventions *to reduce fear and anxiety.*

INTERMEDIATE PHASE

Care of the patient with UGIB during the intermediate phase centers around monitoring for recurrence of bleeding, correction of abnormal laboratory values, and interventions to prevent rebleeding episodes. Length of stay in the critical care unit varies depending upon patient condition and institutional standards (usually 24 to 72 hours), but acute bleeding should be controlled within 24 hours. Intermediate phase monitoring and interventions begin when

Plan of Care (cont'd)

the patient's vital signs and hemodynamic status are stabilized, and the patient is ready for transfer to the general nursing unit. The intermediate phase will extend for approximately 2 to 7 days.

PATIENT CARE PRIORITIES	EXPECTED PATIENT OUTCOMES
High risk for fluid volume deficit *r/t blood volume loss*	Hemodynamic parameters: WNL or within patient norms Absence of recurrent bleeding Urine output: WNL Urine:plasma osmolarity ratio $<2:1$ Specific gravity: WNL Hct: WNL without blood/blood product transfusion
High risk for coagulation defect *r/t multiple transfusions and/or underlying liver disease*	Absence of local and/or diffuse bleeding PT: WNL APTT: WNL Platelets: WNL Bleeding time: WNL Ionized Ca^{++}: WNL
Pain *r/t procedures and/or surgery*	Reports comfort
Self-care deficit *r/t lack of knowledge regarding treatment and/or surgery (i.e., indication, procedure, potential complications, recovery expectations)*	Patient/family acknowledge understanding of: • Indication for treatment and/or surgery • Basic elements of procedure/surgery • Potential complications of procedures/surgery • Recovery process, including post-procedure/surgery, monitoring and expected progression (specific to procedure or surgery), diet therapy, medications, and length of hospitalization

INTERVENTIONS

Monitor HR, BP, CVP, orthostasis, Hct, Hgb, BUN, urine-to-plasma osmolarity ratio, Na^+, K^+, Cl^-, HCO_3^-, peripheral pulses, skin color, T *to assess patient for recurrence of bleeding.*
Monitor PT, APTT, platelets, bleeding time *to assess clotting factor replacement.*
Measure I/O from all sources *to assess fluid balance.*
Administer blood and blood products and monitor for transfusion reaction.
Avoid IM injections *to prevent intramuscular bleeding with coagulation abnormality.*
Administer Ca^{++} and vitamin K *to promote normal coagulation.*
Administer lactulose *to treat elevated serum ammonia of encephalopathy.*
Administer enemas *to clear lower GI tract of blood to avoid absorption.*
Administer pain medication and/or sedatives *to reduce discomfort and anxiety.*
Provide patient/family with information regarding treatment and/or surgery (indication, procedure, potential complications, recovery expectations).

TRANSITION TO DISCHARGE

In preparation for discharge, the nurse must instruct the patient on the overt and subtle signs and symptoms of GI bleeding. These include the signs and symptoms of orthostasis, the presence of bloody or "coffee ground" vomitus or stool, positive occult blood in stool, weakness, lightheadedness, and dizziness. Medication and diet instruction as appropriate is essential information in preparation for discharge. Specific information related to medication and diet is dictated by the short- and long-term therapeutic plan and any procedures or surgery the patient has undergone.

If the patient undergoes any specific interventional procedures such as injection sclerotherapy, decompressive shunt surgery, or gastric or esophageal surgery to control or prevent recurrent bleeding, the nurse must assure that the patient understands potential complications to report to the physician.

Since the leading factor associated with the development of esophageal varices is alcoholic liver disease, the nurse should assess the patient for a current history of alcohol abuse. If the patient is known to be an alcohol abuser, the nurse should consider making a referral to an alcohol counseling program. It is important to emphasize that although there is a frequent association between UGIB and alcohol abuse, it is inappropriate to automatically make the assumption that a patient with UGIB is an alcohol abuser.

REFERENCES

1. Adams A, Soulen MC: TIPS: a new alternative for the variceal bleeder, *Am J Crit Care* 2(3):196-201, 1993.
2. Andrus CH, Ponsky JL: The effects of irrigant temperature in upper gastrointestinal hemorrhage: a requiem for iced saline lavage, *Am J Gastroenterol* 82(10):1062-1064, 1987.
3. Bisonni RS, et al: Colloids versus crystalloids in fluid resuscitation: an analysis of randomized controlled trials, *J Fam Pract* 32(4):387-390, 1991.
4. Burnett DA, Rikkers LF: Nonoperative emergency treatment of variceal bleeding, *Surg Clin North Am* 70:291-305, 1990.
5. Doyle RL: *Healthcare management guidelines, volume 1: inpatient and surgical care,* 1992, Milliman and Robertson.
6. Falk JL, O'Brien JF, Kerr R: Fluid resuscitation in traumatic hemorrhagic shock, *Crit Care Clin* 8(2):323-340, 1992.
7. Farmer JC, Parker RI: Coagulation disorders. In Civetta JM, Taylor RW, Kirby RR, editors: *Critical care,* New York, 1988, JB Lippincott.
8. Fiddian-Green RG, et al: Goals for resuscitation of shock, *Crit Care Med* 21(suppl 2):S25-31, 1993.
9. Gould SA, et al: Hypovolemic shock, *Crit Care Clin* 9(2):239-259, 1993.
10. Grieffel MI, Kaufman BS: Pharmacology of colloids and crystalloids, *Crit Care Clin* 8(2):235-253, 1992.
11. Haupt MT: The use of crystalloidal and colloidal solutions for volume replacement in hypovolemic shock, *Crit Rev Clin Lab Sci* 27(1):1-26, 1989.
12. Hurst JM: Gastrointestinal bleeding. In Civetta JM, Taylor RW, Kirby RR, editors: *Critical Care,* New York, 1988, JB Lippincott.
13. Klein D: Physiologic response to traumatic shock, *AACN Clin Iss Crit Care Nurs,* 1:508, 1990.
14. McCance KL, Huether SE: *Pathophysiology: the biologic basis for disease in adults and children,* St. Louis, 1990, Mosby–Year Book.
15. McQuaid KR, Isenberg JI: Medical therapy of peptic ulcer disease, *Surg Clin North Am* 72(2):285-315, 1992.
16. Quigley EMM: Upper gastrointestinal hemorrhage. In Parrillo JEE, editor: *Current therapy in critical care medicine,* ed 2, Philadelphia, 1991, BC Decker.
17. Shoemaker WC, Appel PL, Kram HB: Oxygen transport measurements to evaluate tissue perfusion and titrate therapy: dobutamine and dopamine effects, *Crit Care Med* 19(5):672-688, 1991.
18. *St Anthony's DRG Guidebook 1995,* Reston, Va, 1994, St Anthony.

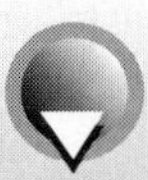

CLINICAL GUIDELINE

49

Gastrointestinal Surgery

Eleanor R. Fitzpatrick, MSN, RN, CCRN
Ann Smith Gregoire, MSN, RN, CCRN

DESCRIPTION

Gastrointestinal (GI) surgery is a broad term for the treatment of diseases and conditions of the GI system. These diseases are numerous and extremely varied, encompassing organs from the esophagus to the anus. Additional organs (such as the gallbladder, pancreas, and liver) play a role in GI function, not in nutrient transit and absorption but in digestion and synthesis of food.

The combined impact of diseases of the GI system is great considering the plethora of organs that are involved and the damage that can ensue with disease entities. Medical treatment is undertaken whenever possible, but surgery is indicated when medical treatment produces suboptimal outcomes or the disease process threatens patient demise. Some of these diseases and the relevant surgical procedures to treat them will be discussed here.

Acute pancreatitis in the United States has an occurrence of 54 to 238 instances per million per year with an overall mortality rate of 10% to 20%.[16] Prompt surgical debridement and resection are necessary for patients in whom vessel erosion, bleeding, and abscess formation are likely. Toxic products are flushed out and sumps are placed for irrigation (See Guideline 43.)

The syndrome of acute mesenteric ischemia has a mortality rate of 70%. This entity can result in a catastrophic emergency requiring vasodilation and revascularization or resection.[14]

Each year at least 500,000 people with irritable bowel disease (diverticulitis, Crohn's disease, ulcerative colitis) are admitted to hospitals in the United States, 30,000 of whom are being treated for the first time.[18] Fistulae are diagnosed preoperatively in this population in 69% of cases and are the primary indication for surgical intervention.[4]

With 140,000 new cases diagnosed each year, colorectal carcinoma remains a major health problem that is responsible for 60,000 deaths annually.[12] Many resection options and sphincter-preserving procedures are employed to treat this disease in addition to the use of radiation and chemotherapy. However, radiation injury to the bowel and colon has been recently reported to occur at a rate of 6.7% in a study of combined adjuvant radiation and chemotherapy for rectal cancer.[9]

The rate of gastric carcinoma occurrence has decreased in recent years with estimated deaths numbering 7.5 per 100,000 population in the United States.[2] Only 30% of patients who present with this entity will have disease that is resectable with curative intent by gastrectomy or subtotal gastrectomy.[17]

Duodenal disease is also less prevalent now in this country. The cause for this decline has not yet been scientifically determined but improvements in medical therapy (such as the use of H_2 blockers) play a role. Most operations are now performed for life-threatening ulcer complications such as hemorrhage, perforation, or obstruction or for recurrences while on medical treatment.[1] Procedures for the treatment of this disorder include pyloroplasty with vagotomy, gastroenterostomy, or antrectomy with vagotomy. Gastric ulcers can also be treated surgically by a subtotal or total gastrectomy with gastroduodenostomy or gastrojejunostomy. (See Guideline 48.)

Gastroesophageal reflux has replaced gastric and duodenal ulcers as the most common upper GI problem.[7] This syndrome can be treated medically. However, if the antireflux barrier is defective to the point where serious reflux and its complications continue, surgical repair is required to restore the antireflux barrier.[7] A Nissen fundoplication is an often-applied surgical technique for this problem.

Esophageal and primary hepatic cancers are less frequently encountered lesions, but they have relatively dismal outcomes when they do occur. There is an approximately 10% survival rate at 5 years for esophageal cancer.[6] Esophagogastrectomy via several approaches is the surgical option for palliation or prolonged survival. It is not curative. Metastases occur in 48% to 73% of cases of primary hepatic carcinoma.[14] Many investigators advocate surgical resection for this and other disorders of the liver parenchyma (abscess, hemangioma, cysts, and granulomas).[14]

The pancreas can be affected by the development of pseudocysts and carcinoma of the periampulla requiring rapid and technically accurate surgical intervention. Surgery in the form of pancreaticoduodenectomy is recommended for carcinoma. Pseudocyst is best managed by internal drainage.[5]

PATHOPHYSIOLOGY

In the GI tract, changes in physiologic function are attributable to altered secretion, altered mobility, inadequate digestion, inadequate absorption, or obstruction. Clinical manifestations of GI disorders include objective demonstrations of pathologic processes. These include abdominal wall tenderness or rigidity, palpable masses, altered bowel sounds, evidence of GI bleeding, poor nutrition, and jaundice.[14] Other symptoms of GI disturbance include nausea, vomiting, anorexia, constipation, diarrhea, dysphagia, and abdominal distension.[14]

There are many disease entities that can cause dysfunction of the GI system and they have a multitude of causes. Acute pancreatitis in the United States is due largely to cholelithiasis or alcohol abuse. The effect is autodigestion of the pancreas by its own enzymes. Pancreatic pseudocysts generally result from a disruption of the ductal system of the pancreas (from pancreatitis, trauma, or surgery).[14] Carcinoma of the pancreas is believed to arise from the ductal system in 90% of the cases; adenocarcinoma is the primary lesion.[14]

When diverticular disease is complicated by an inflammatory response, acute diverticulitis, abscesses, peritonitis, fistulae, and obstruction occur. These sequelae, as well as bleeding complications, must be treated surgically. Elective resection for diverticulosis is preferable to an emergency operation. The actual causes of inflammatory bowel disease remain virtually unknown.

Chronic duodenal ulceration is almost never of neoplastic origin except in rare instances. Chronic gastric ulceration may be caused by benign or malignant lesions. Acute ulcers may occur in a setting of extreme stress. The etiology of acute and chronic duodenal and gastric ulceration is multivariate, including acid secretion and changes in protective factors.[14]

Common factors have been identified in patients who develop esophageal cancer. Heavy alcohol consumption and smoking are two major factors. Stasis due to gastroesophageal acid reflux is another possible cause. Cellular changes associated with the stasis are possible precursors to the development of adenocarcinoma of the esophagus.[15]

Mesenteric vascular occlusion without major vessel involvement may produce localized ischemia. With complete loss of arterial flow, there is infarction, gangrene, and, if untreated, perforation of the involved intestinal segment with peritonitis and death.[14] Arterial occlusions may be caused by a thrombosis or an embolus to a large or distal arterial branch, cardiac abnormalities, a hypercoagulable state, advancing atherosclerosis, conditions of low-flow states, or direct trauma.[13]

Intestinal obstruction can occur as the result of a malignancy, adhesions, volvulus, or hernia. The results range from a simple mechanical obstruction to a strangulated obstruction. Many factors have been implicated in the etiology of colorectal cancer and motility disorders of the GI system, but the causes are as yet unknown.[14]

Primary carcinoma of the liver has been associated with cirrhosis. These lesions, in addition to cysts, granulomas, and metastatic tumors, may require surgery for optimal therapy.

LENGTH OF STAY/ANTICIPATED COURSE

Several DRGs (diagnosis-related groups) are encompassed under the umbrella title of GI surgery. The anticipated length of stay for a GI procedure ranges from 9 to 12 days, with 2 to 3 of those days spent in an ICU or intermediate care unit. Should complications such as wound infection, anastomotic disruption, impaired gas exhange, or fistula formation occur, the average length of stay is increased to 13 to 15 days, with more days spent in the ICU.

Extreme cases of necrotizing pancreatitis can result in greatly prolonged hospital stays of as many as 30 to 60 days or more. Common DRGs associated with GI surgery are summarized in Table 49-1.

MANAGEMENT TRENDS AND CONTROVERSIES

Care of the GI surgical patient in the critical care unit poses a unique challenge to the multidisciplinary team. The responsibility for achieving positive patient care outcomes in this population can be great.

The goal of the preoperative period is to establish the diagnosis, maintain optimal organ function, and correct defects or deficiencies that may be present. Additionally, the patient and significant others must be supported and educated regarding the disease, diagnostic and surgical inter-

TABLE 49-1 Selected DRGs Related to Gastrointestinal Surgery

DRG #	DRG label	Average LOS
148	Major small and large bowel procedures with complications	14.7 days
149	Major small and large bowel procedures without complications	8.2 days
154	Stomach, esophageal, and duodenal procedures, age >17, with complications	17.0 days
155	Stomach, esophageal, and duodenal procedures, age >17, without complications	7.2 days
170	Other digestive system *or* procedures with complications	14.6 days
171	Other digestive system *or* procedures without complications	5.9 days

Source: *St Anthony's DRG guidebook 1995*, Reston, Va, 1994, St Anthony.

ventions, and other therapies. Some patients with malignant tumors of the GI tract may undergo chemotherapeutic and/or radiation therapy to reduce the size of the lesion. These therapies, however, can result in profound weakness, altered wound healing, and a predisposition to infection, all impacting on patient care.

Naturally, in the postoperative phase, wound healing is a primary concern for care givers. Successful transition through the three phases of wound healing depends partly on the presence of adequate nutritional stores. Malnutrition (which can be a pre-illness phenomenon) slows the healing process and can cause wounds to heal inadequately or incompletely.[8] Through appropriate physical assessment and intervention, the critical care nurse can improve and/or maintain a patient's nutrition status, minimizing malnutrition-related complications such as impaired wound healing.[8] Nutritional assessment of the patient in the critical care environment may include an expired gas analysis through a metabolic cart study. This calculates the oxygen consumption index in an effort to assess for hypermetabolism because of increased cellular demand for oxygen in response to increased metabolism.[8] Several formulas are also used to calculate approximate caloric requirements.

In general, patients with a normal preoperative nutritional status suffer no ill effects of a nothing-by-mouth status (NPO) for up to 7 days postoperatively.[14] Following GI surgery, most patients are kept NPO for a period of days until bowel function returns. High-risk patients and those with prolonged NPO status may be placed on total parenteral nutrition or receive enteral feedings. There is controversy over which route is preferable. Some studies have indicated that enteral therapy compared with the parenteral route may have an important role in immunonutrition by maintaining gut integrity, stimulating the immune system, and preventing bacterial translocation from the gut.[11]

ICU-acquired infection in association with progressive organ system dysfunction is an important cause of morbidity and mortality in critical surgical illness.[10] The upper GI tract has been found to be a reservoir of the organisms causing ICU-acquired infection.[10] (See Guideline 48.) Pathologic GI colonization is associated with the development of multiple organ failure in the critically ill surgical patient. A recent study found infections associated with GI colonization to include pneumonia, wound infection, urinary tract infection, recurrent peritonitis, and bacteremia. ICU mortality was greater for patients colonized with *Pseudomonas;* organ dysfunction was most marked in patients colonized with *Candida, Pseudomonas,* or *S. epidermidis.*[10] Close surveillance of preoperative and postoperative GI surgical patients by the entire multidisciplinary team is key in preventing nosocomial infections. Vigilant central line changes, scrupulous assessment and management of wounds and drains, and strict attention to hand washing by all care givers may thwart the development of infectious complications. Early mobilization and aggressive pulmonary toilet are also advantageous in preventing pulmonary complications. With the incidence of infection with antibiotic-resistant organisms, preventing infection before it occurs is essential to minimize morbidity and mortality and reduce length of stay.

The relatively recent advent of the interventional radiology specialty has enabled patients with abnormalities such as abscesses, collections, and pseudocysts to avoid repeat surgical interventions. Special drainage devices (such as locking and nonlocking all-purpose drainage catheters or sumps) and monitoring allow for nonsurgical treatment of these problems.

The challenge of caring for the adult undergoing GI surgery is to meet diverse needs and multisystem problems. In the critical care arena, patients frequently have significant coexisting illnesses that complicate their survival and prolong ICU and hospital stays. It is not uncommon for these patients to experience slower ventilator weans secondary to abdominal incisions, and decreased diaphragmatic excursion. It is imperative that risk factors be addressed proactively to diminish the rate of complications in this population.

Invasive monitoring has added a more comprehensive assessment of cardiovascular status and fluid balance. Epidural and PCA modalities for pain relief afford better tolerance for mobilization and rehabilitative activities. Thus, effective analgesia ensuring optimal patient comfort with minimal side effects may yield positive patient outcomes.

Methods for managing the GI surgical patient have evolved to include planning for same-day surgery and briefer hospital stays. The use of laser technology, laparoscopes, and endoscopy is revolutionizing surgical practice. Laparoscopic vagotomies for treatment of ulcer disease have been proposed and studied.[20] Nissen fundoplication via the laparoscope has been performed successfully. In clinical practice the nurse can anticipate caring for older clients, transplant recipients, or those with GI malignancies. Certainly, a major thrust for the future is to diagnose GI disease early, and more important, institute measures to enhance prevention of these ailments.

ASSESSMENT

PARAMETER	ANTICIPATED ALTERATION
Bowel sounds	Absent *due to immobile bowel, peritonitis, gangrenous bowel* Rare, isolated *due to paralytic ileus, manipulation of the bowel in surgery, or effects of general anesthetic* Loud, high pitched *due to intestinal obstruction*
Percussion of abdomen	Tympanitic sounds with distension and the absence of normal liver dullness *due to perforated viscus*
Palpation of abdomen	Rebound tenderness *due to peritoneal inflammation* Involuntary rigidity or spasm *due to peritonitis* Murphy's sign — RUQ pain on inspiration, possibly referred to shoulder *due to cholecystitis* *Possible masses may be detected*
Pain	Intermittent, crampy, colic *due to intestinal obstruction* "Burning" midepigastric pain *due to penetrating ulcer* Knifelike pain *due to perforated viscus* Dysphagic *due to esophageal tumor or decreased esophageal or stomach motility* Sustained pain *due to strangulated intestinal obstruction or peritonitis* Deep, midepigastric pain radiating to back *due to pancreatitis* Varied levels of pain increasing with movement *due to abdominal surgical incision* Severe, cramping, nonlocalized *due to intestinal ischemia*
NG aspirate, vomitus	Blood *due to rapidly bleeding lesion in the stomach or duodenum* Coffee-ground *due to slower-bleeding lesion (allowing gastric acid to convert Hgb to methemoglobin)* Fecal origin *due to intestinal obstruction*
Chest x-ray	Free abdominal air *due to ruptured abdominal viscus* Distended loops of bowel (air filled) *due to obstruction* Patchy infiltrates *due to atelectasis* Diffuse alveolar infiltrates *due to ARDS*
Stools	Constipation, obstipation *due to obstruction or volvulus* Loose, bloody *due to mesenteric infarction* Melena *due to upper GI bleeding (ulcers, tumors)* Bright red blood per rectum *due to lower GI bleeding (carcinoma, diverticular disease)* Occult blood *due to GI bleeding source* Fatty and foul smelling *due to pancreatic insufficiency or malabsorption* Diarrhea *due to altered bowel motility, malabsorption, intolerance to enteral feedings, increased levels of osmotically active substances, excess intestinal secretion*
Laboratory Tests	
WBC count	Elevated: >10,000/mm³ *due to abscesses, fistulae, sepsis, mesenteric vascular occlusion, bowel obstruction or strangulation, any inflammatory process*
Platelet count	*Decreased: <100,000/m³ due to platelets being activated, aggregating, and being destroyed*
APTT	Prolonged: >30 to 40 seconds

PT	Prolonged: >12.5 seconds Both prolonged *due to decreased circulating levels of coagulation proteins*
Serum electrolytes	May be increased or decreased *due to dehydration, GI losses, decreased renal excretion*
Hgb and Hct	Elevated >18 g/dl; >52% with hemoconcentration *due to decreased intake, fluid losses from drains or vomiting* Decreased with bleeding
Serum amylase	Elevated: >190 IU/L *due to acute pancreatitis, perforated viscera, obstruction, cholecystitis*
Serum Ca^{++}	Decreased: <4.5 mg/dl *due to acute pancreatitis, pancreatic or small bowel fistulae, multiple blood transfusions*
Serum Mg^{+}	Decreased: <1.3 mEq/L *due to GI losses, decreased intake, pancreatitis, alcohol use*
Serum lactate level	Increased: >2.2 mEq/L *due to impaired perfusion in the shock state as a result of the anaerobic metabolism that occurs*
Liver function tests	Elevated *due to biliary tract disease, impaired hepatic function,* or *ischemia with shock liver*
Barium swallow upper GI study with or without small bowel follow-through	Radiographic abnormalities *due to ulcer disease, diverticular disease, esophageal abnormalities, tumors*
Esophagoscopy, gastroscopy, duodenoscopy	Visual identification of site of bleeding or tumor; allows for biopsy
Abdominal radiograph	Dilated loops of bowel *due to intestinal obstruction* Presence of abdominal mass
Barium enema	Irregularities *due to ulcerative colitis, tumors, diverticulitis*
Manometric motility studies	Elevated pressures in affected area *due to disorders of motility*
Angiography	Abnormal *due to site of bleeding or tumor mass*
Radionucleotide imaging	Abnormal uptake *due to site of GI bleeding*
Abdominal ultrasound, CT scan, MRI scan	Identify abnormalities in abdominal vasculature, solid or cystlike lesions or abscesses
Liver biopsy	Abnormal cytology *due to pathologic process*
ERCP (endoscopic retrograde cholangiopancreatography)	Visualized abnormalities of the bilary tree and pancreas (strictures, inflammation, stones, and pancreatitis)

PLAN OF CARE

INTENSIVE PHASE

The length of the ICU course will vary for patients who undergo GI surgery. It depends on the severity and extent of disease, response to therapy, and the existence of postoperative complications. Once stabilized, the patient can be moved to an intermediate care environment.

PATIENT CARE PRIORITIES	EXPECTED PATIENT OUTCOMES
Impaired ventilation *r/t* *Decreased diaphragmatic excursion secondary to abdominal surgery* *Shallow respirations due to pain/anxiety*	Free of pneumonia or infiltrate SaO_2 >92%

Plan of Care (cont'd)

Decreased intravascular volume *r/t* *Interstitial fluid shifts* *Dehydration* *Bleeding*	Euvolemia as evidenced by weight within patient's norm, balanced I/O, preload indices: WNL
Impaired coagulation *r/t* *Vascular disruption* *Repeated transfusions* *Hepatic dysfunction*	Stable coagulation profile
Pain *r/t* *Incision* *Limited mobility*	Patient will be comfortable Able to rest, sleep, and engage in care-related activities
High risk for impaired wound healing *r/t* *Surgical incisions* *Drains* *Altered nutritional status*	Wound edges well approximated without inflammation
Decreased nutrition *r/t dysfunction associated with disease process and surgical intervention*	Positive protein balance
High risk for infection *r/t* *Surgical incision* *Drains* *Preoperative risk factors*	Afebrile WBC count: WNL
Fluid and electrolyte imbalance *r/t* *Interstitial fluid shifts* *NG drainage* *Surgical drains* *Change in perfusion*	Stable electrolyte profile and adequate fluid resuscitation
Self-care deficit *r/t inadequate knowledge about preoperative and postoperative medical illnesses and expectations for recovery while in the critical care unit*	Patient verbalizes comprehension of plan of care
Impaired bowel function *r/t* *Surgical dissection and manipulation* *Altered perfusion* *Anesthetic agents*	Normal bowel sounds with stable GI motility
Impaired renal function *r/t* *Hypovolemia* *Interstitial fluid shifts and effects from medications*	Creatinine and BUN: WNL Urine output: WNL

INTERVENTIONS

Assess V_{Σ} *for respiratory expenditure.*

Monitor for decreased O_2 delivery. Assess VO_2/DO_2 q8h.

Monitor SaO_2 *for adequate O_2 delivery.*

Assess $ETCO_2$ trends *to assist with weaning.*

Measure daily respiratory parameters *to evaluate readiness for weaning.*

Assess risks related to mechanical ventilation (barotrauma, aspiration, tracheoesophageal fistula, iatrogenic infection).

Assess improved diaphragmatic excursion after sedation, especially with use of epidural infusions.

Assess breath sounds *for adventitious sounds.*

Monitor daily chest x-ray *for evidence of infiltrate, pneumonia, ARDS.*

Assess temperature curve, sputum production, and WBC count trend *for evidence of infection.*

Monitor for ectopy or ST, T-wave changes.

Plan of Care (cont'd)

Maintain stable MAP *for adequate tissue perfusion and to prevent end-organ dysfunction.*
Administer fluid replacements *to achieve euvolemic state and to avoid prerenal ischemic insults.*
Administer vasopressors and titrate *to achieve MAP adequate for tissue perfusion.*
Trend CO, CI, and SVR q1h to q4h or as vasopressors are titrated *to assess response.*
Maintain PCWP within limits of patients cardiac status *for adequate myocardial contractility.*
Assess chest x-ray for cardiac enlargement.
Monitor for cardiogenic and septic shock.
Auscultate for murmurs, S_3 or S_4.
Trend SVO_2 *for changes in cellular O_2 delivery.*
Administer blood products based on specific blood losses.
Assess for changes in coagulation factors indicative of DIC. (See Guideline 59.)
Avoid pharmacologic regimens with adverse effects on coagulation factors (such as Inocor decreasing platelet counts).
Assess skin closely for superficial bleeding.
Monitor abdomen for increased abdominal size or retroperitoneal bleeding.
Test all drainage for occult blood.
Assess any decrease in Hgb and Hct *for potential signs of bleeding.*
Assess for abdominal pain, distension, or tenderness.
Monitor response to epidural, PCA, or IV sedation; score patient according to pain intensity scale. (See Figure 49-1.)
Maintain position of comfort based on patient's preference.
Assess for nonverbal cues of discomfort.
Assess for secondary causes of discomfort, such as anxiety or sleep deprivation.
Maintain adequate nutrition *to promote wound healing.*
Assess wound every shift for approximation, erythema, or drainage.
Use sterile technique for wound care.
Assess wound for hematoma, abscess formation, or evidence of infection.
Monitor nutritional needs for enteral or parenteral feedings.
Collaborate with nutritional support team for high-risk patients.
Monitor metabolic requirements weekly with urine urea nitrogen 24 hour collections and metabolic cart studies.
Monitor weight daily.
Assess all wounds for drainage and obtain appropriate cultures.
Monitor all culture reports for appropriate antibiotic therapy.
Assess response to antibiotics and monitor for increased or decreased WBC count, as well as bandemia.
Administer antibiotics as prescribed and assess peak/trough levels for adequacy.
Assess daily laboratory values for appropriate levels and replace electrolytes accordingly.
Assess for peripheral edema.
Monitor serum osmolality and urine osmolality.
If high output NG drainage occurs, replace fluid cc per cc.
Monitor bowel sounds q8h.
Assess for postoperative ileus, bowel perforation, or abdominal distension.
Assess stoma viability.
Monitor for decreased bowel activity caused by postoperative narcotics.
Explore any causes of diarrhea: enteral feeds, ischemic colitis, *C. difficile,* or VRE (vancomycin-resistant enterococcus) infections.
Monitor all drugs for nephrotoxicity.
Strict I/O.
Administer renal dose dopamine to achieve adequate renal perfusion.

Plan of Care (cont'd)

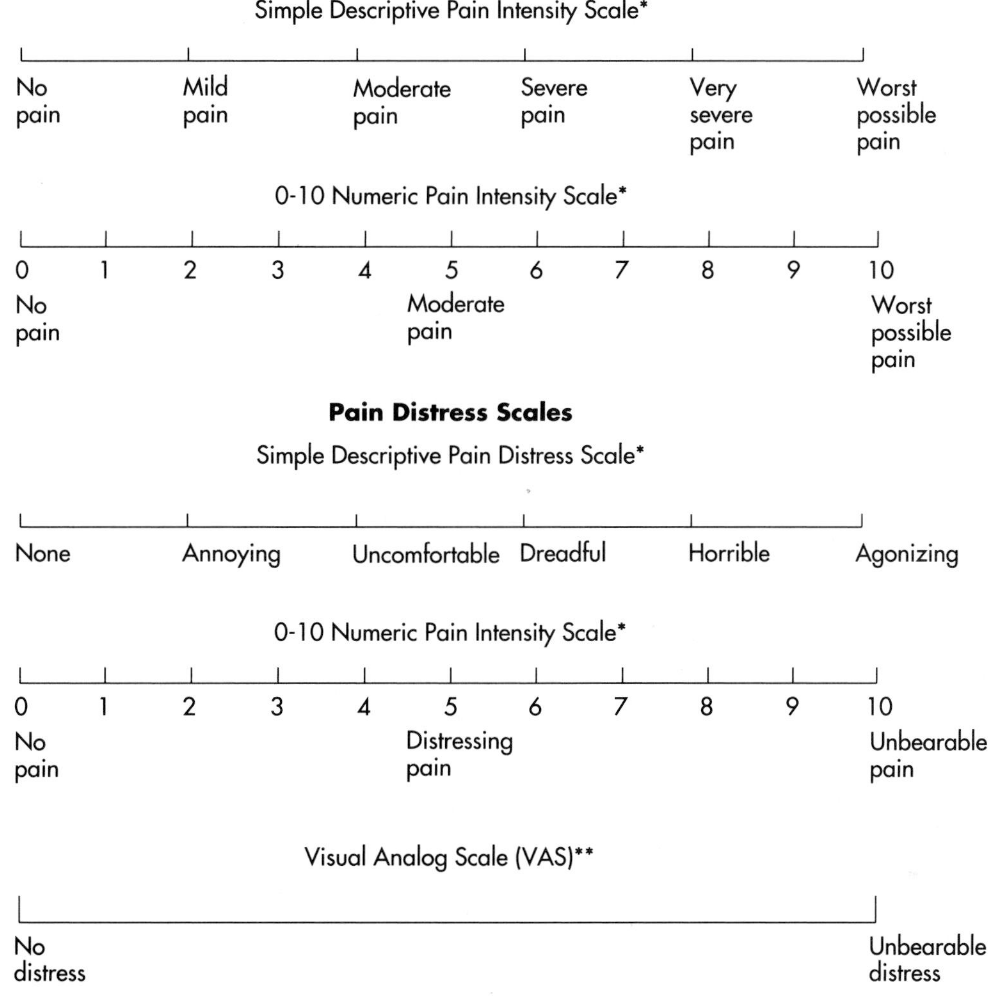

Figure 49-1 Pain intensity scales. (From the Acute Pain Management Guideline Panel: Acute pain management: operative or medical procedures and trauma, *Clinical Practice Guidelines* vol no 92-0032, Rockville, Md, 1992, Agency for Health Care Policy and Research, Public Health Service, U.S. Department of Health and Human Services.

INTERMEDIATE PHASE

The focus of nursing care in the intermediate phase is to continue the plan of care initiated in the ICU, maintain patient stability, and prevent the development of complications. The discharge planning and educational interventions are accelerated and there is increased participation of the patient and family.

PATIENT CARE PRIORITIES	EXPECTED OUTCOMES
High risk for decreased pulmonary function *r/t*	RR: WNL
Decreased ventilatory volume from guarding with incisional pain or abdominal distention	SaO_2 ≥92%; ABG within patient norms
Tachypnea related to fever, pain, or anxiety	

Plan of Care (cont'd)

Decreased intravascular fluid volumes *r/t* *Preoperative volume state* *Intraoperative and postoperative fluid shifts* *Vomiting* *NG suction* *Diarrhea* *Fistula drainage*	Normal volume state No signs or symptoms of hypovolemia
High risk for decreased tissue perfusion *r/t postoperative bleeding*	Prompt recognition and control of bleeding Replenished circulating blood volume
Pain *r/t incision* and *mobilization*	Subjective pain rating of 0 to 2 on a 10-point rating scale (see Figure 49-1) Patient performs preoperative and postoperative activities with well-controlled pain
High risk for impaired wound healing *r/t altered skin integrity*	Normal progression through the three phases of wound healing[3] Free from wound-related complications
Decreased nutritional status *r/t* *NPO status* *GI losses* *Catabolic state*	Optimal nutritional status to promote tissue repair Positive nitrogen balance
High risk for infection *r/t* *Incisions* *Nutritional deficits* *Risk for perfusion deficit*	Free from nosocomial infections
Electrolyte imbalance *r/t* *GI losses* *Decreased intake of nutrients and electrolytes* *Fluid imbalance*	Serum electrolytes: WNL
Self-care deficit *r/t* *Inadequate knowledge about wound management* *Signs of infection* *Dietary changes* *Medications* *Activities* *Follow-up care*	Patient understands and demonstrates appropriate elements of self-care
High risk for decreased bowel function *r/t* *Disease process* *Surgical manipulation* *General anesthesia* *Decreased activity*	Bowel function: WNL Absence of paralytic ileus, correction of obstruction

INTERVENTIONS

Chest physiotherapy and postural drainage q4h and as needed.

Assist patient with incentive spirometry, coughing, and deep breathing exercises *to improve alveolar gas exchange.*

Monitor pulse oximetry continuously or q4h.

Nasotracheal, tracheal, or endotracheal tube suctioning as needed.

Assess for signs of respiratory difficulty (decreased chest wall movement, tachypnea, sternal or intercostal retraction, nasal flaring).

Medicate for pain as needed *to promote maximum diaphragmatic excursion.*

Compression sleeves to lower extremities when not ambulating *to maintain circulation.*

Mobilize as soon as possible to out-of-bed status and ambulation.

Plan of Care (cont'd)

Administer physiologic fluid supplements (balanced salt solutions) *to maintain adequate tissue perfusion.*

Monitor vital signs in conjunction with patient acuity (at least q4h), alert for postoperative or sepsis-related hypotension, tachycardia.

Monitor CVP and maintain WNL.

Monitor intake and output with frequency concomitant with patient acuity.

Maintain cardiac monitoring *to detect potential arrhythmias.*

Monitor Hgb and Hct levels, coagulation profile.

Assess abdomen, any indwelling drains, stools for signs of obvious bleeding *to detect potential coagulopathy.*

Hematest all tube drainage and stools.

Replace blood losses for patients who are symptomatic or if ≥20% of the total circulating blood volume is lost.

Replace other blood factors, administer vitamin K SQ prn.

Monitor pH of gastric drainage and administer antacid for pH <5 to 6 *to protect the GI tract from potential stress ulceration.*

Instruct patient regarding type of analgesia being administered (epidural, patient-controlled, or IV bolus as needed).

Use pain intensity scale to assess effectiveness of pain regimen. (See Figure 49-1.)

Encourage use of analgesia before activities (out-of-bed activity, ambulation, C & DB).

Encourage use of wound-supporting pillow *to decrease splinting with C & DB exercises.*

Monitor status of incisional area, alert for signs of infection, disruption (redness, swelling, drainage, separation of wound edges), or anastomotic leak.

Monitor for other signs of infection (elevated WBC count, confusion, temperature elevation).

Maintain sterile technique with incisional dressing changes.

Maintain patency and assess drainage of abdominal tubes and drains.

Assess for adequate nutritional intake.

Maintain nutritional intake (oral, TPN, enteral feedings) and monitor tolerance.

Monitor weight trends.

Consult nutritional support team for "at-risk" patients.

Monitor effects of nutritional therapies and of nutritional status via hourly urine urea nitrogen measurements and pertinent laboratory values (albumin, transferrin levels).

Monitor temperature at least q4h.

Obtain appropriate culture studies (wound, urine, sputum, drains) for temperature elevations.

Note qualities of all tube or wound drainage.

Strict hand-washing technique.

Administer antibiotic therapy and monitor patient tolerance.

Assess lab values and replace as needed.

Monitor for signs of electrolyte imbalance (arrhythmias, weakness, lethargy, change in mental status).

Assess patient/family knowledge of discharge plan.

Instruct patient and family about wound care, signs of wound infection, medication, postoperative activity, dietary regimen.

Elicit feedback and observe performance of patient in accomplishing self-care activities.

Provide information related to follow-up care.

Provide instruction to patient and family regarding stomal assessment and ostomy care.

Consult appropriate services to provide educational support and home care follow-up (enterostomal therapist, home care coordinator).

Monitor for signs of returning bowel function (normoactive bowel sounds, presence of flatus).

Monitor for signs and symptoms of paralytic ileus or intestinal obstruction.

Monitor for presence of abdominal pain, nausea, vomiting.

Note presence of high gastric output via NG tube *to ensure adequate fluid replacement and detect potential complications.*

Assess stomal characteristics *(if applicable).*

TRANSITION TO DISCHARGE

The GI surgical patient undergoes many system alterations during a hospitalization episode. As the patient moves through the ICU and intermediate phases, many physiologic parameters are assessed and interventions implemented with the goal of positive patient outcomes. The patient has likely undergone some changes in body image or is experiencing anxiety related to a new diagnosis. The nurse can be instrumental in alleviating anxiety by coordinating efforts of the multidisciplinary team, patient, and family. Developing and implementing the education and discharge plans are key in promoting patient acceptance and limiting anxiety related to self-care (wound care, ostomy care, tube management).

REFERENCES

1. Bliss DW, Stabile BE: The impact of ulcerogenic drugs on surgery for the treatment of peptic ulcer disease, *Arch Surg* 127:609-612, 1991.
2. Boring C, Squires T, Tong T: Cancer statistics, 1991, *CA Cancer J Clin* 41(1):19-36, 1991.
3. Cooper DM: Optimizing wound healing: r/t practice within the domain of nursing, *Nurs Clin North Am* 25(1):165-180, 1990.
4. Fabrizio M, et al: Incidence, diagnosis and treatment of enteric and colorectal fistulae in patients with Crohn's disease, *Ann Surg* 218(5):660, 1993.
5. Fromm D, editor: *Gastrointestinal surgery,* New York, 1985, Churchill Livingstone, p 876.
6. Herskovic A, et al: Combined chemotherapy and radiotherapy compared with radiotherapy alone in patients with cancer of the esophagus, *N Engl J Med* 326:1593, 1992.
7. Hill LD, Aye RW, Ramel S: Antireflux surgery, a surgeon's look, *Gastroenterol Clin North Am* 19(3):745-774, 1990.
8. Konstantinides NN: The impact of nutrition on wound healing, *Crit Care Nurs Clin North Am* 13(5):25-33, 1993.
9. Krook JE, et al: Effective surgical adjuvant therapy for high rectal carcinoma, *N Engl J Med* 324:709, 1991.
10. Marshall JC, Christow NV, Meakins JL: The gastrointestinal tract, the undrained abscess of multiple organ failure, *Ann Surg* 218(2):111-119, 1993.
11. McClave SA, Lowen CC, Snider HL: Immunonutrition and enteral hyperalimentation of critically ill patients, *Dig Dis Sci* 37:1153-1161, 1992.
12. Murray JJ: Preface, *Surg Clin North Am* 73(1), 1993.
13. Quinn AD: Acute mesenteric ischemia, *Crit Care Nurs Clin North Am* 5(1):171-175, 1993.
14. Schwartz S, editor: *Principles of surgery,* New York, 1989, McGraw-Hill.
15. Sideranko S: Esophagogastrectomy, *Crit Care Nurs Clin North Am* 5(1):177-184, 1993.
16. Sleisenger M, Fordtran J: *Gastrointestinal disease,* Philadelphia, 1989, WB Saunders.
17. Smith JW, Brennan MF: Surgical treatment of gastric cancer, *Surg Clin North Am* 72(2):381-421, 1992.
18. Stabile BE: Current surgical management of duodenal ulcers, *Surg Clin North Am* 72(2), 1992.
19. *St Anthony's DRG Guidebook 1995,* Reston, Va, 1994, St Anthony.
20. Wolff, BG. Preface, *Surg Clin North Am* 73(5):xi-xii, 1993.

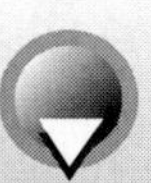

CLINICAL GUIDELINE

50

Abdominal Trauma

Suzanne Wasch Zimmerman, BSN, RN, CCRN

DESCRIPTION

Trauma is the leading cause of death in people under the age of 30. Abdominal injuries account for a large number of trauma-related injuries and 13% to 15% of trauma deaths.[18] This is due largely to the fact that abdominal injury frequently involves multiple organs or organ systems and therefore has increased morbidity and mortality rates.[3]

Abdominal trauma is blunt or penetrating injury to the vascular or visceral structures within the confines of the abdomen and pelvis. It is a frequent sequela of major trauma. Since the abdominal area comprises a large portion of the body's trunk, it has increased vulnerability to injury.

PATHOPHYSIOLOGY

Motor vehicle accidents account for 60% of blunt abdominal injuries,[15] but they also may be the result of falls, sports injuries, or assaults with a blunt object.

Blunt injuries require diligent assessment because most of them are hidden. Fatal wounds can be subtle or masked by more obvious but less threatening injuries. The patient appears to be stable one moment and then rapidly decompensates. Autopsy reports continue to identify undiagnosed abdominal injury as a major preventable cause of trauma death.[3]

The organs most frequently injured in blunt trauma are the spleen, liver, kidneys, and small intestine.[20] Splenic and liver injuries occur due to crushing forces that compress these organs against the vertebral column. A direct blow to the abdomen can transmit forces sufficient to rupture an organ. Lower rib fractures on the right side should increase suspicion of liver injury, and left lower rib fractures carry with them a 20% incidence of splenic rupture.[1] Because the liver and spleen are so vascular, hemorrhage is a serious problem, and patients with these injuries often are taken to the operating room for surgical repair.

Sudden deceleration injuries occur when the body stops but the organs still have velocity.[22] These shearing forces can rip an organ from its fixation point or vascular supply, causing hemorrhage. The kidneys may be badly contused or the renal arteries torn from their attachment to the aorta, causing massive blood loss.[18]

Hollow viscus organs may burst from sudden impact as abdominal pressure rises drastically. The intestines can be transected by a seatbelt worn too high over the abdomen, or they may burst from sudden impact pressure.[18] This causes spillage of intestinal contents into the abdominal cavity, resulting in irritation and probable infection.

Pelvic fractures are caused by direct impact on the pelvic ring. Thirty percent of patients with pelvic fractures have associated abdominal injuries caused by either the force of impact or penetrating injury by the fractures themselves.[20]

Renal and urinary damage are common. Injury to the male urethra should be suspected, and insertion of a Foley catheter may be contraindicated, especially if there is blood at the meatus or a high-riding prostate. Foley insertion could convert a partial tear into a complete transection.[15] If the bladder is full, the chance of rupture is good[22] and will be evidenced by ecchymosis of the flanks or lower back.

Pelvic fractures may be treated with the use of external fixation to stabilize the pelvis and decrease venous and fracture-site bleeding. If arterial bleeding is substantial, the patient may go to vascular radiology for embolization of the vessels.

The pancreas lies deep in the abdomen, protected by other organs and layers of muscle. Therefore, if this organ is injured, it presents as part of a severe multitrauma picture that carries a very high mortality rate.[21] Pancreatic injury is difficult to assess and damage may go undetected for days or weeks. Fistula, abscess, hemorrhage, or pseudocyst may occur late after injury and are equally difficult to treat once discovered.

Penetrating abdominal trauma is most often the result of violence and gunshot or knife wounds; like blunt trauma, it may be deceiving. Often the dramatic external wounds distract from more life-threatening internal damage.

Gunshot wounds tend to be more severe than stab wounds because deflection of the missile by various tissues can create a myriad of internal injuries. A shotgun fired at close range can cause blast wounds as well as missile damage, and fragments of wadding and clothing that enter the wound greatly increase the risk of infection.[22] Gunshot wounds to the abdomen are associated with an 80% to 90% incidence of peritoneal injury[23]; thus exploratory laparotomy is indicated to control hemorrhage and prevent sepsis. Stab wounds are more straightforward and much less likely to lead to serious injury.[11] These wounds may be evaluated by diagnostic peritoneal lavage unless evisceration is obvious or the patient remains hemodynamically unstable. To avoid hemorrhage, an impaled object should be left in place and stabilized until it can be removed in the operating room.[2]

LENGTH OF STAY/ANTICIPATED COURSE

The length of stay for victims of abdominal trauma varies widely depending on mechanism and severity of injury and occurrence of complications. In the acute phase, complications can be devastating. Blood loss and sepsis are the major causes of death.[11] The abdominal-trauma patient often is in hemorrhagic shock and needs aggressive resuscitation. A progressive drop in hematocrit (Hct) can be indicative of unrecognized abdominal injury, and the patient should be taken to the operating room promptly for repair of these injuries.[7]

Sepsis is the most significant hazard of colon or rectal trauma, and occurs when the native microbial flora present in the lumen are allowed to leak into the peritoneal space. The colon is present in all four quadrants of the abdomen, and thus is at risk in almost all patients with an abdominal wound.[8]

Acute respiratory distress syndrome (ARDS) is common in severe trauma and makes oxygen delivery a formidable task (see Guideline 35.) Surgical manipulation of the intestines, shock, and use of anesthesia during surgery can cause an ileus. Because this makes enteral feeding more difficult, nutritional support of the patient may be more challenging.

After the acute phase of injury, wound infection and abscess formation are of concern. Careful assessment, early detection, and prompt intervention are essential to avoid septic shock. Morbidity and mortality are directly related to the failure to diagnose and treat septic shock early.[3]

Abdominal trauma falls within DRG 444: Traumatic injury, age >17 years with complications, and DRG 445: Traumatic injury age >17 years without complications. The average lengths of stay are 6.2 and 4 days, respectively.[17]

MANAGEMENT TRENDS AND CONTROVERSIES

The most important factor in determining patient outcome is prompt recognition of intra-abdominal injury, because morbidity rates decrease when diagnosis is made early. An optimal patient outcome depends on rapid identification of pathology, followed by appropriate surgical intervention. Systematic, repeated assessment by a single caregiver is essential to identify the subtle changes present with abdominal injuries.

A history of the traumatic event can provide valuable clues as to the location and severity of injuries. If a car accident, was the victim belted, unbelted, or thrown from the vehicle? How long was extrication time? What was the mechanism of injury? If a penetrating wound, what type and size of weapon was used? In addition, were drugs or alcohol involved? These details, along with the patient's medical history, can help expedite diagnosis and treatment. All trauma patients should have their immune status verified or made current with administration of a tetanus vaccine.[4]

As with any trauma patient, the first priorities are placed on airway, breathing, and circulation.[15] The patient must have a patent airway and adequate oxygen delivery. Because abdominal trauma is often part of a multitrauma picture, pneumo-hemothorax and other chest trauma may complicate this process. Severe injury may require intubation and mechanical ventilation. Abdominal injuries can impact this problem if there is diaphragmatic rupture with abdominal organs in the thoracic cavity.

Fluid replacement and organ perfusion are immediate concerns.[21] Two large-bore peripheral IV catheters are placed above the diaphragm to provide access for fluid administration.[2] Lower IV lines are contraindicated in patients with abdominal or lower-body injuries, and peripheral sites are preferred initially because they are quicker, easier, and safer than a central line to insert in a hypotensive patient.[7] As soon as the lines are placed, blood is sent for type and cross-match as well as Hct and electrolytes. Crystalloid fluid boluses are infused quickly and may be warmed to prevent hypothermia. If the patient does not stabilize after two liters of IV fluids, blood should be given promptly.[11] If cross-matched blood is not available, type O or uncross-matched blood is used; thus the clinician should be alert for signs of a transfusion reaction.[22] If multiple units of blood are transfused, fresh frozen plasma and platelets may be given to provide clotting components.

Once the patient is stabilized, the entire body is stripped and inspected for signs of injury. Special attention is paid to the flanks, back, and peritoneum for bruising that may indicate internal bleeding. To avoid masking of symptoms that may lead to diagnosis of injury, analgesia is held until the evaluation is complete.[11] It is important to encourage verbalization of pain and give clear explanations as to why pain medication is being withheld temporarily. Information about pain or discomfort from the patient can be invaluable and should never be disregarded.

Peritoneal lavage is a quick, specialized diagnostic procedure used to ascertain the presence of intra-abdominal injury. A small incision is made in the abdomen and a catheter is placed in the peritoneal space. If the physician can immediately aspirate 5 to 10 cc of gross blood, the patient is taken directly to surgery.[2] If no direct blood is present, a liter of lactated Ringer's solution is infused, allowed to equilibrate, drained, and analyzed. The presence of blood, WBCs, and intestinal contents indicates a need for surgical repair.

Controversy exists as to whether diagnostic peritoneal lavage (DPL) or computerized tomography (CT) scan of the abdomen should be the diagnostic tool of choice in abdominal trauma patients. While CT scan is noninvasive and can provide more detailed, organ-specific information, accuracy is highly variable based on many factors, including type of scanner and experience of the radiologist.[13] CT scans are also expensive and relatively time-consuming. As CT scans cannot be performed at the bedside, it may not be a suitable diagnostic test for an unstable patient.

DPL has been shown to be 98% effective in diagnosis of intraperitoneal bleeding, with a low incidence of false positive and false negative results.[13] However, it is not useful for determining the exact cause or severity of injury. It does accurately predict the need for surgery. Some believe these procedures should not be compared directly but viewed as complementary.[13]

Surgical management of abdominal trauma is aimed at stopping hemorrhage, preserving damaged organs, and decontaminating the abdomen. Antibiotics are begun before surgery, preferably in the trauma room, and are continued as needed in the postoperative period.

First, any sites of bleeding are identified and controlled. Sometimes, as in cases of severe liver injury, bleeding is massive and the organ simply will be identified and packed. In these cases, the risk of untreated injuries is weighed against the risk of further blood loss, hypothermia, and anesthesia.[14] The patient is taken to the intensive care unit for stabilization so that further operative treatment will be better tolerated.

Simple perforations and lacerations of the bowel may be closed by suture, while more serious injuries are treated by resection. In this case, a proximal ileostomy or colostomy is made, as well as a distal mucous fistula. This defunctionalizes the bowel and allows it to heal.[8] The ostomy and mucous fistula may be rejoined later after healing has taken place.

Surgical treatment of solid-organ injury consists of repair and resection of the damaged areas and, in very severe cases, removal of the entire organ. The spleen, for example, is often injured but rarely removed. Because of the spleen's immunologic functions, removal may lead to an increased risk of infection and sepsis, especially in children.[5] Splenectomy may become necessary, however, in cases of uncontrolled hemorrhage or if conservative therapy fails. In this case, the patient will receive a pneumococcal vaccine postoperatively. Surgical repair of the pancreas entails drainage and resection to try to preserve as much of the organ as possible. Pancreatectomy is a last resort.[21]

Once bleeding is controlled and areas of injury are repaired, the abdominal cavity is irrigated with several liters of saline to remove blood clots, bowel contents, and other debris.[16] It is critical to remove bacteria and digestive enzymes from the abdomen and allow the injuries to heal.

Critical care of the abdominal trauma patient focuses on ensuring adequate fluid volume to maintain organ and tissue perfusion. Third-spacing is common, so fluid needs may be extensive. Appropriate antibiotics and sterile-dressing techniques reduce incidence of infection. Good pulmonary toilet is essential because painful abdominal wounds inhibit coughing and deep breathing. Analgesia can make the patient more comfortable and more willing to participate in care. Careful and continued assessment remains a cornerstone in the care of the patient with abdominal trauma.

Future trends in abdominal trauma focus on even more aggressive resuscitation to achieve supranormal values of cardiac index, oxygen delivery, and oxygen consumption. The theory is that focusing on normal values as outcome criteria may lead to inadequate resuscitation.[6] Premium importance is placed on oxygen delivery and consumption. Increasing oxygen delivery to compensate for the effects of an increased oxygen debt in the severely injured patient during resuscitation was studied and found to improve survival and decrease morbidity.[6] When compared with a control group receiving standard resuscitation, the experimental patients had less incidence of organ failure, fewer days of mechanical ventilation, and shorter ICU stays. Hyperdynamic state is accomplished through timely and aggressive resuscitation using optimal ventilatory support, rapid infusion of massive amounts of fluid and blood products, and effective pain control.

Providing adequate nutrition to these patients is also a topic of considerable investigation. The latest studies suggest that enteral feedings into the jejunum to decrease incidence of pneumonia and aspiration, as compared to parenteral nutrition, aid in maintaining gut integrity, stimulate the immune system, and prevent the translocation of bacteria from the gut into the systemic circulation.[12] In a study of 98 abdominal trauma patients, enteral feedings caused fewer episodes of septic morbidity than parenteral feedings.[10] Further investigation focuses on a way to determine the exact nutritional needs of the patient and the most therapeutic way to meet those needs.

ASSESSMENT

PARAMETER	ANTICIPATED ALTERATION
Cardiovascular Status	
HR	Tachycardia: >100 bpm *due to low intravascular volume*
MAP	Decreased: <70 mm Hg *due to low intravascular volume*
CI	Decreased: <2.5 L/min/m² *due to low intravascular volume*
Urine output	Decreased: <30 cc/hr *due to inadequate organ perfusion*
Pulmonary Status	
RR	Increased: >20 breaths/min and dyspnea *due to thoracic injury from trauma, or inability to maintain airway due to altered neurological status*
Oxygen consumption	Elevated: >250 cc/min O_2 *due to increased metabolic demand*
Oxygen delivery	Decreased: <900 cc/min O_2 *due to hypovolemia, hypoxia*
Neurological Status	
LOC	Anxiety and confusion *due to possible head injury or effects of drugs or alcohol. Neurological status may be difficult to assess.*
Abdominal Assessment	
Inspection	Abdominal ecchymosis Grey-Turner's sign: discoloration of flanks and abdomen *due to splenic injury* Cullen's sign: discoloration around the umbilicus *due to injury to the duodenum, gallbladder, or pancreas*
Bowel sounds	Decreased or absent *due to injury or stress response* Bowel sounds heard in the thoracic region *may indicate diaphragmatic rupture*
Palpation	Pain/tenderness/guarding *due to peritoneal irritation caused by blood, bile, or feces in the abdominal cavity*
Laboratory Tests	
Hgb Hct	Decreased: <10 g/dl Decreased: <30% *Due to hemorrhage or fluid resuscitation* Serial hematocrits are important for monitoring blood loss
WBC count	Elevated: >12,000 mm³. *Early increases may be due to spleen or liver injury; late increases may be due to infection.*
Urinalysis	Hematuria *due to urinary injury*
Amylase	Elevated: >190 IU/L *due to pancreatitis or duodenal injury*

PLAN OF CARE

INTENSIVE PHASE

Care of the abdominal trauma patient in the intensive phase focuses on ensuring adequate volume replacement to maintain organ and tissue perfusion while determining the exact cause and severity of injury. Early detection of life-threatening internal damage caused by the trauma requires diligent assessment and monitoring.

Plan of Care (cont'd)

PATIENT CARE PRIORITIES	EXPECTED PATIENT OUTCOMES
Impaired gas exchange *r/t* *Chest trauma (hemo-/pneumothorax, rib fracture)* *Atelectasis* *Altered neurological status*	Clear, equal breath sounds Patent airway ABG: WNL Equal chest expansion
Decreased tissue perfusion *r/t* *Hypovolemia* *Vascular injury* *Hypothermia*	Urine output >30 cc/hr Palpable peripheral pulses Capillary refill <3 sec T >36.5° C
Fluid volume deficit *r/t* *Hemorrhage* *Third-spacing*	MAP >70 mm Hg HR <120 bpm Urine output >30 cc/hr Hgb/Hct: WNL
Pain/discomfort *r/t* *Tissue injury* *Invasive procedures*	Verbalizes comfort Able to rest, sleep, and engage in care activities
Impaired skin integrity *r/t* *Penetrating wounds* *Abrasions* *Immobility*	Skin healing Absence of further breakdown
Inadequate nutrition *r/t* *Digestive system injury* *Increased metabolic need*	Albumin: WNL Adequate nutritional intake Anabolic state Positive nitrogen balance
High risk for infection *r/t* *Open wounds* *Invasive procedures* *Lines, tubes, and drains*	WBC count: WNL No redness or swelling, or drainage from wound Afebrile

INTERVENTIONS

Maintain a patent, secure airway *to minimize risk of aspiration and ensure oxygenation.*

Auscultate breath sounds *to assure adequate expansion and ventilation in all lung fields.*

Provide mechanical ventilation/oxygenation therapy as needed.

Monitor ABG with ventilatory changes and changes in patient status.

Encourage patient to cough, deep breathe, and use incentive spirometer *to improve lung expansion.*

Teach patient to splint abdomen during suctioning and coughing *to decrease pain from abdominal wounds and encourage compliance.*

Administer fluids, blood, and blood products *to ensure adequate intravascular volume.*

Warm IV fluids and blood products *to promote normothermia.*

Measure urine output hourly *as urine output is an indicator of fluid status and tissue perfusion.*

Assess dressings/wounds for signs of bleeding.

Repeatedly inspect patient back and front for signs of bruising and other indications of bleeding.

Measure abdominal drains frequently *as increased output can indicate internal hemorrhage.*

Obtain serial Hgb/Hct levels *to monitor blood volume.*

Use blankets or warming device to warm patient to within normal range. *Patient may be hypothermic due to administration of fluids, hypovolemia, or prolonged OR time.*

Administer analgesics/sedatives as needed *to maintain comfort and decrease O_2 demand and/or enable the patient to cooperate with care.*

Plan of Care (cont'd)

Monitor wounds and sites of lines and drains for signs of inflammation or infection.
Perform each dressing change separately *to avoid cross-contamination of wounds.*
Administer antibiotics as ordered.
Collaborate with dietitian daily to determine caloric needs. *Consider enteral nutrition to maintain gut integrity and prevent bacterial translocation.*
Consider a therapeutic mattress to prevent skin breakdown. The patient's skin may be badly contused or frail from massive fluid infusions.
Provide honest, clear explanations about abdominal wounds, surgery, and plan of care *to decrease anxiety and instill trust.*
Encourage patient participation in care as early as possible *to allow patient some control and promote healing.*

INTERMEDIATE PHASE

If the patient survives the intensive phase, care is focused on preventing complications such as ileus and wound infection. Meticuluous wound care and maintenance of adequate nutritional intake are nursing priorities. It is important to encourage patient mobilization and participation in care during this phase.

PATIENT CARE PRIORITIES	EXPECTED PATIENT OUTCOMES
High risk for impaired breathing pattern *r/t abdominal pain, atelectasis, fatigue*	Normal/improved pattern RR 10 to 28 breaths/min Spo_2 >94%
High risk for wound infection/dehiscence *r/t poor nutrition, poor wound healing*	Wound healing Absence of drainage or erythema at wound
Activity intolerance *r/t pain of abdominal wounds, multiple drains*	Activity with increasing independence
Inadequate nutrition *r/t digestive system injury*	Intake meets metabolic demands Increase body mass to pre-injury value

INTERVENTIONS

Encourage coughing and deep breathing with splinting of abdominal wounds.
Provide analgesics *to decrease abdominal pain and increase participation in pulmonary toilet and mobilization.*
Use aseptic technique with all dressing changes.
Assess wound/dressings meticulously for any signs or symptoms of infection (increased or purulent drainage, foul odor, etc.).
Encourage participation in ADL and plan of care.
Ensure adequate sleep/rest periods *to promote physical healing and strength.*
Collaborate with physical therapist *to increase strength and endurance.*
Encourage p.o. intake *to reach nutritional goals.*
Allow patient's significant other(s) to bring favorite foods (within reason) from home *to increase appetite and intake.*

TRANSITION TO DISCHARGE

In preparation for discharge, the patient and significant other(s) will need to learn about wound care and possibly ostomy care. They will need to be able to recognize signs of infection or dehiscence and act appropriately. The need for home health care should be assessed. Gradual activity increases and good nutrition should be outlined and encouraged. Follow-up appointments are arranged and the patient is instructed how to access the resources needed for help in returning to a normal, productive life.

REFERENCES

1. Beal SL, Trunkey DD: Splenic injury. In Blaisdell WF, Trunkey DD, editors: *Abdominal trauma,* New York, 1993, Thieme Medical Publishers, pp 230-249.
2. Berman ML, Ricciardelli CA, Savino JA: Abdominal trauma, *Patient Care* 21(13):105, 1987.
3. Cardona V, et al: *Trauma nursing from resuscitation through rehabilitation,* Philadelphia, 1988, WB Saunders, pp 491-523.
4. Dellinger ED: Prevention and management of infections. In Moore EE, Mattox KL, Feliciano DV, editors: *Trauma,* Norwalk, Conn, 1991, Appleton & Lange, pp 231-244.
5. Feliciano DV, Marx JA, Sclafini SJA: Abdominal trauma, *Patient Care* 26(18):44, 1992.
6. Fleming A, et al: Prospective trial of supranormal values as goals of resuscitation in severe trauma, *Arch Surg* 127:1175-1181, 1992.
7. Halvorsen L, Holcroft JW: Resuscitation. In Blaisdell WF, Trunkey DD, editors: *Abdominal trauma,* New York, 1993, Thieme Medical Publishers, pp 13-31.
8. Harris JE Jr, Trunkey DD: Trauma to the colon and rectum. In Blaisdell WF, Trunkey DD, editors: *Abdominal trauma,* New York, 1993, Thieme Medical Publishers, pp 209-229.
9. Kitt S: Abdominal trauma. In Kitt S, Kaiser J, editors: *Emergency nursing,* Philadelphia, 1990, WB Saunders, pp 283-297.
10. Kudsk KA, et al: Enteral versus parenteral feeding: effects on septic morbidity after blunt and penetrating abdominal trauma, *Ann Surg* 215:503-513, 1992.
11. Lane-Reticker A: Assessment of the injured abdomen, *Topics in Emergency Medicine* 15(1):1-7, 1993.
12. McClave SA, Lowen CC, Snider HL: Immunonutrition and enteral hyperalimentation of critically ill patients, *Dig Dis Sci,* 37:1153-1161, 1992.
13. Merrill CR, Sparger G: Current thoughts on blunt abdominal trauma, *Topics in Emergency Medicine* 12(2):21-28, 1990.
14. Ragsdale J, Trunkey DD: Injuries to the liver and extrahepatic ducts. In Blaisdell WF, Trunkey DD, editors: *Abdominal trauma,* New York, 1993, Thieme Medical Publishers, pp 190-208.
15. Semonin-Holleran R: Critical nursing care for abdominal trauma, *Crit Care Nurs* 8(3):48-52, 1988.
16. Smith M, Christianson N: Small bowel and mesentery. In Blaisdell WF, Trunkey DD, editors: *Abdominal trauma,* New York, 1993, Thieme Medical Publishers, pp 190-208.
17. *St Anthony's DRG guidebook 1995,* Reston, Va, 1994, St Anthony.
18. Thompson NA: Convert your assessment into a care plan for the patient with abdominal trauma, *Nursing* 13(7):26-33, 1983.
19. Trunkey DD, Hill AC, Scheeter WP: Abdominal trauma and indications for celiotomy. In Moore EE, Mattox KL, Feliciano DV, editors: *Trauma,* Norwalk, Conn, 1991, Appleton & Lange, pp 409-426.
20. Unkle D, DeLong WG: Abdominal trauma associated with pelvic fractures, *Orthop Nurs* 8(4):27-30, 1989.
21. Vonfrolio LG, Bacon KA: Abdominal trauma, *RN* 64(6):30, 1991.
22. Wagner MM: The patient with abdominal injuries, *Nurs Clin North Am* 25(1):45-55, 1990.
23. Wisner DH, Lanto DA: Peritoneal lavage, computerized tomography, ultrasound, and magnetic resonance imaging. In Blaisdell WF, Trunkey DD, editors: *Abdominal trauma,* New York, 1993, Thieme Medical Publishers, pp 32-55.

UNIT

V

Renal System

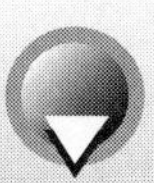

CLINICAL GUIDELINE

51

Acute Renal Failure

Karen K. Carlson, MN, RN, CCRN

DESCRIPTION

Acute renal failure (ARF) is the abrupt reduction of renal function accompanied by the progressive retention of waste compounds (creatinine and urea). It is usually reversible and accompanied by oliguria. Acute renal failure is the most common renal problem that patients in critical care units experience.[1] It is associated with a high mortality, especially when seen as part of multisystem organ dysfunction. It is estimated that there are greater than 10,000 cases per year of ARF, a number that is expected to greatly increase in future years; as the population continues to age and knowledge and technology continue to grow, a greater number of individuals are experiencing more serious and complex diseases.[2] Use of hemodialysis as treatment in the critically ill ARF patient has positively impacted this patient population's mortality.[7]

PATHOPHYSIOLOGY

Multiple causes of ARF exist and are divided into three classifications: prerenal, intrarenal, and postrenal. Each type of ARF has different pathophysiology, laboratory findings, and clinical presentation. Differential diagnosis is important in determining treatment.

Prerenal failure is characterized by physiologic conditions that lead to decreased renal perfusion without intrinsic damage to the renal tubules. Conditions that can predispose a patient to prerenal failure are characterized by hypovolemia, decreased cardiac output, or decreased peripheral vascular resistance (PVR). The decrease in renal arterial perfusion leads to decreased afferent arteriole pressure, ultimately resulting in a decreased glomerular filtration rate (GFR). Decreased flow of fluid through the tubules of the nephron results in secondary release of renin, antidiuretic hormone (ADH), and aldosterone. This release leads to further increases in fluid volume and hypertension. When the pressure in the afferent arteriole drops below 70 mm Hg, autoregulation is also lost. This further decreases GFR.[9] Most forms of prerenal failure are easily reversed by removing the cause and enhancing renal perfusion.

In prerenal failure, renal function is still completely normal, yet the kidneys are unable to filter blood because of the decreased GFR. As a result of the decreased GFR, the filtrate moves more slowly through the renal tubules. The changes seen in diagnostic tests are shown in Table 51-1. Predictable changes occur as a result of this decreased perfusion, regardless of the cause. If the decreased perfusion state persists, it can lead to irreversible damage to the tubules.

The clinical presentation of the patient in prerenal failure differs with the cause. In the patient with decreased circulating volume or altered PVR, the presentation will include tachycardia, hypotension, dry mucous membranes, decreased filling pressures, flat neck veins, and lethargy. As the disease progresses, coma can develop. Patients in cardiac failure have decreased cardiac output, hypotension, tachycardia, cool, clammy skin, and elevated filling pressures.

Actual damage to the renal tubule or blood vessels results in **intrarenal failure**. With a prolonged perfusion deficit, the kidneys gradually suffer damage that restoring perfusion does not improve. **Acute tubular necrosis (ATN)** and **acute glomerulonephritis** are the most common pathologic conditions leading to intrarenal failure. The extent of injury differs with the cause. The causes of intrarenal failure are

TABLE 51-1 Differential Diagnosis of Renal Dysfunction

Test	Prerenal	Intrarenal	Postrenal
Volume	Oliguria	Oliguria	Variable
Specific gravity	>1.020	<1.010	Variable
Osmolality	>500 mOsm/L	<350 mOsm/L	Variable
BUN	>25 mg/dl	>25 mg/dl	>25 mg/dl
Creatinine	Normal	>1.2 mg/dl	>1.2 mg/dl
BUN:creatinine ratio	20:1	10:1	Variable
Na^+	20 mEq/L	>30 mEq/L	Variable

varied and are classified as nephrotoxic, ischemic, or inflammatory.

When the insult to the kidney is nephrotoxic, damage is done primarily to the epithelial layer. Because the epithelial layer has the ability to regenerate, rapid healing often occurs. When the insult is ischemic or inflammatory, the basement membrane is also damaged and regeneration is not possible. These latter types of injury are more resistant to healing and often proceed to chronic renal failure (CRF).

The underlying pathophysiologic abnormality in intrarenal failure is renal cellular damage, leading to functional abnormalities. The glomerulus normally acts as a filter and does not allow large molecules to pass. When damaged, protein and cellular debris are allowed to enter the renal tubules, intraluminal obstruction and backleak of glomerular filtrate occurs.

The diverse causes of intrarenal failure determine the clinical presentation of the patient. Renal failure can cause multiple organ dysfunctions and, therefore, manifests itself in a variety of ways. *Uremia* is the term used to describe the clinical syndrome that accompanies the detrimental effects of renal dysfunction on the other organ systems. The clinical presentation of the patient in uremia reflects the degree of nephron loss and corresponding loss of renal function.

The differential diagnosis of intrarenal failure is shown in Table 51-1. The clinical presentation is determined by the primary or underlying disease. As the renal failure progresses, the patient shows clinical manifestations of uremia. The patient may be confused, lethargic, nauseated, vomiting, experiencing diarrhea or constipation, have deep, rapid, respirations and pulmonary edema, tachycardia, hypotension or hypertension, and dry skin. The patient will also have an increased susceptibility to infection.[1]

Postrenal failure occurs when there is any type of obstruction, partial or complete, of urine flow from the kidney to the urethral meatus. Partial obstruction increases renal interstitial pressure, which, in turn, increases Bowman's capsule pressure, opposing filtration. Diminished urine output is possible. Complete obstruction leads to urine backup into the kidney, eventually compressing the kidney. With complete obstruction, there is no urine output from the affected kidney. Postrenal failure is caused by either mechanical or functional problems. The tests used to diagnose postrenal failure are shown in Table 51-1. The patient with bilateral obstruction displays symptoms of renal failure and has no urine output. Prompt removal of the obstruction usually brings relief of symptoms.

LENGTH OF STAY/ANTICIPATED COURSE

Acute renal failure falls within DRG 316: Renal failure, with an average length of stay of 8.4 days.[8] There are three clinical phases of ARF. The first phase is the oliguric phase, which usually begins within 48 hours of the insult to the kidney and is accompanied by an approximate rise in blood urea nitrogen (BUN) of 20 mg/100 ml/day and rise in creatinine of 1 mg/100 ml/day. The most common complications during this phase are fluid overload and acute hyperkalemia. The oliguric phase may range from a few days to several weeks but on average lasts 12 days.[4] The longer the oliguric phase continues, the poorer the patient's prognosis.

The diuretic phase follows the oliguric phase. During this phase, there is a gradual return of renal function. Although the BUN and creatinine continue to rise, there is an increase in urine output. The urine output is determined by the patient's state of hydration when he or she enters this phase. Fluid overload can lead to diuresis of 5 liters of urine per day.[4] There is marked sodium (Na^+) wasting. The average time in this phase is 2 weeks.[4] Patients must be observed carefully for risk of complications from fluid and electrolyte deficits.

The recovery phase marks the stabilization of laboratory values. It can take 3 to 12 months for the recovery phase to be completed. Often, patients are left with some degree of renal insufficiency. Some patients do not recover and instead progress to CRF.

MANAGEMENT TRENDS AND CONTROVERSIES

Once the patient develops ARF, the goal must be to reestablish homeostasis as quickly as possible. To accomplish this, the insult must be removed before homeostasis can be achieved. Ideally, a collaborative approach to the treatment of patients in ARF begins by focusing on prevention. Both medicine and nursing play a role in recognizing patients at risk for renal failure, developing and implementing plans to maintain perfusion, and taking steps to avoid further renal compromise.

There have been remarkable advances in prevention and treatment over the past 30 years. These advances have focused on prompt correction of hypotension and the early use of dialysis before the development of uremia. Aggressive management includes the appropriate use of medications, nutrition, electrolyte balance, and prevention or prompt treatment of infection.

There are two goals of pharmacologic intervention in the renal failure patient: to prevent or reverse the renal insult before ARF occurs and, once ARF is established, to support the patient to minimize morbidity and mortality. The use of a number of pharmacologic agents in the prevention and treatment of ARF has been proposed. Unfortunately, there is a lack of well-controlled studies to validate their success. As a result, many of these pharmacologic agents are considered to be controversial.[3]

Diuretics and dopamine are commonly used medications for treatment of the ARF patient in the critical care setting. Other medications used in the renal failure patient may include antihypertensive agents, antimicrobial agents, and analgesics.

Diuretics are commonly used both in the prevention and treatment of renal failure. Diuretics are used to challenge a patient when the patient's fluid status is uncertain. Increasing dosages are used in an attempt to determine the dose that will produce an increased urine output. This is often done by doubling the dose (20 mg, 40 mg, 80 mg, and so on) every 30 to 60 minutes until the desired increase in urine output is achieved or a ceiling dose, as determined by the physician, is reached.

Once renal failure is established, diuretics may be used to prevent fluid overload and to potentiate the effects of the patient's antihypertensive medications. It is, however, important to avoid use of potassium (K^+) sparing diuretics because the renal failure patient will have diminished ability to eliminate K^+

Two commonly used diuretics are mannitol and furosemide. Mannitol, an osmotic diuretic, is frequently used in attempts to prevent ARF. It causes vasodilation of the renal vessels and expands vascular volume by enhancing movement of fluid from the interstitial space. Mannitol is often used prophylactically in patients who are at risk of developing ARF, in an effort to protect the kidney. The beneficial use of mannitol after ARF has been established is unclear. It can contribute to fluid overload in the patient who has lost excretory renal function and therefore, should be used cautiously.

Furosemide, a loop diuretic, is more commonly used after ARF has been established. It works by blocking Na^+ reabsorption in the renal tubules, thereby enhancing excretion of Na^+ and water. It is often used in efforts to reduce fluid overload and frequency of dialysis in the ARF patient.

Dopamine is believed to have dose-dependent effects on renal blood flow. At low doses (2 to 5 μg/kg/min), renal vasodilation is believed to occur and at higher doses (>10 μg/kg/min), vasoconstriction. Recently, however, the effects of dopamine use have been questioned.[5] A recent report suggests that the beneficial effect of increased urine output with dopamine use may actually be related to the positive inotropic effect of dopamine rather than a dopaminergic effect. Additionally, there may actually be a direct diuretic effect on the kidney. Care should be used to adequately assess the patient's fluid status before the institution of renal dopamine because any diuretic use in a hypovolemic state could be deleterious to the patient.

Both narcotic and nonnarcotic *analgesics* may be used to treat pain in the ARF patient. Acetaminophen is the drug of choice for the treatment of mild pain. It is metabolized in the liver and requires no dosage alteration. Most narcotic analgesics do not require dosage adjustments and are usually not removed by dialysis. Meperidine is not recommended for use in the ARF patient because its metabolites are eliminated by the kidneys and accumulate in these patients.

Hypertension is a major problem for many renal failure patients as a result of fluid overload and stimulation of the angiotensin-aldosterone system, often requiring concomitant use of several antihypertensive agents. Most antihypertensive agents are not removed by dialysis. It is important to adjust the dosage schedule in the patient who is being dialyzed to avoid undue hypotensive episodes during dialysis. However, some antihypertensive agents are eliminated by the kidney. Therefore, dialysis patients receiving these medications require alterations in their dose or dosing schedule.

Renal failure patients are at high risk for *infection*, secondary to an impaired immune system and altered skin integrity,[1] and are, therefore, commonly treated with antimicrobial agents. The antimicrobial agents need to be carefully selected and monitored, and often require dose adjustment. Careful monitoring of both renal function and drug levels during antimicrobial therapy is imperative to avoid further renal damage.

Maintaining *fluid balance* in the renal failure patient is challenging. A fine balance must be achieved in providing the fluid necessary for adequate renal perfusion while preventing fluid overload. Concurrently, it is often difficult to assess if the patient is volume depleted or overloaded. Correcting fluid balance is crucial in prerenal disease while the underlying problem is being rectified. Fluid replacement must be matched with fluid loss, both in amount and composition, with insensible losses also considered. Volume loading, with normal saline, to the patient who is at risk for renal dysfunction is a widely accepted practice. Additionally, volume expansion is certainly beneficial in preventing a volume-depleted patient from developing ARF.

Managing fluid balance can become even more complex

during the diuretic phase, when the patient may require 1 to 4 L of fluid/day to prevent hypovolemia. Usually, during this phase, the patient is allowed to diurese more fluid than is replaced so that fluid will be pulled from the interstitial and intracellular spaces back into the vascular space. For example, replacement of fluid loss, sensible and insensible, with the exception of 500 to 1000 cc will promote the desired fluid shifts without leaving the patient in a hypovolemic state.

Throughout the care of the ARF patient, careful attention should be paid to accurate intake and output measurement and daily weights. Body weight should be allowed to drop by 0.2 to 0.3 kg per day as a result of catabolism. If the patient's weight is stable or increasing, volume expansion should be suspected. If weight loss exceeds these recommendations, volume depletion or hypercatabolism should be investigated.[3] Once the patient is normovolemic, daily fluid needs must be calculated carefully. It is not uncommon for a patient to be unable to tolerate more than 750 to 1000 cc of fluid per day, placing constraints on other therapies.

There are a number of electrolyte imbalances that can occur in the patient in ARF, the most common being hyperkalemia, hyponatremia, hypocalcemia, hyperphosphatemia, and hypomagnesemia.

Of all of the potential electrolyte disorders, *hyperkalemia* is considered to be the most life threatening secondary to K^+ effect on the heart. Hyperkalemia is also the most common reason for the initiation of dialysis in the ARF patient. Conservative management begins with a dietary restriction of 40 mEq/day. As the K^+ level rises, use of cation-exchange resins such as Kayexalate should be considered. Kayexalate is usually administered by mouth or by enema with sorbitol. The sorbitol acts to draw fluid into the bowel, where the Kayexalate causes an exchange between Na^+ and K^+ions. The K^+ is then eliminated from the body through feces.

When plasma K^+ levels exceed 6 mEq/L, other interventions are usually instituted as temporary measures to protect the heart from the negative effects of hyperkalemia. Hypertonic (50%) glucose infusions may be used with intravenous regular insulin. Insulin, along with carrying glucose into the cells, drives K^+ into the cell on a temporary basis. Sodium bicarbonate infusions may also be used. This infusion also causes movement of K^+ into the cell, encouraging the exchange of hydrogen (H^+) ions inside the cell with the excess K^+ ions outside the cell. Calcium salts, such as calcium gluconate, may be administered to elevate the stimulation threshold, thereby protecting the patient from the negative myocardial effects and potential dysrhythmias. Dialysis is necessary when the patient's K^+ level cannot be controlled by other methods.

Hyponatremia is actually a manifestation of water excess. Mild, asymptomatic hyponatremia is often not treated, or treated only with a water restriction. Dialysis may be instituted to remove excess water if the patient is showing signs or symptoms of water intoxication. If central nervous system signs are present, careful infusions of hypertonic saline may be employed in conjunction with dialysis.

The ARF patient often demonstrates calcium (Ca^{++}) and phosphorous (PO_4^{--}) imbalances within 2 to 3 days of the onset of failure. Hypocalcemia is usually easily corrected by dialysis. If tetany or a positive Chvostek's sign develop, calcium supplementation may be instituted concurrently with the administration of PO_4^{--} binders, such as aluminum hydroxide.

The most common acid–base disorder in the renal failure patient is *metabolic acidosis*. This is due to the inability of the kidney to reabsorb bicarbonate (HCO_3^-) and to excrete H^+. Additionally, patients often develop a mild respiratory alkalosis to compensate. Treatment is usually not instituted until the serum HCO_3^- level drops below 15 mEq/L.[3] Even then, replacement of only half the base deficit is made so as not to overcorrect the pH. Administration of excessive sodium bicarbonate can cause tetany and lead to the development of pulmonary edema.

The challenge in managing the renal failure patient's *nutrition* is to provide a balance between sufficient calories and protein to prevent catabolism, yet not create problems such as fluid and electrolyte imbalances or increased need for dialysis. The typical renal failure patient is often hypermetabolic and, therefore, has increased caloric needs, often as high as twice normal. Additional stresses, related to being critically ill, can further elevate caloric requirements. As a result of their uremia, these patients often experience nausea and vomiting, which results in decreases in oral intake.

Because the kidney is unable to rid the body of wastes, fluid, and electrolytes, the renal failure patient's diet is typically fluid, K^+, Na^+, and protein restricted. The degree of these restrictions depends on the cause and severity of disease. For example, the level of Na^+ restriction is determined by the cause of the renal failure. Some causes lead to Na^+ wasting and others to Na^+ retention. Phosphorus may need to be restricted and Ca^{++} supplemented, if the Ca^{++} level is low in conjunction with normal PO_4^{--} levels. Additionally, supplementation of folic acid, pyridoxine, and water-soluble vitamins is often necessary. Dietary requirements change for patients, depending on their renal status and the severity of their underlying condition.

Patients who are critically ill or have more serious underlying conditions often are hypermetabolic and catabolic. This is associated with a poorer prognosis. Although the precise role of nutrition in ARF is controversial, it is felt that malnutrition increases morbidity and mortality in these patients.[6] It has been shown that total parenteral nutrition used in conjunction with frequent dialysis improves survival[10] and promotes healing of renal tubular cells. The usual nutritional approach in hypercatabolic states is to provide adequate proteins and carbohydrates to provide for resynthesis of damaged or lost tissue elements. Protein requirements may initially be 0.5 to 1.0 g/kg/day, increasing with dialysis to 1.0 to 1.5 g/kg/day.[10] Nonprotein calories, usually in the form of fat, are given for nonanabolic metabolic needs.

Careful monitoring of the patient's weight, fluid balance, and electrolyte balance is important. The nutritional interventions may need to be tailored daily as the patient's status changes. Dialysis treatments need to be taken into consideration when planning a patient's diet.

ASSESSMENT

PARAMETER	ANTICIPATED ALTERATIONS
Cardiovascular Status	
HR	Increased: >100 bpm *due to fluid overload*
Pulse	Bounding *due to fluid overload*
BP	Increased: >140/90 *due to fluid overload, Na^+ retention, and stimulation of the renin-angiotensin system* Orthostatic changes *due to fluid shifts from dialysis treatments*
Rhythm	Dysrhythmias *due to fluid overload, acid–base, and electrolyte imbalances, hypoxia*
PAP	Increased: >25/15/20 mm Hg (PAS/D/M) *due to fluid overload*
PCWP	Increased: >18 mm Hg *due to fluid overload*
CVP	Increased: >12 mm Hg *due to fluid overload*
Peripheral perfusion	Edema (peripheral, pulmonary) *due to fluid overload, Na^+ retention* JVD *due to fluid overload*
Color	Pallor *due to anemia*
Wt	Increased *due to fluid overload*
Other	Pericarditis Fatigue *due to anemia, hypermetabolic state, and decreased nutritional status* Dry mucous membranes
Respiratory Status	
Rate	Increased: >24 breaths per minute *due to fluid overload, acid–base imbalance*
Pattern	Kussmaul breathing *due to acid–base imbalance* Hyperventilation *due to fluid overload and acid–base imbalance* Dyspnea *due to fluid overload*
Breath sounds	Rales *due to fluid overload* Rhonchi *due to consolidation/infection*
Effort	Increased work of breathing *due to fluid overload and acid–base imbalance*
Chest x-ray	Signs of hilar pneumonitis
FiO_2	Increasing % O_2 needed to maintain adequate oxygenation *due to anemia from lack of erythropoietin*
Other	Urine smell on breath *due to uremic toxins*
Genitourinary Status	
Volume	Oliguria, anuria *due to inability to eliminate fluid* Polyuria in postrenal failure and in recovery phase *due to release of obstruction/recovery of eliminating ability*
Urine analysis	Hematuria, proteinuria, pyuria *due to infection* Casts

Urine creatinine clearance	Decreased: <85 ml/min
Urine Na^+	Prerenal: decreased <20 mEq/L *due to increased reabsorption of Na^+ ion in the attempt to increase renal perfusion* Intrarenal: increased >30 mEq/L *due to loss of Na^+ reabsorption by kidney* Postrenal: variable
Specific gravity	Prerenal: increased >1.020 *due to inability to eliminate fluid* Intrarenal: decreased <1.010 *due to loss of concentrating ability* Postrenal: variable depending on the level of diuresis

Neurological Status

LOC	Restlessness Insomnia Drowsiness Disorientation Confusion Lethargy *All due to effect of excess uremic toxins, hypoxia, acid–base imbalance*
Other	Headache Weakness Seizures

Gastrointestinal Status

Appetite	Anorexia *due to uremic toxins* Decreased caloric intake *due to fatigue, stomatitis, dietary restrictions* Nausea, vomiting *due to uremic toxins* Stomatitis *due to uremic toxins* Ammonia taste in mouth *due to urea decomposition in mouth*
Elimination	Constipation *due to hypomotility, electrolyte imbalance, decreased circulating fluid* Diarrhea *due to hypermotility, electrolyte imbalance*

Laboratory Tests

Serum creatinine	Increased: >1.2 mg/dl or doubled baseline *due to decreased renal filtering and excretion*
Serum BUN	Increased: >20 mg/dl *due to decreased renal filtering and excretion*
BUN: creatinine ratio	Prerenal: 20:1 *due to renal hypoperfusion* Intrarenal: 10:1 Postrenal: Variable
Urine osmolality	Prerenal: >500 mOsm/L Intrarenal: <350 mOsm/L Postrenal: variable depending on level of diuresis
Serum Electrolytes	
• K^+	Increased: >5 mEq/L *due to decreased excretion*
• Na^+	Decreased: <130 mEq/L *due to increased excretion*
• Ca^{++}	Decreased: <8.5 mEq/dl *due to increased excretion*
• PO_4^{--}	Increased: >4.5 mEq/dl *due to decreased excretion*
• Mg^{++}	Decreased: <1.5 mEq/L *due to increased excretion*
Coagulation Studies	
• APTT	Increased: >40 seconds *due to uremic toxins*
• PT	Increased: >12.5 seconds *due to uremic toxins*
• Hgb	Decreased: <12 to 14 g/dl *due to lack of erythropoietin*

• Hct	Decreased: <37% *due to lack of erythropoietin*
• Platelets	Decreased: <150,000/mm³ *due to uremic toxins*
• ABG	Initially normal
	Metabolic acidosis *due to kidney's inability to reabsorb* HCO_3^-

PLAN OF CARE

INTENSIVE PHASE

Caring for the patient in ARF can be challenging for the critical care nurse. Dysfunction of the kidney impacts virtually all other body systems. Prevention of renal failure is imperative. Once renal insufficiency is present, the nurse must balance interventions for a wide variety of patient care needs.

PATIENT CARE PRIORITIES	EXPECTED PATIENT OUTCOMES
Fluid volume excess *r/t* *Inability to excrete fluid/*Na^+ *Increased aldosterone release* *Excess administration of fluids*	Normovolemic Decreased edema Urine specific gravity: WNL Balanced intake and output Wt: WNL PAP/PCWP/CVP: WNL
Altered electrolyte balance (hyperkalemia, hypocalcemia hypermagnesemia, hyperphosphatemia) *r/t* *Inability to excrete/reabsorb electrolytes* *Compensatory mechanisms*	Electrolyte values: WNL Cardiovascular status at pre-illness levels
Ineffective breathing pattern *r/t* *Volume overload/pulmonary edema* *Metabolic acidosis* *Electrolyte imbalances* *Uremic toxins*	Intravascular volume: WNL Breath sounds: WNL ABG: WNL Electrolyte levels: WNL Creatinine/BUN: WNL
Decreased tissue perfusion *r/t* *Anemia/bleeding* *Hemolysis* *Coagulation abnormalities resulting from uremia*	Normal peripheral pulses Hgb and Hct values: WNL
Altered acid–base balance *r/t* *Inability to excrete* H^+ *Inability to retain* HCO_3^- *Altered ammonia production*	ABG: WNL HCO_3^-: WNL Anion gap: WNL Serum ammonia: WNL
High risk for infection *r/t* *Accumulation of metabolic wastes* *Compromised skin integrity* *Use of invasive lines/catheters*	Infection free WBC/differential: WNL Creatinine/BUN: WNL Negative cultures
Inadequate nutrition *r/t* *Hypermetabolic state* *Dietary restrictions* *Nausea/vomiting* *Fatigue*	Adequate nutritional status Wt: WNL Appropriate caloric intake
Altered level of consciousness *r/t* *Accumulation of metabolic waste* *Electrolyte imbalances* *Hypoxia*	Oriented to time, place, and person

Plan of Care (cont'd)

Activity Intolerance *r/t*
Anemia
Nutritional deficits
Fluid status
Electrolyte imbalances

Able to assist with daily activities
Increased energy level

INTERVENTIONS

Maintain head of bed ≥45° *to facilitate ventilation.*
Monitor vital signs and LOC q1h to q2h.
Encourage turn, cough, and deep breathing *to assist in mobilizing secretions and promoting ventilation.*
Suction as needed.
Administer O_2 as needed.
Monitor for evidence of adequate oxygenation.
Monitor specific gravity and I/O.
Provide for fluid restriction and/or careful fluid administration.
If hypervolemia occurs, administer diuretics and antihypertensive agents as ordered.
Prepare for renal replacement therapies.
Minimize blood loss from blood draws and waste from indwelling catheters *because patients are already anemic.*
Administer blood and blood products as needed.
Monitor for bleeding from all sites.
Guaiac all stools/emesis/NG drainage.
Institute protective measures, such as maintaining skin integrity, using careful aseptic technique, ensuring good skin and mouth care, ensuring good overall hygiene, and protecting patients from others with infections.
Monitor temperature and note trends.
If fever occurs, administer antipyretics as ordered.
Monitor for signs of infection: malaise, chills, abnormal WBC counts, positive cultures.
Avoid indwelling catheters *because it is preferred to remove Foley catheters as early in ARF as possible to reduce the chance of infection.*
Administer antibiotics carefully *because many are eliminated by the kidneys and will therefore need dose alterations.*
Monitor daily laboratory values (Na^+, K^+, Ca^{++}, PO_4^{--}, Mg^{++}, BUN, creatinine, serum osmolality, urine osmolality, Hgb, Hct, platelet count, WBC with differential ABG).
Monitor electrolyte values and their relationship to sensorium and changes in sensorium.
Treat abnormal laboratory values as needed.
Maintain prescribed diet: restricted protein, Na^+, K^+, fluid; high calorie *because patients are often hypermetabolic.*
Provide small, frequent meals.
Administer enteral or parenteral feedings as ordered.
Provide frequent oral hygiene, using soft toothbrush.
Provide ice chips and hard candy as indicated.
Maximize respiratory status.
Monitor and document changes in LOC.
Institute seizure precautions *because the increase in metabolic waste creates an unstable environment in the brain and patients may have seizures.*
Provide with frequent rest periods.

INTERMEDIATE PHASE

If a patient survives the intensive care phase of ARF, recovery will depend on the cause of renal failure, the length of time in failure, and the condition of other body systems. It is not uncommon for critically ill patients to recover from ARF but retain some degree of renal

Plan of Care (cont'd)

insufficiency. The focus of nursing care during this phase is targeted to enhancing nutrition for continued healing, weaning the patient from dialysis if possible, and assisting the patient to adjust to life-style changes resulting from critical illness.

PATIENT CARE PRIORITIES	EXPECTED PATIENT OUTCOMES
Inadequate nutrition *r/t* *Hypermetabolic state* *Dietary restrictions* *Nausea/vomiting* *Fatigue*	Adequate nutrition to support healing Wt: WNL Appropriate caloric intake
Activity intolerance *r/t* *Anemia* *Nutritional deficits* *Fluid status* *Electrolyte imbalances*	Increased activity progression and toleration Increased energy level

INTERVENTIONS

Increase calories and fluids as renal function will allow *to improve nutritional status and provide for enhanced healing.*

Supplement diet with high-calorie snacks.

Continue to offer small, frequent meals *to assist the fatigued patient to increase caloric intake.*

Increase activity daily (up in chair, ambulation) *to increase strength and activity tolerance.*

Continue to offer explanations of tests, procedures, and activities *to keep patient informed and assist with life-style adjustments.*

Encourage the patient to participate in ADLs and in planning daily schedule *to promote patient involvement in care and future planning.*

TRANSITION TO DISCHARGE

As patients prepare to leave the critical care environment, the focus of care shifts to prepare the patient for discharge. Depending on the patient's degree of renal function, preparations may need to be made for outpatient dialysis. Additionally, the patient and significant others needs to become familiar with any dietary restrictions and any medications, including the action, schedule, and precautions before discharge. Follow-up care will focus on assisting the patient to adapt to the changes caused by this illness.

REFERENCES

1. Baer CL: Acute renal failure. In Kinney MR, et al, editors: *AACN's clinical reference for critical care nursing,* ed 3, St Louis, 1993, Mosby–Yearbook, pp 885-901.
2. Baer CL, Lancaster LE: Acute renal failure, *Crit Care Nurs Q* 14(4):1-21, 1992.
3. Brezis M, Rosen S, Epstein FH: Acute renal failure. In Brenner B, Rector FC, editors: *The kidney,* ed 4, Philadelphia, 1991, WB Saunders, pp 993-1061.
4. Butkus DE: Acute renal failure. In Hudak, Gallo, Benz, editors: *Critical care nursing: a holistic approach,* ed 5, Philadelphia, 1990, JB Lippincott, pp 450-467.
5. Duke GJ, Bersten D: Dopamine and renal salvage in the critically ill patient, *Anaesth Intensive Care* 20(3):277-302, 1992.
6. Hoffart N: Nutrition in renal failure, dialysis, and transplantation. In Lancaster L, editor: *Core curriculum for nephrology nursing,* Pitman, 1993, American Nephrology Nurse's Association, pp 145-166.
7. Owen WF, Lazarus JM: Hemodialysis in acute renal failure. In Lazarus JM, Brenner B, editors: *Acute renal failure,* ed 3, New York, 1993, Churchill Livingston, pp 487-525.
8. *St Anthony's DRG Guidebook 1995,* Reston, Va, 1994, St Anthony.
9. Stark JL: The renal system. In Alspach G, editor: *Core curriculum for critical care nursing,* ed 4, Philadelphia, 1991, WB Saunders, pp 472-608.
10. Wolfson M, Kopple JD: Nutritional management of acute renal failure. In Lazarus JM, Brenner B, editors: *Acute renal failure,* ed 3, New York, 1993, Churchill Livingston, pp 467-485.

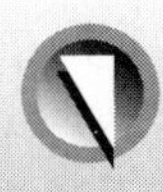

TRANSPLANT GUIDELINE

52

Renal Transplantation

Mandy Bass, MS, RN, CCRN, CNN

DESCRIPTION

As of January, 1994, in the United States 33,394 people were waiting for solid organ transplants and 24,973 registrants were waiting for a kidney transplant. In 1993, 9736 kidney transplants were performed, 2534 from living donors and 7202 from cadaver (brain-dead) donors. There are 239 centers that perform kidney transplants in the United States.[15] The difference between the number of patients waiting for an organ and the number of transplants performed demonstrates the inadequate number of organs currently available for transplantation. Those patients who received a cadaver renal transplant in 1989 waited, on the average, 500 days for an organ to become available for them. These statistics make it apparent that some form of dialysis is necessary in the interim.[16]

End-stage renal disease (ESRD) affects over 160,000 patients nationwide.[16] Without treatment, these people do not survive their end-stage disease. Currently, there are several treatment options for the person with ESRD. These options include (1) hemodialysis, either provided in a dialysis center or at home with a partner; (2) peritoneal dialysis, provided by continuous ambulatory peritoneal dialysis (CAPD), nighttime use of a cycler for peritoneal dialysis, continuous cycling peritoneal dialysis (CCPD), or intermittent peritoneal dialysis (IPD); and (3) renal transplantation. When transplantation is the option of choice, the donor may be either a living donor (related or unrelated) or a cadaver. Transplantation is performed most often for ESRD caused by glomerulonephritis, chronic tubulointerstitial disease, chronic pyelonephritis, or diabetes mellitus.

Renal transplantation offers the best treatment option for many patients with ESRD, for reasons of quality of life and cost-effectiveness. All treatments for ESRD are covered under the Medicare program, and it has been shown that the cost to maintain a transplant patient is one third that of a dialysis patient.[7] Renal transplantation can offer people a more normal life-style, an improved sense of well-being, and a more liberalized medication and dietary regimen than is possible with dialysis. This provides a greater feeling of independence for the patient. Psychosocial problems may be alleviated or avoided altogether.[9]

PATIENT SELECTION

For a renal transplant to be effective, appropriate immunologic assessment and testing must be done. The recipient must have a compatible ABO blood group with the donor. Matching Rh factor is not necessary. In addition to ABO compatibility, tissue compatibility is also considered. This is done by testing HLA, or human leukocyte antigens. These are the antigens primarily responsible for graft rejection. They are genetically determined, by a site on the sixth chromosome. Although there are many identified antigens at this time, the three antigens tested before renal transplantation are named A, B, and DR. Every person has one set of antigens, or one haplotype, from each parent, for a total of two haplotypes. Since there are two haplotypes, each child of the same set of parents has a 25% chance of having the same HLA type as a sibling, a 25% chance of having no similarity with a sibling, and a 50% chance of having one of the same haplotypes as a sibling.[12] Because only A, B, and DR antigens are typed, there are a total of six antigens that are tested for transplantation. The chances of a potential recipient being HLA-identical for all six tested antigens with a cadaveric donor are very slim. The better the match, the better the chance of success for long-term graft survival after renal transplantation. Therefore, if a six-antigen match does occur between a cadaver and a potential recipient (as determined through a computer-generated list of those waiting for a renal transplant), the kidney is given to that person.

A white blood cell cross-match determines if there are preformed antibodies in the recipient's serum to antigens on the donor tissue. If there is a positive cross-match (if the potential recipient's serum reacts to the donor lymphocytes), the transplant is not performed.

PROCEDURE

The renal transplant operation itself usually takes approximately 4 hours. The transplanted organ is placed in the iliac fossa. Usually the right side is chosen because the iliac vessels are better exposed on the right side. The renal artery is anastomosed to the recipient's iliac artery. The renal vein is anastomosed to the recipient's iliac vein. Either a ureteroneocystostomy (donor ureter tunneled into recipient bladder) or a ureteroureterostomy (donor ureter to recipient ureter) is performed.[6] A Jackson Pratt drain is inserted at the site of the incision to prevent fluid collections; this practice varies from one institution to another. Lymphocele, or a collection of lymphatic fluid, can occur after transplantation around the transplanted kidney, but this reportedly occurs in less than 10% of transplant patients.[2]

Bleeding after transplantation seldom occurs and thrombosis of the graft has a reported incidence of 0.5% to 3.5%.[2] Unless the diagnosis of thrombosis is made quickly and the graft repaired immediately, the graft is lost.

LENGTH OF STAY/ANTICIPATED COURSE

A complete evaluation for transplantation can be done on an outpatient basis for all potential recipients. It involves various laboratory studies, tissue typing, urologic studies, and, when necessary, complete cardiac, gastrointestinal, or pulmonary evaluations. Immediately before surgery, particular attention is focused on ensuring a normal range of vital signs and physiological laboratory studies.

In the early postoperative period patients usually are cared for in a specialty care unit, where nurses are familiar with physiologic monitoring and infection control for this population.

The average length of stay for a renal transplant recipient is 8 days, but may vary from 7 to 14 days, depending on graft function.[11] Many centers are now discharging people earlier and monitoring them closely at home, or with frequent clinic visits.

The most common DRG for the renal transplant recipient is 302: Kidney transplant. Other diagnoses that may be used for this population include 304: Kidney, ureter, and major bladder procedure for non-neoplasm age >17; and 331: Other kidney and ureter tract diagnosis age >17. The average length of stay is 14.6 days.[13]

MANAGEMENT TRENDS AND CONTROVERSIES

Management of the renal transplant recipient after surgery includes monitoring the function of the kidney with daily blood work, frequent blood pressure measurements, and careful assessment of the wound for bleeding or infection.[1,3] Hemodialysis or peritoneal dialysis may be indicated if the transplanted kidney is in acute tubular necrosis (ATN) in the immediate postoperative phase. Acute tubular necrosis can be caused by hypotension, hypovolemia, prolonged kidney preservation time, or high-dose cyclosporine. Some studies report a 20% reduction in one-year graft survival when early graft function is impaired. Postoperative ATN can occur in 10% to 70% of the patient population, depending on the transplant program.[2]

One of the greatest threats to the transplanted organ is graft rejection. Accordingly, patients are placed on high-dose immunosuppressive drugs. The immunosuppressive drugs of choice in many centers are steroids (prednisone), azathioprine, and cyclosporine to prevent rejection. Some centers also add OKT_3 to prevent rejection postoperatively. Should rejection occur, steroid doses often are increased and then tapered to a maintenance dose. Monoclonal therapy (OKT_3) is another option for the treatment of rejection. Polyclonal therapy (ATG) may be used instead of monoclonal therapy. Accelerated rejection occurs 5 to 7 days postoperatively; acute rejection usually occurs within 6 weeks after transplantation.[5]

Immunosuppressive medications depress the patient's immunological reaction against the donor tissue. Unfortunately, this therapy decreases the patient's ability to fight infection from bacteria, fungi, and viruses. Measures to prevent infection are an essential component of the postoperative regimen, and immunosuppressed patients must be monitored carefully for signs of infection. Sepsis is a constant concern and can result in life-threatening situations, which at times can be complicated by a rejection episode. Careful monitoring of the patient for signs of infection and rejection while hospitalized includes having cultures done routinely and at the first sign of infection.

Although great advances have been made in transplantation in the past 30 years, there are still problems related to graft rejection, infection, and long-term toxicity of immunosuppressive agents. The goal in transplantation is to alter the host response to the transplanted organ so that it is not recognized as foreign, thereby alleviating the need for immunosuppressive therapy after transplantation.[14] Until the time that occurs, though, pharmacologic interventions will continue to be researched.

The number of patients waiting for a kidney transplant grows proportionately larger than the number of transplants that are done each year. At the current rate, there will never be enough organs for all those who want a transplant. Most of the efforts to increase donations have been aimed at public awareness and education, through local and regional organ procurement agencies. Public awareness, however, has not caused an increase in actual donations.[12] Because of the shortage issue, various groups have elicited discussion about related issues. These groups are considering the following possibilities:

- Using donors that previously have been considered marginal in order to increase the potential donor pool. This may be possible because currently there are better preservation solutions for organs before transplantation, and better immunosuppressive agents for recipients after transplantation.
- Presumed consent for donation in the case of unexpected death (unless the potential donor has made other arrangements). This possibility has generated some ethical debate, because our society expects informed consent when working with the medical community; therefore, it may not be a solution at the present time.
- Provide compensation in the form of money to the family of the donor, either for burial or other benefit. The impact of financial compensation is being studied, as it would detract from the altruistic gesture of donation.

A controversial option to alleviate the organ shortage that is under study at various centers is xenografting, or using organs from species other than humans. As more is understood about the immune process, and how to manipulate it prior to transplantation, this option may become more of a reality.

ASSESSMENT

PARAMETER	ANTICIPATED ALTERATION
Fluid Balance	
UO	Increased: 100 to 1000 cc/hr with good graft function Anuria or oliguria (urine output <30 cc/hr) *due to postoperative ATN or obstructive clot*
Weight	±2 kg of patient's dry weight, or expected weight pretransplant; compare to baseline weight pretransplant
Hct	Elevated: >30% *due to dehydration* Decreased: <20% *due to overload states or bleeding postoperatively* Compare to baseline, as many renal failure patients have Hcts that are in the upper 20s or 30s *due to lack of erythropoeitin.*
Electrolyte Balance	
K^+	Increased: >5.0 mEq/L *due to ATN* Decreased: <3.5 mEq/L *due to large urine outputs and inadequate replacement postoperatively*
Na^+	Increased: >145 mEq/L *due to ATN* Decreased: <135 mEq/L *due to good graft function and inadequate replacement postoperatively*
HCO_3^-	Decreased: <22 mEq/L *due to diuresing kidney losing* HCO_3^- *and inadequate replacement postoperatively*
CO_2	Decreased: <24 mEq/L *due to metabolic acidosis common in renal failure, which has not corrected in the first 24 hrs posttransplantation*
Glucose	Increased: >120 mg/dl *due to steroids in diabetic or overuse of dextrose solutions*
Renal Function	
Creatinine	Increased: >8 mg/dl immediately after transplant Compare to baseline of individual before transplantation Should note postoperative trend toward normal, which is 0.6 to 1.5 mg/dl
BUN	Compare to baseline of individual before transplantation Should note postoperative trend toward normal, which is 10 to 20 mg/dl
Cardiovascular Status	
HR	Increased: >100 bpm *due to dehydration*

Systolic BP	Decreased: <90 mm Hg *due to dehydration or hemorrhage* Increased: >180 mm Hg *due to ATN or underlying hypertensive disease present*
CVP	Decreased: <4mm Hg *due to dehydration or hemorrhage (if occurs)* Increased: >10 mm Hg *due to ATN*
Pulmonary Status	
Breath sounds	Rales *due to fluid overload (if present)*
RR	Increased: >20 breaths/min *due to fluid overload* Decreased: <12 breaths/min *due to effects of anesthesia postoperatively*
Postoperative pain	Present as assessed on a scale of 0 to 10. Also may have associated signs and symptoms: elevated HR, BP, restlessness, splinting, and guarding.
T	Increased: >100° F *due to postoperative atelectasis, urinary tract infection, wound infection*

PLAN OF CARE

INTENSIVE PHASE

Care of the postoperative renal transplant patient in the intensive phase is focused on managing the fluid and electrolyte imbalances that can result, especially if the transplanted kidney is in ATN in the immediate postoperative period. The patient is also at high risk for infection because high-dose immunosuppressive drugs are required to prevent graft rejection of the transplanted organ. Careful assessments and interventions to prevent wound or invasive line infection are a nursing priority.

PATIENT CARE PRIORITIES	EXPECTED PATIENT OUTCOMES
Fluid imbalance *r/t* *Uremic osmotic diuresis* *Fluid overload from postoperative ATN* *Ureter kink or leak* *Renal artery kink* *Vein thrombosis*	Adequate fluid volume state evidenced by adequate blood flow to kidney and UO >30 cc/hr Body weight ±2 kilograms
Electrolyte imbalance *r/t* *Na^+, K^+, HCO_3^- loss with diuresis* *Na^+, K^+ overload with transplant dysfunction or ATN* *CO_2 decrease from residual effects of renal-failure-related acidosis*	Electrolytes: WNL
Urine retention *r/t obstruction postoperatively*	UO >30 cc/hr; absence of urinary retention
Impaired tissue perfusion *r/t* *Postoperative ATN* *Postoperative bleeding* *Postoperative thrombosis*	Creatinine normalizing BUN normalizing Hct comparable to preoperative value, usually in 30% range for patients with renal failure
Impaired oxygenation *r/t* *Fluid overload* *Postoperative atelectasis*	Spo_2 ≥90% ABG: WNL
Excess glucose level *r/t* *High steroid dose* *Endogenous gluconeogenesis secondary to stress*	Fasting glucose: WNL
High risk for infection *r/t* *Uremia* *IV lines* *Tubes*	T <100° F WBC count: WNL C & S of sputum, urine, and drain site negative

Plan of Care (cont'd)

Drains
Immunosuppression
Ineffective airway clearance
Open wound

Pain *r/t postoperative incision* — Pain controlled per patient report
Able to rest, sleep, and engage in care activities

INTERVENTIONS

Monitor I/O, including urine, drainage, and bleeding, q1h in the first 24 hours and administer fluids based on previous hour's output *for ongoing, sufficient fluid administration without overload.*

Monitor for decrease in UO or blood in urine *due to bleeding/clot formation.*

Monitor BP, HR, CVP q1h for first 4 hours or until patient is stable. Then monitor q2h to q4h, depending on patient stability, *to assess for fluid overload.*

Weigh patient daily, starting first postoperative morning, in A.M. Weigh same time every day, with same clothing/hospital attire, and using same scale *to assure accurate comparison to previous day's weight while assessing fluid balance.*

Monitor NA^+, K^+, and HCO_3^- at 1 and 5 hours postoperatively *to assess effects of postoperative osmotic diuresis. Loss of* Na^+, K^+, *and* HCO_3^- *may be significant.*

Monitor creatinine and BUN. *Elevation in BUN/creatinine may signify either ATN or rejection. Acute rejection usually occurs several days postoperatively, while ATN usually occurs in the immediate postoperative period.*

Monitor ABG 1 and 5 hours postoperatively; monitor oxygen saturation continuously. *Because of postoperative atelectasis and usual metabolic acidosis associated with renal failure, acid-base balance and oxygenation may be abnormal.*

Monitor cardiac rhythm for signs of tachycardia, *due to dehydration, or abnormal* K^+ *level. Hyperkalemia will cause peaked T waves, bradycardia.*

Provide chest physiotherapy and encourage patient to cough and deep breathe q4h *to prevent postoperative infection related to atelectasis.*

Instruct patient to splint incision *to control pain during treatments.*

Monitor for signs of rejection, such as fever, decreased UO, edema, tenderness at graft site, elevated BUN, creatinine, malaise, *so that treatment for rejection can be started in a timely fashion to prevent permanent kidney transplant damage.*

Protect patient from infection *due to high risk status on immunosuppression.* Empty drains with meticulous care; do not violate IV lines. Discontinue all drains, Foley catheters, and IVs as soon as possible *to decrease risk of infection;* use aseptic technique wound care; protect wound and skin from tape injury by using paper tape only.

Provide analgesia as needed *to maintain comfort.*

Provide reassurance regarding progress *to decrease anxiety about postoperative progress.*

INTERMEDIATE PHASE

Generally the patient can be considered for intermediate phase care 24 hours postoperatively. Monitoring continues for fluid and electrolyte imbalance, infection, rejection, pain, and fear or anxiety about graft function, but invasive lines and drains will be discontinued as long as the patient is stable. Even if the patient is in fluid overload and ATN, noninvasive assessment is desired over maintaining invasive lines. Nursing assessment depends on skilled physical assessment rather than monitors. As the patient recovers, other concerns become evident, such as change in infection risk related to opportunistic infections, need for proper nutrition, changes in family roles, self-concept related to functioning renal status, ability to return to work, and change in body image related to side effects of medication and nonuremic state. There is also a knowledge deficit related to medications and self-care after transplantation.

Plan of Care (cont'd)

PATIENT CARE PRIORITIES	EXPECTED PATIENT OUTCOMES
Fluid imbalance *r/t* *Dehydration* *Postoperative ATN* *Ureter kink or leak* *Renal artery kink or thrombosis*	Adequate fluid volume evidenced by UO >30 cc/hr Body weight ± 2 kg r/t dry (expected) weight
Electrolyte imbalance *r/t* *Losses with inadequate replacements postoperatively* *Excesses with transplant ATN*	Electrolytes: WNL
Self-care deficit *r/t* *Decreased mobility after surgery* *Inadequate knowledge regarding postoperative medication regimen, control of infection, identification of rejection, long-term self-care*	Performs ADL Pours medications correctly Lists signs and symptoms of rejection and infection post-discharge Describes appropriate plan of care
Altered role performance *r/t changes in health status after transplantation*	Verbalizes feelings Starts to plan rehabilitation and set long-term goals
High risk for rejection *r/t ABO incompatibility*	Absence of rejection evidenced by UO >30 cc/hr, normalization of creatinine and BUN, afebrile, and no sign of pain or swelling at graft site
High risk for rejection *r/t uremia, immunosuppression*	T within patient norms WBC count: WNL C&S of sputum, urine, drain site negative

INTERVENTIONS

Monitor I/O including urine and drainage q4h *to provide sufficient fluid administration without overload.*

Monitor HR, BP q4h and weigh patient daily *to assess fluid status.*

Monitor electrolytes daily for abnormalities. *Deficits may be due to diuresis with inadequate replacement, and excesses may be due to lack of excretion in ATN or early rejection.*

Monitor creatinine and BUN daily *to assess for ATN resolution, if present, or early rejection so timely treatment can be given.*

Discontinue IV lines, drains, Foley catheter, and provide skin and wound care *to prevent infections.*

Provide patient education as early as possible *to assist patient in becoming independent and knowledgeable about self-care after transplantation.*

Collaborate with health care team, including nursing, medicine, dietitian, physical therapy, and social worker *to assist patient to learn/return to a healthy style of living, including activities, medical regime, self-monitoring for rejection and infection, and self-medication of prescription medicines.*

TRANSITION TO DISCHARGE

As the patient moves from the intermediate phase of care toward discharge, it is imperative that postoperative teaching be completed, including knowledge about medications, infection, rejection, diet and fluid prescriptions, activities, sexual activity, schedule for follow-up care to clinics, and any support or home arrangements that may need to be done. Such arrangements may include home IV care for infection or rejection treatment when indicated, information about long-term support groups for people who have received a transplant, vocational rehabilitation, and/or financial planning for long-term immunosuppression treatment.[10] The prognosis for a patient who receives a renal transplant is improving constantly. One-year patient survival is 92.8% for the cadaveric donor recipient and 97.1% for the recipient of a kidney from a living donor, as reported by UNOS.[14] One-year graft survival for the cadaveric recipient is 79% and for the living donor recipient is 90.7%.[14] These statistics indicate better outcomes than those reported for patients on dialysis. Therefore, transplantation is the option of choice for many patients with ESRD. Many posttransplantation issues are ameliorated or prevented by good nursing care and can make the transition from other ESRD treatments to transplantation a positive growth experience.

REFERENCES

1. AACN: *Outcome standards for nursing of the critically ill,* Laguna Niguel, Calif., 1990, AACN.
2. Amend WJC, Vincenti F, Tomlanovich SJ: The first two posttransplant months. In Danovitch GM, editor: *Handbook of kidney transplantation,* Boston, 1992, Little, Brown.
3. ANNA: *Standards of clinical practice for nephrology nursing,* ed 2, Pitman, NJ, 1993, ANNA.
4. Blanford NL: Renal transplantation: a case study of the ideal, *Crit Care Nurs* 13:46-55.
5. Cunningham NL, Boteler S, Windham S: Renal transplantation, *Crit Care Nurs Clin North Am* 4:79-88.
6. Danovitch GM, editor: *Handbook of kidney transplantation,* Boston, 1992, Little, Brown.
7. Eggers PW: Effects of transplantation on the Medicare and end-stage renal disease program, *N Engl J Med* 318:223-229.
8. Haggerty LM, Sigardson-Poor K: Kidney transplantation. In Sigardson-Poor K, Haggerty LM, editors: *Nursing care of the transplant recipient,* Philadelphia, 1990, WB Saunders.
9. Hathaway D, Strong M, Ganza M: Posttransplant quality of life expectations, *ANNA Journal* 17:433-439.
10. Massachusetts General Hospital Transplant Team: *Organ transplants: a patient's guide,* Cambridge, Mass, 1991, Harvard University Press.
11. Pattella PS, Weiskittel PD: Kidney transplantation. In Norris MK, House MA, editors: *Organ and tissue transplantation: nursing care from procurement through rehabilitation,* Philadelphia, 1991, FA Davis.
12. Smith S: Immunologic aspects of transplantation. In Smith S, editor: *Tissue and organ transplantation,* St Louis, 1990, Mosby–Year Book.
13. *St Anthony's DRG guidebook 1995,* Reston, Va, 1994, St Anthony.
14. UNOS: *Annual report of the scientific registry for organ transplantation and the organ procurement and transplantation network, 1990,* Richmond, Va, UNOS; and Bethesda, Md, Division of Organ Transplantation, Health Resources and Services Administration.
15. UNOS: *Update, 1994,* 10:1, Richmond, Va, UNOS; and Bethesda, Md, Division of Organ Transplantation, Health Resources and Services Administration.
16. United States Renal Data System: *1992 Annual Data Report,* Bethesda, Md, Division of Kidney, Urologic, and Hematologic Diseases, The National Institute of Diabetes and Digestive and Kidney Diseases, The National Institutes of Health.

DEVICE GUIDELINE

53

Acute Peritoneal Dialysis

Karen K. Carlson, MN, RN, CCRN

DESCRIPTION

Dialysis is an artificial process that partially replaces renal function (elimination of wastes, fluid, electrolytes, and other toxic substances). The general principles of dialysis are the same for both acute and chronic renal failure patients and can be accomplished through hemodialysis (HD), peritoneal dialysis (PD), or other continuous renal replacement therapies (CRRT). HD is the most prevalent renal replacement therapy used in acute renal failure, but PD is a viable option for patients who cannot tolerate the hemodynamic changes associated with HD. In PD, dialysis is performed using the peritoneal membrane as the semipermeable (dialyzing) membrane[3]; in HD and CRRT, a dialyzer or hemofilter is the dialyzing membrane.

The peritoneum is a serous membrane covering the abdominal organs and lining the abdominal wall. It is divided into two sections, the parietal and visceral. The parietel peritoneum receives its blood supply from the arteries that feed the abdominal wall and drains into the systemic circulation. The visceral peritoneum receives its blood supply from the mesenteric and celiac arteries and drains into the portal vein. The peritoneum also has extensive lymphatic flow and drainage. All or part of the peritoneal membrane can be used for PD.[2]

The peritoneal membrane is a semipermeable membrane.[3] Like the dialyzer in HD or hemofilter in CRRT, this membrane is permeable to substances and water. Substance removal in PD occurs primarily through diffusion (substance movement from an area of greater concentration to lesser concentration). Fluid removal occurs as the result of osmosis (water movement from an area of lesser concentration to greater concentration). Ultrafiltration, or enhanced water movement, can be accomplished through the use of hyperosmolar, usually high in glucose, dialysate solutions. Additionally, substances can be added to the blood through diffusion.

Before acute PD can be initiated, access to the peritoneum is required. Generally, the peritoneal catheter is made of silastic tubing, has multiple perforations to allow for fluid exchange, and has an attached anchor device. This anchor may be a cuff, a soft disk, or a balloon.[2] Occasionally, a rigid stylet, designed for single acute use only, will be used when immediate initiation of PD is necessary. Although immediate initiation of PD may be advantageous, this catheter presents a higher risk of organ perforation and dialysate leak into the peritoneum.[5]

Catheter insertion may be done at the bedside or in the operating room (OR). With either procedure, patient preparation includes an enema to empty the bowel and voiding to empty the bladder to decrease the risk of organ perforation. These patients are at extremely high risk for peritonitis, so prophylactic antibiotics are often administered. Both procedures are performed using strict sterile techniques.

When the catheter is inserted at the bedside, the skin is prepped and local anesthetic administered. A trocar is used to penetrate the abdominal wall. Often, once the trocar is in place, dialysate will be infused to expand the peritoneal cavity, making threading of the catheter easier. Once the catheter has been inserted, the trocar is removed. A stab wound is made and a subcutaneous tunnel created, through which the catheter is threaded. The catheter exits the skin through the stab wound, which is then sutured. The rigid stylet is always placed at the bedside, because, as mentioned, it is designed for acute use only.[5]

If catheter insertion is to be done in the OR, the procedure is similar. The primary difference is that a peritoneoscope is used to allow visualization inside the abdomen. Catheters are more commonly placed using this technique when it is anticipated that the catheter will have chronic use.[2]

The exact composition of the dialysate solution is determined by the patient's condition and desired outcomes. The composition will be designed to create concentration gradients to achieve optimal removal of wastes, acid–base and electrolyte balance, and maintenance of extracellular fluid balance.[1] The composition of peritoneal dialysate solutions commercially available[1,5] are shown in the following Box. These standard solutions may be used initially, but they are often altered to better meet the needs of individual patients. Heparin and potassium chloride are almost always added. When any medication is added to a dialysate bag, it should be added immediately before the bag is hung and mixed well.[3] In diabetic patients, insulin may be added to counteract the effects of the glucose.

PD is accomplished through a series of cycles or exchanges. The dialysate must flow into the peritoneal cavity, remain in the cavity for a preset amount of time (dwell time), and then drained out. Each set of activities is called a cycle or exchange. Dialysate flows into the peritoneal cavity by gravity, using a manual or cycler system. It normally takes approximately 10 minutes for two liters of fluid to infuse. The rate of infusion can be increased by increasing the height of the bag in relationship to the abdomen, using larger or shorter inflow tubing. The dwell time allows for diffusion, osmosis, and ultrafiltration to occur. Ultrafiltration is greatest immediately after infusion of fresh dialysate and decreases as the solution osmolality equilibrates with fluid movement. A typical dwell time ranges from 10 to 30 minutes. With an optimally functioning catheter, it takes 2 liters of fluid 10 minutes to drain from the abdomen. The rate of drainage can be increased by moving the patient from side to side and shortening the distance from the patient to the drainage bag.

Different dialysate delivery systems are available. Manual PD requires that the nurse warm, spike, and hang each bag while controlling each phase of the exchange. When PD is being done manually, a manifold or multipronged infusion set is used. This allows multiple bags of dialysate to be hung simultaneously so that system reopening is minimized.

A cycler, often used in the acute care setting, consists of a heater scale, storage hooks, a drain scale, pump, and the computer system. One bag of dialysate is kept on the heated scale to be warmed and measured. Additional bags of dialysate are hung on the rack. When the bag on the heater is empty, the computer is programmed so that the pump takes a specific amount of dialysate from the storage bags and moves it to the heater bag. Dialysate is pumped from all bags on the rack at the same time. After the dialysate has infused and dwelled for the set amount of time, the computer is programmed to open the correct valves so that drainage will occur. The drain scale weighs the fluid draining from the peritoneum, also called effluent. The computer calculates the ultrafiltrate volume. Once completed, the process begins again.

Commercially Available Peritoneal Dialysate Solutions

pH	5.2
Osmolality	346, 396, 425 mOsm
Glucose	1.5, 2.5, 4.25 g%
D-L-Lactate	35, 40 mEq/L
Magnesium	0.5, 1.5 mEq/L
Calcium	2.5, 3.5 mEq/L
Chloride	95, 96, 192 mEq/L
Potassium	0 mEq/L
Sodium	132 mEq/L

INDICATIONS

The indications for PD include the following:

- Acute volume overload
- Symptomatic uremia
- Pericarditis
- BUN >100 mg/dl
- Uncontrolled acidosis
- Creatinine >10 mg/dl
- Creatinine clearance 5 to 7 ml/min
- Uremic encephalopathy
- Electrolyte imbalances
- Drug overdoses
- HD access failure
- Dialysis is needed but anticoagulation is contraindicated

Most often, PD is indicated for the critically ill patient who needs dialysis but is unable to tolerate the hemodynamic changes associated with HD. PD may also be performed in a critical care unit for a patient who is on chronic PD and presently hospitalized with an acute illness.

PD is generally readily available. It requires less-skilled personnel than HD and has fewer complications. PD is contraindicated in patients who have had recent or extensive abdominal surgery, abdominal adhesions, or peritonitis.

LIMITATIONS

PD may require significant commitment of nursing care time depending on the frequency of the exchanges. In addition, PD is not a common procedure. As a result, it may make more sense to train a core group of staff to perform this intervention. On the other hand, the increase in home PD, with improved cannulation techniques and fairly streamlined exchange systems, may make PD a less intensive intervention than previously assumed. However, PD may not be an

TABLE 53-1 General Nursing Interventions For Acute Peritoneal Dialysis

General Considerations	Recommended Action
Monitoring for Effectiveness	
Fluid balance	Ensure that total fluid volume and intravascular volume are within acceptable limits Careful assessment of all of the following: • Wt: always weigh patient during the same time of a cycle—during dwell time or after drain before fill • If wt is done during dwell time, adjust wt for amount of fluid in abdomen • Fluid status: JVD, peripheral/sacral edema, breath sounds, pulses, CVP, PAPs, PCWP, peripheral circulation (cool, blanched extremities) • BP: lying, sitting, standing • Auscultate heart tones, rhythm, pericardial friction rub • Monitor I/O
Laboratory values	Monitor urine volume, specific gravity, and electrolytes Monitor serum electrolytes: creatinine, BUN, uric acid, Ca^{++}, phosphorus, ABG Monitor liver function studies, especially clotting studies, serum protein, albumin levels Monitor Hgb, Hct, platelets, WBC count Monitor drug levels
Prevention of Complications	
Bleeding	Assess patient history of bleeding, response to previous anticoagulation, prior Hct and clotting studies Be alert to sudden pain in the abdomen, hips, back, or buttocks in the patient with femoral access—sign of retroperitoneal bleeding Closely monitor catheter insertion and stab wound sites for bleeding If local bleeding occurs: • Apply ice packs • Consider local infiltration with epinephrine • Be prepared to assist with surgical repair • Monitor color and Hct of dialysate
Hypervolemia/hypertension	Careful predialysis assessment of all of the following: • Wt (may be done as often as q2h to q4h): compare with previous wts • Fluid status: JVD, peripheral/sacral edema, breath sounds, pulses, CVP, PAPs, PCWP, peripheral circulation (cool, blanched extremities) • BP: lying, sitting, standing Auscultate heart tones, rhythm, pericardial friction rub

Continued.

adequate intervention in all cases of renal failure. Hemodialysis may still be necessary in some cases.

POTENTIAL COMPLICATIONS

Complications seen in the patient receiving PD are most often related to the abdominal catheter required. Meticulous technique while connecting and disconnecting the catheter (coupling and uncoupling) and proper exit site care are essential. Detailed procedures for these activities can be found in the AACN Procedure Manual.[4]

Other complications related to PD are as follows:

- Bleeding
- Hypervolemia/hypertension
- Hypovolemia/hypotension
- Electrolyte/acid–base imbalance
- Peritonitis
- Intra-abdominal perforation
- Catheter obstruction
- Catheter leakage
- Exit site infection
- Inadequate management of renal failure

GENERAL NURSING INTERVENTIONS

The patient on PD requires close monitoring, as does any patient in renal failure. There are many similarities in caring for renal failure patients regardless of their mode of renal replacement therapy. Nursing interventions associated with monitoring the effectiveness of PD, as well as assessing and intervening for complications, are listed in Table 53-1.

TABLE 53-1 General Nursing Interventions For Acute Peritoneal Dialysis—cont'd

General Considerations	Recommended Action
Prevention of Complications—cont'd	
Hypervolemia/hypertension—cont'd	Monitor I/O with each cycle Assess closely for signs of hypervolemia (tachycardia, hypertension, bounding pulses, increasing PAPs, paradoxical pulses) Administer fluid/blood as ordered while being dialyzed Administer O_2 as needed Monitor ultrafiltrate output Increase the osmolality of the dialysate to enhance the fluid removal Increase frequency of exchanges Shorten dwell time
Hypovolemia/hypotension	Careful assessment as listed in hypervolemia Monitor for signs of hypovolemia (tachycardia, hypotension, falling PAPs, PCWP) Monitor amount of ultrafiltrate If hypotension occurs: • Administer O_2 as needed • Administer saline or albumin • Elevate patient's legs • Administer vasopressor medications as ordered
Electrolyte acid–base imbalances	Obtain serum K^+/Na^+/ABG as needed Notify MD and ensure dialysate is ordered appropriately Adjust the dialysate during the treatment as needed Assess for signs of acid–base/electrolyte imbalances Hyperkalemia: wide-absent T wave, depressed ST segment, tall, tented T wave, prolonged QT interval Hypokalemia: elevated P wave, flattened or inverted T wave, prolonged QT interval, PVCs Hypernatremia: dry, flushed skin, thirst, vomiting, weak, crampy, or spastic muscle tone, seizures Hyponatremia: muscle weakness, lethargy, irritability, headaches
Peritonitis	Monitor effluent for turbidity Monitor for abdominal discomfort (especially rebound tenderness), redness, tenderness, or drainage at exit site Utilize scrupulous sterile technique when entering system If peritonitis is suspected, culture dialysate When peritonitis is diagnosed: • Administer intraperitoneal and/or IV antibiotics as ordered • Consider increasing frequency of exchanges • Remove catheter if peritonitis is unresolved in 3 to 5 days from onset
Intra-abdominal perforation	Monitor for sudden-onset abdominal pain, massive watery diarrhea, sudden large diuresis, inadequate drainage Suspect perforation if effluent is cloudy, malodorous, or contains frank fecal material If perforation is suspected, dipstick urine and feces for sugar (if positive, may indicate dialysate is present) Once perforation is confirmed: • Stop PD immediately • Remove PD catheter
Catheter obstruction	Monitor inflow and outflow cycles to evaluate for obstruction Irrigate new catheters with heparinized saline Monitor bowel patterns (constipation is a common cause of obstruction)
Catheter leakage	Monitor exit site for dialysate leakage; if leakage occurs, discontinue PD for prescribed time to allow for tissue seal to develop

TABLE 53-1 General Nursing Interventions For Acute Peritoneal Dialysis—cont'd

General Considerations	Recommended Action
Prevention of Complications—cont'd	
Exit site/tunnel infection	Assess for signs of infection: elevated T, chills, drainage, localized warmth, redness, tenderness, swelling, or pain at insertion and exit sites and along tunnel Assess for signs of tunnel irregularity, thickening along the tunnel, or catheter loose in the tunnel Administer prophylactic antibodies at the time of catheter insertion Monitor laboratory values (WBC count, differential) Administer antibiotics as ordered (usually given intraperitoneally) If tunnel infection is diagnosed, remove the catheter
Inadequate treatment	Ascertain accuracy of dialysis orders based on patient assessment: • Frequency and timing of exchanges • Composition of dialysate If using a cycler: • Monitor inflow and outflow times to evaluate function of computer • Fluid administration and/or replacement

TROUBLESHOOTING

The critical care nurse holds an essential role in troubleshooting problems that may occur with PD. The nurse may need to intervene related to the PD process, the catheter, or the patient's response to treatment. The most common problems, usual causes, and corrective actions for PD are as follows.

Fluid Overload/Hypertension

CAUSE	CORRECTIVE ACTION
Excess fluid administration (patient) Inadequate fluid removal (patient) Poorly functioning catheter (device) Dialysate leak (device)	Monitor amount of ultrafiltrate Replace fluid carefully Administer blood/blood products while patient is being dialyzed to minimize fluid increases Monitor patient's wt daily Increase the osmolality of dialysate and frequency of exchanges Shorten the dwell time Ensure catheter function

Problem: Fluid Volume Deficit/Hypotension

CAUSE	CORRECTIVE ACTION
Excess Na^+ and fluid removal (patient) Inadequate fluid intake (patient)	Closely monitor BP, HR, and peripheral circulation Be aware that fluid may be retained when patient is hypovolemic For mild hypotension: • Open drain clamp and allow for outflow (relieves pressure on vena cava) • Position patient on left side • Notify MD quickly if severe hypotension occurs • Administer fluid as ordered • Administer vasopressor medications as ordered • Decrease the osmolality of dialysate • Lengthen dwell time

Bleeding from insertion site (patient)	Prevent catheter dislodgement by taping securely in place Observe catheter insertion site frequently Monitor serial Hcts; if bleeding occurs: • Monitor VS • Notify MD stat • Hold pressure on sites for 10 to 15 min and apply pressure dressing for 3 to hr • Administer blood/fluids as ordered

Problem: Electrolyte Imbalances

CAUSE	CORRECTIVE ACTION
Inappropriate intake (patient) Inappropriate dialysate (device) Inefficient dialysis (device)	Monitor laboratory values closely Administer electrolyte replacement as needed Adjust electrolyte levels in dialysate

Problem: Inability to Drain and/or Infuse

CAUSE	CORRECTIVE ACTION
Constipation (patient)	If constipation is suspected, administer enema or other cathartic to stimulate bowel movement
Kinked or obstructed catheter (device)	Undress and unkink catheter Check tubing for clamps, kinks, or pressure Anchor tubing to prevent kinks Aspirate to assess for fibrin or blood clot Raise bag to at least 4 feet above patient Apply warm pads to patient's abdomen Ensure adequate nutrition Obtain flat plate and lateral x-ray to rule out internal catheter kinking Administer fibrinolytic agents as ordered Change patient's position Consider adding heparin to dialysate or flush catheter with heparinized saline Prepare to replace catheter if obstruction cannot be relieved

SUMMARY

Caring for the patient requiring PD is very challenging. Although PD is not as common as hemodialysis, critical care nurses still must be familiar with the process of PD and the underlying disease that necessitates renal replacement therapy. (See Guideline 51.) The growing use of PD in the management of acute and chronic renal failure makes knowledge and skill in this support intervention an important capability of the critical care nurse.

REFERENCES

1. Palmer BF: Dialysate composition in hemodialysis and peritoneal dialysis. In Henrich WL, editor: *Principles and practice of dialysis,* Baltimore, 1994, Williams & Wilkins, pp 17-19.
2. Parker J, Ulrich BT: Peritoneal dialysis therapy. In Ulrich BT, editor: *Nephrology nursing: concepts and strategies,* Englewood, NJ, 1989, Appleton & Lange, pp 153-171.
3. Prowant B, Gallagher NM: Concepts and principles of peritoneal dialysis. In Lancaster LE, editor: *Core curriculum for nephrology nursing,* Pitman, NJ, 1990, American Nephrology Nurse's Association, pp 277-322.
4. Robinson KJ, Robinson JA: Peritoneal dialysis. In Boggs RL, Wooldridge-King M, editors: *AACN procedure manual for critical care,* Philadelphia, 1993, WB Saunders, pp 609-618.
5. Smith LJ: Peritoneal dialysis in the critically ill patient, *AACN Clin Iss Crit Care Nurs* 3(3):558-569, 1992.

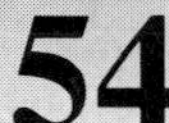

DEVICE GUIDELINE

54

Acute Hemodialysis

Karen K. Carlson, MN, RN, CCRN

DESCRIPTION

Dialysis is an artificial process that partially replaces renal function (i.e., metabolic waste product, fluid, and electrolyte removal) during renal failure. It can also be used to remove toxic substances and in the treatment of drug overdoses.

Hemodialysis (HD) is the most prevalent renal replacement therapy for both acute renal failure and end-stage renal disease (ESRD). Using HD is advantageous because fluid and electrolyte imbalances can be corrected efficiently, usually in 4- to 6-hour treatments. Until the early 1980s, intermittent HD and peritoneal dialysis were the most commonly used modes of dialysis. Since that time, a number of continuous renal replacement therapies (CRRT) have been developed and are utilized in selected patient populations. Using CRRT, many of the desirable outcomes of HD can be accomplished without the hemodynamic instability frequently seen in HD. More details on CRRT modalities are found in Guideline 55.

Access to the bloodstream must be established before dialysis can be performed. Access can be either temporary or permanent and will be determined by the reason for initiation and method of dialysis.

External arteriovenous (AV) shunts (e.g., the Scribner shunt) were the first available access for long-term dialysis but are rarely used for HD today. These catheters, made of Teflon, were surgically placed between the radial artery and an adjacent vein. There were many problems maintaining these shunts, such as clotting and infection, and their life span (6 to 12 months) was relatively short.

Presently, temporary HD access, used in patients with acute renal failure and in patients with ESRD while their graft or fistula is maturing, is generally achieved through percutaneous cannulation of the subclavian or internal jugular veins. A large-bore, double- or single-lumen, central venous catheter (CVC), specifically designed for dialysis, is placed like any other CVC, but is used primarily for dialysis treatments. The double-lumen catheter is used most commonly because recirculation (a portion of the "arterial" blood being aspirated by the "venous" side) is decreased because the openings for inflow and outflow are at different sites. When a single-lumen catheter is used, a Y adaptor is necessary so that blood can be pulled alternately from the patient to the dialyzer and returned to the patient. Femoral catheters, although easy to place and causing few complications, are rarely used for HD. Patients with a femoral HD catheter must remain in the hospital on bed rest, and the catheter must be changed every 5 to 6 days. The most permanent of the temporary catheters is a CVC, described above, which is surgically placed in the operating room. This catheter has a cuff under the skin exit site, which adds to the catheter's stability. The CVC can be left in place for 2 to 3 months (Figure 54-1).

Permanent access, used in patients with ESRD, is in the form of either an AV fistula or AV graft. A fistula is a surgically created anastomosis between an artery (radial, brachial, or femoral) and a vein allowing arterial blood to flow through the vein, causing vein enlargement and engorgement. Preferred location for an AV fistula is an upper extremity. This is the access of choice in patients requiring chronic dialysis.[2]

AV grafts are placed in patients who do not have adequate vessels to create a fistula. A prosthetic graft is implanted subcutaneously and used to anastomose an artery to a vein. A period of maturation, usually 2 to 3 weeks, is necessary before the access can be used.[1] This maturation time allows

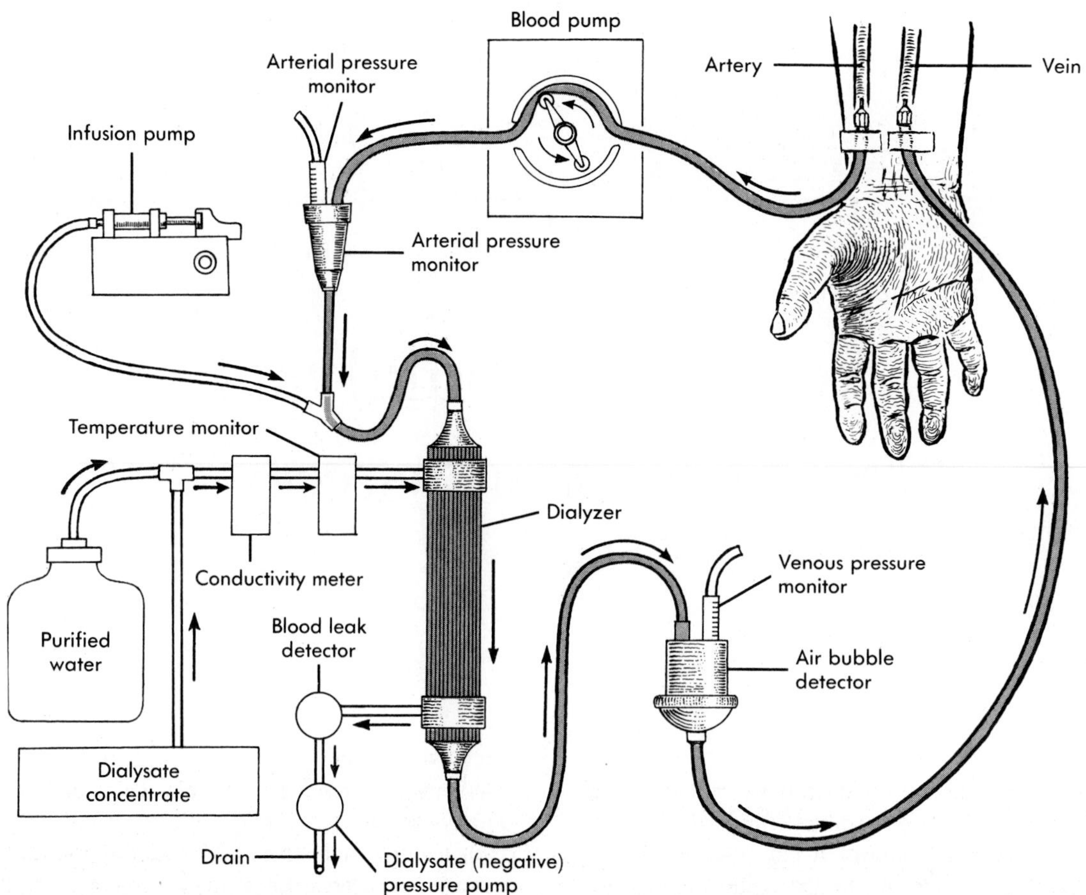

Figure 54-1 Components of a hemodialysis system. (From Thelan LA, et al: *Critical care nursing: diagnosis and management*, ed 2, St Louis, 1993, Mosby–Year Book.)

for the venous side to dilate and the vessel wall to thicken, permitting repeated insertion of dialysis needles.

The type of dialyzer (artificial kidney) used is determined by the patient's condition and desired outcomes of the dialysis treatment. The most commonly used dialyzers are hollow-fiber and parallel-plate dialyzers. All dialyzers have two compartments, a blood compartment and a dialysate compartment, separated by a semipermeable membrane. The dialyzer has two inlet ports and two outlet ports, one each for blood and dialysate. In HD, blood and dialysate are pumped in opposite directions through their individual compartments.

The exact composition of the dialysate solution is, like the dialyzer, determined by the patient's condition and desired outcomes. While standard solutions may be used initially, they often are altered for individual patients and can contain different concentrations of Na^+, K^+, Mg^+, Ca^{++}, Cl^-, glucose and buffers (bicarbonate or acetate).

Different dialysate delivery systems are available. The proportioning system, most commonly used in acute hemodialysis, provides mixing of water with the dialysate to assure the correct concentration before it is delivered to the dialyzer. This concentration is monitored continuously to assure that the dialysate is neither hypertonic nor hypotonic.

Initiation of HD through a temporary access is accomplished using a procedure called coupling. During coupling, the dialysis catheter and dialysis circuitry are connected, using sterile technique.

To initiate dialysis through a permanent access, two 14- or 16-gauge needles are inserted into the dilated vein of the fistula or the graft portion of the synthetic graft. One needle is considered afferent (arterial) and used for blood outflow, while the other is considered efferent (venous) and used for blood return to the body. The needles should be placed at least 5 cm apart to decrease the chance of recirculation. Details of these procedures can be found in the *AACN Procedure Manual for Critical Care*.[3]

The basic components of a hemodialysis system are shown in Figure 54-1. Blood leaves the patient by way of the arterial needle, is pumped through the dialysis circuitry, and returns to the patient through the venous needle. The blood pump—two or more roller heads that squeeze the blood tubing—is used to move the blood through the dialysis circuitry and dialyzer. The heads are calibrated so that different flow rates of blood can be achieved. Both arterial and venous pressures are monitored in the circuitry. The arterial pressure monitor is usually located before the blood pump and assists in guarding against excess suction on the access. The monitor will turn off the blood pump (automatically clamping the venous line) if pressures exceed predetermined limits. Venous pressure monitoring, usually located after the dialyzer, protects against resistance to blood return. The monitor can calculate transmembrane pressure and will also shut off the blood pump if pressure exceeds preset limits. Conductivity monitors also are used to assess the concentration of the dialysate.

Whenever blood comes in contact with a foreign surface, there is an increased risk of clot formation, making anticoagulation a necessary part of dialysis. Heparin is the anticoagulant of choice for dialysis because it has a short half-life and quick onset of action.[1]

Different methods of anticoagulation are used in HD. Systemic anticoagulation provides for anticoagulation of the entire bloodstream and extracorporeal system and is used when dialyzing patients who are at low risk for bleeding. Heparin therapy can be delivered either continuously, by infusion of heparin into the arterial dialysis line, or intermittently, by administering a bolus dose at the onset of treatment and adding doses as necessary throughout the treatment. Additionally, bolus doses of heparin often are administered at the beginning of a continuous infusion.

There are several methods of anticoagulation used in patients who are at high risk for bleeding. Regional heparinization is achieved by infusion of heparin into the arterial line of the dialyzer as the blood leaves the patient to enter the dialysis circuitry.[2] Protamine sulfate is then used in the venous line as the blood leaves the dialyzer before it returns to the patient. Administration of protamine sulfate neutralizes the effect of heparin.

Use of a citrate anticoagulation regime is considered by some to be the method of choice in patients at risk for bleeding.[1] Citrate, administered into the arterial line of the dialysis circuit, combines with Ca^{++} preventing normal progression of the clotting cascade. A simultaneous Ca^{++} infusion is administered into the venous limb of the dialysis circuit to minimize the systemic effects that would result from a lower Ca^{++} level.

Occasionally, dialysis will be performed without any heparin. Heparin-free dialysis requires frequent saline flushes and a higher than usual blood flow through the circuitry.

The degree of anticoagulation is monitored frequently through bedside monitoring of the activated clotting time (ACT). The therapeutic goal is determined individually for each patient.

Fluid is removed from the body by the process of ultrafiltration.[2] A pressure gradient is established by the driving force of the patient's hydrostatic pressure. As the dialysate moves through the dialyzer, negative pressure is generated. The net result of these pressures is removal of excess fluid from the body.

Solutes are removed from the body by the process of diffusion. When substances are present in different concentrations on two sides of a semipermeable membrane, as in the dialyzer, movement of those substances occurs from the side of greater to lesser concentration, as long as the membrane is permeable. For example, in dialyzing a renal failure patient, urea diffuses from the blood into the dialysate and bicarbonate moves from the dialysate into the blood.

INDICATIONS

HD is implemented when aggressive therapy is indicated in acute situations. Indications for HD include:

- Acute volume overload
- Uncontrollable hyperkalemia/acidosis
- Symptomatic uremia
- Pericarditis
- BUN >100 mg/dl
- Uncontrolled acidosis
- Creatinine >10 mg/dl
- Creatinine clearance 5 to 7 ml/min
- Uremic encephalopathy
- Pulmonary edema, refractory to diuretics
- Uremic bleeding
- Compromised nutritional state with anorexia, nausea, and vomiting
- Electrolyte imbalances
- Drug overdoses

HD is contraindicated in the hemodynamically unstable or hypovolemic patient, and in patients in whom adequate vascular access cannot be achieved. CRRT may be instituted simultaneously with measures to improve hemodynamic stability.

LIMITATIONS

Since HD is highly technical, most critical care units have a core group of staff trained in the procedure. This is the preferred method for facilities in which a lower volume of HD patients makes it important to limit the number of trained staff so that staff members have adequate experience to maintain their competence in the procedure. In facilities with a significant HD patient population, entire staffs may be dedicated to treating HD patients. Depending on the facility, ready access to properly trained staff may be a challenge for HD patients.

There may also be clinical conditions that make HD risky, limiting its appropriateness. Hypovolemic or actively septic patients may not be able to withstand the hemodynamic fluctuations that occur with HD as blood volume is directed to the dialysis machine. In other cases, acceptable vascular access may be difficult to achieve. In cases such as this, PD may be a better choice.

POTENTIAL COMPLICATIONS

HD often causes or contributes to the hemodynamic instability of critically ill patients. There are numerous complications associated with HD. The majority of these complications are related to patient response to treatment and require careful monitoring and timely intervention.

Potential complications associated with HD include the following:

- Bleeding
- Infection
- Hypervolemia/hypertension
- Hypovolemia/hypotension
- Electrolyte/acid-base imbalance
- Changes in mentation
- Dysrhythmias
- Air embolus
- Pyrogenic reaction
- Disequilibrium
- Hemolysis
- Inadequate management of renal failure

GENERAL NURSING INTERVENTIONS

There are many similarities in caring for patients who require renal replacement therapy regardless of the type of intervention used. In addition to nursing care related to the technology and process of HD, the critical care nurse must also be aware of the medication profile of the patient, have sound understanding of how the medications may impact a dialysis treatment, and know which medications may be removed via HD. As a result, customizing the medication profile for each HD patient is essential.

General nursing interventions are directed at monitoring the effectiveness of the HD as well as preventing, detecting, and intervening for complications as they arise. These nursing interventions are detailed in Table 54-1.

TABLE 54-1 General Nursing Interventions For Hemodialysis (HD)

General considerations	Related nursing interventions
Monitoring for effectiveness	
Fluid balance	Assure that total fluid volume and intravascular volume are within acceptable limits After HD treatment assess: • Weight: compare with previous and dry weights: weight gain of no more than 1 kg/day between treatments • Fluid status: JVD, peripheral/sacral edema, breath sounds, pulses, CVP, PAPs, PCWP, peripheral circulation (cool, blanched extremities) lying, sitting, standing • Auscultate heart tones, rhythm, pericardial friction rub • Monitor intake and output
Laboratory values	Monitor urine volume, specific gravity, and electrolytes. Monitor electrolytes: creatinine, BUN, uric acid, Ca^{++}, PO_4^{--}, ABG Monitor liver function studies, especially clotting studies, serum protein, albumin levels Monitor Hgb, Hct, platelets, WBC count Monitor drug levels
Prevention of complications	
Bleeding	Assess patient history of bleeding, and response to previous anticoagulation, prior Hct, and clotting studies Assess for bruises, occult bleeding, overt bleeding (skin, NG/tracheal aspirate, insertion sites, urine, stool) Monitor clotting studies as per unit standards Adjust anticoagulation protocol as needed based on clotting times, patient's condition, patency of circuit, and response to previous anticoagulation Be alert to sudden pain in the abdomen, hips, back, or buttocks in patients with femoral access (sign of retroperitoneal bleeding) Closely monitor catheter insertion/needle puncture sites for bleeding After discontinuing dialysis using permanent access, hold pressure at needle puncture sites and 1 inch above arterial site and 1 inch below venous insertion site In preparation for catheter removal, discontinue heparin infusion at least 4 hours prior to MD removal of catheters After catheter removal, hold pressure on catheter insertion sites for 20 to 30 minutes Reapply pressure if bleeding occurs

Continued.

TABLE 54-1 General Nursing Interventions For Hemodialysis (HD)—cont'd	
General considerations	**Related nursing interventions**
Prevention of complications—cont'd	
Infection	Assess for signs of infection: elevated temperature, chills, drainage, localized warmth, redness, tenderness, swelling, or pain at access site Monitor for drainage at insertion sites of catheters/shunts/grafts Monitor laboratory values (WBC count and differential) Administer antibiotics as ordered
Hypervolemia/hypertension	Perform predialysis assessment of: • Weight: compare with previous and dry weights • Fluid status: JVD, peripheral/sacral edema, breath sounds, pulses, CVP, PAP, PCWP, peripheral circulation (cool, blanched extremities) • BP: lying, sitting, standing Auscultate heart tones, rhythm, pericardial friction rub Monitor hourly intake and output Assess closely for signs of hypervolemia (tachycardia, hypertension, bounding pulses, increasing PAP, paradoxical pulses) Administer fluid/blood as ordered while being dialyzed Correctly prime dialysis machine and circuit Administer O_2 as needed Monitor UF output
Hypovolemia/hypotension	Perform predialysis assessment as outlined in hypervolemia (see previous section). Assure that antihypertensive medications are held before treatments Monitor for signs of hypovolemia (tachycardia, hypotension, falling PAPs and PCWP) Monitor UF rate Correctly prime dialysis machine If hypotension occurs: • Slow UF rates • Administer O_2 as needed • Administer normal saline or albumin • Elevate patient's legs • Administer vasopressor medications as ordered
Electrolyte/acid-base imbalances	Obtain serum K^+/Na^+/ABG as needed. Notify MD and assure dialysate order is appropriate Adjust the dialysate during the treatment as needed Assess for signs of acid-base/electrolyte imbalances: • Hyperkalemia: wide-absent T wave; depressed ST segment; tall, tented T wave; prolonged QT interval • Hypokalemia: elevated P wave, flattened or inverted T wave, prolonged QT interval, PVCs • Hypernatremia: dry, flushed skin; thirst; vomiting; weak, crampy, or spastic muscle tone; seizures • Hyponatremia: muscle weakness, lethargy, irritability, headaches
Change in mentation	Assess neurological status initially, q4h and prn while being dialyzed Monitor electrolyte, coagulation, and ABG results Orient patient and family to HD
Dysrhythmias	Assess patient's rhythm pre-, intra-, and postdialysis Administer antidysrhythmic agents as needed Monitor electrolyte values
Air embolus	Ensure that dialysis circuit is primed completely when initiating HD and with all tubing/dialyzer changes Avoid kinks in tubing Tighten and tape all connections Monitor for air in tubing, signs of air embolus (chest pain, cough, cyanosis) Notify MD of any abnormalities and actions taken

Continued.

TABLE 54-1 General Nursing Interventions For Hemodialysis (HD)—cont'd

General considerations	Related nursing interventions
Prevention of complications—cont'd	
Pyrogenic reaction	Assess VS frequently pre-, intra-, and postdialysis Monitor for chills and fever Assure that dialysis machine/circuit is sterile or has been adequately disinfected If pyrogenic reaction is suspected, notify MD stat C & S water, dialysate, and blood Discontinue treatment Administer medications as ordered
Disequilibrium	Monitor laboratory values (BUN, creatinine, creatinine clearance) Monitor VS and weight Monitor for signs of disequilibrium: hypertension, headache, confusion, nausea/vomiting, seizures If disequilibrium is suspected: • Slow blood pump • Monitor BP frequently • Administer volume expanders, antiepileptic medications, mannitol as needed • Apply seizure precautions prn
Hemolysis	Assure dialysate temperature is near body temperature before beginning dialysis Provide for adequate anticoagulation Monitor conductivity of dialysate
Inadequate treatment	Ascertain accuracy of dialysis orders based on patient assessment: • Frequency and length of treatment • Type of dialyzer • Composition of dialysate • Fluid administration and/or replacement • Acceptable flow rates • Degree of UF • Anticoagulation protocol • Laboratory specimens to be sent Assure that all alarms are armed throughout treatment

TROUBLESHOOTING

Nursing plays a major role in troubleshooting problems that can occur in dialysis. Troubleshooting is related to either the device itself or the patient's response to the treatment. General troubleshooting guidelines are provided as follows:

Problem: Air Embolus

CAUSE	CORRECTIVE ACTION
Device • Loose connections • Disarmed air/foam detector • Empty IV bags • Pump set at higher rate than access can deliver • Retained air in dialyzer	Correct any identified circuit problem to prevent embolus If embolus is suspected: • Stop infusion, clamp lines • Position patient on left side with legs elevated • Administer O_2 per unit standards • Assess VS and LOC • Notify MD stat • Identify and correct cause

Problem: Bleeding

CAUSE	CORRECTIVE ACTION
Loss of platelets (patient/device)	Monitor platelet counts Administer platelets as ordered
Overanticoagulation (device)	Adjust anticoagulation routine as indicated by assessment of patient's condition, patency of circuit, previous history of response to anticoagulation, and clotting study results

Problem: Fluid Volume Overload/Hypertension

CAUSE	CORRECTIVE ACTION
Excess fluid administration (patient)	Monitor rate of UF and increase as tolerated Monitor response to changes in UF rate Replace fluid carefully Administer blood/blood products while patient is being dialyzed to minimize fluid increases Monitor patient's weight between treatments (should not exceed 1 kg/day) Monitor for signs of disequilibrium

Problem: Fluid Volume Deficit/Hypotension

CAUSE	CORRECTIVE ACTION
Antihypertensive medication administration (patient)	Review patient's antihypertensive medications Closely monitor BP, HR, and peripheral circulation in patients at risk for hypotension due to their medications Notify MD quickly if hypotension occurs Administer fluid as ordered Administer vasopressor medications as ordered
Diversion of patient's blood to dialysis machine (approximately 200 to 300 cc) (device)	Prime dialysis machine with normal saline, albumin, or blood as ordered Monitor wt loss/ultrafiltration during treatment
Excessive ultrafiltration (device)	Monitor patient's toleration to UF rate Slow UF rate as necessary
Hypertonic dialysate (device)	Assure conductivity alarms and limits are set at appropriate levels Monitor VS carefully throughout treatments If hypertonic dialysate is suspected: • Stop dialysis. Clamp blood tubing. Do not return blood to patient. • Monitor patient for neurologic changes • Notify MD stat Administer IV fluids as ordered Reinstitute dialysis as soon as possible to correct imbalance, using new dialysate
Bleeding from tubing disconnect or catheter/graft insertion site leakage	Prevent needle dislodgement by securely taping needles in place Observe needle insertion sites frequently Position extremity to avoid abrupt movements Monitor serial Hct If needle becomes dislodged, clamp arterial and venous blood lines Monitor VS Notify MD stat Hold pressure on sites for 10 to 15 min, remove needles, and apply pressure dressing for 3 to 4 hr If dialysis needs to be continued, reinsert new needles Administer blood/fluids as ordered

Problem: Hemolysis

CAUSE	CORRECTIVE ACTION
Hypotonic dialysate (device)	Assure conductivity alarms are set at appropriate levels Monitor VS throughout treatments If hypotonic dialysate is suspected: • Stop dialysis • Clamp tubing—do not return blood to patient • Administer O_2 as ordered • Call MD stat • Identify the cause and correct • Restart dialysis using new equipment/dialysate

Problem: Clotting

CAUSE	CORRECTIVE ACTION
Insufficient heparin infusion (device)	Adjust heparin infusion rates Flush needles with heparinized saline
Tubing obstruction (kinked, bent tubing) (device)	Unkink tubing Prepare to change dialyzer as needed

Problem: Electrolyte Imbalances

CAUSE	CORRECTIVE ACTION
Inappropriate dialysate (device)	Monitor laboratory values closely Administer electrolyte replacement as needed

SUMMARY

HD is frequently seen in the care of the critically ill patient. The most common indication for acute HD is acute renal failure, which is discussed in depth in Guideline 51.

Caring for patients who are being treated with HD is challenging and requires careful vigilance by the critical care nurse. In order to best care for a patient needing dialysis, it is important for the nurse to have an understanding of the underlying disease process and its impact on other body systems.

REFERENCES

1. Ismail N, Hakim R: Hemodialysis. In Levine, editor: *Care of the renal patient,* ed 2, Philadelphia, 1991, WB Saunders, pp 220-246.
2. Peeshman P: Acute hemodialysis issues in the critically ill, *AACN Clin Iss Crit Care Nurs* 3(3):545-557, 1992.
3. Robinson KJ, Robinson JA: Acute hemodialysis. In Boggs RL, Wool-ridge-King M, editors: *AACN procedure manual for critical care,* ed 3, Philadelphia, WB Saunders, pp 579-598.
4. Thelan LA, et al: Critical care nursing: diagnosis and management, ed 2, St Louis, 1993, Mosby–Year Book.

DEVICE GUIDELINE

55

Continuous Renal Replacement Therapies

Karen K. Carlson, MN, RN, CCRN

DESCRIPTION

Acute renal failure (ARF) is a common problem in critical care units. Until the late 1970s, intermittent hemodialysis (HD) or peritoneal dialysis (PD) were the primary modes of therapy utilized. As the acuity in critical care units has increased, the acuity of patients with ARF has increased. These patients often have ARF in conjunction with hemodynamic instability, making traditional HD a less viable intervention.

In 1977, continuous arteriovenous hemofiltration (CAVH), an alternative to traditional HD/PD, was introduced.[6] Since that time, the number of continuous renal replacement therapies (CRRT) has increased, offering critical care professionals more viable options for treatment of the critically ill ARF or fluid-overloaded patient.

The goal of CRRT is fluid and uremic toxin removal. Each of the five CRRT available have varying degrees of efficacy in accomplishing those goals. CRRT fall into two categories: those requiring arteriovenous (AV) access and those requiring venous access. These therapies are described in the following Box. Indications for the use and efficacy of each therapy will be discussed later.

Generally, CRRT are prescribed for 8 to 24 hours and provide for extracorporeal blood flow, either from an artery to a vein, using two catheters, or through a single vein, accessed by a single catheter. The blood flows through a highly porous hemofilter, allowing free water and dissolved molecules with a molecular weight of less than 50,000 daltons[9] to drain. The product is a protein-free ultrafiltrate of whole blood.[10] CRRT are basically dependent on the patient's blood flow, determined by the patient's own cardiac output (CO). The system works most efficiently if the mean arterial pressure (MAP) is 60 to 70 mm Hg.[2,10]

The removal or clearance of fluid and solute is based primarily on the principle of convection. Lower-weight molecules are conveyed across the semipermeable membrane of the hemofilter as the result of hydrostatic pressure, determined by the patient's MAP. This pressure pushes fluid across the hemofilter's membrane into the ultrafiltrate compartment. Simultaneously, negative hydrostatic pressure, created by the height of the fluid in the ultrafiltrate compartment, pulls fluid from the blood compartment into the ultrafiltrate compartment. Additionally, oncotic pressure, exerted by the plasma proteins, is working to hold fluid in the intravascular compartment, and therefore opposes filtration. The difference between the hydrostatic and oncotic pressures determines movement across the hemofilter, and, therefore, the rate of ultrafiltration (UF).

The ultrafiltrate is protein free. As more water is removed from the patient's blood, the plasma protein concentration (determining the oncotic pressure) in the blood rises. As a result, the oncotic pressure in the patient's blood begins to balance with the hydrostatic pressure in the ultrafiltrate. If this pressure gradient is entirely removed, UF ceases.

Several strategies can be used to increase the hydrostatic pressure to assist in maintaining an adequate UF rate. Increasing the patient's MAP, decreasing the amount of tubing connecting the hemofilter to the ultrafiltrate collection bag (ideal tubing length is 40 cm without kinks or loops), decreasing blood flow resistance by lowering the collection

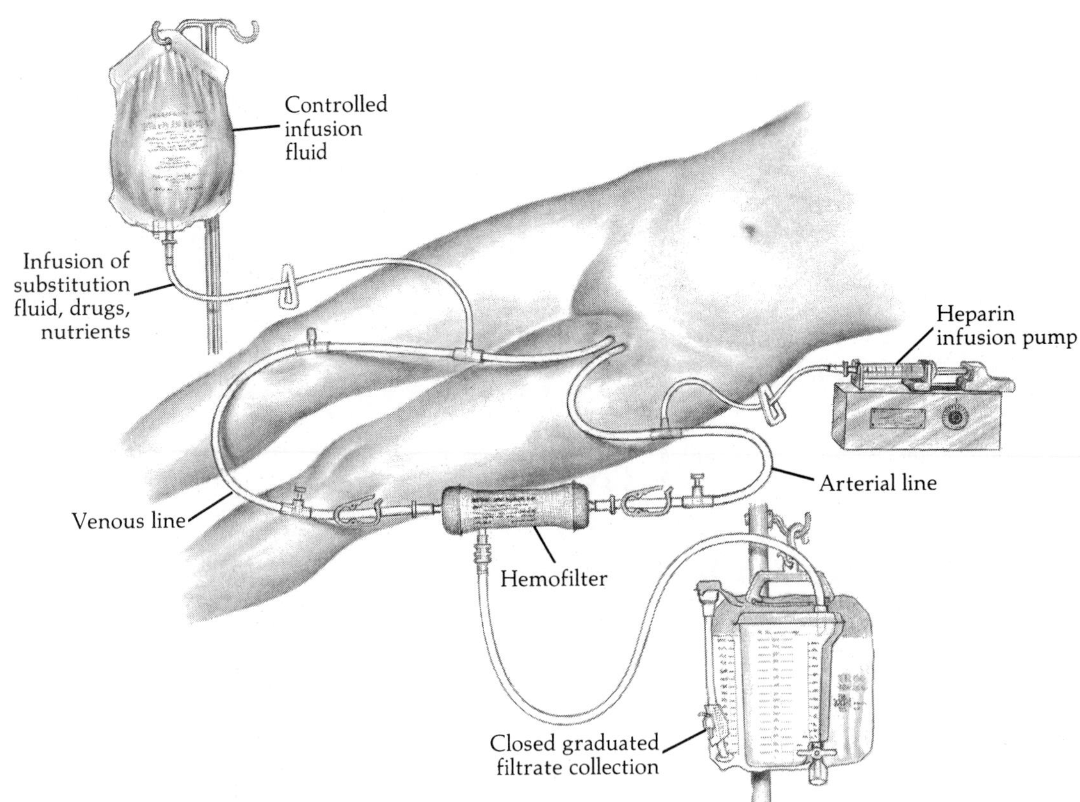

Figure 55-1 Diagram of CAVH system. (From Thompson JM: *Mosby's Clinical Nursing Reference*, ed 3, St Louis, 1993, Mosby–Year Book.)

Types of CRRT

Continuous arteriovenous ultrafiltration (CAVU)
Slow continuous ultrafiltration (SCUF)
Continuous arteriovenous hemofiltration (CAVH)
Continuous arteriovenous hemodialysis (CAVHD)
Continuous venovenous hemofiltration (CVVH)
Continuous venovenous hemodialysis (CVVHD)

bag, attaching suction to the ultrafiltrate bag, or decreasing oncotic pressure by diluting the blood prefilter will all enhance the rate of UF.[3]

Removal of solutes from the body is also accomplished through diffusion. When substances are present in different concentrations on two sides of a semipermeable membrane, as in the hemofilter, movement of those substances occurs from the side of greater-to-lesser concentration, provided the membrane is permeable.

In order to initiate CAVU, CAVH, or CAVHD, vascular access is required. Two 14 to 16-gauge catheters are placed, one in an artery and one in a vein. The femoral artery and vein are commonly used. (See Figures 55-1 and 55-2.) Occasionally, the subclavian vein and the axillary artery are used. In some centers, Schribner shunts are placed as access. Chronic dialysis access, such as internal AV fistulas or AV shunts, can also be used.

When either CVVH or CVVHD are instituted, a 14 to 16-gauge, double-lumen, central venous catheter is placed in the subclavian or femoral vein. (See Figure 55-3.)

In CAVHD and CVVHD, the exact composition of the dialysate solution is, like the dialyzer, determined by the patient's condition and desired outcomes. Standard PD solutions may initially be used, but they are often altered for individual patients and can contain different concentrations of Na^+, K^+, Mg^+, Ca^{++}, Cl^-, glucose, and buffers (bicarbonate or acetate).

Once access has been obtained, CRRT can be initiated by a trained RN or MD. The transport lines are usually primed with a saline-and-heparin solution. The tubing is then attached to the appropriate side of the vascular access. Often, red tubing is used to depict the arterial access and blue tubing is used to depict the venous access. Blood flow begins at the arterial side and passes through the hemofilter. In CVVH and CVVHD, blood flow is augmented by the use of a blood pump.

The hemofilters are made of highly permeable hollow fibers or plates. These fibers or plates are surrounded by a UF space and have both arterial and venous blood ports.

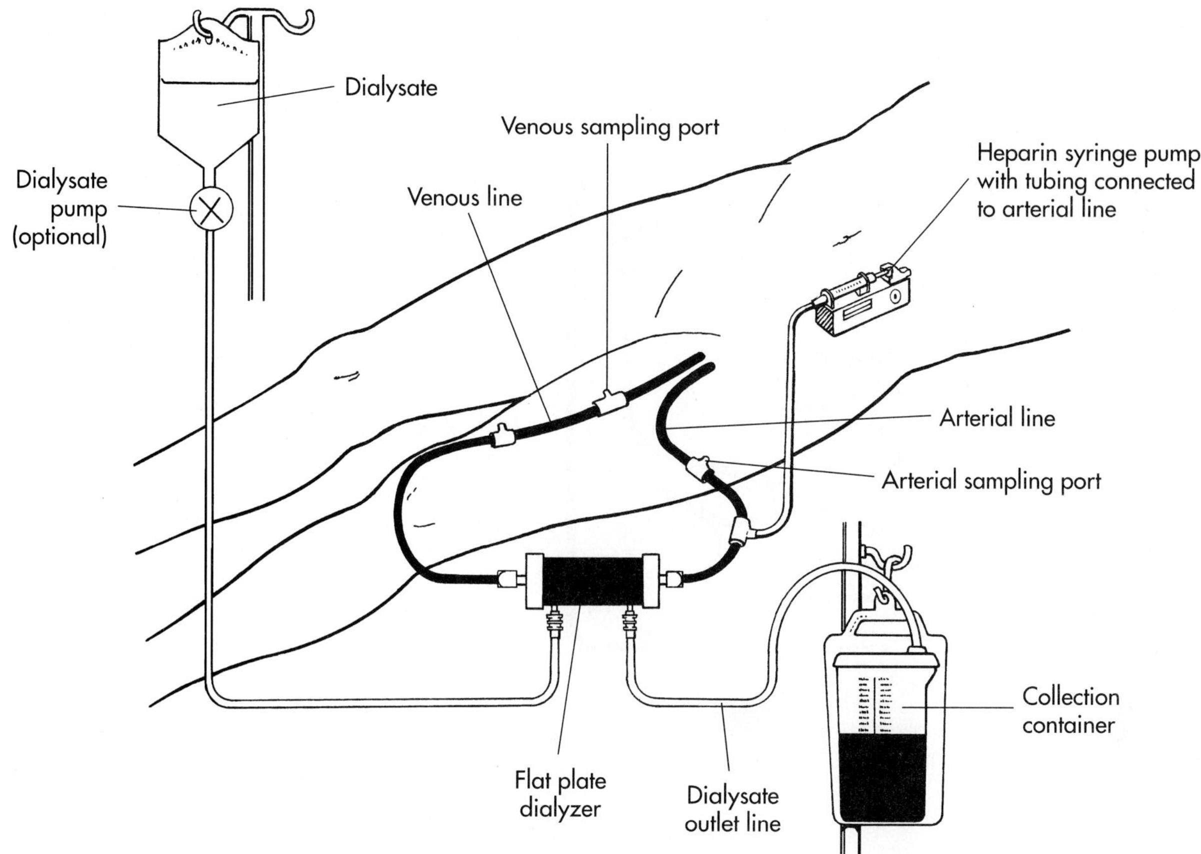

Figure 55-2 Diagram of CAVHD system. (Redrawn from *Critical Care Nurse*. From Lawyer LA, Velasco A: Continuous arteriovenous hemodialysis in the ICU, *Crit Care Nurs* 9(1):29, 1989.)

Plasma water and certain solutes are separated from the blood by the hemofilter and drain into a collection device. The blood, minus the ultrafiltrate, then passes back into the venous tubing and back into the body.

Additionally, in CAVHD and CVVHD, blood leaves the patient through the arterial catheter/arterial side and flows or is pumped through a dialyzer rather than a hemofilter.[7] Wastes and fluid are removed and emptied into an ultrafiltrate bag. The blood is then returned to the body through the venous catheter/venous side. The dialysate is either pumped slowly using an IV pump or is run through the dialyzer by gravity, countercurrent to blood flow.

Anticoagulation is not mandatory in CRRT. If the vascular access provides good blood flow and the patient has an adequate, stable MAP, anticoagulation can be avoided.[2] Frequently, however, these are not consistently present, and anticoagulation is required. The purpose of anticoagulation is to anticoagulate the circuit, avoiding systemic anticoagulation of the patient. When anticoagulation is initiated, a heparin bolus of 1000 to 3000 units may be administered through the prefilter line.[12] A continuous infusion of 200 to 1000 units/hr is then maintained through the same port.

Risk of dialyzer clotting is greater in CAVHD because the blood, moving only by the force of the patient's MAP, moves more slowly than if being pumped. For this reason, CAVHD patients are usually continuously heparinized. If a patient has a serious anticoagulation problem, CAVHD can be performed without heparinizing the patient. Without anticoagulation, the patency of the dialyzer must be assessed frequently.

Clotting times must be assessed frequently to avoid bleeding. The type of coagulation studies that are followed are determined by individual unit protocols. Partial prothrombin times (PTT) performed by the laboratory or bedside activated clotting time (ACT) are monitored. Table 55-1 summarizes the therapeutic goals of anticoagulation.

Fluid replacement can be administered either prefilter (predilution method) or postfilter (postdilution method). Although the method used is determined by physician preference, the predilution method has several advantages. Fluid administered by predilution is generally thought to decrease anticoagulation requirements and enhance the removal of solute.

The need for and type of replacement fluid is determined by the clinical condition of the patient and is influenced by the patient's hemodynamic and metabolic needs.[9] CRRT allow the critical care nurse to calculate necessary adjustments to the patient's fluid status hourly. Generally, hourly

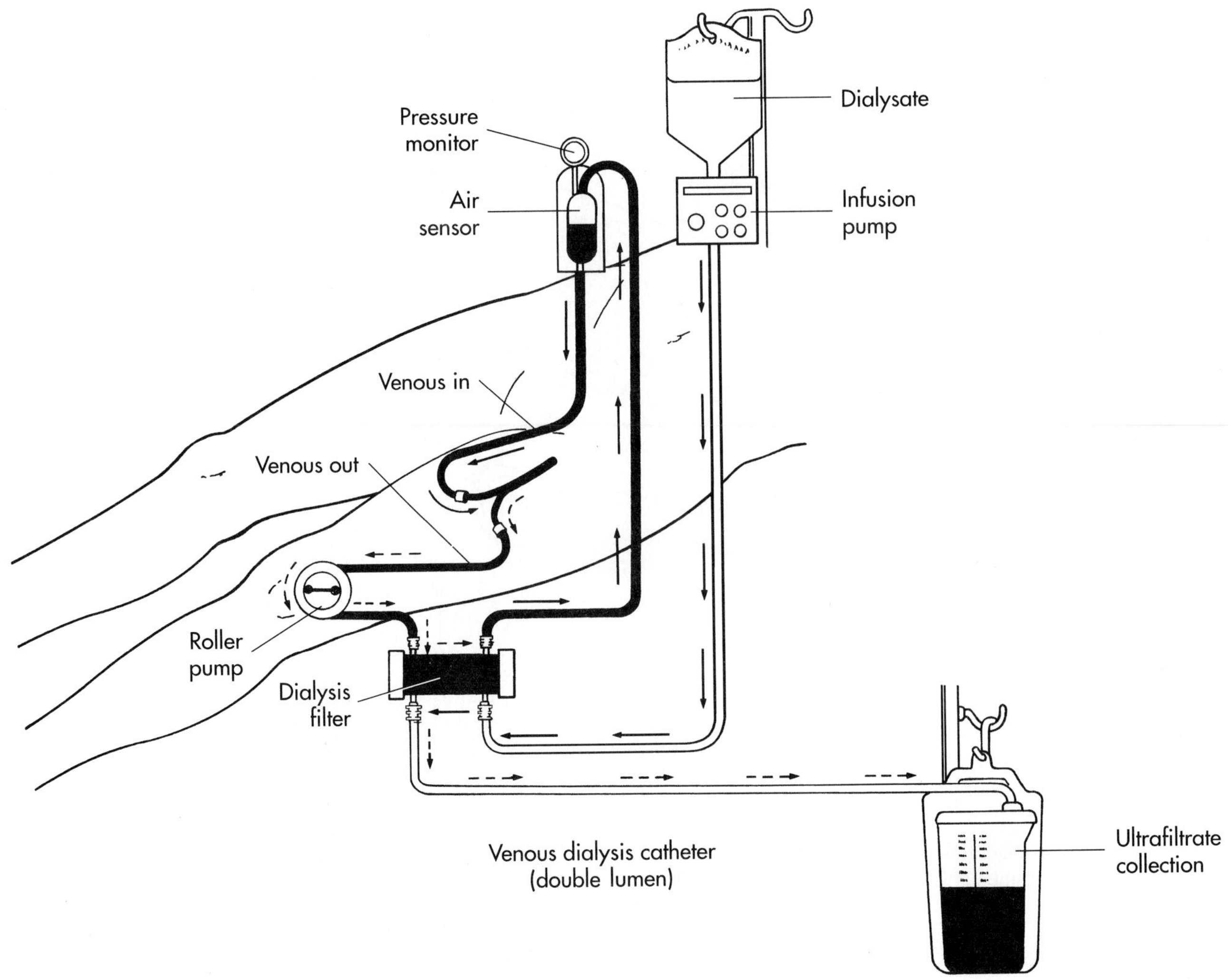

Figure 55-3 Diagram of CVVHD system. (Redrawn from *AJCC*. From Strohschein BL, Caruso DM, Green KA: Continuous venovenous hemodialysis, *Am J Crit Care* 3:95, 1994.)

TABLE 55-1 Goals of Anticoagulation

	Normal	Tight range	Systemic range
PTT	25-40 sec	1.5 times normal (40-60 sec)	2-2.5 times normal (50-100 sec)
ACT	90-100 sec	1.25-1.5 times normal (125-150 sec)	1.5-2.5 times normal (150-250 sec)

net fluid loss is ordered by the physician. Anticipated UF ranges are from 500 to 800 cc/hr.[11] Giving consideration to all sources of intake and output, the nurse will calculate the amount, if any, of fluid replacement needed.

Standard fluid mixtures, such as normal saline or lactated Ringer's, may be used, but more often customized solutions such as ½ normal saline with calcium gluceptate or ¼ normal saline with sodium bicarbonate are used.[11] Patients with electrolyte disorders, with intractable acidosis, or in need of nutritional support benefit from specific fluid replacement. Blood products or total parenteral nutrition (TPN) may be used. However, TPN is more often run at a continuous infusion rate rather than the rate being determined by the previous hour's net fluid loss.

INDICATIONS

Patients appropriate for CRRT are chosen after evaluating their clinical diagnosis, hemodynamic parameters, and metabolic status. The specific type of CRRT is selected after considering the patient's fluid and electrolyte status, metabolic needs, and severity of uremia.[11]

The most commonly used forms of CRRT are CAVU, CAVH, and CAVHD. CVVH and CVVHD are newer therapies and their efficacy is currently being researched.[1,8] Other countries utilize these latter therapies with greater frequency than the United States. Indications for all types of CRRT include:

- Hemodynamically unstable acute renal failure
- Hemodynamically unstable end-stage renal disease
- Massive fluid overload
- Significant azotemia
- TPN restriction due to hypervolemia
- Pulmonary edema refractory to diuretics
- Renal insufficiency with need for large amounts of fluid replacement

Indications for each CRRT are summarized in the paragraphs that follow.

CAVU and SCUF are techniques of slow continuous UF commonly performed without simultaneous fluid replacement.[4] Urea and creatinine are minimally removed. This therapy is used primarily in patients with an extracellular fluid volume excess who retain some degree of renal function.

The main objectives of **CAVH** are moderate fluid removal and solute clearance. Large changes in blood chemistries are not expected, but some removal of solute does occur. Using CAVH, it is possible to maintain stable volume and composition of body fluids. Because the system is capable of removing large amounts of fluid, flexibility is increased in fluid and medication administration. Often, CAVH will be used to enable a patient to receive TPN, establish a positive nitrogen balance, and thus allow for enhanced healing. A CAVH system is shown in Figure 55-1.

In some settings, CAVH has become the treatment of choice not only for the unstable patient but for the patient with serious coagulation disorders, making HD difficult, or with intra-abdominal sepsis, ruling out the use of PD. Patients can be maintained on CAVH for up to several weeks until either long-term HD can be initiated or the patient's renal function returns.

Candidates for CAVH fall primarily into two groups. The first group includes patients who would ideally be treated with HD but are hemodynamically unstable. The second group encompasses patients in uncontrolled congestive heart failure, pulmonary edema, hepatorenal syndrome, or those patients in renal failure who need nutritional support but cannot tolerate the extra fluid required to deliver the nutrition. There are no absolute contraindications for CAVH.

CAVHD is a form of CRRT that combines the principles of hemofiltration with a slow form of dialysis. More aggressive removal of fluid and solute is possible than with CAVH. Dialysate, tailored to the patient's needs, is infused through a dialyzer, countercurrent to the patient's blood flow. A CAVHD system is shown in Figure 55-2.

Although the indications for CAVHD are similar to HD, candidates for continuous rather than intermittent HD are usually selected because they are poor candidates for HD. Often, critically ill, hypotensive patients with renal failure or fluid overload are hemodynamically unstable and are not able to tolerate the rapid fluid and electrolyte shifts that occur during traditional HD. Using CAVHD, fluid and electrolyte balance can be controlled without the hemodynamic instability. Because the technique uses the patient's own MAP, the positive aspects of dialysis can be achieved without compromising the patient's status. A 24-hour period on continuous dialysis with the dialysate running at approximately 1 L/hr is thought to be equal in urea clearance to a traditional 4-hour dialysis treatment performed every other day.[5]

There are no absolute contraindications for CAVHD. However, because the AV pressure difference is influential in determining the success of the dialysis effort, patients with a systolic BP of less than 80 mm Hg are not good candidates. Clotting of the dialyzer is a high risk, so patients with serious coagulation disorders require special precautions.

One of the newer CRRT is **CVVH.** It is similar to CAVH but is a pump-assisted, rather than MAP-assisted, technique of UF. The major advantage to CVVH in comparison with CAVH is a decrease in access-related complications.[1]

CVVHD is similar to CAVHD but is also a pump-assisted, rather than MAP-assisted, technique. It is an excellent alternative for patients who have only venous access and cannot tolerate traditional HD.[14] An example of a CVVHD system is displayed in Figure 55-3.

LIMITATIONS

The greatest limitation of CAVH, CAVHD, and CVVHD is that these interventions may not provide adequate management of the renal failure state. Their effectiveness is primarily related to fluid management. The electrolyte and various metabolite imbalances associated with renal failure may not be adequately controlled with these support devices. Peritoneal or hemodialysis may be better choices for severely compromised patients.

POTENTIAL COMPLICATIONS

The critical care nurse must be vigilant in monitoring for complications in patients receiving CRRT. The initial preparation of the hemofilter and the period immediately following initiation of CRRT are critical times requiring intense scrutiny by the nurse. The potential complications associated with CRRT are as follows:

- Bleeding
- Infection
- Hypervolemia/hypertension
- Hypovolemia/hypotension
- Electrolyte/acid–base imbalance

- Changes in mentation
- Dysrhythmias
- Clotting of the system
- Hypothermia
- Hyperglycemia
- Air embolus
- Loss of access
- Decreased UF rate

GENERAL NURSING INTERVENTIONS

The frequency of CRRT as a therapy in critical care units is increasing daily. Each therapy has unique characteristics, but all require similar nursing interventions.[13] The nurse's careful observations and interventions are essential in maintaining safe, effective CRRT. Accurate fluid management is key in the management of patients receiving CRRT. Hourly calculation of UF rates and the appropriate administration of fluid are essential. Close monitoring of the patient's MAP, urine output, CO, CVP, PCWP, and daily weights is crucial. Of primary concern in nursing care during CRRT is the maintenance of the patient's hemofiltration system with adequate blood flow. Careful monitoring of acid–base and serum chemistries is mandatory. The critical care nurse assumes a primary responsibility for early recognition and initial interventions for patient and system problems. These general nursing interventions are presented in Table 55-2.

TABLE 55-2 General Nursing Interventions For Continuous Renal Replacement Therapies (CRRT)

General considerations	Related nursing interventions
Monitoring for effectiveness	
Fluid balance	Ensure that total fluid volume and intravascular volume are within acceptable limits Calculate net fluid loss q1h or as ordered Careful assessment: pre-CRRT and intra-CRRT • Wt: compare with previous and dry wt • Fluid status: JVD, peripheral/sacral edema, breath sounds, pulses, CVP, PAPs, PCWP, peripheral circulation (cool, blanched extremities) • BP: lying, sitting, standing • Auscultate heart tones, pericardial friction rub, S_3, gallop Monitor I/O
Metabolic stability	Monitor creatinine, urea levels per unit protocol Institute appropriate CRRT based on patient's fluid and metabolic status
Prevention of complications	
Bleeding	Assess patient history of bleeding, response to previous anticoagulation, prior Hct, and clotting studies Assess for bruises, occult and/or overt bleeding, oozing (skin, NG/tracheal aspirate, insertion sites, urine, stool) Monitor clotting studies as per unit standards Adjust anticoagulation protocol as needed based on clotting times, patient's condition, patency of circuit, and response to previous anticoagulation Monitor for decreased CVP, PAPs, PCWP as indication of fluid loss Be alert to sudden pain in the abdomen, hips, back, or buttocks in the patient with femoral access (sign of retroperitoneal bleeding) Closely monitor catheter insertion/needle puncture sites for bleeding In preparation for catheter removal, discontinue heparin infusion at least 4 hr prior to MD removal of catheters After catheter removal, hold pressure on catheter insertion sites for 20 to 30 min; hold pressure 1 inch above arterial insertion site and 1 inch below venous insertion site Keep patient supine for 6 to 8 hr after femoral catheter removal Reapply pressure if bleeding occurs Discontinue CRRT immediately if profuse bleeding occurs
Infection	Ensure sterility of hemofilter, tubing, fluids, and dialysate (if used) Use sterile technique when handling or flushing CRRT circuit Utilize vascular access for CRRT exclusively Assess for signs of infection: elevated T, chills, drainage, localized warmth, redness, tenderness, swelling, or pain at access site

Continued.

TABLE 55-2 General Nursing Interventions For Continuous Renal Replacement Therapies (CRRT)—cont'd

General considerations	Related nursing interventions
Prevention of complications—cont'd	
Infection—cont'd	Monitor for drainage at access insertion sites Monitor laboratory values (WBC count and differential) Administer antibiotics as ordered
Hypervolemia/hypertension	Perform pre-CRRT assessment: • Wt: compare with previous and dry wt • Fluid status: JVD, peripheral/sacral edema, breath sounds, pulses, CVP, PAPs, PCWP, CO/CI peripheral circulation (cool, blanched extremities) • BP: lying, sitting, standing • Auscultate heart tones, pericardial friction rub, S_3, gallop Continuously monitor cardiac rhythm/rate Monitor hourly I/O Assess closely for signs of hypervolemia (tachycardia, hypertension, bounding pulses, paradoxical pulses, increasing PAPs, CO/CI) Administer fluid/blood as ordered Correctly prime CRRT and cricuit Administer O_2 as needed Monitor ultrafiltrate output Calculate hourly fluid replacement and administer fluid as ordered Monitor VS as needed
Hypovolemia/hypotension	Perform pre-CRRT assessment: as outlined in hypervolemia After therapy has been initiated, reevaluate need for antihypertensive medications Monitor UF rate If hypotension occurs, slow UF rates Correctly prime CRRT circuit Monitor for signs of hypovolemia (tachycardia, hypotension, falling PAPs) Administer O_2 as needed Administer normal saline or albumin Position patient with legs elevated Administer vasopressor medications as ordered
Electrolyte/acid–base imbalances	Obtain serum K^+/Na^+/ABG per unit protocols Notify MD and ensure replacement fluid is ordered appropriately Adjust the K^+/Na^+/buffer in the replacement fluid during therapy as needed In CAVHD/CVVHD, adjust dialysate as needed Assess for signs of acid–base/electrolyte imbalances: • Hyperkalemia: wide-absent T wave; depressed ST segment; tall, tented T wave; prolonged QT interval • Hypokalemia: elevated P wave, flattened or inverted T wave, prolonged QT interval, PVCs • Hypernatremia: dry, flushed skin; thirst; vomiting; weak, crampy, or spastic muscle tone • Hyponatremia: muscle weakness, lethargy, irritability, headaches • Hypomagnesemia: prolonged QT interval, broadened T waves with decreased amplitude, positive Chvostek and Trousseau signs, tetany • Hypocalcemia: lengthened ST segment, prolonged QT interval, positive Chvostek and Trousseau signs, tetany
Change in mentation	Assess neurological status initially, q4h, and prn during therapy Monitor electrolyte, coagulation, and ABG results Orient patient and family to CRRT
Dysrhythmias	Assess patient's rhythm pre-CRRT and continuously during CRRT Administer antidysrhythmic agents prn Monitor electrolyte values

Continued.

TABLE 55-2 General Nursing Interventions For Continuous Renal Replacement Therapies (CRRT)—cont'd

General considerations	Related nursing interventions
Prevention of complications—cont'd	
Clotting of system	Administer fluids and medications to maintain adequate CO Avoid rotation, binding, or bending of CRRT tubing and insertion sites Obtain serum clotting studies as ordered Maintain continuous heparin infusion as ordered Monitor setup at least q1h, observing for darkening of filter membrane, appearance of strands of fibrin, or obvious clots Monitor UF output: be alert if output decreases for two consecutive hours because this may be a sign of filter clotting
Hypothermia	Cover patient with warm blankets, offer warm liquids Assess for chilling, pallor, cyanosis, decreased T, ABG Discuss using warmed fluid/dialysate
Hyperglycemia	Monitor serum glucose as ordered Ensure patient compliance to dietary restrictions Alter dialysate as needed to lower blood sugar Administer insulin as ordered
Air embolus	Ensure that all CRRT tubings and filter are primed completely when initiating CRRT and with all tubing/hemofilter changes Avoid kinks in tubing Tighten and tape all connections Monitor for air in CRRT tubing, signs of air embolus (chest pain, cough, cyanosis) Notify MD of any abnormalities and actions taken
Loss of access	Properly care for access, using aseptic technique If graft/shunt is being utilized, assess patency q shift by listening for bruit, feeling for thrill Avoid use of access extremity for blood draws or BPs Use CRRT catheters for CRRT only Assess pulses in cannulated extremity to assess for peripheral circulation
Decreased UF rate	Calculate UF rate q1h or as ordered: $\frac{(\text{hourly output} - \text{hourly fluid input})}{60} = \text{cc/min}$ Administer fluids and medications to maintain adequate CO and MAP Monitor intake and output q1h Monitor serum and ultrafiltrate urea nitrogen levels as ordered Assess for system clotting Change CRRT system per unit protocol

TROUBLESHOOTING

It is important for the critical care nurse to be able to troubleshoot problems as they arise in CRRT. The problems that commonly occur in the patient being treated with CRRT and the nurse's actions are summarized in the following.

Problem: Air Embolus

CAUSE	CORRECTIVE ACTION
Loose connections (device) Retained air in dialyzer (device)	Change hemofilter as needed Correct any identified circuit problem (loose connections, empty bags, disarmed air alarm, use of nonluerlock connections) to prevent embolus

CAUSE	CORRECTIVE ACTION
	If air is visualized: • Withdraw air from tubing ports • Administer O_2 per unit standards • Assess VS and LOC • Notify MD stat • Discontinue CRRT as ordered If embolus is suspected: • Stop infusion, clamp lines • Position patient on left side in Trendelenburg position

Problem: Bleeding

CAUSE	CORRECTIVE ACTION
Overanticoagulation (device)	Adjust anticoagulation routine as indicated by assessment of patient's condition, patency of circuit, previous history of response to anticoagulation, and clotting studies Apply pressure at catheter insertion sites Discontinue heparin infusion Administer protamine sulfate as ordered Discontinue CRRT
Bleeding from tubing disconnect (device)/access insertion site leakage (patient)	Prevent needle dislodgement by securely taping needles in place Have access and connections visual at all times Observe needles and insertion sites frequently Position extremity to avoid abrupt movements Maintain patient on bed rest during therapy Monitor serial Hct If catheter becomes disconnected or needle becomes dislodged, clamp arterial and venous tubing Monitor VS Reconnect tubing to catheter using aseptic technique Hold pressure on sites for 10 to 15 min, remove needles, and apply pressure dressing for 3 to 4 hr Notify MD Administer blood/fluids as ordered

Problem: Fluid Overload/Hypertension

CAUSE	CORRECTIVE ACTION
Excess fluid intake/administration (patient)	Monitor level of UF and increase as tolerated Monitor response to changes in UF rate Replace fluid as prescribed Administer blood/blood products during CRRT to minimize fluid increases Monitor patient's wt between treatments Readjust restrictions of dietary and IV fluids as ordered

Problem: Fluid Deficit/Hypotension

CAUSE	CORRECTIVE ACTION
Antihypertensive medication administration (patient)	Review patient's antihypertensive medications Closely monitor BP, HR, and peripheral circulation in patients at risk for hypotension due to their medications Accurately calculate net hourly fluid loss Notify MD if hypotension occurs Administer fluid as ordered Administer vasopressor medications as ordered

Excessive ultrafiltration (device)	Monitor patient's toleration to UF rate Slow UF rate as necessary by decreasing the distance between the hemofilter and the collection chamber

Problem: Clotting

CAUSE	CORRECTIVE ACTION
Decreased CO (patient)	Administer increased replacement fluids in predilution mode Monitor VS
Insufficient heparin infusion (device)	If hemofilter is suspected to be clotted, flush arterial catheter with heparinized saline and observe hemofilter for clots or dark streaks Adjust heparin infusion rate
Tubing obstruction (kinked, bent tubing) (device)	Unkink tubing Prepare to change hemofilter as needed

Problem: Electrolyte Imbalances

CAUSE	CORRECTIVE ACTION
Inadequate infusion of appropriate replacement fluids (device)	Monitor laboratory values closely Administer electrolyte replacement as needed

SUMMARY

An understanding of the underlying disease process and its impact on other body systems is essential for the critical care nurse caring for a patient being treated with CRRT. Increasingly, CRRT are being selected as the treatment of choice for critically ill patients in ARF. Use of these therapies demands continuous vigilance by the critical care nurse.

REFERENCES

1. Bellomo R, et al: A prospective comparative study of continuous arteriovenous hemodiafiltration and continuous venovenous hemodiafiltration in critically ill patients, *Am J Kidney Dis* 21(4):400-404, 1993.
2. Bosworth C: SCUF/CAVH/ CAVHD: critical differences, *Crit Care Nurs Q* 14(4):45-55, 1992.
3. Coloski D, et al: Continuous arteriovenous hemofiltration patient: nursing care plan. *DCCN* 9(3):130-142, 1990.
4. Dickson DM, Hillman KM: Continuous renal replacement in the critically ill, *Anaesth Intensive Care* 18(1):76-101, 1990.
5. Geronemus RP: Slow continuous hemodialysis, *Trans Am Soc Artif Intern Organs* 34:59-60, 1988.
6. Kramer P, et al: Intensive care potential of continuous arteriovenous hemofiltration, *Trans Am Soc Artif Intern Organs* 28:28-32, 1982.
7. Lawyer LA, Velasco A: Continuous arteriovenous hemodialysis in the ICU, *Crit Care Nurse* 9(1):29-41, 1989.
8. Macias WL, et al: Continuous venovenous hemofiltration: an alternative to continuous arteriovenous hemofiltration and hemodiafiltration, *Am J Kidney Dis* 18(4):451-458, 1991.
9. Nahman NS, Middendorf DF: Continuous arteriovenous hemofiltration, *Med Clin North Am* 74(4):975-984, 1990.
10. Price CA: Continuous arteriovenous ultrafiltration: a monitoring guide for ICU nurses, *Crit Care Nurse* 9(1):12-19, 1989.
11. Price CA: Continuous renal replacement therapy: the treatment of choice for acute renal failure, *ANNA Journal* 18(3):239-244, 1991.
12. Price CA: An update on continuous renal replacement therapies, *AACN Clin Iss Crit Care Nurs* 3(3):597-604, 1992.
13. Price CA: Continuous renal replacement therapies. In Burrows-Hudson S, editor: *Standards of clinical practice for nephrology nursing,* Pitman, NJ, 1993, American Nephrology Nurse's Association.
14. Strohschein BL, Caruso DM, Greene KA: Continuous venovenous hemodialysis, *Am J Crit Care* 3:92-101, 1994.

UNIT VI

Endocrine System

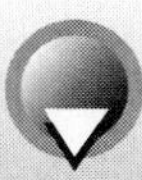

C L I N I C A L G U I D E L I N E

56

Diabetic Ketoacidosis

Karen Clark, MS, RN

DESCRIPTION

Diabetes mellitus is classified by the National Diabetes Data Group into categories that include insulin-dependent diabetes mellitus (IDDM) and non–insulin-dependent diabetes mellitus (NIDDM).[10]

IDDM results when there is absolute or relative lack of endogenous insulin production due to beta-cell destruction in the pancreas. NIDDM is a result of a decreasing number of insulin receptor sites in the body or because these sites become defective and less responsive to insulin.[13]

Diabetic ketoacidosis, DKA, an acute and serious complication of uncontrolled IDDM, is a complex, multisystem disorder. It develops when two hormonal abnormalities occur concurrently—relative or absolute insulin deficiency and an excess in stress (counterregulatory) hormones. DKA is characterized by hyperglycemia, acidosis, and ketosis, all three of which must be present for diagnosis.

DKA affects both children and adults with the average patient age being 43 years.[9] Studies indicate that 2% to 14% of all hospitalizations of diabetic patients involve DKA and coma, or approximately 45,000 to 130,000 episodes per year.[11] The new-onset diabetes mellitus patient represents 20% of the total episodes of DKA and 80% occur in those previously diagnosed. Among the latter group, 20% have multiple annual episodes.[9] Information from the National Diabetes Data Group[10] indicates that 10% of all diabetes-related deaths are from DKA, or 57 per 100,000 per year. These numbers have a profound implication for critical care nurses because the management of the acute phases of this illness occurs in the critical care unit.

PATHOPHYSIOLOGY

The primary problem in DKA is insulin deficiency, which causes abnormalities in the metabolism of carbohydrate and fat. Normally, after eating, insulin is released from the pancreas to assist in the conversion of ingested carbohydrates, protein, and fat to glucose, amino acid, and free fatty acids, respectively. These are stored as glycogen in the liver, protein in the muscle, and triglyceride in the fat cells.[8] Insulin and glucagon, therefore, maintain a molar ratio that provides for a coordinated regulation of blood sugar. When there is an insulin deficiency, these cells are unable to function normally and are thrown into a catabolic state. Also in response to the deficiency of insulin, peripheral tissues, primarily muscle tissue, decrease their uptake of glucose.

In response to stress or to a deficit of insulin, the body releases the counterregulatory hormone glucagon, which elevates the glucagon/insulin ratio. This stimulates the liver to break down stored glycogen in a process called *glycogenolysis* to form glucose. Hyperglycemia and consequently hyperosmolality result. At the same time, the liver forms glucose from amino acids in a process known as *gluconeogenesis*. Glucose is not available for cellular metabolism; therefore, cells use an alternative source of fuel in the form of fat. Lack of insulin allows triglycerides to be released as free fatty acids into the bloodstream. The free fatty acids are then transported to the liver, where ketoacids are produced as a byproduct of their oxidation.[13] This process, and the decreased uptake of ketones by the peripheral tissues, allows ketonemia to develop. As ketoacids (acetoacetic acid, betahydroxybutyric acid, and acetone) dissociate, they yield hydrogen ions, lowering the body's pH and causing the loss of bicarbonate and other body buffers. The result is metabolic acidosis.[11]

In addition to excess glucagon, there can be excessive secretion of the other counterregulatory hormones: catecholamines, corticosteroids, and growth hormone. These hormones may be secreted in response to the metabolic stress of ketosis or as a stress reaction to underlying infection or injury. Each of these hormones can further impair the use of glucose by peripheral tissues and enhance lipolysis, contributing directly or indirectly to ketone production.

Metabolic acidosis then activates the chemoreceptors, which stimulate the respiratory system to increase the rate and depth of respiration, commonly referred to as a Kussmaul breathing pattern. As the acetone is blown off, the patient's breath develops a characteristic "fruity" odor. Additionally, the kidneys respond to the excess ketone anions by excreting this in the urine (ketonuria). The kidneys also increase tubular excretion of hydrogen ions in an attempt to increase the serum pH. These compensatory mechanisms soon fail as the body's buffering system is overwhelmed.

As the serum glucose concentration increases, excessive urination (osmotic diuresis) and glycosuria occurs. Hyperglycemia causes plasma osmolality to increase and water then moves from the intracellular compartment into the extracellular compartment. An osmotic diuresis results. There is a loss of water and electrolytes and eventually depletion of intravascular volume. In response to the diuresis, the body attempts to compensate by stimulation of the thirst center in the brain, causing polydipsia (increased fluid intake).[11] Glycosuria occurs because the excess glucose cannot be reabsorbed at the renal tubule.

The electrolyte loss results in deficits of sodium (Na^+), potassium (K^+), magnesium (Mg^{++}), and phosphorus (PO_4^-). Hyponatremia is found in two thirds of patients with moderate to severe DKA, even in the presence of osmotic diuresis, which would be expected to result in hypernatremia.[9] Hyperglycemia causes excess water to be retained in the extracellular compartment unless hypovolemia becomes extreme. A corrected Na^+, calculated by adding to the measured serum Na^+ 2.75 mEq/L for each 100 mg/dl of plasma glucose over 100 mg/dl, should be used to determine the appropriate fluid to administer to correct the serum Na^+.[3] As hyperglycemia is corrected the reverse should occur with a rise in the serum concentration of Na^+.

The most critical electrolyte imbalance is K^+ deficiency. An initial low serum K^+ is suggestive of a severe total-body depletion and requires immediate intervention.[4] More often, however, the shift from intracellular to extracellular K^+ may give a normal or slightly elevated serum value. Without intervention, serum K^+ drops dramatically at approximately 4 to 12 hours.[9] Lethal cardiac dysrhythmias can follow.

Magnesium deficits develop in most patients with advanced DKA, but signs and symptoms including tetany, seizures, dysrhythmias, and CNS depression are rarely seen. Magnesium deficiency influences the secretion and action of parathyroid hormone, which can lead to hypocalcemia and hypokalemia.[4]

Hypophosphatemia develops in much the same way as hypokalemia. Initially, hyperphosphatemia results from release of phosphate from the cells followed by phosphate deficit as DKA continues. Phosphate is necessary for correcting impaired oxygen dissociation from hemoglobin by regenerating adequate levels of red blood cell 2,3 diphosphoglycerate, thus promoting tissue oxygenation. Severe hypophosphatemia can lead to altered mental status, hemolysis, rhabdomyolysis, and heart failure.[1] These signs and symptoms are rarely seen in patients with DKA.

LENGTH OF STAY/ANTICIPATED COURSE

Length of stay for patients with DKA varies with the severity of the illness, age, and premorbid condition of the patient. Therapy is directed toward management of the precipitating factors and correcting the patient's pH, electrolytes, glucose, and fluid volume status based on the patients' clinical responses and laboratory values. Complications that can arise, such as continued hypotension with minimal urine output, prolonged ileus, no improvement in mental status, and opportunistic infections, can prolong the anticipated course.[7]

DKA falls within DRG 294: Diabetes age >35 years and DRG 295: Diabetes age 0 to 35 years. Average length of stays for this disorder are 6.5 days and 5.1 days, respectively.[14]

MANAGEMENT TRENDS AND CONTROVERSIES

Therapy is directed at correcting the insulin insufficiency and fluid and electrolyte imbalances, mediating the condition triggering the counterregulatory response, and preventing complications of therapy. Optimal management is not equated with rapid normalization of abnormalities. Incremental therapy based on an understanding of the pathophysiology of DKA should be used. The course of management should be reviewed and revised every 3 to 4 hours based on the patient's response.[5]

Administration of insulin should be started with short-acting, low-dose regular insulin as soon as DKA is diagnosed. Controversy has existed regarding insulin protocols, but studies suggest that most patients respond well to low-dose insulin therapy. High-dose insulin therapy is needed for patients who are insulin resistant.[1] Most authorities advise administrating an intravenous (IV) bolus of 0.1 to 0.2 U/kg of insulin initially followed by constant IV infusion of 0.1 U/kg/hr.[4] Insulin may be given by intramuscular injection, but subcutaneous injection is not recommended because of erratic tissue absorption. Human insulin is usually preferred to pork or beef insulin. Although there are no significant differences in therapeutic response, fewer allergic or toxic reactions have been observed with the use of human insulin. The goal of treatment is to lower the serum glucose by approximately 75 to 150 mg/dl/hour. Ketone bodies clear at a slower rate than glucose, so the rate of the insulin infusion should be decreased but not stopped as 5% dextrose is added to the IV fluids. As glucose levels are normalized and acidosis is resolved, subcutaneous insulin should be resumed.[12] Changes in glucose use by the body lag 30 to 60 minutes behind a change in the rate of insulin infusion;[1] therefore, it is important to observe the DKA patient for signs and symptoms of hypoglycemia during therapy (see Box).

Rapid fluid replacement is indicated clinically by Kussmaul breathing, fruity breath, and marked dehydration. Controversy surrounds the most appropriate type of IV fluid and the ideal rate of infusion. Most physicians advocate the use of approximately 1 L of isotonic saline or 10 to 20 ml/kg within the first hour, until the blood pressure is stabilized and urine output of 60 ml/hr has been established.[3] Controversy remains as to whether normal saline or half-normal saline should be the initial IV fluid of choice. The use of normal saline is thought to prevent a rapid decrease in extracellular osmolality. Colloid infusion may be used for severely hypotensive patients. After the serum glucose falls to approximately 250 mg/dl, 5% dextrose should be added to the infusion. Some physicians replace one half of the fluid deficit over the first 8 hours with the balance being replaced over the next 16 hours.[4] Others, if hypotension is not present, replace the estimated fluid deficit evenly over 48 hours.[3] Initially, fluid should be infused peripherally, but early insertion of a central venous line may be indicated for better fluid management, especially in elderly patients or those with underlying renal or cardiovascular disease.

The development of cerebral edema is a serious problem in the management of the patient with DKA, particularly the pediatric patient. Some authors believe that a degree of cerebral edema occurs in all patients with DKA, but only a few cases are clinically significant.[2] Cerebral edema is a serious and potentially fatal complication. It usually occurs within 24 hours of therapy when the patient appears to be improving clinically and biochemically.[3] Many theories have been proposed to explain the pathophysiology of cerebral edema. The movement of water driven across cerebral membranes by osmotic forces is suspected to be integrally involved.[6] As the plasma glucose approaches 250 to 300 mg/dl, glucose should be added to the replacement fluid. This prevents hypoglycemia with insulin therapy and prevents the development of cerebral edema.

Osmotic diuresis with DKA results in a total-body K^+ depletion of approximately 5 to 10 mEq/kg of body weight. Serum K^+ decreases further with rehydration and correction of acidosis as K^+ moves back into the cells from the extracellular spaces. Replacement K^+ therapy should begin immediately, except in the presence of anuria or profound hyperkalemia. Potassium supplements are titrated based on hourly assessments of serum K^+ levels. The average adult requires 80 to 160 mEq over the first 12 hours.[4] If indicated, K^+ is administered at 20 to 40 mEq/L or higher, frequently with one half as KCL and one half as KPO_4.

Hyponatremia is rare in DKA and usually accompanies underlying renal disease. It is generally corrected when the glucose concentration is lowered with insulin. Glucose and Na^+ are the principle determinants of osmolality in DKA. As the serum glucose is reduced, the concentration of serum Na^+ should rise. This will modify the osmolality change and cause a slow, gradual fall to prevent the movement of free water across the membranes of the brain cells.[6] This could potentially decrease the risk of cerebral edema.

Magnesium deficits are normally corrected by normal diet resumption. However, Mg^{++} deficiency interrupts the secretion of parathyroid hormone and can lead to hypocalcemia and hypokalemia.[4] Serum Mg^{++} levels should be monitored and calcium supplements given with necessary Mg^{++} replacement.

Bicarbonate therapy to correct acidosis in DKA is very controversial. Bicarbonate did not alter the recovery or outcome of DKA significantly in a prospective randomized study done in patients with arterial blood pH of 6.9 to 7.14.[8] The use of insulin and fluid therapy is usually adequate unless there is severe acidosis with an arterial pH less than 7.0. If sodium bicarbonate is required, it is given slowly to prevent rebound CNS acidosis, severe hypokalemia, and cardiac dysrhythmias.[1]

Signs and Symptoms of Hypoglycemia

Physiologic		
Tachycardia	Sweating	General weakness
Dilated pupils	Pallor	Slight increase in systolic BP
Faintness	Numbness	
Cerebral manifestations		
Nervousness	Apprehension	Visual disturbances
Headache	Thick speech	Muscle twitching
Convulsions	Unconsciousness	Urinary incontinence
Tonic and clonic spasm		Babinski reflex
Unexpected behavior reaction		
Restlessness	Negativism	

ASSESSMENT

PARAMETER	ANTICIPATED ALTERATION
Laboratory Tests	
Glucose	Increased: >300 to 900 mg/dl (moderate to severe); 300 to 350 mg/dl (mild) *due to absolute or relative insulin deficiency*
pH	Decreased: <7.2 (moderate to severe); <7.35 (mild) *due to production of ketoacids because of insulin deficiency*
HCO_3^-	Decreased: <18 to 19 mEq/L *due to ketoacidosis*
Ketones	Increased: >3 mmol/L *due to ketoacidosis*
K^+	Elevated: >5.0 mEq/L initially *due to hemoconcentration* Decreased: <3.5 mEq/L *due to osmotic diuresis from hyperglycemia (total body stores are depleted because of movement of* K^+ out of cells)
PO_4^-	Decreased: <2.5 mg/dl *due to osmotic diuresis (may initially be elevated due to hemoconcentration)*
Mg^{++}	Decreased: <1.5 mg/dl *due to osmotic diuresis (may initially be elevated due to hemoconcentration)*
Na^+	Decreased: <135 mEq/L *due to fluid shifts, vomiting, lack of insulin, and the shift of extracellular* Na^+ *to intracellular spaces as* K^+ *is depleted*
BUN	Elevated: >20 mg/dl *due to dehydration*
Creatinine	Elevated: >1.2 mg/dl *due to dehydration*
Osmolality	Elevated: >300 Osm/L (hyperosmolar) *due to osmotic diuresis*
Anion gap	Elevated: >20 mmol/L *due to ketoacidosis*
Urine Tests	
Glucose	Increased: >4% *due to insulin deficiency and hyperglycemia*
Ketones	Positive *due to ketoacidosis*
Pulmonary Status	
RR	Increased: >20 breaths/min (Kussmaul breathing) *due to respiratory compensation for metabolic acidosis and fluid deficits*
Cardiovascular Status	
HR	Elevated: >100 bpm *due to fluid volume deficit*
BP	Hypotension *due to fluid volume deficit*
ECG	Peaked T waves *due to hyperkalemia* Flattened T waves with U waves *due to hypokalemia* Ventricular ectopy *due to* K^+ *imbalance*
Neurologic Status	
Mental Status	Confusion, drowsiness, lethargy, visual disturbances, disorientation, coma *due to hyperglycemia, electrolyte imbalance, acidosis*
Other	
GI symptoms	Excessive hunger and thirst *due to dehydration* Nausea and vomiting (in later stages) *due to gastric stasis* Abdominal cramping *due to fluid and electrolyte imbalance*

Bowel sounds	Absent *due to bowel infarction (if present)*
GU status	Polyuria *due to osmotic diuresis*
Wt	Decreased *due to profound diuresis*

PLAN OF CARE

INTENSIVE PHASE

Care of the patient with DKA in the intensive phase is initially focused on reestablishing fluid balance to prevent circulatory collapse. Circulatory overload from the rapid administration of fluid volume is a serious complication that may occur, particularly in the patient with compromised cardiovascular or renal systems. Insulin therapy is initiated simultaneously to promote the cellular use of glucose, reduce the counterregulatory hormone glucagon, and break the ketotic cycle. The replacement of electrolytes lost from the osmotic diuresis is also a priority during this phase.

PATIENT CARE PRIORITIES	EXPECTED PATIENT OUTCOMES
Fluid volume deficit *r/t* *Hyperglycemia-induced osmotic diuresis* *Vomiting* *Total body water loss*	BP within patient norms HR: WNL Hemodynamic profile: WNL Urine output >30 cc/hr Normal skin turgor Moist mucous membranes Wt: within patient's norm
Electrolyte imbalance *r/t* *Lack of insulin* *Acid–base imbalance* *Fluid shifts* *Vomiting*	Serum glucose: WNL Electrolytes: WNL
Metabolic acidosis *r/t hyperglycemia-induced increase in ketone bodies*	ABG: within patient norms Absence of serum and urine ketones Anion gap: WNL
Ineffective breathing pattern *r/t* *Metabolic acidosis* *Changes in mental status*	RR 8 to 16 breaths/min Breathing pattern within patient norms $Paco_2$: WNL
Coma or altered mental status *r/t* *Metabolic and electrolyte abnormalities* *Cerebral edema* *Sepsis* *Meningitis*	Return to baseline mentation
High risk for hypoglycemia *r/t insulin replacement therapy*	Absence and/or resolution of hypoglycemia
High risk for hypoxemia *r/t pulmonary edema caused by reduction in plasma osmotic pressure during therapy in combination with reduced pleural pressure (due to rapid RR and constant tidal volume)*	Pao_2: WNL RR 8 to 16 breaths/min
High risk for cerebral edema *r/t decreased glucose in replacement IV therapy*	Return to baseline mentation
High risk for vascular thrombosis *r/t dehydration and increased viscosity in low-CO state*	Absence of thrombolytic events
High risk for aspiration pneumonia *r/t gastric stasis*	Absence of lung consolidation

Plan of Care (cont'd)

INTERVENTIONS

Monitor I/O q1h *to detect trend in volume deficit correction.*

Insert a Foley catheter when indicated *for accurate measurement of urine output. Note that patients with diabetes mellitus are extremely susceptible to infections and Foley catheter use is strongly linked to nosocomial urinary tract infections.*

Accurate daily wts *because wt gain or loss reflects overall fluid status.*

Monitor VS, including T q1h until stable; note the presence of fever *to identify infection, which is a common predisposing factor in DKA. However, the patient may be hypothermic or normothermic in the presence of infection because of lack of available substrate to generate heat.*[5]

Lab glucose determination q2h *to monitor trends in serum glucose and adjust insulin administration. Fingersticks are commonly used, but hyperosmolarity can affect capillary blood glucose measurement.*

Monitor for signs and symptoms of electrolyte imbalances *to identify/promote early intervention.*

- K^+ deficit may or may not be reflected in serum measurements *because of the extracellular* K^+ shift. ECG changes reflect the K^+ status of the cardiac cell.
- Na^+ levels can have a profound influence on CNS status. *Observe for signs and symptoms of increasing intracranial pressure to prevent cerebral edema.*
- Severe deficits of Mg cause tetany, seizures, dysrythmias, and CNS depression, but these are rarely seen.
- Severe hypophosphatemia can lead to altered mental status, hemolysis, rhabdomyolysis, and heart failure, but these are rarely seen.

Monitor ABG *to evaluate pH changes and respiratory status. Patients with moderate to severe DKA can have pH values below 7.1 and bicarbonate administration is still recommended for use in this population. Note that it is given at a rate of 44 to 50 mEq/hr with the goal of therapy to raise the patient's pH between only 7.10 and 7.15.*[11]

Assist with intubation if mechanical ventilation is indicated and continue to monitor respiratory status.

Monitor for complications of therapy *to prevent problems that can occur rapidly in the patient with DKA, such as hypoglycemia, cerebral edema, aspiration pneumonia, vascular thrombosis.*

Monitor blood glucose levels *to detect hypoglycemia resulting from insulin therapy.*

Observe for signs and symptoms of altered mental status *to detect cerebral edema.*

Place NG tube *to prevent vomiting and aspiration if patient is obtunded.*

Keep other patients NPO until acute phase is ended.

Apply antiembolism devices *to prevent venous stasis.*

Observe for the presence of the precipitating factors to DKA *because treatment can fail and the metabolic status can be further compromised if these are uncorrected.*

INTERMEDIATE PHASE

The key to the initial management of patients with DKA is intensive and continuous monitoring of their physiologic response to therapy and making rapid adjustments appropriately. Identifying the precipitating problem and correcting the insulin, fluid, and electrolyte imbalances continue to be the goal for treatment in the intermediate care phase. Patient teaching or reinforcement of teaching related to the pathophysiology of diabetes mellitus and management of this chronic disease can begin during this phase.

PATIENT CARE PRIORITIES

High risk for altered metabolic status *r/t unstable insulin regulation*

EXPECTED PATIENT OUTCOMES

Serum glucose: WNL

Absence of serum and urine ketones

Plan of Care (cont'd)

High risk for self-care deficit *r/t management of diabetes mellitus*

Verbalize signs and symptoms of early metabolic decompensation in diabetes mellitus
Verbalize importance of stress factors, diet, susceptibility to infection, need for routine medical follow-up, hygiene, and foot care
Demonstrate correct self-care management of therapies prescribed for diabetes mellitus

INTERVENTIONS

Perform glucose monitoring *to provide information for insulin.*
Perform urine ketone monitoring *to detect excretion of ketone bodies in the urine.*
Provide patients with education *to increase knowledge and promote understanding of all aspects of diabetes mellitus.*

TRANSITION TO DISCHARGE

Until there is a cure for diabetes mellitus, patient education about prevention of DKA is vital. Diabetic patients and families need to learn the routine skills necessary for blood glucose monitoring, insulin administration, urine ketone testing, diet and meal planning, and exercise management. These patients must also receive intensive instruction about events that can precipitate a crisis, such as infection, stress, and imbalance in insulin and dietary intake. They must learn to recognize the signs and symptoms of hypoglycemia and hyperglycemia and to notify the physician or nurse practitioner as soon as problems arise.

REFERENCES

1. Cefalu WT: Diabetic ketoacidosis, *Crit Care Clin* 7(1):89-107, 1991.
2. Couch RM, Acott PD, Wong GWK: Early onset fatal cerebral edema in diabetic ketoacidosis, *Diabetes Care* 14(1):78-79, 1991.
3. Ellis EN: Concepts of fluid therapy in diabetic ketoacidosis and hyperosmolar hyperglycemic nonketotic coma, *Pediatr Clin North Am* 37(2):313-321, 1990.
4. Graves L: Diabetic ketoacidosis and hyperosmolar hyperglycemic nonketotic coma, *Crit Care Nurs Q* 13(3):50-61, 1990.
5. Hamblin PS, Topliss DJ, Stockigt JR: Practical management of diabetic ketoacidosis and hyperosmolar coma, *Aust N Z J Med* 20:836-841, 1990.
6. Harris GD, et al: Minimizing the risk of brain herniation during treatment of diabetic ketoacidemia: a retrospective and prospective study, *J Pediatr* 17(1):22-30, 1990.
7. Karam JH, Salber PR, Forsham PH: Pancreatic hormones and diabetes mellitus. In Greenspan FS, editor: *Basic and clinical endocrinology,* Norwalk, Conn, 1991, Appleton & Lange, pp 634-638.
8. Kitabchi AE, Murphy MB: Diabetic ketoacidosis and hyperosmolar hyperglycemic nonketotic coma, *Med Clin North Am* 72(6):1545-1563, 1988.
9. Kreisberg RA: Diabetic ketoacidosis. In Rifkin, Porte, editors: *Diabetes mellitus theory and practice,* ed 4, New York 1990, Elsevier Science Publishing, pp 591-601.
10. National Diabetes Data Group. U.S. Department of Health and Human Services, Public Health Service. National Institutes of Health, National Institute of Arthritis, Diabetes and Kidney Disease. Publication no. NIH 85, p 1468, 1985.
11. Sabo CE, Rush-Michael S: Diabetic ketoacidosis: pathophysiology, nursing diagnosis, and nursing interventions, *Focus Crit Care* 16(1):21-28, 1989.
12. Sanson TH, Levine SN: Management of diabetic ketoacidosis, *Drugs* 38(2):289-300, 1989.
13. Sauve DO, Kessler CA: Hyperglycemic emergencies, *AACN Clin Iss Crit Care Nurs* 3(2):350-360, 1992.
14. *St Anthony's DRG Guidebook 1995,* Reston, Va, 1994, St Anthony.

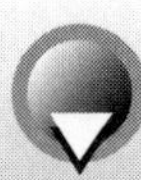

CLINICAL GUIDELINE

57

Hyperosmolar Nonacidotic Diabetes (HNAD)

Karen Clark, MS, RN

DESCRIPTION

Hyperosmolar nonacidotic diabetes (HNAD) is a metabolic emergency and a life-threatening complication of diabetes mellitus. First described over a century ago by Dreschfeld,[2] HNAD was infrequently diagnosed until a 1957 report by Sament and Schwartz.[9] This syndrome is known by many names, including hyperosmolar nonketotic coma, hyperglycemic hyperosmolar nonketotic state or syndrome (HHNK or HHNS), diabetic hyperosmolar state, hyperosmolar coma, and hyperosmolar nonacidotic uncontrolled diabetes. The more descriptive term, uncontrolled diabetes with appropriate modifiers (HNAD),[7] will be used throughout this guideline.

HNAD is diagnosed by the presence of severe hyperglycemia, profound dehydration secondary to osmotic diuresis, marked increase in serum osmolality, mild or undetectable ketonuria, and absence of ketosis. Although there is disagreement, the diagnosis generally is made if serum glucose is greater than 600 mg/dl, and plasma osmolarity is greater than 350 mOsm/L. Both of these values are higher than those associated with diabetic ketoacidosis (DKA). However, many patients show a mix of DKA and HNAD. Uncontrolled diabetes can be thought to represent a spectrum with DKA and HNAD as opposite extremes.[11]

While HNAD can affect children as young as 18 months, it occurs most frequently in patients with undiagnosed non-insulin-dependent diabetes mellitus (NIDDM) over the age of 60 who also have an underlying physiologic disorder such as renal insufficiency or congestive heart failure. For these reasons, the diagnosis of HNAD is frequently missed. Currently, the incidence is figured as one case per 5000 to 6000 persons,[12] but as the American population ages, the incidence of HNAD is expected to rise.

Deaths from DKA and HNAD are approximately 4000 annually.[7] Patient prognosis with HNAD appears directly related to age, with recent studies recording mortality rates between 14% and 17% for those with a mean age of 77 and none under age 50.[7] Mortality is also associated with nursing home residence, decreased mental function, higher plasma osmolarity, and high blood urea nitrogen (BUN) and sodium levels.[11]

Aggressive recognition and treatment of HNAD is vital. Critical care nurses and physicians must consider this a possibility when admitting an older patient who has altered mental status and profound dehydration. Pancreatic beta-cell insufficiency is a natural phenomenon of aging, as is a decline in renal function impairing the body's ability to excrete glucose.[8] These factors place this population at risk for HNAD.

PATHOPHYSIOLOGY

The pathophysiology of HNAD is not completely understood. The hyperglycemia probably results from deficient insulin production and/or decreased tissue responsiveness to insulin. A person with NIDDM who is continuously stressed may not have an adequate supply of endogenous insulin to control serum glucose levels. However, the individual may have enough insulin to prevent production of the ketones seen in DKA.

Metabolic Stressors Associated with HNAD		
Infections		
Urinary tract	Pneumonia	Upper respiratory tract
Enteritis	Gram-negative sepsis	Sinusitis
Tonsillitis	Candidiasis	Diarrhea
Underlying illness/conditions		
Diabetes	Cholecystitis	Pancreatitis
Renal failure	Hypothermia	GI bleeding
Burns	MI	Recent cardiac surgery
Hypertension	Stroke	Thromboembolic disorder
Alcoholism	Trauma	Psychiatric illness
Medications		
Beta-blockers	Steroids	Thiazide and loop diuretics
Phenytoin	Glucocorticoids	Calcium channel blockers
Cimetidine	Immunosuppressive agents	

Metabolic stressors stimulate counterregulatory hormone release (see preceding Box). These hormones (glucagon, catecholamines, corticosteroids, and growth hormone) impair the use of glucose by the peripheral tissue. The resulting hyperglycemia induces an osmotic diuresis in which a disproportionate amount of water is lost in relation to solute, producing a hyperosmolar state and dehydration. The dehydration triggers a sensation of thirst to which the patient responds by drinking high-glucose-containing fluid, further aggravating the hyperglycemia and diuresis.[12] In those patients who cannot recognize the signs of dehydration—including institutionalized, mentally impaired, or comatose persons, or many of the elderly—the dehydration worsens. Often these patients are not able to take fluids due to restraints, sedation, or impairment from strokes.[11]

The severe hyperosmolality also impairs the thirst center in the hypothalamus, thus preventing these patients from responding appropriately to significant water losses. Because these patients do not develop ketoacidosis, signs and symptoms occur later, resulting in more severe hyperglycemia, hyperosmolality and osmotic diuresis. The dehydration gradually progresses over several days or weeks and the patient eventually suffers altered mental status and unresponsiveness. This is frequently the point at which these patients are brought to the hospital for treatment.

LENGTH OF STAY/ANTICIPATED COURSE

The length of stay for patients with HNAD is generally longer than that experienced by those with DKA. This population is compromised due to age and general health status, and the accompanying problems will frequently prolong hospitalization. As previously stated, the mortality rate is high for patients with a mean age of 70 years. Death that occurs during the first 48 hours generally results from dehydration and hyperosmolarity,[12] and beyond 48 hours from the accompanying or precipitating problems. HNAD falls within DRG 300: Endocrine disorders with complication. The average length of stay is 8.3 days.[10]

MANAGEMENT TRENDS AND CONTROVERSIES

The management of HNAD is standardized. The most important aspect of therapy is fluid and electrolyte replacement, as opposed to DKA where insulin replacement is primary.[1] The objective is to complete rehydration and normalize serum glucose levels within 36 to 72 hours.[4] Additionally, steps are taken immediately to correct the precipitating factors such as infection.

Controversy remains about initial fluid replacement and which fluid to use, isotonic saline or half-normal saline. There is debate about whether or not dehydrated cells will take up free water too rapidly with infusion of a hypotonic solution. Whatever the choice of treatment, the volume deficit is corrected at the rate of 1 liter/hour until the central venous pressure or pulmonary capillary wedge pressure begins to rise, or until the blood pressure and urine output are acceptable. Then the rate is reduced to 100 to 200 ml/hour.[12] Patients in HNAD lose an average of 9 to 12 liters of fluid or 24% of their total body water.[6] Most clinicians replace one half of the deficit over the first 12 hours and the second half over the next 36 hours,[12] depending on the condition of the patient. In those patients with unstable hemodynamics who cannot be supported by crystalloids alone, colloid-containing solutions such as albumin are used. When the blood glucose level reaches 250 mg/dl, 5% dextrose is added to the infusion. As soon as the patient is conscious, oral fluids should be encouraged.

Potassium (K^+) is given when a deficit is indicated by laboratory values. All patients with HNAD are hypokalemic though serum K^+ may be high initially due to the shift of K^+ from intracellular to extracellular space. This K^+ loss is less severe than that noted in patients with DKA. Potassium can be added to intravenous fluids at 30 mEq/L, with one half as phosphate and one half as chloride, as soon as renal function is determined.[3]

Insulin therapy is less important in HNAD than in DKA. Fluid replacement alone decreases glucose levels considerably by improving renal perfusion, causing increased excretion of glucose in the urine and thereby decreasing the blood glucose level.[5] If insulin is indicated, intravenous administration is preferred in dehydrated patients because of unpredictable absorption from subcutaneous or intramuscular tissue; the insulin is given at a rate of 5 to 15 units/hour until the serum glucose reaches 250 mg/dl. The therapy then is switched to the subcutaneous route and amounts are adjusted based on blood glucose values.

ASSESSMENT

PARAMETER	ANTICIPATED ALTERATION
Laboratory Tests	
Serum glucose	Increased: >600 mg/dl *due to uncontrolled glucose metabolism*
Osmolality	Increased: >350 mOsm/L *due to hyperglycemia*
Glycosuria	Increased: >1 to 2% *due to uncontrolled glucose metabolism*
Ketones	Absent or modest rise *due to absence of ketoacidosis*
K^+	Increased slightly: >5.0 mEq/L *due to dehydration. Total body* K^+ *is low initially due to shift from intracellular to extracellular compartment.*
PO_4^-	Increased: >6 to 7 mg/dl *due to osmotic diuresis*
Na^+	Slightly decreased: <125 mEq/L *due to fluid shifts and decreased insulin*
BUN	Increased: >20 mg/dl *due to dehydration and insulin deficiency, which leads to protein catabolism*
Creatinine	Increased: >1.2 mg/dl *due to dehydration*
ABG	WNL *due to absence of ketoacidosis*
Physical Assessment	
Mental status	Diminished mental status, stuporous, may be comatose *due to brain cell dehydration and electrolyte imbalance*
RR	Increased: >20 breaths/min *due to hypoxemia*
HR	Increased: >100 bpm *due to osmotic diuresis and fluid losses*
ECG changes	Peaked T waves *due to hyperkalemia*
GI status	Profound dehydration, thirst, nausea (less than DKA), constipation, gastric stasis, ileus, and weight loss *due to fluid volume deficit*
GU status	Polyuria *due to hyperglycemia*

PLAN OF CARE

INTENSIVE PHASE

Care of the patient in the intensive phase of HNAD is focused first on replacing fluid volume and electrolytes lost as a result of the hyperglycemic osmotic diuresis. Because this disorder occurs in an older population, careful assessment of the cardiovascular system is needed during fluid replacement to prevent complications associated with fluid overload. Patients with HNAD usually have some endogenous insulin supplies. However, insulin therapy is needed in this phase to control serum glucose levels and counterregulatory hormone release.

PATIENT CARE PRIORITIES	EXPECTED PATIENT OUTCOMES
Fluid volume deficit *r/t hyperglycemia-induced diuresis*	CO, CVP, and PCWP: all WNL Wt within 5% of patient normal Skin turgor: WNL Mucous membranes moist

Plan of Care (cont'd)

Altered serum electrolytes: • Hyperkalemia *r/t osmotic diuresis* • Hypokalemia *r/t vomiting, diarrhea* • Hypernatremia *r/t dehydration* • Hyponatremia *r/t hyperglycemia* • Hypophosphatemia *r/t osmotic diuresis* • Hypomagnesemia *r/t fluid shifts and decreased insulin*	Electrolytes: WNL
Metabolic imbalance *r/t respiratory alkalosis and hyperglycemia or hypoglycemia associated with insulin therapy*	ABG within patient norms Regular, even respirations Glucose: WNL
Impaired mental status *r/t* *Metabolic/electrolyte imbalance* *Resulting cerebral edema and coma* *Complications of sepsis or meningitis*	Awake, alert, and oriented Correct fluid replacement administered at proper rate
High risk for mortality/morbidity *r/t precipitating factors such as* • *acute MI* • *pancreatitis* • *trauma* • *CNS insult* • *sepsis* • *meningitis* • *pneumonia* • *gastroenteritis* • *influenza*	Stabilization and recovery from precipitating conditions
High risk for ineffective breathing pattern *r/t* *Hypoxemia associated with pulmonary edema caused by decreased plasma oncotic pressure* *Potential aspiration pneumonia associated with gastric stasis and marked dilatation of the stomach*	Pao$_2$: WNL Sao$_2$: WNL Prompt insertion of NG tube when indicated Protected from aspiration
High risk for impaired tissue perfusion *r/t vascular thrombosis associated with dehydration and increased serum viscosity in combination with decreased CO*	Optimal fluid replacement Peripheral perfusion within patient norms
Anxiety (patient and family) *r/t lack of knowledge about disease process and therapy required*	Decreased anxiety Verbalize basic knowledge of disease process and intervention needed

INTERVENTIONS

Monitor I/O hourly *to detect trends in volume deficit correction.*

Insert a Foley catheter when indicated *for accurate measurement of urine output. Note that patients with diabetes mellitus are extremely susceptible to infections and Foley catheter use is strongly linked to nosocomial urinary tract infections. Remove catheter as soon as patient is able to void.*

Record accurate daily wts *because wt gain or loss reflects overall fluid status.*

Monitor VS including T q1h until stable; note the presence of fever *to identify infection, which is a common predisposing factor in HNAD. However, the patient may be hypothermic or normothermic in the presence of infection because of lack of available substrate to generate heat.*[12]

Obtain lab glucose determination q2h *to monitor trends in serum glucose and adjust insulin administration if insulin therapy is instituted. Fingersticks are commonly used, but hyperosmolarity can affect capillary blood glucose measurement.*

Plan of Care (cont'd)

Monitor for signs and symptoms of electrolyte imbalances *to identify and promote early intervention.*

- *K^+ deficit may or may not be reflected in serum measurement due to the extracellular K^+ shift. ECG changes reflect the K^+ status of the cardiac cell.*
- Na^+ *levels can have a profound influence on CNS status.*
- *Observe for signs and symptoms of increasing intracranial pressure to prevent cerebral edema.*
- *Severe deficits of Mg^{++}* cause tetany, seizures, dysrythmias, and CNS depression, but these are rarely seen.
- *Severe hypophosphatemia can lead to altered mental status, hemolysis, rhabdomyolysis, and heart failure, but these are rarely seen.*

Monitor for complications of therapy *to prevent problems that can occur rapidly in the patient with HNAD; i.e., hypoglycemia, cerebral edema, aspiration pneumonia, vascular thrombosis.*

Monitor blood glucose levels *to detect hypoglycemia resulting from insulin therapy.*

Observe for signs and symptoms of altered mental status *to detect cerebral edema.*

Place NG tube *to prevent vomiting and aspiration if patient is obtunded. Keep patient NPO until acute phase is ended.*

Apply antiembolism devices *to prevent venous stasis.*

Observe for the presence of the precipitating factors to HNAD *because treatment may fail and the patient's metabolic status will be further compromised if these are uncorrected.*

INTERMEDIATE PHASE

Management of patients with HNAD is focused on fluid and electrolyte replacement and intervention of any underlying precipitating factor(s). This remains the priority throughout the intermediate phase of care.

PATIENT CARE PRIORITIES	EXPECTED PATIENT OUTCOMES
Metabolic abnormalities *r/t* *Hyperglycemia/hypoglycemia* *Inappropriate fluid* *Electrolyte balance*	Glucose: WNL Correct insulin regulation Adequate fluid intake Decreased thirst sensation
Anxiety *r/t inadequate information regarding importance of stress factors, importance of proper diet, susceptibility to infection, need for routine medical follow-up, hygiene, and foot care*	Patient and family verbalize appropriate management of diabetes mellitus

INTERVENTIONS

Perform self glucose monitoring *to provide information for hyperglycemic management.*

Monitor fluid I/O *to ensure appropriate fluid balance.*

Trend VS *to detect underlying precipitating factors of HNAD and complications of therapy.*

Provide patient with education *to increase knowledge and promote understanding of all phases of diabetes mellitus.*

TRANSITION TO DISCHARGE

Proper diabetic management skills must be taught to patients and their families where possible. However, many of these patients are unable to care for themselves and will be discharged to long-term facilities. In either case, prompt diagnosis and treatment of infections and other precipitating conditions is critical. Education for patients or their primary care giver should be directed toward compliance with therapy and recognition of problem signs and symptoms.

REFERENCES

1. Berger W, Keller U: Treatment of diabetic ketoacidosis and nonketotic hyperosmolar diabetic coma, *Bailliere's Clin Endocrinol Metab* 6(1):1-22, 1992.
2. Dreschfeld J: *British Medical Journal* (2):358-363, 1886.
3. Ellis EN: Concepts of fluid therapy in diabetic ketoacidosis and hyperosmolar hyperglycemic nonketotic coma, *Pediatr Clin North Am* 37(2):313-321, 1990.
4. Hamblin PS, Topliss DJ, Stockigt JR: Practical management of diabetic ketoacidosis and hyperosmolar coma, *Aust N Z J Med* 20:836-841, 1990.
5. Karam JH, Salber PR, Forsham PH: Pancreatic hormones and diabetes mellitus. In Greenspan FS, editor: *Basic and clinical endocrinology,* Norwalk, Conn, 1991, Appleton and Lange, pp 634-638.
6. Levine SN, Sanson TH: Treatment of hyperglycaemic hyperosmolar nonketotic syndrome, *Drugs* 38(3):462-472, 1989.
7. Matz R: Hyperosmolar nonacidotic diabetes. In Rifkin, Porte, editors: *Diabetes mellitus theory and practice,* New York, 1990, Elsevier Science Publishing, pp 604-616.
8. Pope DW, Dansky D: Hyperosmolar hyperglycemic nonketotic coma, *Endocrine and Metabolic Emergencies* 7(4):849-857, 1989.
9. Sament S, Schwartz MB: Severe diabetic stupor without ketosis, *S Afr Med J* 31:893, 1957.
10. *St Anthony's DRG guidebook 1995,* Reston, Va, 1994, St Anthony.
11. Wachtel TJ, et al: Hyperosmolarity and acidosis in diabetes mellitus: a three-year experience in Rhode Island. Presented at 13th annual meeting of the Society of General Internal Medicine, Arlington, Va, May 3, 1990.
12. Wachtel TJ: The diabetic hyperosmolar state, *Clin Geriatr Med* 6(4):797-806, 1990.

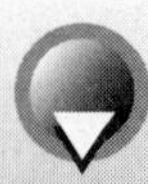

CLINICAL GUIDELINE

58

Hyperthyroidism and Thyroid Storm

Christine Kessler, MN, RN, CCRN, CS

DESCRIPTION

Hyperthyroidism ("thyrotoxicosis") is second only to diabetes mellitus as the most common endocrine disorder encountered. Hyperthyroidism represents a constellation of clinical findings resulting from the body's response to excessive quantities of circulating thyroid hormones, thyroxine (T4), and triiodothyronine (T3). The physiologic effects of T4 and T3 are widespread, affecting nearly every cell in the body. These hormones accelerate cellular metabolic activity, playing a key role in thermal regulation. They are also instrumental in growth and maturation, especially in childhood, by augmenting the effects of growth hormone. Perhaps the most pronounced effect of T3 and T4 is their synergism of catecholamine activity.[22]

Hyperthyroidism is seen predominantly in women, with a female-to-male ratio of 8 to 1, and usually manifests in the third and fourth decades of life. It is rarely seen in children.[3,18] The most common cause of hyperthyroidism is Graves' disease. The exact stimulus for the development of Graves' disease is unclear; however, it is believed to be an autoimmune disorder. Over 90% of patients with Graves' hyperthyroidism have thyroid-stimulating IgG (TSI) in their serum. This antibody reacts with the thyroid-stimulating hormone (TSH) receptors on cells of the thyroid gland, stimulating the gland to produce T3 and T4.[3] As with many autoimmune disorders, other autoimmune disorders (e.g., diabetes mellitus, Addison's disease, and vitiligo) may coexist with Graves' disease.[11] Less common causes of hyperthyroidism are outlined in the following Box.

Thyroid storm (thyrotoxic crisis) is a deadly hypermetabolic state where death can occur within 48 hours without appropriate treatment. The condition generally is caused by inadequately controlled hyperthyroidism or decompensation of the disease due to numerous factors; among them infection (most common), pulmonary embolus, myocardial infarction, surgery, severe physical stress, toxemia, labor and delivery, and hyperglycemic emergencies.[5] In previous years, thyroid storm was a dreaded complication following surgical thyroid gland removal for hyperthyroidism. The current practice of rendering the thyroid gland euthyroid, or nonfunctioning, prior to thyroidectomy has made such a complication a rarity. Thyroid storm is most likely to develop within 2 months to 4 years after the diagnosis of hyperthyroidism is made.[21]

PATHOPHYSIOLOGY

The actual pathophysiology of hyperthyroidism varies slightly depending on the etiology, although all forms of hyperthyroidism share some common characteristics. These include an increase in metabolic rate, heat intolerance, and an increased tissue sensitivity to stimulation by catecholamines. In essence, a "pseudohyperadrenergic" state results that exacts an enormous toll on the body in terms of energy utilization, oxygen consumption, and catabolism. Death is inevitable, unless treatment is initiated.[11]

Normally, thyroid hormone secretion is tightly regulated by a negative feedback mechanism involving the thyroid

Causes of Hyperthyroidism (Thyrotoxicosis)

Graves' disease (most common)
Toxic multinodular goiter
Hyperfunctioning thyroid adenoma
Thyroiditis
Ingestion of excessive amounts of thyroid hormone
TSH-producing pituitary adenomas
Trophoblastic tumors (hydatidiform mole, choriocarcinoma)
Follicular thyroid carcinoma with metastases
Struma ovarii (ovarian teratoma)

gland, the hypothalamus, and the anterior pituitary gland. The initiating hormone is thyrotropin-releasing hormone (TRH) which is synthesized in the hypothalamus and released into the hypothalamic-pituitary portal system in response to low circulating levels of T4 and T3. There is also an increase in TRH in response to a drop in body temperature and high caloric intake. In the presence of TRH, the anterior pituitary gland releases TSH, which in turn stimulates the thyroid gland to synthesize and release T4 and T3 (Figure 58-1). When adequate circulating levels of thyroid hormones are achieved, TRH and TSH release is inhibited, thereby creating an effective system of self-regulation. Of the thyroid hormones produced by the thyroid gland, approximately 90% is T4 and 10% is T3. More than 99% of these hormones are bound by plasma proteins, thus unable to exert physiologic effects. Much of the "free," or unbound, T4 is eventually converted to T3 in the liver and peripheral tissues. Therefore T3 is generally regarded as having the greatest metabolic effects.[5]

In hyperthyroidism, the thyroid gland is stimulated to produce abnormally high amounts of thyroid hormones. In Graves' disease, a circulating antibody (TSI) mimics TSH, causing the thyroid gland to synthesize and release thyroid hormones unchecked by the negative feedback system. Increased circulating levels of T3 and T4 will result in inhibition of TRH and TSH release; however, thyroid hormone secretion continues unabated. A secondary cause of overstimulation of the thyroid gland is excessive TSH release from the anterior pituitary due to central nervous system pathology. Whatever the cause, an overstimulated thyroid gland eventually hypertrophies and a goiter may form. Goiters often are accompanied by a systolic or continuous bruit heard over the thyroid gland, owing to extreme vascularity of the organ. An accompanying thrill may be palpated.[5]

Autoimmune hyperthyroidism (Graves' disease) has been the subject of intense study. It is believed that severe and prolonged hyperthyroidism may exert an adverse effect on generalized suppressor T-lymphocyte function, thus precipitating other associated autoimmune disease, mentioned previously.[21]

Much of the pathophysiology of hyperthyroidism relates

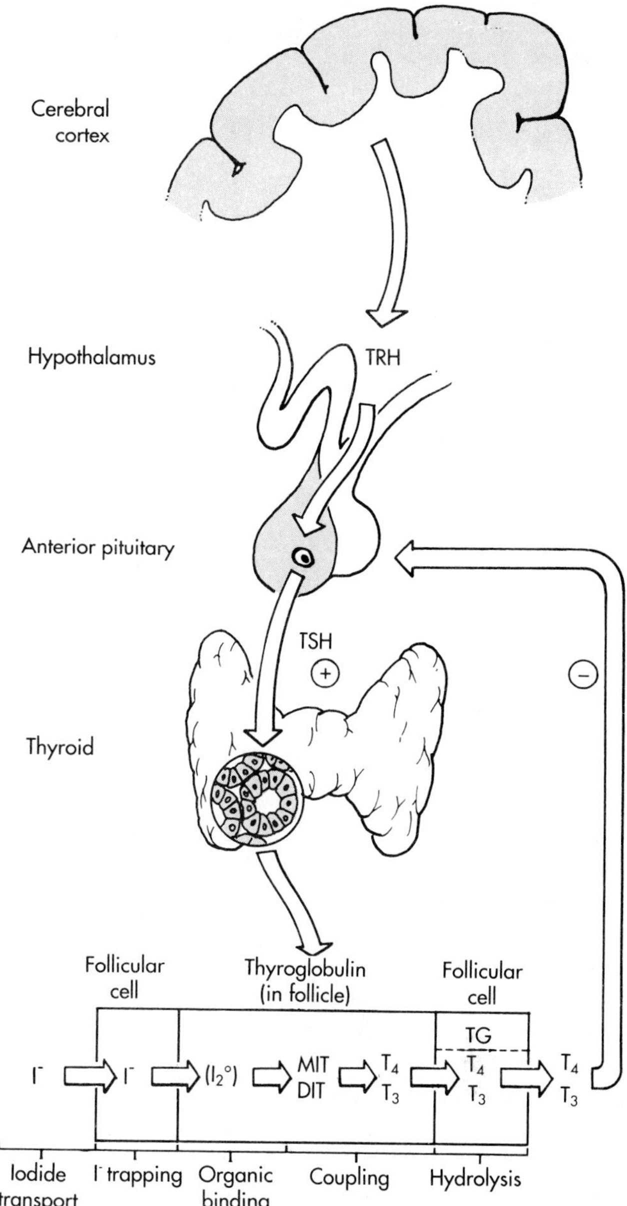

Figure 58-1 The feedback loop between the hypothalamic-pituitary axis and the thyroid gland for production of thyroxine (T4) and triiodothyronine (T3). (From Price SA, Wilson LM, editors: *Pathophysiology: clinical concepts of disease processes,* ed 4, St Louis, 1992, Mosby–Year Book, Fig 59-3, p 850.)

to an exaggeration of the metabolic effects of thyroid hormone. The clinical presentation of the disease reflects these attenuated effects. Although hyperthyroidism impacts every body system, few patients have all the clinical features. Manifestations of hyperthyroidism are summarized in the following Box.

Thyroid storm (acute hyperthyroidism) is a life-threatening syndrome of decompensated hyperthyroidism and presents a clinical picture of exacerbated thyrotoxic manifestations. The synergized effects of catecholamines pre-

Clinical Manifestations of Hyperthyroidism*

Neuromuscular

Fatigue
Fine finger tremor
Hyperreflexia
Proximal muscle weakness

Mentation

Manic behavior
Emotional lability
Confusion
Psychosis

Cardiovascular system

Resting tachycardia
Palpitations
High flow murmur
Exertional dyspnea

Thermoregulatory system

Heat intolerance
Low-grade fever
Diaphoresis

Hematologic system

Normochromic anemia
Megaloblastic anemia†
Granulocytopenia
Lymphocytosis

Gastrointestinal system‡

Increased appetite
Weight loss
Hyperdefecation
Abdominal cramps
Hepatomegaly (may be poor prognostic sign)

Cutaneous system

Smooth, warm, moist, velvety skin
Pruritis
Pretibial dermopathy (myxedema)§
Thinning hair, spotty alopecia
Vitiligo||
Onycholysis (separation of distal third of nail from nail bed)

Ocular¶

Exophthalmos
  Protruding eyeballs
  Lid lag
  Infrequent blinking
Blurred vision (extraocular muscle dysfunction)

Reproductive system

Relative infertility
Oligomenorrhea
Oligospermia
Gynecomastia
Impotence

Other

Hypercalcuria
Osteoporosis
Goiter#

*References 2, 3, 5, 6, 7, 8, 12, 14, 16, 21.
†Pernicious anemia is found in 3% of persons with Graves' disease.
‡Manifestations of celiac disease, an autoimmune disease, may be seen in association with Graves' disease.
§Pretibial dermopathy is an orange-peel thickening and erythema of the skin in the dorsum of foot related to infiltration of mucopolysaccharide. It is associated with Graves' disease.
||Vitiligo is an autoimmune disorder causing areas of depigmentation. It is often associated with Graves' disease.
¶Exophthalmos is a characteristic finding in Graves' disease.
#Goiters are found in persons with Graves' disease, hypothyroidism (e.g., Hashimoto's thyroiditis), or iodine deficiency states.

dominate. Fever is a characteristic finding, ranging between 38° C (100° F) and 41° C (105.8° F). This is accompanied by facial and palmar flushing and profuse diaphoresis, with fluid losses as high as 4 liters in 24 hours.[5] Compensatory mechanisms of peripheral vasodilatation and diaphoresis are no longer adequate to dissipate the excess heat.

Supraventricular tachycardia is almost always seen with ventricular rates near or above 200 beats per minute typical. Tachycardia is common because the conductive system is sensitive to thyroid hormone activity. Although circulating catecholamine levels do not rise, cardiac beta-adrenergic receptors do increase in response to elevated thyroid hormone levels. Rapid atrial fibrillation is found in approximately 30% of patients in thyroid storm. Tachycardia is usually accompanied by some degree of heart failure or pulmonary edema that is relatively refractory to digitalis.[6] Cardiovascular collapse and death are the lethal consequences of thyroid storm.

Pronounced mental status changes are seen, such as extreme agitation, delirium, psychosis, stupor, or coma. Reflexes are generally exaggerated. Gastrointestinal disturbances and hyperdefecation may herald the onset of thyroid storm. Hyperglycemia may ensue due to adrenergic precipitation of gluconeogenesis, glycogenolysis, and relative insulin resistance.[6,11]

Thyroid storm may be more difficult to identify in elderly patients because they may manifest their thyroid disease quite differently. The hyperkinetic manifestations associated with hyperthyroidism may be absent in individuals 70 years of age and older. They more often will display lethargy and apathy, giving rise to the term *apathetic thyrotoxicosis*. Although proximal muscle weakness and weight loss are common, the typical ocular signs are absent. Instead, blepharoptosis (drooping upper eyelid) is seen more often. Many times these patients are monosymptomatic, with isolated cardiovascular disturbances, usually atrial fibrillation and congestive heart failure (CHF).[6,8] The pathogenesis of apathetic hyperthyroidism is not fully understood. However, it should be considered in any elderly patient who has refractory atrial fibrillation with accompanying CHF.

LENGTH OF STAY/ANTICIPATED COURSE

The length of stay for patients experiencing thyroid storm is difficult to predict. Patients' responses to therapy may vary. Thyroid storm may last from 1 to 8 days because of the long half-life of thyroid hormones (6 days for T4 and 22 days for T3). The mortality rate for this disorder is estimated to be between 10% and 20%.[5] Underlying hyperthyroidism may require treatment for up to 2 years. Remission rates, after treatment, range between 30% and 70% depending upon mode of treatment.[2] Hyperthyroidism and thyroid storm fall within DRG 300: Endocrine disorders with complications; and 301: Endocrine disorders without complications. The average lengths of stay are 8.3 days and 4.9 days, respectively.[19]

MANAGEMENT TRENDS AND CONTROVERSIES

In deciding on the correct treatment regimen, it is important to determine how quickly the patient needs to achieve a euthyroid state. Generally, two modes of treatment are available for hyperthyroidism: pharmacologic interventions, and surgical intervention (thyroidectomy).

Pharmacologic therapy for hyperthyroidism can be divided into three classes: (1) agents that inhibit synthesis of thyroid hormone (antithyroid drugs), (2) agents that inhibit the release of thyroid hormone (iodine preparations), and (3) agents that block the effects of thyroid hormone (beta-adrenergic blocking agents).

The thionamides, or antithyroid drugs, constitute this first class of drugs. The two drugs of this type presently used in the United States are propylthiouracil (PTU) and methimazole. These drugs interfere with the synthesis (but not the release) of thyroid hormone by inhibition of thyroid peroxidase.[17,23] The thyroid gland first must be depleted of its hormonal stores before there is a reduction in the supply of hormone at the tissue level. Thus it may take days to weeks for the effects of thionamides to be realized. PTU has an added benefit of blocking the extrathyroid conversion of T4 to T3. For this reason, the acute effects of PTU are more striking than methimazole. After normalization of serum T3 and T4 levels, the dose can be decreased to one half to one third. Methimazole and PTU also have been shown to be immunosuppressive, thus additionally beneficial for the treatment of Graves' disease. The use of these drugs may be limited in some patients with thyroid storm, as only oral forms of the drug exist. Because antithyroid drugs cross the placenta and can harm the fetus, they should be given in reduced doses to pregnant patients.[10,11,23]

Radioiodine 131I is the most common drug prescribed for Graves' hyperthyroidism in the United States. Its ability to acutely block the release of thyroid hormone, allowing circulating levels of T3 and T4 to fall rapidly, makes this a popular form of thyroid ablation therapy. To prevent the utilization of iodine in the production of thyroid hormone, 131I should be administered at least 1 hour following an initial dose of antithyroid drugs. Iodine therapy can be administered orally as saturated sodium iodide (Lugol's solution) or intravenously as sodium iodine. The latter is administered slowly (1 gram q8h to q12h) in the presence of an actual or impending thyroid storm. In chronic therapy, most patients become euthyroid after the first dose. Hypothyroidism is the main complication of the drug and occurs in most patients, often years later.[11,23]

Cholecystographic agents—sodium ipodate (Oragrafin), and iopanoid acid (Telepaque)—are effective in the acute management of hyperthyroidism because they are potent inhibitors of the conversion of T4 to T3 in peripheral tissues. Considering that this mechanism accounts for approximately half of the T3 production in hyperthyroid patients, the usefulness of these drugs can be appreciated. In addition, cholecystographic agents block the release of hormone from the thyroid gland. Administration of the agents in conjunction with antithyroid drugs can cause a rapid improvement of hyperthyroidism. Unfortunately, their effectiveness in the chronic treatment of hyperthyroidism has not been demonstrated.[1,3,10,11]

Beta-adrenergic blocking agents have had considerable impact on the management of the severely ill thyrotoxic patient. The efficacy of these agents is primarily through inhibition of thyroid hormone action on catecholamines, thus quickly ameliorating the signs and symptoms that resemble a hyperadrenergic state (e.g., anxiety, tachycardia, tremor, and sweating). An additional benefit is that they inhibit the conversion of T4 to T3. The use of these agents has dramatically reduced the mortality associated with thyroid storm. Propranolol, although remarkably effective, may be difficult to dose adequately because of the variability in dosage range (from 40 mg to 2 g per day).[9] Esmolol, a cardioselective beta-blocker, is an acceptable alternative to propranolol. In patients who are unresponsive to beta-adrenergic blockers, calcium antagonists (e.g., verapamil) may be effective in treating tachydysrhythmias. Diltiazem has proven to be an effective alternative to propranolol in hyperthyroid outpatients.[9,10,12]

Thyroidectomy can effectively eradicate hyperthyroidism. However, its usefulness is hampered by its side effects and complications. To prevent postoperative thyroid storm, due to intraoperative thyroid manipulation, the patient must be rendered euthyroid using antithyroid drugs and stable iodine. Postoperatively, 30% of patients develop permanent hypothyroidism. Hypoparathyroidism and laryngeal nerve palsy also may be complications of thyroidectomy. These complications and the expense and trauma of the procedure make surgical ablation less acceptable than radioiodine ablation. Thyroidectomy is usually reserved for patients intolerant to antithyroid agents, noncompliant with medical regimens, or who have thyroid neoplasms or obstructing goiters.[3,10,16]

All classes of the previously described drugs are used in the treatment of thyroid storm. Ideally, a loading dose of PTU is given prior to administration of sodium iodide. In addition, a steroid (usually dexamethasone) is administered to acutely inhibit T4 conversion to T3. Beta-adrenergic blocking agents help ameliorate the tachydysrhythmias associated with thyroid storm and minimize other hyperdynamic sequelae. Standard therapy with digitalis preparations generally are ineffective. Beta-blockers can be tried judiciously in the presence of heart failure because many of these patients presumably have "high output" failure, which is rate-dependent. Esmolol may be the drug of choice in these instances, especially when accompanied by angina.[5,16] Verapamil also may be used in resistant tachycardias. Pharmacological management of the hyperthermia is best accomplished with non-aspirin antipyretics, as aspirin is believed to reduce the binding of T3 and T4 with thyroid-binding proteins, thus raising the level of free thyroid hormones in the blood.

ASSESSMENT

PARAMETER	ANTICIPATED ALTERATION
CNS	
Stamina	Fatigue, proximal muscle weakness *due to skeletal muscle catabolism*
Mental status	Restlessness, anxiety, personality changes, labile emotions, insomnia, confusion, coma *due to augmentation of catecholamine effects*
Reflexes	Hyperreflexia, tremors *due to enhanced catecholamine effects*
Cardiovascular Status	
HR	Elevated: >200 bpm (supraventricular tachycardia) *due to increased beta-adrenergic response of heart*
Heart rhythm	Rapid atrial fibrillation (predominates in elderly), palpitations *due to increased beta-adrenergic response of heart*
BP	Elevated: >140 SBP (initially) with wide pulse pressure *due to increased SV and reduced SVR* Hypotension *as cardiovascular decompensation occurs*
SVR	Decreased: <800 dynes/sec/cm^{-5} *due to beta-adrenergic responses*
CO	Elevated: >8 L/min (initially) *due to increased myocardial contractility and reduced SVR*
Heart sounds	S_3 gallop, loud S_1, systolic murmur *due to high output failure*
Chest x-ray	Mildly enlarged heart *due to prolonged increases in myocardial workload*
Pulmonary Status	
Pattern	Exertional dyspnea, reduced vital capacity *due to effects of synergized catecholamines*
RR	Elevated: >20 breaths/min *due to associated anxiety*
Breath sounds	Pulmonary crackles *due to cardiogenic pulmonary edema*
GI Status	
Nutrition	Weight loss, catabolism, muscle wasting *due to excessive metabolic energy expenditures (hypermetabolism)*

Appetite	Increased appetite or anorexia, nausea *due to catecholamine effects*
Bowel function	Abdominal cramps, hypermotility (increased bowel sounds), hyperdefecation, diarrhea (less frequently) *due to exaggerated catecholamine effects*
Thermoregulatory Status	
Temperature	Elevated: >38° C to 41° C *due to thyroid hormone-induced hypermetabolism*
Skin	Profuse diaphoresis (especially hands) *due to hyperadrenergic state* Palmar and facial flushing *due to increased SVR*
Laboratory Tests	
T4	Elevated: >142 nmol/L *due to overstimulation of the thyroid gland*
T3	Elevated: >3.4 nmol/L *due to overstimulation of the thyroid gland (T3 is disproportionately increased relative to T4 in Graves' disease)*
T3 resin uptake (T3RU)	Elevated: >0.35 T3 binding. This value helps determine the level of free T3.
Thyroid-stimulating hormone (TSH)	Decreased: <0.1 uIU/ml *due to increased circulating levels of T3 and T4. Note that TSH will be normal or elevated in TSH-induced hyperthyroidism. TSH levels also may be decreased in some severely ill "normal thyroid" patients—"sick thyroid syndrome."*
Glucose	Elevated: >150 mg/dl *due to stimulation of catecholamines.*

PLAN OF CARE

INTENSIVE PHASE

Care of the patient in the intensive phase focuses on treating the effects of an increased metabolic rate, heat intolerance, and increased tissue sensitivity to stimulation by catecholamines caused by thyrotoxicosis. Intensive monitoring and treatment are required in this phase because catecholamines affect virtually all body systems.

PATIENT CARE PRIORITIES	EXPECTED PATIENT OUTCOMES
Increased CO *r/t hypermetabolic responses*	Premorbid HR and BP Minimized or abolished dysrhythmias Resolution of heart failure as evidenced by no S_3 gallop, clear breath sounds CO: WNL
Ineffective thermoregulation *r/t extreme hypermetabolic state*	Normalization of body temperature Increased tolerance of ambient temperature Decreased diaphoresis and flushing
Ineffective coping (individual) *r/t thyroid hormone-induced anxiety and altered mental status*	Reduced observable nervousness, emotional lability, and hyperkinesis Reports improved sleeping patterns Verbalizes fears or concerns regarding illness, behavior, or hospitalization
High risk for self-injury *r/t fatigue, tremor, osteoporosis, and exophthalmos*	Free from self-injury Able to demonstrate safe mobility (when allowed to move) Exhibits increased activity tolerance No evidence of corneal damage Reduced tremors
Inadequate nutrition *r/t protein catabolism and hypermetabolism*	Wt stabilized Verbal and behavioral evidence of increased physical stamina Albumin: WNL

Plan of Care (cont'd)

Diarrhea *r/t increased GI motility*

Returns to normal defecation patterns
Diminished abdominal discomfort

INTERVENTIONS

Monitor cardiovascular status: HR and rhythm, BP, pulse pressure, PAP, capillary refill, edema, daily wts, and skin color.
Monitor rate, depth, regularity, and effort of respirations.
Assess ABG and/or arterial oxygen saturations as needed.
Auscultate lungs for crackles and evidence of heart failure.
Monitor results of thyroid function tests.
Administer and assess patient response to medications aimed at inhibiting thyroid hormone synthesis and release, and suppressing adrenergic overactivity.
Assess patient's core T, degree of diaphoresis and dehydration, and degree of peripheral vasodilation.
Implement hypothermic measures *to gradually reduce elevated T.*
Prevent shivering *which will increase metabolism and body T.*
Monitor fluid I/O (include diaphoretic losses).
Assess patient's LOC, nervousness, and emotional stability, noting subtle changes.
Reorient patient and confirm reality as necessary.
Promote a tranquil environment as much as possible *to decrease stressful stimuli.*
Assist patient in relaxation techniques; e.g., diaphragmatic breathing *to assist in coping capability.*
Reassure patient and family that any irritable behavior is primarily disease-related and may be controlled with appropriate therapy.
Assess patient's psychophysiologic response to activities.
Clear the environment of potential obstacles and mobility hazards *to prevent injury.*
Schedule activities *to conserve energy.*
Schedule periods of uninterrupted rest.
If patient has exophthalmos, shield eyes from excessive dust, light, and trauma with eyeglasses or eyepatches. Provide cool, moist compresses to soothe irritated eyes. Examine corneas for clarity and intactness.
Assess degree of GI disturbance (abdominal pain, diarrhea, nausea, vomiting, anorexia).
Auscultate bowel sounds for hypermotility.
Monitor degree of catabolism: daily wts, degree of fatigue, muscle wasting, albumin, Hgb, and WBC count.
Provide well-balanced diet high in calories, carbohydrates, vitamins, and protein.
Avoid foods high in roughage *to reduce diarrhea.*

INTERMEDIATE PHASE

The focus of care at this point will be to address the patient's continuing nutritional needs and emotional adaptation to the disease. Unique to this stage of therapy is the need to provide sufficient patient education to prevent a reoccurrence of thyroid storm and long-term side effects of therapy.

PATIENT CARE PRIORITIES

Self-care deficit *r/t inadequate knowledge of the disease, treatment, and future prophylactic care*

EXPECTED PATIENT OUTCOMES

Verbalizes understanding of basic thyroid function, hyperthyroidism, cause and manifestations of thyroid storm
Describes the manifestations of hypothyroidism and need to seek medical assistance if it appears
Discusses importance and benefits of practicing relaxation techniques post-discharge; demonstrates diaphragmatic breathing
Describes the indications, dosages, and side effects of prescribed antithyroid drugs

Plan of Care (cont'd)

INTERVENTIONS

Assess patient's readiness to learn *(include family members)*.

In teaching the patient, include the following:

- Basic functioning of the thyroid gland
- Cause and pathophysiology of hyperthyroidism
- General manifestations of hyperthyroidism and thyroid storm
- Safe use of prescribed antithyroid medications
- The signs and symptoms of hypothyroidism, which are usually insidious, such as exceptional fatigue; dry, cool, scaly skin; hair loss; puffy face; periorbital edema; and cold intolerance
- Benefits of continuing to practice relaxation techniques (assess patient's ability to demonstrate diaphragmatic deep breathing)

TRANSITION TO DISCHARGE

If the patient has a good response to therapy associated with normalization of vital signs, mentation, and laboratory thyroid hormone levels, discharge may occur within 1 week of admission. A plan for chronic therapy and follow-up must be determined. It is important to realize that antithyroid therapy (especially with radioiodine) will ablate the thyroid gland. This may occur months or years after radioiodine therapy, depending on the dose. Therefore, the prospect of eventually developing hypothyroidism and requiring thyroid hormone replacement is very real. The ramifications of hyperthyroidism and its treatment, and the complications of thyroid storm or hypothyroidism, should be discussed at length with the patient.[14]

REFERENCES

1. Allannic H, et al: Antithyroid drugs and Graves' disease: a prospective randomized evaluation of the efficacy of treatment duration, *J Clin Endocrinol Metab* 70:675-679, 1990.
2. Forfar JC, Caldwell GC: Hyperthyroid heart disease, *J Clin Endocrinol Metab* 14:487-494, 1985.
3. Herschman J: Hyperthyroidism: diagnosis and treatment. In *Thyroid diagnosis and management,* 1992, National Health Laboratories.
4. Isley WL: The thyroid. In Civetta JM, Taylor RW, Kirby RR, editors: *Critical care,* Philadelphia, 1988, JB Lippincott.
5. Kessler CA: Endocrine emergencies. In *AACN Instructor's Manual for the Core Curriculum,* Philadelphia, 1991, WB Saunders.
6. Kessler CA: Hyperthyroidism and thyroid crisis. In Dossey BM, Guzzetta CE, Kenner CV, editors: *Critical care nursing: body-mind-spirit,* Philadelphia, 1992, JB Lippincott.
7. Klein I, Levy GS: New perspectives on thyroid hormone, catecholamines, and the heart, *Am J Med* 76:165-170, 1984.
8. McMorrow ME: The elderly and thyrotoxicosis, *AACN Clin Iss Crit Care Nurs* 3:114-119, 1992.
9. Milner MR, Gelman KM, Phillips RA: Double-blind crossover trial of diltiazem versus propranolol in the management of thyrotoxic symptoms, *Pharmacotherapy* 10:97-103, 1990.
10. Orgiazzi J: Management of Graves' hyperthyroidism, *Endocrinol Metab Clin North Am* 16:365-389, 1987.
11. Reasner CA, Isley WL: Thyrotoxicosis in the critically ill, *Crit Care Clin* 57-74, 1991.
12. Roti E, Montermini M, Roti S: The effect of diltiazem, a calcium channel blocking drug, on cardiac rate and rhythm in hyperthyroid patients, *Arch Intern Med* 148:1918-1923, 1988.
13. Sakiyama R: Common thyroid disorders, *Am Fam Physician* 38:227-238, 1988.
14. Schimke N: Hyperthyroidism: the clinical spectrum, *Postgrad Med* 91(5):229-236, 1992.
15. Schleusener H, Peters H, Bogner Y: Immunogenetics in Graves' disease: an overview, *Acta Endocrinol* (suppl 2):123-129, 1989.
16. Solomon DH: Treatment of Graves' hyperthyroidism. In Ingbar S, Braverman LE: *The thyroid,* ed 5, Philadelphia, 1986, JB Lippincott.
17. Solomon G, Lagasse R, Wartofsky L: Current trends in the management of Graves' disease, *J Clin Endocrinol Metab* 70:1518-1524, 1990.
18. Spittle L: Diagnoses in opposition: thyroid storm and myxedema coma, *AACN Clin Iss Crit Care Nurs* 3(2):300-308, 1992.
19. *St Anthony's DRG guidebook 1995,* Reston, Va, 1994, St Anthony.
20. Taylor RW: Endocrine and metabolic issues in critical care: a practitioner's perspective, *Crit Care Nurs Q* 13:1-2, 1990.
21. Volpe R: Autoimmune thyroid disease. In *Thyroid diagnosis and management,* 1992, National Health Laboratories.
22. Wartofsky A, Ingbar S: Diseases of the thyroid. In *Hanson's Principles of Internal Medicine,* 12 ed, New York, 1990, McGraw-Hill.
23. Werner SC, Ingbar SH: *The thyroid,* ed 5, Philadelphia, 1986, JB Lippincott.

U N I T

VII

Hematologic and Immune System

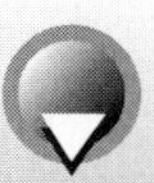

CLINICAL GUIDELINE

59 Disseminated Intravascular Coagulation

Peg Snyder, MN, RN, CCRN

DESCRIPTION

Disseminated intravascular coagulation (DIC), defibrination, and consumptive coagulopathy are all names that have been applied to a heterogeneous group of syndromes characterized by thrombus formation and depletion of select coagulation proteins. The lack of accepted parameters for distinguishing the various syndromes limits determination of DIC prevalence and hampers evaluation of recommended therapies. The following discussion will focus on acute, severe DIC as described by Marder[17] in which thrombin formation causes systemic activation and consumption of selected coagulation proteins and fibrin deposition in the microvasculature.

The reported prevalence of DIC in hospital patients is low. Mant and King[15] identified 47 cases of DIC for a time period when hospital admissions totaled 115,175. Siegal et al.[22] calculated the frequency of DIC as 1 out of every 3127 in newborns and 1 out of every 867 in other hospitalized patients in their review. Zbilut[24] determined the frequency of DIC in patients admitted through the emergency department to be 13 out of every 21,576 cases. However, DIC occurs more frequently in specific patient populations. Fourrier and colleagues[9] reported that 44 of 60 patients with septic shock met laboratory criteria for DIC. Dahmash and associates[7] identified DIC in 11 of 45 patients with septic shock but did not describe the diagnostic criteria used.

DIC is associated with a greater than 50% mortality.[7,9,15,22] Because DIC is not a primary pathology but a complication of a number of illnesses, including sepsis, shock, severe head injury, and trauma, there is disagreement about the relative contribution of DIC to mortality in these critically ill patients. Mant and King[15] concluded that DIC was rarely responsible for patient deaths in their series and should be considered an incidental preterminal event that occurs in a variety of acute catastrophic illnesses. However, Fourrier et al.[10] noted a trend toward decreased mortality in septic shock patients who received therapy that ablated the DIC compared to septic patients with DIC who did not receive the treatment.

PATHOPHYSIOLOGY

Normal blood coagulation occurs through initiation of the intrinsic (contact-activation dependent) pathway by damage to vascular endothelium or the extrinsic (tissue-factor dependent) pathway by tissue injury. Both pathways culminate in the conversion of prothrombin to thrombin, which then cleaves fibrinogen to form soluble fibrin monomers. Factor XIII causes polymerization of the fibrin strands to form insoluble clot. (See Figure 59-1.)

DIC always occurs as a secondary complication of some other disease process. A partial list of the etiologies that may trigger DIC is found in the following Box. Theoretically, DIC is initiated when the underlying disease process results in systemic activation of blood coagulation. The mechanisms by which each of the triggering pathologies may cause DIC are not known. Presumably, substances that initiate blood coagulation gain access to the circulation. These procoagulants may include tissue factor released from injured cells or cells stimulated by cytokines, such as tumor

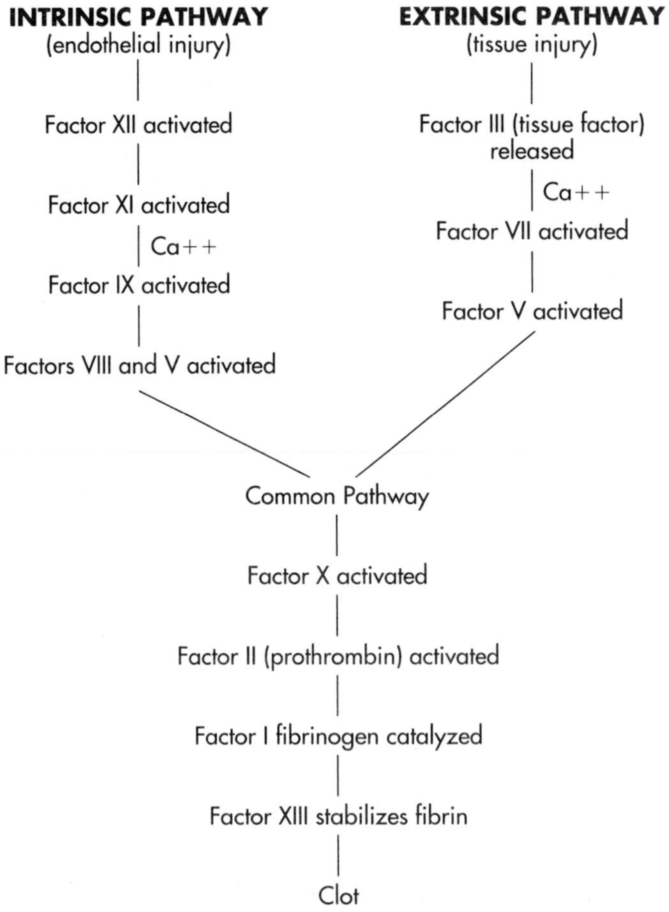

INTRINSIC PATHWAY
(endothelial injury)
Factor XII activated
Factor XI activated
Ca++
Factor IX activated
Factors VIII and V activated

EXTRINSIC PATHWAY
(tissue injury)
Factor III (tissue factor) released
Ca++
Factor VII activated
Factor V activated

Common Pathway
Factor X activated
Factor II (prothrombin) activated
Factor I fibrinogen catalyzed
Factor XIII stabilizes fibrin
Clot

Figure 59-1 Normal blood coagulation system.

necrosis factor.[1] Damage to vascular endothelium during infection or hypotension may expose subendothelial structures that activate the intrinsic pathway of blood coagulation. Regardless of the initiating process, widespread thrombin production occurs. Thrombin contributes to the process of DIC by producing fibrin and promoting platelet stimulation and aggregation.

Blood coagulation is normally regulated by a number of intrinsic mechanisms, including the fibrinolytic system, the protein C–protein S system, and antithrombin III. The activities of these systems may also contribute to the pathogenesis of DIC.

Tissue plasminogen activators, released from injured cells, and activated Factor XII or kallikrein formed during the intrinsic pathway of coagulation convert plasminogen into plasmin. Plasmin causes lysis of fibrin clot as well as digesting circulating fibrin and fibrinogen. The circulating fibrin(ogen) degradation products (FDPs) inhibit polymerization of fibrin monomers, which prevents them from forming stable clots. Traditionally, fibrinolytic system activation in DIC was assumed to occur as a consequence of widespread coagulation. Recent studies indicate that fibrinolytic activity is enhanced in the initial phase of endotoxemia, but

Etiologies of DIC—A Partial Listing

- Infections
  - Bacterial (particularly Gram-negative sepsis)
  - Viral
  - Fungal
- Obstetric
  - Amniotic embolus
  - Retained dead fetus
  - Abruptio placentae
  - Fatty liver of pregnancy
- Neoplasia
  - Solid tumors
  - Leukemia (especially promyelocytic leukemia)
- Snake venoms
- Acute hemolysis (mismatched blood transfusion)
- Malignant hyperthermia
- Trauma
- Shock
- Circulation of ascitic fluid
- ARDS (acute respiratory distress syndrome)
- External circulation devices (e.g., cardio-pulmonary bypass pump, ECHMO)

is rapidly inhibited. This subsequent inhibition of the fibrinolytic system may result in poor clearance of fibrin from the microcirculation.[14]

Activated protein C inhibits coagulation factors V and VIII. This anticoagulant activity is greatly enhanced by protein S. Diminished protein C and protein S activities have been demonstrated in experimental sepsis complicated by DIC.[14]

Antithrombin III is a protein produced in the liver that inactivates thrombin and inhibits several other activated coagulation proteins. Antithrombin III is consumed during DIC, and relative deficiency of antithrombin III may promote ongoing clot formation.

The effects of thrombin and plasmin are believed to be primarily responsible for the clinical manifestations of DIC. Thrombin promotes coagulation and the deposition of fibrin clots in the microvasculature. Tissue beds become ischemic, dysfunctional, and necrotic if oxygen delivery is sufficiently compromised. This widespread microvascular coagulation and compromise of effective tissue perfusion may be an important mediator of multiple organ failure. Theoretically, with DIC, all organ systems are vulnerable to thrombosis. In a pathology review of 29 patients with DIC, autopsy (22 patients) or skin biopsy (7 patients) demonstrated thrombi most frequently in the vasculature of the kidney (68%), skin (52%), and lung (50%); 26 of 29 patients had identifiable thrombus in some organ system.[21]

The ongoing activation of the coagulation proteases and platelets results in demand that exceeds productive capacity—the "consumption" of clotting factors and platelets. Activation of the fibrinolytic system results in lysis of fibrin clots and circulation of FDPs and their intrinsic anticoagulant properties. These aspects of DIC are believed to be responsible for the bleeding manifestations that are often the first symptom of DIC. The most common sites for bleeding are mucous membranes, skin, wounds, gastrointestinal tract, urinary tract, lung, and central nervous system.

Although DIC has been associated with a number of common conditions, it occurs relatively infrequently. The implication is that additional host factors may also be necessary for full expression of DIC. These factors have been reviewed and fall into two main categories: (1) factors causing poor capillary blood flow, such as decreased cardiac output, vasoconstriction, and arteriovenous shunting; and (2) factors that promote hypercoagulability, such as acidosis, increased platelet adhesiveness, and the effects of adrenal hormones.[13] Impaired clearance of activated clotting factors and FDPs by the reticuloendothelial system has also been implicated as contributing to ongoing DIC.[17]

LENGTH OF STAY/ANTICIPATED COURSE

The length of stay for the patient with DIC depends on the precipitating disease and the rapidity and effectiveness with which the primary pathology is recognized and treated. The outcome of patients surviving DIC will depend on the degree of concomitant organ system dysfunction.

DIC falls within DRG 397: Coagulation Disorders. It has an average length of stay of 6.9 days.[23]

MANAGEMENT TRENDS AND CONTROVERSIES

Aggressive, definitive treatment of the precipitating pathology and general supportive measures such as correcting hypoxemia, acidosis, and hypotension are recognized as the foremost therapies for DIC. A high index of suspicion in patients at risk for DIC may aid in early detection. Measures directed specifically at the pathophysiologic mechanisms of DIC are controversial and generally lack prospective, randomized, controlled clinical trials to evaluate efficacy.

Exogenous anticoagulants have been administered in an attempt to disrupt the production of thrombin and terminate the cycle of subsequent events. The greatest body of clinical experience is with heparin, which greatly augments the effects of antithrombin III. Heparin is dosed in therapeutic amounts of 10 to 20 units/kg/hr. Heparin therapy cannot be monitored by the usual laboratory tests, which are altered in DIC. The clinician monitors for a decrease in clinical manifestations of DIC and a gradual normalization of the coagulation profile and platelet count. There is also belief that DIC may result in heparin resistance, perhaps due to decreased antithrombin III activity.[4,10,17] Advocates of heparin therapy cite cases of sharp improvement in DIC symptoms with the initiation of therapy,[6] but heparin therapy has been equivocal in other studies.[2,15] Fatal hemorrhage has also been attributed to the use of heparin in these patients, who are already at risk for bleeding.[12] Heparin has been shown to improve survival in experimental models of DIC and may be useful in DIC of selected etiologies.[8]

A randomized, prospective study evaluated the use of antithrombin III concentrate, heparin, and heparin with antithrombin III in patients with sepsis and DIC.[4] There was no control group. Survival was the same in all groups, and no deaths were attributed to the DIC. Tests of coagulation improved more quickly in the two groups that received antithrombin III, and bleeding complications were more severe in the group that received heparin and antithrombin III. A controlled trial of antithrombin III in patients with sepsis and DIC demonstrated sharp reduction in the duration of DIC and a trend toward improved survival in the treatment group.[10]

Hirudin is a thrombin inhibitor found in the saliva of the leech, *Hirudo medicinalis*. Hirudin can be manufactured through recombinant DNA technology. Nowak and Markwardt studied hirudin in three experimental models of DIC and found that the various triggering mechanisms were blocked by infusion of hirudin.[20]

Blood component therapy to replace depleted plasma proteins and platelets has been somewhat controversial. Opponents believe it adds "fuel to the fire"—providing additional substrate for ongoing thrombus formation. However, blood component therapy to control hemorrhage is now generally accepted as part of the supportive therapies for patients with ongoing DIC, although some authors advocate transfusion only after anticoagulation with heparin.[3,17] The blood components most commonly used are platelets, fresh-frozen plasma (coagulation factors and antithrombin III), and cryoprecipitate (fibrinogen, factor VIII). Red blood cell transfusions are provided as needed to maintain oxygen delivery. Incremental increases in platelet count and fibrinogen levels indicate that consumption has diminished and therapies are effective.

Previously, an antifibrinolytic agent, epsilon-aminocaproic acid, was empirically used to treat DIC. The rationale for antifibrinolytic therapy was based on the contribution of ongoing fibrinolysis and fibrin(ogen) degradation products to hemorrhage. Anecdotal documentation of favorable response exists,[16] but there are also cases of fatal thrombosis following the use of epsilon-aminocaproic acid in DIC, and there is little support for antifibrinolytic therapy in DIC at this time.[11,19] In fact, thrombolytic agents have been suggested as potentially beneficial in managing DIC, although clinical trials have not been done.[13]

Given the broad spectrum of pathologies that may trigger DIC, the variable presentation and severity of DIC in individual patients, and the lack of agreement of a diagnostic definition of DIC, appropriate clinical trials to establish the efficacy of therapies are difficult. There is a growing body of information about DIC in sepsis.[14] Consequently, clinical management of DIC at this time is largely based on a case-by-case judgment of the patient's response to treatments directed at the primary process. Ongoing organ dysfunction due to thrombus-induced ischemia indicates a need for anticoagulation. Currently, heparin is the first choice, although other anticoagulants may provide options in the future. Hemorrhage is managed with blood component therapy.

ASSESSMENT

PARAMETER	ANTICIPATED ALTERATION
Platelet count	Decreased: $<100{,}000/mm^3$ *because circulating platelets are activated, aggregate, and are destroyed*
APTT	Prolonged: >30 to 40 seconds
PT	Prolonged: >12.5 seconds
Thrombin time	Prolonged: >15 seconds or >5 seconds of control *All prolonged because decreased circulating levels of coagulation proteins and circulating fibrin(ogen) degradation products prolong all "timed" tests of blood coagulation*
Fibrinogen	Decreased: <150 mg/dl *due to the potential that the patient's baseline fibrinogen level may be increased as part of the disease process or inflammatory response. Initial measurements of fibrinogen may not be absolutely decreased, but serial readings should reflect diminishing amounts.*
Fibrin degradation products (FDPs)	Increased (normal values vary with measurement method used) *due to ongoing fibrinolysis*
D-dimer	Elevated: usually >500 μg/L *due to plasmin degradation of cross-linked fibrin. Elevated levels indicate both thrombin and plasmin activity*
Soluble fibrin	Increased: (normal values vary with measurement method used) *due to fibrin monomers complex with FDPs in DIC, preventing polymerization and resulting in detectable blood levels. Quantitative analysis of soluble fibrin may be useful for diagnosis of DIC*[5]
Antithrombin III	Decreased: <80% *due to depletion*
Hgb	Decreased: <12 g/dl *due to hemorrhage*
Hct	Decreased: <37 g/dl *due to hemorrhage*
RBC	Fragmented cells, histiocytes *due to red cell damage as red cells pass through small vessels clogged with fibrin strands*
Skin	Ecchymosis, petechiae, purpura, hematoma, and (rarely) necrosis
Other	Overt or occult appearance of blood in urine or gastric aspirate Oozing of blood from mucous membranes Signs and symptoms related to the causative disease process or organ failure caused by DIC

PLAN OF CARE

INTENSIVE PHASE

The intensive care phase of the patient with DIC is directed at identifying and treating the underlying pathology, providing support for dysfunctional organ systems, controlling hemorrhage, and monitoring the progression/regression of DIC. Patient outcome will depend on the primary disease etiology, the rapidity of treatment, and the extent of organ system damage. Fulminant DIC and multisystem organ failure are associated with a high mortality. Patient care during this phase includes emotional support to the patient and family as they face decisions regarding continuance of aggressive therapies.

PATIENT CARE PRIORITIES	EXPECTED PATIENT OUTCOMES
Intravascular volume deficit *r/t uncontrolled hemorrhage and inability to form and maintain protective clot*	Adequate intravascular volume with normal cardiac filling pressures, CO, VS
Decreased tissue perfusion *r/t clot formation in the microvasculature*	Preservation of optimal organ function
Pain *r/t tissue ischemia, bruising, hematoma, invasive procedures*	Relief of pain
Inadequate nutrition *r/t high metabolic needs, intubation*	Sufficient intake to meet needs Maintain lean body wt
Impaired physical mobility *r/t ischemia to limbs and deconditioning from bed rest*	Maintain mobility
High risk for injury *r/t altered hemostasis*	Absence of traumatic bleeding (such as from vascular puncture or repositioning)
Decisional conflict regarding continuing life support measures *r/t desire to sustain patient life in the face of high probability for poor outcome*	Aware of probable outcomes Emotional and spiritual support for decision making
High risk for renal failure, skin breakdown, respiratory failure *r/t organ dysfunction*	Maintenance of organ function Preservation of skin integrity

INTERVENTIONS

Replace lost intravascular volume with crystalloid solutions.

Administer prescribed blood components per institutional protocol.

Minimize trauma, including punctures, suctioning, and transfers, *to reduce blood loss into skin and mucous membranes.*

Use intravascular catheters for blood draws for laboratory analysis *to reduce punctures.*

Use minimun discard volume when drawing blood for laboratory analysis from vascular catheters *to reduce iatrogenic blood loss.*

Use compressible sites (such as brachial or femoral rather than subclavian) for placement of hemodynamic monitoring catheters or other punctures.

Take BP only when necessary and inflate cuff only as needed to obtain accurate reading *to prevent pressure trauma from the cuff.*

When suctioning, do not extend suction catheter beyond the artificial airway *to prevent trauma to the trachea.*

Test all aspirations, secretions, and drainage for occult blood.

Monitor and report changes in Hgb, Hct, and coagulation profile that reflect blood loss or changes in patient's hemostatic capability.

Monitor I/O.

Monitor laboratory tests for signs of decreased renal, respiratory, and hepatic function.

Administer heparin as prescribed.

Monitor fibrinogen levels *to determine effectiveness of heparin and monitor for increased bleeding with initiation of heparin. Traditional monitoring with APTT may not be appropriate in these patients with already prolonged APTT. Increases in fibrinogen levels reflect ablation of ongoing DIC.*

Plan of Care (cont'd)

Monitor for skin breakdown and necrosis.
Position to relieve pressure to skin.
Evaluate for specialty mattress to reduce pressure to skin.
Reposition patient frequently.
Use extreme caution when repositioning, transporting patient *to prevent trauma to soft tissue.*
Pad side rails of bed *to protect against trauma from patient contact with hard surfaces.*
Administer analgesics/sedatives as needed *to relieve pain and promote rest.*
Collaborate with physical therapy to establish activities that prevent deconditioning but minimize patient trauma and fatigue.
Collaborate with nutrition services to determine caloric needs and establish best means of meeting needs.
Provide nutrition via enteral route if possible *to prevent gut mucosal atrophy, reduce risk of stress-related mucosal damage, and prevent constipation.*
Provide frequent, gentle oral care. Avoid alcohol-containing mouthwashes *to prevent mucosal drying and damage.*
Avoid taking temperatures rectally and using suppositories *to prevent damage to rectal mucosa.*
Establish bowel protocol *to prevent constipation.*

INTERMEDIATE PHASE

The patient surviving acute, severe DIC may have few residual effects or may have a prolonged critical illness, depending on the underlying pathology. However, the ongoing cycle of DIC should have been interrupted. Care during this phase is directed at ongoing support of dysfunctional organ systems and efforts to return the patient to a premorbid state of activity and self-care. For a small subset of patients who suffer from symmetrical peripheral gangrene there will also be issues of body image and loss of necrotic digits, limbs, and skin.[18]

PATIENT CARE PRIORITIES	EXPECTED PATIENT OUTCOMES
Inadequate nutrition *r/t high metabolic needs*	Intake of sufficient nutrition to meet needs Wt within patient norms
Activity intolerance *r/t deconditioning*	Increased mobility and endurance
Failure to wean from organ supports such as hemodialysis or mechanical ventilation *r/t deconditioning or permanent organ damage*	Adequate renal and pulmonary function
Altered body image *r/t possible loss of digits, extremeties to ischemia*	Grieve loss of body image, digits, limbs Begins rehabilitative adjustment

INTERVENTIONS

Continue to provide nutrition via parenteral or enteral route until oral intake adequate.
Collaborate with physical therapy *to establish a schedule of increased activity. Patients with symmetrical peripheral gangrene may require special assistive devices, such as splints, casts, or prostheses.*
Talk with patient/family about rehabilitative needs if there is loss of digits or limbs, or if an extended period of reconditioning is necessary.
Identify normal reactions to loss—depression, anger, fear, withdrawal.
Identify and enlist supports for patient and family that will facilitate appropriate grieving, coping, and general recovery.

TRANSITION TO DISCHARGE

The patient who survives the acute and intermediate phases of DIC will usually be cared for outside of the critical care environment. Organ systems, such as the renal and respiratory systems, should be functioning adequately without support. Nursing care focuses on reversal of deconditioning and rehabilitative needs for patients suffering loss of digits or limbs.

REFERENCES

1. Aderka D: Role of tumor necrosis factor in the pathogenesis of intravascular coagulopathy of sepsis: potential new therapeutic implications, *Isr J Med Sci* 27:52, 1991.
2. Al-Mondhiry H: Disseminated intravascular coagulation, *Thrombos Diathes Haemorrh* 34:181, 1975.
3. Bick RL, Baker WF: Disseminated intravascular coagulation syndromes, *Hematol Pathol* 6:1, 1992.
4. Blauhut B, et al: Substitution of antithrombin III in shock and DIC: a randomized study, *Thromb Res* 39:81, 1985.
5. Bredbacka S, et al: Laboratory methods for detecting disseminated intravascular coagulation (DIC): new aspects, *Acta Anaesthesol Scand* 37:125, 1993.
6. Colman RW, Robboy SJ, Minna JD: Disseminated intravascular coagulation (DIC): an approach, *Am J Med* 52:679, 1972.
7. Dahmash NS, Chowdhury MNH, Fayed DF: Septic shock in critically ill patients: etiology, management, and outcome, *J Infect* 26:159, 1993.
8. Dutoit HJ, Coetzee AR, Chalton DO: Heparin treatment in thrombin-induced disseminated intravascular coagulation in the baboon, *Crit Care Med* 19:1195, 1991.
9. Fourrier F, et al: Septic shock, multiple organ failure, and disseminated intravascular coagulation, *Chest* 101:816, 1992.
10. Fourrier F, et al: Double-blind, placebo-controlled trial of antithrombin III concentrates in septic shock with disseminated intravascular coagulation, *Chest* 104:882, 1993.
11. Gralnick HR, Griepp P: Thrombosis with epsilon aminocaproic acid therapy, *Am J Clin Pathol* 56:151, 1971.
12. Green D, et al: The role of heparin in the management of consumptive coagulopathy, *Med Clin North Am* 56:193, 1972.
13. Hardaway A, Adams WH: Blood clotting problems in acute care, *Acute Care* 14-15:138, 1988-1989.
14. Levi M, et al: Pathogenesis of disseminated intravascular coagulation in sepsis, *JAMA* 270:975, 1993.
15. Mant MJ, King EG: Severe, acute disseminated intravascular coagulation, *Am J Med* 67:557, 1979.
16. Marder VJ, Matchett MO, Sherry S: Detection of serum fibrinogen and fibrin degradation products, *Am J Med* 51:71, 1971.
17. Marder VJ, et al: Consumptive thrombohemorrhagic disorders. In Colman RW, et al, editors: *Hemostasis and thrombosis*, Philadelphia, 1987, JB Lippincott, pp 975-1015.
18. Molos MA, Hall JC: Symmetrical peripheral gangrene and disseminated intravascular coagulation, *Arch Dermatol* 121:1057, 1985.
19. Naeye RL: Thrombotic state after a hemorrhagic diathesis, a possible complication of therapy with epsilon aminocaproic acid, *Blood* 19:694, 1962.
20. Nowak G, Markwardt G: Hirudin in disseminated intravascular coagulation, *Haemostasis* 21(suppl):42, 1991.
21. Robboy SJ, Colman RW, Minna JD: Pathology of disseminated intravascular coagulation (DIC), *Hum Pathol* 3:327, 1972.
22. Siegal T, et al: Clinical and laboratory aspects of disseminated intravascular coagulation (DIC): a study of 118 cases, *Thromb Haemost* 39:122, 1978.
23. *St Anthony's DRG guidebook 1995*, Reston, Va, 1994, St Anthony.
24. Zbilut JP: Incidence of disseminated intravascular coagulation in patients admitted through the emergency department: a 5 year retrospective study, *Heart Lung* 9:833, 1980.

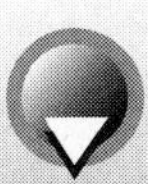

CLINICAL GUIDELINE

60

Human Immunodeficiency Virus (HIV) and Acquired Immunodeficiency Syndrome (AIDS)

Debbie Tribett, MS, RN, CCRN

DESCRIPTION

In the early 1980s, health care professionals were introduced to a new, ultimately fatal syndrome of severe immune system compromise. This syndrome was called the acquired immunodeficiency syndrome (AIDS). Subsequent years of intensive scientific research resulted in the discovery of the cause of this syndrome: infection by a virus, which eventually was designated human immunodeficiency virus (HIV or HIV-1). A second strain of HIV has been identified and is indicated as HIV-2.

Today, health care workers often erroneously use the term AIDS interchangeably with HIV infection. Although all patients with AIDS are infected with HIV, all patients infected with HIV do not have AIDS. HIV represents a spectrum of disease from the acute onset of primary infection, asymptomatic seroconversion, a latent yet contagious period of variable length, manifestation of declining immune function, to the development of severe opportunistic infection, cancer, and/or deterioration of the nervous system.

The first manifestations of AIDS were seen in male homosexuals in the United States. However, HIV has become a worldwide epidemic affecting all ages and races, and both sexes. Transmission does not occur by casual contact, but through sexual intercourse via semen and vaginal secretions, use of intravenous (IV) needles contaminated with HIV-infected blood, transfusion of HIV-contaminated blood or blood products, or from mother to baby either during the perinatal period or by way of breast milk. Transmission through transplantation of tissue and organs from HIV-infected individuals has occurred.

High-risk groups for the development of HIV infection include homosexual or bisexual males, IV drug users, and participants in unprotected heterosexual, bisexual, or homosexual intercourse with a known HIV-positive person.

The number of cases associated with IV drug use and heterosexual transmission has been increasing in this country.[5] A disproportionate number of AIDS patients in the United States continue to be black and Hispanic.[5] Transmission of HIV via blood or blood product transfusion has been limited since the 1985 implementation of HIV testing of all donated blood and stringent donor screening processes.[5] There are geographical differences in the distribution of cases of AIDS in this country. Urban areas with large populations have a higher prevalence than rural areas.[6]

In 1989, the latest year for which final mortality data are

available, the third leading cause of death for persons ages 25 to 44 was HIV infection.[22] HIV was the second leading cause of death in men and the sixth leading cause of death in women in this age group.[22]

From 1981 to 1989, 100,000 cases of AIDS were reported in the United States.[5] In the two-year period from 1990 through 1991, an additional 100,000 cases were reported, dramatically increasing the total number of AIDS cases.[5] In 1993, the Centers for Disease Control (CDC) revised the classification of HIV infection (Table 60-1). This is likely to increase the statistics for 1993 due to the expanded inclusion criteria.

Projections from the CDC indicate that by 1994, a cumulative total of between 415,000 and 535,000 cases of AIDS will be diagnosed; 134,000 to 228,000 people will be living with AIDS; and between 330,000 and 385,000 deaths from AIDS will have occurred.[4] An estimated 500,000 to 900,000 people were HIV seropositive as of January 1991.

HIV infection and AIDS have raised profound moral, ethical, legal, social, political, and scientific dilemmas. Because the disease is associated with behaviors that are not generally socially acceptable, the psychological effects on its victims are as overwhelming as the pathophysiological. The economic effects can be devastating to persons with HIV, and the burden on the limited health care budgets of this country is huge. However, identification of HIV and over a decade of clinical experience with this disease have

TABLE 60-1 1993 Revised CDC Categories for HIV Infection and Expanded Case Definitions for AIDS

CD4+ T lymphocyte counts

Category	CD4+ absolute count	CD4+ percentage (%)
1	>500 cells/μL	>29
2	200-499 cells/μL	14-28
3	<200 cells/μL	<14
Normal reference	600-1200 cells/μL	34-67

Clinical condition categories

Category A

Asymptomatic HIV infection
Persistent generalized lymphadenopathy
Acute primary HIV infection with accompanying illness or history of acute infection

Category B

Bacillary angiomatosis
Candidiasis, oropharyngeal (thrush)
Candidiasis, vulvovaginal: persistent, frequent, or poorly responsive to therapy
Cervical dysplasia (moderate or severe)/cervical cancer in situ
Constitutional symptoms, such as fever (38.5° C) or diarrhea lasting >1 month
Oral hairy leukoplakia
Herpes zoster (shingles) involving at least two distinct episodes or more than one dermatome
Idiopathic thrombocytopenic purpura
Listeriosis
Pelvic inflammatory disease, particularly if complicated by tubo-ovarian abscess
Peripheral neuropathy

Category C

Candidiasis of esophagus, bronchi, trachea, or lungs
Invasive cervical cancer

Category C—cont'd

Coccidioidomycosis, disseminated or extrapulmonary
Cryptococcosis, extrapulmonary
Cryptosporidiosis, chronic intestinal (>1 month duration)
Cytomegalovirus disease (other than liver, spleen, or nodes)
Cytomegalovirus retinitis with loss of vision
HIV-related encephalopathy
Herpes simplex: chronic ulcers >1 month duration, bronchitis, pneumonitis, or esophagitis
Histoplasmosis, disseminated or extrapulmonary
Isosporiasis, chronic intestinal >1 month duration
Kaposi's sarcoma
Lymphoma: Burkitt's, immunoblastic, or primary of brain
Mycobacterium avium complex, or *M. kansasii,* disseminated or extrapulmonary
M. tuberculosis, any site pulmonary or extrapulmonary
Mycobacterium, other species or unidentified species, disseminated or extrapulmonary
Pneumocystis carinii pneumonia
Recurrent pneumonia
Progressive multifocal leukoencephalopathy
Recurrent salmonellosis septicemia
Toxoplasmosis of brain
HIV wasting syndrome

Center for Disease Control: 1993 revised classification for HIV infection and expanded surveillance case definition for AIDS among adolescents and adults. *MMWR*, 41:RR-17, 1992.

demonstrated the risk of occupational transmission of HIV to health care workers to be extremely small, less than 1%.[16]

Since 1982 the CDC has recommended precautions when handling blood and body fluids. In 1987 the CDC issued guidelines for universal precautions in treating all patients.[8] Federal mandates from the Occupational Safety and Health Administration (OSHA) specify the types of protective equipment to be used and the responsibility of employees and employers in prevention of occupational spread of blood-borne pathogens.[13]

Although the majority of opportunistic infections seen in patients with HIV and AIDS are not transmissible to health care workers with a normal immune system, there is one infection that may be transmitted via inhalation of droplet nuclei to those caring for HIV/AIDS patients—*M. tuberculosis* (TB).

The CDC guidelines addressing prevention of transmission of TB in hospitals include respiratory isolation for suspected or known cases, use of personal respirators by persons involved in the care of such patients, and specific environmental considerations.[9] Nurses who have frequent contact with patients with TB should be skin tested every 6 months; otherwise annual testing is required.[9]

Any patient admitted to an intensive care unit (ICU) for any reason may be HIV-infected. Therefore, following universal precautions is of the utmost importance in the highly unpredictable setting of the ICU, and with the frequent use of invasive procedures in care of the critically ill patient.

Testing for HIV should not be used as a substitute for the implementation of universal precautions or other infection-control measures.[10] However, when obtaining an assessment nursing data base, the health care team should ask patients about their risks for HIV infection. Patients at risk should be offered HIV counseling and testing. Maintaining patient confidentiality is essential, and patients should provide informed consent for testing in accordance with local laws.[10]

PATHOPHYSIOLOGY

HIV is classified as a retrovirus. A retrovirus must invade a cell and use its nucleic acids for replication. The HIV has an affinity for cells with the CD4 surface marker. The T4 or helper lymphocyte carries the CD4 surface marker and thus becomes the primary target for HIV in the human body. Once the target cell is invaded by HIV, it remains infected for the lifetime of the cell. Macrophages/monocytes also may be invaded by HIV, but seem to survive, thus contributing to lifetime infection with HIV.

Normal CD4+ T lymphocytes coordinate many important immune system functions. They regulate cell-mediated immunity protecting against viral, fungal, protozoal, and slow-growing bacterial infection. These cells are also responsible for immunological surveillance and subsequent destruction of abnormal or tumor cells that are detected within the body. The T lymphocytes also activate B lymphocytes, which are responsible for antibody production or humoral immunity.

CD4+ T lymphocytes infected with HIV eventually die as the virus replicates itself. Loss of CD4+ T lymphocytes causes impaired immune system function. Gradual, progressive, irreversible immunodeficiency manifests in the development of opportunistic viral, fungal, protozoal, and slow-growing bacterial infections. Kaposi's sarcoma, lymphomas, and invasive cervical cancer are malignancies that develop. Increased antibody production may occur due to loss of the modulating effects of the T4 lymphocytes on B lymphocytes. These antibodies may be nonspecific and lead to the development of autoimmune disease. T lymphocyte dysfunction may increase the risk for development of hypersensitivity reactions to medications seen in the HIV patient.[20]

Nervous system tissue such as neurons, microglial cells, Schwann cells, and dendritic cells are infected by HIV. Central and peripheral nervous system deterioration can result from HIV infection, leading to a wide range of neurological manifestations that include dementia, peripheral neuropathy, paresthesias, and muscle weakness. Autonomic nervous system effects may result in disruptions in regulatory mechanisms of heart rate and blood pressure.[20]

After initial infection with HIV, production of HIV-specific antibody usually occurs within 6 to 12 weeks. Nearly all patients will seroconvert within 3 to 6 months after HIV transmission.[2] Testing during the period between acute infection and antibody production may be negative, but the individual is infected and considered contagious. Repeated positive HIV testing with the enzyme-linked immunosorbent assay (ELISA) and confirmation with a Western Blot or immunofluorescence assay (IFA) is the most common test for HIV infection. However, the CDC also includes viral isolation, HIV antigen detection, or a positive result on any other highly specific licensed test for HIV as criteria for HIV infection.[11]

Studies have shown that less than 5% of HIV-positive patients develop AIDS within 2 years of infection, 20% to 25% develop AIDS within 6 years, and 50% progress to AIDS in 10 years.[7] The advantage of knowing HIV status is to institute early medical management of the condition, thus potentially slowing the effects of HIV, and to begin prophylaxis for opportunistic infections. Informing HIV-positive patients of their status and counseling them on high-risk behaviors may prevent further HIV transmission.

The CDC recently revised its classification for HIV of infected adolescents (>13 years old) and adults to include three CD4+ T lymphocyte categories, and three categories of clinical conditions associated with HIV infection (Table 60-1). These categories create a matrix of nine mutually exclusive groups for classification purposes. Patients with absolute CD4+ T lymphocyte counts of <200/μL or a percentage of <14 who manifest clinical conditions in category A, B, or C meet the case definition of AIDS.[11] The new classification reflects the importance of the loss of CD4+ T lymphocytes in predicting the risk and severity of opportunistic infection.

Physical wasting also may occur in the HIV patient. The wasting syndrome is characterized by profound loss of greater than 10% of baseline body weight, chronic weakness with intermittent or constant fever, and chronic diarrhea (two or more loose stools per day for 30 days or more) that cannot be attributed to any other cause.[11] It is the second most commonly reported AIDS diagnosis. The wasting syndrome may precede the manifestation of opportunistic infection or malignancy. However, past attempts to reverse cachexia in AIDS patients by the use of drugs and nutritional therapy generally have been unsuccessful.[21]

Complications of HIV infection begin to surface as immune system dysfunction progresses. Table 1 lists the multitude of medical diagnoses that are indicative of AIDS. Some of these conditions may result in admission to an ICU. Opportunistic pulmonary infection or cancer may lead to respiratory failure. Opportunistic infection may lead to sepsis and progress to septic shock. Gastrointestinal (GI) problems may lead to severe fluid and electrolyte imbalances, causing dysrhythmias or hypovolemia. Opportunistic infection, HIV infection, or cancer may cause acute deterioration in neurological status, coma, or seizures. Congestive heart failure may develop secondary cardiomyopathy. Because of increased incidence of IV drug abuse and its connection to the spread of HIV infection, many HIV patients admitted to the ICU may be IV drug abusers. Endocarditis and cardiac valve dysfunction may lead to cardiovascular compromise, necessitating ICU admission. AIDS is a multisystem disease that may involve every organ system. Critical care admission is most likely to be required for pulmonary infections, central nervous system infections, and bacterial sepsis.[2]

LENGTH OF STAY/ANTICIPATED COURSE

In the 1990s, HIV-AIDS has evolved into a more manageable chronic disease process as antiviral drugs have been developed to slow the process of the infection, and drugs to treat some of the opportunistic infections have become available.[17]

The anticipated length of stay or clinical course of the HIV patient is determined by the condition of the individual patient and the specific type of problems manifested. HIV falls within DRG 488: HIV with extensive OR procedure, with an average length of stay of 21.5 days; DRG 489: HIV with major related conditions, with an average length of stay of 12.5 days; and DRG 490: HIV with or without related conditions, with an average length of stay of 8.0 days.[24]

In general, severe or life-threatening opportunistic infections are rare with CD4 cell counts $>300/mm^3$, uncommon with CD4 cell counts $>200/mm^3$, common with CD4 cell counts $<100/mm^3$, and associated with lethal complications when CD4 cell counts are $<50/mm^3$.[2]

Response to the primary onset of an infection may be more favorable than if the patient has suffered multiple exacerbations of an infection. Patients exhibiting HIV wasting syndrome with loss of 20% of their baseline body weight have a significant decrease in survival.[21] The type and location of infection may affect the outcome of the patient. Some opportunistic infections, such as cytomegalovirus, do not have FDA-approved drug therapy available for treatment (other than for retinitis). The increased incidence of severe side effects from medication regimens also influences length of stay and patient outcome.

MANAGEMENT TRENDS AND CONTROVERSIES

The goals of research related to HIV disease and AIDS over the past 10 years have included development of effective antiviral therapies for HIV, development of drug therapies for opportunistic infections, and HIV-related malignancies, restoration of normal immune system function, and development of a vaccine effective in preventing HIV infection. Much has been learned about HIV, and many new drug therapies have emerged. Encouraging progress remains overshadowed by the fact that no cure is available for HIV, transmission is on the rise, and vaccine development is still in early trials. The new drugs designed for treating HIV and opportunistic infections seem only to slow or suppress disease manifestation, eventually becoming ineffective, and they are not without significant side effects or toxicities. These new drugs also are very expensive and often have limited routes of administration.

Because of increased survival rates among patients with AIDS-related diseases treated in ICUs, each patient should be informed of the potential benefits of ICU admission and therapies for the individual's specific condition.

Although the cause of patient problems may be unique to HIV or unusual opportunistic infections, medical care provided in the ICU to treat the patient is generally the same as it would be for other causes of the same problem. For example, congestive heart failure is treated with digitalis, diuretics, vasodilators, and limited activity. Acute respiratory failure may be treated with oxygen, intubation, mechanical ventilation, and positive end-expiratory pressure. If an infection is present, its etiology is identified, and appropriate antimicrobial therapy is instituted for the microorganism. Unfortunately, for patients with HIV, fewer choices of therapies exist to treat their infections.

Antiretroviral therapy (anti-HIV drugs) approved by the FDA at the time of publication include zidovudine (formerly known as AZT), dideoxyinosine (ddI), and dideoxycytidine (ddC). All HIV-positive patients with a CD4 cell count of $<500/mm^3$ should receive zidovudine. As the patient's immunologic condition worsens, combination therapy with ddC is recommended. When patients develop dose-limiting toxicity to zidovudine or significant clinical or immunological deterioration, ddI may be instituted. Research continues on a variety of new anti-HIV agents as well as combination therapies with the currently approved agents.

The major dose-limiting toxicity of zidovudine is on bone marrow, producing anemia, neutropenia, or thrombocytopenia. Each may occur singly or in combination. Therapy with recombinant human erythropoietin is approved for use in HIV patients with zidovudine-induced anemia. Myopathy also may be seen from zidovudine. Side effects of ddI include pancreatitis and peripheral neuropathy. An increased sodium load from the buffers in the drug may cause fluid and electrolyte imbalances. Moderate to severe peripheral neuropathy and pancreatitis result from ddC.

Kaposi's sarcoma (KS) was one of the first clinical manifestations of AIDS. Its incidence has decreased to about 11% to 15% for reasons that are not clear.[2,18] It may range from a few cutaneous lesions affecting the patient's body image to a fulminant spread involving the viscera such as the GI tract, respiratory system, and heart. Critical care of patients with KS may be related to respiratory obstruction or failure, or to GI obstruction or bleeding. KS of internal organs is associated with a poor prognosis.[14]

Treatment varies with the stage and location of lesions. Local treatment with laser therapy, cryotherapy, intralesion injection of vinblastine, or radiation may be effective.[12] However, systemic therapy with alpha interferon in combination with zidovudine or IV chemotherapy with vinblastine, bleomycin, and/or adriamycin may be required with multiple, large, or extensive internal lesions.[12] Systemic treatment with chemotherapy has the associated risks of bone marrow suppression with a negative impact on immune and hematologic system function. Current research includes therapies with inhibitors of new blood vessel growth called angiogenesis inhibitors, and gentler methods of chemotherapy administration in the form of liposomes.[12]

AIDS-related lymphomas seem to develop systemically in patients with CD4+ counts of <200 cells/mm^3, and in the central nervous system with counts of approximately 30 cells/mm^3.[12] These malignancies are aggressive, high-grade, and usually of B-cell origin. Systemic chemotherapy and radiation have been used with some initial success, but most patients relapse and have a poor overall survival rate.[23]

These patients differ from other patients receiving systemic chemotherapy in that they have little chance of regaining normal immune system function after chemotherapy due to their underlying HIV disease. Their risk for opportunistic infection persists. Research continues to identify mechanisms for the triggering of HIV-related lymphomas and in chemotherapy regimens in combination with zidovudine.

Opportunistic infection (OI) caused by a variety of organisms is the most likely reason for ICU admission for patients with HIV and AIDS. The infection will likely be severe, affecting the respiratory, neurological, and GI systems, or producing sepsis and/or septic shock. Table 60-2 lists the most frequent types of organisms causing OI and the sites where these infections most often occur.

Prevention of OI is difficult because many of the organisms are ubiquitous, and previous infection may be reactivated secondary to the impaired immune function in this patient population. Nonetheless, prevention of OI is a major

TABLE 60-2 Opportunistic Infection Seen in HIV/AIDS Patients

Organism	Clinical presentation
Viral	
Herpes simplex type I and II	Mucocutaneous Esophagitis Bronchitis Pneumonitis
Herpes zoster	Dermatomal skin
Cytomegalovirus (CMV)	Retinitis Pneumonia Colitis
JC-type Polyomavirus	Progressive multifocal leukoencephalopathy (PML)
Fungal	
Candida albicans	Oropharyngeal (thrush) Vaginitis Esophagitis Bronchitis Tracheitis Pneumonia
Cryptococcus neoformans	Meningitis Disseminated
Coccidioidomycosis	Disseminated
Histoplasmosis	Disseminated
Protozoal	
Pneumocystis carinii	Pneumonia
Toxoplasma gondii	Encephalitis
Cryptosporidium	Enteritis
Isospora belli	Enteritis
Bacterial	
M. tuberculosis	Pneumonia Disseminated
M. avium complex (MAC)	Disseminated
Salmonella	Diarrhea Sepsis

TABLE 60-3 Relationship of CD4+ Count and Opportunistic Infection (OI) in HIV Patients

Absolute CD4+ lymphocyte count	Type of OI
>500 cells/μL	*M. tuberculosis*
200 cells/μL	*Pneumocystis carinii* pneumonia (PCP)
100-200 cells/μL	Toxoplasmosis
>100 cells/μL	*Cryptococcal* meningitis Candidiasis Cytomegalovirus retinitis
>50 cells/μL	*M. avium* complex (MAC)

concern in managing HIV-infected patients. The total number of CD4+ lymphocytes is often helpful in predicting occurrence of a particular OI[15] (Table 60-3). Prophylaxis for infections likely to occur can be instituted as CD4+ counts decrease.

Pneumocystis carinii pneumonia (PCP) has been and continues to be the most common lethal OI in patients with AIDS. Without preventative measures, approximately 80% of patients with advanced HIV disease will develop PCP.[1] Any HIV-positive patient with a CD4 cell count of <200/mm^3 should receive primary prophylaxis, and any patient with a history of PCP should be on secondary prophylaxis.[1] The drug of choice is trimethoprim-sulfamethoxazole (TMP-SMX). Alternative therapy with aerosolized pentamidine or dapsone is an option when TMP-SMX side effects are not tolerated by the patient.

The ubiquitous protozoa *P. carinii* gains entry to the body by inhalation into the lungs. The immunocompromised state of the patient with AIDS allows previously acquired PCP to grow unchallenged by normal host defenses in the alveoli. Cysts of *P. carinii* form and lodge in the alveoli and interstitial spaces of the lung, producing a barrier to perfusion of alveoli and disrupting normal surfactant production. Respiratory failure similar to that seen in the adult respiratory distress syndrome (ARDS) can develop.

Respiratory failure with refractory hypoxemia is treated with standard interventions used for ARDS. The PCP infection requires antibiotic therapy with TMP-SMX. Alternative drugs include TMP and dapsone, pentamidine, clindamycin, or clindamycin and primaquine. Patients with moderately severe or severe disease with Po_2 less than 70 mm Hg should receive adjunctive corticosteroids early in the course of treatment rather than as a salvage therapy later in the disease process. The anti-inflammatory effects of steroids on the alveoli improve oxygenation, and this benefit outweighs the potential dangers of giving steroids to an immunocompromised patient.

Mycobacterium tuberculosis (TB) is on the increase in the HIV patient population. It is most likely to occur early in the disease process when CD4+ cell counts are 500 or greater,[15] and especially in IV drug abusers.[2] Patients with HIV and a high risk for TB, such as IV drug users, the homeless, and migrant farm workers, are recommended to receive prophylaxis with isoniazid (INH) against TB.[2]

Treatment for HIV patients with confirmed TB includes polypharmacy with INH, rifampin, ethambutol, and pyrazinamide. If the strain of TB is susceptible to these drugs, patients respond well to standard therapy. There have been epidemic outbreaks of resistant strains of TB. Multiresistant strains of TB require aggressive therapy with drugs such as ciprofloxacin or olfoxacin.[1] Most HIV patients with resistant TB expired at a mean time of 4 to 16 weeks following the diagnosis.[1]

Mycobacterium avium complex (MAC) is a group of ubiquitous acid-fast bacilli occurring worldwide in soil, water, and animals. The bacterium gains entry into the body via the GI tract or respiratory tract. In 40% to 50% of persons with AIDS, it becomes a disseminated infection spreading to the liver, spleen, kidneys, bone marrow, or lymph nodes.

Prophylaxis against this infection is advocated with a CD4+ cell count of <100 to 150/mm^3.[1] Rifabutin is a drug recommended as prophylaxis for MAC.[19] Treatment of active infection with MAC requires multidrug therapy with at least three drugs mentioned in treating TB, which are active against the *Mycobacterium* species.[1]

The most frequently encountered CNS opportunistic infection is toxoplasmosis gondii, which affects an estimated 5% to 15% of patients with AIDS.[2] When the CD4+ count drops to 100 to 200, toxoplasmosis is likely to occur.[15] This is most likely a reactivation of a latent primary infection.

The infection manifests itself as encephalitis with focal intracerebral lesions. Patient symptoms may include headache, seizures, and mental status changes. Definitive diagnosis can be made only with a brain biopsy. Due to the inherent risks of this procedure, a presumptive diagnosis is made from magnetic resonance imaging (MRI) testing revealing multiple ring-enhancing lesions.

Empiric therapy with oral sulfadiazine and pyrimethamine are used with good patient response within 2 weeks.[2] Clindamycin also has shown promising results. Treatment of this infection is suppressive rather than curative. The patient must be maintained on suppressive therapy for life.

With CD4+ cell counts of 100 or less, cryptococcal meningitis is likely to occur.[15] The patient may experience typical meningitis symptoms; however, due to the patient's immunocompromised state, it is just as likely that they will be absent.[3]

Initial therapy is with IV amphotericin B, and 5-flucytosine is effective in the majority of cases. Because of frequent relapse, long-term maintenance therapy with fluconazole is required.

Although they are not diagnostic for AIDS, the role of acute bacterial infections generally has been underappreciated in HIV disease.[2] Many studies have shown that, collectively, bacterial infections are the most common cause of a fatal outcome in HIV patients.[2]

The most common pulmonary pathogens early in HIV disease are *S. pneumoniae* and, less commonly, *Haemophilus influenzae* and *Pseudomonas aeruginosa*. Infections associated with fatal outcome include pneumococcal pneumonia, salmonellosis, or infection by *P. aeruginosa* or *S. aureus*. Diagnosis, care, and drug therapy for the HIV patient with bacterial infection are analogous to those methods used to treat the same infection in other patient populations.

Diagnosis and management of OI in patients with AIDS is a challenge for health care professionals. This discussion is not inclusive of all the possibilities of OI, but reviews those most frequently occurring and that may directly relate to an ICU admission. Table 60-2 is a comprehensive listing of OI in patients with HIV and AIDS. Experience with the disease and new discoveries related to HIV infection and its sequelae require constant updating of treatment protocols for this patient population. This dynamic state will continue until a cure for HIV can be found.

ASSESSMENT

PARAMETER	ANTICIPATED ALTERATION
History	
HIV exposure	Sexually transmitted diseases Type and frequency of sexual activity (homosexual, bisexual, heterosexual, partner and IV drug user) Use of condoms during sexual activity Use of IV drugs Occupational injury related to blood, body fluids, or contaminated needle stick Blood or blood product transfusion and date received Organ/tissue transplant recipient and date received
Laboratory and Radionucleotide Tests	
CBC with differential	Anemia, leukopenia, leukocytosis, thrombocytopenia
Total lymphocyte count	Decreased: <500 cells/mm^3 *due to HIV infection*
CD4+ lymphocyte count	Decreased: <500 cells/mm^3 or $<29\%$ *due to HIV infection*
T4:T8 ratio	Decreased: <1 *due to loss of T4 cells*
HIV serology	Positive ELISA confirmed by Western Blot
PPD skin test	Positive or anergic
Electrolytes	Decreased Na^+, K^+, Cl^-, Mg^{++} *due to severe diarrhea*
Culture reports from sputum, blood, CSF, urine, tissue, and/or bronchoalveolar lavage	Positive for opportunistic organisms, TB, and/or other bacteria
Antibody titers	Positive for cryptococcal antigen Positive for hepatitis B antigen
ABG	Respiratory acidosis *due to effects of lung infection (i.e., PCP) and result of tachypnea* • Pa_{O_2} <80 mm Hg • Pa_{CO_2} <35 mm Hg Increased A-a D_{O_2}
Sp_{O_2}	Decreased: $<90\%$ with exertion
Chest x-ray	Bilateral interstitial infiltrates, lower lobe infiltrates, pleural effusion, consolidated lobar or bronchial pneumonia, cavitary lesions
Gallium scan	Diffuse uptake with PCP
MRI	Multiple ring-enhanced lesions *due to toxoplasmosis gondii*

General Status	
Wt	Decreased: >10% body wt
Temperature	Chronic fever >30 days, night sweats
Energy level	Chronic fatigue
Neurological Status	
Cognitive	Slowed verbal response, difficulty with problem solving, complex sequencing, and/or concentration, and memory loss
Motor	Imbalance, incoordination, difficulty with complex motor tasks, proximal muscle weakness, problems with rapid alternating movements, hypo-/hyperreflexia, flaccid paraparesis
Sensory	Painful peripheral neuropathy, cranial nerve palsies, visual disturbances/blindness
Psychological	Change in mood, decreased energy level, apathy, anorexia, morning insomnia, decreased libido, flat affect, social withdrawal
LOC	Reduced awareness, acute onset delirium, incoherent speech, coma
Other symptoms	Headache, nuchal rigidity, seizures, papilledema
Pulmonary Status	
RR	Tachypnea, dyspnea
Breath sounds	Bibasilar crackles, diffuse rales
Cough	Dry, nonproductive with PCP, may be productive with other infections
Pain	Pleuritic chest pain *due to lung infection, pleural effusion*
Cardiovascular Status	
HR	Tachycardia, irregular rhythm
ECG changes	Nonspecific ST and T wave changes, atrial ectopy, ventricular ectopy, electrical alternans
Heart sounds	S_3, murmurs, pericardial friction rub, muffled heart tones *due to CHF*
Peripheral vascular	Evidence of systemic thromboemboli, JVD, dependent edema
Hemodynamic changes	Hypotension must be differentiated as to its etiology (hypovolemia, sepsis, obstruction, congestive heart failure) by its association with other abnormal parameters (CVP, PCWP, CO/CI, SVR)
GI Status	
General	Anorexia, nausea, vomiting, dysphagia, chronic diarrhea
Oral mucosa	White patches, ulcers, red-purple nodules *due to opportunistic fungal infection*
Other	
Skin	Red-/purple-/brown-black nodules *due to KS* Vesicles *due to HS* Maculopapular lesions *due to drug reactions* Petechiae Fungal nail infection
Genitourinary	Ulcers *due to sexually transmitted disease, toxicities of drugs, Candida vaginitis* Proteinuria with increased BUN and decreased creatinine clearance
Lymphoreticular	Lymphadenopathy in two noncontiguous sites other than inguinal, hepatomegaly, splenomegaly

PLAN OF CARE

INTENSIVE PHASE

The intensive phase of management of a patient with HIV/AIDS will vary based on the multitude of reasons for ICU admission. The major goals of care in this phase are also based on the specific problems or conditions that the patient has regardless of the fact that the HIV infection may have been the precipitating factor. Therefore, refer to the specific guidelines associated with the appropriate priorities for more details. This care plan will provide an overview based on the underlying HIV/AIDS problem.

PATIENT CARE PRIORITIES	EXPECTED PATIENT OUTCOMES
Infection *r/t decreased immune capacity*	Resolution/remission of signs and symptoms of opportunistic infection Free of nosocomial infection
Impaired gas exchange *r/t* *Pneumonia* *Respiratory muscle weakness*	Lungs clear Respiratory pattern: WNL Spo_2 and ABG: WNL
Impaired skin integrity *r/t* *Poor nutrition* *Opportunistic infections*	Skin intact and free of infection, or infection controlled
Pain/general discomfort *r/t* *Disease process* *Multiple complications* *Infections*	Verbalizes acceptable comfort Able to sleep, rest, eat, and engage in ADL to optimal level Able to maintain social interactions
Inadequate nutrition *r/t* *Poor appetite* *Oral infection and pain* *GI distress* *Catabolic state*	Wt stable Oral intake maintains anabolic state Positive nitrogen balance Albumin: WNL
High risk for social isolation *r/t* *Stigma associated with HIV/AIDS* *Unrealistic fear of transmission of infection* *Need for extensive support*	Maintains interactions with friends and family Support systems are identified and integrated into patient care

INTERVENTIONS

Monitor for signs/symptoms of inflammation/infection.

Check T at regular intervals *to monitor for trend indicative of systemic inflammatory response.*

Interpret CBC with differential for elevations or decreases in WBC count with increased percentage of bands, neutropenia, or lymphopenia, *which indicate presence of acute infection or immunocompromise.*

Review trends in hemodynamic parameters to detect sepsis/septic shock, *such as increased HR, decreased BP, increased CO/CI, and decreased SVR.*

Observe for tachypnea, dyspnea, change in sputum characteristics, hypoxia, decreased Pco_2, and chest x-ray for infiltrates or consolidation *to detect respiratory infection.*

Observe LOC for changes or decreased mental status or decreased total Glasgow coma score, *which may indicate sepsis or neurological infection.*

Assess for UO <0.5 ml/kg/hr and increased lactic acid levels *to detect impaired tissue perfusion.*

At least once a day, inspect insertion sites of all invasive devices used in care and monitoring of patient *to detect localized signs of inflammation, infection, or tissue trauma.*

Inspect skin folds, axilla, groin, and perineal areas at least once a day *to detect skin irritation, breakdown, or infection.*

Plan of Care (cont'd)

Inspect oral cavity at least once a day *to detect lesions.*

Inspect any wounds or surgical incisions at least once a day *to detect changes in drainage or signs of infection.*

Palpate cervical, axillary, and inguinal lymph nodes at least once a day *to assess for enlargement or tenderness.*

Examine all secretions/excretions for changes causing suspicion of infection.

Assess patient for the presence of pain. *New onset of pain may be an early sign of infection in the immunocompromised host.*

Institute infection control measures *to prevent nosocomial infection.*

- Enforce handwashing before and after patient contact for all health care workers and visitors.
- Screen all health care workers and visitors for infectious illness prior to contact with patient. No one with fever, upper respiratory symptoms, diarrhea, open skin lesions, or recent exposure to childhood contagious diseases should care for or visit the patient.
- Institute isolation appropriate for any known or suspected patient infections.
- Adhere to strict aseptic technique in all invasive procedures and care of invasive IVs and monitoring devices *to prevent/detect infection.*
- Prohibit fresh flowers and plants from patient room *to limit reservoirs for organism growth.*
- Change fluids used in care of patient, or IV solutions, q24h *to minimize organism growth.*
- Collaborate with physicians and other health care workers to avoid unnecessary or minimize invasive procedures and venipunctures, *thus decreasing the risk for iatrogenic infection.*
- Obtain cultures of any suspicious drainage or patient secretions *to detect and differentiate organisms that may be a source of infection.*

Support adequate nutritional intake.

- Collaborate with dietitian, family, significant others to maximize oral intake of diet appropriate for patient condition, using HIV-specific nutritional supplements *to increase caloric intake, prevent wasting, and enhance immune system function.*
- Eliminate fresh uncooked fruits and vegetables from diet of neutropenic patients *to minimize introduction of potentially harmful organisms into the GI tract.*
- If patient condition prevents eating, attempt enteral nutrition, even at very low flow rates, *to attempt to prevent translocation of gut microorganisms into the circulation.*
- Collaborate with physician to institute peripheral or total parenteral nutrition *to supply adequate caloric intake in patients who cannot use their GI tract.*
- Monitor trend in daily wts *to assess fluid balance versus true wt gain/loss.*

Institute measures to support first-line or natural defenses *to minimize portals of entry for microorganisms into the internal environment of a compromised host.*

Maintain integrity of the skin.

- Reposition patient q2h.
- Lubricate skin *to prevent dryness.*
- Use protective devices (such as a special mattress or bed).
- Use skin protectants prior to using tape.
- Use adhesive remover prior to dressing removal.
- Use skin barriers for incontinent patients.
- Provide perineal care, and cleansing of axilla and other skin folds daily and as necessary.
- Use a blow dryer *to eliminate moisture from skin folds as needed.*
- Avoid using incontinence pads/diapers.
- Use scissors, electric razors, or depilatories for hair removal.

Avoid trauma to mucous membranes.

- Provide frequent oral care to NPO patient and after meals to those able to eat.
- Avoid alcohol-containing solutions for mouth care.

Plan of Care (cont'd)

- Use chlorhexadine mouth rinses in neutropenic patients.
- Cleanse nares and secure any nasal tubes to prevent pressure necrosis.
- Reposition oral endotracheal tubes daily and secure to prevent pressure necrosis.
- Do not use rectal T probes, rectal tubes, or suppositories. Avoid digital rectal exams to prevent trauma and potential site of infection.
- Collaborate with physicans for administration of gastric mucosa prophylaxis.

Maintain pulmonary toilet *to enhance normal cleansing function and minimize risk of iatrogenic respiratory infection.*

- Have non-intubated patient deep breathe and use incentive spirometer q2h while awake and immobilized.
- Follow deep breathing with coughing to mobilize secretions.
- Maintain airway humidification when administering O_2.
- Encourage patient hydration.

Maintain normal bowel and bladder elimination *to minimize risk for iatrogenic GI or genitourinary infection.*

- Implement individualized regimen *to prevent constipation or control diarrhea.*
- Encourage high fluid intake unless contraindicated by other patient problems.
- Provide activity as appropriate to patient condition.
- Use condom catheters and frequent scheduled offering of bedpan to incontinent patients rather than resorting to bladder catheterization or diapers.

Use patient-specific strategies to minimize stress/pain *to prevent increases in endogenous corticosteroid production, which decreases normal immune system function.*

Tailor visiting to encourage interaction with friends and family *to maintain sense of belonging and social acceptance.*

INTERMEDIATE PHASE

If the patient survives the intensive phase, recovery will depend on the event precipitating the ICU admission, the length of time in the intensive phase, the complications arising during the intensive care phase, and the patient's underlying immunological state. Maintaining pulmonary and hemodynamic stability with increasing activity will be the priorities for nursing care during the intermediate phase.

PATIENT CARE PRIORITIES	EXPECTED PATIENT OUTCOMES
Activity intolerance *r/t hypoxemia and deconditioning*	RR, HR, rhythm, BP within patient norms Absent diaphoresis Expresses tolerance of activity

INTERVENTIONS

Collaborate with physical therapist to gradually increase patient activity *to enhance exercise tolerance.*

Set realistic goals with patient and provide feedback regarding patient progress *to decrease patient anxiety.*

Monitor patient during and after activity *to detect evidence of onset of signs of hypoxemia/intolerance* (RR, dyspnea, dysrhythmias, diaphoresis, significant change in BP) and terminate activity at signs of intolerance.

Schedule activities to decrease energy expenditure and allow for rest periods after meals and between activities *to promote rest and regain strength.*

Maintain supplemental O_2 during activity *to enhance O_2 delivery.*

Collaborate with dietitian in planning caloric intake adequate for patient *to prevent increasing CO_2 production to reduce the stress of the pulmonary system for CO_2 removal.*

TRANSITION TO DISCHARGE

As the patient is transferred out of the critical care setting, the focus of nursing care will shift to prepare the patient for discharge and for future management of HIV-related disease. Often HIV patients have limited financial resources and psychosocial support systems. Collaboration with social services to identify available resources based on individual patient needs is necessary. In addition to HIV problems, the patient may require a drug rehabilitation program.

Preparation for home care may include planning for assistance with basic activities of daily living in addition to home management of HIV-related problems. Patient, family, and/or significant others may need extensive education regarding spread of HIV infection (e.g., safe sex practices, refraining from IV drug use), detection of opportunistic infection, and administration of a variety of medications with high risk of side effects. Some medication administration may require insertion of semipermanent venous access devices and use of continuous infusion pumps.

If the patient with HIV and AIDS has survived an ICU admission, and the subject of advance directives has not been addressed previously, it is appropriate to discuss these issues with the patient. If mentally competent to make such determinations, the patient should be provided information in order to make decisions regarding future care before his or her condition deteriorates any further. In states with health care proxy initiative, the patient may choose a surrogate decision maker instead of the legal next of kin. This is especially important with homosexual patients, where the patient's significant other would otherwise have no legal rights.

For some patients, transfer from the ICU setting may mean that the individual's condition is terminal and the focus of care is for comfort and emotional support of a dying person, the family, and significant others. It may be appropriate to involve hospice or specific local groups committed to the support of the terminal HIV patient. Collaboration with social services to find appropriate resources is necessary.

REFERENCES

1. Bartlett JG: *The Johns Hopkins Hospital guide to medical care of patients with HIV infection,* ed 3, Baltimore, Md, 1993, Williams & Wilkins.
2. Bartlett JG: Human immunodeficiency virus infection, *New Horizons* 1(2):20-21,24, 1993.
3. Beckham MM: Neurologic manifestations of AIDS, *Crit Care Nurs Clin North Am* 2(1):29-32, 1990.
4. Carr G: Opportunistic infections and pharmacology, *Crit Care Nurs Clin North Am* 4(3):395-400, 1992.
5. Centers for Disease Control: The second 100,000 cases of acquired immunodeficiency syndrome—United States, June 1981-1991, *MMRW Morb Mortal Wkly Rep,* Jan 17, 1992, pp 28-29.
6. Centers for Disease Control: Quarterly AIDS map, *MMRW Morb Mortal Wkly Rep* 42(3), January 29, 1993.
7. Centers for Disease Control: Projections of the number of persons diagnosed with AIDS and the number of immunosuppressed HIV-infected persons—United States, 1992-1994, *MMRW Morb Mortal Wkly Rep* 41(RR-18), 1992.
8. Centers for Disease Control: Recommendations for prevention of HIV transmission in health-care settings, *MMRW Morb Mortal Wkly Rep* 36(3S), 1987.
9. Centers for Disease Control: Guidelines for preventing the transmission of tuberculosis in health-care settings, with special focus on HIV-related issues, *MMRW Morb Mortal Wkly Rep* 39(RR-17), 1990.
10. Centers for Disease Control: Recommendations for HIV testing services for inpatients and outpatients in acute-care hospital settings, *MMRW Morb Mortal Wkly Rep* 42(RR-2), 1993.
11. Centers for Disease Control: 1993 revised classification system for HIV infection and expanded surveillance case definition for AIDS among adolescents and adults, *MMRW Morb Mortal Wkly Rep* 41(RR-17), 1992.
12. Coulter A: Treating Kaposi's sarcoma with angiogenesis inhibitors and other chemotherapies, *AIDS Patient Care* 6(6):270-272 1992.
13. Federal Register: Occupational exposure to bloodborne pathogens: final rule, 29 CFR Part 1910.1030, 1991.
14. Flaskerud JH, Ungvrski PJ: *HIV/AIDS: a guide to nursing care,* ed 2, Philadelphia, 1992, WB Saunders.
15. Fuerst ML: Current trends in the treatment and prevention of opportunistic infection, *AIDS Patient Care* 7(1):38-39, 1993.
16. Henderson DJ: HIV infection: risks to health care workers and infection control, *Nurs Clin North Am* 23:767-777, 1988.
17. Hessol NA, Buchbinder SP: Predictors of HIV disease progression in the era of prophylactic therapy. In Volberding P, Jacobson MA, editors: *AIDS clinical review 1992,* New York, 1992, Marcel Dekker.
18. Kahn JO, Nothfelt DW, Miles SA: AIDS-associated Kaposi's sarcoma. In Volberding P, Jacobson MA, editors: *AIDS clinical review 1992,* New York, 1992, Marcel Dekker.
19. Karpen M: Rifabutin prophylaxis for MAC infection, *AIDS Patient Care* 6(6):276-277, 1992.

20. Lovejoy NC, Rumley R: AIDS epidemiology and pathology implications for intensive care units, *Crit Care Nurs Clin North Am* 4(3):383-393, 1992.
21. Nahlen BL, et al: HIV wasting syndrome in the United States, *AIDS* 7(2):183-188, 1993.
22. National Center for Health Statistics: *Monthly Vital Statistics Report* 41(1), 1992.
23. Stanley H, Fluetsch-Bloom M, Bunce-Clyma M: HIV-related non-Hodgkin's lymphoma, *Oncol Nurs Forum* 18(5):875-880, 1991.
24. *St Anthony's DRG guidebook 1995*, Reston, Va, 1994, St Anthony.

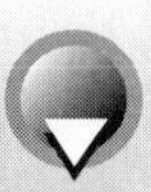

CLINICAL GUIDELINE

61

Oncologic Crises

Jan Foster, MSN, RN, CCRN

DESCRIPTION

There are numerous acute medical emergencies related to cancer and cancer therapy. The emergencies can be classified in a variety of ways: by system; as metabolic, obstructive, or infiltrative; and by prevalence (see Box). This chapter focuses on four conditions—septic shock, hypercalcemia, cardiac tamponade, and acute tumor lysis syndrome (ATLS)—on the basis of their high incidence in prevalent cancers, rapid progression, and devastating and irreversible effects. Because septic shock is discussed in another chapter of this book (see Guideline 63), only its specific relationship with cancer patients will be addressed in this guideline.

Septic shock is a syndrome that involves complex interactions of hemodynamic, humoral, cellular, and metabolic abnormalities resulting from both host- and treatment-related factors. Septic shock remains a major cause of death among critically ill patients and is the most common cause of shock in cancer patients.[2] Immune deficiencies, neutropenia, integumentary disruption, malnutrition, and necroses caused by tumor obstruction are host-related factors that increase cancer patients' risk for infection and sepsis, the systemic response to infection. Treatment-related factors include chemotherapy, radiotherapy, surgery, steroids, antimicrobials, and invasive procedures, all of which lower the body's resistance to infection. Many invasive pathogens cause infection in cancer patients, including bacteria, viruses, fungi, and protozoa. The most common cause of septic shock is Gram-negative bacteria. Septic shock is defined as sepsis with sustained hypotension despite adequate fluid resuscitation, with evidence of perfusion abnormalities.[2] It generally progresses rapidly and often results in multiorgan dysfunction syndrome (see Guideline 64) and disseminated intravascular coagulation (see Guideline 59). The mortality rate for septic shock exceeds 75% in cancer patients.[2]

Hypercalcemia, which was first identified in the 1920s, occurs in 10% to 20% of all cancer patients and is the most common life-threatening metabolic disorder associated with cancer.[4] Hypercalcemia occurs in 30% to 40% of women with breast cancer and in 12.5% to 35% of patients with lung cancer.[7] It is the most frequent complication of breast cancer[3] and is also commonly associated with multiple myeloma, head and neck cancer, renal cell carcinoma, and lymphoma. Immobilization, dehydration, diuretics, and generalized wasting are additional factors that play a role in the pathogenesis of malignancy-related hypercalcemia. Investigators report that the serum level of calcium does not correlate with the manifestation of symptoms. Some individuals show symptoms at much lower levels than others; however, levels that are consistently 16 mg/dl or higher will inevitably trigger cardiac abnormalities.[4] Early detection of hypercalcemia allows prompt intervention and prevention of serious complications, including cardiac dysrhythmias, sensory-perceptual alterations, renal failure, and gastrointestinal ileus.

Cardiac tamponade is a life-threatening complication of cancer in which excessive fluid collects in the pericardial space. As many as 21% of all patients with cancer have pericardial effusion on autopsy, and 16% of those have cardiac tamponade.[2] Pericardial effusion resulting from pericardial metastases is the most common cause of cardiac tamponade. Cancers most frequently associated with pericardial metastasis are lung cancer (37%), breast cancer (22%), leukemia, and lymphoma (17%).[5] Other causes of pericardial effusions are pericarditis resulting from radio-

Oncologic Crises
Superior vena cava syndrome
Intestinal obstruction
Syndrome of inappropriate antidiuretic hormone
Third space syndrome
Disseminated intravascular coagulation
Spinal cord compression
Cerebral herniation
Seizures
Toxic epidermal necrolysis
Graft-versus-host disease

therapy, infectious pericarditis, and uremic pericarditis associated with renal failure.[3]

Acute Tumor Lysis Syndrome (ATLS) is a metabolic emergency that occurs in cancer patients when a large number of rapidly proliferating tumor cells are lysed. ATLS occurs in patients who have large tumor burdens and with tumors that have high growth fractions; it is triggered by the induction of chemotherapy and radiotherapy. This group includes patients wth high-grade lymphomas and acute lymphoblastic leukemia. ATLS is also associated with acute myelogenous leukemia, chronic myelogenous leukemia in blast crisis, and non-Hodgkins lymphoma. Rarely, solid tumors such as small-cell lung cancer, metastatic breast cancer, and metastatic medulloblastoma have been associated with ATLS.[11] Acute renal failure, cardiac dysrhythmias, neurological irritability, and seizures can be fatal.

PATHOPHYSIOLOGY

The pathophysiology of **septic shock** involves a complex series of hemodynamic alterations triggered by bacterial endotoxins, neutrophil oxygen-derived free radicals, hormonal mediators, and cytokine immune mediators released during the immune response.[6,8] Cancer patients are at risk for infection because of neutropenia and immunosuppressive effects of the tumor, chemotherapy, radiotherapy, steroids, and other immunosuppressive agents for graft-versus-host disease in patients who have bone marrow transplants; poor nutritional status; and many invasive procedures, indwelling lines, and catheters. Cancer patients develop septic shock most frequently in response to infections caused by Gram-negative bacteria; however, immunosuppression makes them overly susceptible to fungal, bacterial, and viral infections, which also lead to septic shock.

The pathophysiology of **hypercalcemia** is unclear, but three mechanisms have been identified. The first is metastatic hypercalcemia, most commonly linked with breast cancer. Osteoclastic activity triggered by the release of osteoclastic activating factor, prostaglandins, parathyroid-related protein from tumor cells, and the administration of estrogen and antiestrogen hormone therapy causes an elevation in serum calcium (Ca^{++}). Hypercalcemia associated with breast cancer without bone metastasis is reported, and presumably is due to the release of these same osteoclastic factors. Humoral hypercalcemia of malignancy, the second type, is associated with nonmetastatic squamous-cell lung cancer, head and neck cancer, and renal cell carcinoma. Humoral mediators released by tumor cells stimulate osteoclastic activity. Hypercalcemia in hematologic malignancies occurs in lymphoma and multiple myeloma and is the result of osteoclastic activity caused by the release of several cytokines by the malignant cells.[4]

Cardiac tamponade, caused by an increase in pericardial pressure, results from pericardial fluid accumulation. Pericardial fluid accumulation in metastatic cancers arises from direct venous or lymphatic obstruction by tumor, and from excessive production of pericardial fluid caused by tumor cells irritating pericardial membranes.[5] As the fluid collects, pericardial pressure increases and eventually equilibrates with right- and left-ventricular end-diastolic pressure. A decrease in diastolic filling leads to a decrease in stroke volume, which results in a decrease in cardiac output. When compensatory mechanisms such as tachycardia and peripheral vasoconstriction are exhausted, intracardiac and intrapericardial pressures equalize and cardiac standstill results.[5] The hallmark physical assessment findings of cardiac tamponade are hypotension/pulsus paradoxus, muffled heart sounds, and jugular venous distension.

ATLS involves a complex series of events related to the release of high levels of intracellular contents into the serum after massive destruction of tumor burden by chemotherapy and radiotherapy. Hallmark signs of ATLS are hyperkalemia, hyperphosphatemia, hypocalcemia and hypomagnesemia resulting from hyperphosphatemia, and hyperuricemia. Potassium (K^+) is relatively concentrated intracellularly, and when lysis occurs, the K^+ is released into the serum, resulting in hyperkalemia. Phosphorous (PO_4^-) and Ca^{++} maintain an inverse relationship intracellularly and extracellularly, respectively. When intracellular PO_4^- spills out into the extracellular space with cell lysis, the serum level increases and forces the serum Ca^{++} level to go down. Magnesium (MG^{++}) levels fall as Ca^{++} levels fall. The lymphoblasts in leukemia contain excessive phosphate, accounting for gross elevation of serum PO_4^-. The cell contains nucleic acids, or purines, that form DNA and RNA. Because uric acid is a purine metabolite, purine release ultimately results in hyperuricemia when cell lysis occurs. Renal failure may result from hyperuricemia progressing to intratubular precipitation of uric acid, Ca^{++} crystallization, and obstructive uropathy.[11]

LENGTH OF STAY/ANTICIPATED COURSE

The length of stay after an oncologic crisis depends on the crisis itself, the patient's response to treatment, the underlying malignancy and its extent, and general vital organ function. The literature reports that death from septic shock occurs within 30 days for 35% of patients and within 180 days for 50% of patients.[9] Early interventions to maintain organ perfusion and prevention of iatrogenic complications play a key role in affecting mortality and length of stay. Hypercalcemia is often a chronic problem that requires ongoing treatment. Discharge from the intensive care unit (ICU) is generally appropriate when the patient's Ca^{++} level is stabilized (even though it may still exceed normal values), and the patient is free from potentially lethal cardiac dysrhythmias. The patient with cardiac tamponade must remain in the ICU until hemodynamic stability is evident, which may not occur until after definitive treatment of the cause of tamponade. Resolution of ATLS depends on the tumor's responsiveness to therapy. Because cytolysis generally occurs within 7 days following treatment, ATLS usually resolves in 4 to 7 days after treatment is initiated, as long as renal function has been preserved and electrolyte abnormalities have been corrected. Patients with ATLS should remain in the ICU until danger of serious cardiac dysrhythmias and unstable central nervous system irritability, secondary to electrolyte abnormalities, passes. If renal function fails to improve with appropriate therapy and hemodialysis is necessary, patients will generally stay in the ICU until renal function studies and serum K^{+} levels are within a safe range.

Patients will be assigned a DRG based on the specific crisis with an average LOS based on that crisis. When a more specific DRG can not be identified, DRG 413: Other Myeloproliferative Disorders with Poorly Differentiated Neoplasm with Complications may be used. This DRG has been noted to average an LOS of 9.9 days.[10]

Calculation of Estimated Ionized Serum Calcium to Correct for Changes in Serum Albumin Concentrations

Corrected serum calcium = measured total serum calcium value (mg/dl) + [4.0 − serum albumin value (g/dl)] × 0.8

Example: serum calcium = 10.0
serum albumin = 2.0

$10.0 + ([4 - 2] \times 0.8)$
$2 \times 0.8 = 1.6$
$10.0 + 1.6 = 11.6$ corrected calcium level

MANAGEMENT TRENDS AND CONTROVERSIES

Treatment of septic shock currently focuses on supporting organ perfusion and tissue oxygenation, preventing complications of therapy, and treating the underlying cause. Inotropes, vasopressors, and fluids are administered to support cardiovascular function and hemodynamic stability. Patients are mechanically ventilated to improve tissue oxygenation, which is often compromised because of adult respiratory distress syndrome. Measures are taken to prevent introduction of secondary microbes through broken skin and mucous membranes. Treatment for infectious sources usually includes a host of antimicrobial agents, including antibiotic coverage for both Gram-negative and Gram-positive organisms and antifungal and antiviral agents. Future directions in the treatment of septic shock depend on the success of current experimentation with agents such as anticytokines to block the release or the effects of humoral and cellular mediators; nitric oxide inhibitors to block vasodilation and damaging effects to tissue; and colony-stimulating factors to promote proliferation and differentiation of hematopoietic cells for neutropenic and immunosuppressed patients. Development of new and refinement of current technology to detect early organ hypoperfusion, such as gastric tonometry for measuring gastric pHi to monitor gastric tissue hypoxia, may facilitate early intervention and full resolution of the shock state and its sequelae.

The most effective method of achieving long-term correction of the serum Ca^{++} level in cancer patients with hypercalcemia is to treat the underlying malignancy. Because Ca^{++} exists both in a free, ionized form and in a form bound to albumin, and because many cancer patients are hypoalbuminemic, Ca^{++} levels may be underestimated. The preceding Box illustrates the calculation for estimating the ionized serum Ca^{++}. Elevated serum Ca^{++} interferes with the action of antidiuretic hormone on the renal collecting tubules, which causes excessive water loss in the urine. Symptomatic hypercalcemia necessitates aggressive therapy with IV saline fluids to restore intravascular fluid volume and to increase glomerular filtration rate; diuretics, such as furosemide, to promote renal excretion of calcium; and antiosteoclastic medications. Several antiosteoclastic drugs may be used concomitantly because the onset and duration of action vary for each drug. Calcitonin is used for its rapid onset of action; duration of effectiveness is short, so its use should be combined with drugs such as pamidronate or gallium nitrate, which maintain normocalcemia for 5 to 7 days.[7]

Treatment for cardiac tamponade is largely palliative, to promote comfort and prevent hemodynamic instability. Treatment includes removing fluid from the pericardial sac, obliterating the pericardial space to prevent fluid accumulation, and treating the underlying malignancy. Pericardiocentesis is emergency treatment for acute cardiac tamponade and decompensation, but it is also done to prevent cardiac tamponade at the onset of symptoms of pericardial effusion. To avoid repeated pericardiocentesis, a pericardial catheter may be inserted for continuous drainage of pericardial fluid. The pericardial sac may be obliterated to prevent reaccumulation of fluid by instilling sclerosing agents through a pericardial catheter. The sclerosing agent stimulates an inflammatory response, followed by fibrosis. Commonly used agents include tetracycline, quinacrine, thiotepa, nitrogen mustard, and 5-fluorouracil.[2]

Chemotherapy instillation is also done to treat the malignancy rather than to sclerose the pericardium. Tumor-sensitive chemotherapy and radiotherapy may be given to destroy the cancer cells and to prevent accumulation of pericardial fluid and cardiac tamponade. A pericardial window may be created if the patient is a surgical candidate. This procedure involves surgical resection of a portion of the pericardium, which prevents fluid accumulation and, in turn, relieves pressure. Generally, the procedure to create a pericardial window is undertaken when excessive (>1 L/day) fluid reaccumulation occurs. Emergency treatment of cardiac tamponade includes oxygen, aggressive fluid therapy, and avoidance of diuretics to increase ventricular filling pressure. Vasoactive medications may be helpful; however, alpha-adrenergic stimulants may increase afterload and further impede cardiac output.[3]

The primary goal for management of ATLS is to prevent renal failure and electrolyte imbalances. Aggressive fluid therapy, loop diuretics, low-dose dopamine, alkalinization of the urine with continuous infusion of sodium bicarbonate, and administration of allopurinol to excrete and decrease the formation of uric acid crystals is the treatment of choice for the prevention of renal failure. Caution is advised with the administration of sodium bicarbonate because alkalinization of the urine may promote the formation of calcium phosphate deposits in the renal tubules and thus obstruct them. Alkalinization may predispose the patient to hypocalcemia, which will further aggravate hyperphosphatemia.[11] Hyperkalemia is usually corrected as a secondary response to diuretic therapy, but if hyperkalemia is severe, insulin and glucose may be given to promote an intracellular shift of K^+. Also, a cation-exchange resin such as sodium polystyrene sulfonate may be given orally or rectally.[2] Aluminum-based antacids are given orally to correct the hyperphosphatemia, hypocalcemia, and hypomagnesemia. Because aluminum binds phosphate, as PO_4^- levels decrease, Ca^{++} and Mg^{++} levels increase.

ASSESSMENT

PARAMETER	ANTICIPATED ALTERATION
Septic Shock	
Neurological status	Change in LOC, behavior, mentation *due to decreased brain perfusion and altered tissue oxygenation*
Temperature	Elevated: >38° C *due to hypermetabolism associated with the systemic inflammatory response*
Lactic acid	Elevated: >2.2 mEq/L *due to anaerobic metabolism from defective tissue perfusion*
ABG	Metabolic acidosis *due to lactic acidosis*
UO	Decreased: >30cc/hr *due to reduction in renal blood flow*
BUN	Elevated: >20 mg/dl *due to rapid muscle wasting, negative nitrogen balance, decreased intravascular volume, and renal dysfunction*
RR	Elevated: >20 breaths/min *due to compensation for metabolic acidosis*
BP	Decreased: <100 systolic, with widened pulse pressure *due to vasodilating effects of mediators and hormones*
HR	Tachycardia: >100 bpm *due to reflexive response to hypotension and in response to fever*
SVR	Decreased: <800 dynes/sec *due to a response to the vasodilating properties of cellular and humoral mediators and hormones*
CO	Elevated: >8.0 L/min (initially) *due to a reflexive response to vasodilation* Decreased: <4.0 L/min (later) *due to the cardiodepressant properties of cellular mediators*
Coagulation Factors	
PT	Prolonged: >14 sec *due to DIC*
APTT	Prolonged: >25 sec *due to DIC*

Plan of Care (cont'd)	
Fibrinogen	Decreased: <60 mg/dl *due to DIC*
Platelets	Decreased: <150,000/mm^3 *due to DIC*
Hypercalcemia	
HR	Tachycardia: >100 bpm *due to the cardiac stimulating effects of* Ca^{++}
Pulse quality	Bounding *due to the cardiac stimulating effects of* Ca^{++}
Rhythm	Prolonged PR and QRS intervals, bradycardia, heart block and asystole *due to the effects of excessive* Ca^{++} *on the action potential of the cardiac muscle cell*
Neuromuscular status	Lethargy, confusion, coma, convulsions, weakness, and hyporeflexia *due to the effects of excessive* Ca^{++} *on the neuromuscular junction in the central and peripheral nervous system*
Renal status	Polyuria and polydipsia *due to the interference of antidiuretic hormone on renal reabsorption of fluid by excessive* Ca^{++}
GI Status	Absent bowel sounds, constipation, ileus and abdominal pain *due to the effect of excessive* Ca^{++} *on smooth muscle of the GI tract*
Cardiac Tamponade	
HR	Tachycardia: >100 bpm *due to decreased stroke volume*
BP	Decreased: <100 systolic or below patient norm *due to decreased SV* Pulsus paradoxus *due to pooling of blood in the pulmonary vasculature during inspiration*
Heart sounds	Muffled *due to decreased transmission of sound because of fluid* Friction rub *due to tumor encroachment or constrictive pericarditis because of fluid surrounding the heart*
CO	Decreased: <4.0 L/min *due to decreased SV*
CVP	Elevated: >8 mm Hg
PCWP	Elevated: >12 mm Hg *All are due to increased pericardial pressure preventing adequate filling of the ventricle and venous congestion*
Chest pain	Dull *due to tumor encroachment or constrictive pericarditis because of fluid surrounding the heart*
Venous system	JVD, edema, abdominal distension, hepatomegaly, hepatojugular reflex *due to resistance of venous return to the right atrium followed by pooling of blood peripherally*
UO	Decreased: <30 cc/hr *due to decreased renal perfusion*
Mental status	Anxiety, sense of doom *due to sense of impending arrest*
ATLS	
Cardiac rhythm	Dysrhythmias, prolonged QT interval, heart block, asystole *due to the effects of increased* K^+ *and decreased* Ca^{++} *and* Mg^{++} *on the cardiac muscle cell*
Neuromuscular status	Twitching, tetany, Trousseau's sign, Chvostek's signs, carpopedal spasm, seizures, muscle weakness, paresthesias *due to the effects of decreased* Ca^{++} *and* Mg^{++} *on the neuromuscular junction in the nervous system*
Renal status	Oliguria, anuria, cloudy urine, sediment, flank pain, *due to the effects of decreased* PO_4^- *levels*
GI status	Nausea, vomiting, anorexia, diarrhea *due to the effects of elevated uric acid levels*

PLAN OF CARE

INTENSIVE PHASE

Care of the patient during the intensive phase of an oncologic crisis is focused on the treatment of the major complications of the cancer process. Stabilization of cardiopulmonary status and treatment of infection are the primary priorities.

PATIENT CARE PRIORITIES	EXPECTED PATIENT OUTCOMES
Septic Shock	
High risk for infection *r/t* *Decreased immune response* *Multiple invasive procedures*	Absence of fever, chills, shivering, tachycardia, or tachypnea Absolute neutrophil count >500/mm^3 Absence of infection Platelet count >20,000/mm^3 Absence of bleeding
Decreased tissue perfusion *r/t* *The interaction of endotoxin, humoral and cellular mediators* *Clotting system factors on the capillary membranes*	HR within 10% of patient norms Hemodynamic profile: WNL Absence of edema RR 12 to 20 breaths/min Lungs clear ABG within patient norms Lactic acid, BUN, and creatinine: WNL UO >30 cc/hr Alert, oriented, responsive
High risk for impaired ventilatory weaning process *r/t* *Pulmonary interstitial edema* *Prolonged mechanical ventilation*	Successfully weaned with maintenance of ABG within patient norms RR<30 breaths/min VT and VC: WNL Absence of pneumothorax Comfortable or sedated, particularly if inverse inspiratory/expiratory ratio and/or pressure-controlled modes of ventilation are used Airway clear and patent Communication of needs through writing, pointing, gesturing, or lip reading if tracheostomy in place
Hypercalcemia	
Decreased CO *r/t dysrhythmias*	ECG rhythm stable within patient norms CO and VS within patient norms CA^{++} level: WNL
Sensory-perceptual alteration *r/t decreased serum* Ca^{++}	Accurate perception of environmental events Alert and oriented
Decreased tissue perfusion *r/t renal output producing dehydration*	I/O balanced CVP and PCWP: WNL CO and CPP: WNL UO >30 cc/hr BUN, creatinine, bilirubin, AST, and ALT: all WNL Peripheral pulses within patient norms Skin color and T: WNL
Constipation *r/t decreased gastric motility*	Stool soft and at reasonable intervals

Plan of Care (cont'd)

Cardiac Tamponade

Decreased CO *r/t impaired diastolic filling pressure associated with neoplastic invasion of pericardial area*	Hemodynamic profile: WNL
Decreased tissue perfusion *r/t decreased CO*	Peripheral pulses within patient norms Capillary refill time <3 sec Skin color within patient norms Mentation within patient norms UO >30 cc/hr ABGs within patient norms
Anxiety *r/t decreased CO and associated sense of impending doom*	Verbalizes general comfort Free of S/S of sympathetic stimulation: HR and VS are WNL, skin warm and dry, pupillary response: WNL Free of restlessness and agitation

ATLS

Decreased CO *r/t dysrhythmias*	ECG rhythm stable within patient norms CO and VS within patient norms Serum K^{+}, Ca^{++}, Mg^{++}: WNL
High risk for injury *r/t paresthesia, seizures*	Free of injury, seizures Serum Ca^{++} and PO_4^{-}: WNL Airway clear, patent
Impaired urinary elimination *r/t uric acid nephropathy, acute renal failure*	UO >300 cc/hr I/O balanced Uric acid, BUN, creatinine and urine pH: WNL

INTERVENTIONS

Septic Shock

Use aseptic technique and hand-washing precautions *to prevent introduction of microbial contaminants and infection.*

Assess for fever *because fever may be the only indication of infection in the neutropenic patient and may signal a metabolic emergency.*

Monitor neutrophil and platelet counts *to anticipate risk for infection and bleeding.*

Administer platelets promptly *to maximize effectiveness in reducing the risk of bleeding.*

Culture blood and other potential sources of infection *to identify the organisms and facilitate appropriate antibiotic coverage.*

Initiate antimicrobial therapy promptly at the onset of fever or other signs of infection *to reduce microbial multiplication, and, in turn, to release fewer toxic substances.*

Administer fluids aggressively *to fill the dilated vascular bed and maintain adequate tissue perfusion.*

Administer vasopressors *to maintain* MAP *and promote vital organ perfusion.*

Administer furosemide and mannitol *to promote renal perfusion and stimulate urine output.*

Administer O_2 *to meet increased tissue demands and relieve dyspnea.*

Initiate mechanical ventilation *to provide adequate gas exchange when the patient cannot maintain oxygenation and respiratory compensation for metabolic acidosis.*

Use reorientation strategies such as clocks, calendars, and family visitation *to assist with reality orientation during lengthy ICU stays.*

When cardiopulmonary and hemodynamic stability are evident, patient is afebrile, and nutritional support is acceptable, establish a protocol *to promote weaning from mechanical ventilation as soon as possible without jeopardizing tissue oxygenation and perfusion.*

Plan of Care (cont'd)

Facilitate tracheostomy if mechanical ventilation is predicted to last more than 10 days *to limit trauma to tracheal mucous membranes, enhance communication and comfort, facilitate oral care, and reduce risk of infection.*

Assess for barotraumatic pneumothorax and facilitate chest tube insertion and maintenance *to prevent tension pneumothorax.*

Administer anxiolytics and analgesics as continuous infusions *to maximize sedation and comfort; use less medication overall; and minimize hypotension, respiratory depression, and decreased LOC, which are frequent side effects of the drugs when they are given in repeated bolus doses.*

Suction the endotracheal or tracheostomy tube when needed *to maintain a clear airway, improve oxygenation, and reduce infection.*

Provide writing tablets, picture boards, and so on *to assist with communication.*

Hypercalcemia

Monitor for ECG changes and dysrhythmias.

Administer isotonic saline (generally 3 L/day) *to restore extracellular fluid volume and promote* Ca^{++} excretion.

Administer diuretics after intravascular volume has been replenished *to promote calciuresis.*

Monitor I/O.

Weigh daily.

Administer drugs that inhibit bone osteoclastic activity, such as calcitonin, mithramycin, gallium nitrate, pamidronate disodium, and glucocorticoids *to reduce serum* Ca^{++} *level.*

Orient to time, place, and events *to assist with reality orientation and accurate perception of events.*

Cardiac Tamponade

Assess for pulsus paradoxus >10 mm Hg, muffled heart sounds, JVD, narrow pulse pressure, hypotension, and tachycardia *because these are classic signs and symptoms of cardiac tamponade.*

Monitor for electrical alternans on ECG *because this may be a sign of cardiac tamponade.*

Monitor CO, CVP, and PCWP *because rising pressures and decreasing CO may signify impending cardiac arrest.*

Administer IV fluids *to maximize ventricular filling pressure.*

Monitor I/O *to assess renal tissue perfusion.*

Administer inotropes *to augment decreasing CO.*

Monitor acid–base balance because decreased CO may produce lactic acidosis.

Assist with pericardiocentesis *to relieve intrapericardial pressure.*

ATLS

Assess serum K^+, PO_4^-, Ca^{++}, Mg^{++}, uric acid levels, BUN, and creatinine levels *to determine need for aggressive therapy and assess renal function.*

Monitor for cardiac dysrhythmias *to initiate early intervention.*

Administer insulin *to promote intracellular shift of* K^+.

Administer a cation-exchange resin (sodium polysterene sulfonate) *to lower serum* K^+ *level.*

Administer aluminum-based phosphate-binding antacid *to lower serum* PO_4^- level and increase serum Ca^{++} level.

Assess for CNS irritability *to anticipate and prevent seizure activity.*

Ensure safe environment *to protect from injury in case of seizure activity.*

Administer allopurinol *to reduce uric acid formation.*

Administer IV fluids aggressively *to promote excretion of uric acid and prevent uric acid nephropathy.*

Administer sodium bicarbonate as a continuous IV infusion *to alkalinize the urine, promote excretion of uric acid, and reduce serum* K^+ *level by causing an intracellular shift.*

Plan of Care (cont'd)

Administer loop diuretics and low dose dopamine *to promote diuresis and K^+* and PO_4^- *excretion.*

INTERMEDIATE PHASE

Anticipation, thorough assessment, and prompt intervention of each oncologic crisis plays a key role in patients' survival and their quality of life following such events. Each crisis requires ongoing monitoring of vital signs and hemodynamic parameters; attention to fluid and electrolyte balances; and maintenance of cardiovascular, neurological, renal, and gastrointestinal functions. As the patient stabilizes from the emergency event, treatment of the underlying malignancy usually resumes, and nursing care appropriate to each treatment modality becomes an important part of patient management.

PATIENT CARE PRIORITIES	EXPECTED PATIENT OUTCOMES
Septic Shock	
High risk for decreased tissue perfusion *r/t* *Vasoconstriction* *Impaired capillary permeability* *Disseminated intravascular coagulation*	Hemodynamic profile: WNL Skin color pink Absence of petechiae and ecchymoses ABG within patient norms SVo_2 and lactic acid: WNL UO >30 cc/hr BUN and creatinine: WNL *with dialysis if necessary* Awake and responsive within patient norms
High risk for decreased CO *r/t* *Tachycardia* *Inadequate oxygenation* *Myocardial depressant factor*	CO: WNL HR within 10% of normal Peripheral pulses within patient norms
Inadequate nutrition *r/t increased metabolic needs and inability to ingest orally*	Absence of diarrhea *due to enteral feedings* Wt within 10% of preshock state Total protein, pre-albumin, transferrin, and total iron binding capacity: all WNL
Hypercalcemia	
Impaired mobility *r/t bone fractures*	Maintains maximum mobility Performs ADLs as independently as possible
Pain *r/t bone fractures*	Indicates acceptable level of comfort Absence of sympathetic stimulation associated with acute pain: tachycardia, hypertension, pupils >2 to 3 mm Absence of signs and symptoms of chronic pain: depression, inertia and fatigue, inability to concentrate, restlessness
Altered urinary elimination *r/t polyuria*	Maintains continence Intact skin and urinary tract mucous membranes Maintains urinary catheter drainage system if necessary Free of infection: afebrile, absence of leukocytes, mucus, and bacteria in urine
Constipation *r/t decreased bowel motility*	Soft stool at reasonable intervals Free of discomfort

Plan of Care (cont'd)

Cardiac Tamponade

Nursing Diagnosis	Expected Outcomes
High risk for infection *r/t* *Hemodynamic monitoring lines* *Intravenous lines* *Pericardial catheter* *Chest drainage system*	Afebrile Absence of drainage, redness, swelling at catheter insertion sites
Ineffective breathing pattern *r/t chest tubes or postanesthesia for pericardial window*	RR 12 to 20 breaths/min VT and VC: WNL Airway clear and patent Equal bilateral breath sounds

ATLS

Nursing Diagnosis	Expected Outcomes
Fluid volume excess *r/t aggressive administration of IV fluids to prevent uric acid nephropathy*	Fluid output equal to intake Free of pulmonary crackles, JVD, peripheral edema Wt stable

INTERVENTIONS

Titrate vasopressors and wean as soon as possible *to maximize CO and minimize vasoconstriction for improved perfusion to vital organs.*

Avoid high-dose dopamine, norepinephrine, and epinephrine *to avoid potentiating vasoconstriction and perfusion failure.*

Use nonsympathomimetic drugs such as digoxin and phosphodiesterase inhibitors *to support CO when response to sympathomimetic drugs is exhausted.*

Administer crystalloids and colloids *to maintain an end-diastolic ventricular filling pressure of 8 to 12 mm Hg and SV 65 to 100 ml/minute.*

Use care during potentially traumatizing procedures, such as oral care, endotracheal suctioning, and catheter insertions, *to reduce the risk of bleeding.*

Provide renal dialysis *to maintain fluid and electrolyte balance and excrete metabolites if renal failure occurs.*

Monitor fluid balance, electrolytes, BUN, and creatinine *to evaluate renal function or dialysis effectiveness, choice of dialysate, and frequency needed for dialysis.*

Assess LOC and responsiveness *to evaluate cerebral perfusion and sedation needs.*

Facilitate enteral feedings *to provide adequate nutrients and energy for diaphragmatic movement while patient is unable to take oral feedings.*

Monitor wt, serum protein levels, and diarrhea *to guide enteral feeding adjustments.*

Monitor pH, CO_2 levels, and RR *to assess tolerance to carbohydrate load.*

Use physical therapy devices and transfer techniques *to assist with mobility and reduce the risk of bone fractures.*

Implement pharmaceutical and nonpharmaceutical methods of pain control *for acute pain related to surgery, if the patient has undergone pericardial window, and for chronic pain resulting from bone demineralization or malignancy.*

Maintain sterile technique for urinary catheter care and for all invasive lines, chest tubes, and dressings *to prevent infection.*

Collaborate with dietitians and pharmacists to provide adequate nutrition, fluid balance, and bowel elimination through parenteral and enteral routes *to meet the special nutritional needs of cancer patients recovering from acute fluid and electrolyte imbalances and from cardiac compromise.*

TRANSITION TO DISCHARGE

When the patient's cardiovascular status, fluid and electrolyte balance, central nervous system, and renal function stabilize, the patient is ready to be discharged from the ICU. Preparation for discharge includes continued attention to fluid and electrolyte balances, oral nutrition, and patient education with instructions to report signs and symptoms of recurrent impending crisis and information pertinent to treatment for the malignancy. Because cancer survival for many malignancies is increasing, patients may experience these problems repeatedly and may require management after discharge from the hospital.

Patients who have recovered from septic shock may need long-term technological organ support and much professional and skilled nursing care because of multiple organ dysfunction, which often accompanies septic shock and requires weeks to months for recovery. Patients may require mechanical ventilation, renal dialysis, physical therapy, and enteral feedings after discharge to home or an intermediate care facility. Management issues for patients requiring technological support are great and include ventilation needs, airway integrity, nutritional support, mobility alterations, skin integrity, patient and family coping strategies, patient and family education needs, role changes, social support, and financial needs. Patients who recover from septic shock who do not need organ support have many educational needs, especially if they remain neutropenic, because infection-control issues will need to be stressed.

Hypercalcemia may be a long-term problem. Management of hypercalcemia requires thorough patient education, including reporting changes in levels of consciousness and energy, irregular pulse, and polyuria; the presence of these symptoms may indicate that the Ca^{++} level has risen to critical levels and that the patient requires urgent therapy. Changes in health care delivery may result in patients receiving IV administration of Ca^{++}-reducing agents and cardiac monitoring in the home rather than in the hospital, requiring the expertise of critical care oncology nurses. Patients with chronic hypercalcemia may require mobility-assist devices because of, or to prevent, bone fractures. A comprehensive bowel management program may be indicated, along with nutritional management, including frequent follow-up on serum protein and albumin levels, weight assessment, and dietary supplementation.

Patients at risk for cardiac tamponade need instructions to report increasing fatigue, shortness of breath, dyspnea, and other symptoms that may indicate fluid has reaccumulated in the pericardium. Serial pericardiocentesis for palliation of recurrent effusions, or to treat the malignancy, infection, or other source of effusion or pericarditis, may be part of the long-term care for patients at risk for cardiac tamponade.

Generally, ATLS is unlikely to occur once patients are discharged. Patients at risk for this problem would not undergo outpatient or home cancer therapy because of rapid onset of potentially devastating complications and the monitoring needs and medical and nursing care required.

REFERENCES

1. Members of the American College of Chest Physicians/Society of Critical Care Medicine Consensus Conference Committee. American College of Chest Physicians/Society of Critical Care Medicine Consensus Conference: Definitions for sepsis and organ failure and guidelines for the use of innovative therapies in sepsis, *Crit Care Med* 20(6):864-874, 1992.
2. Dietz KA, Flaherty AM: Oncologic emergencies. In Groenwald SL, et al, editors: *Cancer nursing principles and practice,* ed 3, Boston, 1993, Jones and Bartlett, pp 800-839.
3. Joiner GA, Kolodychuk GR: Neoplastic cardiac tamponade, *Crit Care Nurse* 11(2):50-58, 1991.
4. Lang-Kummer JM: Hypercalcemia. In Groenwald SL, et al, editors: *Cancer nursing principles and practice,* ed 3, Boston, 1993, Jones and Bartlett, pp 644-661.
5. Mangon CM: Malignant pericardial effusions: pathophysiology and clinical correlates, *Oncol Nurs Forum* 19(8):1215-1221, 1992.
6. McCord JM: Oxygen-derived free radicals, *Crit Care Med* 1(suppl 1):70-75, 1993.
7. Schulmeister L: Managing cancer-related hypercalcemia, *Office Oncol Nurs* 6(2), 1992.
8. Shapiro L, Gelfand JA: Cytokines and sepsis: pathophysiology and therapy, *Crit Care Med* 1(suppl 1):13-19, 1993.
9. Spooner C, Markowitz NP, Saravolatz L: The role of tumor necrosis factor in sepsis, *Clin Immunol Immunopathol* 62(1):511-517, 1992.
10. *St Anthony's DRG Guidebook 1995,* Reston, Va, 1994, St Anthony.
11. Stucky L: Acute tumor lysis syndrome: assessment and nursing implications, *Oncol Nurs Forum* 20(1):49-57, 1993.

U N I T

VIII

Multisystem

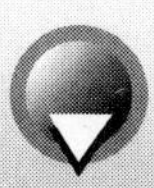

CLINICAL GUIDELINE

62

Hypovolemic Shock

Kathleen Kerber, MSN, RN, CCRN, CS

DESCRIPTION

Shock can be defined as a complex syndrome of decreased blood flow to body tissues resulting in inadequate delivery of oxygen and nutrients to body cells.[6] Cellular dysfunction occurs because of the imbalance between oxygen supply and demand in the microcirculation. Prolonged hypoperfusion results in progressive organ failure and possible death. Despite research and advanced technology, mortality from most forms of shock remains high.[8] Rapid detection and appropriate intervention are critical to survival.

Hypovolemic shock occurs as a consequence of decreased intravascular volume. While hemorrhage is the most common cause, the loss of large amounts of any body fluid can lead to hypovolemic shock.[6] External fluid loss may occur with continuous gastrointestinal suctioning, vomiting, diarrhea, fistulas, and ostomies. Excessive diuretic use, diabetes insipidus, Addison's disease, and hyperglycemic osmotic diuresis may result in severe dehydration and subsequent hypovolemia. Internal shifting of fluid out of the vascular compartment can occur with internal hemorrhage and the pooling of fluid in the interstitial space (third spacing). Third spacing occurs in the presence of edema, peritonitis, pancreatitis, burns, ascites, and large soft-tissue injury.

PATHOPHYSIOLOGY

An intravascular volume deficit of 15% of total blood volume (approximately 750 ml) can occur without a significant effect on arterial blood pressure or cardiac output.[2] As volume deficit exceeds 15% of total blood volume, venous return to the heart is reduced and stroke volume decreases. Arterial blood pressure and cardiac output decline. Blood flow through capillaries is diminished and oxygen delivery to cells is inadequate.

The shock syndrome can be divided into three major stages: nonprogressive, progressive, and refractory. The evolution of each stage depends on the severity and rate of development of hypovolemia.

During the nonprogressive stage of shock, compensatory mechanisms are activated to restore arterial blood pressure and increase circulating blood volume. As cardiac output decreases, pressure receptors located in the aorta and carotid arteries stimulate the vasomotor center of the medulla of the brain, activating the sympathetic nervous system. This activation increases heart rate and contractile force to improve cardiac output and raise arterial blood pressure. In response to sympathetic stimulation, blood vessels in the skin, lungs, kidneys, and GI tract constrict to redistribute blood flow to the heart and brain. Generalized venous constriction improves venous return and prevents pooling of blood in the venous circulation.

The kidneys secrete renin in response to decreased renal perfusion. Renin, when converted to angiotensin II, increases arteriolar vasoconstriction and stimulates the adrenal cortex to secrete the hormone aldosterone. Aldosterone increases blood volume by decreasing sodium and water excretion by the kidneys. Atrial baroreceptors sense low atrial pressure and stimulate the hypothalamus to release antidiuretic hormone (ADH) from the posterior pituitary gland. In response to ADH, the distal tubules and collecting ducts of the kidneys increase the reabsorption of water.

While compensatory mechanisms are redirecting blood flow to vital organs and increasing blood volume, adverse responses develop. Gastrointestinal motility diminishes in response to decreased blood flow. Prolonged vasoconstriction can lead to ischemia and ulceration of the luminal surface of the stomach and intestine.[4] Decreased pulmonary blood flow increases alveolar dead space. The rate and depth of breathing must increase to maintain adequate arterial oxygenation. The increase in ventilation may result in alkalosis, impairing oxygen delivery to the tissues.

The progressive stage of shock occurs when compensatory mechanisms are unable to maintain perfusion to the heart and brain. There is a marked reduction in cardiac output and arterial blood pressure despite intense vascular constriction. As arterial blood pressure falls, coronary perfusion is inadequate and myocardial contractility is depressed. Dysrhythmias and myocardial infarction can occur.

As the shock syndrome progresses, tissue anoxia and acidosis reverse arteriole constriction.[3] Loss of autoregulation in the microcirculation and increased capillary permeability allow fluid to shift out of the vascular space. Severe hypoperfusion results in multiple system failure.

The refractory stage of shock is characterized by profound hypotension unresponsive to therapy. The inability to restore blood volume and reestablish circulation ultimately leads to total body failure. Death is inevitable.

LENGTH OF STAY/ANTICIPATED COURSE

The length of stay for patients with hypovolemic shock depends on the precipitating cause, response to therapy, and the development of multiple organ dysfunction syndrome (MODS). HCFA does not have a DRG that specifically addresses hypovolemic shock. However, this condition could be coded under several DRGs, including DRG 127: Heart failure and shock, with an average LOS of 7.1 days;[7] or DRG 144: Other circulatory system disorders with complications, with an average LOS of 6.4 days.[7] "Unspecified shock," which could include hypovolemic shock, is listed under many of the cardiac DRGs related to acute MI, as well as under the DRGs that address sepsis.[7]

MANAGEMENT TRENDS AND CONTROVERSIES

The ultimate objective in the management of hypovolemic shock is to meet the oxygen needs of the cell. Variables that influence oxygen delivery to the cell include cardiac index (cardiac output/body surface area), hemoglobin level, and arterial oxygen saturation.[1] Immediate management priorities include (1) control of fluid loss or correction of the precipitating event, (2) repletion of intravascular volume, and (3) restoration of oxygen-carrying capacity.

Fluid resuscitation is a fundamental part of the treatment of hypovolemic shock. Restoration of intravascular volume increases venous return to the heart and improves cardiac output and cardiac index. The amount and rate of fluid replacement depends on the severity of the intravascular volume depletion and the patient's response to fluid resuscitation. General assessment of a patient's response to fluid resuscitation includes blood pressure, hourly assessments of urine output, level of consciousness, capillary refill, and serial hematocrits. A pulmonary artery catheter or central venous pressure catheter provides information about intravascular volume, as well as monitoring of the patient's hemodynamic response to fluid replacement.

The rapid fluid challenge is a simple intervention that can be used in the management of hypovolemic shock. A small bolus of 0.9% saline is administered intravenously. If an increase in blood pressure is noted, a second bolus is repeated. This procedure is repeated until no further increment in blood pressure is noted. The recommended starting volume is 400 ml of normal saline, infused over 5 minutes, followed by repeated boluses of 200 ml infused over 5 minutes each.[8]

Controversy exists as to the most beneficial fluids to use in the patient with hypovolemic shock.[3] Colloids can be used to increase colloidal osmotic pressure to draw fluid into the vascular compartment and rapidly expand intravascular volume. Crystalloid solutions are recommended by others because they are cost effective, nonallergenic, and reduce blood viscosity, leading to improved microcirculation.[2] Normal saline or Ringer's lactate are common crystalloid solutions used during initial fluid resuscitation.

The oxygen-carrying capacity of the blood depends on adequate levels of hemoglobin. Patients experiencing hypovolemic shock secondary to blood loss may require transfusions of whole blood or packed red blood cells to maintain a hematocrit of 30%. Autotransfusion may be useful for the replacement of blood lost from hemothorax or other intrathoracic injuries.

If the cardiac index remains low after the administration of fluids and blood components to restore intravascular volume, pharmacologic intervention is necessary. Inotropic agents, vasopressors, and vasodilators for reduction of afterload may be used to optimize cardiac performance and control vascular tone to improve tissue perfusion.

Supplemental oxygen is administered to prevent hypoxemia during the compensatory and progressive stages of shock. The amount and route of oxygen administration vary according to the patient's needs. As shock progresses, the use of artificial airways and mechanical ventilation may be required to ensure adequate ventilation.

The pneumatic antishock garment (PASG), also known as medical antishock trousers (MAST), can be used in the treatment of hypovolemic and traumatic shock. Inflation of the device provides compression to the legs, pelvis, and abdomen. Bleeding below the chest level is reduced and arterial blood pressure elevates due to the increased peripheral vascular resistance.[5] The use of the PASG is contraindicated in patients with pulmonary edema and congestive heart failure. Controversy exists regarding the use of the device with trauma patients where intrathoracic or abdominal injury is suspected, and patients with head injury with increased intracranial pressure.[2,5]

ASSESSMENT

PARAMETER	ANTICIPATED ALTERATION
Cardiovascular	
HR	Tachycardia: >100 bpm
BP	Decreased: MAP <70 mm Hg *Initial blood pressure response to volume loss is a slight elevation in diastolic pressure, and normal to slight elevation in systolic pressure. As more volume is lost, the blood pressure decreases.*
CI	Decreased: <2.5 L/min/m^2
SVR	Increased: >1200 dynes/sec/cm^{-5}
PCWP	Decreased: <8 mm Hg
RAP or CVP	Decreased: <2 cm H_2O or mm Hg
Peripheral pulses	Rapid, weak, thready, may be absent
Skin	Cool, moist, pale, CRT <3 sec Cold, cyanotic, mottled
Hgb	Decreased: <12 g/dl *due to hemorrhage, hemodilution*
Hct	Increased or decreased. *May appear normal or elevated in the hypovolemic patient. After fluid resuscitation, the hematocrit will decrease.*
Pulmonary	
Respirations	Tachypnea Increased depth of respiration (early) Decreased depth of respiration (late)
ABG	Early changes: Hyperventilation with respiratory alkalosis *due to compensatory mechanisms* • pH increased: >7.45 • P_{CO_2} decreased: <35 mm Hg Late changes: Hypoventilation with respiratory acidosis *due to exhaustion of compensatory mechanisms* • pH decreased: <7.35 • P_{CO_2} decreased: <45 mm Hg Metabolic acidosis with a fall in HCO_3 <22 mm Hg *due to decreased organ perfusion with organ damage and failure* Hypoxemia with Pa_{O_2} <90 mm Hg *due to hypoventilation and hypoperfusion*
Renal	
UO	Decreased: <30 ml/hr
Urine specific gravity	Increased: >1.030 *due to dehydration*
Urine osmolality	Increased: >800 mOsm/kg H_2O *due to dehydration*
Urine Na^+	Increased: >220 mEq/L *due to Na^+ reabsorption secondary to aldosterone*
Serum Na^+	*Increased: >145 mEq/L due to increased renal retention of Na^+ secondary to aldosterone*
Serum K^+	Decreased: <3.5 mEq/L (early) *Increased aldosterone causes renal excretion of K^+.*

BUN	Increased: >20 mg/dl. *Rises both in hypovolemia and in renal failure. The normal BUN to serum creatine ratio is 10:1 to 20:1. If BUN:creatine ratio is increased hypovolemia is suspected. If BUN:creatine ratio stays the same, along with rises in BUN, renal failure is suspected.*
Neurologic	
LOC	Apprehension Confusion Lethargy Coma
Other	
Bowel sounds	Hypoactive, absent *due to dehydration*
Serum glucose	Increased (early): >110 mg/dl *due to sympathetic stimulation* Decreased (late): <70 mg/dl *due to depletion of body glycogen stores and decreased liver function*
Serum lactate	Increased: >2.2 mEq/L *due to decreased tissue perfusion and anaerobic metabolism*

PLAN OF CARE

INTENSIVE PHASE

The intensive phase of treating hypovolemic shock is aimed at preserving organ perfusion and oxygenation by replacing appropriate fluids aggressively. Hypovolemic shock must be treated with fluid resuscitation. Use of vasopressor agents or inotropic support will not yield the needed return of perfusion pressure without fluid replacement. The type of fluid used should be based on the cause of the hypovolemia. For example, hemorrhaging patients require blood replacement since isotonic or hypertonic fluids lack oxygen-carrying capacity. While isotonic or hypertonic fluids may be used initially to maintain organ perfusion pressure, organ perfusion without oxygenation will not preserve organ viability and, ultimately, will not save the patient's life. Vigilant monitoring of Hgb/Hct and oxygen delivery are essential during this phase of care to ensure optimal patient outcome.

PATIENT CARE PRIORITIES	EXPECTED PATIENT OUTCOMES
Fluid volume deficit *r/t external fluid losses:* *Hemorrhage* *Severe vomiting* *Diarrhea* *Gastrointestinal bleeding and internal fluid losses (losses of intravascular fluid volume to the interstitial and intracellular spaces):* *Ileus* *Intestinal obstruction* *Burns* *Peritonitis*	Hemodynamic stability: • Systolic BP >90 mm Hg • MAP ≥70 mm Hg • HR ≤110 bpm • PCWP 8 to 12 mm Hg Hgb 12 to 14 g/100 ml Hct ≥30% Serum electrolytes: WNL UO ≥30 ml/hr
Decreased CO *r/t* *Decreased intravascular volume* *Myocardial depressant factors*	CI 2.5 to 4 $L/min/m^2$ MAP ≥70 mm Hg UO ≥30 ml/hr Absence of dysrhythmias, angina pectoris or ST segment, T wave changes Skin warm, dry CRT ≤3 sec

Plan of Care (cont'd)

	Follows simple commands, or sensorium comparable to preshock state Clear lungs
Impaired gas exchange *r/t ventilation perfusion mismatch*	ABG: WNL Respiratory function sufficient for adequate oxygenation and ventilation
Pain/discomfort *r/t precipitating event:* *Trauma* *Burns* *Surgery* *Peripheral ischemia, invasive procedures*	Indicates feeling of comfort Able to sleep, rest, and participate in care activity
Inadequate nutrition *r/t increased metabolic demands of the shock state*	Positive nitrogen balance

INTERVENTIONS

Maintain patent airway.
Administer supplemental oxygen; ventilatory support if indicated.
Monitor Sp_{O_2} *to ensure adequate oxygenation.*
Monitor ABG. *Acid-base balance maintains a favorable oxyhemoglobin dissociation curve.*
Administer fluid, electrolytes, blood, and blood products to *restore normal blood volume, maintain adequate CO, and ensure organ oxygenation.*
Administer vasopressors as ordered (only after blood volume deficit is corrected). *Dobutamine may be administered to increase CO in the presence of myocardial depressant factors.*
Keep patient supine until signs of hypovolemia resolve *to maximize blood flow to central organs.*
Monitor I/O, including loss from gastrointestinal tract, wounds, drains, suction *to ensure adequate fluid replacement.*
Monitor the patient for signs of fluid and electrolyte imbalance.
Monitor weight daily.
Monitor Hgb/Hct levels *to ensure adequate organ oxygenation.*
Monitor BUN: creatine ratio.
Maintain temperature WNL. *Hypothermia impairs O_2 delivery to the tissue.*
Provide analgesia and sedation as needed *to maintain comfort and decrease oxygen demand/consumption.*
Position and turn patient q2h *to mobilize secretions and maintain skin integrity.*
Collaborate with dietitian regarding caloric needs.
Administer enteral feedings or total parenteral nutrition as ordered.

INTERMEDIATE PHASE

If the patient survives the intensive phase, recovery will depend on the precipitating event and the development of complications related to decreased organ perfusion, including multiple organ dysfunction syndrome (MODS). During the intermediate phase, the goal is to assist the individual to adapt to changes resulting from traumatic injury or acute illness, and to reestablish activity tolerance.

PATIENT CARE PRIORITIES	EXPECTED PATIENT OUTCOMES
Decreased activity tolerance *r/t* *Decreased CO* *Prolonged bedrest* *Lack of uninterrupted sleep* *Electrolyte imbalance*	Demonstrates increasing physical endurance Able to perform ADL

Plan of Care (cont'd)

High risk for inadequate nutrition *r/t* *Stress response* *Wound/tissue repair requirements*	Positive nitrogen balance Decreased fatigue Improved skin integrity (wound healing)
High risk for fluid volume deficit *r/t underlying disease or injury that precipitated hypovolemia*	Maintain hourly fluid intake within 30 ml of hourly fluid output from urine, wound drainage, or blood loss Weight returns to normal Serum electrolyte balance: WNL

INTERVENTIONS

Collaborate with physical therapy and occupational therapy to increase patient's physical strength and endurance and gradually return patient to activities of daily living.

Ensure adequate sleep/rest periods *to promote wound healing and strength.*

Collaborate with the dietitian to determine caloric needs.

Provide supplemental or enteral feedings to meet caloric needs.

Administer fluids as necessary.

Weigh daily.

TRANSITION TO DISCHARGE

Preparation for discharge includes assisting the patient to regain activity tolerance and establish self-care regimes. If the precipitating event, such as trauma, results in physical disability, the patient is instructed in adaptive techniques to increase independence. If the potential exists for recurrent hypovolemia, such as in gastrointestinal hemorrhage, patient education is focused on management of the underlying condition or illness. Successful discharge planning is the result of the collaborative efforts of the nurse, physician, dietitian, physical therapist, occupational therapist, social worker, and patient. Together, the interdisciplinary team can facilitate a successful transition to discharge.

REFERENCES

1. Barone JE, Snyder AB: Treatment strategies in shock: use of oxygen transport measurements, *Heart Lung* 20(1):81-86, 1991.
2. Cardona VD, et al: *Trauma nursing: from resuscitation through rehabilitation,* ed 2, Philadelphia, 1994, WB Saunders.
3. Falk JL, O'Brien JF, Kerr R: Fluid resuscitation in traumatic hemorrhagic shock, *Crit Care Clin* 8(2):323-337, 1992.
4. Hartmann M, et al: Tissue oxygenation in hemorrhagic shock measured as transcutaneous oxygen tension, subcutaneous oxygen tension, and gastrointestinal intramucosal pH in pigs, *Crit Care Med* 19(2):205-210, 1991.
5. Pepe PE: Antishock garments: more harm than good? *J Crit Illness* 7(2):166-168, 1992.
6. Rice V: *Shock, a clinical syndrome: an update,* New York, 1991, Cahners Publishing.
7. *St Anthony's DRG guidebook 1995,* Reston, Va, 1994, St Anthony.
8. Suhl J: Patients with shock. In Clochesy JM, et al, editors: *Critical Care Nursing,* Philadelphia, 1993, WB Saunders.

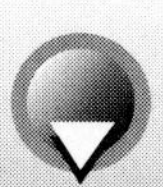

CLINICAL GUIDELINE

63

Systemic Inflammatory Response Syndrome, Sepsis, and Septic Shock

Myra F. Ellis, MSN, RN, CCRN, CS

DESCRIPTION

Sepsis is a systemic inflammatory response to infection. The hematologic, hemodynamic, and metabolic derangements that occur are a result of the human body's response to cellular mediators and toxins triggered by infection. The manifestations of sepsis include tachypnea, tachycardia, fever or hypothermia, and inadequate organ perfusion (shock) or organ dysfunction/failure.[8]

A consensus conference of clinicians and investigators was held in August of 1991 to agree on a set of definitions to define and describe the clinical manifestations and progression of sepsis.[1] Approximately 50% of the patients with a clinical syndrome consistent with sepsis do not have an identifiable infection.[26] The committee agreed to use the term *sepsis* only in the presence of an identified infection; the diffuse inflammatory response to something other than infection, such as trauma, pancreatitis, or burns, would be termed *systemic inflammatory response syndrome* (SIRS). Thus, sepsis is a subset of the larger entity, SIRS. The presence of any two of the following criteria is diagnostic of SIRS: altered temperature (>38° C or <36° C), tachycardia (heart rate >90 bpm), tachypnea (respiratory rate >20 breaths/min or $Pa{CO_2}$ <32 torr), and altered white blood cell count (WBC >12,000 cells/mm^3, <4000 cells/mm^3, or 10% immature [band] forms). This definition should be used in combination with an evaluation of the severity of the illness, which may progress along a continuum of increasing severity to septic shock, characterized by perfusion abnormalities, and culminate in multiple organ dysfunction syndrome. The use of standardized definitions and descriptions of this disease process decreases the reliance on blood culture results to initiate treatment and allows for earlier bedside detection and intervention. Additionally, research protocols and application of information derived from studies can be standardized.

Sepsis has become a common disease, with a 137% increase in incidence in the last decade.[6] Annually, more than 400,000 patients develop sepsis,[9] or approximately 1 out of every 100 hospitalized patients.[26] Septic shock develops in 40% of these patients and adversely affects prognosis.[8] Sepsis and septic shock is the most common cause of death in noncardiac critical care units.[26] Despite development of more potent and broader-spectrum antimicrobial agents, mortality and morbidity from sepsis is unchanged or increasing, especially in the immunocompromised, elderly, and critically ill patient.[3] Septic shock had a 41% mortality rate in 1909,[22] and the death rate continues to be 40% to 60%.[13] Five to ten billion dollars are spent annually for health care in the treatment of sepsis.[9] Experts predict that infections, sepsis, and septic shock will continue to increase in numbers and importance for the next several years and possibly even decades.[26]

PATHOPHYSIOLOGY

The pathophysiologic changes that occur with severe infections are numerous and complex. A nidus of infection can lead to a bloodstream infection. The microorganisms or the toxins they produce can cause the release of chemical mediators, triggering an inflammatory reaction. The local inflammatory response is followed by systemic multisystem derangements. The result is the clinical picture referred to as SIRS.

Mediators of the Septic Cascade

Cellular damage or microbial invasion initiates an acute inflammatory response. This inflammatory response is designed to increase blood flow and enhance capillary permeability, which results in accumulation of fluid (edema) and delivery of leukocytic cells to the site of injury. Granulocytes accumulate in 30 to 60 minutes and function primarily to destroy any intruder. If the source of inflammation continues, within 5 to 6 hours the area will be infiltrated with macrophages and lymphocytes. Macrophages are circulating phagocytic monocytes that also participate in the processing and presentation of antigen to lymphocytes. Lymphocytes participate in the production of antibodies (and initiation of the complement cascade) and cell-mediated immunity.[4]

In addition to the initial inflammatory response, a number of chemotactic mediators activated by cellular injury have been identified. The mediators and their actions are summarized in Table 63-1. In general, these chemotactic substances cause systemic effects in three ways: (1) peripheral vasodilation, (2) maldistribution of blood flow, and (3) myocardial depression.[2]

Cardiovascular Effects

The predominant cardiovascular effect of SIRS is vasodilation of arterial and venous blood vessels. Peripheral vasodilation results from the release of vasoactive metabolites of the arachidonic acid cascade and complement cascades. Initially, patients may compensate by increasing cardiac output with tachycardia and endogenous catecholamines. This results in the characteristic cardiovascular pattern of a high cardiac index (CI), low systemic vascular resistance (SVR), decreased left ventricular ejection fraction (LVEF), dilated left ventricle, and normal stroke volume.[26]

In addition to vasodilation, chemical mediators of SIRS cause an increase in vascular permeability, which leads to loss of intravascular fluid, creating a decrease in the effective circulating volume. This creates an ongoing need for fluid replacement and a tendency toward fluid retention with edema formation.[18]

About one third of the patients with SIRS will develop septic shock.[30] Much of the early literature on septic shock divided it into two phases: warm (hyperdynamic) shock and cold (hypodynamic) shock. Researchers have reviewed much of this literature and now attribute the cold phase of septic shock to volume depletion and inadequate preload. Early aggressive fluid replacement and vasoactive therapy are essential in improving outcomes because the patient's survival is jeopardized within the first hour of shock.[14]

An anti-inotropic substance has been identified in SIRS patients and may be responsible for the impaired cardiac output in later shock stages. The liver and spleen may become ischemic as blood is shunted to vital organs during septic shock. Myocardial depressant factor is released from ischemic pancreatic tissue and may be at least partially responsible for myocardial depression associated with septic shock.[21,26]

Respiratory

Dyspnea and tachypnea are classic early symptoms of SIRS. This early hyperventilation is of unknown cause, although direct stimulation of the respiratory centers has been implicated.[18] Endotoxin release causes bronchoconstriction, which may lead to increased respiratory muscle work, muscle fatigue, and ventilatory failure.[21]

The two predominant pulmonary manifestations of progression of SIRS are decreased lung compliance and impaired gas exchange.[20] Increased capillary permeability in the lungs causes an increase in interstitial edema. The lungs become stiffer and gas exchange is impaired.

Central Nervous System

The most common central nervous system (CNS) findings in SIRS are fever or hypothermia and disturbed level of consciousness, ranging from confusion and agitation to lethargy, obtundation, and coma. Release of interleukin-1 (IL-1), cachectin, and other endogenous pyrogens from macrophages involved in the inflammatory response is responsible for fever. Elderly patients and patients who have impaired muscle heat production due to low muscle mass, neuromuscular disease, or drugs that inhibit shivering are more prone to hypothermia. The cause of this is less well understood, but is probably related to respiratory and cutaneous heat loss caused by hyperventilation and peripheral vasodilation.[18]

Renal

Oliguria, defined as urine output <0.5 ml/kg/hr, is almost always present in early SIRS and can generally be attributed to low functional blood volume. Fluid replacement will correct this initially. However, the glomerular filtration rate tends to be low in septic patients even if serum creatinine and BUN levels are normal. This is especially important in patients treated with aminoglycosides.[40] In patients with more severe sepsis, oliguria may continue in spite of an adequate blood pressure and volume. If shock ensues, oliguria may progress to acute tubular necrosis or anuria.[18]

Hematologic

The early hematologic effect of SIR is usually leukocytosis, although a transient leukopenia may be present. Endotoxins and chemical mediators adhere to the surface of WBCs,

TABLE 63-1 Chemical Mediators of Septic Cascade[2]

Mediator	Source	Effects
Endotoxin	Gram-negative bacterial cell walls	Activates monocytes and stimulates the release of TNF, IL-1, interleukin 6, and platelet-activating factor Has direct effects on the coagulation cascade and the complement system
Oxygen radicals	Macrophages	Creation of extremely destructive hydroxyl radicals In sepsis, alveolar epithelial cells are especially susceptible to this reaction
Interleukin-1 (IL-1) and interleukin-2 (IL-2)	Macrophages and (to a lesser degree) endothelial cells, epithelial cells, dendritic cells, neutrophils, and B-lymphocytes	IL-1 • Facilitates movement of white blood cells toward injured, ischemic, or infected cells • Stimulates release of arachidonic acid from phospholipids in plasma membranes • Produces fevers, hypotension, and a decreased SVR • Breaks down muscle protein IL-2 • Decreased blood pressure and SVR • Decreased left ventricular ejection fraction • Increased cardiac output • Increased heart rate
Histamines	Mast cells	Vasodilation Capillary leak
Tumor necrosis factor (TNF), also known as cachectin	Macrophages	Stimulates platelet-activating factors, as well as prostaglandin and IL-1 production Contributes to smooth muscle contraction and endothelial cell adhesion
Arachidonic acid prostaglandins	Membrane phospholipids	Potent vasodilators, they attempt to balance the adverse effects created by other chemical mediators
• Thromboxane		Maldistribution of blood flow by potent vasoconstriction and platelet-aggregating effects
• Prostacyclin		Vasodilation and antiaggregant; causes initial decrease in SVR
• Leukotrienes		Increased tissue permeability, bronchoconstriction, and increased activation of neutrophils
Complement cascade	Activated by bacterial products, endotoxin, or interaction with antigen–antibody complex	Cell lysis, stimulation of smooth-muscle contraction, mast cell degradation, neutrophil chemotaxis, and activation of phagocytosis
Coagulation and fibrinolysis cascade	Activated by injury to vascular endothelium	Fibrin clot formation and fibrinolysis
Bradykinin	Activation of Hageman factor in the coagulation cascade or complement activation	Vasodilation and capillary leak
Myocardial depressant factor (MDF)	Ischemic pancreas cells	Decrease in the degree and velocity of contractions in myocardial cells
Beta-endorphins	Pituitary and hypothalamus	Peripheral vasodilation and a decrease in cardiac contractility

Used with permission from Allen C, Clochesy J: Patients with sepsis. In Clochesy J, et al, editors: *Crit Care Nurs*, Philadelphia, 1992, WB Saunders, pp 1245-1257.

tagging them and causing their removal from circulation by the reticuloendothelial system (RES) (macrophages, Kupffer cells of the liver, reticular cells of the lungs, spleen, and lymph nodes). This process results in a decrease in the number of circulating WBCs. As the disease progresses, the bone marrow is stimulated to produce more WBCs, and some immature neutrophils are released into circulation. The result is reflected in the complete blood count, which shows a WBC count >10,000 cells/mm^3 with a shift to the left.[2]

Anemia may occur in the septic patient due to hemodilution after fluid resuscitation for hypotension. If the patient remains ill from SIRS for more than a few days, the anemia may become progressive due to shortened red blood cell survival, blood letting for laboratory testing, and impaired hematopoiesis accompanying any systemic inflammatory response.[18]

Coagulation abnormalities are often present in SIRS. Thrombocytopenia may result from the adherence of platelets to damaged microvascular endothelium, and is usually reversed when SIRS is controlled. Mild to moderate elevations of the prothrombin time and the partial thromboplastin time are also common in sepsis.[18] Some patients may progress to disseminated intravascular coagulopathy (DIC).

Hepatic/Metabolic

The rapid development of hypoalbuminemia is a classic sign of SIRS. Cachectin and IL-1 cause redistribution of albumin into the extravascular space, presumably to provide a source of amino acids for wound healing, and the shift in hepatic protein synthesis to acute-phase-reactant proteins. Amino acids from protein breakdown become a major energy source in SIRS, and this results in a negative nitrogen balance and rapid loss of body mass.[18]

Hepatic and RES function in the liver is impaired in SIRS, especially if it progresses to shock. Patients tend to develop high bilirubin and liver transaminase levels, often referred to as *septic jaundice* or *ischemic hepatitis*. Although the liver enzyme levels can reach extremely high levels, this tends to subside in a few days.[22]

Glucose utilization is impaired in SIRS due to increased levels of endogenous catecholamines, glucocorticoids, and glucagon.[18] Hyperglycemia is common, and there is often a concurrent insulin resistance. Late in sepsis, hypoglycemia develops as glycogen stores are depleted and peripheral supplies of amino acids and fats are not adequate to supply metabolic demands.[19]

LENGTH OF STAY/ANTICIPATED COURSE

The length of hospitalization for patients with sepsis depends on the presence of chronic disease,[26] immunosuppression,[26] early recognition and treatment of SIRS,[8,26] appropriate antibiotic therapy,[17] and the development of septic shock.[8,17,39] However, when sepsis or septic shock is the primary diagnosis, DRG 416: Septicemia, age greater than 17 would apply.[35] The average LOS for this DRG is listed as 9.5 days.[35]

MANAGEMENT TRENDS AND CONTROVERSIES

Many critically ill patients are predisposed to the development of sepsis and will benefit from continuous monitoring for its onset. This is especially true of patients who are immunosuppressed, who have undergone long surgical procedures, who have underlying chronic diseases, or who have invasive medical devices such as urinary catheters, endotracheal tubes, or hemodynamic lines. Despite numerous laboratory tests available, the early diagnosis of SIRS is usually made on clinical grounds. The critical care nurse plays an important role in the recognition of trends in patient status. Prompt recognition of SIRS may prevent progression of the disease and improve patient outcome.

The critical care setting and hemodynamic monitoring are important parts of the management of the patient with SIRS. The patient's chances of survival are increased when hemodynamic monitoring guides the treatment.[34,36] The diagnosis of SIRS is often made or confirmed by a hemodynamic profile obtained from a thermodilution pulmonary artery catheter, which reveals a decreased systemic vascular resistance (SVR), an increased (or decreased, late in sepsis) cardiac output/index (CO/CI), a low pulmonary artery wedge pressure (PAWP), and a narrow arterial–mixed venous oxygen saturation difference.[21,26] Arterial lines are beneficial because they allow continuous monitoring of systolic, diastolic, and mean arterial pressure and access for frequent diagnostic testing to monitor metabolic parameters without subjecting the patient to venipunctures. Cuff blood pressure Korotkoff sounds may be inaccurate in shock states.[10] Continuous electrocardiographic monitoring is beneficial because the patient may develop atrial or ventricular tachyarrhythmias that require treatment.

Treatment of the patient in SIRS is aimed at three goals: (1) identify and eradicate the precipitating infection, (2) ensure fluid resuscitation, and (3) maintain adequate ventilation and oxygenation. Aggressive, optimal therapy has been shown to reduce mortality in septic shock.[26]

If a patient develops the features of SIRS in the absence of evident infection, patient cultures (urine, blood, sputum, cerebrospinal fluid, and wound drainage) and sensitivities should be obtained and antimicrobial therapy instituted. Empiric therapy with a broad-spectrum third-generation cephalosporin in combination with an aminoglycoside is recommended.[26,31] The prognosis of the septic patient is significantly better if antibiotics that kill the microorganism are used.[38] It is important to realize that 50% of patients with symptoms of septic shock will have negative cultures and a causative organism will never be identified, even with the use of computerized tomography.[26] Even when the responsible pathogen is identified, 48 to 72 hours are needed before the antibiotics become effective, and other treatment must also be aimed at the consequences of the toxic component of the disease.

Some degree of hemodynamic instability is usually present in SIRS. Septic patients tend to become hypovolemic due to the increased permeability of capillaries and vasodilation. Volume infusion, preferably guided by hemodynamic monitoring, is the first step in the management of the hypotensive patient. There is some disagreement among clinicians over the type of fluids to administer. No studies have demonstrated that any form of fluid is superior in performance or reduction of mortality.[21] Based on experience with more than 700 septic patients at the National Institutes of Health, Parrillo recommends the following guidelines for fluid resuscitation[26]: (1) if the patient's hematocrit is <30%, blood is the preferred volume expander; (2) if the albumin is <2.0 g/dl, salt-poor albumin should be infused (50 to 100 g); and (3) if the patient has a satisfactory hematocrit and serum albumin, a crystalloid solution that corrects any electrolyte abnormalities can be used. Generally, volume infusion is continued until a PAWP of 12 to 18 mm Hg is reached. Individual patient response should guide the actual goal of therapy.

When fluid resuscitation has increased the PAWP to 18 mm Hg and fails to maintain an adequate blood pressure (MAP >60 mm Hg), vasopressor therapy is indicated.[26] Dopamine at low dose (2 to 5 μg/kg/min) is the best initial agent because it increases cardiac performance and increases renal and mesenteric blood flow.[21,26] The dopamine may be titrated up to 20 μg/kg/min if necessary to maintain an adequate arterial pressure. If this fails to maintain a MAP >60 mm Hg, levateronal, a powerful alpha-adrenergic agonist with moderate β-adrenergic activity, is added at 2 to 8 μg/min, and the dopamine is decreased to renal dose (2 to 5 μg/kg/min).[26] Epinephrine infused at 1 to 8 μg/min or phenylephrine at 20 to 200 μg/min are potent vasoconstrictors that may be useful when other therapies fail. Phenylephrine is a pure alpha agonist and is sometimes useful for patients experiencing serious atrial or ventricular tachyarrhythmias.[2,26]

Oxygen therapy is indicated to maintain an arterial oxyhemoglobin saturation above 95%.[18] Adequate ventilation in the septic patient is a minute volume at least 1½ to 2 times normal.[40] Endotracheal intubation and ventilatory support may be necessary when inspired oxygen fails to maintain an adequate saturation, when level of consciousness threatens airway integrity, or in patients with persistent hypotension who are at risk to develop acute respiratory failure. Often, patients require the addition of positive end-expiratory pressure (PEEP) to aid oxygenation. This helps improve oxygenation by increasing the alveolar diameter or by redistributing the intra-alveolar fluid in the interstitial

spaces of the
before using
venous retu

Althoug
comes her
therapy. T
caused by
metaboli
feedings
immun
ter util
intesti
flora.
been show
ative patients.[24] If paren
glucose is minimized initially and adv
ery. Lipid intake is limited to 10% to 15% of calori
to avoid elevated serum triglycerides and further activation of the arachidonic acid cascade.[2]

Corticosteroid therapy in SIRS remains controversial. Recent studies have shown that it did not enhance survival or reverse shock[7,25] and may increase mortality.[37] Currently, corticosteroid treatment is reserved for patients with suspected or documented adrenal insufficiency.[27]

New therapies aimed at inhibiting the mediators of the inflammatory response are currently undergoing clinical trials. Ibuprofen[12] and indomethicin have shown promise as inhibitors of prostaglandin, thromboxane, and prostacyclin (metabolites of the arachidonic acid cascade), and are presently undergoing large clinical trials.[11,20] Nitric oxide has been implicated as a mediator of the hyperdynamic state and the low systemic vascular resistance of SIRS, and drugs aimed at its inhibition are under investigation.[28] Genetic engineering has been useful in the development of monoclonal antibodies to inactivate the mediators that induce the septic cascade: bacterial endotoxin, tumor necrosis factor, and IL-1.[5,15]

The concept of titrating hemodynamic therapy to supranormal levels and therefore augmenting oxygen delivery (DO_2) has recently been investigated and may reduce mortality in septic shock.[33,34,36] Many therapies tested have shown some improvement in outcome in sepsis, but the best result will probably be obtained with combination therapy that augments the body's natural compensations and interrupts the inflammatory cascade at multiple points.[5,16]

The key to reducing the mortality rate associated with sepsis is early detection and intervention.[29] Proper management of the patient with sepsis may limit the destructive progression of the disease. Nurses who are able to recognize trends in patient status play an important role in proper early management. Delays in therapy may lead to a fatal outcome. It is vital for the critical care nurse to have an understanding of the pathophysiologic changes, suggestive clinical and laboratory findings, and current treatment modalities in order to offer patients optimal care.

	ANTICIPATED ALTERATION
	Tachypnea, >20 breaths/min *due to endotoxins*[30] Dyspnea, respiratory distress Ventilatory effort may involve use of accessory muscles if not mechanically ventilated[19]
[illegible] ventilation	May increase to 1.5 to 2 times normal *to meet metabolic demands in a patient not mechanically ventilated*[40]
HR	Increased: >90 bpm *due to increased metabolic demands and sympathetic stimulation due to decreased circulating volume*
ECG	Sinus tachycardia; patient may develop atrial or ventricular tachyarrhythmias
BP	Hypotension with systolic BP <90 mm Hg, MAP <60 mm Hg, or a decrease of 40 mm Hg from baseline *due to vasodilation and reduced venous return* *MAP is the best indicator of overall perfusion to organs, but trends are more important than isolated measures* *Hypotension in late SIRS may be attributed to low CO*
CO/CI	Early SIRS is characterized by an increased CO >8 L/min or CI >4.5 L/min/m^2 *due to tachycardia and endogenous sympathetic stimulation* *Low CO/CI in early stages is usually a sign of severe hypovolemia*[26] *May remain high in late stages* *Low CO/CI with poor response to volume and vasoactive drugs is an indicator of poor prognosis in advanced SIRS*
PCWP	Initially, low to normal: <8 to 12 mm Hg, *due to vasodilation* Elevated >16 mm Hg *as cardiac function declines*
SVR	Decreased: <800 dynes/sec/cm^{-5}, initially *due to vasodilation and by chemical mediators of the septic cascade* *A very elevated SVR due to a low cardiac output state with resultant sympathetic overactivity may develop late in septic shock*[19]
LVSW	Decreased: <35 g/m^2/beat *due to myocardial depression*
CVP	Decreased: <2 mm Hg, *due to hypovolemia*
Do_2	Increased: >1100 ml/min *due to elevated cardiac output*
Vo_2	Initially increased: >250 ml/min *due to increased cardiac output* *A low Vo_2 carries a poor prognosis in sepsis*[33]
Svo_2	Increased: >75 mm Hg *due to increased cardiac output and oxygen delivery* As sepsis progresses, Svo_2 may fall *due to compromised oxygen delivery* Late in sepsis, Svo_2 may increase *due to impaired oxygen extraction in low-perfusion states*[13]
Neurologic Status	
Mentation	Restlessness, anxiety, confusion, or obtundation; acute changes in mental status or LOC *due to hypoxia, decreased cerebral perfusion, or elevated plasma amino acid levels associated with protein catabolism*[18] Confusion is one of the earliest signs of impending septic shock[19] Stupor and coma are late signs of septic shock
Renal	
UO	Oliguria *due to poor organ perfusion, which may result in acute tubular necrosis and anuria*

Urine Na^+	Decreased: <40 mEq/L/day as renal perfusion falls Excreted Na^+ falls as Na^+ is conserved[19]
Skin	
Color	Flushed appearance *due to peripheral vasodilation caused by vasoactive mediators*
Temperature	Altered: >38° C or <36° C, *due to the presence of endogenous pyrogens released from WBCs in the inflammatory response* *Elderly patients and patients who have burns, spinal cord injuries, or extensive soft tissue injuries may lose the skin's thermoregulatory ability and experience hypothermia*[2]
Edema	Present *due to capillary leak and increased ADH and aldosterone production, which cause water and* Na^+ *retention*
Laboratory Values	
Glucose	Elevated: >110 mg/dl *due to glucagon released in the stress response* *Glucagon causes gluconeogenesis by stimulating the liver to convert glycogen to glucose* Hypoglycemia <70 mg/dl may occur in later stages *due to depletion of glucose stores*
ABG	Initial ABG often reveal a pattern of hyperventilation (mild hypoxemia and hypocarbia) As sepsis progresses, there is a standard progression of acid–base changes from respiratory alkalosis, compensated metabolic acidosis, uncompensated metabolic acidosis, and combined metabolic and respiratory acidosis[40]
Albumin	Decreased: <3.2 g/dl *due to increased gluconeogenesis, movement of albumin into the interstitial fluid space, and impaired hepatic production of albumin*[40]
Electrolyte	
Na^+	Decreased: <135 mEq/L *due to limited water excretion ability and excretion of antidiuretic hormone*[18]
Ca^{++}	Decreased: <8.5 mg/dl *due to movement of* Ca^{++} *into the cytoplasm; associated with decreased myocardial performance and hypotension*[18,40]
Hematologic	
WBC count	Elevated: >10,000 cells/mm^3, or decreased: <5000 cells/mm^3, or 10% immature band forms (shift to the left) Transient leukopenia may develop in early stages *due to aggregation of white cells* May be low in advanced stages *and is an ominous prognostic sign*
Platelets	Decreased: <150,000/mm^3 or increased: >400,000/mm^3 *due to adherence to damaged microvascular endothelium*[18] Progressive thrombocytopenia *due to sequestration of platelets in the lungs and some capillary beds*[19]

PLAN OF CARE

INTENSIVE PHASE

A patient may be admitted to the ICU for this syndrome or already be present in the ICU and experiencing sepsis as a secondary diagnosis or complication. Frequent monitoring and aggressive management can improve patient outcomes from this devastating syndrome.

PATIENT CARE PRIORITIES	EXPECTED PATIENT OUTCOMES
Alteration in cardiac output *r/t vasodilation and fluid shift*	BP, CO, CI, SVR: all WNL

Plan of Care (cont'd)

Interstitial edema *r/t*
Increased capillary permeability
Excessive fluid replacement
Stress adaptation

UO >fluid intake as edema is mobilized
CVP and PCWP: both WNL

Impaired gas exchange *r/t ventilation perfusion imbalance and diffusion defect*

ABG: within patient norms
Lactic acid level <2.2 mmol/dl
Breath sound clear or improving

Altered thought processes *r/t*
Decreased cerebral perfusion
Hypoxia
Disturbances in neurotransmitter function

Return to previous LOC

Decreased tissue perfusion *r/t cellular shunting*

Skin warm/dry
Strong peripheral pulses
Capillary refill ≤3 seconds
Absence of cyanosis or mottling in extremities
Absence of edema

High risk for inadequate nutrition *r/t catabolic state*

Albumin: WNL
Nitrogen balance negative
Body weight maintained
No evidence of muscle mass loss

INTERVENTIONS

Monitor respiratory rate and depth. *In early SIRS, a pattern of hyperventilation is common. As patient tires or condition deteriorates, respiratory failure may ensue.*

Assess for use of accessory muscles or cyanosis.

Continuous pulse oximetry to determine oxygenation.

Obtain ABG if SpO_2 ≤95% or if other sign or symptom of hypoxemia is present. Evaluate ABG for trends and abnormalities.

Monitor breath sounds q1h to q2h. *Absence of breath sounds may indicate the development of a pneumothorax or atelectasis. Adventitious sounds may indicate fluid accumulation in the lungs.*[19]

If the patient is mechanically ventilated, monitor PIP q1h to q2h. *Elevated PIP with normal plateau pressures may reflect narrowing airways or presence of secretions. Elevated PIP and plateau pressures may indicate fluid overload or ARDS.*

Assess the consistency, color, and quantity of secretions in mechanically ventilated patient. Hyperventilate and suction as needed. *Thick purulent secretions indicate a pulmonary infection, and thin foamy secretions may indicate pulmonary edema.*[19]

Provide frequent position changes *to promote optimal chest expansion and drainage of secretions.*

Assess BP q1h if stable; q15min if unstable. *Narrowing of pulse pressure may indicate progression of shock.*[19]

Continuously monitor ECG for HR and arrhythmias.

Monitor CVP and PCWP q1h; more frequently if unstable.

Measure cardiac output q4h and after changes in therapy, and calculate minimum CI, SVR, PVR, SVI, and LVSWI.

Assess peripheral pulses q1h rating presence, equality, rate, and quality. *Weak or declining pulses may indicate a decreasing cardiac output.*

Monitor core temperature q1h to q2h.

Administer IV fluids as ordered. *Large volumes of fluid may be needed due to vasodilation and capillary leak.*

Assess hemodynamic parameters frequently during fluid administration to *prevent fluid overload. PCWP >18 mm Hg may indicate overhydration.*[26]

Plan of Care (cont'd)

Administer vasoactive and inotropic medications as prescribed and titrate to achieve the desired results.

Assess skin color and capillary refill. *Cool skin, cyanosis (especially around mucous membranes), and prolonged capillary refill indicate poor perfusion.*[19]

Reduce potential for increased V_{O_2} by reducing fever, promoting rest, and reducing pain and anxiety.

Monitor level of consciousness every hour. *Deteriorating LOC may indicate decreased perfusion, hypoxia, or impaired neurotransmitters.*[22]

Control blood glucose levels *to enhance nitrogen balance and avoid the potential of increased incidence of infection during hyperglycemia.*[32]

Administer enteral[24] or parenteral nutrition as ordered if patient is unable to eat.

Weigh patient daily.

Monitor laboratory values, especially albumin, transferrin, electrolytes, nitrogen balance studies, glucose, liver function tests, and total lymphocyte count for adequacy of intake.

INTERMEDIATE PHASE

Patients are not transferred from the intensive care unit until they become hemodynamically stable. The following criteria are helpful in evaluating patients for transfer: MAP >60 mm Hg without IV inotrope or vasoactive support; pulse and ventilatory rate within normal limits; normal acid–base balance; adequate oxygenation without ventilator support; urine output >0.5 ml/kg or >30 cc/hr; and no evidence of organ failure. Nursing care priorities will vary greatly from patient to patient depending on the degree of sepsis experienced and the length of stay in the intensive care unit. Specific nursing care plans can be generated based on individual assessment of the patient's condition.

PATIENT CARE PRIORITIES	EXPECTED PATIENT OUTCOMES
Activity intolerance *r/t prolonged bed rest*	Participates in conditioning/rehabilitation program to enhance exercise tolerance Patient verbalizes increased comfort while performing activities
Self-care deficit *r/t reconditioning regimen*	Patient demonstrates ability to intersperse activity with appropriate rest periods. Performs self-care activities within level of own ability
High risk for ineffective breathing pattern *r/t exacerbation of pulmonary complications.*	Patient maintains effective breathing pattern, clear airway, stable pulmonary status

INTERVENTIONS

Encourage deep breathing every hour while awake and assist with incentive spirometry as ordered.

Assist with frequent position changes if necessary.

Gradually elevate the head of bed for increasing periods of time *to promote the return of the orthostatic reflex. Exercises for arms and legs with HOB >45° will also promote the return of reflex.*[23] *Exercises performed while patient is supine do not contribute to maintaining orthostatic reflex.*[41]

Introduce ambulation at times when most likely to succeed. Avoid the following times:

- Early morning *because receptors are sluggish after prolonged periods of sleep*
- After a warm bath *because peripheral vasodilation may contribute to orthostatic hypotension*
- After meals *because blood is shunted to the gastrointestinal tract and may contribute to orthostatic hypotension*[23]

Maintain adequate caloric intake with sufficient fluid intake.

Contract with patient regarding the increase or maintenance of activities.

Include family in planning and implementing activities of daily living.

TRANSITION TO DISCHARGE

Planning for discharge varies according to individual patient needs. Depending on length of hospitalization and severity of illness, plans for discharge may need to include care in a rehabilitation facility. Begin assessment and planning regarding probable discharge status and needs from the initial day of admission. As patient recovery progresses, a multidisciplinary team approach will be most effective in ensuring a timely and effective discharge process whether the patient is discharged to a rehabilitation facility or directly home with outpatient rehabilitation.

REFERENCES

1. AACP/SCCM Consensus Conference Committee: American College of Chest Physicians/Society of Critical Care Medicine Consensus Conference: definitions for sepsis and organ failure and guidelines for the use of innovative therapies in sepsis, *Crit Care Med* 20:864-874, 1992.
2. Allen C, Clochesy J: Patients with sepsis. In Clochesy J, et al, editors: *Critical care nursing,* Philadelphia, 1992, WB Saunders, pp 1245-1257.
3. Balk R, Bone R: The septic syndrome: definition and clinical implications, *Crit Care Clin* 5:1-8, 1989.
4. Benjamini E: The cells of the immune system. In Benjamini E, Leskowitz S, editors: *Immunology: a short course,* ed 2, New York, 1991, Wiley-Liss, pp 17-36.
5. Bone R: A critical evaluation of new agents for the treatment of sepsis, *JAMA* 266:1686-1691, 1991.
6. Bone R: Sepsis and its complications: clinical definitions and therapeutic prospects. In *SCCM 1993 educational and scientific symposium—symposia highlights* Anaheim, Calif, 1994, Society of Critical Care Medicine, pp 1-2.
7. Bone R, et al: A controlled clinical trial of high-dose methylprednisolone in the treatment of severe sepsis and septic shock, *N Engl J Med* 317:653-658, 1987.
8. Bone R, et al: Sepsis syndrome: a valid clinical entity, *Crit Care Med* 17:389-393, 1989.
9. Centers for Disease Control: Increase in national hospital discharge survey rates for septicemia—United States, 1979-1987, *MMWR Morb Mortal Wkly Rep* 39(2):31-34, 1990.
10. Cohn JN: Blood pressure measurement in shock: mechanisms of inaccuracy in auscultatory and palpatory methods. *JAMA* 199:972-976, 1967.
11. Demling R: Adult respiratory distress syndrome: current concepts, *New Horizons* 1:388-401, 1993.
12. Haupt M, et al: Effect of ibuprofen in patients with severe sepsis: a randomized, double-blind, multicenter study, *Crit Care Med* 19:1339-1347, 1991.
13. Hazinski M, et al: Epidemiology, pathophysiology, and clinical presentation of Gram-negative sepsis, *Am J Crit Care* 2:224-235, 1993.
14. Hoyt N: Host defense mechanisms and compromises in the trauma patient, *Crit Care Nurs Clin North Am* 1:753-762, 1989.
15. Klein D, Witek-Janusek L: Advances in immunotherapy of sepsis, *Dimensions Crit Care Nurs* 11:75-89, 1992.
16. Knox J: Oxygen consumption–oxygen delivery dependency in adult respiratory distress syndrome, *New Horizons* 1:381-387, 1993.
17. Kreger BE, Craven DE, McCabe WR: Gram-negative bacteremia IV: re-evaluation of clinical features and treatment in 612 patients, *Am J Med* 68:344-355, 1980.
18. Light RB: Sepsis syndrome. In Hall JB, Schmidt GA, Wood L, editors: *Principles of critical care,* New York, 1992, McGraw-Hill, pp 645-655.
19. Littleton M: Pathophysiology and assessment of sepsis and septic shock, *Crit Care Nurs Q* 11(1):30-47, 1988.
20. Littleton M: Trends in agents used for the management of sepsis, *Crit Care Nurs Q* 15(4):33-46, 1993.
21. Luce J: Pathogenesis and management of septic shock, *Chest* 91:883-888, 1987.
22. Marino P: *The ICU book,* Philadelphia, 1991, Lea & Febiger.
23. Memmer M: Acute orthostatic hypotension, *Heart Lung* 17:134-141, 1988.
24. Moore F, et al: Early enteral feeding, compared with parenteral, reduces postoperative septic complications, *Ann Surg* 216(2):172-183, 1992.
25. Parrillo J: High dose glucocorticoid therapy: two prospective randomized, controlled trials find no efficacy, *Update Crit Care Med* 2:1, 1987.
26. Parrillo J: Septic shock in humans: clinical evaluation, pathogenesis, and therapeutic approach. In Shoemaker WC, et al, editors: *Textbook of critical care,* Philadelphia, 1989, WB Saunders, pp 1006-1024.
27. Parrillo J, et al: Septic shock in humans: advances in the understanding of pathogenesis, cardiovascular dysfunction, and therapy, *Ann Intern Med* 113(3):227-242, 1990.
28. Petros A, Bennett D, Vallance P: Effect of nitric oxide synthase inhibitors on hypotension in patients with septic shock, *Lancet* 338:1557-1558, 1991.
29. Rackow E, Weil M: Systemic response to sepsis, *Crit Care Med* 17:483, 1989.
30. Rice V: The clinical continuum of septic shock, *Crit Care Nurse* 4(5):86-109, 1984.
31. Roach AC: Antibiotic therapy in septic shock, *Crit Care Nurs Clin North Am* 2(2):179-186, 1990.
32. Schlichtig R, Ayres S: *Nutritional support of the critically ill,* Chicago, 1988, Year Book Medical.
33. Shoemaker W, Appel P, Kram H: Role of oxygen debt in the development of organ failure, sepsis, and death in high-risk patients, *Chest* 102:208-214, 1992.
34. Shoemaker W, et al: Prospective trial of supranormal values of survivors as therapeutic goals in high risk surgical patients, *Chest* 94:1176-1186, 1988.
35. *St Anthony's DRG guidebook 1995,* Reston, Va, 1994, St Anthony.
36. Tuchschmidt J, et al: Elevation of cardiac output and oxygen delivery improves outcome in septic shock, *Chest* 102:216-220, 1992.
37. Veterans Administration Systemic Sepsis Cooperative Study Group: Effects of high-dose glucocorticosteroid therapy on mortality in patients with clinical signs of systemic sepsis, *N Engl J Med* 317:659-665, 1987.

38. Young L, et al: Gram-negative rod bacteremia: microbiologic, immunologic and therapeutic considerations, *Ann Intern Med* 86:456-469, 1977.
39. Weil M, Shubin H, Biddle M: Shock caused by Gram-negative microorganisms, *Ann Intern Med* 60:384-400, 1964.
40. Wilson R, Wilson J: Sepsis. In Kinney M, Packa D, Dunbar S, editors: *AACN's clinical reference for critical-care nursing,* ed 2, New York, 1988, McGraw-Hill, pp 1519-1555.
41. Winslow E: Cardiovascular consequences of bedrest, *Heart Lung* 14:326-346, 1985.

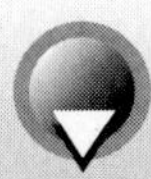

CLINICAL GUIDELINE

64

Multiple Organ Dysfunction Syndrome

Karen K. Carlson, MN, RN, CCRN

DESCRIPTION

Multiple organ failure (MOF) is a relatively new entity. It has evolved as technology and science have improved, allowing health care professionals to be more successful in treating single organ failures. The increasing morbidity and mortality related to MOF has paralleled these advances in technologies,[1] as well as the fact that patients of higher risk are now part of the population being treated. With increased knowledge about MOF, it is apparent that there are no universally accepted definitions of any given organ failure, leading researchers to call this syndrome multiple organ dysfunction syndrome (MODS) rather than MOF. The term dysfunction implies a continuum of physiological derangements rather than the presence or absence of organ failure.[1]

MOF has been defined as the failure of two or more organ systems as a result of malignant intravascular inflammation.[7] Malignant intravascular inflammation refers to an abnormal host response to a generalized, persistent activation of the immune response. Early in the MOF research, numerous studies demonstrated that infection was an important part of the syndrome. More recent studies show that not only can organ system dysfunction occur in the absence of infection, it can be produced experimentally by infusing the spectrum of mediators of inflammation.[11]

MODS is viewed as either primary or secondary. Primary MODS is the direct result of a well-defined insult where organ dysfunction occurs early and is directly related to the insult.[1] The abnormal and excessive inflammatory response is less evident than in secondary MODS. Conversely, secondary MODS results from the effects of the persistent presence and actions of the inflammatory response mediators on the body, rather than the injury.

The patient populations who develop MODS are survivors of major surgery or a traumatic event to the body. Those affected fall generally into three categories: patients with hypoperfusion with or without sepsis, patients with a persistent inflammatory focus, and patients with a continued hypermetabolic state.

The prevalence of MODS in this country is difficult to ascertain. In 1985, approximately 15% of all intensive care admissions were MODS patients.[6] Another study reported that MODS is the cause of death in >90% of surgical intensive care patients who remain in the unit more than 5 days.[2] As more and more consumers are without health care access and delay seeking care, the incidence of MODS may greatly increase, providing a future of critical care units filled entirely with MODS patients.

Mortality related to MODS is linked to the patient's prior state of health, the patient's age, the duration of the systems failure, and the number of systems that have failed. According to one study, in patients with systems in failure for more than 3 days, the mortality rate was 40% with one system involved, 60% when two systems were involved, approaching 100% when three systems were involved, and 100% when four or more systems were involved.[7] A recent study, utilizing a simple scoring system based on systems in failure on day 1 of ICU stay, found that mortality could be accurately predicted approximately 75% of the time.[5]

PATHOPHYSIOLOGY

When the body receives an insult of any type, a number of interrelated systems in the body are activated to protect the host, limit the extent of injury, and promote rapid healing. These systems are all designed to be beneficial. MODS results when these protective mechanisms are initiated, host defense fails, and the body is overwhelmed by the impact of the inflammatory responses.

The process of inflammation includes the envelopment, suppression, and elimination of infectious organisms and the clearance of cellular debris and foreign materials. When the organisms are uncontrolled, generalized activation of the inflammation systems occur.[10] The outcome of this uncontrolled or "malignant" intravascular inflammation is damaged endothelium and direct cytotoxicity, impairing organ function. The malignant intravascular inflammation occurs either because the body is overrun by bacteria and their byproducts, or because the inflammatory responses are unregulated by the body. Widely diverse processes, such as massive transfusions, pancreatitis, trauma, infection, and aspiration, will initiate the inflammatory response.

With injury to the body, five systems of inflammation are simultaneously activated. These systems are summarized in the following Box. The first system to be activated is the complement system. As a result of this activation, neutrophil aggregation is stimulated and white blood cells (WBCs) move to the area of injury. Leukotaxis and leukoagglutination are promoted, and the foreign cells are lysed and opsonized. Cellular components also are activated, play a major role in host defense, and are the source of many different mediators. Polymorphonuclear (PMN) cells are the dominant neutrophil present in the body. Their primary function is to phagocytize foreign particles. During phagocytosis, PMN cells undergo increased metabolic activity at which time mediators are released. These mediators include leukotrienes, thromboxane, and interleukin-1. Mast cells are stimulated, releasing histamine. Histamine, also released by platelets and basophils after complement stimulation or direct cell trauma, causes vasodilation, increased capillary permeability, myocardial depression, and smooth muscle contraction. A summary of the action of many of the mediators seen in the MODS patient are described in Table 64-1.

Monocytes and macrophages are the body's primary defense against foreign invasion of the tissue and are a major source of mediator release. These cells act to rid the invasion site of all foreign materials and cell debris. The primary mediators released by these cells include tumor necrosis factor (TNF), interleukin-1, thromboxane, and coagulation factors.

TNF is produced primarily by the macrophages after activation by the presence of endotoxin. Endotoxin is released from cell walls of bacteria as the cells are destroyed. TNF is thought to mediate the toxic effects of endotoxin, producing many of the signs and symptoms seen in the patient in shock. It has been shown that TNF produces hypotension, tachycardia, tachypnea, hyperglycemia, metabolic acidosis, third spacing, and gastrointestinal (GI) ischemia.[12] It also produces alveolar thickening, acute tubular necrosis, and profound changes in temperature. Therefore, it is thought that TNF is the major mediator of septic shock and MODS. There has been extensive animal research into TNF synthesis, metabolism, activity, and treatment potential. Actions in the body that are believed to be TNF-mediated include enhanced PMN function, fever induction, decreased vascular responsiveness to catecholamines, and the production of anorexia and wasting, probably secondary to the effect on the hypothalamus and gastric emptying.

Interleukin-1 is another mediator released by PMN cells, macrophages, B cells, and others when activated by endotoxin. It acts to stimulate leukocytosis, and enhances both B- and T-cell activity. It causes fever and a decreased responsiveness to catecholamines.

Lymphocytes, a major cellular component of lymph nodes and the spleen, act to regulate, stimulate, or suppress

Summary of Inflammation Systems

Complement system

Stimulation of cellular components (WBCs, platelets, mast cells)
- Neutrophil aggregation
- Leukotaxis/leukoagglutination
- Opsonization
- Phagocytosis

Mediator release: histamine

Monocytes/macrophages
- Eliminate foreign materials and cell debris

Mediator release: TNF and interleukin-1

Lymphocytes
- T cells: direct cytotoxicity and enhanced B-cell activity
- B cells: antibody production

Platelets
- Role in coagulation and inflammation

Kinin system

Mediator release: Bradykinin

Renin-angiotensin-aldosterone system

Renin splits angiotensin from angiotensinogen which is converted to angiotensin II

Clotting system

Factor VII stimulation, leads to hypercoagulability and microemboli formation

Sympathetic nervous system

Epinephrine/norepinephrine release
Renin-angiotensin-aldosterone system stimulation

TABLE 64-1 Mediators of Inflammation

Mediators	Actions
Histamine	Vasodilation Increased capillary permeability Myocardial depression Smooth muscle contraction
Leukotrienes	Increased capillary permeability Activation of phagocytosis Potentiation of inflammatory response Pulmonary vasoconstriction
Thromboxane A_2	Myocardial depression
Interleukin-1	Stimulate leukocytosis Enhanced B- and T-cell activity Fever induction Decreased vascular responsiveness to catecholamines
TNF	Enhanced PMN function Fever induction Decreased vascular responsiveness to catecholamines Production of anorexia
Bradykinin	Vasodilation Increased capillary permeability Bronchoconstriction

as needed in an injury situation. The two types of lymphocytes, T cells and B cells, have different functions. T-cell lymphocytes act to cause direct cytotoxicity, enhance B-cell activity, regulate immune response through activation and suppression, and release mediators. B-cell lymphocytes are responsible for antibody production and the cloning of memory cells.

Platelet release is also stimulated. Platelets play an important role in both coagulation and inflammation processes and also release mediators, thromboxane, and complement activator.

The second system activated by injury is the kinin system. When stimulated, the kinin system releases a peptide called bradykinin. Bradykinin causes vasodilation and increased capillary permeability. This action is augmented by adhesion of the activated leukocytes to blood vessel walls, which potentiates local inflammation, facilitates fluid exudate, and increases vascular compliance.

Renin-angiotensin-aldosterone system activation is stimulated in response to low volume or low renal perfusion states. When renin is released from the juxtaglomerular apparatus on the afferent arteriole of the kidney, it circulates and splits angiotensin from angiotensinogen, which has been released by the liver. Angiotensin travels to various tissues where converting enzyme converts it to angiotensin II, a powerful vasoconstrictor. Additionally, angiotensin II stimulates the release of aldosterone, resulting in increased sodium reabsorption from the renal tubules.

The clotting system is also activated. Factor VII, the Hageman factor, is stimulated, resulting in hypercoagulability and the formation of microemboli. Decreased blood flow and tissue perfusion, secondary to thrombosis, results in microemboli and leads to tissue ischemia and hemolysis. Consumption of platelets and clotting factors is not uncommon.

In addition to the system activation already described, the sympathetic nervous system (SNS) is stimulated. Epinephrine and norepinephrine are released and cause vasoconstriction. Antidiuretic hormone release is stimulated, causing decreased water reabsorption in the renal tubule. The renin-angiotensin-aldosterone system as already described is also activated by the SNS.

There is a release of endogenous opiates called endorphins. Endorphins are found in the brain and are morphine-like substances, having receptor sites in both the central and peripheral nervous system. When these receptors are stimulated, vasodilation results.

Myocardial depressant factor is released from the pancreas following any period of hypotension-induced pancreatic ischemia. Circulating to the heart, it has a negative inotropic effect.

All of these systems are interrelated and communicate cell-to-cell, which adds to the "malignant" intravascular inflammation origin of MODS. All of the pathophysiologic mechanisms activated by injury manifest into systemic consequences. These include the maldistribution of blood flow, oxygen supply and demand imbalance, and a variety of metabolic abnormalities.

The *maldistribution of blood flow* is the result of the vasodilation, vasoconstriction, and vascular occlusion that occurs secondary to system and mediator activation. Vasodilation is the primary abnormality resulting from histamine and bradykinin release. While many vascular beds dilate, others vasoconstrict from epinephrine, norepinephrine, and angiotensin II release, as well as from compensatory mechanisms activated in response to the insult. Vascular occlusion adds to the maldistribution of blood flow. When the clotting systems are activated, microemboli result, causing vascular occlusion. Complement activation causes damage to the endothelial wall, enhancing emboli formation. With the increased capillary permeability that results from histamine and bradykinin release, fluid leaks into the interstitial space, decreasing circulating volume, increasing blood viscosity, and enhancing emboli formation. Neutrophil and platelet aggregation also slow blood flow, adding to the possibility of vascular occlusion.

The changes in blood flow occurring as a result of the mediator release attempt to match circulation with oxygen need. Initially, these mediators are successful, but as the inflammation continues, compensatory mechanisms are exhausted, resulting in an oxygen supply and demand imbalance. After suffering an injury, the body has an increased demand for oxygen. Metabolism becomes hypermetabolic as the body gears up to defend itself. Depending on the injury, the body's demand for oxygen may be further increased due to fever, pain, and increased work of breathing. As a result of the injury, supply frequently is diminished. Many patients experience decreased cardiac output (CO) and hemoglobin (Hgb) levels, decreasing oxygen-carrying sites. Pulmonary edema and ventilation/perfusion mismatch or shunt decrease available oxygen. Additionally, there is strong evidence that cellular deficits occur, leading to decreased cellular utilization of oxygen. Additionally, there may be an oxygen extraction deficit at the tissue level.

Carbohydrate, fat, and protein metabolism are altered when intracellular enzyme systems fail. In response to the body's hypermetabolic state, the liver initially increases the amount of glucose released from glycogenolysis. As the cells become depleted and glucose stores are decreased, the ability to synthesize new sugar is inhibited, and the patient becomes hypoglycemic. Resistance to exogenous administration of substrate may also occur. As a result of these metabolic abnormalities, catabolism occurs and protein stores are used for fuel.

The interrelationships between the mediators of the inflammatory response are extremely sophisticated and difficult to interrupt when host defense fails. There is little agreement in the literature on exact definitions to explain the individual system effects of this host defense. Bone and colleagues suggest that a comprehensive and continuously updated data base is necessary to clinically validate criteria for describing how MODS can be identified in each system.[1]

LENGTH OF STAY/ANTICIPATED COURSE

The anticipated course for a patient with MODS is difficult to predict. The length of stay is heavily dependent on the patient's pre-injury state of health, age, number of systems in failure, and duration of failure. Early recognition and treatment of individual organ system failure theoretically will shorten the length of stay in the ICU, as will positive response to therapy. Patients with MODS are typically classified in accordance with the system most in failure, with the anticipated length of stay calculated consistent with the specific DRG classification.

MANAGEMENT TRENDS AND CONTROVERSIES

There is no treatment for MODS per se. Instead, the therapy focuses on treatment of individual system failures. The three primary foci of care are to treat the cause, remove the initial insult, and support failing systems aggressively. There is some evidence that MODS can be reversed if infection is prevented or controlled, and if tissue oxygenation remains adequate.[8] Treatment for patients with MODS must be tailored to fit the patient as a whole since therapy aimed at supporting one system may damage another. Treatment also must be individually tailored since different patients will have different affected systems.

Immediate attention must be given to prevention of infection. Surgical debridement of wounds may be required. Immediate stabilization of fractures is advised to prevent further tissue injury. Prophylactic antibiotics may be used, depending on the injury.

There has been controversy about the appropriateness of selective decontamination of the GI tract to avoid bacterial translocation from the gut. Such therapy generally utilizes broad-spectrum antibiotics and thus may contribute to colonization, so it has not been universally recommended.[8] Current studies have shown that selective decontamination has no impact on reducing mortality or cost.[4,14]

Maintaining adequate tissue oxygenation in MODS patients is often difficult. The maintenance of adequate cardiac function, adequate Hgb, and adequate O_2 saturation are primary goals. Treatment objectives for the patient in respiratory failure are focused on achieving acceptable gas exchange while minimizing damage to the lungs. Early, aggressive ventilation, often with positive end expiratory pressure (PEEP), is aimed at keeping the PaO_2 greater than 80 mm Hg. Some centers are utilizing inverse ratio ventilation (IRV) in the severely hypoxic, PEEP-resistent MODS patient. IRV reverses the inspiratory and expiratory phases of the respiratory cycle, making the inspiratory time long and the expiratory time short. Concurrently, these patients are ventilated utilizing pressure control ventilation to maintain the mean airway pressures as low as possible. Use of IRV may be uncomfortable, so sedation and paralysis should be considered.

Fluid balance is a challenge in the MODS patient. Attempts are made to avoid fluid overload. Use of diuretics and low-dose dopamine may be instituted to minimize pulmonary edema. At the same time, consideration must be given to adequate fluid balance to support renal function. Hemodialysis or hemofiltration may be initiated to allow additional fluid or parenteral nutrition administration. Pulmonary artery monitoring is essential to evaluate fluid balance and the success of interventions. There is continued debate over the use of crystalloids or colloids in management of these patients. While hypoalbuminemia is common in the MODS patient, albumin and other colloids must be administered with extreme caution. In the presence of increased capillary permeability, colloid administration may exacerbate vascular fluid movement into the insterstitium. Fluid therapy must be individualized to each patient.

Therapies directed at cardiac failure will be focused on the patient's symptoms, which will vary depending upon whether the patient is also septic. Vasopressor agents, dopamine, phenylephrine, and levarterenol are commonly used when patients are hypotensive despite fluid interventions. Dobutamine, isoproterenol, or amrinone may be indicated, and use is determined by individual patient situations. Generally, patients who maintain high CO and low systemic vascular resistance (SVR) will not require vasodilator therapy. However, in MODS and sepsis, patients may progress to low CO states with a high SVR. In this situation, agents such as nitroprusside may be helpful. Antidysrhythmic agents should be used as indicated. Frequently, however, patients in MODS continue to have dysrhythmias despite what appears to be adequate antidysrhythmic therapy.

Patients in hepatic failure often have acid-base disturbances. These should be treated aggressively with sodium bicarbonate and dialysis as needed. Encephalopathy, with or without increased intracranial pressure (ICP), is an ominous sign. Efforts to decrease ICP may include hyperventilation, and use of mannitol or furosemide (see Guideline 41). Coagulation disturbances are also grave indicators, because disseminated intravascular coagulation (DIC) will further complicate treatment (see Guideline 59).

Early institution of nutritional support may minimize catabolism. Some centers are using slow drip (for example, 5 to 10 cc/hr) enteral feedings to maintain GI integrity while using total parenteral nutrition to meet the balance of nutritional needs.

Much energy is being focused on researching new therapies in the treatment of MODS. Our knowledge of appropriate interventions will continue to change as research and technology advance. The use of monoclonal antibodies offered promise but has been shown to be ineffective in MODS and sepsis patients.[15] A recent study suggests that the use of human recombinant interleukin-1 receptor antagonist may prove favorable.[3] Investigation of the use of anti-TNF antibodies is being suggested.[13]

ASSESSMENT

PARAMETER	ANTICIPATED ALTERATIONS
Cardiovascular Status	
HR	Tachycardia: >100 bpm *due to fluid overload, hypoxia*
Pulse	Bounding or diminished *due to fluid status*
MAP	Decreased: <70 mm Hg *due to acid-base imbalances, TNF, fluid shifts, myocardial depressant factor, vasodilation from mediators*
Rhythm	Intractable dysrhythmias *due to electrolyte imbalances, acidosis, hypoxia*
PAP	Decreased: <25/15/20 mm Hg (PAS/D/M) *May be elevated initially*
PCWP	Decreased: <12 mm Hg *due to fluid shifts to interstitium*
CVP	Decreased: <2 mm Hg *due to fluid shifts to interstitium*
CO	Elevated: >8.0 L/min (initially) *due to inflammatory mediators and systemic vasodilation* Decreased: <4.0 L/min *due to decreased sympathetic stimulation, myocardial ischemia, hypoxia*
CI	Elevated: >4.0 L/min *due to inflammatory mediators and systemic vasodilation* Decreased: <2.5 L/min *due to decreased sympathetic nervous system stimulation, myocardial ischemia, hypoxia*
SVR	Decreased: <800 dynes/sec/cm^{-5} *due to circulating endotoxin, acidosis, inflammatory mediators*
Peripheral perfusion	Initially warm then cool, clammy skin Peripheral pulses variable Peripheral edema *due to fluid movement into interstitial space*
Color	Pallor Refractory cyanosis *due to hypoxia, cellular oxygen utilization deficits*
Wt	Increased *due to fluid overload, often in interstitial space*
Heart sounds	S_3 *due to fluid overload* Murmur
Respiratory Status	
RR	Decreased or increased: <10 or >20 breaths/min *due to fluid overload, acid-base imbalance, hypoxia*

Pattern	Dyspnea *due to fluid overload, acid-base imbalance, hypoxia*
Breath sounds	Crackles/wheezes *due to fluid overload, acid-base imbalance, hypoxia* Increased work of breathing *due to fluid overload, acid-base imbalance, hypoxia*
Chest x-ray	Diffuse infiltrates *due to consolidation, infection, and possible ARDS*
Pao_2	Decreased: <60 mm Hg on Fio_2 >50% *due to hypermetabolism and decreased O_2* carrying sites
$Paco_2$	Elevated: >45 mm Hg *due to inadequate air exchange*
Fio_2	Increase % needed to maintain adequate oxygenation, often with PEEP >5 cm H_2O
Pulmonary compliance	Decreased
ABG	Refractory hypoxia/hypercarbia *due to cellular utilization deficits, poor gas exchange*

GI Status

UO	Decreased: <30 cc/hr *due to renal dysfunction from hypoxia, decreased perfusion*
Serum Osmolality	Elevated: >295 mOsm/kg *due to fluid shift into interstitial space*
Creatinine clearance	Decreased: <30 cc/min *due to renal dysfunction from hypoxia, decreased perfusion*
Urine Na^+	Prerenal: Decreased: <20 mEq/L *due to increased reabsorption of Na^+ ion in the attempt to increase renal perfusion* Intrarenal: Elevated: >30 mEq/L *due to loss of Na^+ reabsorptive ability by the kidney*
Specific gravity	Prerenal: Elevated: >1.030 *due to inability to eliminate fluid* Intrarenal: Decreased: <1.010 *due to loss of concentrating ability*

Neurological Status

LOC	Disorientation Unconsciousness Coma Glasgow coma scale <6 ICP >15 mm Hg Respiratory depression Hypothermia/hyperthermia Weakness/fatigue/malaise Vertigo Headache *All are due to effects of hypoxia, acid-base imbalance, hypoperfusion, and uremic toxins*

GI Status	Anorexia Nausea, vomiting Stress ulcers Ileus with NG output >600 cc/24 hr Constipation/diarrhea Decreased caloric intake Hematemesis Melana Guaiac positive NG output/stool Jaundice Bleeding tendencies All are *due to GI tract hypoxia, decreased motility, and decreased use*

Laboratory Tests

Creatinine	Increased: >2.0 mg/dl, or doubling of admission creatinine *due to decreased renal filtering and excretion*
BUN	Increased: >20 mg/dl *due to decreased renal filtering and excretion*
Electrolytes (dependent on individual system in failure)	
• K^+	Increased: >5 mEq/L *due to decreased excretion*
• Na^+	Decreased: <130 mEq/L *due to increased excretion*
• Ca^{++}	Decreased: <8.5 mg/dl *due to increased excretion*
• PO_4^-	Increased: >4.5 mg/dl *due to decreased excretion*
• Mg^{++}	Decreased: <1.5 mEq/L *due to increased excretion*
Coagulation studies	
• PT	Elevated: >25% above normal
• APTT	Elevated: >25% above normal
• Fibrin-split products	Elevated: >10 μg/ml
• Fibrinogen	Decreased: <60 mg/dl
• Hgb	Decreased: <12 g/dl
• Hct	Decreased: <33% without blood loss
• Platelets	Decreased: <100,000/ml *All are due to liver dysfunction, activation of the clotting system by mediators, and/or DIC associated with MODS*
WBC count	Increased: >10,000/mm³ initially *due to inflammatory mediators, infection, and circulatory catecholamines* Decreased: <5000/mm³ later *due to bone marrow exhaustion*
ABG	Initially normal Metabolic acidosis *due to maldistribution of blood flow* Respiratory alkalosis *due to compensation for metabolic acidosis*
Bilirubin	Increased: >2.0 mg/dl *due to loss of bilirubin conjugation with liver failure*
LDH	Increased: >50% above normal
SGOT (AST)	Increased: >50% above normal
Albumin	Decreased: <2.8 g/dl
Glucose	Refractory hyperglycemia *due to SNS activation and effects of intravascular inflammation*

PLAN OF CARE

INTENSIVE PHASE

Nursing Care of the MODS patient is challenging. Interventions that benefit one system may harm another system. The four primary goals of this phase are to assure adequate oxygenation, maximize the effectiveness of the heart as a pump, assure appropriate circulating volume, and prevent or control infection.

PATIENT CARE PRIORITIES	EXPECTED PATIENT OUTCOMES
Ineffective airway clearance *r/t* *Intubation* *Mechanical ventilation* *Retained secretions*	ABG within patient norms Patent airway

Plan of Care (cont'd)

Nursing diagnosis	Expected outcomes
Impaired gas exchange *r/t* *Pulmonary edema* *Ventilation/perfusion mismatch* *Shunting* *Alveolar collapse* *Inadequate Hgb* *Inadequate CO*	ABG: within patient norms Hgb: WNL Breath sounds within patient norms
Ineffective breathing pattern *r/t* *Increased work of breathing* *Anxiety* *Acid-base disturbances* *Volume overload* *Hypoxemia* *Uremic toxins* *Electrolyte imbalances*	PCWP: WNL Breath sounds within patient norms Creatinine and BUN: WNL ABG: within patient norms Electrolytes: WNL
Decreased tissue perfusion *r/t* *Circulating volume status* *Vasoconstriction* *Bleeding* *Microemboli*	Peripheral pulses within patient norms Hgb: WNL Skin warm and dry VS: WNL
Decreased CO *r/t* *Dysrhythmias* *Decreased contractility* *Myocardial depressant factor* *Endotoxin*	CO: WNL ECG rhythm stable, within patient norms
Fluid volume excess *r/t* *Altered renal function* *Excessive fluid administration*	Normovolemic Decreased edema Urine specific gravity: WNL Balanced I/O Wt: WNL PCWP and CVP: WNL
Relative fluid volume deficit *r/t impaired capillary permeability and resulting third spacing*	Urine specific gravity: WNL Balanced I/O Wt: WNL PCWP and CVP: WNL
High risk for infection *r/t* *Use of invasive lines/catheters* *Compromised defense mechanisms* *Decreased nutritional state* *Compromised skin integrity* *Accumulation of metabolic wastes*	Afebrile WBC count: WNL Negative cultures Creatinine and BUN: WNL
Inadequate nutrition *r/t* *Hypermetabolic state* *Nausea/vomiting* *GI dysfunction* *Intubation* *Fatigue* *Prolonged NPO status* *Liver dysfunction*	Wt: stable Albumin: WNL Transferrin saturation: WNL Positive nitrogen balance
Electrolyte and acid-base imbalance *r/t* *Altered renal function* *Altered respiratory function* *Compensatory mechanisms*	Electrolytes: WNL ABG within patient norms Anion gap: WNL

Plan of Care (cont'd)

Altered LOC *r/t*
Hypoxemia
Electrolyte imbalances
Uremia
Decreased cerebral perfusion

Oriented to time, person, and place
Cerebral perfusion pressure: WNL

INTERVENTIONS

Maintain patent airway *to maximize air exchange.*

Implement pulmonary hygiene such as suctioning, chest physiotherapy, incentive spirometer; and turning, coughing, and deep breathing as needed *to assist in mobilizing secretions and promoting ventilation.*

Intubate patient early during care *to increase the patient's functional residual capacity before alveoli collapse; and to promote O_2 delivery.*

Institute mechanical ventilation including PEEP *to increase the patient's functional residual capacity before alveoli collapse; and to maximize ventilation.*

Monitor patient ventilatory compliance and minute ventilation.

Consider use of reverse inspiration: expiration ventilatory ratios *to recruit additional alveoli for enhanced ventilation.*

Monitor oxygenation closely using ABG, oximetry, or oximetric catheter. When evaluating ABG assess $Pao_2/Paco_2$ ratio and Fio_2/Pao_2 relationship.

Evaluate patient for need of restraints *to maintain intact endotracheal tube.*

Calculate and trend alveolar-arterial oxygen gradient.

Monitor respiratory status q1h, including RR, effort and pattern, breath sounds, and presence of adventitious sounds.

Use bronchodilators as needed *to enhance ventilation.*

Position patient *to maximize blood flow to lungs.*

Evaluate impact of any position change on patient's hemodynamic status and oxygenation *to identify position of maximal ventilation without hemodynamic compromise.*

Suction as needed *to maintain patent airway, and to maximize O_2 and CO_2 exchange.*

Consider use of paralytic agents when an acceptable Pao_2 cannot be reached *to decrease O_2 consumption by respiratory muscles and decrease the pressure needed to ventilate.*

If paralytic agents are used, assure that the patient is adequately sedated *to minimize anxiety.*

Institute PA monitoring early in care *to follow fluid status carefully and avoid fluid overload and pulmonary edema.*

Monitor CO, CI, and SVR q4h and as needed *to evaluate the effect of PEEP and maximize fluid status.*

Use colloids rather than crystalloids in fluid replacement *to minimize movement of fluid into interstitial space.*

Administer diuretics as needed *to avoid fluid overload and manage heart failure.*

Institute continuous cardiac and VS monitoring.

Administer antidysrhythmic agents as needed.

Monitor distal pulses as well as temperature, color, and capillary refill *to monitor peripheral perfusion.*

Administer inotropic and/or vasopressor medications as ordered *to maximize cardiac function.*

Maintain mechanical assist devices as necessary (pacemaker, IABP) *to enhance cardiac function.*

Monitor for bleeding from all sites.

Administer blood and blood products as needed *to maximize tissue perfusion.*

Strict attention to aseptic technique is required in all procedures *to minimize patient's risk of infection.*

Institute measures to prevent infection:

- Maintain skin integrity
- Careful aseptic technique

Plan of Care (cont'd)

- Skin and mouth care
- Overall hygiene measures
- Protect from visitors or other patients who are infected

Monitor for signs of infection: malaise, abnormal WBC, positive cultures.

Pan-culture (sputum, urine, blood, catheter tips, etc.) before instituting antibiotics *to assure that correct antibiotics are used.*

If fever occurs, administer pyretics/hypothermia blanket as ordered.

Administer antibiotics carefully *because dose alterations may be necessary if renal function is diminished.*

Monitor BUN and creatinine when administering renal toxic antibiotics.

Monitor daily laboratory values (ABG, electrolytes, BUN, creatinine, Hgb, Hct, platelet count, PT, APTT, WBC with differential and treat as needed).

Monitor skin turgor and mucous membranes.

Monitor daily wts and note trends.

Monitor I/O hourly.

Maintain fluid restriction or provide for careful fluid administration.

Institute low-dose dopamine (2 to 5 μg/kg/min) *to enhance renal blood flow.*

Prepare for dialysis or CRRT if indicated. See Guideline 55.

Maintain Foley catheter with closed drainage system *to enable more accurate measurement of output.*

If hypervolemia occurs, administer diuretics and antihypertensives as ordered.

Monitor specific gravity q shift *to monitor concentrating ability of kidney, and fluid status.*

Initiate NG tube and attach to low intermittent suction *to monitor gastric output (color, amount).*

Guaiac all stools/emesis/NG drainage *to assess for occult bleeding.*

Provide for gastric alkalinization (antacids, H_2 blockers) according to pH.

Maintain prescribed diet, high calorie, frequent feedings.

If patient is NPO, institute enteral (if the GI tract is functional) or total parenteral nutrition *to prevent tissue catabolism.*

Provide frequent oral hygiene, using soft toothbrush and ice chips/hard candy as indicated *to maintain intact oral membranes.*

Monitor changes in LOC q1h.

Reorient to person, place, and time.

Keep bed in low position and side rails up *to enhance patient safety.*

Institute seizure precautions as needed.

Calculate CCP every shift, if ICP catheter is in place.

INTERMEDIATE PHASE

If a patient survives the intensive phase of MODS, recovery will depend upon the patient's age and pre-injury health status. There may be a prolonged rehabilitation time of up to 10 months or longer.[9] The rehabilitation time will be spent regaining muscle mass and neuromuscular function. Nursing care will focus on assisting the patient to adjust to a nonintensive care environment, and increasing independence in activities.

PATIENT CARE PRIORITIES	EXPECTED PATIENT OUTCOMES
Activity intolerance *r/t* *Prolonged bed rest* *Fatigue* *Muscle wasting* *Poor nutritional status*	Able to perform ADL independently
Ineffective breathing pattern *r/t* *Muscle weakness* *Prolonged intubation*	Breathing pattern: WNL ABG: within patient norms

Plan of Care (cont'd)

High risk for fluid and electrolyte imbalance *r/t residual renal insufficiency*	Balanced I/O Stable wt Breath sounds clear Electrolytes: WNL

INTERVENTIONS

Collaborate with physical and occupational therapy *to design and implement a plan for progressive activity and for patient participation in ADL.*
Provide for adequate rest and nutrition *to promote strength and healing.*
Institute measures as needed (such as incentive spirometry) *to maintain breathing pattern.*
Monitor fluid I/O *to evaluate renal function.*
Monitor electrolyte balance and intervene appropriately.

TRANSITION TO DISCHARGE

When it becomes apparent that a patient will survive MODS, plans for discharge should begin. The intensive phase of MODS is often prolonged, and gradual transition is needed to assist the patient and family in moving from this environment to an intermediate care unit and then to home. Patients may be faced with a lengthy rehabilitation phase once they leave the critical care unit. The goals and expected outcomes of this rehabilitation phase should be openly discussed with the patient and family so that they may begin the psychological adjustments necessary.

REFERENCES

1. Bone RC, et al: Definitions for sepsis and organ failure and guidelines for the use of innovative therapies in sepsis, *Chest* 101(6):1644-1655, 1992.
2. Carrico CJ, et al: Multiple organ failure syndrome, *Arch Surg* 121:196-208, 1986.
3. Fisher CJ, et al: Initial evaluation of human recombinant interleukin-1 receptor antagonist in the treatment of sepsis syndrome: a randomized, open-label, placebo-controlled multicenter trial, *Crit Care Med* 22(1):12-21, 1994.
4. Hammond JMJ, Potgieter PD, Saunders L: Selective decontamination of the digestive tract in multiple trauma patients—is there a role? Results of a prospective, double-blind, randomized trial, *Crit Care Med* 22(1):33-39, 1994.
5. Herbert PC, et al: A simple multiple system organ failure scoring system predicts mortality of patients who have sepsis syndrome, *Chest* 104:230-235, 1993.
6. Knaus WA, et al: Prognosis in acute organ system failure, *Ann Surg* 202:685-693, 1985.
7. Knaus WA, Wagner DP: Multiple systems organ failure: epidemiology and prognosis, *Crit Care Clin* 5(2):221-232, 1989.
8. Macho JR, Luce JM: Rational approach to the management of multiple systems organ failure, *Crit Care Clin* 5(2):379-392, 1989.
9. Madoff RD, et al: Prolonged surgical intensive care, *Arch Surg* 120:698, 1986.
10. Pinsky MR, Matuschak GM: Multiple systems organ failure: failure of host defense homeostasis, *Crit Care Clin* 5(2):199-220, 1989.
11. Sculier JP, et al: Multiple organ failure during interleukin-2 and LAK cell infusion, *Intensive Care Med* 14:666-667, 1988.
12. Tracey KJ, Cerami A: Tumor necrosis factor: an updated review of its biology, *Crit Care Med* 21(10):S415-S422, 1993.
13. Wherry JC, Pennington JE, Wenzel RP: Tumor necrosis factor and the therapeutic potential of anti-tumor necrosis factor antibodies, *Crit Care Med* 21(10):S436-S440, 1993.
14. Vandenbroucke-Grauls CM, Vandenbroucke J: Effect of selective decontamination of the digestive tract on respiratory tract infections and mortality in intensive care, *Lancet* 338:859-862, 1991.
15. Ziegler EJ, et al: Treatment of gram-negative bacteremia and septic shock with HA-1A human monoclonal antibody against endotoxin, *New Engl J Med* 324:429-436, 1991.

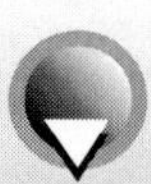

CLINICAL GUIDELINE

65

Multiple Trauma

Jocelyn Farrar, MS, RN, CCRN

DESCRIPTION

Multiple trauma is the leading cause of death in people between the ages of 1 and 44 years.[29] It is a significant health care problem in the United States and contributes to more potential life lost per year than cancer and heart disease combined. Approximately 140,000 trauma-related deaths occur per year. The economic impact is substantial: trauma costs society more than $100 billion dollars per year ($227 million dollars per day) in lost wages, medical expenses, losses in work productivity, insurance expenses, and rehabilitation costs.[21]

In general, males are more at risk for trauma injury than females, with 70% of drivers in automobile crashes being male. Females are at greater risk for injury from domestic violence.[25]

Mechanism of injury for multiple trauma is either blunt or penetrating. Blunt trauma is a result of motor vehicle or bicycle crashes, falls, assaults, sports accidents, industrial accidents, or explosions. Penetrating trauma is caused by guns, knives, or impalement.[27] The pattern of organ injury is determined by the mechanism of injury, the force and type of energy applied to the organ, the age of the patient, and the agent of injury.[14]

PATHOPHYSIOLOGY

Following multiple traumatic injury, the patient experiences a multitude of metabolic, neuroendocrine, and immunologic responses intended to provide energy for restoration, support, and short-term survival, and to reestablish homeostasis (Table 65-1).[10,16] Initially, these responses are life sustaining. Later in the trauma cycle, however, these same physiologic responses have the potential to contribute to detrimental complications. These potential complications include sepsis, due to alterations in immunocompetence, protein catabolism and inappropriate utilization of substrates, sodium and water retention, and decreased clearance of metabolites.[10]

Metabolic and Neuroendocrine Responses

The physiologic responses to traumatic injury can be classified into three phases: the ebb phase, characterized by physiologic instability; the acute flow phase, characterized by hypermetabolism and catabolism; and the adaptive flow, or reparative, phase, characterized by anabolism and tissue repair.[5,16,22] The duration of these phases is determined by the severity of the injury, the prior health of the patient, and the impact of further surgeries and complications.[16]

The Ebb Phase

The ebb phase, that is, the time from injury to physiologic stabilization, represents the first phase of the metabolic response to trauma. Acute tissue injury and volume loss initiate this phase, as cellular perfusion diminishes and local tissue acidosis results.[16] The ebb phase generally lasts from 24 to 48 hours.

It is believed that during this phase increased levels of the catecholamines epinephrine and norepinephrine are released into the general circulation. Inadequate tissue perfusion produces anaerobic glycolysis and acidosis, reflected by rising serum lactate, pyruvate levels, and potassium levels. Serum glucose increases, which produces an increase in the serum osmolarity. The resultant osmotic effect causes a shift of the extravascular fluid into the intravascular space, contributing to an increase in circulating volume.[22]

Reestablishment of adequate circulating volume and oxy-

TABLE 65-1 Post-Traumatic Changes in the Normal Functions of Hormones

Hormone	Normal function	Change after injury
Insulin	Promotes fat storage	Decreased
	Promotes protein anabolism	Decreased
	Decreases blood sugar	Decreased
Glucagon	Promotes lipolysis	Increased
	Promotes proteolysis	Increased
	Promotes gluconeogenesis	Increased
	Increases blood sugar	Increased
Aldosterone	Sodium retention	Increased
	Potassium excretion	Increased
	Increases blood volume	Increased
	Increases blood pressure	Increased
Glucocorticoids	Increases blood sugar	Increased
	Promotes gluconeogenesis	Increased
	Promotes proteolysis	Increased
	Promotes fatty acid mobilization	Increased
	Anti-inflammatory effect	Increased
Antidiuretic hormone	Increases water retention	Increased
	Increases blood volume	Increased
	Increases blood pressure	Increased
Catecholamines Epinephrine	Increases heart rate	Increased
	Increases cardiac output	Increased
	Increases blood pressure	Increased
Norepinephrine	Vasoconstriction	Increased
	Increases blood pressure	Increased
Growth hormone	Promotes protein anabolism	Increased
	Decreases utilization of glucose	Increased
	Increases use of fatty acids for energy	Increased
Thyroid hormone	Increases rate of chemical reactions in all cells	Increased or unchanged
	Increases basal metabolic rate	Increased or unchanged
Gonadal hormones	Promotes secondary sexual characteristics	Decreased
	Promotes anabolism on specific cells	Decreased
	Increases body musculature (testosterone)	Decreased

Used with permission from Howell E, Widra L, Hill M: *Comprehensive trauma nursing: theory and practice,* Boston, 1988, Scott, Foresman, p 298.

gen during the ebb phase is essential. Failure to do so may result in impairment of glucose production (because of inadequate perfusion of the liver), depletion of energy stores, loss of cell membrane function, and death.[16] Inadequate perfusion and oxygenation of vital organs may result in life-threatening sequelae such as multiple organ failure syndrome, adult respiratory distress syndrome, and renal failure.[16]

Other complex neuroendocrine responses are initiated during the ebb phase. These responses include the release of regulatory hormones such as cortisol, glucagon, and growth hormone. The maximal metabolic effects of these hormones are seen following resuscitation after restoration of circulating volume, reduction of acidosis, and improvement of oxygen delivery.[16] Therefore, these hormones will be discussed during the discussion of the flow phase.

The Flow Phase

The acute flow phase begins with stabilization of the patient and return of adequate circulating volume and oxygen delivery.[16] Cellular requirements for glucose as an energy substrate increase substantially during this phase, as vital organs utilize it for energy production.[16] Increased glucose utilization also is seen in the wound, in inflammatory tissues,

TABLE 65-2 Effects of Malnutrition on Target Organs and Systems

Heart	Decreased cardiac mass Decreased volume Dilation of all four chambers Decreased cardiac reserve
Kidney	Decreased mass Decreased glomerular filtration rate Metabolic acidosis Renal failure
Liver and spleen	Decreased mass Subtle changes in hepatic synthetic capacity
Lungs	Decreased vital capacity Decreased response to hypoxia Respiratory muscle decrease Emphysema
Skeletal muscle	Up to 50% loss in mass with corresponding weakness
Gastrointestinal tract	Reduction in mass with atrophy and loss of surface area Malabsorption Diarrhea Sepsis from enteric organisms
Hematologic system	Depression of the immune system Decreased cell-mediated immunity Impaired neutrophil response Anemia

Used with permission from Howell E, Widra L, Hill M: *Comprehensive trauma nursing: theory and practice,* Boston, 1988, Scott, Foresman, p 299.

in the kidney, and in the reticuloendothelial system.[16] Characteristic of this phase are hypermetabolism and hypercatabolism. The metabolic rate may increase by 10% to 30% above the resting basal metabolic rate.[22] The increase is believed to be in proportion to the severity of the injury. Because metabolism is accelerated, the patient demonstrates an elevation of the core body temperature by 1 to 2° C, hyperglycemia, hyperinsulinemia, hypertriglyceridemia, increased cardiac output, and negative nitrogen balance.[16,22] Negative nitrogen balance results from accelerated demand and inadequate protein synthesis. Branched-chain amino acids are catabolized in skeletal muscle and in the liver, resulting in enhanced glucose production. Immobilization and starvation often decrease the necessary protein synthesis. This negative nitrogen balance is manifested in the trauma patient as progressive wasting of skeletal muscle and weakness.[16] Inadequate replacement of protein and calories following traumatic injury may have serious negative effects on the function of vital organs (Table 65-2).[5] Because protein catabolism is enhanced, labile protein stores such as albumin and transferrin are depleted, thus reducing plasma oncotic pressure. Consequently, fluid may leave the intravascular space to sequester in interstitial spaces. This produces systemic edema, which is known as "third spacing of fluid."[5]

Maximal neuroendocrine response occurs during the flow phase.[16] Catecholamine release continues. In addition, adrenocorticotropic hormone (ACTH), from the anterior pituitary gland, causes the release of adrenocortical hormones, primarily cortisol. Cortisol promotes gluconeogenesis, proteolysis, and mobilization of fatty acids. In addition, cortisol decreases extrahepatic protein synthesis and storage. As a result, there is enhanced catabolism of peripheral proteins and increased serum glucose levels.[5,12]

Decreased circulating volume and increased plasma osmolality causes ADH to be elaborated from the posterior pituitary.[19] In an attempt to replenish volume, ADH causes free water to be reabsorbed from the distal tubules and collecting ducts. Consequently, the patient demonstrates a decrease in urine output and an increase in urine specific gravity. Furthermore, ADH also promotes glucose production in the liver.[19]

During the flow phase, glucagon levels rise, even in the presence of elevated serum glucose levels.[16] Glucagon acts to promote glycogenolysis and stimulate gluconeogenesis.[16] The net effect is an increase in blood glucose levels, lipolysis in liver and peripheral tissue, and ketogenesis.[5]

Insulin levels show a diphasic pattern following multiple trauma. Initially, insulin levels fall below normal despite elevations in serum glucose concentrations.[16] Following resuscitation, insulin levels rise. An insulin resistance develops in skeletal muscle and in the liver.[16]

Decreased blood pressure results in diminished glomerular filtration rate (GFR), which stimulates the renin-angiotensin-aldosterone (RAA) reaction.[12] Renin, released by the juxtaglomerular apparatus of the kidney, activates the conversion of angiotensinogen (a plasma protein) to angiotensin I. Angiotensin I is converted in the lung to angiotensin II, a potent vasoactive substance. Angiotensin II causes systemic peripheral vasoconstriction and an increase in aldosterone release.

Aldosterone, in turn, promotes sodium and water retention. The combined effect of the RAA reaction is to increase the blood pressure through enhanced peripheral arteriolar vasoconstriction and retention of water and sodium.[12]

The Adaptive Flow, or Reparative, Phase

The adaptive flow phase (also referred to as the reparative phase) is characterized by an anabolic response following injury. The beginning of a positive nitrogen balance is seen during this phase. Levels of insulin, growth hormone, and thyroid hormone rise. Glucagon levels decrease. The net effect of these changes promotes protein synthesis, restores fat deposits, stimulates the immune system, and facilitates cell proliferation and tissue repair.[19,22]

Immunologic Response

Multiple trauma significantly alters the immunocompetence of the patient. As a result of immunosuppression, the trauma patient may be at risk for generalized infection or overwhelming sepsis 7 to 10 days after injury.[5,10]

Some mediators of inflammation, particularly prostaglandin E_2, may cause a reduction of T-cell production.[3] As a result, anergy is common following trauma.[5,10] Deactivation of neutrophils and a reduction in chemotaxis may be seen. Prostaglandins may produce vasodilation, decreased peripheral resistance, decreased leukocyte metabolism, and alterations in phagocytosis. The level of circulating glucocorticoids after trauma may further contribute to depression of the T lymphocytes and impair wound healing.[5]

The hypermetabolic response associated with protein catabolism and protein/calorie malnutrition also contributes to alterations in immune response by decreasing phagocytosis, depressing T-cell function, and causing complement and neutrophic deficiency.[5] Restoration of proteins and calories to offset the protein/calorie malnutrition drastically improves immune function.[5]

Iatrogenic factors also can contribute to the loss of immunocompetence following traumatic injury. These include anesthesia, use of antibiotics, administration of blood products, and massive fluid resuscitation.[2]

Prior medical conditions may complicate and compound the degree of injury associated with multiple trauma. Preexisting conditions found to have the greatest impact of morbidity and mortality include cardiac disease, pulmonary disease, diabetes mellitus, osteoporosis, hepatic disease, renal disease, cancer, and alcoholism.[25] For example increased mortality following trauma has been found for patients with two or more preexisting medical conditions and for patients experiencing renal or cardiac disease or a malignancy before the traumatic injury.[20]

The trauma itself, as well as the possible surgeries following injury, contribute to the pathophysiology associated with multiple trauma. Potential complications include skin or wound breakdown, muscle atrophy or weakness, contractures, pulmonary emboli, fat emboli, acute respiratory distress syndrome (ARDS), acute renal failure, disseminated intravascular coagulation (DIC), liver failure, multiple organ dysfunction syndrome (MODS), and myocardial failure.[4]

LENGTH OF STAY/ANTICIPATED COURSE

The length of stay for the patient experiencing a traumatic injury depends on multiple factors. First, the severity of the initial injuries may dictate the course of recovery. The more severe the injuries, the longer the patient may need invasive monitoring or respiratory, renal, or cardiovascular support.

The variable nature of multiple trauma is reflected in the DRG classifications for this condition. DRG 484 refers to significant multiple trauma that requires craniotomy with an average LOS of 20.2 days.[26] In the event that limb reattachment is a focus, DRG 485: Limb Reattachment, Hip and Femur Procedures for Multiple Significant Trauma may apply with an average LOS of 14.4 days.[26] DRG 486: Other OR Procedures for Multiple Significant Trauma carries an average LOS of 16.8 days.[26] Finally, multiple trauma that can be managed medically is classified as DRG 487: Other Multiple Significant Trauma with an average LOS of 10.2 days.[26]

Factors That Contribute to Tissue Hypoxia in the Trauma Patient

- Shifts to the left of the oxyhemoglobin dissociation curve secondary to (1) infusion of large volumes of banked blood, (2) hypocarbia or alkalosis, (3) hypothermia
- Reduced hemoglobin secondary to hemorrhage
- Reduced cardiac output in the presence of cardiovascular insults
- Impaired cellular oxygen consumption associated with metabolic alterations of sepsis
- Increased metabolic demands associated with the stress response to injury

From Neff J, Kidd P: *Trauma nursing: the art and science*, St Louis, 1993, Mosby–Year Book, p 683.

MANAGEMENT TRENDS AND CONTROVERSIES

The overall goal in the treatment of the multiple trauma patient is to reestablish effective perfusion of tissues to deliver an adequate supply of oxygen to the cells.[18] Thus, the injured patient is considered to be in shock until proven otherwise. Equally important, interventions to restore oxygen delivery to the tissues must be instituted within a finite period of time.[18] Multiple factors may contribute to tissue hypoxia in the trauma patient (see the preceding Box).

To restore adequate oxygen delivery to the tissues, it is essential to immediately establish a secure, patent airway. Administration of high-flow oxygen is necessary for all trauma patients to satisfy increased oxygen demand.[17] Supplemental oxygen may be provided via a face mask or endotracheal intubation with mechanical ventilation.

Once a secure airway is established and supplemental oxygen provided, the focus turns to transporting oxygen to the tissues.[18] Immediate vascular access is established with large-bore IV catheters. Large peripheral veins such as the antecubital fossa, saphenous vein, jugular vein, or subclavian vein are utilized.[1,17] Extremities with injuries proximal to an intended IV site should not be used because of the risk of venous extravasation.[17]

Active, ongoing bleeding must be controlled by direct pressure, splints, or traction. Pneumatic shock trousers, a source of controversy in trauma care,[18] may be used temporarily to minimize bleeding from unstable pelvic fractures or to provide tamponade for other sources of bleeding.[11,17]

The choice of crystalloids versus colloids as the ideal resuscitation fluid is the subject of ongoing debate.[24] Central to this debate is the concern that the use of certain fluids for resuscitation exacerbates the accumulation of lung water and the development of acute respiratory distress syndrome (ARDS). Opponents of colloidal resuscitation argue that, because capillary permeability increases significantly following local trauma or infection (because of the effect of circulating mediators), colloidal fluids, such as albumin, may escape across the pulmonary capillary membrane. This accumulation of albumin increases the colloidal osmotic pressure within the lung tissue and causes fluid to seep into the interstitial space.[24] On the other hand, opponents of crystalloid resuscitation state that significantly greater volumes of crystalloids are needed to restore hemodynamic stability for the trauma patient. This massive influx of crystalloid reduces the intravascular colloidal osmotic pressure, allowing fluid to leave the intravascular space and accumulate in lung tissue.[24] Currently, there are insufficient data to resolve the debate.

Replacement of blood lost following injury also is of concern. A healthy adult can sustain a blood loss of approximately 15% and demonstrate few clinical symptoms.[18] For this patient population, crystalloid or colloid fluid resuscitation can effectively restore circulating volume. A patient sustaining a greater blood loss, or a previously compromised patient, typically requires blood and/or clotting factor replacement. The type and amount of blood products required vary depending on patient status, physician preference, and institution policy. The use of autotransfusion to replace lost blood is a source of debate. Of concern is the potential for septic or coagulopathic complications following the administration of autologous blood.[23]

Regardless of the type of resuscitation fluid used, the effectiveness of volume resuscitation is indicated by evidence of adequate organ perfusion.[17] Clinical indicators of effective organ perfusion include adequate urine output, return to baseline or improvement of mentation, and improved skin perfusion.[17] Trends in hemodynamic parameters can be assessed to evaluate the continued effectiveness of the resuscitation efforts.

Following initial resuscitation, stabilization, and early therapeutic intervention, the severely injured trauma patient is transferred to a critical care setting. The importance of a complete, ongoing assessment cannot be overemphasized.[13] The impact of the injury, along with consequences of resuscitation, can result in multisystem dysfunction. In addition, hidden injuries may have been missed inadvertently during the resuscitation phase. Subtle changes in assessment findings or inappropriate response to treatment may be the first indicators of missed injuries. Hemodynamic monitoring is indicated to ensure the balance between oxygen supply and demand.[13]

If the patient is breathing spontaneously, aggressive pulmonary toilet, chest physiotherapy, oropharyngeal suctioning, and incentive spirometry are useful to prevent respiratory complications. Supplemental, humidified oxygen may be ordered. A fall in the arterial oxygen pressure (PaO_2) below 60 mm Hg or an arterial carbon dioxide pressure ($PaCO_2$) greater than 45 mm Hg is generally considered an indication of respiratory compromise and the need for endotracheal intubation and mechanical ventilation.[13]

Assessment of trends in neurologic parameters is of importance in the management of the trauma patient. Alterations in level of consciousness may be the result of multiple factors, including neurologic insult, inadequate tissue perfusion, the effects of alcohol or drugs, or consequences of therapeutic intervention. Refer to the chapters on neurologic injury for a more detailed discussion.

The trauma patient is at risk for development of renal dysfunction and oliguric renal failure. Many conditions contribute to this, including preexisting chronic renal disease, decreased renal perfusion related to the injury, the effects of nephrotoxic drugs, or myonecrosis with myoglobinemia due to massive tissue injury.[13] A urine output of 0.5 to 1.0 ml/kg/hr is satisfactory for the trauma patient.[13] Urine specific gravity and the presence of hematuria are also assessed. Refer to the chapter on renal failure for a more detailed discussion.

The hypermetabolic trauma patient is at risk for life-threatening complications of trauma, including infection, vital organ dysfunction, translocation of bacteria due to bowel mucosal atrophy, and malnutrition.[19] Nutritional support must be instituted before these complications of protein/calorie deficiency occur.

Parenteral nutrition can be utilized to meet the nutritional needs of the trauma patient. A highly concentrated carbohydrate source (dextrose) is used to supply an energy source, and amino acids are utilized for protein synthesis. An infusion of lipids can be used to supply fats for energy and reduce the amount of carbon dioxide produced by excessive carbohydrate metabolism.[19] Parenteral nutrition, however, is not without controversy and is being investigated as a contributor to the development of gut mucosal deterioration, sepsis, and multiple organ failure.[9,19]

Currently, the use of enteral nutrition, rather than parenteral nutrition, is advocated.[9,15,19] Early use of the gut reduces the potential for gastrointestinal mucosal thinning and translocation of bacteria across the damaged mucosa into the systemic circulation, enhances substrate use, and requires less energy for nutrient utilization.[9,19] A significantly lower incidence of septic consequences and morbidity has been found in patients fed enterally following trauma.[15]

Ongoing research in trauma care includes investigation

TABLE 65-3 Primary and Secondary Assessment Components

Primary assessment

Airway

Assess airway patency.
Use chin left and/or jaw thrust maneuver to establish a patent airway.
Never use hyperextension of the patient's head and neck to establish an airway because of the potential for cervical spine injury.

Breathing

Expose patient's chest.
Assess for adequate breathing.
Look for signs of tension pneumothorax, open pneumothorax, and/or flail chest.

Circulation and bleeding

Assess pulses for quality, rate, regularity.
Note: If radial pulse is palpable the systolic pressure will be >70 mm Hg.
Check capillary refill.
Control obvious hemorrhage by utilizing the following:

1. Direct pressure
2. Elevation
3. Pressure points
4. PASG, if indicated

Brief neurological evaluation

Assess level of consciousness (Glasgow coma scale).
Check pupillary size and response.
Remove all clothing from patient.
Draw baseline laboratory studies.
Insert Foley catheter and nasogastric tube.
Perform emergency diagnostic studies as indicated (peritoneal lavage and/or radiographic studies).

Secondary survey

Head

Check scalp for cuts, bruises, swelling, and other signs of injury.
Examine skull for deformities and depressions.
Inspect eyes and eyelids. Determine pupil size, equality, and reaction to light.
Note color of inner surfaces of eyelids.
Look for presence of blood and/or serous fluid in the nose and ears.
Examine mouth for presence of blood, vomitus, loose teeth, dentures.

Neck

Palpate for point tenderness over cervical spine region.
Stabilize neck using a cervical collar and backboard if cervical spine injury is suspected.

Chest

Examine chest for lacerations, contusions, entrance and exit wounds, and/or impaled objects.
Look for equal expansion, deviated trachea, and presence of sucking wounds and/or flail chest.
Palpate rib cage, sternum, and clavicles.

Abdomen

Examine for lacerations, contusions, penetrating wounds, and/or impaled objects.
Perform light and deep palpation.
May apply PASG if intra-abdominal hemorrhage is suspected to slow blood loss while waiting for surgical intervention.
Note: PASG are contraindicated in patients with the following:

1. Bleeding thoracic wounds
2. An impaled object in the abdomen
3. Abdominal evisceration
4. Tension pneumothorax
5. Cardiac tamponade

It remains controversial whether PASG should be utilized for patients with a closed head injury.
Note: If patient arrives with PASG in place, physician should remove per established procedure. Inadvertent removal without proper procedure may cause profound shock and/or cardiac arrest.

Lower back

Palpate for point tenderness, deformities, and other signs of injury.

Pelvis

Use compression to check for presence of fractures.

Genital region

Note obvious injuries.
Assess for obvious bleeding.

Lower extremities

Inspect for deformities, swelling, dislocations, bleeding, bone protrusions, and obvious fractures.
Palpate for point tenderness at suspected fracture sites.
Assess pedal pulses bilaterally.
Be alert for presence of compartment syndrome if severe injuries are present.

Upper extremities

Inspect for deformities, swelling, bleeding, discoloration, bone protrusions, and obvious fractures.
Palpate for point tenderness at suspected fracture sites.
Assess radial pulses bilaterally.
Assess for neurovascular compromise.

Back surfaces

Examine for obvious injury.
Palpate for point tenderness over thoracic and lumbar spinal region.

Used with permission from Cardona V, et al: *Trauma nursing: from resuscitation through rehabilitation,* Philadelphia, 1988, WB Saunders, p 78.

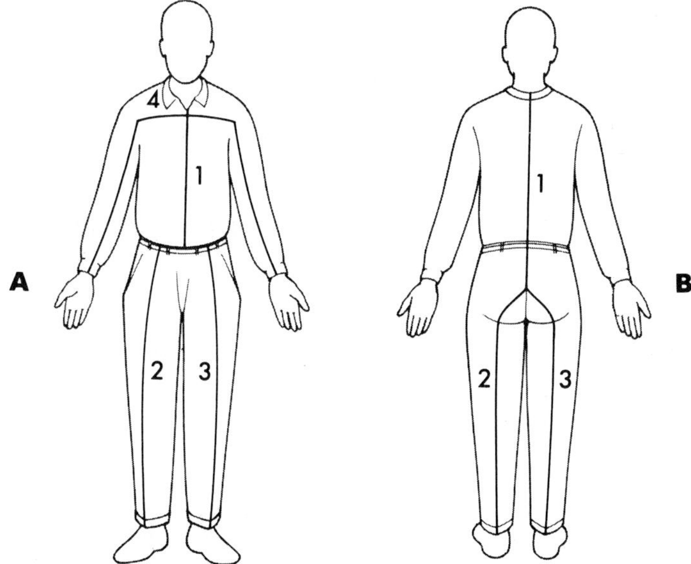

Figure 65-1 Technique for clothing removal in the supine and prone positions, also called "strip and flip." In the supine position: **A,** *1*, Cut down midline of shirt, which exposes any emergent anterior chest injuries; *2* and *3*, cut down legs of pants, which exposes any pelvic cavity, lower abdomen, thigh, or leg injuries. Cut through belt twice, keeping wide distance from genitals. *4*, Cut up arms, which will expose any peripheral injuries. Clothes will now fall away completely, allowing examination of back during logroll. In the prone position: **B,** *1*, Cut down midline of shirt, which exposes any emergent posterior chest injuries; *2* and *3*, starting at center, cut belt once, then continue down one leg. Finish by cutting down other leg by starting at midbuttocks. After patient is rolled onto backboard, clothes can be gently pulled away from front. (Redrawn from Bull G: Strip and flip, *Emergency Medical Services* 14(6):14-16, 1985. From Neff J, Kidd P: *Trauma nursing: the art and science,* St Louis, 1993, Mosby–Year Book, p 131.)

of the administration of glutamine, an amino acid used by the gut for fuel. Glutamine is thought to increase gut mucosal thickness and integrity and decrease the risk of bacterial translocation.[9,19] The most advantageous route for administration (parenteral versus enteral) is a source of debate.

ASSESSMENT OF MULTIPLE TRAUMA

The initial assessment of the multiple trauma patient consists of a rapid primary survey and a more thorough secondary survey. In addition, it is important to collect information regarding the patient's history and history of the events surrounding the injury.

Primary Survey

The goal of the primary survey is to rapidly identify and treat conditions that pose an immediate threat to the life of the patient. The primary survey and initial resuscitation are performed simultaneously. This survey should take 30 to 60 seconds (see Table 65-3). The mnemonic A, B, C, D, E may assist the nurse in organizing the survey.[6]

- A Airway and cervical spine control
- B Breathing
- C Circulation and hemorrhage control
- D Disability (neurologic exam)
- E Exposure of the patient

Because clothing restricts the assessment of the trauma patient, it is removed in a safe and rapid manner (Figure 65-1). In particular, clothing must be removed from patients who have severe trauma or gunshot wounds or who are unconscious without obvious etiology.[14] It is important to take measures to protect the patient from hypothermia during exposure and assessment.

Secondary Survey

The secondary survey begins when the primary survey and resuscitation have been completed.[6] The goals of the secondary survey are to evaluate the interventions performed during resuscitation and to identify other injuries not identified during the primary survey. The secondary survey consists of a thorough head-to-toe assessment of the patient (see Table 65-3). During this time, specific diagnostic procedures are initiated to further assess the patient.

Patient History

Early in the initial management of the multiple trauma patient, a brief history can be obtained from prehospital care providers, witnesses, family, or friends. Because of the severity of the injury, or alterations in level of consciousness due to neurologic injury or drug or alcohol use, it may not be feasible to depend on the patient to provide reliable information. The mnemonic AMPLE, shown in the preceding Box, may help the nurse in eliciting important information.[8,14]

AMPLE Mnemonic

A Allergies
M Medications
P Past medical and surgical history
L Last meal and last tetanus immunization
E Events leading to injury

Used with permission from Kidd P: Assessment of the trauma patient. In Neff J, Kidd P: *Trauma nursing: the art and science,* St Louis, Mosby–Year Book, 1993.

In a less urgent manner, the following information also can be obtained: family and social history, routine demographic information, and insurance information.[8]

Ongoing Assessment

Following resuscitation and therapeutic intervention, it is essential that the multiple trauma patient be thoroughly assessed on an ongoing basis.

ASSESSMENT

PARAMETER	ANTICIPATED ALTERATION
Cardiovascular Status	
HR	Initially Tachycardia: >100 bpm *in response to sympathetic nervous system stimulation, hypermetabolic response, hypovolemia* Subsequent WNL *with hemodynamic stabilization* Bradycardia: <60 bpm *due to conduction defects or toxic effects of mediators on myocardium, spinal cord injury, or increased ICP*
Cardiac rhythm	Dysrhythmias *due to metabolic or electrolyte abnormalities*
Pulse pressure	Initially Narrowed: ≤30 mm Hg *in response to shock, decreased circulating volume, and effects of sympathetic nervous system and endocrine stimulation* Subsequent WNL *with hemodynamic stabilization*
MAP	Initially Hypotension: MAP <70 mm Hg *due to decreases in circulating volume or effects of vasoactive mediators* Subsequent WNL *with hemodynamic stability*
CO	Initially Decreased: <4 L/min *due to decreased circulating volume, reduced contractility, decreased preload* Subsequent WNL *with hemodynamic stabilization, increased preload, inotropic and vasoactive drug therapy*
CI	Initially Decreased: <2.7 L/min/m^2 *in response to decreased circulating volume, reduced contractility, reduced preload* Subsequent WNL *in response to vasoactive and inotropic drug therapy, optimized preload, optimized fluid volume*
SVR	Initially Increased: >1200 dynes/sec/cm^{-5} *in response to sympathetic vasoconstriction* Subsequent WNL *with hemodynamic stability* Decreased: <800 dynes/sec/cm^{-5} *in response to infection or vasodilation due to circulating mediators*
PCWP	Initially Decreased: <8 mm Hg *due to decreased circulating volume, decreased preload* Subsequent WNL *in response to optimized circulatory volume, optimized preload, sympathetic vasoconstriction, vasoactive drug therapy* Elevated: >12 mm Hg *in response to overaggressive fluid resuscitation with compromised myocardium or complications of pulmonary pathology*
Pulmonary Status	
Airway patency	Wheezes, gasping, stridor hoarseness, altered gag reflex, intolerance of supine position, subcutaneous emphysema, *when compromised by debris, facial fractures, blood, teeth, laryngeal or tongue edema, laryngeal injury, decreased LOC*

Chest excursion	Restricted excursion *with chest trauma*
Symmetry of breathing	Paradoxical chest wall movement *with flail chest*
Work of breathing	Retractions, increased work of breathing *with chest trauma, compromised airway*
Breath sounds	Absent, unilateral, or diminished *with chest trauma, airway compromise, pneumothorax, hemothorax*
Respiratory rate	Decreased: <8/min or increased: >40/min *with chest trauma, head injury, metabolic alterations, or airway compromise*
Tracheal location	Deviated *with chest trauma*
ABG	WNL *with hemodynamic and respiratory stability* • pH <7.35 *with uncompensated metabolic or respiratory acidosis* • Pao_2 <60 mm Hg or Sao_2 <95% *with inadequate oxygenation* • $Paco_2$ >45 mm Hg *with inadequate ventilation*
Do_2	Initially Decreased: <900 ml/min *in response to decreased circulating volume, decreased cardiac output, decreased hemoglobin levels, decreased arterial oxygen content, peripheral shunting* Subsequent WNL: 900 to 1100 ml/min *in response to adequate cardiac output, normal arterial oxygen content, normal hemoglobin levels*
Vo_2	Initially Increased: >275 ml/min *due to hypermetabolic response to trauma* Subsequent WNL: 225 to 275 ml/min *with normalized cardiac output and metabolic rate*

Serum Laboratory Values

Serum lactate	Elevated: >2.2 mEq/L *with disturbances in oxygen transport, inadequate tissue perfusion, and anaerobic metabolism*
Serum glucose	Initially Elevated: >110 mg/dl *in response to sympathetic, metabolic, and neuroendocrine stimulation, as a source of energy* Subsequent Elevated: >110 mg/dl *in response to TPN therapy or insulin resistance*
Na^+	Increased: >145 mEq/L *in response to aldosterone release*
K^+	Initially Transient increase *in response to tissue/cellular destruction* Decreased: <3.5 mEq/L *in response to effects of aldosterone* Subsequent Increased: >5.0 mEq/L *in response to metabolic acidosis or renal failure* Decreased: <3.5 mEq/L *in response to inadequate replacement*
Ca^{++}	Decreased: <8.5 mEq/L *due to massive citrated blood transfusions*
Serum osmolality	Initially Increased: >295 mOsm/kg *with hemoconcentration, hyperglycemia, shock, rising lactate levels* Subsequent WNL *with normalized circulating volume, normal glucose and lactate levels* Decreased: <285 mOsm/kg *with overaggressive fluid therapy*
Hgb	Initially WNL, *which may not reflect acute bleeding* Subsequent Decreased: <12 g/dl *with hemorrhage and fluid resuscitation or the dilutional effect of aggressive IV therapy*

Hct

Initially
WNL *with whole blood loss, which may not reflect acute bleeding*
Subsequent
Decreased: <37% *with hemorrhage and fluid resuscitation or the dilutional effect of aggressive IV therapy*

Platelets

Initially
Increased: >400,000/mm^3 *due to stress response*
Subsequent
Decreased: <150,000/mm^3 *with continued whole blood loss and inadequate replacement of platelets*

Fibrinogen

Initially
Increased: >356 mg/dl *due to stress response*
Subsequent
Decreased: <195 mg/dl *with continued whole blood loss or inadequate replacement of clotting factors, development of DIC*

Infectious Status

WBC

Initially
Increased: >10,000/mm^3 *due to stress response*
Subsequent
Increased: >10,000/mm^3 *due to infective process*

Temperature

Initially
Hypothermic: <35° C *due to effects of environment or cold fluid resuscitation*
Subsequent
Increased: 1 to 2° C *due to hypermetabolic state*

Skin Status

Color

Pale *due to effects of vasoconstriction*

Peripheral pulses

Weak, thready *due to decreased circulating volume*

Capillary refill

Slowed: >3 sec *due to vasoconstriction and shunting of blood to vital organs*

Nutritional Parameters

Serum albumin

Initially WNL
Subsequent
Decreased: <3.2 g/dl *due to hypercatabolic state, protein/calorie malnutrition, decreased synthesis*

Transferrin

Initially WNL
Subsequent
Decreased: <200 mg/dl *due to decreased total iron, blood loss, transfusions, depletion*

Creatinine height index

Initially WNL
Subsequent
Decreased: <90% standard *due to negative nitrogen balance, hypermetabolic state*

Total lymphocyte count

Initially WNL
Subsequent
Decreased: <20% *due to immunosuppression*

Renal Status

UO

Initially
WNL *due to effects of ADH, decreased circulating volume*
Subsequent
Decreased: <0.5 ml/kg/hr or 30 cc/hr *with adequate restoration of circulating volume and normal kidney function*

PLAN OF CARE

INTENSIVE PHASE

The need for ICU admission in the presence of multiple trauma depends primarily on the risk or actual presence of hemodynamic instability. Additionally, the need for frequent monitoring and aggressive management may require intensive nursing care and admission to a critical care unit.

PATIENT CARE PRIORITIES	EXPECTED PATIENT OUTCOMES
Ineffective airway clearance *r/t:* *Oral debris* *Teeth* *Foreign bodies* *Blood* *Altered LOC* *Laryngeal or tongue edema* *Maxillofacial trauma* *Intubation* *Mechanical ventilation*	Patent airway Bilateral breath sounds ABG within patient norms Secretions removed/managed Clear lungs Secure natural or artificial airway Absence of respiratory distress
Ineffective breathing pattern *r/t:* *Airway obstruction* *Chest trauma* *Pain* *Anxiety* *Maxillofacial trauma* *Altered LOC* *Increased work of breathing*	Breathing pattern: WNL/improved Anxiety relief Pain relief/reduction to optimize respiration, rest, sleep Improved LOC Normal/improved work of breathing Symmetrical chest expansion with respiration No complaints of dyspnea
Impaired gas exchange *r/t:* *Impaired oxygen delivery* *Altered pulmonary capillary bed* *Ventilation/perfusion mismatch* *Shunting* *Retained secretions*	Hgb: WNL ABG within patient norms Ventilation perfusion relationship within patient norms A-a gradient: WNL Shunt fraction: WNL Improved pulmonary compliance CXR: WNL Svo_2: WNL
High risk for aspiration *r/t:* *Oral bleeding* *Altered gag reflex* *Altered LOC* *Vomiting* *Reflux of enteral feedings* *Artificial airway*	CXR: WNL Airway protected Breath sounds clear bilaterally Feeding tubes patent/in position Absence of enteral feeding in airway ABG: WNL Gastric residual: WNL
High risk for fluid volume deficit *r/t:* *Hemorrhage* *Fluid shifts* *Decreased vascular tone r/t increased vascular permeability*	Pulse pressure improved Palpable pulses MAP: WNL CVP: WNL CI: WNL SVR: WNL No evidence of hemorrhage UO: WNL Skin turgor: WNL Coagulation profile: WNL

Plan of Care (cont'd)

Nursing diagnosis	Outcome criteria
High risk for decreased cardiac output *r/t:* *Cardiac trauma* *Thoracic trauma* *Decreased circulating volume* *Decreased preload* *Increased afterload*	CI: WNL SVR: WNL CVP: WNL PCWP: WNL Full, equal pulses UO: WNL Cardiac rhythm within patient norms Do_2: WNL Svo_2: WNL
High risk for hypothermia *r/t:* *Environmental exposure* *Cold resuscitation fluids* *Impaired thermoregulation*	Core temperature: WNL Shivering absent or controlled Verbalize comfort
Decreased peripheral perfusion *r/t:* *Decreased circulating volume* *Peripheral vasoconstriction* *Hypothermia* *Edema* *Fluid shifts* *Thrombus formation* *Compartment syndrome* *Unstable fractures*	Capillary refill $\leq$3 sec Full, equal pulses Extremities warm, pink LOC within patient norms BUN: WNL Serum creatinine: WNL UO: WNL No evidence DVT or PE Compartment pressures: WNL
High risk for acid–base abnormalities *r/t:* *Anaerobic metabolism* *Metabolic abnormalities* *Respiratory abnormalities*	ABG within patient norms Serum lactate levels: WNL Serum potassium levels: WNL Do_2: WNL Svo_2: WNL
Decreased nutrition *r/t:* *Hypermetabolism* *Catabolism* *Preexisting nutritional deficiencies* *Inability to utilize nutrients* *Altered nutrient metabolism* *Inadequate protein/calorie replacement*	Adequate calorie/protein intake CO_2: WNL Serum albumin: WNL Serum glucose: WNL Transferrin: WNL Prealbumin: WNL Total lymphocyte count: WNL Greater than 90% ideal body weight Trace elements: WNL Serum magnesium: WNL Serum phosphorus: WNL Muscle mass maintained
High risk for infection *r/t:* *Impaired immune response* *Invasive procedures* *Bacterial translocation* *Wounds and lacerations* *Malnutrition* *Exposure to nosocomial infections* *Tissue ischemia*	WBCs: WNL Normothermic No evidence of infection Clear, dry wound and drain sites Clear CXR Negative cultures
Risk for neurovascular compromise *r/t:* *Unstable fractures* *Elevated compartment pressures* *Edema/hematoma formation* *Decreased vascular flow*	Compartment pressures: WNL Stable fractures Improved edema Full, equal peripheral pulses Sensation within patient norms Motion within patient norms

Plan of Care (cont'd)

Pain *r/t:* *Tissue trauma* *Edema* *Invasive procedures* *Nerve injury* *Fracture movement*	Report decreased pain Exhibit less restlessness Exhibit no sympathetic indicators of pain
Anxiety/fear *r/t:* *Unexpected injury* *Loss* *Fear of death* *Therapeutic regimen*	Verbalize concerns and fears Exhibit no complications of stress Demonstrate effective coping strategies
High risk for inadequate patient/family coping *r/t:* *Fear* *Lack of knowledge of therapeutic regimen* *Potential death* *Loss of control* *Inadequate supports* *Inappropriate perception*	Verbalize concerns and fears Demonstrate effective coping Utilize support systems Have knowledge of therapeutic regimen Realistic perception of injury and potential recovery

INTERVENTIONS

Open airway using jaw thrust or chin lift method. *Cervical spine must be protected and maintained in alignment at all times.*

Suction debris or blood from airway *to preserve airway patency and adequately assess/monitor potential injuries.*

Secure adequate airway using nasopharyngeal or oropharyngeal airway *to facilitate suctioning and relieve obstruction.*

Prepare for nasotracheal or orotracheal intubation, cricothyroidotomy, or tracheostomy. *Patients with possible cervical spine or facial fractures must be intubated via the nasal route.*

Secure artificial airway.

Monitor respiratory rate, pattern, depth, work of breathing, symmetry, use of accessory muscles, breath sounds.

Monitor secretions.

Maintain patency of airway via suctioning, humidification of oxygen, hydration of patient, positioning.

Insert and maintain patency of gastric tube *to prevent aspiration of stomach contents or vomiting.*

Administer sedation or paralytics as ordered *to control ventilation.*

Administer analgesia as ordered *to provide pain relief and improve lung expansion.*

Monitor hemoglobin, cardiac output, $Sa{O_2}$ *to maximize oxygen delivery.*

Assess oxygen utilization/evaluate $Sv{O_2}$ *as an indication of cellular oxygen utilization and adequacy of oxygen delivery.*

Elevate head of bed during tube feeding infusion or place patient in side-lying position *to prevent aspiration.*

Control external hemorrhage using manual pressure, MAST trousers, tourniquet as appropriate. *Extreme caution is required with tourniquet use because tissue necrosis and death may occur.*

Prepare for and assist in the insertion of large-bore peripheral or central intravenous catheters. *Rapid fluid resuscitation necessitates the use of large-bore catheters.*

Monitor/maintain autotransfusion system *to minimize volume of banked blood needed.*

Prepare for and assist in utilization of rapid infusion systems *to optimize massive volume resuscitation.*

Administer blood replacement as ordered and note response to therapy.

Plan of Care (cont'd)

Monitor Ca^{++} levels *to prevent tetany and cardiac dysrthythmias associated with hypocalcemia, citrate in banked blood may cause hypocalcemia in the patient.*

Monitor clotting factors including PT, PTT, fibrinogen, platelets, FDPs. *Coagulopathies may result from massive blood resuscitation and impact of trauma on coagulation system.*

Replace clotting factors. *Continued hemorrhage and administration of blood products deficient in clotting factors may place patient at risk for inappropriate clotting and prolonged hemorrhage.*

Observe for bleeding at venipuncture and catheter insertion sites, incisions or wounds, or mucous membranes; note hematuria or occult blood in stool, and report promptly. *Coagulopathies may result after trauma as a result of massive blood transfusions, inadequate replacement of clotting factors, suppression of coagulation system, development of DIC.*

Maintain crystalloid and/or colloid infusion *to maximize preload and promote hemodynamic stability and renal function.*

Monitor hemodynamic parameters, including HR, BP, MAP, CO, CI, PAP, PCWP, CVP, SVR.

Monitor skin color, warmth, UO, BUN, creatinine. *Changes in skin color, temperature, or renal function may indicate centralization of circulating volume with shunting of blood to vital organs.*

Monitor Hgb and Hct. *Recognize that changes in both are delayed indications of hemorrhage.*

Prepare for and assist in transport of patient to radiology, angiography, OR, and so on *for further evaluation and definitive treatment.*

Administer inotropic and vasoactive medications as appropriate and monitor effects *to optimize CO and* Do_2.

Administer pharmacologic agents *to optimize SV, CO,* Do_2 *and to reduce afterload.*

Monitor core body temperature and maintain at $\geq 37°$ C. *Hypothermia can result in life-threatening complications, and hyperthermia increases tissue oxygen consumption.*

Administer warmed IV and peritoneal fluids and humidified oxygen *to prevent reduction of core temperature.*

Utilize warming lights, rescue blanket, or other warming device *to maintain core temperature* $\geq 37°$ *C.*

Avoid exposure to cold.

Monitor ABGs for evidence of metabolic or respiratory acid–base abnormalities.

Maximize CO_2 removal. *Ineffective ventilation with accumulation of* CO_2 *will promote acidosis.*

Monitor for hyperventilation. *Anxiety and pain may cause hyperventilation and transient respiratory alkalosis in the early trauma period.*

Monitor serum lactate levels. *Rising serum lactate may indicate worsening anaerobic metabolism.*

Judiciously administer sodium bicarbonate as ordered. *Inappropriate use of sodium bicarbonate may shift the patient into metabolic alkalosis.*

Monitor basal energy expenditure (BEE). *Indicates estimated energy needs taking into consideration the activity factor and injury factor.*

Monitor skeletal muscle mass, albumin, urinary nitrogen loss, lymphocyte count, transferrin, iron-binding capacity. *Abnormal values are indications of inadequate protein/calorie replacement for the hypermetabolic, catabolic trauma patient.*

Provide adequate enteral or parenteral nutrition *to meet nutritional demands.*

Monitor serum laboratory values of patient on TPN or PPN, including glucose, electrolytes, trace elements, creatinine, blood urea nitrogen, liver enzymes, osmolality. *Abnormal values may indicate potential complications of therapy.*

Monitor urine specific gravity, glucose, ketones, and protein.

Monitor for signs and symptoms of hyperglycemia or hypoglycemia.

Assess for signs and symptoms of infection of wounds and invasive sites, including redness, swelling, purulent drainage, pain, heat.

Plan of Care (cont'd)

Monitor WBC and differential *to detect early evidence of infection.*

Provide wound and invasive line care using aseptic technique according to unit policy. *Immunosuppression of trauma patient increases risk of infection.*

Maintain sterile technique during all invasive procedures. *Immunosuppression of trauma patient increases risk of infection.*

Monitor sputum color, amount, odor, viscosity.

Monitor results of all cultures.

Monitor patient response to antibiotics.

Administer tetanus toxoid vaccine as ordered. *Open, contaminated wounds pose a potential risk for tetanus to the trauma patient.*

Monitor peripheral pulses utilizing Doppler checks as appropriate. *Vascular trauma, edema, unstable fractures, increased compartment pressures, hematoma formation, or constricting casts or splints may impinge on peripheral flow, causing tissue necrosis.*

Assess capillary refill.

Elevate injured extremity as appropriate *to reduce edema.*

Assess for motor and sensory function of all extremities and notify physician immediately of alterations in sensation or motion. *Sensory or motor loss may indicate decreased vascular flow resulting in tissue ischemia and necrosis.*

Prevent constrictive dressings, casts, splints, or restraints.

Assess and report increasing or unrelieved pain or burning in casted extremity. *May indicate increasing pressure that can result in skin breakdown, tissue ischemia and necrosis, or nerve damage.*

Avoid administration of pain medication until injuries have been identified and evaluated. *Elimination of pain may mask injury; sedation effects may mask head injury.*

Explain rationale for avoiding oversedation with pain medication to patient and family. *Pain management goals focus on ensuring basic comfort, and ability to rest, sleep, and participate in care. Oversedation may result in vascular or pulmonary complications.*

Assess for objective (sympathetic nervous system responses) and subjective (grimacing, restlessness, verbal reports) signs of pain *due to possibility that patient may not be able to speak as a result of intubation or decreased LOC.*

When appropriate, medicate for pain as ordered and assess effectiveness of pain medication and document.

Use alternative pain relief measures, including guided imagery, breathing techniques, music, presence of significant others.

Collaborate with health care team to develop pain relief regimen for patient.

Assess patient and family concerns, fears, and understanding of injuries, therapy, and prognosis.

Maximize communication with patient and family regarding therapies and changes in patient status.

Assess patient/family's understanding of health care team members' explanations.

INTERMEDIATE PHASE

The intermediate care phase beings when the life-threatening physiologic abnormalities have been stabilized. It is important to note that although the trauma patient is no longer critically ill, he or she must continue to be closely observed for the development of complications such as sepsis, infection, and the consequences of immobility.

PATIENT CARE PRIORITIES	EXPECTED PATIENT OUTCOMES
Inadequate wound healing *r/t*	Development of wound granulation tissue
Infection	Free of infection
Nutritional deficiencies	Tolerate adequate nutrition to promote healing
Immune suppression	Negative wound cultures

Plan of Care (cont'd)

Impaired mobility *r/t* *Pain* *Impaired motor function* *External splints and orthopedic devices* *Orthopedic trauma* *Mobility restrictions of therapeutic regimen*	Mobilize within limits of injury Perform ADLs within limits of injury Maximal ROM of all joints within limits of injury Safely use mobilization devices
High risk for injury *r/t hazards of immobility, including* *Thrombus formation* *Pulmonary embolus* *Skin breakdown* *Contracture formation*	Passive/active exercise as allowed No evidence of thrombus formation No pulmonary compromise Maximal ROM of all joints within limits of injury Intact, irritation-free skin
High risk for body image and/or self-esteem disturbances *r/t* *External wounds and scars* *Loss of control* *Changes in functional ability*	Verbalize concerns regarding body image and/or self-esteem changes Perform self-care activities Participate in rehabilitation program Identify personal strengths and abilities
Anxiety *r/t therapeutic care needs and discharge plan*	Verbalize knowledge of post-discharge care needs Demonstrate therapeutic regimen required after discharge Describe when to call for medical support Obtain durable goods/supplies necessary for care after discharge

INTERVENTIONS

Assess for risk factors of impaired wound healing, including inadequate nutrition, history of poor peripheral perfusion, immobility, age, infection.

Assess wound for evidence of granulation tissue.

Observe for signs and symptoms of wound infection, including redness, pain, purulent drainage, heat.

Apply appropriate dressing as ordered using strict aseptic technique.

Monitor for signs and symptoms of inadequate protein and calorie replacement, including weight loss, negative nitrogen balance, low serum albumin and low transferrin, decreased total lymphocyte count, fatigue, decreased strength, decreased endurance, muscle wasting.

Encourage oral intake of high-protein, high-calorie diet. *During the continued catabolic state, the trauma patient requires high-protein and high-calorie intake to maintain muscle mass and promote granulation and healing.*

Collaborate with dietitian to develop an adequate diet for the patient.

Teach patient the principles of good nutrition as they relate to wound healing and the increased nutritional demands as a result of trauma. *Teenage patients may be hesitant to consume a high-calorie diet for fear of weight gain.*

Consult with physical therapist for a mobilization program.

Perform passive/active ROM.

Assist with mobilization within limits of injury.

Teach safe use of mobilization devices.

Use pneumatic pressure devices as ordered.

Assess for signs and symptoms of deep vein thrombosis.

Assess for signs and symptoms of pulmonary embolus.

Prevent factors that contribute to impairment of skin integrity, including shearing, pressure, and wetness, by using sheepskin padding, propping heels off bed at all times, padding elbows, maximizing hygiene.

Use pressure relief devices, including specialty beds or mattresses.

Encourage expression of concerns regarding changes in body image.

Provide patient and family realistic information about potential for recovery or reconstruction of damage.

Plan of Care (cont'd)

Convey acceptance of patient's body image changes.

Encourage self-care activities and emphasize patient progress regardless of its magnitude.

Collaborate with psychologist, social worker, or other resource to develop a plan to address body image and self-esteem changes.

Assist family in adjusting to patient's body image or self-esteem changes.

Collaborate with appropriate members of health care team to develop a discharge plan for the patient.

Instruct patient/family regarding discharge regimen, including activity, medications, wound care, mobilization, weight-bearing, diet, when to seek medical attention, and follow-up care.

Assess patient/family understanding of discharge regimen.

Obtain durable goods and supplies needed for discharge regimen.

Link patient/family with appropriate community supports.

TRANSITION TO DISCHARGE

Multiple trauma affects the physical, emotional, social, and vocational status of the patient and family. Often, the patient recovers from injuries with deficits in basic self-care skills or a changed self-image. The goal of rehabilitation after injury is to help the patient optimize functional abilities and adjust to an altered self-image.

Rehabilitation starts in the emergency and intensive care phases as the critical care nurse implements strategies, such as range of motion, skin care, and prevention of hypoxia, to reduce the chance of functional disability. As the patient moves to the intermediate care phase, plans are often made to discharge the patient to an acute rehabilitation setting. Patients most in need of acute rehabilitation include those experiencing spinal cord injury, head injury, hypoxic and anoxic brain injury, peripheral nerve injury, traumatic amputations, or alterations in mobility. It is essential to include the patient, the family, and the multidisciplinary health care team in planning for discharge to a rehabilitation facility.

The less disabled trauma patient will be discharged directly to home. Early patient and family education is needed to address learning needs. Financial assistance may be needed to obtain durable goods or nursing support in the home.

REFERENCES

1. Beaver BM: Care of the multiple trauma victim: the first hour, *Nurs Clin North Am* 25:11-20, 1990.
2. Berry CG: Infection. In Bayley E, Turcke S, editors: *A comprehensive curriculum for trauma nursing,* Boston, 1992, Jones & Barlett.
3. Bone RC: The pathogenesis of sepsis, *Ann Intern Med* 115(6):457-469, 1991.
4. Bucher N, Osborne MJ: Medical sequelae to trauma. In Bayley E, Turcke S, editors: *A comprehensive curriculum for trauma nursing,* Boston, 1992, Jones & Barlett.
5. Bullock B: Metabolic and immunologic responses to trauma. In Howell E, Widra L, Hill M, editors: *Comprehensive trauma nursing: theory and practice,* Glenville, Conn, 1988, Scott, Foresman.
6. Collicott PE: Initial assessment of the trauma patient. In Moore EE, Mattox KL, Feliciano DV, editors: *Trauma,* ed 2, Norwalk, Conn, 1991, Appleton & Lange.
7. Committee on Trauma Research, Commission of Life Sciences, National Research Council, and the Institute of Medicine: *Injury in America: a continuing public health problem,* Washington, DC, 1985, National Academy Press.
8. Espisito B: Nursing assessment. In Bayley E, Turcke S, editors: *A comprehensive curriculum for trauma nursing,* Boston, 1992, Jones & Barlett.
9. Fischer JE: Nutritional support of the intensive care unit patient. In Najarian JS, Delaney JP, editors: *Progress in trauma and critical care surgery,* St Louis, 1992, Mosby–Year Book.
10. Fontaine D: Physical, personal, and cognitive responses to trauma. In *Critical care nursing clinics of North America,* vol 1, Philadelphia, 1989, WB Saunders.
11. Gares D: Shock. In Bayley E, Turcke S, editors: *A comprehensive curriculum for trauma nursing,* Boston, 1992, Jones & Barlett.
12. Gotch P: The endocrine system. In Alspach J, editor: *Core curriculum for critical care nursing,* ed 4, Philadelphia, 1991, WB Saunders.
13. Johnson K: Critical care of the trauma patient. In Neff J, Kidd P, editors: *Trauma nursing: the art and science,* St Louis, 1993, Mosby–Year Book.
14. Kidd P: Assessment of the trauma patient. In Neff J, Kidd P, editors: *Trauma Nursing: the art and science,* St Louis, 1993, Mosby–Year Book.
15. Kudsk KA, et al: Enteral versus parenteral feeding. Effects on septic morbidity after blunt and penetrating abdominal trauma, *Ann Surg* 215:503-513, 1992.
16. Lowe D: Metabolic effects of trauma. In Trunkey D, Leris F, editors: *Current therapy of trauma,* ed 2, Philadelphia, 1991, BC Decker.
17. Maier RV: Evaluation and resuscitation. In Moore EE, editor: *Early care of the injured patient,* ed 4, Toronto, 1990, BC Decker.

18. McQuillan KA: Initial management of traumatic shock. In Cardona V, et al, editors: *Trauma nursing: resuscitation through rehabilitation,* ed 2, Philadelphia, 1993, WB Saunders.
19. McLeod K, McLeod W, Neff J: Relationships and physiologic processes: anticipating complications. In Neff J, Kidd P, editors: *Trauma nursing: the art and science,* St Louis, 1993, Mosby–Year Book.
20. Milzman DP, et al: Preexisting disease in trauma patients: a predictor of fate independent of age of injury severity score, *J Trauma* 32:236-244, 1992.
21. Morgan T: Trauma care systems. In Bayley E, Turcke S, editors: *A comprehensive curriculum for trauma nursing,* Boston, 1992, Jones & Barlett.
22. Nact A, Kahn R, Ramanathan S: Metabolic endocrine response to trauma and nutritional support. In Caplan L, Miller S, Turndorff H, editors: *Trauma anesthesia and intensive care,* Philadelphia, 1991, JB Lippincott.
23. Plaisier BR, et al: Autotransfusion in trauma: a comparison of two systems, *Am Surg* 58:562-566, 1992.
24. Robertson C, Redmond AD: *The management of major trauma,* Oxford, UK, 1991, Oxford University Press.
25. Stein D: Epidemiology of trauma. In Bayley E, Turcke S, editors: *A comprehensive curriculum for trauma nursing,* Boston, 1992, Jones & Barlett.
26. *St Anthony's DRG guidebook 1995,* Reston, Va, 1994, St Anthony.
27. Vanore M: Mechanism of injury. In Bayley E, Turcke S, editors: *A comprehensive curriculum for trauma nursing,* Boston, 1992, Jones & Barlett.
28. Von Rueden KT: Cardiopulmonary assessment of the critically ill trauma patient, *Crit Care Nurs Clin North Am* 1(1): 33-44, 1989.
29. Walsh P: Prevention of trauma. In Bayley E, Turcke S, editors: *A comprehensive curriculum for trauma nursing,* Boston, 1992, Jones & Barlett.

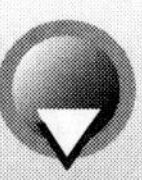

CLINICAL GUIDELINE

66

Burns

Hilary S. Blackwood, MSN, RN, CCRN

DESCRIPTION

A burn injury is a direct alteration in tissue integrity. Causative factors include thermal (flame); exposure to caustic chemicals or radiation; contact with an electrical current; and contact with hot liquids, steam, hot metal, or grease. Each year approximately 2.5 million people in the United States suffer burns that require medical attention.[12] Each year, 100,000 people are hospitalized and 12,000 die as a result of their injuries.[14] The direct and indirect costs of burn care are enormous, including physical, emotional, and financial losses for the patient, family, and society.

PATHOPHYSIOLOGY

Skin Anatomy and Physiology

The skin is the largest organ of the body. It is composed of two layers, the epidermis and the dermis. The epidermis is a thin, avascular layer of stratified squamous epithelial cells, which functions as a barrier against environmental hazards. The thicker dermis consists of a closely interwoven layer of dense areolar connective tissue, blood vessels, hair follicles, and sweat and sebaceous glands. The dermis also contains sensory fibers for pain, touch, pressure, and temperature. The subcutaneous tissue lies beneath the dermis. It is a layer of connective tissue and fat (Figure 66-1).

The skin has multiple functions. It provides a protective barrier between the body's internal and external environments and plays an active role in the prevention of trauma. It also protects the body from excessive fluid loss, yet permits elimination of excess water and other waste products. It assists in thermoregulation, prevents the damaging effects of sunlight (ultraviolet light), secretes oil to soften and lubricate, produces vitamin D, and is an important sensory organ. Finally, the skin determines appearance, thus serving to give each of us a sense of identity and individuality. Each of these functions is threatened following a burn injury.

Burn Severity

The severity of a burn is determined by estimating the depth and extent of the injury. Historically, the most commonly used classification to describe the depth of burn injury has been first-, second-, and third-degree burn. Current terminology to describe burns is superficial partial thickness, deep partial thickness, and full thickness burns. Both sets of classifications use the same criteria to describe the extent of tissue destruction (Table 66-1). The degree of tissue destruction is affected proportionally by the heat source, its temperature, and its duration of contact with the skin.

The extent of injury indicates the percentage of the total body surface area (TBSA) involved. Accurate calculation of TBSA involvement is required in order to estimate fluid losses and replacement needs. The "rule of nine" is a convenient and clinically practical guide used to make a rapid assessment of the extent of body surface involved by dividing the body into multiples of nine (Figure 66-2). This formula is simple to use, but accurate only for adult patients because it does not take into account proportional differences related to age. The most widely used method of determining the extent of burn injury for all age groups is the Lund and Browder chart. It employs a table with a relative anatomic scale to estimate TBSA involvement by age and body size (Figure 66-3).

In addition to depth and extent of burn injury, other severity factors must be considered. If the burn involves

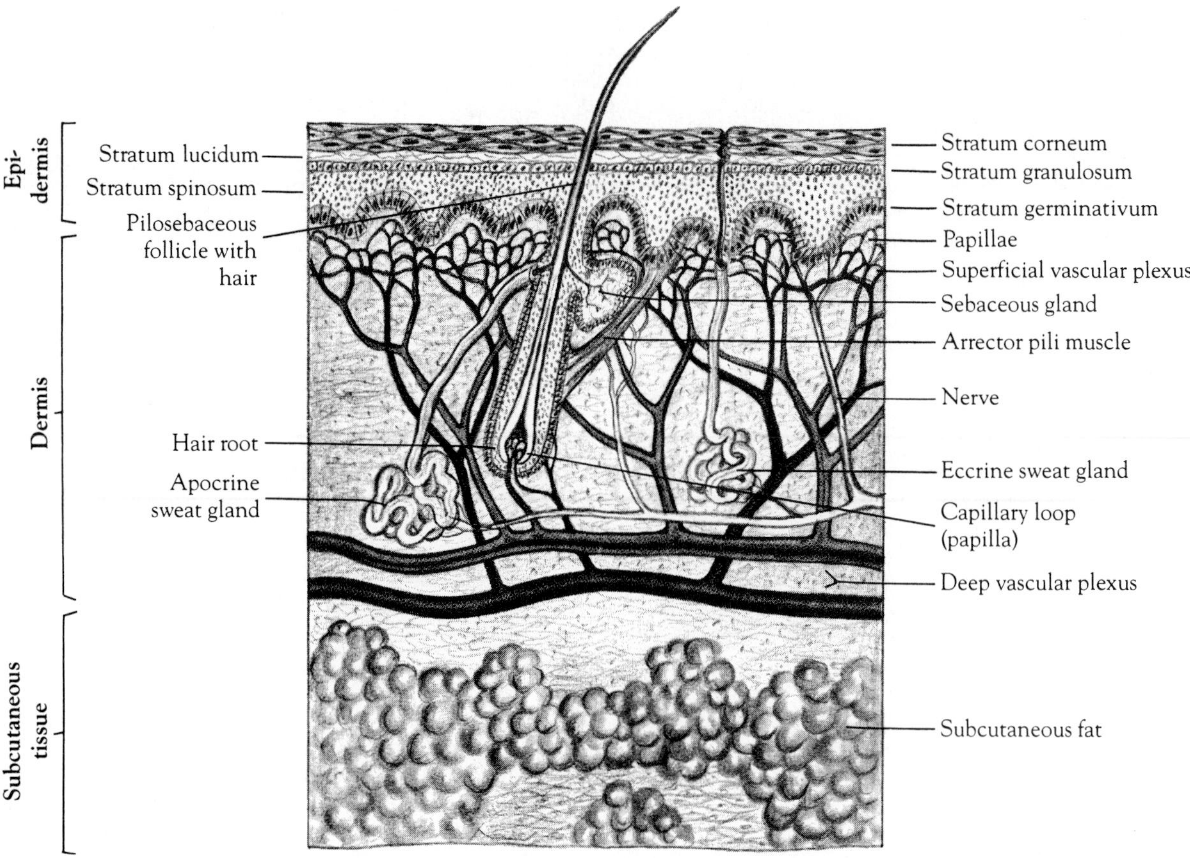

Figure 66-1 Anatomy of the skin. (From Thompson JM, et al, editors: *Mosby's manual of clinical nursing,* ed 3, St Louis, 1993, Mosby–Year Book.)

any special care areas, which include the hands, face, feet, or genitalia, the burn is considered to be a more serious injury due to the functional and cosmetic complications possible in these areas. Concomitant injuries such as inhalation burns or other traumas sustained at the time of injury are common and must be carefully evaluated and treated. Patients who abuse alcohol or drugs may present an additional management problem. Preexisting conditions such as cardiovascular disease, diabetes, sickle cell anemia, pulmonary conditions, and AIDS also complicate wound management and healing.

The patient's age is important. Children have a larger body surface area in proportion to their weight. Infants have immature kidneys and immune systems and may have unstable peripheral circulation, thus making them less tolerant of large fluid shifts associated with the burn injury and its treatment. Burns in the elderly often are complicated by preexisting medical problems such as congestive heart failure or diabetes.

Finally, the etiology of the burn is an important consideration in determining treatment. Chemical and electrical burns may need additional management in the emergent phase of care. Burns as a result of neglect or abuse will require social service consultation.[16]

Burns can potentially result in multiple organ system dysfunction throughout the period of management. Loss of skin integrity leads to increased capillary permeability and thrombosis, cellular necrosis, massive fluid shifts with increased evaporative losses of heat and water, increased metabolic expenditures of energy (calories), constant threat of invasive sepsis, and altered defense mechanisms with generalized immunosuppression. Therefore, a burn injury presents a clinical profile that demands a thorough understanding of fluid and electrolyte balance, cardiopulmonary physiology, renal function, gastrointestinal integrity, metabolic alterations, sepsis, and neurological/psychological management.

The American Burn Association (ABA) has identified several types of burn injuries that usually require referral to a burn center.[1] This list is presented in Table 66-2 as a guide to assist practitioners in determining which patients require referral to a specialized burn care facility after initial assessment and treatment at an emergency room.[7]

The pathophysiology of burns can be classified into three periods: emergent period (shock phase), acute period (phase of eschar separation/healing), and rehabilitation period (phase of reconstruction and social reentry).

The emergent period is characterized by increased cap-

TABLE 66-1 Classification of Burns/Tissue Destruction

Burn depth	Skin involvement	Sensation	Appearance	Course
Superficial PT (first degree)	Epidermis	Pain Tingling	Mild erythema Slight edema Blanching on compression	Spontaneous regeneration within 1 week Peeling No residual scarring
Deep PT (second degree)	Entire epidermis, varying depths of dermis Sweat glands and hair follicles intact	Increased sensitivity to pain and temperature Sensitive to deep pressure, may or may not be sensitive to pinprick	Dry or blistered Erythema Edema Moist wound Cherry red or dull white	May regenerate spontaneously within 2 weeks if infection is prevented Depigmentation and scarring
Full thickness (third degree)	Entire epidermis and dermis May involve varying depths of subcutaneous tissue	Painless Sensitive only to deep pressure	Wet or dry leathery surface Cherry red to white or black	No chance of spontaneous regeneration; requires grafting Scarring Decreased function Alteration of appearance
Fourth degree	Entire epidermis, dermis, and subcutaneous fat Varying depths of fascia, muscle, and bone	Complete anesthesia	Blackened and depressed Dull, dry Bones and ligaments may be exposed	Usually requires amputation of involved body part

PT: partial thickness

illary permeability, caused by vasoactive substances such as histamine that are released by the damaged cells. This response is localized in burns less than 25% TBSA, and generalized in burns greater than 25%.[4] Due to increased capillary permeability, plasma protein, fluid, and electrolytes seep into the interstitial tissue causing edema and decreased circulating blood volume. This results in a concurrent increase in hematocrit and viscosity of the circulating blood. Systemically the patient experiences an initial marked increase in peripheral vascular resistance and a decreased cardiac output.[18] The greatest interstitial loss of plasma occurs during the first 12 hours with spontaneous sealing of capillary integrity within 24 to 72 hours postburn. Repair and survival of injured cells and restoration of vital organ function depend on rapid and adequate fluid resuscitation to correct hypovolemia and promote optimal cardiac output, and renal and tissue perfusion.

The acute period of burn recovery is the phase of eschar separation. This period lasts until the wound, if partial thickness, heals spontaneously; or, if full thickness, is excised and covered with autografts. During this time it is essential to prevent complications. The most common complications are cardiopulmonary and renal failure, and infection leading to septicemia. Inadequate caloric and protein intake leading to muscle wasting or delayed wound healing, contractures, and scarring are also concerns during this phase.

The rehabilitation period begins when the patient is admitted and may continue for years. This period is concerned with functional physical restoration, and psychosocial reentry of the patient into society. Vigorous rehabilitation including physical and occupational therapy helps prevent contractures and hypertrophic scarring, and correlates with achievement of maximal functioning and mobility of affected body parts. Surgical intervention to restore function and improve cosmetic appearance may be necessary from a physical and emotional standpoint.

Fluid Resuscitation

Fluid replacement is based on the patient's weight (in kilograms) and the TBSA burned. Numerous fluid resuscitation formulas are in use at various burn units (See Table

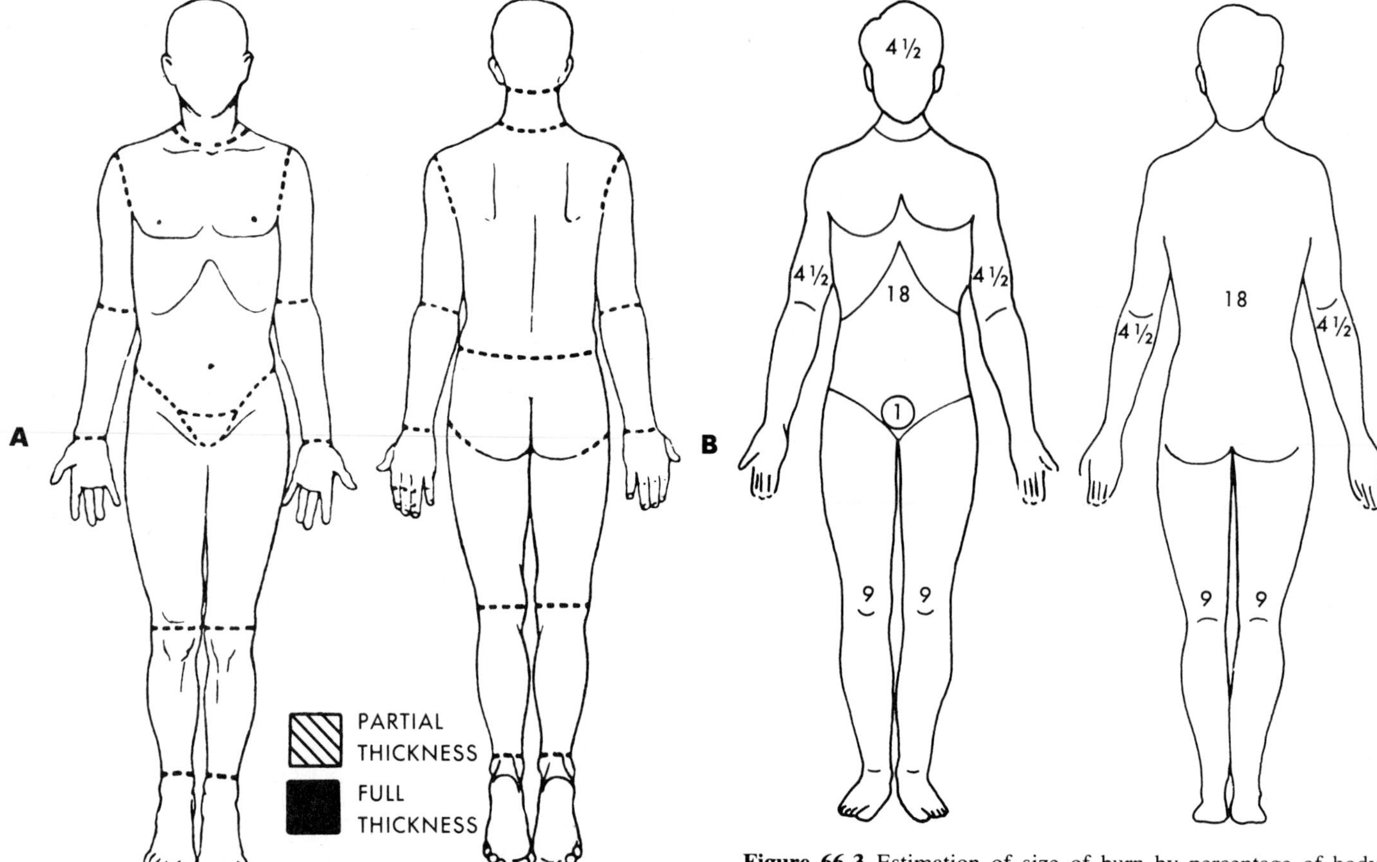

Figure 66-2 Estimate of size of burn (percentage of body surface involved) by rule of nine. **A,** anterior; **B,** posterior. Nines are assigned to specific areas (anterior and posterior) and may be summed as follows:

Head	9
Right upper extremity	9
Left upper extremity	9
Torso	36
Perineum	1
Right lower extremity	18
Left lower extremity	18
TOTAL	100

It is advisable to color code depth of burns for estimated size to give a better picture of the injury to the patient. (Used with permission from DiMola MA, Acres CA, Winkler JB: Burns. In Kinney MA, editor: *AACN's clinical reference for critical care nursing,* New York, 1988, McGraw-Hill.)

Figure 66-3 Estimation of size of burn by percentage of body surface. (From Lund CC, Browder NC: The estimation of areas of burns, *Surg Gynecol Obstet* 79:352-358, 1944.)

66-3). The formula selected depends on physician preference and is intended to serve only as a guide to the initiation of resuscitation. The Parkland formula, developed by Baxter in the 1950s, has been adopted by the American Burn Association and is the most widely used resuscitation formula in the United States.[3]

The Parkland formula for calculating fluid resuscitation in the first 24 hours postburn is: 2 to 4 ml lactated Ringer's solution, per percent burn, per body weight in kilograms (ml/%/kg). Fluid needs are calculated from the time of injury, *not* the time of the patient's entry into the hospital system. One half of this volume is given in the first 8 hours and an additional one fourth in each of the next 8-hour periods. The volume of fluid given is adjusted to the individual's response to the burn and its treatment. Urine output of 30 to 50 ml/hr in adults and 1 ml/kg in children is the hallmark sign of adequate renal perfusion and the adequacy of fluid resuscitation. If the burn totals less than a 10% to 15% TBSA, oral replacement of fluid deficits may be possible. Urine output and fluid balance must still be carefully monitored.

After the first 24 hours, fluid treatment varies; typically 5% dextrose in water, or half-normal salines are used as maintenance fluids. It is important to note that 5% dextrose in water is given to maintain serum sodium greater than 130 mEq/L. Potassium is replaced as needed to meet physiologic need. During the second 24 hours, when capillary integrity is beginning to reestablish, the administration of colloids is also recommended, in the form of albumin or plasma, 0.3 to 0.5 ml/kg/% burn. Resuscitation may last anywhere from 48 hours to several days. It ends with the mobilization of fluid (diuresis) and the reestablishment of cardiopulmonary and renal stability.

It is essential to remember that any resuscitation formula

TABLE 66-2 Burn Center Referral Criteria

Type of burn		
Partial thickness	**Full thickness**	**Miscellaneous**
>10% TBSA in patients <10 and >50 years old >20% TBSA in other age groups Burns with threat of functional loss or cosmetic impairment that involve face, hands, feet, genitalia, perineum, and major joints	>10% TBSA in patients <10 and >50 years old >20% TBSA in other age groups Burns with threat of functional loss or cosmetic impairment that involve face, hands, feet, genitalia, perineum, and major joints >5% TBSA in any age group	All electrical burns including lightning injury Chemical burns that may cause functional or cosmetic impairment Inhalation injury with conjunction of burn injury Circumferential burns of the extremities and chest Burn injury in patients with preexisting medical disorders that would complicate management, prolong recovery, or affect mortality Any burn patient with concomitant trauma in which the burn injury poses the greatest risk of morbidity or mortality Hospitals without qualified personnel or equipment for the care of children should transfer such patients to a burn center with these capabilities

Adapted from American Burn Association Guidelines with permission.

is intended to be used only as a guideline to initiate fluid therapy. The patient must be monitored hourly, as individual reaction may vary considerably. Response to fluid resuscitation is judged by hourly urine output, in conjunction with vital signs, electrolyte balance, hemodynamic pressures, and level of consciousness.

Specific Types of Burns

Chemical and electrical burns need additional management during the emergent period. The severity of a chemical burn depends on the duration of contact, as well as the concentration and type of offending agent. Although fluid resuscitation remains the same as for thermal injuries, it must be accompanied by copious amounts of external water irrigation for prolonged periods in an effort to flush away the offending chemical. Attempts to neutralize the chemical should be avoided due to the possibility of generating heat and increasing tissue destruction. Irrigation is continued until the patient reports decreased pain in the wound. Ophthalmological damage necessitates irrigation with water and/or saline. Special attention must be given to oropharyngeal and tracheobronchial involvement resulting from possible ingestion and aspiration. Finally, patients with chemical injuries must be carefully monitored for the added danger of systemic toxicity.

Electrical injuries occur as a result of electrical energy being converted to heat. They often involve what is known as the "iceberg effect"—that is, damage to tissue, muscle, and internal organs is frequently more extensive than what appears on the surface. The greatest transfer of heat is at the point of contact with the electrical source. The characteristic "entry" and "exit" wounds are indicative of local destruction of underlying tissue. Hands and wrists are common entry points and typically have a charred and depressed appearance. Feet are common exit points, with dry depressed edges and an appearance as though the electrical current "exploded" as it made its exit. Internally, the greatest tissue damage occurs directly under and adjacent to the contact points. The extensive underlying tissue damage is evidenced by intense and immediate edema proximal to the entry wound.

Initial treatment for electrical injuries involves assessing and managing cardiac dysrhythmias, particularly ventricular fibrillation. The patient also must be treated for respiratory paralysis or arrest, fractures (especially of the long bones), neurological trauma, and compartment syndrome or various forms of vascular compromise. Depending on the extent and depth of the tissue and visceral damage, early debridement, escharotomy or fasciotomy, and even amputation of necrotic limbs may be necessary. Fluids must

TABLE 66-3 Resuscitation Formulas to Prevent Burn Shock

	Evans formula	Brooke formula	Modified Brooke formula	Artz formula	Parkland formula	Hypertonic formula
First 24 hours:						
Electrolyte solution	Normal saline	Ringer's lactate	Ringer's lactate	Ringer's lactate	Ringer's lactate	Hypertonic lactated saline (sodium, 250 mEq/L)
ml/kg/% burn	1.0	1.5	2.0	3.0	4.0	Rate based on urine output of 70 ml/hour in adults
Colloid	1 ml whole blood plasma, or plasma expanders/kg/% burn	0.5 ml/kg/% burn	None	None	None	None
Free water (D_5W)	2000 ml	2000 ml	None	None	None	None
Second 24 hours:						
Solution	One-half first 24-hour dose; same amount D_5W	One-half first 24-hour dose; same amount D_5W	D_5W, and colloid	D_5W, and colloid	Only D_5W to maintain urine output; colloid, 0.5 to 2 L	Continued at rate to maintain urine output >30 ml

be infused to maintain adequate urine output and hemodynamic stability.

An important potential complication of electrical injuries is renal tubular necrosis resulting from the myoglobinuric and hemoglobinuric by-products of generalized muscle breakdown. Fluid resuscitation needs for electrical injuries may be difficult to calculate accurately because of the practitioner's inability to completely assess the extent of the burn and underlying tissue destruction. Fluids are increased to maintain an initial urine output of 75 to 100 ml/hr until the urine is grossly clear. Some physicians add 50 mEq of sodium bicarbonate to each liter of lactated Ringer's to alkalinize the urine and increase myoglobin excretion. If urine output and pigment do not respond to fluid administration, the use of mannitol may be considered.

LENGTH OF STAY/ANTICIPATED COURSE

The length of stay for a burn patient is heavily dependent on the size and severity of the burn, as well as the patient's age and preexisting medical problems. A patient with a small burn (<10% TBSA) who does not require grafting, or who requires only one surgical procedure, may be ready for discharge to home within 1 to 2 weeks postburn. At the other end of the spectrum, a patient with a large burn (>50% TBSA) may require multiple surgical procedures, necessitating a four- to six-month hospital stay, followed by discharge to a long-term rehabilitation facility. Complications encountered during recovery, such as sepsis, pneumonia, or renal failure also significantly affect the hospital course and length of stay. Aggressive surgical treatment, including early excision and grafting of deep partial and full thickness burns, has dramatically decreased the required hospital stay (see Table 66-4).

TABLE 66-4 Common DRGs Associated with Burns

DRG #	DRG label	Average LOS
456	Burns, transferred to another acute care facility	10.2 days
457	Extensive burns without OR procedure	5.6 days
460	Nonextensive burns without OR procedure	8.0 days
458	Nonextensive burns with skin graft	19.8 days
459	Nonextensive burns with wound debridement or other OR procedure	12.5 days
472	Extensive burns with OR procedure	30.4 days

Information from *St Anthony's DRG guidebook 1995*, Reston, Va, 1994, St Anthony.

MANAGEMENT TRENDS AND CONTROVERSIES

Hydrotherapy is used once or twice daily to assist in fighting infection, and to cleanse the wound surface, remove nonviable tissue, and provide patient hygiene. Wound care and debridement during hydrotherapy thus serve to prevent an outgrowth of bacteria, promoting healing, and, if necessary, prepare the wound bed for grafting.

A wide variety of methods are used in the treatment of burn wounds.* Depending on the extent, type, and location of the injury, a single treatment or a combination of therapies may be used at the discretion of the burn team.

Microorganisms in a burn wound usually are controlled with the use of topical agents. Ideally, a topical antimicrobial should be bacteriostatic; actively penetrate burn eschar; lack significant side effects or systemic toxicity; be painless and easy to apply and remove; prevent wound desiccation; and promote re-epithelialization.[15] Unfortunately, no one topical agent meets all these requirements. Several topicals are commonly used, depending on the wound care protocols of particular units, and unit-specific pathogens. Proof of a particular agent's effectiveness can be judged in part by wound infection rates and the incidence of sepsis.

*References 1, 2, 4, 5, 6, 8, 9, 18, 20.

Silver sulfadiazine (Silvadene) is the most widely used topical antimicrobial.[4,5,18] It provides coverage against gram positive and gram negative organisms, as well as yeast. Silvadene is easy to apply, nontoxic, and has very few side effects. It is not recommended for use on patients with known sulfonamide sensitivity. Temporary leukopenia is a side effect of the use of Silvadene, resolving without treatment even when the drug is continued. Silvadene does not penetrate eschar well, and is not particularly effective against *Pseudomonas,* a common burn-wound pathogen.

Mafenide acetete (Sulfamylon) is a popular topical antimicrobial for use in treating extensive, full thickness burns, as well as avascular areas such as the ears and nose.[4,5,6,18] It penetrates eschar well and is effective against gram positive and gram negative organisms. Sulfamylon is water soluble and rapidly absorbed by the body. It is a carbonic anhydrase inhibitor, which results in a metabolic acidosis and requires respiratory compensation. One side effect that should be taken into consideration is that Sulfamylon frequently causes transient burning and stinging upon application.

Polymyxin B (Polysporin) is a widely used ointment for superficial burns or healing deep burns and grafts.[4,5,6,18] It provides gram positive and gram negative coverage only and does not penetrate eschar. Polysporin is painless on application and may be used with or without occlusive dressings. Long-term use of the drug has been associated with rashes and inflammation in some patients.

These topical ointments, creams, and lotions may be applied directly to the burn and left open, or covered with an occlusive dressing. The open method allows for constant observation of the wound to assess healing and monitor for infection. This method is generally not as popular as the closed method of wound care because of problems with hypothermia, increased pain, and the need for frequent reapplication of dressings. The closed method of wound care offers the wound protection from environmental pathogens, allows absorption of exudate from the wound into the dressing, reduces evaporative losses, and increases patient comfort.

In addition to traditional gauze, two other types of dressings are commonly used.* Biologic dressings consist of tissue harvested from human or pig cadavers. They can be used to prepare a wound bed for grafting, cover a donor site, or cover a partial thickness burn and promote healing. Biologic dressings adhere to the wound surface, providing a water and thermal barrier, while remaining air-permeable. These dressings serve only as a temporary skin substitute. They slough off spontaneously, or are removed and replaced with autografts within 14 to 21 days. The use of pigskin has decreased over the last 5 to 8 years. Use of human cadaver skin has also decreased, secondary to the fear of transmission of communicable diseases such as AIDS, and the associated increased cost of harvesting and storing of the tissue prior to use.

Synthetic dressings are a second type of covering available for use in partial thickness burns. They generally are made of nylon fabric bonded to collagen fibers and they are permeable to air and fluids. The advantages to this type of dressing are that it is less expensive than biologic dressings, readily available, and not associated with any fear of disease transmission.

Closure of the burn wound within 2 to 3 weeks is the goal of burn care, in order to decrease the risk of infection and sepsis. Surgical excision and grafting therefore is the definitive treatment for deep partial and full thickness burns.

Excision is the surgical debridement of necrotic tissue. In addition to removal of devitalized tissue, excision removes most of the bacteria invading the wound, thereby providing a clean wound bed for the placement of autografts. Excision is done in a tangential (sequential) or fascial method.[18]

Tangential excision involves the sequential shaving of thin layers of necrotic tissue until a layer of viable tissue is reached, as evidenced by profuse bleeding. Tangential excision is the preferred method for partial thickness burns and areas where cosmesis and function are of primary importance (except hands and face).[1,6] Excision in a single operative procedure is usually limited to less than 20% TBSA, primarily because of large volumes of blood loss during tangential excision. Once homeostasis is achieved, skin grafts can be applied.

Fascial excision is performed on full thickness burns.[5,6,19] It is generally limited to the trunk, arms and thighs. The hands, face, lower legs, and feet are rarely excised to fascia due to cosmetic appearance. Fascial excision produces minimal blood loss, and usually has a greater graft success rate than tangential excision, but provides poor long-term cosmetic results.

Following excision, autografting is performed to remove definitive closure of the wounds.[5,6,18,19] Grafts are applied in meshed (expanded) or sheet form. Meshed grafts are used most frequently because they adhere well to the wound bed, allowing escape of bodily fluids through the interstices of the graft. Meshed grafts also require a smaller donor site than the size of the wound that they are harvested to cover. Sheet grafts are used over the face and hands because they provide a better cosmetic appearance.

All grafts must remain in constant contact with the excised wound bed in order to receive oxygen and nutrients. They are secured to the wound bed in the operating room with staples, sutures, or steristrips at the periphery of the graft and must be protected from shearing and desiccation. Meshed grafts usually are covered with an occlusive dressing and immobilized for 2 to 5 days postop. Splints may be utilized over joints to prevent movement. Sheet grafts generally are left open to air after surgery in order to provide visualization of the graft.[20] Any exudate or serum that accumulates under the graft must be evacuated to prevent graft sloughing. All grafts and donor sites should be monitored for color, odor, drainage, erythema, and stages of healing at each dressing change.

The most controversial alternative for providing permanent wound coverage for full thickness burns is the use of cultured epithelial cells, or "cultured skin."[8,18,19] This technique has gained popularity during the past 10 years, and is used primarily to provide autografts for patients with extensive burns and limited donor sites (greater than 85% TBSA). The process requires harvesting of a full thickness skin biopsy. Epithelial cells are then spun off and grown in a culture medium for approximately 3 weeks, then applied to a clean wound bed in sheet grafts. The advantages of this method are coverage of large burns with improved cosmetic appearance, and lack of need for large donor site areas. Disadvantages include high cost, fragility, and frequent blistering of the cultured skin.

*References 4, 5, 6, 9, 13, 18.

ASSESSMENT

PARAMETER	ANTICIPATED ALTERATION
Burn history	Time of burn, *to assess fluid resuscitation* Open or closed space, *to assess possibility of inhalation injury* Type of injury: thermal, electrical, chemical, radiation Concomitant trauma
Allergies	Especially sulfa *(an ingredient found in the topical antimicrobial Silvadene)*
Psychosocial history	Whether or not the accident involves other losses (family, home, car, pet) What the injury means to the patient's family and occupation Whether or not other people were injured or killed in the accident Whether or not the accident implicates the patient in a criminal way Whether or not the burn history coincides with the type and pattern of injury. *If not, abuse/neglect must be considered. Approximately 10% of child abuse cases are burn injuries.*[16] *Younger children are at greater risk for abuse due to their inability to protect themselves. Intentional burns may be inflicted by the parent or other caregiver, and must be assessed carefully because the etiologies for intentional and accidental burns are the same.*[18]
Burn Assessment	
Extent of injury	Determine percentage of surface involvement using rule of nine or Lund and Browder chart
Depth of injury	Full thickness burns sensitive only to deep pressure *due to destruction of nerve endings* Pain may be significant in partial thickness burns *due to exposure of nerve endings*
Location of burns	Circumferential thoracic burns may require an escharotomy (a linear incision extending through necrotic burn tissue to subcutaneous fat) *to allow for chest expansion and ventilation and permit the flow of blood to affected extremities*
Pulmonary Status	
Evidence of inhalation injury	Burns of the face and/or neck Singed facial or nasal hairs Burns of the lips and/or mouth Hoarseness, stridor Cough, carbonaceous sputum Cyanosis
RR	Tachypnea Dyspnea Use of accessory muscles
Fio_2	100% oxygen until carboxyhemoglobin level is normal (0 to 2% normal, up to 15% normal in heavy smokers)[18] Half-life of carboxyhemoglobin is 1 hour on 100% Fio_2, 4 hours on room air
ABG	Metabolic acidosis *due to decreased circulation, poor peripheral circulation, and CO poisoning*
Carboxyhemoglobin levels	15%: indicative of inhalation injury 15 to 35%: confusion, dizziness, irritability, weakness, shortness of breath >35%: cardiopulmonary instability, dysrhythmias, tissue ischemia, organ ischemia and dysfunction, semicomatose to comatose >60%: usually fatal

Chest x-ray	Usually normal in early postburn period, even in presence of inhalation injury Assess for presence of blunt or penetrating trauma associated with circumstances of injury
Bronchoscopy	Edema, erythema, carbonaceous sputum visible in the airway (upper and lower) *due to inhalation injury* Epithelial sloughing of the trachea and mainstem bronchus *due to inhalation injuries* Partial or complete occlusion of the airway *seen in inhalation injuries and/or circumferential neck burns*

Cardiovascular Status

HR	Tachycardia *due to pain, anxiety, increased metabolic rate, hypovolemia or iatrogenic hypervolemia*
Rhythm	Dysrhythmias *due to electrical injuries and hypoxia*
BP	Decreased during shock phase *due to hypovolemia* Increased *with acute pain*
CO	Decreased during shock phase *due to fluid shifts and hemoconcentration* Decreased filling pressures (CVP, PCWP) Decreased stroke volume
SVR and PVR	Initial increase after injury *due to catecholamine release*
Peripheral pulses (in the presence of deep or circumferential burns to arms, hands, fingers, legs, feet, or toes)	Decreased pulses Dusky color in distal extremities Decreased capillary refill Cold extremities Decreased SaO_2 on fingers, toes Numbness of fingers, toes Swollen extremity, tight skin Deep pain *These parameters are clinical indications of the circulatory status of affected extremities. Tissue damage and possible necrosis result quickly in the face of decreased O_2 supply to tissues*

Neurologic Status

LOC	Anxiety *due to pain* Restlessness, confusion *due to pain, hypoxia, hypovolemia* Decreased LOC *seen in patients with intoxication, overdose, associated trauma, hypovolemia*
C spine series	C spine fracture *secondary to trauma (fall) or tetanic muscle contractions due to contact with electrical current*
GI status	Abdominal distension *due to swallowing* Absent bowel sounds *due to paralytic ileus* Coffee-ground emesis or rectal bleeding *due to Curling's ulcer, common in burns*

Renal Status

UO	Decreased: $<$30 cc/hr *due to decreased renal blood flow in hypovolemia, hypoperfusion, or acute tubular necrosis secondary to nephrotoxic antibiotics, vasopressors, electrical injuries, and excretion of metabolic toxins*
BUN	Increased: 720 mg/dl *due to decreased renal perfusion and catabolism of proteins from injury*
Urine myoglobin	Positive *due to electrical injuries*

Laboratory Tests

K^+	Increased: >4.5 mEq/L in early postburn period *due to hemolysis of RBCs and loss of intracellular potassium* Decreased: <3.5 mEq/L as resuscitation progresses *due to aldosterone release and loss of potassium in the urine*
Na^+	Normal or slightly decreased in early postburn period *due to loss of extracellular body fluids or trapping of sodium in interstitial edema in the burn wound* Decreased: <135 mEq/L *due to renal excretion*
Hct and Hgb	Hct increased: >52% early postburn *due to hemoconcentration; then decreased: <37% as resuscitation progresses* Hgb falsely increased early postburn *due to hemolysis of RBCs and release of free Hgb into bloodstream*
WBC count	Increased: >10,000/mm^3 *early. Leukocytopenia is a poor prognostic sign of the patient's inability to fight infection*
Albumin	Decreased: <4.5 g/dl *due to loss of protein from the wound*

PLAN OF CARE

INTENSIVE PHASE

The intensive phase of care for critically ill burned patients focuses on preservation of vital body functions such as respiration and hemodynamic homeostasis. The potential for respiratory injury, either from the burn or from physiologic and immune responses to severe burns elsewhere, requires vigilant monitoring and swift intervention. Hemodynamically, severely burned individuals require aggressive fluid management to preserve optimal tissue perfusion/oxygenation essential for eventual recovery. Multiple organ dysfunction syndrome (MODS) is a significant risk in this phase of care. Intervention must provide swift stabilization and begin restorative support if the patient is to survive.

PATIENT CARE PRIORITIES	EXPECTED PATIENT OUTCOMES
Interruption in skin integrity with high risk for infection *r/t* *Open burn wounds* *Wound colonization* *Immobility* *Decreased resistance to infection* *Multiple invasive lines/catheters*	Absence or resolution of infection Healing of wounds, spontaneously or with surgical intervention Maintains normal temperature
Ineffective airway clearance *r/t* *Airway obstruction* *Edema of the face, neck* *Smoke inhalation injury* *Pulmonary edema*	Adequate oxygenation: PaO_2 >80 mm Hg Clear lung sounds in all lobes Unlabored respirations SaO_2 >90%
Impaired gas exchange *r/t* *Atelectasis* *Pneumonia* *Pulmonary emboli* *Smoke inhalation injury* *Pneumothorax* *Circumferential burns of the neck/thorax* *Pulmonary edema* *ARDS*	Absence of adventitious breath sounds PaO_2 >80 mm Hg $PaCO_2$ 35 to 45 mm Hg Effective mobilization of secretions

Plan of Care (cont'd)

Decreased tissue perfusion *r/t* *Decreased circulation volume from plasma/fluid shifts* *Blood loss with decreased cardiac output and decreased tissue perfusion from circumferential burns of the extremities* *Inadequate or delayed fluid resuscitation*	Positive peripheral pulses HR: WNL for age Adequate UO for age CVP: WNL ABG: within patient norms LOC: within patient norms CRT: ≤3 sec Warm extremities
High risk for fluid volume deficit *r/t* *Burn shock* *Evaporative fluid loss from wound surface* *Decreased fluid intake* *Excessive fluid losses due to diarrhea, fever*	Sensorium within patient norms CVP: WNL HR: WNL UO: WNL for age Absence of paralytic ileus HCT: WNL Weight within patient norms Electrolytes: WNL
Impaired renal function *r/t* *Decreased circulating blood volume* *Myoglobinuria and ATN* *Nephrotoxic antibiotics*	UO: WNL for age
Inadequate nutrition *r/t* *Inadequate intake and digestion of nutrients* *Increased basal metabolic rate* *Protein losses from wound, bowel dysfunction* *Hepatic pancreatic dysfunction* *Stress ulcers* *GI bleeding* *Increased urinary nitrogen losses* *Altered glucose, fat, protein metabolism*	Positive nitrogen balance Consumes required caloric and protein requirements Weight maintenance or gain Wound healing Hair and nail growth Menses per patient norm Albumin/prealbumin levels: WNL
High risk for impaired elimination *r/t* *Paralytic ileus* *Opiate consumption*	Maintain adequate gastric functioning and bowel elimination
Pain, pruritis *r/t* *Damaged and exposed nerve endings with partial thickness burns* *Debridement procedures* *Dressing changes* *Donor sites* *Stretching of extremities during exercise, ROM*	Pain will be minimized or controlled per patient report, VS, and nonverbal behaviors
Sleep pattern disturbance *r/t* *Pain* *Hospital environment*	Expresses feelings of refreshment after sleep Experiences increased feeling of well-being

INTERVENTIONS

Wash hands and wear gloves when caring for patient.

Use gown, mask, goggles, hat, and gloves when performing wound care.

Observe strict aseptic technique when performing wound care.

Administer agents to support immune system as ordered *(tetanus toxoid, gamma globulin, etc.)*.

Encourage personnel or visitor with upper respiratory, GI, or skin infections to avoid visiting while contagious.

Plan of Care (cont'd)

Perform daily wound care as ordered, to include bathing with antimicrobial soap, and debridement of necrotic tissue. *Broken blisters and loose necrotic tissue should be debrided because the moist burn wound will harbor bacteria. Management of intact blisters is controversial. Some burn unit protocols dictate breaking and debriding all blisters, secondary to the risk of infections; others debride only blisters located over mobile areas such as joints, believing that the intact blister serves as a protective barrier that assists in wound healing and reepithelialization.*[15] *Some burn unit protocols dictate the shaving of hair from burned areas to prevent wound colonization around hair follicles. Other units do not shave hair, believing that this practice damages the epithelial barrier at the wound margin, lending an increased risk of contamination.*

Monitor wound for changes in appearance.

- Exudate, swelling
- Odor, tenderness, redness
- Appearance of wound margins and healthy skin around the wound
- Graft breakdown, wound breakdown

Apply topical antimicrobial agents to wounds as ordered.

Culture wounds for aerobic and anaerobic organisms by swabbing the wounds with a culture cath tip as ordered.

Monitor indwelling lines and catheters; change catheters as per unit protocol *to prevent infection.*

Monitor for signs/symptoms of local/systemic infection including:

- Leukocytosis
- Headache, chills, malaise, decreased sensorium
- Nausea/vomiting
- Decreased BP, hemodynamic instability
- Decreased urine output
- Hypo-/hyperthermia
- Decreased bowel sounds/ileus
- Positive culture results from wound, blood, urine, stool, sputum

Collaborate with physician and the patient regarding activities to prevent contractures and deformities.

- Apply splints to extremities as ordered
- Maintain burned area in position of physiological function
- Keep burned extremities elevated above the level of the heart
- Abduct arms 90° and keep slightly above shoulder level if axilla are burned
- Avoid use of pillows if neck or ear burns are present
- Active range of motion (ROM) activities q1h to q2h

Intervene to avoid the complications of immobility.

- Turn patient side to side in bed, or assist patient out of bed as condition permits
- Discuss need for therapeutic mattress/bed with physician to prevent skin breakdown
- Ambulate as tolerated if appropriate
- Auscultate lung sounds q4h and prn, including character, rate, and depth of respirations.

Encourage patient to turn, cough and deep breathe and/or use incentive spirometer q2h to q4h.

Monitor for signs/symptoms of respiratory distress.

- Tachypnea, dyspnea, wheezing, stridor
- Adventitious breath sounds
- Pallor, cyanosis

Implement guidelines for the care of patients requiring mechanical ventilation.

Monitor patient's ability to cough and effectively clear secretions.

Monitor quantity and quality of pulmonary secretions, including color, amount, odor, viscosity.

Monitor results of ABG, noting acid-base balance and oxygenation. Report abnormal results to physician.

Plan of Care (cont'd)

Prepare for and assist in escharotomy procedure *if the patient has circumferential, full thickness, or constricting burns of the neck, chest, or any extremities.*

Provide respiratory treatments: chest PT, ROM exercises, O_2 therapy, nebulization as ordered.

Assess peripheral perfusion hourly, including:

- Pulses, edema
- Color, capillary refill
- Motion, sensation

Monitor cardiac rhythm.

Obtain 12-lead ECG daily times three, and cardiac isoenzymes q8h times three in the presence of electrical injuries.

Obtain admission weight and daily weights until patient's condition stabilizes.

Use Parkland Formula (or other burn resuscitation formula) as basis for calculating fluid resuscitation needs.

Monitor I/O hourly during resuscitation period.

Titrate fluid replacement with hourly UO and hemodynamic parameters.

Monitor for signs/symptoms of vascular depletion *caused by third-space fluid shifts during emergent phase.*

Monitor for signs/symptoms of hypovolemia, including:

- Hypotension, orthostatic hypotension
- Decreased CVP, CO, PAP, PCWP
- Decreased UO, hemoglobinuria, myoglobinuria
- Increased Hct
- Poor skin turgor, dry mucous membranes
- Extreme thirst
- Gross bleeding or fluid loss from wound, NG tube
- Restlessness and disorientation

Monitor for signs/symptoms of hypervolemia or cardiogenic shock associated with excessive fluid administration.

- Increased BP, tachycardia
- Increased CVP, PAP, PCWP, and decreased CO
- Increased systemic vascular resistance and O_2 consumption
- Inadequate UO
- Marked weight gain, edema in dependent body areas
- Dyspnea, wheezes, rales
- "White out" appearance in lung fields per chest x-ray
- Disorientation

Restrict sodium and fluid intake as necessary *if fluid overload is present. Fluid overload may be iatrogenic and related to the patient's past medical history (e.g., coronary artery disease).*

Administer diuretic and/or mannitol as ordered. *Diuretic therapy is generally avoided during the resuscitative phase due to the risk of intravascular volume depletion. Mannitol may be necessary in severe electrical injuries to assist in the renal clearance of myoglobin.*

Insert Foley catheter as ordered *for patients with burns greater than 20% TBSA (patients requiring fluid resuscitation).*

Monitor urine output qh for the first 24 to 48 hours postburn, then q2h to q4h. Maintain adequate UO for age.

Monitor urine specific gravity q2h while patient is being fluid resuscitated, then q shift.

Insert NG tube as ordered for patient with greater than 20% TBSA burn; place to low continuous suction.

Measure amount, color, heme content, and pH of NG aspirate.

Plan of Care (cont'd)

Assess cultural and social dietary habits, food preferences, and nutritional status. Set nutritional requirements accordingly in collaboration with nutritionist and physician.

Advance dietary intake to goal levels based on calorie, protein, and fat requirements, and patient tolerance.

Ensure required caloric and fluid intake.
- List foods taken daily
- Allow home-cooked food within set limits
- Provide supplementary nourishment with snacks
- Accurate intake and output
- Daily weights
- Vitamin supplements

Provide conditions conducive to eating.
- Frequent oral hygiene
- Assist with eating or feed patient as needed
- Position for comfort
- Avoid painful procedures close to eating times

Provide tube feeding as ordered. *Hyperalimentation is not recommended for burn patients secondary to high risk of infection and decreased absorption of nutrients via this route.*

Monitor abdominal cramping, diarrhea, nausea, vomiting, aspiration, gastric distension.

Administer antacids and H_2 blockers as ordered, *to maintain gastric pH* <5.

Monitor nutritional status and therapy.
- Albumin and prealbumin as ordered
- 24-hour urine nitrogen studies as ordered
- State of muscle mass, weight loss/gain
- Patient's energy level
- Glucose levels
- Calorie counts

Promote bowel movements as per patient's norm.
- Administer fluids including juices, coffee
- High-fiber diet
- Laxatives prn or as ordered
- Ambulation, exercise as tolerated

Assess the nature, location, quality, intensity, and duration of pain. Accept individual responses to pain.

Have patient rate pain on a visual analog scale.

Administer analgesics as ordered and monitor efficacy of medications given. Utilize nonpharmacologic methods of pain relief. Collaborate with physician to achieve successful pain control.

Administer antihistamines as ordered for relief of pruritis

Utilize nonpharmacologic methods of pain relief.
- Relaxation
- Guided imagery
- Biofeedback
- Hypnosis
- Music therapy
- Distraction: visitors, TV, music, books, games

Explain all procedures prior to enactment and allow patient time for questions and to verbalize concerns.

Maximize efforts to allow patient opportunities to sleep/rest.
- Maintain day/night routine when possible
- Provide quiet, darkened room at night and during rest periods
- Group patient care activities to allow for uninterrupted periods
- Position for comfort when possible

Plan of Care (cont'd)

INTERMEDIATE PHASE

This phase of burn recovery begins after the resuscitation period is complete (48 to 72 hours) or when the patient is hemodynamically stable. It continues until the patient's wounds are predominantly healed and the patient is increasingly able to participate in personal care.

PATIENT CARE PRIORITIES	EXPECTED PATIENT OUTCOMES
Fear anxiety *r/t* *Pain* *Crisis of injury and hospitalization* *Fear of death* *Hospital environment and protocols* *Separation from parents* *Knowledge deficit about burn care recovery*	Verbalizes decreased apprehension Demonstrates ability to cope with emotions
Decreased physical mobility *r/t* *Burn dressings* *Pain* *Stiffness* *Shortening of tendons* *Development of scars or contractures*	Returns to optimal level of functioning through adherence to individualized rehabilitation program
Disturbance in self-concept *r/t* *Loss of role function* *Body image changes* *Disfigurement* *Loss of persons and/or possessions during burn injury* *Alteration in motor or sensory abilities*	Able to verbalize feelings related to self-concept Progresses through stages of grief and loss at individual pace Ultimately feels comfortable with self-concept
Social isolation *r/t* *Loss of previous life-style and role functions* *Alterations in appearance* *Impaired sensory motor functions* *Infection control protocols*	Engages in positive interactions with family and caregivers Interacts with the environment in a way that is comfortable to self and socially acceptable to others
High risk for powerlessness *r/t* *Hospitalization* *Unit schedules and routines* *Loss of control over self*	Participates in care Expresses feeling of control for self and future
Post-traumatic stress response *r/t* *Burn injury*	Expresses decreased anxiety when flashbacks occur Sleeps without nightmares
Self-care deficit *r/t* *Knowledge* *Physical limitation due to burns* *Pain and discomfort* *Psychologic limitations*	Sufficient knowledge to care for burns on discharge: • Performs remaining wound care at time of discharge • Demonstrates correct application of splints, special equipment • Describes dietary, medication, and activity regimes Describes signs and symptoms of infection Describes plan for follow-up care

INTERVENTIONS

Explain all interventions to patient/family prior to and during care.

Explain noises and equipment in use for patient care that are unfamiliar to the patient/family.

Encourage verbalization of questions and concerns. Common concerns may include:

- Stages of wound healing

Plan of Care (cont'd)

- Anticipate degree of scarring
- Long-term disabilities, body changes

Encourage patient to identify source of stressors and minimize when possible.

Be consistent in caring for the patient.

Monitor physical symptoms of stress:

- Tachycardia, palpitations, sweating
- Increased blood pressure, respiratory rate

Assess coping and defense mechanisms. Assist the patient to develop new methods of dealing with stress if previous ones are ineffective. Build on methods used successfully by the patient in the past.

Set limits on maladaptive behaviors.

Allow the patient control over care decisions.

Allow the patient to determine schedule of activities when possible.

Provide positive reinforcement for progress/accomplishments.

Encourage patient and family to become involved in patient care activities.

Allow for flexible visiting hours when possible.

Consult ancillary services to assist patient and family deal with concerns as appropriate (social work, psychiatry, school teachers).

Medicate patient prn with antianxiety agents and/or analgesics and antipyretics.

Promote occupational therapy activities and ADL that increase activity/exercise levels.

Promote an atmosphere of acceptance.

Offer environmental stimuli through contact with other patients and families as appropriate.

Encourage patient and family to participate in an appropriate support group if available.

Assist the patient in identifying self-care deficits and anticipated needs in the home environment.

Explain burn care with return demonstration and verbalization of rationale for procedures by patient, prior to discharge.

- Wound cleansing, application of dressings
- Application of sunscreen, emollients
- Application of splints, compression garments
- Signs and symptoms of infection
- Physical/occupational therapy exercise regime
- Diet regimen
- Medication schedule
- Appointments to return to clinic

TRANSITION TO DISCHARGE

Any major burn is viewed by a patient and family members as a crisis. It is a sudden and traumatic event that permanently alters their lives. The patient's and family's response to the burn depends on age, culture, socioeconomic status, coping mechanisms, body image, family support systems, and previous experience with pain.[15]

As the patient's burns heal, the patient and family gradually assume more responsibility for wound care and activities of daily living. Prior to discharge, they must become familiar and comfortable with dressing changes, prescribed nutritional regimes, activity levels, exercises, and the use of pressure garments to control scarring. They also must be prepared to take steps to control the pain and itching frequently associated with the healing process. The family will need careful evaluation of their ability to provide support. The patient will need evaluation of his or her anticipated level of compliance with the rehabilitation program.

All members of the burn team should be involved in rehabilitation of the patient. This includes physicians, nurses, therapists, nutritionists, psychologists, social workers, vocational rehabilitationists, school teachers, and recreation therapists. Each patient will respond in a unique manner, and therefore should have input into an individualized plan for care and recovery. Nursing assessment of rehabilitation needs should focus on evaluation of the patient's wound healing, mobility level, pain level, nutritional status, and psychological functioning.

Recent advances in burn care have greatly increased the survival rate for burn victims. Due to the devastating physical and psychological changes incurred from the burn and recovery process, planning of discharge and the beginning of the rehabilitative phase of recovery must begin on admission and continue throughout the patient's stay.

REFERENCES

1. *Advanced Burn Life Support Course Manual,* Omaha, Neb, 1987, Nebraska Burn Institute.
2. Artz CP, Moncrief JA, Priutt BA: *Burns: a team approach,* Philadelphia, 1979, FA Davis.
3. Baxter CR: Fluid volume and electrolyte changes in the early postburn period, *Clin Plast Surg* 1(4):693-709, 1974.
4. Berkowitz RL: Burns. In Krupp MA, et al: *Current medical diagnosis and treatment,* Norwalk, Conn, 1987, Appleton and Lange.
5. Bernstein NR: *Comphrensive approaches to the burned person,* New York, 1983, Medical Examination Publishing Company.
6. Boswick JA: *The art and science of burn care,* Rockville, MD., 1987, Aspen Publications.
7. Committee on Education: *Protocols for burn and transfer agreements,* Galveston, Tex., 1984, American Burn Association.
8. Compton CC: Skin regenerated for cultured epithelial autografts on full thickness burn wounds from 6 days to 5 years after grafting, *Lab Invest* 60:600, 1987.
9. Demling RH: Management of the burn patient. In Shoemaker WC, et al: *Textbook of critical care,* Philadelphia, 1989, WB Saunders.
10. DiMola MA, Acres CA, Winkler JB: Burns. In Kinney MA, editor: *AACN's clinical reference for critical care nursing,* New York, 1988, McGraw-Hill.
11. Lund CC, Browder NC: The estimation of areas of burns, *Surg Gynecol Obstet* 79:352-358, 1944.
12. Martin LM: Nursing implications of today's burn care techniques, *RN* 5:26-33, 1989.
13. McLaughlin EG: *Critical care of the burn patient: a case study approach,* Rockville, Md, 1990, Aspen Publications.
14. National Center for Health Statistics: *National health interview survey,* Washington, DC, 1990, DHHS.
15. Sadowski DA: Care of the child with burns. In Hazinski MF, et al: *Nursing care of the critically ill child,* St Louis, 1992, Mosby–Year Book.
16. Schmitt BD, Kempe CH: Abuse and neglect of children. In Behrman RE, et al: *Nelson textbook of pediatrics,* Philadelphia, 1987, WB Saunders.
17. *St Anthony's DRG guidebook 1995,* Reston, Va, 1994, St Anthony.
18. Trofino RB: *Nursing care of the burn injured patient,* Philadelphia, 1991, FA Davis.
19. Wachtel TL, Kahn V, Frank HA: *Current topics in burn care,* Rockville, Md, 1983, Aspen Publications.
20. Wallace AB: The exposure treatment of burns, *Lancet* 1:501, 1951.

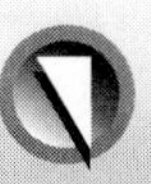

TRANSPLANT GUIDELINE

67

Obstetrical Events in Critical Care

Marge Zerbe, BS, RNC

DESCRIPTION

The pregnant patient in the critical care setting presents a unique challenge to her care givers. Normal physiology is altered due to the pregnancy, and the fetus is profoundly affected by changes in maternal condition. Therefore, assessment protocols and management interventions must be adapted to meet the needs of the gravid patient in the ICU.[2]

Normal physiologic changes of pregnancy affect every organ system. All of the normal adaptations of pregnancy are the result of either increased maternal and fetal requirements for tissue growth or preparation for delivery. A pregnancy is typically between 38 and 42 weeks in duration. Most systemic changes begin early in the first trimester and become more profound as the pregnancy advances. Therefore, gestational age will affect assessment parameters. The systems that undergo the most profound changes include the cardiovascular, hematologic, respiratory, renal, endocrine, and reproductive.

PHYSIOLOGIC CHANGES OF PREGNANCY

Cardiovascular

Dramatic anatomic and hemodynamic changes occur within the cardiovascular system. Blood volume, cardiac output, stroke volume, and heart rate increase, and blood pressure, pulmonary vascular resistance, and systemic vascular resistance decrease.[3,4,7,8] The physiologic basis for these changes involves the provision of adequate blood flow to the uteroplacental unit and protection from delivery-related hypovolemia. Blood volume increases up to 50% above nonpregnant levels. Plasma volume increases proportionately more then red cell mass, leading to the so-called physiologic anemia of pregnancy.[3] Most of the increased blood volume and cardiac output is distributed to the uterus, kidneys, skin, and breasts.[3,5] Cardiac output increases as a result of increased stroke volume and heart rate.[5] Variations in cardiac output can occur, however, related to maternal position. The gravid uterus can obstruct the inferior vena cava when the mother is in the supine position. Significant blood volume can be trapped in her lower extremities thereby decreasing cardiac return and cardiac output. Decreased uterine perfusion results as blood is diverted to the maternal central circulating volume.[3,5,7]

Blood pressure tends to decrease somewhat in the second trimester because of the physiologic vasodilation caused by progesterone.[5] Systemic vascular resistance (SVR) is decreased during pregnancy because of the dilation of peripheral blood vessels and the presence of the low-resistance placental vascular system.[5] The heart is displaced upward and rotated forward because of increased intra-abdominal pressure.[5] ECG changes commonly associated with pregnancy include a left-axis deviation and transient ST and T changes. An inverted T in lead II is not uncommon.[3,7] Benign ectopy is also frequently noted during pregnancy. The left ventricle enlarges, but this does not seem to alter function during normal pregnancy.[3] Systolic ejection murmurs are common and usually benign.[3,5] The first heart sound is often louder with exaggerated splitting, and the second heart sound is more intense in later pregnancy. A third heart sound can be elicited in 90% of all pregnant women after 30 weeks gestation.[1,3]

Hematologic

Changes in the white blood cell (WBC) count are mediated by estrogen and plasma cortisol. WBC counts can be greatly elevated during labor as a result of stress.[1,3] Bone marrow is hyperplastic during pregnancy and for 2 months postpartum, causing a dramatic increase in phagocytes, especially neutrophils.

Coagulation profiles are also altered. The pregnant woman functions in a state of enhanced coagulopathy because of an increase in most of the coagulation factors and a decrease in the fibrinolytic factors.[1] This coagulopathy protects the mother from blood loss during delivery, but also puts her at increased risk for thromboembolytic complications.

Significant adaptive responses to pregnancy result in laboratory values that would appear abnormal and pathologic to those unfamiliar with pregnancy profiles.

Respiratory

Respiratory modifications during pregnancy are necessary to meet both maternal and fetal needs. Mechanical and biochemical alterations enhance oxygen delivery and carbon dioxide excretion. Maternal oxygen requirements increase by approximately 32% in response to the increased growth and metabolism associated with pregnancy. The diaphragm is elevated by 4 to 7 cm as the uterus expands. Compensation for the shortening of the thoracic cavity occurs as the anteroposterior and the thoracic diameters of the chest enlarge. The transverse diameter increases by 2 cm with flaring of the lower rib cage.[1,3] Breathing tends to be diaphragmatic rather than costal during pregnancy. Vital capacity remains unchanged, but tidal volume and minute ventilation increase significantly. Alveolar ventilation is typically increased by 65% to 70%.[3,5] Maternal plasma levels of carbon dioxide and bicarbonate are both decreased, and plasma oxygenation is slightly increased. The pregnant woman therefore functions in a state of compensated respiratory alkalosis.[3,5] Hemoglobin saturation levels below 90% are critical.[3] Oxygen consumption increases progressively during pregnancy and the decrease in functional residual capacity lowers oxygen reserve. Therefore, short periods of impaired respirations or apnea can induce critical changes in saturation and arterial blood gases and can contribute to substantial fetal damage. Ventilatory support of the pregnant patient must be based on a thorough understanding of the respiratory physiology. Nasal mucosa often become very vascular and edematous. Nosebleeds are common and accidental trauma during intubation and suctioning procedures can cause significant bleeding.[1] Airway edema may also require the use of smaller-lumen tubes and catheters.

Gastrointestinal

Gastrointestinal motility is greatly decreased during pregnancy because of progesterone. Emptying time is prolonged because of hormonal influence and mechanical obstruction by the expanding uterus; relative incompetence of the esophageal spinchter is common.[5] The pregnant patient is consequently at much higher risk for reflux, regurgitation, and aspiration of undigested food and stomach acid. The hormone gastrin, produced by the placenta, increases the acidity of gastric acid, making acid aspiration an extremely critical potential.[5] Liver function is enhanced, but gallbladder activity is decreased, increasing risk during pregnancy for the development of gallstones.[3,5] The small intestines are displaced by the enlarging uterus and are compartmentalized in the upper abdominal quadrants.[1]

Renal

Renal function is enhanced during pregnancy due to increased demands for filtration and excretion. Both renal perfusion flow (RPF) and glomerular filtration (GFR) may increase by as much as 50%.[3,5] The increase in RPF and GFR improves the renal clearance of many substances, with a corresponding decrease in serum levels. Urea, creatinine, and uric acid are excreted more efficiently during pregnancy, and the complete reabsorption of some substances may not occur because of the inability of the tubules to handle the high flow. Drugs are also rapidly excreted. Subtherapeutic blood and tissue levels may require dosage adjustments to maintain optimal clinical responses. Progesterone is responsible for the progressive dilation of the ureters and relaxation of the bladder. Dilation and rotation of the right ureter is particularly prominent, leading to an increased incidence of ascending right pyelonephritis.[5] The bladder is relaxed, very vascular, and anatomically displaced out of the pelvis and into the abdominal cavity. Stasis, incomplete emptying, and bladder trauma are common.

Endocrine

Changes occurring within the endocrine system during gestation are quite profound. The pituitary gland doubles in size and weight and requires an enormous blood supply during pregnancy. Situations involving decreased perfusion or hemorrhage into the pituitary can cause significant damage and subsequent impairment of hormone production. Thyroid function increases, causing an increased basal metabolic rate. The hyperplastic islets of Langerhans increase production of insulin in early pregnancy, but peripheral resistance to insulin increases due to pregnancy hormones, making the gravid woman more insulin resistant. Glycogen storage during gestation is limited, and patients whose pancreatic reserve is also marginal may develop gestational or even true diabetes. Hyperglycemic situations are critical to fetal development, especially during the first trimester. Fasting and nocturnal hypoglycemia are also relatively common during pregnancy.[5]

Reproductive

The reproductive system undergoes enormous changes during gestation. Uterine enlargement is accomplished by hyperplasia, hypertrophy, and stretching. Blood vessels and lymphatics increase, and hypertrophy of the peripheral nerves supplying the uterus occurs. The uterus moves up and out of the pelvis after the twelfth gestational week. The uterus is very mobile because the lower segment is the only portion firmly anchored to the cervical connections. Uterine perfusion increases dramatically during pregnancy. The

TABLE 67-1 DRGs Associated with Obstetrical Events in Critical Care

DRG #	DRG label	Average LOS
370	Cesarean section with complications	5.9 days
372	Vaginal delivery with complicating diagnoses	3.4 days
378	Ectopic pregnancy	3.0 days
383	Other antepartum diagnoses with medical complications	4.0 days

Information from *St Anthony's DRG guidebook 1995*, Reston, Va, 1994, St Anthony.

uterine arteries are the major blood supply for the uterus. They lie along the broad ligaments and enter the uterus close to the level of the internal os of the cervix and then ascend on each side of the uterus to form a network of spiral arterioles. These blood vessels increase considerably in both size and number during gestation. The cervix is primarily made up of connective tissue and is also very vascular. Bleeding from cervical and vaginal lacerations can be extensive.

Continuous monitoring of the viable fetus is an important part of care because compromised heart tones may be the first sign of maternal deterioration. Fetal heart tones are assessed as to baseline, variability, and periodic changes. Normal baselines are considered to be 120 to 160 bpm and an increasing fetal baseline is typically associated with early intrauterine hypoxia. It is generally accepted that decreased fetal variability indicates intrauterine hypoxia. Periodic changes include both accelerations and decelerations. Accelerations are usually considered to be a reassuring sign. Decelerations are characterized as early, late or variable, and, depending on the characteristics, may be of more concern. A full discussion of fetal monitoring is beyond the scope of this chapter and the reader is referred for further study to a more in-depth text.[2,5]

LENGTH OF STAY/ANTICIPATED COURSE

The LOS for uncomplicated vaginal delivery is fast becoming an outpatient event. However, there can be obstetrical events that may require critical care level intervention. DRGs that reflect complications with a potential for critical care intervention are summarized in Table 67-1.

MANAGEMENT TRENDS AND CONTROVERSIES

Preeclampsia/Eclampsia

The preeclamptic/eclamptic patient would most likely require critical care interventions as a result of hemodynamic instability, neurologic complications, or situations involving major coagulation derangements. Preeclampsia is being shown to have varying hemodynamic characteristics and invasive monitoring is increasingly being used to differentiate pathophysiology. Some individuals are profoundly intravascularly dehydrated because of critical fluid shifts, and others are unstable because of hyperdynamic cardiac outputs with potential for left ventricular failure and pulmonary edema. Still others require interventions for refractory hypertension. The varying and complicated aspects of the pathophysiology have increased the need for invasive hemodynamic monitoring techniques to guide management decisions.

Seizure activity associated with preeclampsia is termed *eclampsia*. Etiology remains unclear, but the potential consequences are well documented. The greatest danger associated with preeclampsia/eclampsia is cerebral hemorrhage. Seizure activity can occur antepartum, intrapartum, or postpartum. The seizure is typically tonic/clonic, although EEG seizure activity has been documented. The patient seldom has a preliminary aura. The tonic phase will last 20 to 30 seconds followed by a 60- to 90-second clonic phase and a 1- to 2-hour postictal phase.[1] Careful neurologic assessment and management of drug therapies is mandatory. Magnesium sulfate is often used to provide peripheral nervous system control. Although conflicting reports exist concerning the efficacy of this drug in the treatment of preeclampsia/eclampsia, most treatment therapies will include both bolus and maintenance dosages. Critical assessments during magnesium administration include decreased respiratory rate and decreased deep tendon reflexes.

Coagulation derangements occur in preeclampsia/eclampsia related to endothelial wall damage and stimulation of the coagulation cascade. HELLP syndrome, a related disorder, usually has vague symptoms suggestive of gallbladder or liver pathology. Pathology involves RBC hemolysis, elevated liver enzymes, and profound thrombocytopenia.[4,6] Treatment will most likely include stabilization with either vaginal or surgical delivery of the infant and blood product replacement.

Hemorrhage

Critical hemorrhage during pregnancy is most commonly associated with abruptio placentae, severe postpartum hemorrhage, and DIC. Placental abruption occurs when the normally implanted placenta suddenly detaches from the uterine wall. The bleeding is predominately maternal. Bleeding can be obvious or concealed. As blood loss continues, perfusion to the placenta will decrease as the uterine arteries vasoconstrict and blood is diverted to the maternal circulating volume. Definitive symptoms of shock may therefore be delayed because of physiologic placental compromise. The fetus is more likely to demonstrate early signs of maternal hypovolemia, as evidenced by deteriorating fetal heart tone patterns. Hemodynamic instability can occur as a result of massive blood loss. Excessive postpartum bleeding is usually associated with uterine atony, major lacerations, uterine rupture, or uterine inversion. DIC is associated as a secondary diagnosis with certain obstetrical triggers such as abruptio, preeclampsia, and amniotic fluid embolism. The intrinsic system can be activated by damage to blood vessel walls. The extrinsic system can be activated by the release of tissue thromboplastin. Physiologic coagulation modifications related to the pregnancy affect the assessment of laboratory data.

Amniotic Fluid Embolism

Amniotic fluid debris may reach the maternal circulation through tears in the maternal cervix, vagina, or uterine walls. It has been suggested that the vasoactive debris causes dramatic pulmonary artery spasm and organ damage. Primary symptoms involve respiratory collapse, rapidly followed by cardiac failure and possibly DIC.[3] Mortality is extremely high and management is directed to resuscitation and supportive care. All advanced cardiac life support protocols should be followed during resuscitation, with special attention to aggressive ventilation and displacement of the gravid uterus by a right hip wedge to decrease inferior vena cava compression. Defibrillation is not contraindicated during pregnancy. ACLS drugs in the usual dosages are considered appropriate. Although these drugs do cross the placenta, the effects of the profound maternal hypoxia and cardiac arrhythmias are thought to be more harmful than drug therapy to the fetus.

Trauma

Trauma in the pregnant individual can be extremely difficult to manage, again because of the physiologic changes that affect assessment and management. Motor vehicle accidents are the most common reason for admission into a critical care setting. Blunt trauma can cause serious damage to both mother and fetus, and fetal death is most often the result of maternal death. The intrauterine pressures generated during impact are enormous. Abruptio placentae, in which bleeding can be either obvious or concealed, can occur following an incident involving blunt trauma. Delayed abruptio, in which there is increasing retroplacental bleeding, can have devastating consequences. Penetrating trauma can also cause serious consequences of the pregnancy. Knife wounds, generally located in the fundal region, may or may not require surgical repair. Gunshot injuries are more common than stab injuries, and are usually surgically explored. Thermal trauma is most commonly associated with house fires, particularly those involving kitchen accidents. The fetus is not actually burned, but may experience serious consequences related to changes in maternal oxygenation. The release of prostaglandins from traumatized tissues can initiate labor contractions. Any complaints of abdominal cramping following trauma must be seriously investigated.

ASSESSMENT

The following details significant laboratory normals and the changes that occur during pregnancy. The critical care provider must be aware that certain parameters, which would normally indicate pathology in the nonpregnant individual, are within normal limits for the gravid patient.

PARAMETER	ANTICIPATED ALTERATION IN PREGNANCY
Hgb Hct	Decreased: Hgb <10 to 14 g/dl, Hct 32% to 42% *due to the natural hemodilution of pregnancy*
WBC with differential	Increased: >25,000/mm^3, *due to stress response or in labor; increase primarily neutrophils*
Sed rate	Increased: >30 to 90 mm/hr *due to the increased level of fibrinogen*
Glucose	WNL
PO_4^-	WNL
Na^+	Decreased: <132 to 140 mEq/L *due to natural hemodilution*
Cl^-	Decreased: <90 to 105 mEq/L *due to hemodilution*
BUN	Decreased: <4 to 12 mg/100 ml *due to enhanced renal function*
Serum creatinine	Decreased: <0.4 to 0.9 mg/100 ml *due to enhanced renal function* *Levels >1.0 may indicate significant pathology during pregnancy*
Alk Phos	Increased: >2 to 3 times during last trimester and for 4 weeks postpartum *due to placental production*
pH	WNL in compensated respiratory alkalosis
Pao_2	Increased: >104 to 107 mm Hg *due to increased alveolar ventilation*
$Paco_2$	Decreased: <28 to 32 mm Hg *due to increased alveolar ventilation*

HCO_3^-	Decreased: <18 to 22 mEq/L *to compensate for decreased CO_2 levels*
Fibrinogen	Increased: >600 mg/dl natural hypercoagulable state
Platelets	WNL
SVR	25% decrease to 600 to 900 dynes/sec/cm^{-5}
PVR	25% decrease to 15 to 90 dynes/sec/cm^{-5}
CO	30% to 45% increase to 5.6 to 9.8 L/min
BP	Decreased slightly in normal pregnancy, returning to prepregnancy levels at week 36 of gestation Hypertension is associated with preeclampsia
Urinalysis	Proteinuria in the presence of preeclampsia
RR	Increased with normal pregnancy If dyspnea and cyanosis are present, suspect amniotic fluid embolism Monitor for fluid overload until spontaneous diuresis occurs, usually 24 to 36 hours after delivery
Skin	Petechiae and oozing from venipuncture sites may provide early warning of the development of DIC and impending hemorrhage

PLAN OF CARE

INTENSIVE PHASE

The following priorities and interventions are specifically pregnancy related and should be considered in addition to the usual assessment and management protocols appropriate in critical care situations.

PATIENT CARE PRIORITIES	EXPECTED PATIENT OUTCOMES
High risk for altered family process *r/t situational crisis of pregnancy complication*	Supportive and cohesive family and friends Appropriate information and counseling concerning maternal, fetal, and neonatal outcomes
High risk for altered placental perfusion *r/t* *Hypovolemia* *Inferior vena cava compression*	Maternal vital signs and hemodynamic parameters remain within normal pregnancy parameters Fetal monitoring remains within normal limits for baseline, variability, and periodic changes
High risk for ineffective breathing pattern *r/t* *Postictal status* *Hemorrhagic decompensation* *ARDS associated with amniotic fluid embolism*	Normal respiratory pattern with saturations remaining >90% and with normal pregnancy ABG (compensated respiratory aklalosis)
High risk for altered renal perfusion *r/t decreased tissue perfusion associated with vascular changes or hemorrhagic shock*	Normal pregnancy renal lab parameters and maintenance of urinary output of at least 30cc/hr
High risk for aspiration *r/t* *Decreased gastric motility* *Relaxation of gastric sphincter*	Gastric acid will remain less acid with pH of >2.5 Patient will maintain patent and unobstructed airway
High risk for ileus and constipation *r/t decreased GI motility*	Active postoperative bowel sounds and/or regular bowel habits will be maintained
Pain *r/t injuries or surgical interventions*	Absence of subjective and objective signs and symptoms of pain
High risk for altered cerebral perfusion *r/t seizure activity associated with preeclampsia and/or neurologic hypoperfusion*	Normal neurologic function with client appropriately awake, alert, and oriented with absence of seizure activity

Plan of Care (cont'd)

INTERVENTIONS

Provide information and reassurance to patient and family *to facilitate cohesive and effective support system.*

Maintain uterine displacement by left lateral position or right hip wedge *to avoid vena caval compression and maintain uterine perfusion.*

Monitor ABG *to assess and manage acid–base status.*

Provide supplemental oxygen to maintain Sao_2 of at least 90% *to facilitate oxygen delivery to uterine circulation.*

Monitor I/O and assess renal labs *to monitor for symptoms of decreasing renal function.*

Administer clear antacids as ordered *to neutralize gastric acidity.*

Monitor bowel sounds and function *to intervene appropriately with ileus and maintain bowel function.*

Provide analgesia and sedation as needed *to maintain comfort level and decrease oxygen demand/consumption.*

Monitor neurologic function *to assess for cognitive changes.*

TRANSISTION TO DISCHARGE

The pregnant patient in critical care who survives the life-threatening complication that brought her to the ICU typically progresses rapidly to a state of recovery after treatment for pathology leading to ICU hospitalization or, in eclampsia, after delivery of the infant. Discharge planning, therefore, focuses on meeting the physical and educational needs of the new mother and promoting wellness in the newborn. Assessing the postpartum parameters of uterine involution and lochia help determine the mother's physical readiness for discharge. Providing information about the infant's condition and maintaining liberal family visitation will help provide important emotional and social support at this time. Consultation with obstetric nurses can maximize professional nursing care and promote the health of both mother and infant.

REFERENCES

1. Cunningham FG, MacDonald PC, Gant NF: *Williams obstetrics,* ed 18, Norwalk, Conn, 1989, Appleton & Lange.
2. Datta S: *Anesthetic and obstetric management of high-risk pregnancy,* St Louis, 1991, Mosby–Year Book.
3. Diaz JH: The physiologic changes of pregnancy have anesthetic implications for both mother and fetus. In Diaz JH, editor: *Perinatal anesthesia and critical care,* Philadelphia, 1991, WB Saunders.
4. Harvey CJ, Burke ME: Hypertensive disorders in pregnancy. In Mandeville LK, Nroiano NH, editors: *High-risk intrapartum nursing,* Philadelphia, 1992, JB Lippincott.
5. Harvey MG: Physiologic changes of pregnancy. In Harvey CJ: *Critical care obstetrical nursing,* Gaithersburg, 1991, Aspen.
6. Shannon DM: HELLP syndrome: a severe consequence of pregnancy induced hypertension, *J Obstet Gynecol Neonatal Nurs* 11:395-402, 1987.
7. Smith LG: The pregnant trauma patient. In Cardona VD, et al, editors: *Trauma nursing from resuscitation through rehabilitation,* Philadelphia, 1988, WB Saunders.
8. Waserstrum N, Cotton DB: Hemodynamic monitoring in severe pregnancy induced hypertension, *Clin Perinat* 12:781-797, 1986.

Appendices

APPENDIX

A

Hemodynamic Parameters, Formulas, and Normal Ranges

Nancie Urban, MSN, RN, CCRN

Parameter	Abbreviation	Indicator	Formula	Normal range
Cardiac output	CO	Cardiac performance	HR × SV	4-8 L/min
Cardiac index	CI	Adequacy of CO for individual	$\frac{CO}{BSA}$	2.5-4 L/min/m^2
Central venous pressure	CVP	Preload Right ventricle	—	2-8 cm H_2O 2-6 mm Hg
Left ventricular stroke work index	LVSWI	Contractility Left ventricle	$\frac{(MAP\text{-}PCWP)SV}{BSA} \times 0.0136$	35-85 g/m^2/beat
Oxygen delivery	Do_2	Delivery of O_2 to tissues	$CO \times Sao_2 \times Hgb \times 1.34 \times 10$	900-1100 ml/min (at rest)
Oxygen consumption	Vo_2	Consumption of O_2 by tissues	$CO \times (Sao_2 - Svo_2) \times Hgb \times 1.34 \times 10$	225-275 ml/min (at rest)
Pulmonary capillary wedge pressure	PCWP	Preload Left ventricle	—	5-12 mm Hg 14-16 mm Hg*
Pulmonary vascular resistance	PVR	Afterload Right ventricle	$\frac{PAM\text{-}PCWP}{CO} \times 80$	37-97 dynes/sec/cm^{-5}
Pulmonary vascular resistance index	PVRI	Afterload Right ventricle for individual	$\frac{PAM\text{-}PCWP}{CI} \times 80$	255-285 dyne · sec/m^2 · cm^{-5}
Right ventricular stroke work index	RVSWI	Contractility Right ventricle	$\frac{(PAD\text{-}CVP)SV}{BSA} \times 0.0136$	7-12 gm/m^2/beat
Stroke volume index	SVI	Contractility general indicator	$\frac{SV}{BSA}$	33-47 ml/m^2/beat
Systemic vascular resistance	SVR	Afterload Left ventricle	$\frac{MAP\text{-}CVP}{CO} \times 80$	800-1200 dynes/sec/cm^{-5}
Systemic vascular resistance index	SVRI	Afterload Left ventricle for individual	$\frac{MAP\text{-}CVP}{CI} \times 80$	1970-2390 dyne · sec/m^2 · cm^{-5}

*Normal range for cardiac patients who need higher filling pressure for optimal CO.
PAD may be substituted for PCWP as long as values demonstrate close correlation

APPENDIX

B

Normal Reference Values

Joanne M. Krumberger, MSN, RN, CCRN

BLOOD, PLASMA, OR SERUM VALUES

Test	Reference range: Conventional values	Reference range: SI units*
Acetoacetate plus acetone	0.30-2.0 mg/dl	3-20 mg/L
Acetone	Negative	Negative
Acid phosphatase	Adults: 0.10-0.63 U/ml (Bessey-Lowry)	28-175 nmol/s/L
	0.5-2.0 U/ml (Bodansky)	
	1.0-4.0 U/ml (King-Armstrong)	
Activated partial thromboplastin time (APTT)	30-40 sec	30-40 sec
Adrenocorticotropic hormone (ACTH)	6 AM 15-100 pg/ml	10-80 ng/L
	6 PM <50 pg/ml	<50 ng/L
Alanine aminotransferase (ALT)	5-35 IU/L	5-35 U/L
Albumin	3.2-4.5 g/dl	35-55 g/L
Alcohol	Negative	Negative
Aldosterone	Peripheral blood:	
	Supine: 7.4 ± 4.2 ng/dl	0.08-0.3 nmol/L
	Upright: 1-21 ng/dl	0.14-0.8 nmol/L
Alkaline phosphatase	Adults: 30-85 ImU/ml	
Alpha-aminonitrogen	3-6 mg/dl	2.1-3.9 mmol/L
Alpha-1-antitrypsin	>250 mg/dl	
Ammonia	Adults: 15-110 μg/dl	47-65 μmol/L
Amylase	56-190 IU/L	25-125 U/L
	80-150 Somogyi units/ml	
Angiotensin-converting enzyme (ACE)	23-57 U/ml	
Antinuclear antibodies (ANA)	Negative	
Antistreptolysin O (ASO)	Adults: ≤160 Todd units/ml	
Antithyroid microsomal antibody	Titer <1:100	
Antithyroglobulin antibody	Titer <1:100	
Ascorbic acid (vitamin C)	0.6-1.6 mg/dl	23-57 μmol/L

BLOOD, PLASMA, OR SERUM VALUES—cont'd

Test	Reference range: Conventional values	Reference range: SI units*
Aspartate aminotransferase (AST, SGOT)	12-36 U/ml 5-40 IU/L	0.10-0.30 μmol/s/L 5-40 U/L
Australian antigen (hepatitis-associated antigen, HAA)	Negative	Negative
Barbiturates	Negative	Negative
Base excess	Men: −3.3 to +1.2 Women: −2.4 to +2.3	0 ± 2 mmol/L 0 ± 2 mmol/L
Bicarbonate (HCO_3^-)	22-26 mEq/L	22-26 mmol/L
Bilirubin		
Direct (conjugated)	0.1-0.3 mg/dl	1.7-5.1 μmol/L
Indirect (unconjugated)	0.2-0.8 mg/dl	3.4-12.0 μmol/L
Total	0.1-1.0 mg/dl	5.1-17.0 μmol/L
Bleeding time (Ivy method)	1-9 min	
Blood count (see Complete blood count)		
Blood gases (arterial)		
pH	7.35-7.45	
PCO_2	35-45 mm Hg	4.7-6.0 kPa
HCO_3^-	22-26 mEq/L	21-28 nmol/L
PO_2	80-100 mm Hg	11-13 kPa
SaO_2	95%-100%	
Blood urea nitrogen (BUN)	5-20 mg/dl	3.6-7.1 mmol/L
Bromide	Up to 5 mg/dl	0-63 mmol/L
Bromosulfophthalein (BSP)	<5% retention after 45 min	
CA 15-3	<22 U/ml	
CA-125	0-35 U/ml	
CA 19-9	<37 U/ml	
C-reactive protein (CRP)	<6 μg/ml	
Calcitonin	<50 pg/ml	<50 pmol/L
Calcium (Ca)	9.0-10.5 mg/dl (total) 3.9-4.6 mg/dl (ionized)	2.25-2.75 mmol/L 1.05-1.30 mmol/L
Carbon dioxide (CO_2) content	23-30 mEq/L	21-30 mmol/L
Carboxyhemoglobin (COHb)	3% of total hemoglobin	
Carcinoembryonic antigen (CEA)	<2 ng/ml	0-2.5 μg/L
Carotene	50-200 μg/dl	0.74-3.72 μmol/L
Chloride (ClI)	90-110 mEq/L	98-106 mmol/L
Cholesterol	150-250 mg/dl	3.90-6.50 mmol/L
Clot retraction	50%-100% clot retraction in 1-2 hrs, complete retraction within 24 hrs	
Complement	C_3: 70-176 mg/dl C_4: 16-45 mg/dl	0.55-1.20 g/L 0.20-0.50 g/L
Complete blood count (CBC)		
Red blood cell (RBC) count	Men: 4.7-6.1 million/mm^3 Women: 4.2-5.4 million/mm^3	
Hemoglobin (Hgb)	Men: 14-18 g/dl Women: 12-16 g/dl (pregnancy: >11 g/dl)	8.7-11.2 mmol/L 7.4-9.9 mmol/L
Hematocrit (Hct)	Men: 42%-52% Women: 37%-47% (pregnancy: >33%)	
Mean corpuscular volume (MCV)	80-95 μ^3	80-95 fl
Mean corpuscular hemoglobin (MCH)	27-31 pg	0.42-0.48 fmol
Mean corpuscular hemoglobin concentration (MCHC)	32-36 g/dl	

Continued.

BLOOD, PLASMA, OR SERUM VALUES—cont'd

Test	Reference range	
	Conventional values	SI units*
Complete blood count (CBC)—cont'd		
White blood cell count (WBC)	5000-10,000/cm^3	
Differential count		
Neutrophils	55%-70%	
Lymphocytes	20%-40%	
Monocytes	2%-8%	
Eosinophils	1%-4%	
Basophils	0.5%-1%	
Platelet count	150,000-400,000/mm^3	
Coombs' test		
Direct	Negative	Negative
Indirect	Negative	Negative
Copper (Cu)	70-140 μg/dl	11.0-24.3 μmol/L
Cortisol	6-28 μg/dl (AM)	170-635 nmol/L
	2-12 μg/dl (PM)	82-413 nmol/L
CPK isoenzyme (MB)	<5% total	
Creatinine	0.7-1.5 mg/dl	<133 μmol/L
Creatinine clearance	Men: 95-104 ml/min	<133 μmol/L
	Women: 95-125 ml/min	
Creatinine phosphokinase (CPK)	5-75 mU/ml	12-80 units/L
Cryoglobulin	Negative	Negative
Differential (WBC) count		
Neutrophils	55%-70%	
Lymphocytes	20%-40%	
Monocytes	2%-8%	
Eosinophils	1%-4%	
Basophils	0.5%-1%	
Digoxin	Therapeutic level: 0.5-2.0 ng/ml	40-79 μmol/L
	Toxic level: >2.4 ng/ml	>119 μmol/L
Erythrocyte count (see Complete blood count)		
Erythrocyte sedimentation rate (ESR)	Men: up to 15 mm/hr	
	Women: up to 20 mm/hr	
Ethanol	80-200 mg/dl (mild to moderate intoxication)	17-43 mmol/L
	250-400 mg/dl (marked intoxication)	54-87 mmol/L
	>400 mg/dl (severe intoxication)	>87 mmol/L
Euglobulin lysis test	90 min-6 hrs	
Fats	Up to 200 mg/dl	
Ferritin	15-200 ng/ml	15-200 μg/L
Fibrin degradation products (FDP)	<10 μg/ml	
Fibrinogen (factor I)	200-400 mg/dl	5.9-11.7 μmol/L
Fibrinolysis/euglobulin lysis test	90 min-6 hrs	
Fluorescent treponemal antibody (FTA)	Negative	Negative
Fluoride	<0.05 mg/dl	<0.027 mmol/L
Folic acid (Folate)	5-20 μg/ml	14-34 mmol/L
Follicle-stimulating hormone (FSH)	Men: 0.1-15.0 ImU/ml	
	Women: 6-30 ImU/ml	
	Castrate and postmenopausal: 30-200 ImU/ml	
Free thyroxine index (FTI)	0.9-2.3 ng/dl	

BLOOD, PLASMA, OR SERUM VALUES—cont'd

Test	Reference range	
	Conventional values	**SI units***
Galactose-1-phosphate uridyl transferase	18.5-28.5 U/g hemoglobin	
Gammaglobulin	0.5-1.6 g/dl	
Gamma-glutamyl transpeptidase (GGTP)	Men: 8-38 U/L Women: <45 years: 5-27 U/L	5-40 U/L 37°C
Gastrin	40-150 pg/ml	40-150 ng/L
Glucagon	50-200 pg/ml	14-56 pmol/L
Glucose, fasting (FBS)	Adults: 70-115 mg/dl	3.89-6.38 mmol/L
Glucose, 2-hour postprandial (2-hour PPG)	<140 mg/dl	
Glucose-6-phosphate dehydrogenase (G-6-PD)	8.6-18.6 IU/g of hemoglobin	
Glucose tolerance test (GTT)	Fasting: 70-115 mg/dl 30 min: <200 mg/dl 1 hr: <200 mg/dl 2 hrs: <140 mg/dl 3 hrs: 70-115 mg/dl 4 hrs: 70-115 mg/dl	
Glycosylated hemoglobin	Adults: 2.2%-4.8% Good diabetic control: 2.5%-6% Fair diabetic control: 6.1%-8% Poor diabetic control: >8%	
Growth hormone	<10 ng/ml	<10 μg/L
Haptoglobin	100-150 mg/dl	16-31 μmol/L
Hematocrit (Hct)	Men: 42%-52% Women: 37%-47% (pregnancy: >33%)	
Hemoglobin (Hgb)	Men: 14-18 g/dl Women: 12-16 g/dl (pregnancy: >11 g/dl)	8.7-11.2 mmol/L 7.4-9.9 mmol/L
Hemoglobin electrophoresis	Hgb A_1: 95%-98% Hgb A_2: 2%-3% Hgb F: 0.8%-2% Hgb S: 0 Hgb C: 0	
Hepatitis B surface antigen (HB_3AG)	Nonreactive	Nonreactive
Heterophil antibody	Negative	Negative
HLA-B27	None	None
Human chorionic gonadotropin (HCG)	Negative	Negative
Human placental lactogen (HPL)	Rise during pregnancy	
5-Hydroxyindoleacetic acid (5-HIAA)	2.8-8.0 mg/24 hrs	
Immunoglobulin quantification	IgG: 550-1900 mg/dl IgA: 60-333 mg/dl IgM: 45-145 mg/dl	5.5-19.0 g/L 0.6-3.3 g/L 0.45-1.5 g/L
Insulin	4-20 μU/ml	36-179 pmol/L
Iron (Fe)	60-190 μg/dl	13-31 μmol/L
Iron-binding capacity, total (TIBC)	250-420 μg/dl	45-73 μmol/L
Iron (transferrin) saturation	30%-40%	
Ketone bodies	Negative	Negative
Lactic acid	0.6-1.8 mEq/L	
Lactic dehydrogenase (LDH)	90-200 ImU/ml	0.4-1.7 μmol/s/L

Continued.

BLOOD, PLASMA, OR SERUM VALUES—cont'd

Test	Reference range	
	Conventional values	SI units*
LDH isoenzymes	LDH-1: 17%-27% LDH-2: 28%-38% LDH-3: 19%-27% LDH-4: 5%-16% LDH-5: 6%-16%	
Lead	120 μg/dl or less	<1.0 μmol/L
Leucine aminopeptidase (LAP)	Men: 80-200 U/ml Women: 75-185 U/ml	
Leukocyte count (see Complete blood count)		
Lipase	Up to 1.5 U/ml	0-417 U/L
Lipids		
Total	400-1000 mg/dl	4-8 g/L
Cholesterol	150-250 mg/dl	3.9-6.5 mmol/L
Triglycerides	40-150 mg/dl	0.4-1.5 g/L
Phospholipids	150-380 mg/dl	1.9-3.9 mmol/L
Lithium		
Long-acting thyroid stimulating hormone (LATS)	Negative	Negative
Magnesium (Mg)	1.6-3.0 mEq/L	0.8-1.3 mm/L
Methanol	Negative	Negative
Mononucleosis spot test	Negative	Negative
Nitrogen, nonprotein	15-35 mg/dl	10.7-25.0 mmol/L
Nuclear antibody (ANA)	Negative	Negative
5′-Nucleotidase	Up to 1.6 units	27-233 nmol/s/L
Osmolality	275-300 mOsm/kg	
Oxygen saturation (arterial)	95%-100%	0.95-1.00 of capacity
Parathormone (PTH)	<2000 pg/ml	
Partial thromboplastin time, activated (APTT)	30-40 sec	
P_{CO_2}	35-45 mm Hg	
pH	7.35-7.45	7.35-7.45
Phenylalanine	Up to 2 mg/dl	<0.18 mmol/L
Phenylketonuria (PKU)	Negative	Negative
Phenytoin (Dilantin)	Therapeutic level: 10-20 μg/ml	
Phosphatase (acid)	0.10-0.63 U/ml (Bessey-Lowry) 0.5-2.0 U/ml (Bodansky) 1.0-4.0 U/ml (King-Armstrong)	0.11-0.60 U/L
Phosphatase (alkaline)	Adults: 30-85 ImU/ml	20-90 units/L
Phospholipids (see Lipids)		
Phosphorus (P, PO_4)	2.5-4.5 mg/dl	0.78-1.52 mmol/L 1.29-2.26 mmol/L
Platelet count	150,000-400,000/mm^3	
P_{O_2}	80-100 mm Hg	
Potassium (K)	3.5-5.0 mEq/L	3.5-5.0 mmol/L
Progesterone	Men, postmenopausal women: <2 ng/ml Women, luteal: peak >5 ng/ml	6 nmol/L >16 nmol/L
Prolactin	2-15 ng/ml	2-15 μg/L
Protein (total)	6-8 g/dl	55-80 g/L
Albumin	3.2-4.5 g/dl	33-55 g/L
Globulin	2.3-3.4 g/dl	20-35 g/L

BLOOD, PLASMA, OR SERUM VALUES—cont'd

Test	Reference range: Conventional values	Reference range: SI units*
Prothrombin time (PT)	11.0-12.5 sec	11.0-12.5 sec
Pyruvate	0.3-0.9 mg/dl	34-103 μmol/L
Red blood cell count (see Complete blood count)		
Red blood cell indexes (see Complete blood count)		
Renin		
Reticulocyte count	0.5%-2% of total erythrocytes	
Rheumatoid factor	Negative	Negative
Rubella antibody test		
Salicylates	Negative	
	Therapeutic: 20-25 mg/dl (to age 10: 25-30 mg/dl)	1.4-1.8 mmol/L
	Toxic: >30 mg/dl (after age 60: >20 mg/dl)	>2.2 mmol/L
Schilling test (vitamin B_{12} absorption)	8%-40% excretion/24 hrs	
Serologic test for syphilis (STS)	Negative (nonreactive)	
Serum glutamic oxaloacetic transaminase (SGOT, AST)	12-36 U/ml	0.10-0.30 μmol/s/L
	5-40 IU/L	
Serum glutamic-pyruvic transaminase (SGPT, ALT)	5-35 IU/L	0.05-0.43 μmol/s/L
Sickle cell	Negative	
Sodium (Na^+)	136-145 mEq/L	136-145 mmol/L
Sugar (see Glucose)		
Syphilis (see Serologic test for, Fluorescent treponemal antibody, Veneral Disease Research Laboratory)		
Testosterone	Men: 300-1200 ng/dl	10-42 nmol/L
	Women: 30-95 ng/dl	1.1-3.3 nmol/L
Thymol flocculation	Up to 5 units	
Thyroglubulin antibody (see Antithyroglobulin antibody)		
Thyroid-stimulating hormone (TSH)	1-4 μU/ml	5 mU/L
Thyroxine (T_4)	Murphy-Pattee: 4-11 μg/dl	
	Radioimmunoassay: 5-10 μg/dl	
Thyroxine-binding globulin (TBG)	12-28 μg/ml	129-335 nmol/L
Transaminase (see Serum glutamic-oxaloacetic transaminase, Serum glutamic-pyruvic transaminase)		
Triglycerides	40-150 mg/dl	0.4-1.5 g/L
Triiodothyronine (T_3)	110-230 ng/dl	1.2-1.5 nmol/L
Triiodothyronine (T_3) resin uptake	25%-35%	
Tubular phosphate reabsorption (TPR)	80%-90%	
Urea nitrogen (see Blood urea nitrogen)		
Uric acid	Men: 2.1-8.5 mg/dl	0.15-0.48 mmol/L
	Women: 2.0-6.6 mg/dl	0.09-0.36 mmol/L
Venereal Disease Research Laboratory (VDRL)	Negative	Negative
Vitamin A	20-100 g/dl	0.7-3.5 μmol/L

Continued.

BLOOD, PLASMA, OR SERUM VALUES—cont'd

	Reference range	
Test	**Conventional values**	**SI units***
Vitamin B_{12}	200-600 pg/ml	148-443 pmol/L
Vitamin C	0.6-1.6 mg/dl	23-57 μmol/L
Whole blood clot retraction (see Clot retraction)		
Zinc	50-150 μg/dl	

*The use of the System of International Units (SI) was recommended at the 30th World Health Assembly in 1977 to implement an international language of measurement. Because this system is being adopted by many laboratories, many of the common values are expressed in both conventional and SI units. SI units are calculated by multiplying the conventional unit by a number factor. The SI measurement system uses *moles* as the basic unit for the amount of a substance, *kilograms* for its mass, and *meters* for its length.

From Pagana KD, Pagana TJ: *Diagnostic testing and nursing implications,* ed 3, St Louis, Mosby–Year Book.

URINE VALUES

Test	Reference range	
	Conventional values	**SI units***
Acetone plus acetoacetate (ketone bodies)	Negative	Negative
Addis count (12-hour)	WBCs and epithelial cells: 1.8 million/12 hrs	Negative
	RBCs: 500,000/12 hrs	
	Hyaline casts: Up to 5000/12 hrs	
Albumin	Random: ≤8 mg/dl	Negative
	24-hour: 10-100 mg/24 hrs	10-100 mg/24 hrs
Aldosterone	2-16 μg/24 hrs	5.5-72 nmol/24 hrs
Alpha-aminonitrogen	0.4-1.0 g/24 hrs	28-71 nmol/24 hrs
Amino acid	50-200 mg/24 hrs	
Ammonia (24-hour)	30-50 mEq/24 hrs	30-50 nmol/24 hrs
	500-1200 mg/24 hrs	
Amylase	≤5000 Somogyi units/24 hrs	6.5-48.1 U/hr
	3-35 IU/hr	
Arsenic (24-hour)	<50 μg/L	<0.65 mol/L
Ascorbic acid (vitamin C)	Random: 1-7 ng/dl	0.06-0.40 mmol/L
	24-hour: >50 mg/24 hrs	>0.29 mmol/24 hrs
Bacteria	None	None
Bence Jones protein	Negative	Negative
Bilirubin	Negative	Negative
Blood or hemoglobin	Negative	Negative
Borate (24-hour)	<2 mg/L	<32 μmol/L
Calcium	Random: 1+ turbidity	1+ turbidity
	24-hour: 1-300 mg (diet-dependent)	
Catecholamines (24-hour)	Epinephrine: 5-40 μg/24 hrs	<55 nmol/24 hrs
	Norepinephrine: 10-80 μg/24 hrs	<590 nmol/24 hrs
	Metanephrine: 24-96 μg/24 hrs	0.5-8.1 μmol/24 hrs
	Normetanephrine: 77-375 μg/24 hrs	
Chloride (24-hour)	140-250 mEq/24 hrs	140-250 mmol/24 hrs
Color	Amber-yellow	Amber-yellow
Concentration test (Fishberg test)	Specific gravity: >1.025	>1.025
	Osmolality: 850 mOsm/L	>850 mOsm/L
Copper (CU) (24-hour)	Up to 25 μg/24 hrs	0-0.4 μmol/24 hrs
Coproporphyrin (24-hour)	100-300 μg/24 hrs	150-460 nmol/24 hrs
Creatine	<100 mg/24 hrs or <6% creatinine	
Creatinine (24-hour)	15-25 mg/kg body wt/24 hrs	0.13-0.22 nmol/kg^{-1} body wt/24 hrs
Creatinine clearance (24-hour)	Men: 90-140 ml/min	90-140 ml/min
	Women: 85-125 ml/min	85-125 ml/min
Crystals	Negative	Negative
Cystine or cysteine	Negative	Negative
Delta-aminolevulinic acid (ΔALA)	1-7 mg/24 hrs	10-53 μmol/24 hrs
Epinephrine (24-hour)	5-40 μg/24 hrs	
Epithelial cells and casts	Occasional	Occasional
Estriol (24-hour)	>12 mg/24 hrs	
Fat	Negative	Negative
Fluoride (24-hour)	<1 mg/24 hrs	0.053 mmol/24 hrs

Continued.

URINE VALUES—cont'd

Test	Reference range: Conventional values	Reference range: SI units*
Follicle-stimulating hormone (FSH) (24-hour)	Men: 2-12 IU/24 hrs Women: During menses: 8-60 IU/24 hrs During ovulation: 30-60 IU/24 hrs During menopause: >50 IU/24 hrs	
Glucose	Negative	Negative
Granular casts	Occasional	Occasional
Hemoglobin and myoglobin	Negative	Negative
Homogentistic acid	Negative	Negative
Human chorionic gonadotropin (HCG)	Negative	Negative
Hyaline casts	Occasional	Occasional
17-Hydroxycorticosteroids (17-OCHS) (24-hour)	Men: 5.5-15.0 mg/24 hrs Women: 5.0-13.5 mg/24 hrs	8.3-25 μmol/24 hrs 5.5-22 μmol/24 hrs
5-Hydroxyindoleacetic acid (5-HIAA, serotonin) (24-hour)	Men: 2-9 mg/24 hrs Women: lower than men	10-47 μmol/24 hrs
Ketones (see Acetone plus acetoacetate)		
17-Ketosteroids (17-KS) (24-hour)	Men: 8-15 mg/24 hrs Women: 6-12 mg/24 hrs	21-62 μmol/24 hrs 14-45 μmol/24 hrs
Lactose (24-hour)	14-40 mg/24 hrs	41-116 μm
Lead	<0.08 g/ml or <120 g/24 hrs	0.39 μmol/L
Leucine aminopeptidase (LAP)	2-18 U/24 hrs	
Magnesium (24-hour)	6.8-8.5 mEq/24 hrs	3.0-4.3 mmol/24 hrs
Melanin	Negative	Negative
Odor	Aromatic	Aromatic
Osmolality	500-800 mOsm/L	38-1400 mmol/kg water
pH	4.6-8.0	4.6-8.0
Phenolsulfonphthalein (PSP)	15 min: at least 25% 30 min: at least 40% 120 min: at least 60%	At least 0.25 At least 0.40 At least 0.60
Phenylketonuria (PKU)	Negative	Negative
Phenylpyruvic acid	Negative	Negative
Phosphorus (24-hour)	0.9-1.3 g/24 hrs	29-42 mmol/24 hrs
Porphobilinogen	Random: negative 24-hour: up to 2 mg/24 hrs	Negative
Porphyrin (24-hour)	50-300 mg/24 hrs	
Potassium (K^+) (24-hour)	25-100 mEq/24 hrs	25-100 nmol/24 hrs
Pregnancy test	Positive in normal pregnancy or with tumors producing HCG	Positive in normal pregnancy or with tumors producing HCG
Pregnanediol	After ovulation: >1 mg/24 hrs	
Protein (albumin)	Random: ≤8 mg/dl 10-100 mg/24 hrs	 >0.05 g/24 hrs

URINE VALUES—cont'd

Test	Reference range: Conventional values	SI units*
Sodium (Na^+) (24-hour)	100-260 mEq/24 hrs	100-260 nmol/24 hrs
Specific gravity	1.010-1.025	1.010-1.025
Steroids (see 17-Hydroxycorticosteroids and 17-Ketosteroids)		
Sugar (see Glucose)		
Titratable acidity (24-hour)	20-50 mEq/24 hrs	20-50 mmol/24 hrs
Turbidity	Clear	Clear
Urea nitrogen (24-hour)	6-17 g/24 hrs	0.21-0.60 mol/24 hrs
Uric acid (24-hour)	250-750 mg/24 hrs	1.48-4.43 mmol/24 hrs
Urobilinogen	0.1-1.0 Ehrlich U/dl	0.1-1.0 Ehrlich U/dl
Uroporphyrin	Negative	Negative
Vanillylmandelic acid (VMA) (24-hour)	1-9 mg/24 hrs	<40 µmol/day
Zinc (24-hour)	0.20-0.75 mg/24 hrs	

APPENDIX

C

Temperature Conversion Chart

FAHRENHEIT AND CELSIUS EQUIVALENTS: BODY TEMPERATURE RANGE

F°	C°	F°	C°	F°	C°	F°	C°	F°	C°
94.0	34.44	97.0	36.11	100.0	37.78	103.0	39.44	106.0	41.11
94.2	34.56	97.2	36.22	100.2	37.89	103.2	39.56	106.2	41.22
94.4	34.67	97.4	36.33	100.4	38.00	103.4	39.67	106.4	41.33
94.6	34.78	97.6	36.44	100.6	38.11	103.6	39.78	106.6	41.44
94.8	34.89	97.8	36.56	100.8	38.22	103.8	39.89	106.8	41.56
95.0	35.00	98.0	36.67	101.0	38.33	104.0	40.00	107.0	41.67
95.2	35.11	98.2	36.78	101.2	38.44	104.2	40.11	107.2	41.78
95.4	35.22	98.4	36.89	101.4	38.56	104.4	40.22	107.4	41.89
95.6	35.33	98.6	37.00	101.6	38.67	104.6	40.33	107.6	42.00
95.8	35.44	98.8	37.11	101.8	38.78	104.8	40.44	107.8	42.11
96.0	35.56	99.0	37.22	102.0	38.89	105.0	40.56	108.0	42.22
96.2	35.67	99.2	37.33	102.2	39.00	105.2	40.67		
96.4	35.78	99.4	37.44	102.4	39.11	105.4	40.78		
96.6	35.89	99.6	37.56	102.6	39.22	105.6	40.89		
96.8	36.00	99.8	37.67	102.8	39.33	105.8	41.00		

To convert Centigrade or Celsius degrees to Fahrenheit degrees: multiply the number of Centigrade degrees by $9/5$ and add 32 to the result. *To convert Fahrenheit degrees to Centigrade degrees:* Subtract 32 from the number of Fahrenheit degrees and multiply the difference by $5/9$.

APPENDIX

D

Drug Overdose

Arlene Gordovez Agra, RN, CCRN
Mary Ann Jarachovic, BSN, RN

Drug overdose is the inadvertent or deliberate consumption of a much larger quantity of drugs than an individual typically uses, resulting in serious toxic reaction or death.[4] This phenomenon often is seen in those who are young and do not wish to die, or those who are lonely, isolated, and/or bereaved.[7] The incidence of drug overdose is more prominent in those who are substance abusers and those with psychological disorders. It tends to occur more often with women than men. Drugs commonly seen in overdose situations are analgesics, sedatives, hypnotics, antidepressants, and alcohol; less frequently seen are barbituates and benzodiazepines.[7]

Diagnosis of overdose is confirmed by history, signs/symptoms, and laboratory values. History includes time of drug ingestion, amount ingested, drug used, and any recent significant life events and prior psychiatric support. If histories are conflicting or absent, diagnosis is contingent on symptomology and laboratory data.

Signs and symptoms of drug overdose vary with the drug ingested. Central nervous system (CNS) involvement ranges from lethargy and coma to confusion and convulsion. Respiratory depression or stimulation and cardiac dysrhythmias can lead to cardiopulmonary arrest. Fluid and electrolyte imbalances, aspiration pneumonia, and disturbances in acid-base balance complicate the clinical picture. Thorough physical assessment of the cardiac, renal, respiratory, and central nervous systems must be accomplished immediately to determine baseline functions. The system with the most life-threatening symptoms receives the highest priority in assessment and treatment.[5]

Toxicology screens of blood, urine, and gastric contents are important values in early management. Serial serum levels are evaluated to follow the progress of drug effects. Liver function tests, complete blood count (CBC), electrolyte levels, and ABG measurements are observed throughout the clinical course to assess systemic complications of drug ingestion.

Treatment is aimed initially at life support. This includes maintaining a patent airway, adequate blood pressure, and stable heart rate; preventing convulsion; and removing the ingested substance. Administration of other medications during the acute phase should be avoided; an individual with a drug-related problem can have unpredictable drug-drug interactions.[8] However, if the ingested drug is known, prompt administration of an antidote may reverse toxic effects. In the conscious patient, emesis is induced (if not contraindicated). For the comatose or seizing patient, lavage through a large-bore gastric tube (i.e., a 36 French) is indicated.[2] Gastric lavage will prevent absorption of a drug in early stages of ingestion. In addition, pill fragments obtained from the lavage can determine actual ingestion. Charcoal administration after gastric lavage or emesis binds toxic metabolites. Ionic cathartics also facilitate removal of drug by-products. Hemodialysis and hemoperfusion are other options in treatment of toxic substance removal. Forced alkaline diuresis and forced diuresis are effective methods for eliminating certain drugs. Close monitoring of fluid and electrolytes prevents shock and renal damage due to diuretic therapy. Early consideration should be given to administration of oxygen, glucose, and naloxone.[7] Increasing oxygen

Drug	Neurological Effects	Respiratory Effects	Cardiovascular Effects	Metabolic Effects
Acetaminophen	Hypothermia Depression	Normal	Normal	Hepatocellular necrosis GI irritability Prolonged prothrombin time Diaphoresis Nausea, vomiting
Amphetamines Amphetamine (Benzedrine) Pamoline (Cylert) Phentermine (Fastin) Mazindol (Sanorex) Phenmetrazine (Preludin) Methyphenidate (Ritalin) Clortermine (Voranil)	Hyperthermia Nervousness Dilated pupils Convulsion Muscle spasms	Stimulation	Tachycardia Hypertension Dysrhythmias Myocardial ischemia	Nausea, vomiting
Anticholinergics Antihistamines Antiparkinsonism medication Belladonna alkaloids Butyrophenones (e.g., Haldol) Local mydriatics Over-the-counter cold remedies Phenothiazines Tricyclic antidepressants	Hyperthermia Hallucinations Stimulation Dilated pupils Seizures Hyperreflexia Coma	Compromise caused by cardiovascular collapse Decreased rate	Tachycardia Hypotension Ventricular dysrhythmias	Low potassium serum Urinary retention Ileus Dry, flushed skin Dry mucous membranes
Barbiturates Short-acting: Thiopental Methohexital Hexobarbital Pentobarbital Secobarbital Intermediate-acting: Amobarbital Aprobarbital Butabarbital Long-acting: Barbital Mephobarbitol Phenobarbital Primidone	Abnormal deep tendon reflexes Nystagmus CNS depression Hypothermia Coma Pupil constriction or dilation	Depression Respiratory arrest Pneumonia Pulmonary edema	Cardiovascular collapse Hypotension Tachycardia Dilatation of circulatory tree Shock	Skin blisters Hypoglycemia Oliguria

Lavage	Antidote	Nursing Management	Treatment
Gastric lavage with normal saline Ipecac 30 cc with 200-300 cc H_2O	Mucomyst in 10% or 20% solution po; initial loading dose 140 mg/kg, 70 mg/kg q4h N-acetylcysteine IV; 150 mg/kg over 15 min then 50 mg/kg over 4 hrs. Must be initiated within 8 hrs for effectiveness.	Avoid steroids, antihistamines, phenobarbital, which increase toxicity of metabolites. Protect airway during lavage.	Treat for hepatic encephalopathy
Forced emesis or lavage if in a coma	Sedation: usually diazepam (Valium) for extreme agitation as ordered Activated charcoal 30-100 g initially; repeat q12h with 20-60 g Saline cathartic	Observe for dysrhythmias, seizures	Phentolamine, propanolol as adrenergic blockers Forced acid diuresis Hemodialysis or peritoneal dialysis
Gastric lavage with normal saline	Activated charcoal as above Physostigmine 2 mg over 5 min; repeat q15min until reversed (use with caution, may cause seizures) Physostigmine is contraindicated if patient is bradycardic or asthmatic or has urinary bladder obstruction	Lidocaine and procainamide quinidine are contraindicated because they depress the myocardium and enhance toxicity Monitor ECG changes Seizure precautions	Sodium bicarbonate Hyperventilate if on ventilator Propranolol for tachycardia
Ipecac as above if conscious Lavage with normal saline Ewald tube with short-acting barbiturate	Activated charcoal as above Saline cathartic	Fluid replacement for hypotension One ampule of D50%, as ordered for hypoglycemia Cardiac and respiratory support	Osmotic alkaline diuresis for short-acting barbiturates Forced alkaline diuresis for long-acting barbiturates Hemodialysis or hemoperfusion as ordered

Continued.

Drug	Neurological Effects	Respiratory Effects	Cardiovascular Effects	Metabolic Effects
Benzodiazepines Lorazepam (Ativan) Clonazepam (Clonopin) Flurazepam (Dalamane) Chloriazepoxide (Librium) Oxazepam (Serax) Chlorazepate (Tranxene) Diazepam (Valium) Prazepam (Verstran)	Hypothermia Dilated pupils Slow pupil response Depression Coma	Depression	Irritable myocardium Hypotension Tachycardia	Vomiting Dry mouth
Cholinergics Neostigmine Physostigmine	Normothermia Tremors Headache Convulsions Coma	Dyspnea Pulmonary edema	Bradycardia Complete heart block	Anorexia Diarrhea Cramping
Cocaine	Coma Convulsions Hallucinations Dilated pupils Restlessness Hyperreflexia	Tachypnea Dyspnea Cyanosis	Shock Irregular tachycardia Blood pressure fluctuation Hypertension Cardiac arrest	Pallor
Digoxin	Muscle weakness Headache Facial neuralgia Hallucinations Confusion Drowsiness Agitation Dizziness	Normal	Arrhythmias Hypotension	Normal
Ethanol	Decreased reflex Visual disturbance Slurred speech Lethargy	Hypoventilation	Vasodilation Cardiac dysrhythmias Tachycardia	Hypoglycemia Low serum phosphate and magnesium Respiratory acidosis Gastritis
Hallucinogens Phencyclidine (PCP) LSD DMT DET MDA Philocbin Peyote	Disoriention Agitation Paranoia Muscle rigidity Nystagmus Blank stare Coma Psychosis Ataxia Hyperreflexia Tremors	Depression Tachypnea	Hypertensive crisis	Nausea Vomiting Renal failure Rhabdomyolysis Temp elevation

Lavage	Antidote	Nursing Management	Treatment
Ipecac as above if conscious Lavage with normal saline	Activated charcoal as above Saline cathartic	Respiratory support Maintain airway	Hydration
Lavage with normal saline	Atropine 0.2-0.4 mg IV; repeat as needed	Observe for seizures and arrest	Atropine as ordered
Not indicated	Sedation as ordered	Observe for respiratory distress and convulsions	Fluids and vasopressors for shock Diazepam as ordered for agitation or convulsions
Not indicated	Digibind	Observe for dysrhythmias	Treat low potassium and magnesium If bradycardic, use a pacer
Ipecac or gastric lavage useful if within 2 hrs of ingestion		Seizure precautions Prevent aspiration Thiamine IM Consider dextrose 25 g	Correct electrolyte imbalances
Ipecac as above Gastric lavage via nasogastric tube with normal saline	Activated charcoal as above; repeat saline cathartic q4-6h until charcoal-laden stool is produced	Reduce sensory stimuli Protect from injury Monitor vital signs	Acid diuresis For agitation give diazepam or ativan Treat HTN with nipride, nifedipene, labetolol For increased temperature give Tylenol

Continued.

Drug	Neurological Effects	Respiratory Effects	Cardiovascular Effects	Metabolic Effects
Inhalants Fluorinated hydrocarbons Nitrous oxide Gasoline Kerosene Carbon tetracloride	CNS excitation and depression Headache Dizziness Intracranial pressure elevated Cerebral edema Seizures	Tachypnea Dyspnea Cyanosis Rales Hemoptysis Pulmonary edema Asphyxiation Hypoxia	Hypotension Arrhythmias Ventricular fibrillation Sudden death	Nausea Vomiting Diarrhea Acute renal failure Metabolic acidosis Thrombocytopenia Megaloblastic anemia
Phenytoin (Dilantin)	Disorientation Hallucinations Headache Ataxia Nystagmus Lethargy Seizures Dystonia	Arrest Aspiration secondary to seizure	and ventricular conduction defects Ventricular fibrillation	Nausea Vomiting Hyperglycemia Acute renal failure
Narcotics Codeine Propoxyphene Hydromorphone Dephenoxalate Heroin Loperamide Levorphanol Meperidine Methadone Morphine Pentazocine	Hypothermia Pinpoint pupils Stupor Spinal cord stimulation Spasticity Hyperreflexia	Apnea Depression Acute respiratory distress syndrome (ARDS)	Bradycardia Hypotension Dilated periphery Syncopy	Dry mouth
Salicylates Aspirin Cold preparations	Hyperthermia Convulsions Stimulation Tinnitus Lethargy Disorientation Coma	Respiratory alkalosis Tachypnea Pulmonary edema	Hypertension Asystole Conduction abnormalities	Nausea Vomiting GI hemorrhage Ketosis Hypokalemia Dehydration Hypoglycemia Hyperglycemia Increased liver enzymes Hepatic encephalopathy
Sedatives/Hypnotics Benzodiazepines Chloral hydrate Meprobamate Glutethimide Methyprylon Ethchlorvynol Methaqualone	Hypothermia Lethargy Coma Hyporeflexia Headache Vertigo	Depression Cyanosis	Collapse Hypotension Tachycardia	Nausea Vomiting
Tranquilizers Prochlorperazine Haldol Loxopine Thioridazine Thiothixene Promethazine Fluphenazine Chlorpromazine Thiethylperazine Perphenazine Trifluoperazine	Delirium Hallucinations Hyperthermia Hypothermia Variable pupils Lethargy Seizures Coma	Arrest secondary to shock	Tachycardia Hypotension Dysrhythmias Shock	Urinary retention

Lavage	Antidote	Nursing Management	Treatment
N/A	None	Monitor for respiratory distress 100% O_2 humidified with assisted ventilations as required Monitor cardiovascular and renal function Monitor serum electrolytes	Anticonvulsants such as diazepam for seizures Treat cerebral edema with hyperventilation, mannitol, or dexamethasone
Ipecac as above Gastric lavage via nasogastric tube with normal saline	Activated charcoal as above Repeat saline cathartic q4-6h until charcoal-laden stool is produced	Observe for dysrhythmia, convulsions, and hyperglycemia	Insulin prn as ordered
Lavage with normal saline	Naloxone 0.4 mg IV repeat q5min until 3.2 mg total is given May induce vomiting Activated charcoal with saline cathartic as above	Maintain airway Check for pulmonary edema	Observe for cardiac or respiratory arrest Observe for withdrawal symptoms—rhinorrhea cramps, dilated pupils, nausea, and vomiting
Lavage with NS up to several hours after ingestion	Activated charcoal with saline cathartic; aluminum hydroxide, and syrup of ipecac as above	Induce emesis if gag reflex is present and patient is conscious Transfuse prn Vitamin K for abnormal clotting factors	Forced alkaline diuresis K^+ supplement Hemodialysis
Lavage with normal saline	Activated charcoal with saline cathartic	Support compromised systems Be aware the excretion route is the kidneys	Hydration
Lavage with normal saline	Activated charcoal with saline cathartic and physostigmine as above	Maintain respiratory function and body temperature, and monitor for dysrhythmias	Anticonvulsants such as diazepam for seizures Norepinephrine, not epinephrine, for hypotension

supply can limit secondary hypoxemic injury. Hypoglycemia may cause neurological symptoms similar to drug overdose situations. Administration of naloxone reverses narcotic effects. The variety and combinations of drug-induced emergencies demand close observation throughout hospitalization. Organ compromise may be delayed or prolonged because of drug interaction, concurrent alcohol intake, or prior system failure.

Patient care in the acute setting has three goals: life support, provision of a safe environment, and reversing the effects of the ingested substance(s). A safe environment includes offering the patient and family emotional support, especially for lingering self-harm tendencies if ingestion was intentional. Throughout hospitalization, it is essential to provide consistent, calm interactions and reassurance and nonjudgmental support. These approaches lead to successful verbalization and staff management of the crisis. The emotional, psychological, and family issues require expert care, and the nurse is urged to consult with a specialist in developing a plan of care for these patients.

The following table presents information on the effects of various drugs, and guidelines for treatment and management of drug-overdose patients.

REFERENCES

1. Reference deleted in proofs.
2. Budassi SA, Barber J: *Mosbys' manual of emergency care: practices and procedures,* St Louis, 1984, Mosby–Year Book.
3. Reference deleted in proofs.
4. Kinney J: *Clinical manual of substance abuse,* St Louis, 1991, Mosby–Year Book.
5. Mathewson MK: *Pharmacytheropeutics: a nursing process approach,* second printing, Philadelphia, 1986, FA Davis.
6. Reference deleted in proofs.
7. Raper RF, Fisher MM: *Critical care,* Philadelphia, 1988, JB Lippincott.
8. Schuckit MA: *Drug and alcohol abuse, a clinical guide to diagnosis and treatment,* New York, 1989, Plenum Medical Co.

APPENDIX

E

Organ Donation

Joan Littel-Conrad, RN, CCRN, CPTC

In the past 20 years, the transplantation of human organs and tissues has evolved from an experimental field of medicine to an accepted method of treatment for people afflicted with end-stage organ disease. Advances in surgical techniques, improved immunological drug therapy, and refined means of organ preservation have resulted in the unprecedented success of organ transplantation.[9] As a result, the number of people listed on the National Transplant Registry has grown at an extraordinary rate. By the year 1995, an estimated 45,000 people will be waiting in the United States for organ transplants.[8]

Unfortunately, while the number of people waiting for transplants has soared, the number of organ donors has remained relatively static. Each year, on average, only 4500 of the estimated 20,000 to 25,000 medically suitable potential donors actually donate.[2] To date, the lack of available donors remains a major deterrent toward providing transplant to those in need. According to the United Network for Organ Sharing, it is estimated that 7 people die in the United States each day while waiting for life-saving organs to become available.[9] In view of the success of transplantation, these deaths become even more tragic.

An important step toward eliminating the donor shortage is for health care professionals to begin to identify each situation in which there is a possibility of donation. The challenge associated with the identification and medical management of the potential organ donor requires the critical care nurse to have an in-depth knowledge of the donation process. In addition, experts in the field of donation believe that a sensitive and coordinated interaction with the potential donor's family increases the likelihood of consent for donation. Therefore, it is important for the nurse to provide accurate and consistent information about donation to the potential donor's family in a manner that allows for the exploration and discussion of the family's feelings, questions, and concerns.

ORGAN AND TISSUE DONOR IDENTIFICATION

In the past, organ donation was limited to situations where the deceased tended to be a young victim of trauma. Prolonged hypotension, high-dose vasopressor therapy, or infection often were considered contraindications for donation. Today, with the improvement of organ procurement and preservation, there are fewer restrictions for organ donation. For example, transplant programs may consider organs for transplant from donors with stable organ function who are upwards of 75 years of age.[1] Cases in which the donor requires high-dose or multiple vasopressor therapy are being evaluated, and organs are being recovered and successfully transplanted from these donors. The absence of HIV infection, current cancer (other than primary brain tumor), or active hepatitis, coupled with adequate organ function at the time of death declaration, makes organ donation a possibility. General guidelines for organ and tissue donation are summarized in Table E-1. It is important to evaluate each donor situation on a case-by-case basis. Because criteria change frequently, it is recommended that one contact the appropriate procurement agency in one's area to assist in determining individual suitability.

DECLARATION OF DEATH

Organ donation requires the maintenance of intact circulation and oxygenation. Therefore, donation of the heart,

TABLE E-1 Donor Criteria Chart[6]

	Heart	Lung	Kidney	Liver	Pancreas	Intestine	Bone and tissue	Heart valves	Eye
Age	Newborn to 70 yrs	Newborn to 70 yrs	Newborn to 70 yrs	Newborn to 70 yrs	Newborn to 70 yrs	Newborn to 70 yrs	15 to 65 yrs	Newborn to 55 yrs	No age limit
Resuscitated Cardiac Arrest	Does not rule out organ donation. Reviewed on an individual basis.						OK		
Hypotension	Does not rule out organ donation. Reviewed on an individual basis.						OK		
Vasopressors; e.g., dopamine-sensitive	High-dose vasopressor therapy does not rule out organ donation.						OK		
Additional lab data required	The coordinator on call will order specific lab tests.						Obtained by tissue program		
Previous disease of organs that alters function	Does not rule out donation. Past and current medical conditions are reviewed on an individual basis.								
Infection	Does not rule out organ and tissue donation. Reviewed on an individual basis.								
Cancer	No *current* cancer other than primary brain tumor.								OK
High-risk behavior for AIDS/hepatitis	Reviewed on an individual basis. Recovering agency will perform testing.						No	No	No
Declaration of death	Present or pending declaration of brain death. Intact circulation with oxygenation maintained by mechanical ventilation.						Recovered after asystole		
Medical examiner/coroner cases	Does not rule out donation. The procuring agency will assist with obtaining release of the body.								

Organ, bone and eye donation does not interfere with funeral arrangements or services.
No costs directly related to organ or tissue donation are passed on to the family or the donor hospital.
If required, autopsy can be coordinated with donation.

lungs, liver, pancreas, intestine, and kidneys is dependent on the declaration of brain death.

Brain death is diagnosed when all brain function has irreversibly ceased.[6] Virtually any seriously injured head-trauma patient should be considered a potential donor, and the possibility of donation should always be considered as a logical step in the algorithm of care.[4] The most common causes of brain death include:

- Cerebral anoxia
- Cerebral vascular accident
- Trauma
- Nonmetastatic primary brain tumor

The following Box provides information relating to the diagnosis of brain death.

While organ donors must meet the criteria for brain death and have vital organ function maintained, tissue donors need not be heart-beating. Following asystole, there is the potential for tissue donation. Bone, skin, cardiovascular tissue, and eye donation are options to be considered. Tissue donation can occur hours after death. Many individuals benefit through tissue transplants that restore sight, improve mobility, prevent amputation and correct cardiac function. Though not as widely publicized as organ transplants, procedures using donated human tissue affect about a half-million people annually in the United States.[5] As with organ donation, the demand for tissue far exceeds the supply available and many people requiring tissue transplants remain untreated.

CLINICAL MANAGEMENT OF THE ORGAN DONOR

Once brain death occurs, maintenance of vital organ function becomes a priority. Declining systemic perfusion occurs as the result of loss of autonomic function.[7] The goal of medical management is to achieve and preserve organ oxygenation and perfusion. Table E-2 outlines the goals for maintenance of optimal organ function. For specific management guidelines, contact your local organ procurement program.

Brain Death Criteria*

Known cause of condition

Diagnosis made in absence of hypothermia (temperature <32.2° C) and absence of central nervous system depressants

Cerebral unresponsiveness

Areflexic

Except for simple spinal cord reflexes; pupillary, extraocular, corneal, gag, and cough reflexes are absent

No spontaneous respiration

Condition irreversible

Duration of observation depends on clinical judgment; recommend 12 hours when an irreversible condition is well established and no confirmatory test; recommend 24 hours for anoxic brain damage and no confirmatory test

Flat EEG (if performed)

Absence of blood flow by cerebral radionuclide scan or arteriogram (if performed)

*President's Commission for the Study of Ethical Problems in Medicine and Biomedical and Behavioral Research. Printed with permission, UNOS 1994.

DISCUSSING THE OPTION OF DONATION WITH FAMILIES

Many states have laws that make offering the option to donate mandatory. However, offering donation as an option to a grieving family can be a difficult task for the healthcare professional. In some cases, discussing donation may seem an imposition upon a bereaved family. It is natural for the nurse to feel some anxiety and uneasiness when faced with the responsibility of discussing donation with a family. Yet, if handled in a coordinated and sensitive manner, discussing donation does not have to cause the family discomfort. Moreover, the discussion of donation can be an opportunity for the nurse to aid the family in their grieving process.

It is helpful to consider the following guidelines before offering the option of donation to a bereaved family.

- Before beginning the discussion, contact your local procurement organization to assist in assessing the potential for donation. Criteria change frequently, and knowing what options exist may prevent offering donations that are not possible.
- Consider the family's understanding of brain death. Explanations of brain death should be repeated until the family can verbalize understanding of the concept. When appropriate, review with the family test results that con-

TABLE E-2 Goals for Maintenance of Organ Function

Problem	Common etiology	Interventions	Desired outcome
Hypotension	Sympathetic nervous system destruction results in vasodilation	Administer vasopressors (e.g., dopamine hydrochloride)	Hemodynamic stability; systolic blood pressure >100 mm Hg
	Therapeutic dehydration to decrease cerebral edema	Volume replacement with colloids, crystalloids	Adequate fluid volume; CVP 5-10 mm Hg or PCWP 6-12 mm Hg
	Hypovolemia related to blood loss, DIC	Blood product administration	Hct approximately 30%
Poor oxygenation	Inappropriate ventilatory support	Adjust ventilator settings to achieve maximum oxygenation Verify tube placement	ABG within normal limits
	Neurogenic pulmonary edema	Avoid overhydration PEEP as tolerated Consider diuretics	
	Pulmonary secretions	Frequent sterile suctioning	
Impaired thermoregulation	Destruction of the hypothalamus	Heating/cooling mattress Adjust room temperature Cool/warm IV fluids	Normothermic
Fluid and electrolyte imbalance	Destruction of pituitary resulting in impaired ADH secretion	Administer synthetic vasopressin to control excessive urine output	Urine output 100-200 cc/hr
	Therapeutic dehydration	Volume replacement Replenish electrolytes	Adequate fluid volume Normal serum electrolyte values

Adapted from Sammons B, Pietroski R: *Organ donor management: pathophysiologic principles*, East Hanover, NJ, 1990, Sandoz Pharmaceuticals Corporation.

TABLE E-3 Common Questions of Donor Families and Possible Responses

Common questions	Possible responses
Will donation prevent an open-casket funeral?	Eye, bone, or organ donation does not prevent an open-casket service.
What are the costs for donation?	Any costs associated with the donation are paid by the program that recovers the organs and tissues.
Are there religious objections to donation?	Most of the major religions in the United States approve of donation.
Will we know who receives the organs?	You will receive a letter that will share with you some general information about the transplant recipients.

firm brain death. Pictures and drawings also may facilitate understanding.[8]

- The discussion of brain death must be coordinated among health care staff. It is important that the family receive consistent and accurate information. Use clear and simple terms to explain that death has occurred. Be aware of the terminology used to discuss brain death. For example, refer to the ventilator as a "breathing machine," rather than "life support." Use the phrase "supporting organ function" rather than saying "keeping the patient alive."[8] In addition, inform the family that when support is stopped, "the patient's heart will stop," rather than saying "the patient will die." Reinforce that brain death is medically, ethically, and legally death. Brain death is not a coma.
- Consider the timing of the discussion. According to a study conducted in the service area of the Kentucky Organ Donor Affiliates, when the conversation about organ donation was separated from the discussion of death, 53 of 82 families consented (64.6%).[3] When the explanation of death and the option of donation were approached in the same conversation, 11 of 61 instances resulted in consent (18%).[3] This indicates that timing of the approach is critical to the success of the approach.
- Remember to choose a quiet, private place to have the discussion about donation. Avoid conducting the conversation at the patient's bedside.
- When the family is ready, begin the discussion about donation. It may be helpful to remember that you are not actually asking the family to donate. Rather, the purpose of the donation conversation is to allow the family to discuss how they *feel* about donation. Keeping this in mind allows you to address their concerns, clarify misconceptions, and provide correct information. Additionally, a discussion allows the family to explore their feelings and make a decision with which most are comfortable.

There are several ways to approach the discussion of donation. Most organ donation programs have a coordinator available to assist you in approaching the family. Involving the coordinator in the discussion can be extremely helpful.

You may wish to begin by extending your sympathy to the family and then explain that you are there to provide the family with some information for them to consider. At this time, discussing their choice of a funeral home, involvement by the medical examiner or coroner (if indicated), and determining who will take the patient's belongings home may be appropriate. Once the family has worked through these issues, introduce the topic of donation. One possible approach is simply to tell the family that you would like to share with them some information about their option of donation. Offer them some basic information and allow them some time to share their thoughts with you. Anticipate questions they may have and provide them with the information they require. (Table E-3.) During the discussion, take your time and use simple explanations. Avoid using the term "harvest," as some families may find this term to be disrespectful. Instead, refer to the process as an organ recovery or a donation. Do not be afraid of silence. The family may need some time to consider what has been discussed. If necessary, offer to give them some time alone. Avoid rushing them into a decision.

In the event that the family chooses not to donate, thank them for considering donation. Reinforce that they are making the best decision for their family and support their decision. If the family chooses to donate, determine what organs and tissues they are comfortable donating. Assist them with signing the consent and answer any questions that they may have. Notify the appropriate procurement program of the family's decision. In a case where the family is undecided, gently explore and address their concerns. Offer them any additional information and support they may need and allow them more time to make their decision.

Whatever decision the family makes, give them adequate time to say good-bye. Other comfort measures may include contacting a chaplain, offering the family a lock of their loved one's hair, or giving family members a chance to hold their loved one. Some families hesitate to ask for these things because of a fear of imposing upon the hospital staff. Give them permission to grieve in a manner that brings them comfort.

CONCLUSION

The nurse plays a key role in facilitating the donation process. Remember that the purpose of the donation discussion is to invite the family to consider their feelings about donation. Whether they decide to donate or decline the option, a sensitive approach can be an opportunity for the nurse to aid and support a family in grief.

REFERENCES

1. Alexander JW, Vaughn WK: The use of "marginal" donors for organ transplantation: The influence of donor age on outcome, *Transplantation* 51(1), 135-141, 1991.
2. Cate FH, Laudicina SS: Current statistical information about transplantation in America, *Transplantation White Paper,* Richmond, Va, 1991, United Network for Organ Sharing.
3. Garrison NR, et al: There is an answer to the shortage of organ donors, *Surg Gynecol Obstet* 173:391-396, 1991.
4. Gill BA: *Transplant challenge: a role for healthcare professionals,* E. Hanover, N.J., 1988, Sandoz Pharmaceuticals Corporation.
5. Koch MC, et al: *Medical school curriculum advocacy guide,* Richmond, Va, 1993, United Network for Organ Sharing.
6. Report of the Medical Consultants on the Diagnosis of Death to the President's Commission for the Study of Ethical Problems in Medicine and Biomedical and Behavioral Research: "Guidelines for the Determination of Death," *JAMA* 246:2184, 1981.
7. Sammons B, Pietroski R: *Organ donor management: pathophysiologic principles,* East Hanover, NJ, 1990, Sandoz Pharmaceuticals Corporation.
8. The Partnership for Organ Donation: *Hospital education package,* ed 2, Boston, Mass, 1993.
9. UNOS: *Annual report of the U.S. Scientific Registry for Transplant Recipients and the Transplantation Network-Transplant Data: 1988-1991,* Richmond, Va, UNOS; and Bethesda, Md, Division of Organ Transplantation, Bureau of Health Resources Development, Health Resources and Service Administration, U.S. Department of Health and Human Services, 1993.

APPENDIX

F

Postanesthesia Care in Critical Care

Richard A. Beastrom, MN, RN, CPAN

The purpose of this appendix is to guide the critical care nurse in caring for the patient during "Phase I" of the postanesthesia period. This term is used to indicate the critical phase of recovery from anesthesia and correlates with the time spent in the Postanesthesia Care Unit (PACU).[1]

The most common and anticipated problems are discussed. Nausea/vomiting and pain are obviously not unique problems in the PACU; however, the medications used in anesthesia practice reflect subtle interactions with anesthetic agents already "on board."[9] Pharmacological treatments may differ from those used in the Surgical Intensive Care Unit (SICU).

Common problem	Etiology	Assessment	Intervention	Discharge
Delayed awakening: failure to awaken rapidly after general anesthesia. Also referred to as "prolonged emergence" and "inability to arouse."[2]	Prolonged action of anesthetic drugs, such as high concentrations of inhaled anesthetic, narcotics, benzodiazepines, insufficient reversal agents, or the development of hypoxia or hypothermia will delay arousal. Metabolic encephalopathy can be caused by the following disorders: hepatic, renal, endocrine, neurologic, hypoxia and hypercapnia, acidosis, hypoglycemia, hyperosmolar syndrome, electrolyte imbalance and water intoxication and hypothermia or neurotoxic drugs.[3] Neurologic injury is associated with intracranial hemorrhage, cerebral edema, cerebral embolism, or cerebral ischemia.	Oxygen saturation by pulse oximetry (Spo_2): <90% while on oxygen Pulmonary status: ≤10 breaths per minute, shallow breaths, partial airway obstruction Neurologic status: cannot be aroused or has difficulty staying responsive	Monitor respiratory rate Monitor Spo_2 values Maintain temperature within normal range Stimulate patient to deep breathe and cough Maintain patent airway with adjuncts or jaw support Administer oxygen at 40% by humidified mask or 3 L/min by nasal prongs Monitor cognitive abilities of patient Position patient to promote ease in respiratory effort Control and manage environment to promote safety Orient patient to person, place, and time Be prepared to administer reversal agents, such as naloxone (Narcan), Fluoranzenil (Romazicon), or physostigmine (Antilirium)	The patient may continue to be drowsy by slipping easily back to sleep, yet readily responding appropriately to verbal instructions. During these periods of sleep, Spo_2 values will remain at or greater than 90% while on room air. The patient will be able to respond in an oriented manner and follow instructions appropriately and consistently.

Continued.

Common problem	Etiology	Assessment	Intervention	Discharge
Emergence delirium: state of postanesthetic excitement characterized by increased motor activity, disorientation, and vocalization.[4] The excitement displays itself upon awakening as restlessness, agitation, thrashing of arms and legs, pulling on tubes, and talking incoherently.	Hypoxia is the most common etiology and should always be considered first. Other etiologies include hypercarbia, hyponatremia, hypochloremia, and acid-base changes.[5] Discomfort can trigger emergence delirium. Pain, bladder, and gastric distension, or claustrophobia from an oxygen mask on the face are some examples. Adverse drug reactions, such as central anticholinergic syndrome related to atropine, scopolamine, diazepam (Valium),[6] and low doses of droperidol (Inapsine)[7] have been known to cause excitement. Ketamine (Ketalar) in proper doses may easily stimulate emergence delirium.[8]	Neurological: agitation, confusion, disorientation, and vocalization Skeletal muscular: thrashing of extremities, pulling objects, and sitting up	Restrain as necessary to promote safety Orient to person, place, and time Comfort with a calming tone of voice Monitor Spo_2 values, monitor cognitive abilities of patient, and administer antagonistic drugs when indicated If there is some recall of the delirious episode, the patient may require emotional reassurance for a short time.	Once the underlying etiology is treated, it is not uncommon for the patient to relax, fall back to sleep, and awake shortly afterward very alert and oriented.

Nausea/vomiting: Nausea is the awareness of the urge to vomit. Vomiting is the forceful expulsion of gastrointestinal contents through the mouth. Retching is the rhythmic spasmodic activity that usually precedes vomiting.	Vomiting is controlled by the bilateral vomiting center in the medulla, which receives input from four major routes: • Irritation or distension of the GI tract • Chemoreceptor trigger zone (CTZ) on the floor of the fourth ventricle of the brain, caused by drugs or metabolic situations • The labyrinthine apparatus of the inner ear (motion) via the vestibular nerve to the cerebellum and CTZ • Visual and psychic input from disturbing sights and thoughts or distasteful odors[10]	A history of the following make nausea/vomiting more likely: prior repeat episodes; prone to motion sickness; females having abdominal surgery; children ages 3 to puberty; food in the stomach less than 6 hours before surgery; metabolic or drug toxicities; prolonged preoperative fasting; or patients with renal failure. Some surgical procedures increase risk of nausea/vomiting: appendicitis; ileus after surgery involving the stomach, duodenum, or gall bladder; increased intracranial pressure; ear, nose, and throat surgery; uterine procedures; strabismus surgery; or intravenous radiologic contrast media. Anesthetics such as narcotics, nitrous oxide with laparoscopy procedures, and etomidate (Amidate) also may precipitate nausea/vomiting. Postoperative conditions may cause nausea/vomiting: pain, patient movement, hypotension, hypoxia, or hypovolemia. Visual and audible signs such as retching; gagging or coughing is an indication. Verbally, the patient complains of feeling nauseated.	Administer antiemetics as needed: droperidol (Inapsine), metrodopramide (Reglan), dimenhydrinate (Dramamine) or ondansetron (Zafran) Minimize unnecessary patient movement Avoid oropharyngeal stimulation Provide adequate pain control Administer supplemental oxygen Encourage slow, deep breathing	Retching and vomiting are subdued before leaving the PACU. Nausea may persist if pain is not brought under control. Increase efforts and/or use alternate pain management strategies.

Continued.

Common problem	Etiology	Assessment	Intervention	Discharge
Pain: Postoperative pain perception is a subjective phenomenon influenced by tissue damage caused by incision, manipulation, retraction, and excision. In addition, responses to pain are influenced by myriad other factors, including age, personality, mood, culture, and emotional state.[11] It is almost an inevitable consequence of surgery.[12] This experience is highly individualized. For patients undergoing surgical procedures, postoperative pain is an anticipated and, often, feared consequence.[13]	Pain stimuli travel from the peripheral receptor sites and are transmitted by two classes of nerve fibers, where two types of pain are recognized. The sharp, transient prickling pain associated with skin trauma is classified as fast pain, as it is transmitted by myelinated A fibers. The more prolonged and unpleasant burning pain, classified as slow pain, results from tissue damage and is mediated by unmyelinated L fibers. Pain transmission continues as the fibers cross over to the other side of the spinal cord before traveling to the brain. The brain then modulates and interprets the incoming pulse.	A preoperative history that reveals fear of pain from either a previous experience or the unknown. The patient is grimacing, frowning, or crying. There are verbal complaints of pain sensation, moaning, or even screaming. Anxiousness, restlessness, or confusion may be present. Physiological signs include tachycardia, tachypnea, dyspnea, hypertension, or nausea.	Administer analgesics as needed: Morphine, meperidine (Demerol), fentanyl citrate (Sublimaze), dezocine (Dalgan) or ketorolac tromethamine (Toradol) Monitor pulse, respirations and blood pressure Position patient comfortably Provide external warmth to prevent shivering	Ideal pain relief during Phase I recovery may not always occur. Goals include preventing or reducing severe pain and transfering the patient in order for long-term pain therapy to be initiated. More aggressive use of the AHCPR guidelines for management of surgical pain during phase I recovery may be indicated.
Hypothermia: low central body temperature, less than 96.8° F. (36° C).[14] May occur unintentionally when profound heat loss overwhelms the patient's ability to generate or recover heat.[15]	Body heat is exchanged with the environment by four mechanisms: radiation, conduction, convection, and evaporation. Decreases in metabolic rate may impair thermoregulation; hypothyroidism, hypoadrenalism, circulatory failure, and central nervous system disorders may be present. Decreases in muscle mass and activity such as paralysis and chronic arthritis can have negative effects on heat production.	Temperature <96.8° F (36° C). The patient will verbally complain about feeling cold. There may be shivering by the patient. The skin will feel cool to touch and/or there is presence of "gooseflesh."	Monitor the patient's temperature by tympanic membrane thermometer. Apply infrared lamps to males <95° F (35.0° C). Apply warm air cover to females <95° F (35.0° C).[16] Apply warm blankets to patients whose temperature is between 95° F (35.0° C) and 96.8° F (36.0° C).	Rapid warming of cold patients quickly reduces the risks associated with hypothermia and with no apparent side effects. The goal temperature for discharge from the critical care area is ≥96.8° F (36.0° C). Ideally, the patient will also feel less cold, but by itself this would not be a reason to delay transfer from Phase I recovery.

	Anesthetics complicate the body's attempt to save heat by depressing central heat-regulating mechanisms and vasodilation.			
Shaking (shivering): Postanesthesia shaking (PS) is characterized by the spontaneous and unpredictable appearance of tremors occurring during early recovery from anesthesia. PS manifests as a rhythmic, intermittent tremor that starts in the head and neck and progresses into the extremities "to generalized shaking."[17]	PS was first observed following ether and Pentothal anesthesia, but because the tremors closely resemble cold-induced shivering, the term shivering is commonly used. One group of researchers suggest that a heightened state of spinal cord reflex activity occurs when the spinal cord "awakens" from anesthesia before the brain does. A possible triggering mechanism such as stimulation of cutaneous cold receptors sets off the spinal reflex, which results in shaking.[18] PS and cold-induced shivering are two different phenomena, characterized by differences in electromyelogram.	Visually the patient will be shaking, shivering, or tremoring. The patient may or may not complain of feeling cold. Hypothermia may or may not be present. The skin of the patient may be cool to the touch, there may be the presence of gooseflesh, or neither may exist.	Apply infrared lamps, warm air cover, or warm blankets as indicated by the patient's temperature. Administer meperidine (Demerol) as needed to reduce or stop tremors. Monitor the patient's temperature by tympanic membrane thermometer. Prevent hypothermia if the patient is normothermic. Provide reassurance to the patient that the shaking has short duration.	Regardless of the presence of hypothermia or not, heat application (active: infrared lamps and warm air cover; or passive: warm blankets) can reduce or prevent shaking. The patient should not be discharged from the PACU until all shaking has stopped.

Continued.

REFERENCES

1. *Standards of postanesthesia nursing practice,* Richmond, Va, 1992, The American Society of Postanesthesia Nurses, p 4.
2. Zelcer J, Wells DG: Anesthetic-related recovery room complications. In Vender JS, Spiess BD, editors: *Post Anesthesia Care,* Philadelphia, 1992, WB Saunders, p 10.
3. Denlinger JK: Prolonged emergence and failure to regain consciousness. In Orkin FK, Cooperman LH, editors: *Complications in anesthesiology,* Philadelphia, 1983, JB Lippincott, pp 368-380.
4. Borchardt AC, Fraulini KE: Postanesthetic problems. In Fraulini KE, editor: *After anesthesia,* East Norwalk, Conn, 1987, Appleton and Lange, p 188.
5. Zelcer J, Wells DG: Anesthesia-related recovery room complications, *Anesthesia Intensive Care* 15:108, 168-174, 1987.
6. Eckenhoff JE, Kneale PH, Dripps RD: The incidence and etiology of post-anesthetic excitement, *Anesthesiology* 22:667-673, 1961.
7. Melnick BM: Extrapyramidal reactions to low-dose droperidol, *Anesthesiology* 69:424-426, 1988.
8. Katz NM, et al: Delirium in surgical patients under intensive care, *Arch Surg* 104:310-313, 1972.
9. Bresson VL: Postoperative nausea and vomiting. In Jacobsen WK, editor: *Manual of post anesthesia care,* Philadelphia, 1992, WB Saunders, pp 180-186.
10. Gunton AC: *Textbook of medical physiology,* ed 6, Philadelphia, 1981, WB Saunders, pp 832-834.
11. Drain CB, Christoph SS: *The recovery room: a critical care approach to post anesthesia nursing,* ed 2, Philadelphia, 1987, WB Saunders, p 26.
12. Prys-Roberts C: Treatment of postoperative pain. In Frost EM, editor: *Post anesthesia care unit,* ed 2, St Louis, 1990, Mosby–Year Book, pp 9-18.
13. Wild L: Pain Management, *Crit Care Nurs Clin North Am* 2(4):537-547, 1990.
14. Natonson RA: Managing perioperative hypothermia and hyperthermia. In Vender JS, Spiess BD, editors: *Post anesthesia care,* Philadelphia, 1992, WB Saunders, p 206.
15. Holtzclaw BJ: Temperature problems in the postoperative period, *Crit Care Nurs Clin North Am* 2(4):579-587, 1990.
16. Beastrom RA, Rickbeil P, Kepner J: Postoperative hypothermia, shaking, and complications: effects of two warming methods. Unpublished research, 1993.
17. Glinieckiam AM: Post anesthesia shaking: a review, *Journal of Post Anesthesia Nursing* 7(2):89-93, 1992.
18. Sessler DI, et al: Spontaneous post anesthetic tremor does not resemble thermalregulatory shivering, *Anesthesiology* 68:843-850, 1988.

Index

Q

R